Endometriosis: Science and Practice

Endometriosis

Science and Practice

EDITED BY

LINDA C. GIUDICE

MD, PhD, MSc

Distinguished Professor and Chair, Department of Obstetrics, Gynecology and Reproductive Sciences
The Robert B. Jaffe Endowed Professor in the Reproductive Sciences
University of California, San Francisco
San Francisco, CA, USA

JOHANNES L. H. EVERS

MD, PhD, FRCOG (ad eundem)

Professor and Chair, Centre for Reproductive Medicine and Biology
GROW, School for Oncology and Developmental Biology
Maastricht University Medical Centre
Maastricht, the Netherlands

DAVID L. HEALY

BMedSci, MBBS, PhD, FRANZCOG, CREI, FRCOG (ad eundem)

Professor and Chair, Department of Obstetrics and Gynecology
Monash University
Melbourne, Australia

WILEY-BLACKWELL

A John Wiley & Sons, Ltd., Publication

This edition first published 2012, © 2012 by Blackwell Publishing Ltd

Blackwell Publishing was acquired by John Wiley & Sons in February 2007. Blackwell's publishing program has been merged with Wiley's global Scientific, Technical and Medical business to form Wiley-Blackwell.

Registered Office
John Wiley & Sons, Ltd, The Atrium, Southern Gate, Chichester, West Sussex, PO19 8SQ, UK

Editorial Offices
9600 Garsington Road, Oxford, OX4 2DQ, UK
The Atrium, Southern Gate, Chichester, West Sussex, PO19 8SQ, UK
350 Main Street, Malden, MA 02148-5020, USA

For details of our global editorial offices, for customer services and for information about how to apply for permission to reuse the copyright material in this book please see our website at www.wiley.com/wiley-blackwell

Library of Congress Cataloging-in-Publication Data

Endometriosis : science and practice / edited by Linda C. Giudice, Johannes L.H. Evers, David L. Healy.
    p.   cm.
  Includes bibliographical references and index.
  ISBN-13: 978-1-4443-3213-1 (hardcover : alk. paper)
  ISBN-10: 1-4443-3213-9 (hardcover : alk. paper)
1. Endometriosis.   I. Giudice, Linda.   II. Evers, Johannes Leonardus Henricus, 1949–
III. Healy, D. L. (David Lindsay)
  [DNLM: 1. Endometriosis. WP 390]
  RG483.E53E556 2012
  618.1'42–dc23
                                    2011027301
A catalogue record for this book is available from the British Library.

Wiley also publishes its books in a variety of electronic formats. Some content that appears in print may not be available in electronic books.

Set in 9.25/12pt Minion by SPi Publisher Services, Pondicherry, India
Printed and bound in Singapore by Markono Print Media Pte Ltd

1   2012

Contents

v

Contents

List of Contributors

Jason Abbott BMed (Hons) MRCOG
FRANZCOG PhD
Associate Professor of Obstetrics and Gynaecology
University of New South Wales
Sydney, Australia

Maurício S. Abrão MD
Associate Professor, Director, Endometriosis
Division
Department of Obstetrics and Gynecology
University of São Paulo Medical School
São Paulo, Brazil

G. David Adamson MD, FRCSC,
FACOG, FACS
Director, Fertility Physicians of Northern California
Adjunct Clinical Professor, Stanford University
Associate Clinical Professor, University of
California San Francisco
San Francisco, CA, USA

Marco Alifano MD, PhD
Professor of Thoracic Surgery
Department of Thoracic Surgery
Cochin-Hôtel-Dieu Hospital
Paris V University
Paris, France

Marwa K. Al-Sabbagh
Research Fellow
Institute of Reproductive and Developmental
Biology
Imperial College London
London, UK

Ayman Al-Talib MD
Department of Obstetrics and Gynecology
McGill University
Montreal, Canada

Erkut Attar MD, PhD
Professor
Division of Endocrinology and Infertility
Department of Gynecology
Istanbul University
Istanbul Medical School
Istanbul, Turkey

Kurt T. Barnhart MD, MSCE
Professor Obstetrics and Gynecology and
Epidemiology
Assistant Dean, University of Pennsylvania School
of Medicine
Director, Women's Health Clinical Research Center
University of Pennsylvania
Philadelphia, PA, USA

Regina G. H. Beets-Tan
Professor in Radiology
Department of Radiology
Maastricht University Medical Center
Maastricht, The Netherlands

Giuseppe Benagiano
Department of Gynecology and Obstetrics
Sapienza
University of Rome
Rome, Italy

Marina Berbic BMedSc, MScMed (RHHG)
Senior Research Fellow
Department of Obstetrics, Gynaecology and
Neonatology
Queen Elizabeth II Research Institute for Mothers
and Infants
The University of Sydney
Sydney, Australia

Karen J. Berkley PhD
Professor Emeritus
Program in Neuroscience
Florida State University
Tallahassee, FL USA

Tommaso Bignardi MD
Department of Obstetrics and Gynaecology
Nepean Clinical School
University of Sydney
Sydney, Australia

Antonio Bobbio MD, PhD
Senior Surgeon
Department of Thoracic Surgery
Cochin-Hôtel-Dieu Hospital
Paris V University
Paris, France

Ivo Brosens MD PhD FRCOG (ad eundem)
Professor Emeritus
Department of Obstetrics and Gynaecology
Catholic University of Leuven
Leuven, Belgium

Jan J. Brosens MD FRCOG PhD
Professor of Reproductive Medicine & Sciences
Honorary Consultant Gynaecologist
Institute of Reproductive and Developmental
Biology
Imperial College London
London, UK

Kaylon L. Bruner-Tran PhD
Assistant Professor
Department of Obstetrics and Gynecology
Women's Reproductive Health Research Center
Vanderbilt University School of Medicine
Nashville, TN, USA

Germaine M. Buck Louis PhD, MS
Director and Senior Investigator
Division of Epidemiology, Statistics & Prevention
Research
Eunice Kennedy Shriver National Institute of
Child Health and
Human Development
National Institutes of Health
Bethesda, MD, USA

Serdar E. Bulun MD
George H. Gardner Professor of Clinical
Gynecology
Chief, Division of Reproductive Biology Research
Department of Obstetrics and Gynecology
Northwestern University
Feinberg School of Medicine
Chicago, IL, USA

Richard O. Burney MD, MSc, FACOG,
LTC, MC, USA
Division of Reproductive Endocrinology and
Infertility
Department of Obstetrics and Gynecology
Madigan Healthcare System
Tacoma, WA, USA

Hakan Cakmak MD
Department of Obstetrics, Gynecology and
Reproductive Sciences
Yale University School of Medicine
New Haven, CT, USA

You-Hong Cheng
Division of Reproductive Biology Research
Department of Obstetrics and Gynecology
Northwestern University
Feinberg School of Medicine
Chicago, IL, USA

Jeris Cox MD
Program in Reproductive and Adult Endocrinology
Eunice Kennedy Shriver National Institute of
Child Health and Human Development
National Institutes of Health
Bethesda, MD, USA

Hilary O. D. Critchley MBChB, MD,
FRCOG, FMedSci
Professor of Reproductive Medicine
and Honorary Consultant in Obstetrics and
Gynaecology
MRC Centre for Reproductive Health
University of Edinburgh
Edinburgh, UK

Diane Damotte MD, PhD
Professor
Department of Pathology
Cochin-Hôtel-Dieu Hospital
Paris V University
Paris, France

Alan DeCherney MD
Program in Reproductive and Adult
Endocrinology
Eunice Kennedy Shriver National Institute of
Child Health and Human Development
National Institutes of Health
Bethesda, MD, USA

Thomas M. D'Hooghe MD, PhD
Director, Leuven University Fertility Center
Department of Obstetrics and Gynaecology
University Hospitals Leuven
Leuven, Belgium

Michael P. Diamond MD
Kamran S. Moghissi Professor and Associate Chair
of Obstetrics and Gynecology
Director, Division of Reproductive Endocrinology
and Infertility
Assistant Dean, Clinical and Translational
Research
Wayne State University School of Medicine
Detroit, MI, USA

Daniela Dinulescu PhD
Assistant Professor
Division of Women's and Perinatal Pathology
Harvard Medical School
Boston, MA, USA

Jacques Donnez
Department of Gynecology
Université Catholique de Louvain
Institut de Recherche Expérimentale et Clinique
Brussels, Belgium

Olivier Donnez
Department of Gynecology
Université Catholique de Louvain
Institut de Recherche Expérimentale et Clinique
Brussels, Belgium

Caroline Dowling MS, FRACS (Urol)
Urologist, Southern Health
Senior Lecturer Department of Surgery
Monash University
Melbourne, Australia

Antoni J. Duleba MD
Professor of Obstetrics and Gynecology
University of California Davis
Sacramento, CA, USA

Gerard A. J. Dunselman MD, PhD
Associate Professor, Centre for Reproductive
Medicine and Biology
GROW, School of Oncology and Developmental
Biology
Maastricht University Medical Center
Maastricht, The Netherlands

Johannes L. H. Evers MD, PhD, FRCOG
(ad eundem)
Professor and Chair, Centre for Reproductive
Medicine and Biology
GROW, School of Oncology and Developmental
Biology
Maastricht University Medical Centre
Maastricht, The Netherlands

Henrik Falconer MD, PhD
Department of Women's and Children's Health
Division of Obstetrics and Gynecology
Karolinska Institute
Stockholm, Sweden

Asgerally T. Fazleabas PhD
Professor and Associate Chair
Department of Obstetrics, Gynecology and
Reproductive Biology
Director, Center for Women's Health Research
Michigan State University
Grand Rapids, MI, USA

Luiz Flávio Cordeiro Fernandes
Department of Obstetrics and Gynecology
University of São Paulo Medical School
São Paulo, Brazil

Ian S. Fraser MD, FRANZCOG
Professor in Reproductive Medicine
Department of Obstetrics, Gynaecology and
Neonatology,
Queen Elizabeth II Research Institute for Mothers
and Infants
University of Sydney
Sydney, Australia

Luca Fusi MD FRCOG
Consultant Gynaecologist
Institute of Reproductive and Developmental
Biology
Imperial College
London, UK

Caroline E. Gargett PhD
Deputy Director (Women's Health)
The Ritchie Centre
Monash Institute of Medical Research;
Department of Obstetrics and Gynaecology
Monash University
Melbourne, Australia

Linda C. Giudice MD, PhD, MSC
Distinguished Professor and Chair
The Robert B. Jaffe, MD Endowed Professor in the
Reproductive Sciences
Department of Obstetrics,
Gynecology and Reproductive Sciences
University of California, San Francisco
San Francisco, CA, USA

Anne Gompel MD, PhD
Professor
Department of Medical Gynaecology
Cochin-Hôtel-Dieu Hospital
Paris V University
Paris, France

List of Contributors

Patrick G. Groothuis PhD
Senior Research Scientist
Department of Women's Health
Merck Sharp and Dohme
Oss, The Netherlands

Ruth Grümmer PhD
Professor
Institute of Molecular Biology
University Hospital Essen
University of Duisburg- Essen
Essen, Germany

Sun-Wei Guo PhD
Professor
Shanghai Obstetrics and Gynecology Hospital
Fudan University Shanghai College of Medicine
Shanghai, People's Republic of China

Bilgin Gurates
Firat University Faculty of Medicine
Division of Reproductive Endocrinology and Infertility
Department of Obstetrics and Gynecology
Istanbul University
Istanbul Medical School
Istanbul, Turkey

David L. Healy BMedSci, MBBS, PhD, FRANZCOG, CREI, FRCOG (ad eundem)
Professor and Chair
Department of Obstetrics and Gynecology
MonashUniversity
Melbourne, Australia

Alison J. Hey-Cunningham BAppSc (Hons), PhD
Senior Research Fellow
Department of Obstetrics, Gynaecology and Neonatology
Queen Elizabeth II Research Institute for Mothers and Infants
The University of Sydney
Sydney, Australia

Jennifer Hirshfeld-Cytron MD, MSCI
Division of Reproductive Endocrinology and Infertility
Department of Obstetrics and Gynecology
Feinberg School of Medicine
Northwestern University
Chicago, IL, USA

Andrew Horne MBChB, PhD, MRCOG
Clinician Scientist and Consultant Gynaecologist
MRC Centre for Reproductive Health
University of Edinburgh
Edinburgh, UK

Daniela Hornung MD, PhD
Vice-Chair
Department of Obstetrics and Gynecology
University of Schleswig-Holstein
Lübeck, Germany

M. Louise Hull BSc, MBChB, PhD, FRANZCOG
Senior Lecturer
Research Centre for Reproductive Health
School of Paediatrics and Reproductive Health
University of Adelaide
Adelaide, Australia

Neil P. Johnson MD, CREI, FRANZCOG, FRCOG
Fertility Plus
Green Lane Clinical Centre;
Department of Obstetrics and Gynaecology
University of Auckland
Auckland, New Zealand

Shirin Khanjani MD, PhD
Clinical Research Fellow
Institute of Reproductive and Developmental Biology
Imperial College London
London, UK

Su-Yen Khong MB, ChB, MRCOG, FRANZCOG
Department of Obstetrics and Gynaecology
Nepean Clinical School
University of Sydney
Sydney, Australia

J. Julie Kim PhD
Assistant Professor
Department of Obstetrics and Gynecology
Division of Reproductive Biology Research
Robert H. Lurie Comprehensive Cancer Center
Northwestern University
Chicago, IL, USA

Petra A. B. Klemmt PhD
Senior Research Scientist
Institute for Cell Biology and Neuroscience
Johann Wolfgang Goethe University
Frankfurt, Germany

Jennifer L. Kulp
Instructor
Department of Obstetrics, Gynecology and Reproductive Sciences
Yale University School of Medicine
New Haven, CT, USA

Alan Lam MBBS, FRCOG, FRANZCOG
Department of Obstetrics and Gynaecology
Nepean Clinical School
University of Sydney
Sydney, Australia

Jolande A. Land MD, PhD
Professor of Reproductive Medicine
Department of Obstetrics and Gynaecology
University Medical Center Groningen
Groningen, The Netherlands

Brigitte Leeners MD, Dr, PD
Head of Psychosomatic Gynaecology
Clinic for Reproductive Endocrinology
University Hospital Zürich
Zürich, Switzerland

Bruce A. Lessey MD, PhD
Director, Reproductive Endocrinology and Infertility
Department of Obstetrics and Gynecology
University Medical Group
University of South Carolina,
Greenville Campus
Greenville, SC, USA

Gerhard Leyendecker Prof. Dr. med
Kinderwunschzentrum (Fertility Center)
Darmstadt
Darmstadt, Germany

Jean-Christophe Lousse
Department of Gynecology
Université Catholique de Louvain
Institut de Recherche Expérimentale et Clinique
Brussels, Belgium

Hirotaka Masuda MD, PhD
The Ritchie Centre
Monash Institute of Medical Research
Melbourne, Australia

Melinda E. McConaha MS
Department of Obstetrics and Gynecology
Women's Reproductive Health Research Center
Vanderbilt University School of Medicine
Nashville, TN, USA

Diana Monsivais
Division of Reproductive Biology Research
Department of Obstetrics and Gynecology
Northwestern University
Feinberg School of Medicine
Chicago, IL, USA

Grant W. Montgomery PhD
Principal Research Fellow
Molecular Epidemiology
Queensland Institute of Medical Research
Brisbane, Australia

Kimberly Moon MD
Program in Reproductive and Adult
Endocrinology
Eunice Kennedy Shriver National Institute of
Child Health and Human Development
National Institutes of Health
Bethesda, MD, USA

Annemiek W. Nap MD PhD
Gynaecologist
Department of Obstetrics and Gynaecology
Rijnstate Hospital
Arnhem, The Netherlands

Camran Nezhat MD
Deputy Chief
Department of Obstetrics and Gynecology
Stanford University Medical Center;
Clinical Professor of Obstetrics and Gynecology
University of San Francisco;
Clinical Professor of Surgery
Stanford University Medical Center
Stanford, CA, USA

Cecilia H. M. Ng BSc, MHIM
Senior Research Fellow
Department of Obstetrics, Gynaecology and
Neonatology
Queen Elizabeth II Research Institute for Mothers
and Infants
The University of Sydney
Sydney, Australia

Kevin G. Osteen PhD
Professor and Director
Department of Obstetrics and Gynecology
Women's Reproductive Health Research Center
Vanderbilt University School of Medicine
Nashville, TN, USA

Jodie N. Painter
Molecular Epidemiology
Queensland Institute of Medical Research
Brisbane, Australia

Chandhana Paka
Center for Special Minimally Invasive and
Robotic Surgery
Stanford University Medical Centre
Palo Alto, CA, USA

Fabio Parazzini MD
Assistant Research Professor
Prima Clinica Ostetrico Ginecologica
Università di Milano
Milan, Italy

Srinu Pathivada MSc
Department of Obstetrics and Gynaecology
University Hospitals Leuven
Leuven, Belgium

Mary Ellen Pavone
Division of Reproductive Biology Research
Department of Obstetrics and Gynecology
Northwestern University
Feinberg School of Medicine
Chicago, IL, USA

Claudio Pelucchi MSc
Department of Epidemiology
Istituto di Ricerche Farmacologiche Mario Negri
Milan, Italy

Oswald Petrucco
The Robinson Institute
University of Adelaide
Adelaide, Australia

Sérgio Podgaec MD
Department of Obstetrics and Gynecology
University of São Paulo Medical School
São Paulo, Brazil

Cristin G. Print
Associate Professor
Department of Molecular Medicine and Pathology
School of Medical Sciences
Co-director
New Zealand Bioinformatics Institute
University of Auckland
Auckland, New Zealand

Peter A. W. Rogers PhD
Professor of Women's Health Research
Department of Obstetrics and Gynaecology
Monash University
Melbourne, Australia

Luk J. F. Rombauts MD, PhD,
FRANZCOG, CREI
Research Director, Monash IVF;
Associate Professor
Department of Obstetrics and Gynecology
Monash University
Melbourne, Australia

Anna Rosamilia MBBS,
FRANZCOG, CU, PhD
Department of Obstetrics and Gynaecology
Monash University
Melbourne, Australia

Lois A. Salamonsen PhD
Senior Principal Research Fellow
Prince Henry's Institute of Medical Research
Melbourne, Australia

Beata E. Seeber MD, MSCE
Department of Gynecologic Endocrinology and
Reproductive Medicine
Medical University Innsbruck
Innsbruck, Austria

Valerie I. Shavell MD
Fellow
Division of Reproductive Endocrinology and
Infertility
Department of Obstetrics and Gynecology
Wayne State University School of Medicine
Detroit, MI, USA

Steven Simoens BA, MSc, PhD
Professor
Research Centre for Pharmaceutical Care and
Pharmaco-economics
Catholic University of Leuven
Leuven, Belgium

Anna Sokalska MD, PhD
Assistant Research Professor
Department of Obstetrics and Gynecology
University of California Davis
Sacramento, CA, USA;
University of Medical Sciences
Poznan, Poland

Edgardo Somigliana MD
Department of Obstetrics, Gynecology and
Neonatology
Fondazione Cà Granda
Ospedale Maggiore Policlinico
Milan, Italy

Jean Squifflet
Department of Gynecology
Université Catholique de Louvain
Institut de Recherche Expérimentale et
Clinique
Brussels, Belgium

Anna Starzinski-Powitz PhD
Full Professor
Head of Molecular Cell Biology and Human
Genetics
Institute for Cell Biology and
Neuroscience
Johann Wolfgang Goethe University
Frankfurt, Germany

Andrew N. Stephens PhD
Prince Henry's Institute of Medical Research
Melbourne, Australia

Pamela Stratton MD
Chief, Gynecology Consult Service
Program in Reproductive and Adult
Endocrinology, Intramural Program
Eunice Kennedy Shriver National Institute of
Child Health and Human Development
National Institutes of Health
Bethesda, MD, USA

Hugh S. Taylor MD
Professor and Director
Department of Obstetrics, Gynecology and
Reproductive Sciences
Yale University School of Medicine
New Haven, CT, USA

Claire Templeman MD
Assistant Professor
Department of Obstetrics and Gynecology and
Surgery
University of Southern California;
Chief of Gynecology
Children's Hospital Los Angeles
Los Angeles, CA, USA

Candace Tingen PhD
Director of Research Programs
Coordinator, Illinois Women's Health Registry
Center for Reproductive Science
Northwestern University
Evanston, IL, USA;
Department of Obstetrics and Gynecology
Division of Fertility Preservation
Feinberg School of Medicine
Northwestern University
Chicago, IL, USA

Hideki Tokunaga
Department of Obstetrics and Gynecology
Tohoku University School of Medicine
Sendai, Japan

Natsuko Tokushige PhD
Senior Research Fellow
Department of Obstetrics, Gynaecology and
Neonatology
Queen Elizabeth II Research Institute for Mothers
and Infants
The University of Sydney
Sydney, Australia

Jim Tsaltas MBBS FRCOG FRANZCOG
Head of Gynaecological Endoscopy
Monash Medical Centre
Southern Health Care Network;
Department of Obstetrics and Gynaecology
Monash University
Melbourne, Australia

Togas Tulandi MD, MHCM
Professor of Obstetrics and Gynecology
Milton Leong Chair in Reproductive Medicine
McGill University
Montreal, Canada

Arathi Veeraswamy MD
Stanford University Medical Center
Center for Minimally Invasive and Robotic
Surgery
Palo Alto, CA, USA

Paolo Vercellini MD
Associate Professor of Obstetrics and Gynaecology
Prima Clinica Ostetrico Ginecologica
Università di Milano
Milan, Italy

Paola Viganò PhD
Senior Principal Investigator
Scientific Institute San Raffaele;
Center for Research in Obstetrics and Gynecology
Milan, Italy

Ursula von Wussow PhD
Scientist
Department of Obstetrics and Gynecology
University of Schleswig-Holstein
Lübeck, Germany

Gareth C. Weston MBBS, MPH, PhD,
FRANZCOG, CREI
Senior Lecturer
Department of Obstetrics and Gynaecology
Monash University
Melbourne, Australia

Ludwig Wildt Prof. Dr. med
Director
Department of Gynecological Endocrinology and
Reproductive Medicine
Medical University Innsbruck
Innsbruck, Austria

Elke Winterhager PhD
Full Professor
Institute of Molecular Biology
University Hospital Essen
Essen, Germany

Teresa K. Woodruff PhD
Thomas J. Watkins Professor of
Obstetrics and Gynecology
Director, Institute for Women's Health Research
Chief, Division of Fertility Preservation
Department of Obstetrics and Gynecology
Feinberg School of Medicine,
Northwestern University
Chicago, IL, USA

Xunqin Yin PhD
Department of Obstetrics and Gynecology
Division of Reproductive Biology Research
Robert H. Lurie Comprehensive Cancer Center
Northwestern University
Chicago, IL, USA

Steven L. Young MD, PhD
Division of Reproductive Endocrinology and
Infertility
Department of Obstetrics and Gynecology
University of North Carolina at Chapel Hill
Chapel Hill, NC, USA

Krina T. Zondervan
Wellcome Trust Centre for Human Genetics
University of Oxford
Oxford, UK

Preface

Endometriosis is a multifaceted disease that affects the quality of life of millions of women and their families worldwide. Its diagnosis is complex, and treatments of associated chronic pelvic pain and infertility, which have evolved through multiple disciplines, have unpredictable and often limited effectiveness. Over the past 20 years, studies on the pathogenesis and pathophysiology of endometriosis have increased our understanding of the roles of steroid hormones, genetics, the environment, the immune system, and the peripheral and central nervous systems in disease establishment, progression/regression, and associated signs and symptoms and co-morbidities. Medical and surgical therapies have been informed by some of these biological mechanisms, and clinical trials testing the efficacies of these therapies, along with evaluating risks and alternatives, offer much promise to improve the quality of life of women with endometriosis.

In this book, we have aimed to provide a comprehensive approach to the biology, diagnosis and treatment of endometriosis. We showcase the latest in molecular, genetic and epigenetic research underlying its pathophysiology, the effects of endometriosis on pregnancy outcomes, insights into its pathogenesis from laboratory studies, animal models, and epidemiologic studies, and rigorous evaluation of clinical diagnostics and therapeutics - past, present, and future - to alleviate pain and suffering associated with this disorder. We have engaged leading surgeons, physicians, established researchers, as well as emerging leaders with fresh ideas and approaches, to achieve these goals.

For the cover illustration we have chosen a detail of the fresco "Events from the Life of Moses" (1481) by Sandro Boticelli in the Sistine Chapel in Rome. The young girl is obviously in pain, as reflected by the red glow on her cheeks. She is wearing a girdle consisting of apples (symbolizing fertility) and acorns (symbolizing slow growth and long duration), probably to fend off two of the most important manifestations of endometriosis, infertility and chronic pelvic pain. We hope that learners of all ages and from multiple disciplines, clinicians, researchers, and patients will take an opportunity to see the entire fresco for its beauty and symbolism and will benefit from the knowledge imparted in the pages of this book, which we hope will stimulate new knowledge, so one day we can cure endometriosis or, perhaps, even better, prevent it.

Linda C. Giudice
Johannes L.H. Evers
David L. Healy

List of Abbreviations

2D PAGE	two-dimensional polyacrylamide gel electrophoresis	ccf	circulating cell-free	DIE	deep infiltrating endometriosis
AAGL	American Association of Gynecologic Laparoscopists	CCOC	continuous combined oral contraceptives	DIGE	differential in-gel electrophoresis
ABMS	American Board of Medical Specialities	CCR	cognate chemokine receptor	Dll	d-like ligand-4
		CDKN	cyclin-dependent kinase inhibitor	DMA	demethylation agent
ACh	acetylcholine	CFU	colony-forming unit	DMPA	depot medroxyprogesterone acetate
aCL	anticardiolipin	CGRP	calcitonin gene-related peptide		
ADC	5-aza-2'-deoxycytidine			DNMT	DNA methyltransferases
AEAB	antiendometrial antibodies	CHM	Chinese herbal medicine	DOF	degrees of freedom
AFC	antral follicle count	CI	confidence interval	DRG	dorsal root ganglia
AFS	American Fertility Society	CNS	central nervous system	DUB	dysfunctional uterine bleeding
AI	aromatase inhibitor	CoA	coenzyme A		
AMH	anti-müllerian hormone	COC	combined oral contraceptives	DZ	dizygotic
ANA	antinuclear autoantibodies	COH	controlled ovarian hyperstimulation	E	estrogen
APC	antigen-presenting cell			EAOC	endometriosis-associated ovarian cancer
AR	androgen receptor	COX	cyclooxygenase		
ART	assisted reproductive technology	CP	catamenial pneumothorax	EBAF	endometrial bleeding associated factor
		CPP	chronic pelvic pain		
ATP	adenosine triphosphate	CPR	clinical pregnancy rate	E-cadherin	epithelial cadherin
BDNF	brain-derived neurotropic factor	CREB	cAMP response element binding protein	ECM	extracellular matrix
				EDC	endocrine disrupting chemical
bFGF	basic fibroblast growth factor	CRP	C-reactive protein		
		CRPS	complex regional pain syndrome	EEC	endometrial epithelial cell
BlyS	B-lymphocyte stimulator			EFI	Endometriosis Fertility Index
BMD	bone mineral density	CS	cesarean section		
BMI	Body Mass Index	CT	computed tomography	EGCG	epigallocatechin gallate
BM-MSC	bone marrow-derived mesenchymal stem cells	DC	dendritic cell	EGF	epidermal growth factor
		DCE MRI	dynamic contrast-enhanced magnetic resonance imaging	ELISA	enzyme-linked immunosorbent assay
bp	base pair				
BPA	bisphenol A	DDE	dichlorodiphenyldichloroethylene	EMMPRIN	extracellular matrix metalloproteinase inhibitor
BrdU	bromodeoxyuridine				
CA	cyproterone acetate, carbonic anhydrase	DDT	dichlorodiphenyltrichloroethane	EMT	epithelial-mesenchymal transition
		DES	diethylstilbestrol	EMX2	empty spiracles homolog 2
CAM	chorio-allantoic membrane, cell adhesion molecule	DEXA	dual-energy x-ray absorptiometry	END-AD	endometriosis and adenomyosis
cAMP	cyclic adenosine monophosphate	DHT	dihydrotestosterone	EP	estrogen-progestin

EpCAM	epithelial cell adhesion molecule	hCG	human chorionic gonadotropin	KIR	killer immunoglobulin-like receptors
ER	estrogen receptor	HDAC	histone deacetylase	K-RAS	Kirsten rat sarcoma viral oncogene homolog
ERBB	erythroblastic leukemia viral oncogene homolog	HDACI	histone deacetylase inhibitor	LCS	laparoscopic coagulating shear
ERE	estrogen response element	H&E	hematoxylin and eosin	LD	linkage disequilibrium
ERK	extracellular signal-regulated kinase	HGF	hepatocyte growth factor	LF	least function
ERRFI1	erythroblastic leukemia viral oncogene homolog receptor feedback inhibitor 1	HIF	hypoxia-inducible factor	LFA	leukocyte function antigen
		HLA	human leukocyte antigen	LH	luteinizing hormone
		HMG	human menopausal gonadotrophin	LHCGR	luteinizing hormone/chorionic gonadotropin receptor
ESC	endometrial stromal cell	HMG-CoA	3-hydroxy-3-methyl glutaryl-coenzyme A		
ESE	early secretory	HMT	histone methyltransferase	LNG-IUS	levonorgestrel-releasing intrauterine system
ESHRE	European Society of Human Reproduction and Embryology	HPA	hypothalamic-pituitary-adrenal	LOD	logarithm of odds
		HPRT	hypoxanthine-guanine phosphoribosyl transferase	LOH	loss of heterozygosity
ESR	estrogen receptors	HRT	hormone replacement therapy	LPD	luteal phase defect
EST	expressed sequence tags			LPS	lipopolysaccharide
FACS	fluorescence activated cell sorting	hsCRP	high-sensitivity C-reactive protein	LR	likelihood ratio
				LRC	label-retaining cell
FasL	Fas ligand	HSD	hydroxysteroid dehydrogenase	LSE	late secretory
FDA	Food and Drug Administration	hsp	heat shock proteins	LUNA	laparoscopic uterine nerve ablation
FGF	fibroblast growth factor	ICAM	intercellular adhesion molecule	MAC	membrane attack complex
FIH	factor inhibiting hypoxia-inducible factor	iCAT	isotope-coded affinity tags	MAPK	mitogen-activated protein kinase
FLL	first-look laparoscopy	ICD	*International Classification of Diseases*	MAPKKK	mitogen-activated protein kinase kinase kinase
FPP	farnesyl pyrophosphate				
FS	fat suppression	ICSI	intracytoplasmic sperm injection	Mb	megabase
FSE	fast spin echo			MBR	Medical Birth Register
FSH	follicle-stimulating hormone	IDC	indwelling catheter	MCP	monocyte/macrophage chemotactic protein
		IEC	International ENDOGENE Consortium		
FTase	farnesyltransferase			MCSF	macrophage colony-stimulating factor
GFP	green fluorescent protein	Ig	immunoglobulin		
GGPP	geranylgeranyl-pyrophosphate	IGF	insulin-like growth factor	MDCK	Madin-Darby canine kidney
		IGFBP	insulin-like growth factor binding protein	MET	mesenchymal-epithelial transition
GGTase	geranylgeranyltransferase				
GIFT	gamete intrafallopian tube transfer	IL	interleukin	MFR	monthly fecundity rate
		ILT	immunoglobulin-like transcript	MHC	major histocompatibility complex
Glut	glucose transporter				
GM-CSF	granulocyte macrophage-colony stimulating factor	IMS	imaging mass spectrometry	MIF	migration inhibitory factor
		INF	interferon	miRNA	microRNA
GnRH	gonadotropin releasing hormone	IPA	ingenuity pathway analysis	MIS	minimally invasive surgery
		IRS	insulin receptor substrate, immunoreactive scores	MMIF	macrophage migration inhibitory factor
GnRHa	gonadotropin-releasing hormone agonist				
		iTRAQ	isobaric tags for relative and absolute quantitation	MMP	matrix metalloproteinase
GO	gene ontology			MPA	medroxyprogesterone acetate
GWA	genome-wide association	IUI	intrauterine insemination		
GWAS	genome-wide association study	IVF	*in vitro* fertilization	MRI	magnetic resonance imaging
		IVP	intravenous pyelography		
HA	hyaluronic acid	JNK	c-Jun NH2-terminal kinase		
HAT	histone acetylase	Kb	kilobases	mRNA	messenger RNA

Abbreviation	Definition
MRU	magnetic resonance urography
MS	mass spectrometry, multiple sclerosis
MSC	mesenchymal stem cells
MSE	midsecretory
mtDNA	mitochondrial DNA
mTORC2	mammalian target of rapamycin complex 2
MVD	microvessel density
MZ	monozygotic
NA	norethisterone (norethindrone) acetate
NADPH	nicotinamide adenine dinucleotide phosphate
NCAM	neural cell adhesion molecule
NCoR	nuclear receptor co-repressor
nDNA	nuclear DNA
NEA	norethindrone acetate
NF	neurofilament
NFκB	nuclear factor-κ-B
NGF	nerve growth factor
NHP	non-human primates
NK	natural killer
NLR	neutrophil/lymphocyte ratio
NMDA	N-methyl-D-aspartate
NOG	NOD/SCID/γ_c null
NPV	negative predictive value
NPY	neuropeptide Y
Nrarp	notch-regulated ankyrin repeat protein
NSAID	non-steroidal anti-inflammatory drug
nt	nucleotide
NT	neurotropin
OC	oral contraceptive
OCP	oral contraceptive pill
ODS	ovarian dysgenesis syndrome
OR	odds ratio
OT	oxytocin
OTR	oxytocin receptor
P	progesterone
p38K	p38 kinase
PAI	plasminogen activator inhibitor
PAR	protease-activated receptor
PB	peripheral blood
PBS	phosphate buffer saline
PCB	polychlorinated biphenyl
PCDD	polychlorinated-dibenzo-dioxin
PCDF	polychlorinated-dibenzo-furan
PCOS	polycystic ovarian syndrome
PCR	polymerase chain reaction
PDGF	platelet-derived growth factor
PDGF-BB	platelet-derived growth factor-BB
PDGFR	platelet-derived growth factor receptor
PDK1	3-phosphoinositide dependent protein kinase-1
PE	proliferative
PECAM	platelet endothelial cell adhesion molecule
PF	peritoneal fluid
PG	prostaglandin
PGR	progesterone receptor
PHA	phytohemagglutinin
PHD	prolyl hydroxylase domain
pI	isoelectric point
PID	pelvic inflammatory disease
PIP2	phosphatidylinositol (4,5) bisphosphate
PIP3	phosphatidylinositol (3,4,5) trisphosphate
PKA	protein kinase A
PKC	protein kinase C
PlGF	placental growth factor
PMC	peritoneal mesothelial cells
PMN	polymorphonuclear neutrophil
PMS	premenstrual syndrome
PNS	peripheral nervous system
POF	premature ovarian failure
POI	premature ovarian insufficiency
PPAR	peroxisome proliferator-activated receptor
PPROM	premature preterm rupture of membranes
PPV	positive predictive value
PR	progesterone receptor
PRDX	peroxiredoxin
PRL	prolactin
PTM	post-translational modification
QALY	quality-adjusted life-years
Q-RT-PCR	quantitative real-time polymerase chain reaction
RA	rheumatoid arthritis
rAFS	revised American Fertility Society
rag2γ(c)	recombinant activating gene 2/common cytokine receptor γ chain (γ_c) double null
RANTES	regulated on activation normal T-cell expressed and secreted
rASRM	revised American Society for Reproductive Medicine
RCOG	Royal College of Obstetricians and Gynaecologists
RGS1	regulators of G protein signaling 1
ROC	receiver operating characteristic
ROS	reactive oxygen species
RR	relative risk
RTK	receptor tyrosine kinase
RT-PCR	real-time (reverse transcriptase) polymerase chain reaction
SAA	serum amyloid A
SAGE	serial analysis of gene expression
SCID	severe combined immunodeficient
SD	standard deviation
SDF	stromal-derived factor
SE	spin echo
SEAN	size exclusion/affinity nanoparticles
SELDI-	surface-enhanced laser
SEM	standard error of the mean
SERM	selective estrogen modulators
SF	steroidogenic factor
SFRP	secreted frizzled-related proteins
SGA	small for gestational age
SHBG	sex hormone binding globulin
sICAM	soluble intercellular adhesion molecule

SIR	standardized incidence ratios	StAR	steroidogenic acute regulatory protein	Treg	regulatory T-cells
siRNA	small interfering RNA	STARD	Standards for Reporting of Diagnostic Accuracy	TSA	trichostatin A
SLE	systemic lupus erythematosus			TSSS	total symptom severity score
SLL	second-look laparoscopy	T	Thomsen–Friedenreich-like	tTgase-2	tissue transglutaminase 2
SMA	smooth muscle actin	TCDD	tetrachlorodibenzo-p-dioxin	TTP	time to pregnancy
SMRT	silencing mediator for retinoid and thyroid hormone	TDF	testis-determining factor	TURE	transurethral resection of endometriosis
		TDS	testicular dysgenesis syndrome	TVS	transvaginal sonography
SNP	single nucleotide polymorphism	TES	thoracic-endometriosis syndrome	TVUS	transvaginal ultrasound
SP	side population, substance P	TF	tissue factor	UNC	ureteroneocystostomy
SPARC	secreted protein, acidic, cysteine-rich, osteonectin	TFI	tubal factor infertility	uPA	urokinase-type plasminogen activator
		TGF	transforming growth factor		
SPRM	selective progesterone modulator	TGF-βR2	transforming growth factor-β receptor 2	UTR	untranslated regions
				VAS	visual analog scores
SRC	steroid receptor co-activator	TFIF	transforming growth factor-β-induced factor	VCAM	vascular cell adhesion molecule
SRM	selected reaction monitoring	TIAR	tissue injury and repair	VEGF	vascular endothelial growth factor
		TIMP	tissue inhibitor of metalloproteinases	vHL	von Hippel–Lindau
SRY	sex-determining region on the Y chromosome	TNF	tumor necrosis factor	VIM	vimentin
		TOF-MS	desorption/ionization time of flight mass spectrometry	VIP	vasointestinal peptide
SS	Sjögren syndrome			VPA	valproic acid
				WBC	white blood cell
				WMD	weighted mean difference

1   History, Epidemiology, and Economics

1 History of Endometriosis: A 20th-Century Disease

Ivo Brosens[1] and Giuseppe Benagiano[2]

[1]Department of Obstetrics and Gynaecology, Catholic University of Leuven, Leuven, Belgium
[2]Department of Gynecology and Obstetrics, Sapienza, University of Rome, Italy

Introduction

A reconstruction of the history of progress made in identifying, describing, and treating the condition we call endometriosis is neither simple nor easy because for almost 90 years endometriosis and adenomyosis, with the possible exception of ovarian endometrioma, were considered as one disease called "adenomyoma." As such, historians must deal first of all with a controversy over who was the first to identify the benign, non-neoplastic presence of ectopic endometrium within the uterine wall or in the peritoneal cavity and structures. In addition, they must be aware that the early history of endometriosis is interwoven with the early history of adenomyosis, since it was not until the mid 1920s that the two conditions were finally separated.

Who identified endometriosis?

The history of medicine is full of controversies over who "discovered" a specific disease. In certain cases this is due to a desire to attribute the discovery to a researcher from a given country; in others, it is due to conflicting evidence, as sometimes disagreement focuses on the criteria utilized to attribute the discovery.

The latter situation is typical of endometriosis, a condition that does not lend itself to a purely clinical diagnosis. This is why, before embarking on a search for who "discovered" (a better word is definitely "identified") it, it is necessary to fix a set of criteria, first and foremost what constitutes the "essence" of endometriosis. Some favor clinical descriptions, rather than histology or pathogenesis. Knapp, for instance, believed that the first descriptions of endometriosis can be found in *Theses and Dissertations* published in Belgium and The Netherlands during the second half of the 17th century [1], whereas Batt believes that

endometriosis was discovered when the presence of heterotopic endometrial tissue was first described, even though the conditions were all labeled "sarcomas" [2].

We are of the opinion that the identification of the conditions we today distinguish in *peritoneal* and *ovarian endometriosis* and in *adenomyosis* (globally here called END-AD) must be based on the observation of the presence of endometrial glands and stroma outside the uterine cavity and on the specification that this invasion was "benign" in nature. Using these criteria, we will critically examine published information on the history of endometriosis.

The first information that needs to be evaluated is contained in a publication by Vincent Knapp [1]. In it, he explained that the disease we name endometriosis was already identified 300 years ago. His conclusion was based on a series of 11 inaugural dissertations presented at European universities between 1690 and 1795. The *Disputatio Inauguralis Medica de Ulceribus Uteri* by Daniel Christianus Schrön presented at the University of Jena in 1690 is now sometimes cited as the first description of endometriosis [3]. However, close scrutiny of some of the original manuscripts from this period has shown that the descriptions evidenced signs of inflammation such as pus, uterine wounds or erosions that were linked to manipulation, an abortion or a syphilitic lesion. The symptoms described were those of an infection and included pain, insomnia, fever, vaginal lesions, dysuria, purulent urine (if the lesion involved the bladder) or purulent stool (if the lesion involved the intestines). There were no descriptions in the *Disputatio Inauguralis* or in the other later dissertations that could be interpreted as being indicative of endometriosis. Sadly, Vincent Knapp passed away a few months after publication of his manuscript and a letter to the Editor of *Fertility and Sterility* remained without response [4].

A point that has been overlooked is that, without a microscope, these early authors had no way to even predict the presence of endometrial tissue outside the uterus. Therefore, applying the

Endometriosis: Science and Practice, First Edition. Edited by Linda C. Giudice, Johannes L.H. Evers and David L. Healy.
© 2012 Blackwell Publishing Ltd. Published 2012 by Blackwell Publishing Ltd.

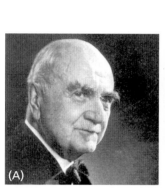
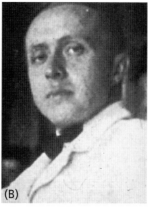
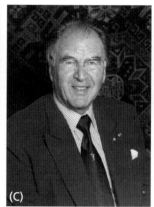
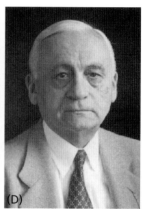

Figure 1.1 Gallery of pioneers in the study of endometriosis. (A) Thomas S. Cullen (1868–1953). Courtesy of Lippincott, Williams & Wilkins. (B) John A. Sampson (1873–1946). Courtesy of Albany Medical College, New York. (C) Kurt Semm (1927–2003). Courtesy of Liselotte Mettler. (D) Emil Novak (1884–1957). Courtesy of Lippincott, Williams & Wilkins.

above-mentioned criteria, it becomes a physical impossibility for endometriosis to have been described during the 17th and 18th centuries. In addition, in those days abdominal surgery could not be performed and so, either the lesions were superficialm and therefore could not be "endometriotic" in nature, or they could have been observed only at macroscopic autopsy examination and there is no trace of this having been the case.

More complex is the situation with regard to Carl Rokitansky, who in 1860 described what Batt called "three phenotypes of endometriosis containing endometrial stroma and glands" [2]. The first consisted of two varieties labeled *Sarcoma adenoids uterinum* (invading the uterine muscular wall) and *Cystosarcoma adenoids uterinum* (a cystic variety associated to myometrial hypertrophy). The second, named *Cystosarcoma adenoids uterinum polyposum*, invaded the endometrial cavity forming a polyp and the third *Ovarian-Cystosarcom* invaded the ovary [5]. In an early paper on the history of endometriosis [6] we omitted any reference to Rokitansky on the basis of the "malignant nature" of his descriptions. Indeed, Rokitanski specifically mentioned:

> … a sarcoma tissue in the form of papillary excrescences grow into the space of the cyst-like degenerated tubules. The slit-like, lacunar clefts scattered within the sarcoma produce on cross-section a granular appearance. The circumscribed nodes, which can be shelled-out, and appear incorporated in the sarcoma mass, doubtless originate from the filling of the great cyst spaces by intruding tumor tissue – a common appearance, which is especially pronounced in *cystosarcoma adenoids mammarium*.

To us, this is the description of a malignant tissue. Batt, however, insists that, in spite of the nomenclature, Rokitansky was aware of the benign nature of these invasions and that therefore he was the first to identify "the benign invasion of endometrial glands and stroma into the peritoneal cavity and organs" [2].

Setting aside the question of the nature of the lesions observed by Rokitansky, it is their origin that created a fierce controversy, with pathologists of the fame of von Recklinghausen [7] contend-

ing that lesions that were then called "adenomyoma" were the result of displacement of Wolffian or mesonephric vestiges.

When we examine the many and detailed descriptions of "mucosal invasions" of the peritoneal cavity and organs published at the end of the 19th and during the early part of the 20th century, we must conclude that the majority of pathologists rejected the hypothesis that the glands they observed were "endometrial." As late as 1918, Lockyer, in detailing the various theories on the origin of epithelial glands and stroma found in the pelvis outside the uterine cavity, was unable to resolve the question of their origin. He wrote: "Nothing but the topography of the tumor, nothing but laborious research entailing the cutting of serial sections in great numbers, can settle the question as to the starting point of the glandular inclusions for many of the cases of adenomyoma" [8]. Therefore, earlier researchers who described mucosal invasions in the abdominal cavity, but failed to consider these invasions as being made of endometrial cells, cannot be considered as having "discovered" END-AD.

It was the surgeon Thomas Cullen (Fig. 1.1A) who described for the first time both the morphological and clinical picture of END-AD. In the preface to his book *Adenomyoma of the Uterus*, Cullen [9] wrote in 1908:

> One afternoon in October 1882, while making the routine examination of the material from the operating room I found a uniformly enlarged uterus about four time(s) the natural size. On opening it I found that the increase in size was due to a diffuse thickening of the anterior wall … Examination of the(se) sections showed that the increase in thickness was due to the presence of a diffuse myomatous tumor occupying the inner portion of the uterine wall, and that the uterine mucosa was at many points flowing into the diffuse myomatous tissue.

Over the following years Cullen collected 90 uteri with adenomyomata and described the various presentations of "adenomyomata" in the myometrial wall, uterine horn, subserosa and uterine ligaments and showed in the uterus the continuity between the endometrial glands and the glandular structures

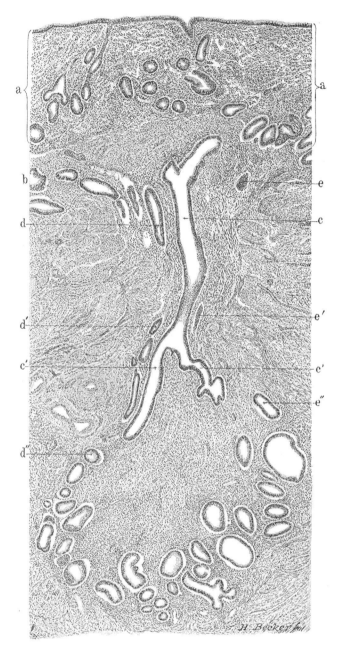

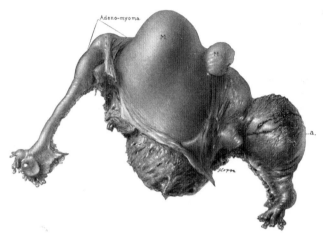

Figure 1.3 Hysterectomy specimen with tubal pregnancy on the right side and deciduoma in the left uterine horn. Sections showed no connection between the cornual deciduoma and the endometrium. Reproduced from Cullen [9] with permission from Elsevier.

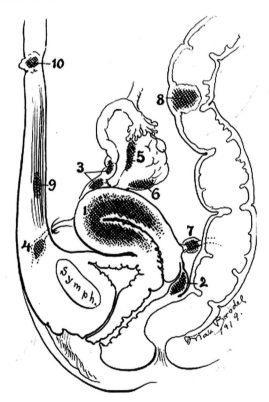

Figure 1.2 Histological demonstration of the continuity between the endometrium layer and the adenomyotic tissue in the myometrium. Reproduced from Cullen [9] with permission from Elsevier.

Figure 1.4 Scheme with the classic sites of adenomyotic lesions in the pelvis according to Cullen (1921). 1 Myometrium; 2 rectovaginal septum; 3 fallopian tube; 4 round ligament; 5 ovarian hilus; 6 ovarian surface; 7 sacrouterine ligament; 8 bowel; 9 abdominal wall; 10 umbilicus. Reproduced from Cullen [10] with permission from Elsevier.

deep in the myometrium (Fig. 1.2). In addition, he was the first to describe decidualization of the stromal cells during pregnancy, providing the functional proof that the cells were of endometrial origin (Fig. 1.3). He was also the first to describe the symptoms of the uterine adenomyoma, and concluded rather optimistically:

> I cannot help feeling that anyone who reads the chapter on symptoms will agree with us that diffuse adenomyoma has a fairly defined clinical history of its own and that in the majority of cases it can be diagnosed with a relative degree of certainty.

In 1920 Thomas Cullen [10] drew a scheme with the classic sites of adenomyotic lesions in the pelvis (Fig. 1.4). Adenomyoma involved ectopic endometrial-like tissue in the myometrial wall, rectovaginal septum, hilus of the ovary, uterine ligaments, rectal

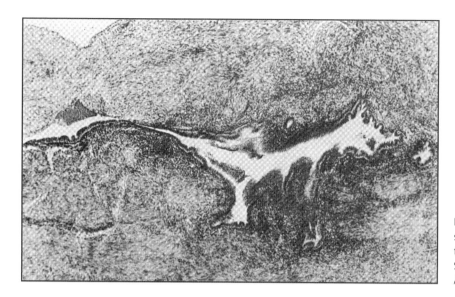

Figure 1.5 Endometriotic implant on the ovary showing shedding and bleeding of the endometrium-like tissue at the time of menstruation. Reproduced from Sampson [11] with permission from American Medical Association.

wall, and umbilicus. There is no doubt that Cullen considered uterine adenomyoma, ovarian endometriosis, and deep endometriosis as one disease characterized by the presence of adenomyomatous tissue outside the uterine mucosa.

It is customary to consider John A. Sampson (see Fig. 1.1B) as the discoverer of endometriosis and indeed, his work on peritoneal and ovarian endometrioma provided the first theory on the pathogenesis of the disease. His original observation came when he operated on women at the time of menstruation and found that the peritoneal lesions were bleeding similarly to what happens in eutopic endometrium (Fig. 1.5) [11]. This proved to him that the tissue outside the uterus was of endometrial origin. In 1927 Sampson postulated that the presence of endometrial cells outside the uterus was due to tubal regurgitation and dissemination of menstrual shedding [12].

Clearly, peritoneal endometriosis became the signature of the disease and with the introduction of laparoscopy in the 1960s, a golden tool became available for visual diagnosis and surgical therapy. As a result, endometriosis was divorced from the uterus and research became focused on how fragments of menstrual endometrium implant on peritoneal surfaces and invade the underlying tissues. Since menstrual regurgitation and implantation could not explain a variety of ectopic localizations, other mechanisms were proposed, such as peritoneal metaplasia, transportation through veins or lymphatics, embryonic vestiges, transformation of bone marrow and stem cells.

Clinical issues

Awareness in the clinic

During the mid-20th century, endometriosis became a major clinical issue. In 1932 Hill Jr [13] reported on a series of 1200 patients who, between 1927 and 1931, were operated upon for pelvic pathology. In 135 women (11%), aberrant endometrium

was detected at microscopy. Amongst these cases, 20 had adenomyomata of the uterus and 115 peritoneal endometriosis. The majority of the patients were between 20 and 45 years of age, with the youngest being 16 years old and the oldest 61. Thirty percent of the patients were sterile. As menstrual problems were absent in 51%, the aberrant endometrium was assumed to have caused little if any of the menstrual disorders and the symptoms were believed to have been caused principally by the associated pathology. The most important individual symptom was pain and tenderness over the site of the growths during the menstrual period; this, however, was the exception and not the rule. On the other hand, acute complications of endometriosis were also described during this period, such as the spontaneous rupture of an endometrial ovarian cyst [14] and obstructing rectovaginal endometriosis [15].

Pelvic pain related to menstruation was, according to Counseller [16], the principal reason for seeking relief through surgery. There was usually a 10-year history from the onset of disease and the symptoms were progressive. Surgical treatment was either radical or conservative, depending on the extent. In cases of uterine adenomyosis, conservative treatment was performed by complete excision of the lesions from the myometrium plus a presacral neurectomy when the lesion was limited to the uterus. Other heterotopic lesions were treated by complete excision whenever possible or by surgical loop diathermy or partial resection when the lesions were located in the sigmoid or the rectovaginal septum.

In the 1940s endometriosis was described as a not uncommon disease, with various clinical appearances. At times a widespread distribution of lesions within the peritoneal cavity was noted. The majority of the lesions occurred on the peritoneum, cul-de-sac, rectovaginal septum, and ovaries. Less frequent locations included the umbilicus, the round ligaments, rectosigmoid, and laparotomy scars. Larger lesions may consist of a more or less solid tumor, an adenomyoma, or may be in the nature of a hemorrhagic cyst. Surgery was the treatment of choice. In this connection,

Benson and Sneeden argued in 1958 that confusion had developed because of the unfortunate and illogical inclusion of uterine adenomyosis with pelvic endometriosis, which, according to them, only occasionally co-exist [17].

In terms of pathogenesis, Javert [18] developed a composite theory of benign metastasis on the basis of his surgical experience with 1371 patients over a period of 17 years. He observed that the spread of benign endometrium is essentially the same as for endometrial carcinoma, with direct extension into lymphatics or blood vessels of the myometrium, or between the muscle bundles, thereby producing adenomyosis uteri, while exfoliation and implantation of endometrial cells at menstruation, during curettage or from a nidus in the tube produced lesions on peritoneal surfaces; finally, lymphatic and venous spread produced lesions in adjacent or distal organs. He explained the increase in the number of cases during the last 4 years of his observation by the tendency towards smaller families, widespread use of contraception, fewer cervical dilations, fewer uterine suspension operations and the use of more intravaginal tampons during menstruation. He believed that pregnancy was the best prophylactic and curative treatment for endometriosis, since it interrupts the cyclical homeoplasia during which time the endometrium lies dormant. Javert favored hysterectomy and bilateral salpingo-oophorectomy as the procedure of choice in older women.

In 1955, Henriksen [19] presented a review of 1000 cases of proven endometriosis. The disease was diagnosed on an awareness of the possibility of its existence, a careful history and a thorough retropelvic examination. Although the disease tended to regress following castration, some patients exhibited clinical and histological evidence of continued activity following ovariectomy. Henriksen also noted a frequent involvement of the bowel and concluded that endometriosis is an important possible factor in problems affecting both the small and large bowel. Proper management is based on the surgeon's appreciation of the natural history of the disease, the evaluation of factors such as age, severity of symptoms, extent of disease, desire for children, and the patient as a whole. He concluded that fortunately, the value of conservatism in the surgical management of the disease was becoming more widely appreciated.

Introduction of endoscopic techniques

New pelvic endoscopic techniques were introduced in gynecology in the late 1940s, whereas peritoneoscopy has been utilized in gastroenterology and general surgery since the late 1930s. Initial clinical applications of the new technique were made in the 1940s, soon widened to include differentiating between causes of intra-abdominal bleeding (including bleeding from rupture of a follicular cyst), between appendicitis and salpingitis and in order to decide whether or not gunshot or stab wounds were penetrating into the abdominal cavity.

In 1944 Decker and Cherry [20] proposed culdoscopy as a new procedure for pelvic visualization in gynecology and claimed that the procedure was invaluable in the investigation of pelvic tumors, small ovarian disease, endometriosis, ectopic pregnancy and especially helpful in the detailed study of primary and secondary sterility in women. Starting in 1967, Semm (see Fig. 1.1C) transformed peritoneoscopy into modern laparoscopy by improving the optical system, removing the source of light from the abdominal cavity and creating an automatic control of gas insufflation into the abdomen [21]. Technical improvements in laparoscopy quickly produced new information on endometriosis and expanded gynecological application of endoscopic surgery, to the extent that in the early 1970s leading gynecologists in Europe and the US concluded that laparoscopy was the preferred tool for diagnosis and surgery of endometriosis.

Attempts to create a classification of endometriosis

In an editorial published in *Obstetrics and Gynecology* in 1966, Beecham [22] claimed that a tedious effort to detail endometriotic location and lesion "would serve no purpose." He therefore presented a simple classification scheme of four stages that used physical and operative findings and stated that such a scheme would be appropriate to follow patients being managed by medical or surgical therapies. Others tried staging systems similar to those used for malignancy staging, but these classification methods were unable to correlate staging with clinical outcome. As a result, none of the attempts to classify endometriosis made before 1978 received widespread acceptance.

In a collaborative effort Acosta and co-workers [23] proposed a classification that divided the disease into mild, moderate, and severe based on surgical findings. Using this staging system with retrospective data, a direct relationship was established between initial stage of the disease and pregnancy rates. Disease also was automatically classified as severe in the presence of an endometrioma larger than 2 cm in size. Peritubal and periovarian adhesions separated mild from moderate disease, because ovarian adhesions were recognized as having a damaging effect on fertility. Many physicians objected that this classification system had several disadvantages, because of the arbitrariness of the staging and the inability to distinguish unilateral from bilateral disease. Buttram, then, in 1979 [24], proposed an expanded classification based on the Acosta scheme that allowed for more flexibility and less ambiguity. Despite modifications, none of the classifications received widespread acceptance or use; this prompted the American Fertility Society (AFS) to create a panel to design a classification system for endometriosis; its recommendations were published in 1979 [25].

The AFS classification scheme stratified endometriosis into mild, moderate, severe, and extensive disease and for the first time used a weighted point score that included assessment of the extent of endometriosis (two-dimensional) and presence of adhesions in the peritoneum, ovaries, and tubes. It also allowed for assessment of unilateral versus bilateral disease. The size of endometriomas was weighted differently, as was the presence of filmy versus dense adhesions. An anatomical drawing was included to aid in surgical finding documentation and a cumulative score was attained. From the outset, critics began to point out the shortcomings of the new classification: the point scores were recognized as arbitrarily assigned and it was anticipated that changes in the assignment would be based on clinical studies and disease progression or response to treatment. The evaluation of pregnancy success suggested that the AFS classification revealed significant differences only if categories were combined (mild plus moderate versus severe plus excessive). Pregnancy success was also significantly reduced if an ovarian endometrioma was greater than 3 cm or had ruptured [26]. While the features of infertility were emphasized, they were not necessarily related to pelvic pain.

In 1985, in response to all the problems identified, a revised scheme of the AFS classification was presented (the so-called rAFS) [27]. As the new system still had flaws similar to its predecessor, the AFS stated that the system would be subject to revision as clinical data became available. In 1996, Vercellini *et al* [28] concluded that the endometriosis stage was not consistently related to pain symptoms, while in 1997, Guzick *et al* [29] stated that the use of an arbitrary weighted system for assigning scores to individual categories of disease, or for computing a total score, has limited the overall effectiveness of the classification system to predict pregnancy. Limitations of the rAFS classification include arbitrariness of the scoring system, limited reproducibility, failure to consider the morphological type of the lesion and a limited value of the system to aid in the evaluation and management in the setting of pelvic pain. These and other critical opinions led in 1997 to the publication of a Revised American Society for Reproductive Medicine classification of endometriosis: 1996 [30].

Diversity of lesions
Peritoneal endometriosis
In the 1980s it became evident that peritoneal endometriosis has multiple appearances including microscopic foci, early-active (red, glandular or vesicular), advanced (black, puckered), and healed (white, fibrotic) forms. These lesions may represent replacement of mesothelium by an endometrial epithelium or endometrial polyp formation [31,32]. However, the anatomical distribution of ectopic endometrium, as assessed by laparoscopy in a series of 182 consecutive patients, supported Sampson's hypothesis of retrograde menstruation as the primary model of development of endometriosis [33]. Laparoscopic observations [34] suggested that early lesions appear and disappear "like mushrooms on the peritoneal surface." The importance of even very small lesions became evident when, in a prospective study of artificial insemination in women with minimal endometriosis, Jansen [35] found reduced fecundability. Awareness of the existence of subtle endometriosis produced an increase in the diagnosis of endometriosis, although clinical significance of early lesions remained controversial [36–38]. From all published evidence, Evers [39] concluded that peritoneal endometriosis appears to be a dynamic disease, especially in the early phase, with subtle, atypical lesions emerging and vanishing again. The dynamic phase of the disease may involve a varying interval of each patient's life (e.g. a period of amenorrhea or pregnancy). Laparoscopy at the end of medical suppression of the activity of the implants may

lead to the erroneous conclusion that treatment has been effective. The final answer to the question of whether endometriosis is a progressive disease will have to come from long-term prospective investigations studying spontaneous evolution of peritoneal lesions without therapeutic interference.

Vercellini *et al* [28] analyzed the prevalence and severity of dysmenorrhea, intermenstrual pain and deep dyspareunia in relation to morphological features of peritoneal endometriosis. A statistically significant association was observed only with deep dyspareunia. Fresh, papular, atypical lesions might cause functional pain, whereas "old," black nodules immersed in infiltrating scars might provoke mainly organic pain. Belasch *et al* [40] found a high prevalence of superficial endometriosis in biopsies from the uterosacral ligaments in both patients with chronic pelvic pain and asymptomatic (fertile and infertile) women.

Rectovaginal endometriosis
As in the case of infertility, investigators found poor correlation between lesion characteristics or stage of disease and pelvic pain. Cornillie *et al* [41] noted a strong correlation between pelvic pain and the depth of invasion, with severe pelvic pain in the presence of implants more than 10 mm deep. Lesions more than 5 mm deep were also found to be histologically more active than superficial lesions. Koninckx *et al* [42] found no correlation between types of endometriotic lesions, total surface area of endometriosis-invaded areas, and amount of pain.

Three subgroups of deep endometriosis were suggested by Koninckx and Martin [43]: *type I* is conically shaped and seems to be formed by infiltration; *type II* is deeply located, covered by adhesions and probably formed by retraction; *type III* is a spherical nodule located in the rectovaginal septum and causes the most severe and largest lesion. They considered type III as a form of adenomyosis.

In the late 1990s, rectal endoscopic ultrasonography was proposed to diagnose the presence of deep bowel infiltration and select patients for surgery [44,45].

In recognition of some of the shortcomings of the rAFS classification in the evaluation of pelvic pain, the American Society for Reproductive Medicine (formerly the AFS) formed a subcommittee which developed a form for the preoperative assessment of pain quality and location on examination and their correlation with operative findings, including adhesion type, description of peritoneal lesion type by morphological appearance and the mean diameter and depth of invasion [46].

Ovarian endometrioma
Ovarian endometriosis can present itself as chocolate cysts of various size, deep non-cystic lesions, surface pits and plaques, and very early lesions. In an detailed study of 29 ovary specimens with chocolate cysts, Hughesdon [47] found that in all except three cases, the ovarian endometrioma was a pseudocyst with an essentially similar structure: the ovary is adherent to the posterior side of the parametrium, the inside is constituted by invaginated ovarian cortex, endometriotic tissue is found at the site of adhesion

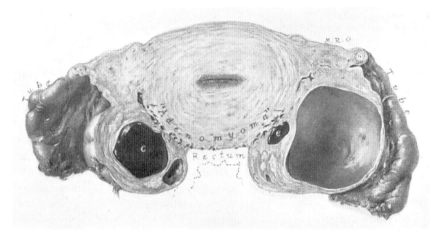

Figure 1.6 Cross-section of the uterus and ovaries. Both ovaries were adherent to the posterior surface of the uterus. Sampson interpreted the adhesions as sequelae of perforation of the endometriotic cysts and the adenomyoma on the posterior side of the uterus as spreading of the endometrioma over the surface of the uterus and early invasion. Reproduced from Sampson [11] with permission from American Medical Association.

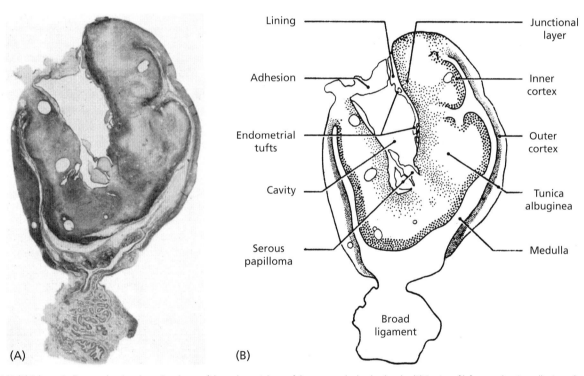

(A)

(B)

Figure 1.7 (A) Schematic diagram showing the various layers of the endometrial cyst of the ovary and other landmarks. (B) Section of left ovary showing adhesions above, cavity below, surrounded successively by thickened invaginated cortex, U-shaped medulla, and remainder of cortex, with broad ligament below. Reproduced from Hughesdon [47] with permission from Elsevier.

and a thin layer of superficial endometrium-like tissue extends to cover partially or fully the invaginated cortex (Fig. 1.6).

Hughesdon described four further characteristic features of ovarian endometriomas (Fig. 1.7). First, primordial and ripening follicles are found in the wall of the cyst. Second, the ovary does not invaginate uniformly, but remains on one side more or less normal. Third, on the extended side the wall is relatively thin and the attenuation of layers on this side is usually too great to reveal the original structure. Fourth, the identity of the cortex on the inner side is frequently obscured by smooth muscle metaplasia.

Hughesdon concluded that ectopic endometrium does not simply erode its way into the ovary: the ovary is actively invaginated, thus providing a pseudouterus. The structure demonstrated that the relation to the surface is primary and not secondary, such as would have been implied by Sampson's [11] original title of "perforating hemorrhagic cysts of the ovary" and by Halban's lymphatic theory [48]. Hughesdon also discussed the few cases with so-called "deep" ovarian endometriosis and demonstrated on serial sections that although deep, non-cystic lesions are, in a gross sense, in the ovary, the associated layering shows that they have originated at the surface. He concluded that the findings weigh heavily against the benign lymphatic metastasis theory and favor a surface origin by implantation or metaplasia.

Using an endoscopic technique, Brosens *et al* [49] investigated a series of endometriotic cysts *in situ* in young women with infertility and confirmed that the wall of the cyst is cortex. In a few cases ovulation has occurred in the cyst and both cavities were linked. In such cases the endometrial tissue colonized the luteal cyst, showing that, under such circumstances, endometriosis can invade the ovary. They distinguished two types of endometriotic cysts: the *red type* which is lined by a surface epithelium and a thin layer of highly vascularized stroma without glands covering partially or completely the whitish or slightly pigmented wall, and the *black type* where the wall is lined by dark, pigmented and fibrotic tissue with scanty vascularization. They also found that at the site of invagination and adhesions, the cortical wall was retracted and the implants were of the mucosa type with glandular structures. They suggested that surgery should be adapted to the type of endometrioma by ablation of the superficial endometriotic lining for the whitish wall and excision of the fibrotic wall for the black wall and the implants at sites of inversion and adherence.

In the 1980s imaging techniques such as magnetic resonance imaging [50–52] and transvaginal ultrasonography [53–55] were used to differentiate ovarian endometriomas from other non-endometriotic masses. While ovarian endometriomas are easily detected at laparoscopy and ultrasonography, small ovarian endometriomas may go unnoticed unless they are detected by puncture [56]. Nezhat *et al* [57] have proposed to distinguish between three types of ovarian endometriomas according to size, cyst contents, ease of capsule removal, adhesion of the cyst to other structures, and location of the superficial endometrial implants relative to the cyst wall. Nisolle *et al* [58] suggested that peritoneal, ovarian, and rectovaginal endometriosis are three different entities with a different structure and pathogenesis, respectively implantation, metaplasia, and mesodermal müllerian differentiation.

Stage V endometriosis

Canis *et al* [59] proposed to add a most severe stage of endometriosis to include patients with extensive disease, especially with bilateral dense adhesions; the addition of this stage is justified in their view by the fact that poor results in terms of restoring fertility are consistently obtained with conservative therapy alone. Using their revised classification scheme, a plan to proceed quickly toward *in vitro* fertilization (IVF) would be uniformly recommended for all stage V patients. It must be stressed that in patients with severe endometriosis, Pal *et al* [60] found with IVF a reduced fertilization potential of preovulatory oocytes.

Malignancy

In 1990, Heaps *et al* [61] reviewed a series of 205 cases reported in the English literature of malignant neoplasms arising from endometriotic foci. The ovary was the primary site (79%), whereas extragonadal sites represented 21%. Endometroid carcinomas accounted for 69% of the lesions and the remaining cases included clear cell carcinomas, sarcomas, and rare cell types. Heaps suggested that the actual frequency of malignancy arising in endometriosis may be higher than reported.

Modern therapeutic approaches

Hormonal therapy

The hormonal management of the symptoms associated with endometriosis was made possible almost 70 years ago, by the availability of the first synthetic steroid hormones and, interestingly enough, androgens preceded estrogens as therapeutic agents.

Androgen therapy

The first suggestion to utilize the newly identified steroid hormones as therapeutic agents came from Geist and Salmon [62] who, in 1941 in an article in *JAMA*, advocated the use of androgens in gynecological disorders. Following this lead, in 1943 Hirst [63] reported the results obtained with the use of testosterone propionate in two cases of women with severe endometriosis: treatment resulted in a reduction in swelling and relief of pain and he recommended the use of this form of treatment when radical surgical excision was contraindicated or refused by the patient.

The following year, Miller [64] published a case of endometriosis of the rectal wall and ovaries, treated preoperatively with testosterone propionate. He stated: "Testosterone propionate can be used in diminishing the activity and decreasing the size of the lesions in endometriosis so that radical surgery can be performed with less danger."

In spite of the positive results obtained, the undesirable side-effects of hirsutism, acne, and deepening of the voice occurred sufficiently often to cause the clinician and patient considerable concern. For this reason, androgen therapy never really took off and other avenues began to be explored. In 1958, commenting on the use of androgens, Kistner [65] noted that "androgenic substances, while adequately documented as having produced desirable results in endometriosis, probably exert their effect through inhibition of gonadotrophic substances although direct effect of the substance upon the endometriotic area has been suggested." This awareness prompted endocrinologists and gynecologists to test other gonadotropin-inhibiting substances.

Estrogens

In the late 1940s, the availability of a non-steroidal, synthetic estrogen, diethylstilbestrol (DES), prompted another line of experimental treatment for severe endometriosis.

We know today that estrogens are intimately involved with the growth of ectopic endometrial foci and therefore, with today's wisdom, estrogens would be, if anything, contraindicated. Indeed, although in all likelihood not an endocrine disease, endometriosis does not manifest itself in the absence of estrogens. Indeed, even when the disease manifests itself in postmenopausal patients, usually it appears in women treated with estrogens [66,67] and, in the rare occurrence in non-treated postmenopausal patients [67], it is believed that symptoms are the consequence of the progression of the estrogen-independent fibrosis, not of the growth of new foci [68]. At the same time, there is evidence that estrogens are not necessary for the endometrium to implant itself ectopically and indeed, grafting studies in nude mice and rabbits have shown that estrogens are required for the success of the implantation process [69,70]. Also, the recently reported presence of endometriotic foci in human fetuses [71] may be evidence of an estrogen-independent process.

In contradistinction to this, proliferation and growth of ectopic implants need the presence of estrogen. For instance, in castrated monkeys, hyperplastic-decidualized endometrial tissue transplanted into the peritoneum retains viability for more than 4 weeks, even without exogenous hormonal support, but the administration of supplemental estrogen and/or progesterone is required to sustain these endometrial plaques for periods of up to 16 weeks [69]. In addition, in a rat animal model experimentally implanted with human endometrial cells, following ovariectomy there is a complete regression of the implants, to the point that, 2 months later, no viable endometrial cells can be detected, even histologically. However, administration of estradiol cypionate to these animals leads to the recurrence of implants [72].

Finally, although endometriosis has been observed in the urinary bladder of men with prostatic carcinoma [73,74], in the case of pure gonadal dysgenesis [75] and Turner syndrome [76,77], streak gonads [78] and in a woman with a Rokitansky-Kuster-Hauser syndrome [79], all these patients had endogenous or exogenous estrogens, alone or in combination with a progestin. Therefore, the concept that estrogens are necessary in order to have active ectopic endometrial foci so far goes unchallenged.

This large body of knowledge did not exist and could not even be guessed when the first attempts were made to treat women with severe endometriosis with estrogens. The first to do so was Karnaky [80] who, in 1948, reported apparently good results with increasing daily doses of up to 100 mg/day of DES to obtain amenorrhea. In his report he reached an intriguing conclusion: "Endometriosis is not stimulated to grow by large continuous doses of stilbestrol, but small doses of stilbestrol may stimulate it." In his series, five patients became pregnant after stilbestrol was discontinued. With today's knowledge, the offspring of those pregnancies should have been followed very closely, although second-generation clear cell vaginal cancer has been usually attributed to use of DES in pregnancy, not before it [81].

In spite of the enthusiasm of its proponents, estrogen treatment of endometriosis did not last, and for reasons only partially related to modern knowledge. In 1958 Kistner [65] wrote: "the unpredictability of permanent relief in endometriosis following the use of estrogenic substances alone" and the fact that "estrogen therapy also has the disadvantage of occasionally resulting in rather profuse break-through bleeding, endometrial hyperplasia and hypermenorrhea at the time of withdrawal of the hormone" make this treatment unwise.

Under the circumstances, a rational approach to the hormonal treatment of endometriosis must involve the use of steroid hormones with the ability of either modulating or antagonizing that of endogenous estrogens.

"Pseudo-pregnancy"

There is indeed a solid rationale for the use of estrogen-progestin combinations for the treatment of symptoms associated with endometriosis and the obvious difficulty in understanding how the administration of an estrogen, especially at high doses, could be beneficial, in particular to patients with advanced endometriosis, the situation is different when we consider the association of an estrogen and a progestin. In this respect, it is well established that the contemporary administration of an estrogen and a progestin results in a partially inactive endometrium.

Although we have ample evidence that ectopic endometrium does not behave in the same way as eutopic endometrium [82] and that, in the same patient, the two can be out of phase with each other at any given time during the menstrual cycle [83], the basic principle of controlled growth under the combined effect of the estrogen-progestin combination remains true.

Historically, knowledge gained during the 1940s and early 1950s allowed the creation of a new concept that went under the name of "pseudo-pregnancy," the artificial creation of a hormonal situation mimicking that occurring naturally during pregnancy. Meigs [84] was the first to come up with this new idea. He wrote: "It is the author's belief that avoidance of endometriosis through early marriage and frequent childbearing is the most important method of prophylaxis." The concept bears striking similarity to the approach taken by Gregory Pincus in creating hormonal contraception [85].

Two researchers share the credit for the advent of "pseudo-pregnancy" as a treatment for endometriosis: Kistner [65] and Andrews [86]. Since "in many patients with this disease, conception is not always possible, either because of unknown factors producing infertility or because marriage is not contemplated," an artificial situation mimicking pregnancy was able to resolve the impasse [65]. The first experiments by Kistner involved 12 patients to whom large doses of a number of estrogenic compounds (diethylstilbestrol, Estinyl, estradiol valerate) and two progestins (17α-hydroxyprogesterone caproate and norethynodrel) were administered in a "graduate scale" for periods of up to 7 months to produce amenorrhea, as well as a decidual reaction in the endometrium. The pseudo-pregnancy regimen resulted in an improvement of the condition, both subjectively and objectively, except for occasional side-effects like uterine cramps or hypermenorrhea.

Andrews and his group [86] went a step further and, starting from the same observation of beneficial effects of pregnancy on endometriosis, they administered Enovid (norethynodrel plus mestranol) to 23 women with endometriosis. Decidual transformation was consistently demonstrated in the endometrial cavity and was present in the ectopic endometrium in all of the five instances in which it was obtained for study. Clinical improvement during therapy was observed in 14 of 17 patients treated because of pain.

To improve the effectiveness of the pseudo-pregnancy regimen, in 1960 Thomas [87] introduced long-acting steroid hormones. He treated 28 women with established endometriosis with an injectable preparation (Delalutin), containing 250 mg of 17α-hydroxyprogesterone caproate and 5 mg of estradiol valerate (administered twice weekly). He recommended that treatment be continued for a minimum of 4–6 months. All patients developed amenorrhea, which persisted throughout the period of hormone administration, and most of the women experienced considerable to complete relief of their symptoms.

The "pseudo-pregnancy" regimen has been used extensively since then for the treatment of endometriosis, although the last paper on the subject was published in 1975. Symptomatic relief of the disease was reported in a majority of cases; pregnancy rates in women who complained of infertility in addition to endometriosis ranged from 10% to 53% [88].

Recently, studies have begun to appear on the use of estrogen-progestin (EP) combinations in the treatment of endometriosis [89,90] and it has been shown that increasing the abnormally low apoptotic activity of the endometrium of patients with endometriosis, while at the same time achieving anovulation, decidualization, amenorrhoea and the establishment of a steady EP milieu, contribute to disease quiescence [90].

Other hormonal regimens

During the second part of the 20th century, a number of additional hormonal regimens have been proposed, the first being an antigonadotropic steroid, *danazol*. Its introduction in 1971 by Greenblatt [91] turned back the clock, since this compound has definite androgenic properties and may produce symptoms not very different from those reported in the 1940s. In 1990, Barbieri published an informative review of the use of danazol [92].

Interesting results have been obtained with the introduction of *gestrinone*, a steroid with androgenic, antiprogestinic and antiestrogenic activities [93]. Fedele and co-workers [94] were the first to compare the clinical effects of gestrinone and danazol, observing a significant decrease of pain-related symptoms (dysmenorrhea, pelvic pain, deep dyspareunia) in both groups, without any significant differences between the two components. The same year, Venturini and co-workers [95] showed that gestrinone significantly reduces serum concentrations of total testosterone and sex-steroid hormone binding globulin (SHBG), whereas free testosterone is slightly but significantly increased. Finally, estradiol is not significantly lowered in comparison with pretreatment follicular phase values.

Given results obtained with a mild antiprogestin like gestrinone, it was logical to expect even better results with the first "real antiprogestin," *mifepristone* [96], widely known as the "abortion pill." Unfortunately, its use in medical abortion has created a situation where, after very promising early clinical studies, for over 20 years no large-scale experimentation has been published. The early studies, conducted by Yen and his group [97,98], demonstrated a significant improvement not only in pelvic pain and dysmenorrhea but also in the rAFS score and therefore, a great potential for the cure of symptoms associated with endometriosis. Today, however, a second antiprogestin, *ulipristal*, has been marketed (as an emergency contraceptive) and work has resumed on possible applications of antiprogestins in the treatment of a number of proliferative disorders of the female reproductive tract.

Conservative surgery

During the second half of the 20th century, conservative surgery gained momentum and popularity [19] for the treatment of endometriosis as management became based on the surgeon's appreciation of the natural history of the disease and the evaluation of factors such as age, severity of symptoms, extent of disease, desire for children, and the patient as a whole. For instance, as already mentioned, it was noted that endometriosis tends to regress following surgical castration or spontaneous menopause, although in some patients it continues to exhibit clinical and histological evidence of activity.

Conservative surgery had the obvious advantage of theoretically preserving fertility and, in 1975 Kistner [99] noted that approximately 40–50% of patients who are desirous of child bearing and who had had conservative surgical treatment would become pregnant. Such pregnancy usually occurs within the first 24 months, although in a few patients, the delay may last 3 or 4 years. Kistner observed that pregnancy rates were influenced by five factors: the extent of disease; the age; having had previous surgery for endometriosis; the duration of infertility before surgery; and the length of postsurgical follow-up. To improve results, he advocated short postoperative periods of pseudo-pregnancy induced by hormonal treatment (see above), if all areas of endometriosis could not be excised. A few years later, Buttram [100] reported pregnancy rates of 73%, 56%, and 40% respectively for patients with mild, moderate, and severe endometriosis. As surgery was most beneficial in the early postoperative period, he recommended that if medical suppressive therapy is to be used in conjunction with conservative surgery to enhance fertility, it should be used preoperatively rather than postoperatively.

Laparoscopy

A major departure from classic gynecological surgery occurred in the early 1970s when Kurt Semm [101] introduced endoscopic methods for hemostasis during surgical pelviscopy, including endocoagulation, Roeder loop ligation, endoligature and endosuture with intra- and extracorporeal knotting. Then, in 1983, he performed the first endoscopic appendectomy. Further advances occurred when Nezhat *et al* [102] introduced carbon dioxide laser for the removal of endometriotic implants, excision of endometrioma capsules, and lysis of adnexal adhesions. In a series of 102 patients, they reported a pregnancy rate of 60% within 24 months after laser surgery without additional hormonal therapy. Laparoscopic vaporization with carbon dioxide laser became a popular treatment modality for endometriosis-associated infertility, yet few data existed regarding the effectiveness of such an approach.

In the 1980s, laparoscopic surgery became the preferred approach for the treatment of ovarian endometrioma [103] and infiltrating cul-de-sac endometriosis [104]. Laparoscopic techniques were further promoted for the treatment of endometriosis by several pioneers and in 1994 Adamson and Pasta [105], combining their data with the results reported by Hughes *et al* [106], carried out a meta-analysis and concluded that either no treatment or surgery is superior to medical treatment for minimal and mild endometriosis associated with infertility; in addition, in moderate and severe disease, surgery seems to yield comparable results with both operative laparoscopy or laparotomy. They recommended that prospective randomized trials be performed to confirm these findings but unfortunately, in surgery prospective, double-blind randomized studies are extremely difficult to perform, although Sutton *et al* were able to conduct such a study and published it in 1994 [107]. They concluded that laser laparoscopy was a safe, simple, and effective treatment in alleviating pain in women with stage I, II, and III endometriosis. A second randomized, controlled trial was published in 1997 by Marcoux *et al* [108], reaching the conclusion that laparoscopic surgery enhanced fecundity in infertile women with minimal and mild endometriosis.

Ovarian endometrioma

Ovarian endometriomas have represented a major challenge for reconstructive surgery, carrying the risk of inadequate as well as excessive surgery. Nezhat *et al* [109] noted that in small endometriomas, the cyst wall is superficial and very difficult to remove, while a large endometrioma may develop as a result of secondary involvement of functional ovarian cysts by endometriotic tissues. Donnez *et al* [110] proposed a combined therapy using a gonadotropin-releasing hormone agonist and carbon dioxide laser laparoscopy. The hormone treatment and drainage after 12 weeks provoked a reduction of the endometrioma size up to 50% of the initial size before surgery was performed. In a large series, they reported, after the combined treatment, a cumulative pregnancy rate of 51% and a recurrence rate of 8% during a follow-up period of 2–11 years.

Bowel endometriosis

Surgical treatment of bowel endometriosis has been controversial, because this localization tends to be limited to the serosa and the muscular coats without penetrating the mucosa, and causes obstruction by fibrosis and kinking of the bowel [111]. Weed and Ray [112] reported on 163 cases of bowel endometriosis, noting that colon and rectal surgeons perform resections of the colon and the ileum and/or cecum, while gynecological surgeons prefer resection of bowel implants, even when they are multiple. In their experience, the bowel mucosa was opened in 15% of implant resection and resection of intestinal implants appeared to be a safe procedure.

Adhesions

The first reports on the use of intraperitoneal adjuncts to reduce postoperative adhesion formation appeared in the literature during the 1980s and gave varying results [113,114]. Reviewing available evidence, DiZerega [115] concluded that although barriers were shown to be safe and effective in human trials, their use did not eliminate adhesions on all patients. At second-look laparoscopy, Canis *et al* [116] found absence of deep ovarian endometriosis in 92%, but *de novo* adhesion formation existed in 21% of the treated adnexae and 17% of the contralateral adnexae; they concluded that laparoscopic cystectomy is effective in treating large endometriomas, but that operative difficulties may be encountered explaining the persistence of some endometriomas and postoperative adhesions.

Assisted reproductive technologies

In a prospective study of artificial insemination by a donor program, Jansen [35] reported reduced fecundability in the presence of minimal endometriosis. This observation was confirmed by Simon *et al* [117] in a retrospective analysis: in comparison with patients with tubal infertility, women with endometriosis have a poor IVF outcome in terms of reduced pregnancy rate per cycle, reduced pregnancy rate per transfer, and reduced implantation rate. Results from oocyte donations showed that patients who received embryos derived from endometriotic ovaries showed a significantly reduced implantation rate as compared to the remaining groups. All these observations suggest that infertility in endometriosis patients may be related to alterations within the oocyte, which in turn result in embryos with decreased ability to implant. From the results of a case–control study from the Yale University IVF-ET program, Arici *et al* [118] concluded that, in patients with endometriosis, implantation rate is low. Abnormal implantation, which may be secondary to endometrial dysfunction or embryotoxic environment, is a factor in endometriosis-associated subfertility.

In search of the pathogenesis

Initial theories

After the publication of his famous 1927 paper [12], Sampson continued the search for morphological clues to prove his thesis. In 1928 he reported on endometriosis in and about the tubal stumps in women who had undergone salpingectomy or tubal sterilization. He found bits of tubal and uterine mucosa that may have been transplanted by the surgeon both in the immediate field and also in remote areas and reasoned that if such transplanted endometrial or tubal epithelia could grow, they should also grow if transplanted during other types of operations and even in circumstances other than surgical interventions [119]. When transplanted tissue becomes differentiated into a structure resembling endometrium, Sampson defined it as "endometriosis" [120]. His view was supported by several publications on postoperative or scar endometriosis following cesarean section, episiotomy and laparotomy for uterine surgery [121,122].

Not everyone agreed with Sampson and in 1932, Novak (see Fig. 1.1D) developed a different theory: he postulated that the occurrence of differentiation anomalies in the epithelium of various segments of the genital canal indicated the tendency towards variability of these genital epithelia under certain conditions [123]. He argued that this tendency reflected their common origin from the same mother tissue, the coelomic epithelium. In his view, it seemed unnecessary to invoke the doctrine of "transplantation" to explain endometriosis, since types of differentiation transitions may be seen in ovarian endometriosis, including a tubal epithelium with or without stroma, a uterine epithelium with or without glands and with or without stroma, an endometrium with or without physiological reactivity, with or without hemorrhage. Novak believed that his theory would support the germinal epithelium origin of serous cystadenomas and explain how tubal pregnancies could develop.

Besides the above-mentioned two theories, during the following decades several additional hypotheses were presented to explain the pathogenesis of endometriosis, though no single theory could explain all presentations.

Peritoneal environment

While early studies concentrated on the histogenesis of endometriotic lesions, during the 1980s interest shifted to changes in the peritoneal, ovarian, and uterine microenvironments observed in the presence of endometriosis.

Halme et al [124] demonstrated that retrograde menstruation through the fallopian tubes into the peritoneal cavity is a very common physiological event in menstruating women with patent tubes and concluded that specific factors must be implicated for successful transplantation and the establishment of endometriosis. They noted the increased activation of peritoneal macrophages in infertile women with mild endometriosis [125].

In 1980, Dmowski and collaborators [126] were the first to point to modifications of the immune system in the pathogenesis of endometriosis. This team demonstrated that rhesus monkeys with spontaneous endometriosis have an altered cellular immune response to autologous antigens, suggesting that endometrial cells translocated from their normal location may implant only in women with specific alteration in cell-mediated immunity. The following year, Haney et al [127] demonstrated that endometriosis is accompanied by a chronic intraperitoneal inflammatory process evidenced by an increased number of peritoneal macrophages in infertile women with endometriosis, when compared to normal women or to women with other causes of infertility. Since the peritoneal fluid is in contact with both peritoneal endometriotic implants and the tubal microenvironment in which fertilization occurs, subtle alterations of this fluid and/or its cellular constituents might adversely influence reproduction independently of anatomical compromise of the ovaries or oviducts.

Today, a number of modifications in the peritoneal environment of women with endometriosis have been identified: Oosterlynck et al [128] found that natural killer (NK) activity and cytotoxicity against autologous endometrial cells were both decreased in women with endometriosis and such decrease correlated well with the severity of the disease. Rana et al [129] demonstrated an increased synthesis of cytokines by peritoneal macrophages in women with endometriosis and Oosterlynck et al [130] found that the peritoneal fluid of women with endometriosis contains more angiogenic factors than peritoneal fluid from unaffected women. Shifrin et al [131] and McLaren et al [132] found that peritoneal fluid concentrations of vascular endothelial growth factor (VEGF) were significantly higher in women with moderate-to-severe endometriosis than in women with minimal-to-mild endometriosis or no disease.

In a review of the peritoneal environment in endometriosis, Oral et al [133] concluded that the etiology is likely to be multifactorial, and that the most widely accepted explanation for peritoneal endometriosis is a composite theory of retrograde menstruation with implantation of endometrial fragments in the presence of peritoneal factors able to stimulate cell growth.

Endometrial dysfunctions

In the late 1990s several reports were published suggesting that endometriosis is associated with endometrial dysfunction. Patients with severe endometriosis were found to have defects in endometrial receptivity, including aberrant integrin expression, suggesting decreased cycle fecundity [134]. In 1996, Noble et al [135] demonstrated that both eutopic endometrial tissues and endometriotic implants from patients with endometriosis are biochemically different from normal endometrial tissues of disease-free women. They speculated that the presence of aromatase expression in eutopic endometrial tissues from patients with endometriosis might be related to the capability of implantation of these tissues on peritoneal surfaces. On the other hand, Shifrin et al [131] have shown that VEGF may be important in the active angiogenesis of human endometrium (both physiological and pathological), as it is an estrogen-responsive angiogenic factor that varies throughout the menstrual cycle and is elevated in women with endometriosis. Donnez et al [136] found that VEGF content was higher in the eutopic glandular epithelium of women with endometriosis during the late secretory phase, possibly suggesting a more likely tendency to implant. On the other hand, similarities in VEGF content were observed in the glandular epithelium of the eutopic endometrium of women with endometriosis and red lesions, suggesting that endometriosis probably arises from the peritoneal seeding of viable endometrial cells during retrograde menstruation and that red lesions can be considered as the first stage of implantation. Finally, Leyendecker et al [137] consider hyperperistalsis and dysperistalsis to be responsible for both reduced fertility and the development of endometriosis.

Conclusion

There seem to be three general concepts that evolved during late 20th-century research in endometriosis. First, the evidence of a local peritoneal inflammatory process, supported by the findings of elevated cytokine and growth factor concentrations in the peritoneal fluid of affected patients. Second, a role for angiogenic factors in the establishment of heterotopic implants. Third, evidence for biochemical differences of eutopic and ectopic endometrium in endometriosis patients; this may contribute to both the pathogenesis and sequelae of this important disorder [138].

References

1. Knapp VJ. How old is endometriosis? Late 17th- and 18th-century European descriptions of the disease Fertil Steril 1999;72:10–14.
2. Batt RE. Emergence of endometriosis in North America: a study in the history of ideas. Dissertation submitted to the Faculty of the Graduate School of the University of Buffalo, State University of New York, 2008, pp.109–113.
3. Schrön DC. Disputatio Inauguralis Medica de Ulceribus Uteri. Thesis presented at the University of Jena, Literis Krebsianis, 1690.
4. Brosens I, Steeno O. A compass for understanding endometriosis. Fertil Steril 2000;73:179–180.
5. Rokitansky C. Über Uterusdrüsen-Neubildung in Uterus- und Ovarial-Sarcomen. Zeitschr Gesellschaft der Aerzte in Wien 1860;16:577–581.
6. Benagiano G, Brosens I. The history of endometriosis: identifying the disease. Hum Reprod 1991;6:963–968.
7. Von Recklinghausen F. Die Adenomyomata und Cystadenomata der Uterus und Tubenwandung: Ihre Abkunft von Resten des Wolffischen Koerpers. Berlin: August Hirschwald Verlag, 1896.
8. Lockyer C. Fibroids and Allied Tumours (Myoma and Adenomyoma). London: MacMillan, 1918.
9. Cullen TS. Adenomyoma of the Uterus. Philadelphia: WB Saunders, 1908.
10. Cullen TS. The distribution of adenomyomata containing uterine mucosa Arch Surg 1921;1:215–283.
11. Sampson JA. Perforating hemorrhagic (chocolate) cysts of the ovary Arch Surg 1921;3:245–323.
12. Sampson JA. Peritoneal endometriosis due to the menstrual dissemination of endometrial tissue into the peritoneal cavity. Am J Obstet Gynecol 1927;14:422–469.
13. Hill Jr LL. Aberrant endometrium Am J Surg 1932;18:303–321.
14. Novak E. Pelvic endometriosis. Spontaneous rupture of endometrial cysts, with a report of three cases. Am J Obstet Gynecol 1931;22:826–837.
15. Graves WP. The treatment of obstructing rectovaginal endometriosis Am J Obstet Gynecol 1927;13:728–731.
16. Counseller VS. The clinical significance of endometriosis. Am J Obstet Gynecol 1939;37:788–797.
17. Benson RC, Sneeden VD. Adenomyosis: a reappraisal of symptomatology. Am J Obstet Gynecol 1958;76:1044–1061.
18. Javert CT. Observations on the pathology and spread of endometriosis based on the theory of benign metastasis. Am J Obstet Gynecol 1951;62:477–487.
19. Henriksen E. Endometriosis. Am J Surg 1955;90:331–337.
20. Decker A, Cherry TH. Culdoscopy. A new method in the diagnosis of pelvic disease – preliminary report. Am J Surg 1944;64:40–44.
21. Semm K. Laparoscopy in gynecology [Die Laparoskopie in der Gynäkologie.] Geburts Frauenheilk 1967;27:1029–1042.
22. Beecham CT. Classification of endometriosis. Obstet Gynecol 1966;28:437.
23. Acosta AA, Buttram VC Jr, Besch PK. A proposed classification of pelvic endometriosis. Obstet Gynecol 1973;42:19–25.
24. Buttram VC Jr. An expanded classification of endometriosis. Fertil Steril 1978;30:240–242.
25. American Fertility Society. Classification of endometriosis. Fertil Steril 1979;32:633–634.
26. Rock JA, Guzick DS, Sengos C. The conservative surgical treatment of endometriosis: evaluation of pregnancy success with respect to the extent of disease as categorized using contemporary classification systems. Fertil Steril 1981;35:131–137.
27. Buttram VC Jr. Evolution of the revised American Fertility Society classification of endometriosis. Fertil Steril 1985;43:347–352.
28. Vercellini P, Trespidi L, de Giorgi O, Cortesi I, Parazzini F, Crosignani PG. Endometriosis and pelvic pain: relation to disease stage and localization. Fertil Steril 1996;65:299–304.
29. Guzick DS, Silliman NP, Adamson GD et al. Prediction of pregnancy in infertile women based on the American Society for Reproductive Medicine's revised classification of endometriosis. Fertil Steril 1997;67:822–829.
30. Canis M, Donnez JG, Guzick DS et al. Revised American Society for Reproductive Medicine classification of endometriosis: 1966. Fertil Steril 1997;67:817–821.
31. Vasquez G, Cornillie F, Brosens IA. Peritoneal endometriosis: scanning electron microscopy and histology of minimal pelvic endometriotic lesions. Fertil Steril 1984;42:696–703.
32. Murphy AA, Green WR, Bobbie D. Unsuspected endometriosis documented by scanning electron microscopy in visually normal peritoneum. Fertil Steril 1986;46:522–524.
33. Jenkins S, Olive DL, Haney AF. Endometriosis: pathogenetic implications of the anatomic distribution. Obstet Gynecol 1986;67:335–338.
34. Wiegerinck MAHM, van Dop PA, Brosens IA. The staging of peritoneal endometriosis by the type of active lesion in addition to the revised American Fertility Society classification. Fertil Steril 1993;60:461–464.
35. Jansen RPS. Minimal endometriosis and reduced fecundability: prospective evidence from an artificial insemination by donor program. Fertil Steril 1986;46:141–143.
36. Jansen RPS, Russel P. Nonpigmented endometriosis: clinical, laparoscopic, and pathologic definition. Am J Obstet Gynecol 1986;155:1154–1159.
37. Stripling MC, Martin DC, Chatman DL, van der Zwaag R, Poston WM. Subtle appearance of pelvic endometriosis. Fertil Steril 1988;49:427–431.
38. Martin DC, Hubert GD, van der Zwaag R, El-Zeky FA. Laparoscopic appearances of peritoneal endometriosis. Fertil Steril 1989;51:63–67.
39. Evers JLH, Land JA, Dunselman GAJ, van der Linden PJQ, Hamilton CJCM. 'The Flemish Giant': reflections on the defense against endometriosis, inspired by Professor Emeritus Ivo A. Brosens. Eur J Obstet Gynecol Reprod Biol 1998;81:253–258.

40. Balasch J, Creus M, Fabregues F et al. Visible and non-visible endometriosis at laparoscopy in fertile and infertile women and in patients with chronic pelvic pain: a prospective study. Hum Reprod 1996;11:387–391.

41. Cornillie FJ, Oosterlynck D, Lauweryns JM, Koninckx PR. Deeply infiltrating pelvic endometriosis: histology and clinical significance Fertil Steril 1990;53:978–983.

42. Koninckx PR, Meuleman C, Demeyere S, Lesaffre E, Cornillie FJ. Suggestive evidence that pelvic endometriosis is a progressive disease, whereas deeply infiltrating endometriosis is associated with pelvic pain. Fertil Steril 1991;55:759–765.

43. Koninckx PR, Martin DC. Deep endometriosis: a consequence of infiltration or retraction or possibly adenomyosis externa? Fertil Steril 1992;58:924–928.

44. Chapron C, Dumontier I, Dousset B et al. Results and role of rectal endoscopic ultrasonography for patients with deep pelvic endometriosis. Hum Reprod 1998;13:2266–2270.

45. Fedele L, Bianchi S, Portuese A, Borruto F, Dort AM. Transrectal ultrasonography in the assessment of rectovaginal endometriosis. Obstet Gynecol 1998;91:444–448.

46. Canis M, Bouquet de Jolinieres J, Wattiez A et al. Classification of endometriosis. Baillière's Clin Obstet Gynaecol 1993;7:759–774.

47. Hughesdon PE. The structure of endometrial cysts of the ovary. J Obstet Gynaecol Br Emp 1957:44:481–487.

48. Halban J. Metastatic hysteroadenosis. Wien Klin Wochenschr 1924;37:1205.

49. Brosens IA, Puttemans PJ, Deprest J. The endoscopic localization of endometrial implants in the ovarian chocolate cyst. Fertil Steril 1994;61:1034–1038.

50. Hricak H, Alpers C, Crooks LE, Sheldon PE. Magnetic resonance imaging of the female pelvis: initial experience. Am J Roentgenol 1983;141:1119–1128.

51. Nishimura K, Togashi K, Itoh K. Endometrial cysts of the ovary: MR imaging. Radiology 1987;162:315–318.

52. Togashi K, Nishimura K, Kimura I et al. Endometrial cysts: diagnosis with MR imaging. Radiology 1991;180:73–78.

53. Mais V, Guerriero S, Ajossa S, Angiolucci M, Paoletti AM, Melis GB. The efficiency of transvaginal ultrasonography in the diagnosis of endometrioma. Fertil Steril 1993;60:776–780.

54. Kurjak A, Kupesic S. Scoring system for prediction of ovarian endometriosis based on transvaginal color and pulsed Doppler sonography. Fertil Steril 1994;62:81–88.

55. Alcázar JL, Laparte C, Jurado M, López-García G. The role of transvaginal ultrasonography combined with color velocity imaging and pulsed Doppler in the diagnosis of endometrioma. Fertil Steril 1997;67:487–491.

56. Candiani GB, Vercellini P, Fedele L. Laparoscopic ovarian puncture for correct staging of endometriosis. Fertil Steril 1990;53:994–997.

57. Nezhat F, Nezhat C, Allan CJ, Metzger DA, Sears DL. Clinical and histologic classification of endometriomas: implications for a mechanism of pathogenesis. J Reprod Med Obstet Gynecol 1992;37:771–776.

58. Nisolle M, Donnez J. Peritoneal endometriosis, ovarian endometriosis, and adenomyotic nodules of the rectovaginal septum are three different entities Fertil Steril 1997;68:585–596.

59. Canis M, Pouly JL, Wattiez A, Manhes H, Mage G, Bruhat MA. Incidence of bilateral adnexal disease in severe endometriosis (revised American Fertility Society [AFS], stage IV): should a stage V be included in the AFS classification? Fertil Steril 1992;57:691–692.

60. Pal L, Shifren JL, Isaacson KB, Chang Y, Leykin L, Toth TL. Impact of varying stages of endometriosis on the outcome of in vitro fertilization-embryo transfer. J Assist Reprod Genet 1998;15:27–31.

61. Heaps JM, Nieberg RK, Berek JS. Malignant neoplasms arising in endometriosis. Obstet Gynecol 1990;75:1023–1028.

62. Geist SH, Salrnon UJ. Androgen therapy in gynecology. JAMA 1941;117:2207–2215.

63. Hirst JC. Favorable response of advanced endometriosis to testosterone propionate therapy. Am J Obstet Gynecol 1943;46:97–102.

64. Miller JR. Preoperative use of testosterone propionate as an aid to surgical treatment of endometriosis. JAMA 1944;125:207–208.

65. Kistner RW. The use of newer progestins in the treatment of endometriosis. Am J Obstet Gynecol 1958;74:264–278.

66. Kempers RD, Dockerty MB, Hunt AB et al. Significant post menopausal endometriosis. Surg Gynecol Obstet 1960;111:348–353.

67. Legros R, Fain-Giono J. Endomètriose paraménopausique et post-ménopausique. A propos de 20 cas sur 351 d'endomètriose. Rev Française Gynécol 1973;63:25–35.

68. Bergqvist IA. Hormonal regulation of endometriosis and the rationales and effects of gonadotrophin-releasing hormone agonist treatment: a review. Hum Reprod 1995;10:446–452.

69. DiZerega GS, Barber DL, Hodgen GD. Endometriosis: role of ovarian steroids in initiation, maintenance, and suppression. Fertil Steril l980;33:649–653.

70. Bergqvist A, Jeppsson S, Kullander S et al. Human uterine endometrium and endometriotic tissue transplanted into nude mice. Am J Pathol 1985;121:337–311.

71. Signorile PG, Baldi F, Bussani R, d'Armiento MR, de Falco M, Baldi A. Ectopic endometrium in human foetuses is a common event and sustains the theory of müllerianosis in the pathogenesis of endometriosis, a disease that predisposes to cancer. J Exper Clin Cancer Res 2009;28:49–53.

72. Rajkumar K, Schott PW, Simpson CW. The rat as an animal model for endometriosis to examine recurrence of ectopic endometrial tissue after regression. Fertil Steril 1990;53:921–925.

73. Oliker AJ, Harris AE. Endometriosis of the bladder in a male patient. J Urol 1971;106:858–859.

74. Pinkert TC, Catlow CE, Straus R. Endometriosis of the urinary bladder in a man with prostatic carcinoma. Cancer 1979;13:1562–1567.

75. Doty DW, Gruber JS, Wolf GC et al. 46xy pure gonadal dysgenesis: report of two unusual cases. Obstet Gynecol 1980;55(suppl):61S.

76. Peress MR, Sosnowski JR, Mathur RS et al. Pelvic endometriosis and Turner's syndrome. Am J Obstet Gynecol 1982;144:474–476.

77. Binnis BO, Banerjee R. Endometriosis with Turner's syndrome treated with cyclical oestrogen/progestogen: case report. Br J Obstet Gynaecol 1983; 90:581–582.

78. Bosze P, Gaal M, Toth A et al. Endometriosis and streak gonad syndrome. Arch Gynecol 1987;240:253–254.

79. Rosenfeld DL, Lecher BD. Endometriosis in a patient with Rokitansky-Kuster-Hauser syndrome. Am J Obstet Gynecol 1981;139:105.

80. Karnaky KJ. The use of stilbestrol for endometriosis. South Med J 1945;41:1110–1111.

81. Greenwald P, Barlow JJ, Nasca PC, Burnett WS. Vaginal cancer after maternal treatment with synthetic estrogens. N Engl J Med 1971;285:390–392.

82. Bergqvist A, Ljungberg O, Myhre E. Human endometrium and endometriotic tissue obtained simultaneously; a comparative histological study. Int J Gynecol Pathol 1984;3:135–145.

83. Schweppe KW, Wynn RM. Ultrastructural changes in endometriotic implants during the menstrual cycle. Obstet Gynecol 1981;58:465–473.

84. Meigs JV. Endometriosis. Etiologic role of marriage age and parity: conservative treatment. Obstet Gynecol 1953;2:46–53.

85. Rock J, Pincus G, Garcia C-R. Effects of certain 19-nor steroids on the human menstrual cycle. Science 1956;124:891–893.

86. Andrews MC, Andrews WC, Strauss AF. Effects of progestin-induced pseudopregnancy on endometriosis: clinical and microscopic studies. Am J Obstet Gynecol 1959;78:776–785.

87. Thomas HH. Conservative treatment of endometriosis. Use of long-acting ovarian steroid hormones. Obstet Gynecol 1960;15:498–503.

88. Moghissi KS. Treatment of endometriosis with estrogen-progestin combination and progestogen alone. Clin Obstet Gynecol 1988;31:823–828.

89. Vercellini P, Crosignani PG, Somigliana E, Berlanda N, Barbara G, Fedele L. Medical treatment for rectovaginal endometriosis: what is the evidence? Hum Reprod 2009;24:2504–2514.

90. Daguati R, Somigliana E, Viganò P, Vercellini P. [Progestogens and estroprogestins in the treatment of pelvic pain associated with endometriosis.] Minerva Ginecol 2006;58:499–510.

91. Greenblatt RB, Dmowski WP, Mahesh VB et al. Clinical studies with an antigonadotropin – danazol. Fertil Steril 1971;22:102–112.

92. Barbieri RL. Danazol: molecular, endocrine and clinical pharmacology. Prog Clin Biol Res 1990;323:241–252.

93. Tamaya T, Fujimoto J, Watanabe Y, Arahori K, Okada H. Gestrinone (R2323) binding to steroid receptors in human uterine endometrial cytosol. Acta Obstet Gynecol Scand 1986;65:439–441.

94. Fedele L, Bianchi S, Viezzoli T et al Gestrinone versus danazol in the treatment of endometriosis. Fert Steril 1989;51:781–785.

95. Venturini PL, Bertolini S, Marre-Bruneghi MC et al. Endocrine, metabolic and clinical effects of gestrinone in women with endometriosis. Fertil Steril 1989;52:589–595.

96. Ulmann A, Tcutsch G, Philibert D. RU 486. Sci Am 1990;262:1824.

97. Kettle ML, Murphy AA, Mortal JF et al. Treatment of endometriosis with the anti-progesterone mifepristone (RU 486). Fertil Steril 1996; 65:23–28.

98. Yen SSC. Use of antiprogestins in the management of endometriosis and leiomyoma. In: Donaldson MS, Dolfinger L, Brown SS et al (eds) Clinical Applications of Mifepristone (RU486) and Other Antiprogestins. Washington, DC: National Academy of Medicine, 1993.

99. Kistner RW. Management of endometriosis in the infertile patient. Fertil Steril 1975;26:1151–1166.

100. Buttram VC Jr. Conservative surgeries for endometriosis in the infertile female: a study of 206 patients with implications for both medical and surgical therapy. Fertil Steril 1979;31: 117–123.

101. Semm K. Laparoscopy in gynecology [Die Laparoskopie in der Gynäkologie.] Geburts Frauenheilk 1967;27:1029–1042.

102. Nezhat C, Crowgey SR, Garrison CP. Surgical treatment of endometriosis via laser laparoscopy. Fertil Steril 1986;45:778–783.

103. Reich H, McGlynn F. Treatment of ovarian endometriomas using laparoscopic surgical techniques. J Reprod Med Obstet Gynecol 1986;31:577–584.

104. Martin DC. Laparoscopic and vaginal colpotomy for the excision of infiltrating cul-de-sac endometriosis. J Reprod Med Obstet Gynecol 1988;33:806–808.

105. Adamson GD, Pasta DJ. Surgical treatment of endometriosis-associated infertility: meta-analysis compared with survival analysis Am J Obstet Gynecol 1994;171:1488–1505.

106. Hughes EG, Fedorkow DM, Collins JA. A quantitative overview of controlled trials in endometriosis-associated infertility. Fertil Steril 1993;59:963–970.

107. Sutton CJG, Ewen SP, Whitelaw N, Haines P. Prospective, randomized, double-blind, controlled trial of laser laparoscopy in the treatment of pelvic pain associated with minimal, mild, and moderate endometriosis. Fertil Steril 1994;62:696–700.

108. Marcoux S, Maheux R, Bérubé S. Laparoscopic surgery in infertile women with minimal or mild endometriosis. N Engl J Med 1997;337:217–222.

109. Nezhat F, Nezhat C, Allan CJ, Metzger DA, Sears DL. Clinical and histologic classification of endometriomas: implications for a mechanism of pathogenesis. J Reprod Med Obstet Gynecol 1992;37:771–776.

110. Donnez J, Nisolle M, Gillet N, Smets M, Bassil S, Casanas-Roux F. Large ovarian endometriomas. Hum Reprod 1996;11:641–646.

111. Martimbeau PW, Pratt JH, Gaffey TA. Small bowel obstruction secondary to endometriosis. Mayo Clin Proc 1975;50:239–243.

112. Weed JC, Ray JE. Endometriosis of the bowel. Obstet Gynecol 1987;69:727–730.

113. Buttram VC, Malinak R, Cleary R. Reduction of postoperative pelvic adhesions with intraperitoneal 32% dextran 70: a prospective, randomized clinical trial. Fertil Steril 1983;40:612–619.

114. Jansen RPS. Failure of intraperitoneal adjuncts to improve the outcome of pelvic operations in young women. Am J Obstet Gynecol 1985;153:363–371.

115. DiZerega GS. Contemporary adhesion prevention. Fertil Steril 1994;61:219–235.

116. Canis M, Mage G, Wattiez A, Chapron C, Pouly JL, Bassil S. Second-look laparoscopy after laparoscopic cystectomy of large ovarian endometriomas. Fertil Steril 1992;58:617–619.

117. Simon C, Gutierrez A, Vidal A et al. Outcome of patients with endometriosis in assisted reproduction: results from in-vitro fertilization and oocyte donation. Hum Reprod 1994;9:725–729.

118. Arici A, Duleba A, Oral E, Olive DL, Bukulmez O, Jones EE. The effect of endometriosis on implantation: results from the Yale University in vitro fertilization and embryo transfer program. Fertil Steril 1996;65:603–607.

119. Sampson JA. Endometriosis following salpingectomy. Am J Obstet Gynecol 1928;16:461–494.

120. Sampson JA. Pelvic endometriosis and tubal fimbriae Am J Obstet Gynecol 1932;24:497–542.

121. Williams PH. Endometriosis of an abdominal scar following cesarean section Am J Obstet Gynecol 1929;17:102–104.

122. Wyrens RG, Randall LM. Endometriosis (adenomyoma) in postoperative scars. An analysis of thirty-one cases. Am J Surg 1942;56:395–403.

123. Novak E. Pelvic endometriosis. Spontaneous rupture of endometrial cysts, with a report of three cases Am J Obstet Gynecol 1931;22:826–837.

124. Halme J, Becker S, Hammond MG. Increased activation of pelvic macrophages in infertile women with mild endometriosis. Am J Obstet Gynecol 1983;145:333–337.

125. Halme J, Hammond MG, Hulka JF. Retrograde menstruation in healthy women and in patients with endometriosis. Obstet Gynecol 1984;64:151–154.

126. Dmowski WP, Steele RW, Baker GF. Deficient cellular immunity in endometriosis. Am J Obstet Gynecol 1981;141:377–383.

127. Haney AF, Muscato JJ, Weinberg JB. Peritoneal fluid cell populations in infertility patients. Fertil Steril 1981;35:696–698.

128. Oosterlynck DJ, Cornillie FJ, Waer M, Vandeputte M, Koninckx PR. Women with endometriosis show a defect in natural killer activity resulting in a decreased cytotoxicity to autologous endometrium. Fertil Steril 1991;56:45–51.

129. Rana N, Braun DP, House R, Gebel H, Rotman C, Dmowski WP. Basal and stimulated secretion of cytokines by peritoneal macrophages in women with endometriosis. Fertil Steril 1996;65:925–930.

130. Oosterlynck DJ, Meuleman C, Sobis H, Vandeputte M, Koninckx PR. Angiogenic activity of peritoneal fluid from women with endometriosis. Fertil Steril 1993;59:778–782.

131. Shifren JL, Tseng JF, Zaloudek CJ et al. Ovarian steroid regulation of vascular endothelial growth factor in the human endometrium: implications for angiogenesis during the menstrual cycle and in the pathogenesis of endometriosis. J Clin Endocrinol Metab 1996;81:3112–3118.

132. McLaren J, Prentice, A, Charnock-Jones DS et al. Vascular endothelial growth factor is produced by peritoneal fluid macrophages in endometriosis and is regulated by ovarian steroids. J Clin Invest 1996;98:482–489.

133. Oral E, Olive DL, Arici A. The peritoneal environment in endometriosis. Hum Reprod Update 1996;2:385–398.

134. Lessey BA, Castelbaum AJ, Sawin SW et al. Aberrant integrin expression in the endometrium of women with endometriosis. J Clin Endocrinol Metab 1994;79:643–649.

135. Noble LS, Simpson ER, Johns A, Bulun SE. Aromatase expression in endometriosis. J Clin Endocrinol Metab 1996;81:174–179.

136. Donnez J, Smoes P, Gillerot S, Casanas-Roux F, Nisolle M. Vascular endothelial growth factor (VEGF) in endometriosis. Hum Reprod 1998;13:1686–1690.

137. Leyendecker G, Kunz G, Wildt L, Beil D, Deininger H. Uterine hyperperistalsis and dysperistalsis as dysfunctions of the mechanism of rapid sperm transport in patients with endometriosis and infertility. Hum Reprod 1996;11:1542–1551.

138. Ryan IP, Taylor RN. Endometriosis and infertility: new concepts. Obstet Gynecol Surv 1997;52:365–371.

2 Endometriosis: Epidemiology, and Etiological Factors

Fabio Parazzini[1], Paolo Vercellini[1] and Claudio Pelucchi[2]
[1]Prima Clinica Ostetrico Ginecologica, Università di Milano, Milan, Italy
[2]Department of Epidemiology, Istituto di Ricerche Farmacologiche Mario Negri, Milan, Italy

Introduction

Endometriosis is a common condition with an impact on women's health during their fertile years.

To date, at least 1000 papers have been published on the epidemiology of endometriosis. These studies have consistently indicated that nulliparous women and women reporting short and heavy menstrual cycles are at an increased risk [1]. Other factors have been studied, but findings are less consistent. In this chapter we summarize the findings on the descriptive and analytical epidemiology of endometriosis.

Frequency

Only a few well-conducted studies have reported data on the prevalence of endometriosis and no data are available on the frequency of onset of the disease in a given period (incidence), among women without a previous diagnosis.

Differences in the prevalence of the disease in various studies vary up to 30–40 times [1–7]. Studies that have analyzed the frequency of endometriosis in the general population showed prevalence rates of about 3–6% and incidence rates of about 2–7/1000 women per year (Table 2.1). Studies that analyzed the frequency of endometriosis in women who underwent surgery for fibroids suggested a prevalence of about 10% [8], but women with fibroids may share some risk factors with endometriosis. The differences observed among studies may partly be explained by different indications for laparoscopy and laparotomy or merely the different attention paid by surgeons to identifying endometriotic lesions and by selective mechanisms drawing patients with suspected endometriosis towards specialized centers. It is worth noting that most published studies have not been conducted on representative samples of the general population. In general, it is difficult to compare prevalence estimates from studies including women with different conditions and conducted in centers applying different diagnostic criteria and with different levels of clinical interest in endometriosis. Selective mechanisms may also be involved in interpreting temporal trends of the frequency of the disease, suggesting an increase in the incidence of pelvic endometriosis among women of reproductive age. Otherwise there are some theoretical considerations that support the hypothesis of an increasing frequency of endometriosis.

Retrograde menstruation seems the most probable pathogenetic mechanism for the development of endometriosis [1–3,9,10]. If this is true, the likelihood of implantation of regurgitated endometrium could be influenced by the recent major increase in the number of retrograde menstruations [11–13]. In fact, the reproductive patterns of women in today's affluent Western nations differ greatly from those of our ancestors. Decrease in age at menarche, in number of pregnancies, in duration of breast feeding and increase in age at first birth all lead to an increase in the overall number of ovulations and menstruations a woman has within a reproductive lifespan [11–16]. These changes appear even more dramatic during the decade at highest risk for endometriosis, i.e. between 25 and 35 years of age. All the above factors are strongly associated with the risk of developing endometriosis [1–3,17]. In Italy, age at first birth increased from 24.9 years in 1974 to 29.6 in 2004, whereas the mean number of children per woman progressively decreased from 2.7 in 1964 to 1.3 in 2004. Mean duration of lactation was only 6.2 months in 2000 [16].

A major rise in the number of ovulations and menstruations may augment pelvic contamination by regurgitated endometrium. Indeed, the risk of endometriosis appears to increase with greater lifetime number of ovulatory cycles [17]. Moreover, the role of ovulation in the genesis of ovarian endometriosis has been confirmed, demonstrating that endometriomas develop from follicles immediately after ovulation [18], and by direct transition from hemorrhagic corpora lutea [19].

Endometriosis: Science and Practice, First Edition. Edited by Linda C. Giudice, Johannes L.H. Evers and David L. Healy.
© 2012 Blackwell Publishing Ltd. Published 2012 by Blackwell Publishing Ltd.

Table 2.1 Estimated incidence of clinically diagnosed endometriosis among women aged 15–44 years: selected studies.

Source	Observation period	Annual rate/1000
Cases		
Houston et al, 1987 [82]	1970–1979	2.49
Leibson et al, 2004 [83]	1987–1999	2.46
Missmer et al, 2004 [29]	1989–1999	2.37
General population		
Houston et al, 1987 [82]	1987	2.5–3.3
Vessey et al, 1993 [42]	1993	1.8

Monthly menstruation for decades on end is not the historical norm. Current menstrual patterns are new and their health effects unproven [15]. Specifically, the likelihood of developing a disease directly caused by ovulation and menstruation, such as endometriosis, might be greater nowadays.

Left:right side ratio of endometriotic implants in the pelvis

The transplantation theory is commonly offered to explain the pathogenesis of endometriosis. This suggests that endometriotic implants are a consequence of reflux of menstrual blood into the pelvis. If this is true, physical factors should influence the site of implants, because the right and left hemipelvis are anatomically different, so asymmetry in the distribution of lesions could be expected. Supporting this, Vercellini et al showed that ovarian endometriomas are more common in the left than the right ovaries [20]. Similar results also emerged in other studies [21–23]. In particular, marked differences in frequency between left and right side are observed for less frequent sites of endometriosis such as diaphragmatic and ureteral endometriosis [24,25].

In etiopathogenetic terms, the findings have been explained in the light of the reflux hypothesis [26]. The probability of peritoneal and ovarian implantation of menstrual cells may be different in the two sides of the pelvis. The asymmetry may be due to the barrier role of the sigma in the left side of the pelvis. Further, the endometrial cells regurgitated through the left tube are not exposed to the clockwise peritoneal current that is believed to keep peritoneal fluid circulating [27], and which may involve cells regurgitated through the right tube.

In addition, the cecum, which is anatomically more cranial than the sigma, may not create a "hidden" microenvironment on the right side of the pelvis. This could make implants of menstrual cells less probable in the right hemipelvis. However, other mechanisms may explain the right:left distribution, such as differences in blood flow, lymphatic drainage or local growth factors. These anatomical and functional considerations may explain the higher rate of endometriotic implants in the left hemipelvis, thus, from an anatomical point of view, supporting the reflux theory in the pathogenesis of endometriosis.

Table 2.2 Risk factors for endometriosis.

Factor	Findings
Perinatal exposure	↑, limited data
Sociodemographic characteristics and socio-economic status	↑, limited data
Constitutional factors	
Family history	↑↑
Weight	↓, inconsistent
Peripheral body fat distribution	↑, limited data
Personal habits	
Smoking	↓, limited data
Alcohol and coffee drinking	inconsistent
Diet (fruit and vegetables)	↓, limited data
Regular exercise	↓, limited data
Reproductive health factors	
Age at menarche (early)	↑↑, consistent
Menstrual cycle length (short)	↑↑, consistent
Duration of flows	↑, limited data
Parity	↓↓, consistent
Contraception	
OC use	–, inconsistent
Enviromental factors	
PCB, dioxin exposure	–, inconsistent
Medical history of immunological related diseases	↑, inconsistent

OC, oral contraceptive; PCB, polychlorinated biphenyl.

Risk factors

Table 2.2 shows the main risk factors suggested or confirmed for endometriosis.

Age

Age is the main determinant of risk of endometriosis: the condition is rare before the menarche and after the menopause, being a condition of fertile age. Studies conducted before the 1950s suggested that the frequency of endometriosis increased with age from menarche to menopause, but more recent studies have not confirmed this finding [3,5,28]. Different selection criteria can explain part of these discrepancies. For instance, in the last few years more young women have undergone laparoscopy for infertility than 20 years ago, when laparotomy was necessary to diagnose endometriosis.

Social class and race

A greater frequency of endometriosis among women of higher social class has been reported [8]. However, this might be the result of a diagnostic "bias," i.e. greater attention towards pelvic pain or infertility among women of higher social class. The role of social-related selective mechanisms in the diagnosis of benign gynecological conditions is well recognized. The same diagnostic "bias" might explain the higher frequency of the disease among white than black women [4,29]. In fact, data on the prevalence in different races often do not take into account the reason for admission for surgical procedures (that may be selectively associated with a higher or lower likelihood of the disease being diagnosed). In the United States, where most studies have been conducted, black women have lower socio-economic conditions. The few studies that evaluated populations comparable for indication to diagnostic procedures and socio-economic class did not find substantial differences in terms of prevalence of the disease among women of different races [30].

In utero exposure

A paper by Missmer *et al* [17] has suggested that *in utero* exposures may be associated with the risk of development of endometriosis. In that study, women born by multiple pregnancies and those exposed to diethylstilbestrol (DES) *in utero* were at higher risk of endometriosis. No association emerged with birthweight and breast-feeding status. Although a potential role of *in utero* exposure may have some biological interpretations, the data are scanty and no conclusion can be drawn on the relation with the risk of endometriosis.

Menstrual and reproductive factors

Age at menarche and menstrual characteristics

Epidemiological studies in the different populations have suggested that women with early menarche are at a higher risk of endometriosis [31–34]. With regard to the characteristics of menses, a regular lifelong menstrual pattern and heavy flows were associated with an increased risk of endometriosis [30,31,35,36]. This may be explained as a higher likelihood of pelvic contamination from menstrual endometrial material – the reflux hypothesis. However, in the interpretation of these findings, caution has been suggested in consideration of potential biases which may act in epidemiological studies of this condition [30].

Infertility

Infertility and pelvic pain are clinical findings in endometriosis [37], and are often the reason for diagnostic procedures. This selective mechanism raises the frequency of infertile women or women with abnormal menstrual pattern among the cases. In order to take this selection bias into account, some studies have analyzed only cases in which the diagnosis of endometriosis was a incidental finding in women who underwent surgery for other benign gynecological conditions [35]. However, this methodological approach may introduce other potential bias so the issue is still under discussion.

Parity

With regard to obstetric history, clinical data suggest that parity is inversely associated with the risk of endometriosis [4,31,35,36,38] and adenomyosis [31,35,39,40]. Further, the risk of endometriosis decreases with increasing number of births. This finding suggests a direct protective effect of pregnancy. There was no relation with age at first and last birth, suggesting that the protection given by pregnancy persists at least in the middle period. In contrast to most clinical data, epidemiological studies have not generally shown any relationship between age at first pregnancy and endometriosis [31,41].

Spontaneous and induced abortions

Few studies have analyzed the relation between previous spontaneous abortions and risk of endometriosis, showing in general no association. On the other hand, a reduced risk of endometriosis in women reporting a history of induced abortion has been reported [41]. This latter finding can likely be explained by a higher fertility in women reporting induced abortions. This suggests that infertility more than pregnancy itself may be associated with a risk of the disease. Data on the issue are, however, scanty and controversial.

Oral contraceptive use

Data regarding any association between oral contraceptive (OC) use and endometriosis are conflicting (see Table 2.3 for a review of selected studies). In some studies, the risk of the disease was lower among current OC users [36]. In a large cohort study (the Oxford Family Planning Association study), the rate of endometriosis was lower among current or recent users than among never-users (relative risk (RR) 0.4, 95% confidence interval (CI) 0.2–0.7), whereas women who had stopped the pill much earlier (i.e. >2–4 years) had a higher risk (RR 1.8, 95% CI 1.0–3.1) [42]. A similar pattern of risk, i.e. lower rate of the disease in current but higher in ex-OC users, was reported from three other cohort studies: the Royal College of General Practitioners study, the Walnut Creek study, and the Nurses' Health Study II [43–45].

Table 2.3 Main results from studies on oral contraceptive use and endometriosis.

Source (country, year)	No. of cases	Current	Past
Cross-sectional			
Moen (Norway, 1987) [84]	19	NE	0.8
Kirshon and Poindexter (US, 1988) [85]	42	0.7	0.7
Mahmood and Templeton (UK, 1991) [7]	227	0.9	–
Moen (Norway, 1991) [86]	42	1.0	–
Italian Endometriosis Study Group (Italy, 1999) [87]	345	1.8	1.6
Case–control studies			
Strathy *et al* (US, 1982) [6]	25	0.1	–
Parazzini et al. (Italy, 1989) [38]	114	1.1	2.3
Parazzini *et al* (Italy, 1994) [88]	377	0.9	1.7
Matorras et al (Spain, 1995) [89]	174	1.3	–
Sangi-Haghpeykar and Poindexter (US, 1995) [36]	126	0.4	–
Cohort			
RCGP (UK, 1974) [43]	43	0.5	1.4
Ramcharan *et al* (US, 1981) [90]	104	0.6	1.4
Vessey (UK, 1993) [42]	138	0.4	1.8
Missmer *et al* (US, 2004) [45]	1340	0.8	1.7

NE, not estimated.

Likewise, in a case–control study conducted in Italy, ever-users had a higher risk of pelvic endometriosis but the risk was restricted to past users [35]. However, other studies reported different results [32–34].

Oral contraception may temporarily suppress endometriosis, but previous OC use could increase the risk of the disease. Probably, treatment with OC does not cure endometriosis, and ectopic endometrial implants survive, although in atrophic form, ready for reactivation when treatment is stopped [46].

There are various biological interpretations of the possible role of OC in endometriosis. OC may reduce the risk by suppressing ovulation, since regular menses increase the risk of endometriosis. However, in castrated monkeys, endometrial tissue seeded into the peritoneum did not require steroid supplementation, but estradiol and/or progesterone were indispensable for the survival of implants [47]. Thus, OC may favor the persistence of endometriosis.

Dysmenorrhea is a frequent symptom of endometriosis and also an important indication for OC use. Thus, the higher risk for ever and past users of OC may be due to selective mechanisms and indication bias. Women with endometriosis-induced dysmenorrhea may to some extent be selectively excluded from the never OC users category, thus raising the risk for past OC users. On the other hand, OC use may reduce the likelihood of diagnosis of endometriosis, since OC reduces dysmenorrhea so current users tend not to be investigated and diagnosed with endometriosis. Women with undiagnosed endometriosis could thus swell the number of controls who use OC, leading to an apparent protective effect for current users. In any case, the lack of relation between total duration of OC use and endometriosis and the pattern of risk with time since last use does not support a causal relationship.

It appears, therefore, that the risk of endometriosis is reduced only among current (or recent) OC users, and any causal inference is hampered by the question of indication bias, apart from the absence of a duration/risk relationship. Thus, before drawing any causal inference, the role of selection and other biases must be considered in the interpretation of epidemiological data regarding OC use and endometriosis. Some of these uncertainties are attributable to the methodological difficulties of epidemiological studies on endometriosis, specifically the problem of identification of the control group. To overcome this problem, studies using different methodological approaches and different control groups are needed.

Family history

It has been consistently shown that the risk of endometriosis is higher in women whose mother or sisters have the disease [48–51]. For example, the first-degree relatives of affected women were at 3–9 times increased risk of developing the disease compared with first-degree relatives of controls in a study conducted by Zondervan et al [52]. However, these findings should be considered cautiously, since information bias cannot be excluded. Cases of endometriosis may tend to recall a family history of the disease more accurately than controls. Studies

concerning family history of cancer have shown that in general, the recall of cancer in first-degree relatives is satisfactory and comparable for cases and controls, whereas recall in second-degree relatives is much less reliable. However, although available data consider only first-degree relatives in a family history of endometriosis, recall bias may be more important for benign conditions. Further research, particularly focused on genetic analyses, is needed to clarify the role of family involvement on the risk of endometriosis [53].

Smoking

Another interesting finding is the protective effect of current smoking on endometriosis. Smoking has an antiestrogenic effect [28]. A protective effect of smoking has also been observed in other benign and malignant gynecological estrogen-related conditions, such as endometrial cancer and fibroids. Available data on the relationship between smoking and endometriosis risk are, however, limited and controversial [3,4,42]. Therefore, we cannot draw any conclusion regarding this association which, if any, is limited and of no clinical relevance.

Diet

The relationship between dietary factors and risk of endometriosis has been analyzed in epidemiological studies, but findings are controversial [3,54]. Moderate intake of alcohol is related to increased levels of estrogens, but the few data on the relation between alchool intake and endometriosis did not show any association [29].

The role of a diet rich in fats in the development of hormone-related diseases has become a topic of interest. For example, diet may have some influence on ovarian and endometrial carcinogenesis and on the development of benign gynaecological conditions, such as fibroids and ovarian cysts [55–57]. Endometriosis is a hormone-related condition, so diet may play a role in its etiopathogenesis. A case–control study in the USA suggested that the risk of endometrioid cysts was elevated for high intake of total, vegetable, non-saturated and polyunsaturated fats [55]. The results of an Italian case–control study suggested that higher intake of green vegetables and fresh fruit can lower the risk of endometriosis [54]. Conversely, intake of beef or red meat in general and ham increased the risk.

In biological terms, fats may influence prostaglandin concentrations, which may affect ovarian function [58]. Hormonal factors are a potential link between diet and endometriosis, since the risk may be increased by exposure to unopposed estrogens, and a diet rich in fat increases circulating unopposed estrogens [59]. More difficult to explain, in biological terms, is the protective effect of a diet rich in green vegetables and fruits. However, similar findings emerged for the risk of breast and endometrial cancer, two estrogen-related diseases. A diet rich in green vegetables and fruits includes high levels of vitamin C, carotenoids, folic acid and lycopene, micronutrients which may help to protect against cell proliferation [60].

Physical activity

Regular physical activity may be linked with lower levels of estrogens and reduce endometriosis risk. Data on this issue are, however, scanty [61].

Body Mass Index

Overweight women had a lower risk of endometriosis in some studies [17,31–33]. This association may be explained by potential biases, including an inverse relationship between bodyweight and socio-economic status, weight gain with child bearing, and loss of appetite as a result of disease. Further, women with higher Body Mass Index have more irregular menstrual cycles and increased rates of anovulatory infertility.

With regard to the association between endometriosis and body fat distribution, the risk of endometriosis by tertiles of waist-to-hip and waist-to-thigh ratios in women aged <30 years has been analyzed [62], showing an increased risk among women with lower waist-to-hip ratio and waist-to-thigh ratio.

Recently it has been suggested that being overweight at 16 years increases the risk of endometriosis [63].

Dioxin

Some studies conducted in the 1990s suggested that exposure to dioxins may be a cause of endometriosis [64]. This finding is of speculative interest, since it suggests that environmental factors, besides hormonal ones, may be associated with the risk of endometriosis.

Studies conducted in non-human primates showed that exposure to the dioxin 2,3,7,8-tetrachlorodibenzo-p-dioxin (TCDD) increases prevalence and severity of endometriosis. Rodent studies support the plausibility of a role of environmental contaminants in the pathophysiology of endometriosis [65]. However, more recent studies did not consistently confirm the association. A recent large review of the literature has shown no significant evidence to support a link between dioxins and endometriosis in women. This observation has been explained by the author by positive publication bias and by significant methodological problems associated with these studies, or by the absence of such a link. There is insufficient evidence in support of the hypothesis that dioxin exposure may lead to increased risk of developing endometriosis in women [66].

History of immune disorders

Some epidemiological data have also linked the risk of endometriosis with the frequency of immune disorders. In particular, in the Endometriosis Family Study the prevalence of rheumatoid arthritis, systemic lupus erythematosus, hypo- or hyperthyroidism and multiple sclerosis was higher in women with endometriosis than in controls. An association with non-Hodgkin lymphomas has been also suggested [67–69]. This potential association is of particular interest in speculative terms, since these findings may support the hypothesis that the cause of endometriosis includes immunological mechanisms.

Other factors

Of interest, there are some isolated but intriguing data supporting a possible association of the disease with pigmentary traits or sun habits. A link between endometriosis and melanoma, a cancer known to be triggered by ultraviolet exposure, has been repeatedly reported [68,70–72]. Moreover, the presence of specific phenotypical traits such as red hair, nevi, freckles, and sensitivity to sun exposure has been shown to be more common in women with endometriosis [73–78]. These data are, however, still scanty and difficult to interpret.

We do not consider the relationship between endometriosis and ovarian cancer since a specific chapter is dedicated to this association in this book.

Differences in risk factors between deep ovarian and superficial endometriosis

In this chapter we have summarized the main evidence on risk factors for endometriosis. However, this disease includes different clinical conditions. In particular, in recent years great attention has been paid to deep endometriosis, which is characterized by a stronger relation with pelvic pain and dyspareunia than cases with endometriosis in other anatomical sites. These clinical characteristics have suggested that deep endometriosis may recognize different etiopathological mechanisms in comparison with pelvic and ovarian endometriosis. Thus, ovarian/peritoneal and deep endometriosis can be considered potential conditions, in terms of both etiopathogenetic mechanisms and clinical findings. For example, it has been suggested that deep endometriosis lesions of the posterior cul-de-sac originate from metaplasia of müllerian remnants located in the rectovaginal septum, thus constituting an entity different from peritoneal endometriosis. Alternatively these forms could be the most severe manifestation of peritoneal disease [79].

In epidemiological terms, if deep endometriosis represents a different condition, it should recognize different risk factors in comparison with endometriosis in other sites. Few data are available from epidemiological studies on risk factors for endometriosis in different sites [35,80]. Some studies have shown no difference between pelvic and ovarian endometriosis [81], but the epidemiological profile of women with deep endometriosis in comparison with women with peritoneal-ovarian endometriosis is substantially unknown. A study conducted by Bérubé et al on 329 infertile cases with endometriosis and 262 infertile controls without endometriosis has shown that age ≥30 was positively associated with the presence of deep endometriotic lesions and not with other types of lesions. The authors interpreted the age-related findings as suggesting that deep endometriosis is a consequence of infiltrating endometriosis and that this process requires some years [80].

The general results of an Italian study suggest that women with deep and pelvic-ovarian endometriosis share a similar epidemiological profile [81]. This finding, in turn, supports the hypothesis that these conditions share similar etiopathogenetic mechanisms. Along this line, several epidemiological data have shown that ovarian and peritoneal endometriosis share similar risk factors.

Conclusion

Conclusions regarding the main epidemiological evidence of endometriosis can be summarized as follows.

• Findings regarding menstrual and reproductive factors consistently support the role of pelvic endometrial contamination as the major determinant of disease development. Along this line, available data on OCs use suggest that ovulation is the major determinant of disease progression.

• Future studies should verify if the actual manifestations of endometriosis are partly due to dramatic modifications in modern women's reproductive habits.

• Future epidemiological investigations should also focus on risk factors that are biologically plausible, are preventable, and have high impact on the population.

References

1. Vigano P, Parazzini F, Somigliana E, Vercellini P. Endometriosis: epidemiology and aetiological factors. Best Pract Res Clin Obstet Gynaecol 2004;18:177–200.
2. Eskenazi B, Warner ML. Epidemiology of endometriosis. Obstet Gynecol Clin North Am 1997;24:235–258.
3. Missmer SA, Cramer DW. The epidemiology of endometriosis. Obstet Gynecol Clin North Am 2003;30:1–19, vii.
4. Houston DE. Evidence for the risk of pelvic endometriosis by age, race and socioeconomic status. Epidemiol Rev 1984;6:167–191.
5. Houston DE, Noller KL, Melton LJ 3rd, Selwyn BJ. The epidemiology of pelvic endometriosis. Clin Obstet Gynecol 1988;31:787–800.
6. Strathy JH, Molgaard CA, Coulam CB, Melton LJ 3rd. Endometriosis and infertility: a laparoscopic study of endometriosis among fertile and infertile women. Fertil Steril 1982;38:667–672.
7. Mahmood TA, Templeton A. Prevalence and genesis of endometriosis. Hum Reprod 1991;6:544–549.
8. Gruppo Italiano per lo studio dell'endometriosi. Risk factors for pelvic endometriosis in women with pelvic pain or infertility. Eur J Obstet Gynecol Reprod Biol 1999;83:195–199.
9. Chapron C, Chopin N, Borghese B et al. Deeply infiltrating endometriosis: pathogenetic implications of the anatomical distribution. Hum Reprod 2006;21:1839–1845.
10. Farquhar C. Endometriosis. BMJ 2007;334:249–253.
11. Thomas EJ. Endometriosis. BMJ 1993;306:158–159.
12. Evers JL, Dunselman GA, Land JA, Bouckaert PX, van der Linden PJ. Management of recurrent endometriosis. In: Coutinho EM, Spinola P, Hanson de Moura L (eds) Progress in the Management of Endometriosis. Carnforth, UK: Parthenon Publishing, 1995, pp. 291–297.
13. Vercellini P, Somigliana E, Viganò P, de Matteis S, Barbara G, Fedele L. Postoperative endometriosis recurrence: a plea for prevention based on pathogenetic, epidemiological, and clinical evidence. Reprod Bio Med Online 2010;21(2):259–265.
14. Eaton SB, Pike MC, Short RV et al. Women's reproductive cancers in evolutionary context. Q Rev Biol 1994;69:353–367.
15. Thomas SL, Ellertson C. Nuisance or natural and healthy: should monthly menstruation be optional for women? Lancet 2000;355:922–924.
16. Italian National Institute of Statistics. Tavole di Fecondità Regionale. www.demo.istat.it.
17. Missmer SA, Hankinson SE, Spiegelman D, Barbieri RL, Michels KB, Hunter DJ. In utero exposures and the incidence of endometriosis. Fertil Steril 2004;82:1501–1508.
18. Jain S, Dalton ME. Chocolate cysts from ovarian follicles. Fertil Steril 1999;72:852–856.
19. Vercellini P, Somigliana E, Vigano P, Abbiati A, Barbara G, Fedele L. 'Blood On The Tracks': from corpora lutea to endometriomas. Br J Obstet Gynaecol 2009;116:366–371.
20. Vercellini P, Aimi G, de Giorgi O, Maddalena S, Carinelli S, Crosignani PG. Is cystic ovarian endometriosis an asymmetric disease? Br J Obstet Gynaecol 1998;105:1018–1021.
21. Al-Fozan H, Tulandi T. Left lateral predisposition of endometriosis and endometrioma. Obstet Gynecol 2003;101:164–166.
22. Ciavattini A, Montik N, Baiocchi R, Cucculelli N, Tranquilli AL. Does previous surgery influence the asymmetric distribution of endometriotic lesions? Gynecol Endocrinol 2004;19:253–258.
23. Parazzini F. Left:right side ratio of endometriotic implants in the pelvis. Eur J Obstet Gynecol Reprod Biol 2003;111:65–67.
24. Vercellini P, Abbiati A, Vigano P et al. Asymmetry in distribution of diaphragmatic endometriotic lesions: evidence in favour of the menstrual reflux theory. Hum Reprod 2007;22:2359–2367.
25. Vercellini P, Pisacreta A, Pesole A, Vicentini S, Stellato G, Crosignani PG. Is ureteral endometriosis an asymmetric disease? Br J Obstet Gynaecol 2000;107:559–561.
26. Jenkins S, Olive DL, Haney AF. Endometriosis: pathogenetic implications of the anatomic distribution. Obstet Gynecol 1986;67:335–338.
27. Rosenshein NB, Leichner PK, Vogelsang G. Radiocolloids in the treatment of ovarian cancer. Obstet Gynecol Surv 1979;34:708–720.
28. Gruppo Italiano per lo studio dell'endometriosi. Prevalence and anatomical distribution of endometriosis in women with selected gynaecological conditions: results from a multicentric Italian study. Hum Reprod 1994;9:1158–1162.
29. Missmer SA, Hankinson SE, Spiegelman D, Barbieri RL, Marshall LM, Hunter DJ. Incidence of laparoscopically confirmed endometriosis by demographic, anthropometric, and lifestyle factors. Am J Epidemiol 2004;160:784–796.
30. Mangtani P, Booth M. Epidemiology of endometriosis. J Epidemiol Comm Health 1993;47:84–88.
31. Cramer DW, Wilson E, Stillman RJ et al. The relation of endometriosis to menstrual characteristics, smoking, and exercise. JAMA 1986;255:1904–1908.
32. Signorello LB, Harlow BL, Cramer DW, Spiegelman D, Hill JA. Epidemiologic determinants of endometriosis: a hospital-based case-control study. Ann Epidemiol 1997;7:267–741.
33. Darrow SL, Vena JE, Batt RE, Zielezny MA, Michalek AM, Selman S. Menstrual cycle characteristics and the risk of endometriosis. Epidemiology 1993;4:135–142.
34. Han M, Pan L, Wu B, Bian X. A case-control epidemiologic study of endometriosis. Chin Med Sci J 1994;9:114–118.

35. Parazzini F, Ferraroni M, Fedele L, Bocciolone L, Rubessa S, Riccardi A. Pelvic endometriosis: reproductive and menstrual risk factors at different stages in Lombardy, northern Italy. J Epidemiol Commun Health 1995;49:61–64.

36. Sangi-Haghpeykar H, Poindexter AN 3rd. Epidemiology of endometriosis among parous women. Obstet Gynecol 1995;85:983–992.

37. Olive DL, Schwartz LB. Endometriosis. N Engl J Med 1993;328: 1759–1769.

38. Parazzini F, La Vecchia C, Franceschi S, Negri E, Cecchetti G. Risk factors for endometrioid, mucinous and serous benign ovarian cysts. Int J Epidemiol 1989;18:108–112.

39. Parazzini F, Vercellini P, Panazza S, Chatenoud L, Oldani S, Crosignani PG. Risk factors for adenomyosis. Hum Reprod 1997;12: 1275–1279.

40. Parazzini F, Mais V, Cipriani S, Busacca M, Venturini P. Determinants of adenomyosis in women who underwent hysterectomy for benign gynecological conditions: results from a prospective multicentric study in Italy. Eur J Obstet Gynecol Reprod Biol 2009;143: 103–106.

41. Parazzini F, di Cintio E, Chatenoud L, Mezzanotte C, Crosignani PG. Previous abortions and risk of pelvic endometriosis. Hum Reprod 1998;13:3283–3284.

42. Vessey MP, Villard-Mackintosh L, Painter R. Epidemiology of endometriosis in women attending family planning clinics. BMJ 1993;306:182–184.

43. Royal College of General Practitioners. Oral Contraceptives and Health: An Interim Report from the Oral Contraceptive Study of the Royal College of General Practitioners. London: Pitman Medical Publishing, 1974.

44. Walnut Creek Contraceptive Drug Study. A Prospective Study of the Side Effects of Oral Contraceptives, vol. 3. Bethesda, MD: National Institutes of Health, 1981.

45. Missmer SA, Hankinson SE, Spiegelman D et al. Reproductive history and endometriosis among premenopausal women. Obstet Gynecol 2004;104:965–974.

46. Nisolle-Pochet M, Casanas-Roux F, Donnez J. Histologic study of ovarian endometriosis after hormonal therapy. Fertil Steril 1988;49: 423–426.

47. Dizerega GS, Barber DL, Hodgen GD. Endometriosis: role of ovarian steroids in initiation, maintenance, and suppression. Fertil Steril 1980;33:649–653.

48. Simpson JL, Elias S, Malinak LR, Buttram VC Jr. Heritable aspects of endometriosis. I. Genetic studies. Am J Obstet Gynecol 1980;137: 327–331.

49. Lamb K, Hoffmann RG, Nichols TR. Family trait analysis: a case-control study of 43 women with endometriosis and their best friends. Am J Obstet Gynecol 1986;154:596–601.

50. Moen MH, Magnus P. The familial risk of endometriosis. Acta Obstet Gynecol Scand 1993;72:560–564.

51. Moen MH. Endometriosis in monozygotic twins. Acta Obstet Gynecol Scand 1994;73:59–62.

52. Zondervan KT, Cardon LR, Kennedy SH. What makes a good case-control study? Design issues for complex traits such as endometriosis. Hum Reprod 2002;17:1415–1423.

53. Treloar S, Hadfield R, Montgomery G et al. The International Endogene Study: a collection of families for genetic research in endometriosis. Fertil Steril 2002;78:679–685.

54. Parazzini F, Chiaffarino F, Surace M et al. Selected food intake and risk of endometriosis. Hum Reprod 2004;19:1755–1759.

55. Britton JA, Westhoff C, Howe G, Gammon MD. Diet and benign ovarian tumors (United States). Cancer Causes Control 2000;11: 389–401.

56. Britton JA, Westhoff C, Howe GR, Gammon MD. Lactose and benign ovarian tumours in a case-control study. Br J Cancer 2000;83: 1552–1555.

57. Bosetti C, Negri E, Franceschi S et al. Diet and ovarian cancer risk: a case-control study in Italy. Int J Cancer 2001;93:911–915.

58. Smith MF. Recent advances in corpus luteum physiology. J Dairy Sci 1986;69:911–926.

59. Gorbach SL, Goldin BR. Diet and the excretion and enterohepatic cycling of estrogens. Prev Med 1987;16:525–531.

60. Bosetti C, Altieri A, La Vecchia C. Diet and environmental carcinogenesis in breast/gynaecological cancers. Curr Opin Obstet Gynecol 2002;14:13–18.

61. Vitonis AF, Hankinson SE, Hornstein MD, Missmer SA. Adult physical activity and endometriosis risk. Epidemiology 2010;21:16–23.

62. McCann SE, Freudenheim JL, Darrow SL, Batt RE, Zielezny MA. Endometriosis and body fat distribution. Obstet Gynecol 1993;82:545–549.

63. Nagle CM, Bell TA, Purdie DM et al. Relative weight at ages 10 and 16 years and risk of endometriosis: a case-control analysis. Hum Reprod 2009;24:1501–1506.

64. Koninckx PR, Braet P, Kennedy SH, Barlow DH. Dioxin pollution and endometriosis in Belgium. Hum Reprod 1994;9:1001–1002.

65. Rier S, Foster WG. Environmental dioxins and endometriosis. Semin Reprod Med 2003;21:145–154.

66. Guo SW, Simsa P, Kyama CM et al. Reassessing the evidence for the link between dioxin and endometriosis: from molecular biology to clinical epidemiology. Mol Hum Reprod 2009;15:609–624.

67. Sinaii N, Cleary SD, Ballweg ML, Nieman LK, Stratton P. High rates of autoimmune and endocrine disorders, fibromyalgia, chronic fatigue syndrome and atopic diseases among women with endometriosis: a survey analysis. Hum Reprod 2002;17:2715–2724.

68. Somigliana E, Vigano P, Parazzini F, Stoppelli S, Giambattista E, Vercellini P. Association between endometriosis and cancer: a comprehensive review and a critical analysis of clinical and epidemiological evidence. Gynecol Oncol 2006;101:331–341.

69. Matalliotakis I, Cakmak H, Fragouli Y, Zervoudis S, Neonaki M, Arici A. Association of endometriosis with family history of non-Hodgkin's lymphoma: presentation of 10 cases. J BUON 2009;14:699–701.

70. Brinton LA, Westhoff CL, Scoccia B et al. Causes of infertility as predictors of subsequent cancer risk. Epidemiology 2005;16:500–507.

71. Kvaskoff M, Mesrine S, Fournier A, Boutron-Ruault MC, Clavel-Chapelon F. Personal history of endometriosis and risk of cutaneous melanoma in a large prospective cohort of French women. Arch Intern Med 2007;167:2061–2065.

72. Melin A, Sparen P, Bergqvist A. The risk of cancer and the role of parity among women with endometriosis. Hum Reprod 2007;22:3021–3026.

73. Kvaskoff M, Mesrine S, Clavel-Chapelon F, Boutron-Ruault MC. Endometriosis risk in relation to naevi, freckles and skin sensitivity to sun exposure: the French E3N cohort. Int J Epidemiol 2009;38: 1143–1153.

74. Frisch RE, Wyshak G, Albert LS, Sober AJ. Dysplastic nevi, cutaneous melanoma, and gynecologic disorders. Int J Dermatol 1992;31: 331–335.

75. Woodworth SH, Singh M, Yussman MA, Sanfilippo JS, Cook CL, Lincoln SR. A prospective study on the association between red hair color and endometriosis in infertile patients. Fertil Steril 1995;64: 651–652.

76. Hornstein MD, Thomas PP, Sober AJ, Wyshak G, Albright NL, Frisch RE. Association between endometriosis, dysplastic naevi and history of melanoma in women of reproductive age. Hum Reprod 1997;12: 143–145.

77. Wachter RF, Briggs GP, Pedersen CE Jr. Precipitation of phase I antigen of Coxiella burnetii by sodium sulfite. Acta Virol 1975;19:500.

78. Somigliana E, Vigano P, Abbiati A et al. 'Here comes the sun': pigmentary traits and sun habits in women with endometriosis. Hum Reprod 2010;25:728–733.

79. Vercellini P, Frontino G, Pietropaolo G, Gattei U, Daguati R, Crosignani PG. Deep endometriosis: definition, pathogenesis, and clinical management. J Am Assoc Gynecol Laparosc 2004;11: 153–161.

80. Berube S, Marcoux S, Maheux R. Characteristics related to the prevalence of minimal or mild endometriosis in infertile women. Canadian Collaborative Group on Endometriosis. Epidemiology 1998;9:504–510.

81. Parazzini F, Cipriani S, Bianchi S, Gotsch F, Zanconato G, Fedele L. Risk factors for deep endometriosis: a comparison with pelvic and ovarian endometriosis. Fertil Steril 2008;90:174–179.

82. Houston DE, Noller KL, Melton LJ 3rd, Selwyn BJ, Hardy RJ. Incidence of pelvic endometriosis in Rochester, Minnesota, 1970–1979. Am J Epidemiol 1987;125:959–969.

83. Leibson CL, Good AE, Hass SL et al. Incidence and characterization of diagnosed endometriosis in a geographically defined population. Fertil Steril 2004;82:314–321.

84. Moen MH. Endometriosis in women at interval sterilization. Acta Obstet Gynecol Scand 1987;66:451–454.

85. Kirshon B, Poindexter AN 3rd. Contraception: a risk factor for endometriosis. Obstet Gynecol 1988;71:829–831.

86. Moen MH. Is a long period without childbirth a risk factor for developing endometriosis? Hum Reprod 1991;6:1404–1407.

87. Italian Endometriosis Study Group. Oral contraceptive use and risk of endometriosis. Br J Obstet Gynaecol 1999;106:695–699.

88. Parazzini F, Ferraroni M, Bocciolone L, Tozzi L, Rubessa S, La Vecchia C. Contraceptive methods and risk of pelvic endometriosis. Contraception 1994;49:47–55.

89. Matorras R, Rodiquez F, Pijoan JI, Ramon O, Gutierrez de Teran G, Rodriguez-Escudero F. Epidemiology of endometriosis in infertile women. Fertil Steril 1995;63:34–38.

90. Ramcharan S, Pellegrin FA, Ray R, Hau J-P. The Walnut Creek Contraceptive Drug Study: A Prospective Study of the Side Effects of Oral Contraceptives. Monograph No. 81-564. Bethesda, MD: National Institutes of Health, Center for Population Research, 1981.

3

Economic Perspective on Diagnosis and Treatment of Endometriosis

Steven Simoens[1] and Thomas M. D'Hooghe[2]

[1]Research Centre for Pharmaceutical Care and Pharmaco-economics, Catholic University of Leuven, Leuven, Belgium
[2]Leuven University Fertility Center, Department of Obstetrics and Gynaecology, University Hospitals Leuven, Leuven, Belgium

Introduction

In a context of spiraling healthcare costs and limited resources, public policy makers and healthcare payers are concerned about the costs of endometriosis. Cost estimates can underline the importance of endometriosis to society when considered alongside its impact on morbidity and mortality and when compared with the economic burden of other diseases. Furthermore, cost studies may allow the identification of the drivers of diagnosis and treatment costs. Finally, cost data can be fed into economic evaluations, so that decision makers can ascertain the cost-effectiveness of various approaches to diagnosing and treating endometriosis by examining their effectiveness in relation to their costs.

The aim of this chapter is to provide an economic perspective on the diagnosis and treatment of endometriosis. To this effect, a literature review is conducted to assess the theory and the evidence relating to the costs of endometriosis and to the cost-effectiveness of the diagnosis and treatment of endometriosis.

Costs

Theory

A cost study of endometriosis can take the form of a cost-of-illness analysis or a cost analysis. A cost-of-illness analysis quantifies the economic burden of endometriosis to society by measuring the costs of diagnosing and treating endometriosis as well as the costs arising as a result of endometriosis (for instance, productivity loss due to time taken off work). Such studies measure direct costs related to healthcare resource use (e.g. medication, contacts with healthcare professionals and hospitalization), direct non-healthcare costs (e.g. transportation to the healthcare professional), and indirect costs arising from time lost from work or reduced productivity at work. A cost analysis compares two or more approaches to diagnosis and treatment of endometriosis (for instance, medical versus surgical therapy).

When carrying out a cost study of endometriosis, multiple methodological issues arise relating to the sample, epidemiological approach, data collection, design, scope of included costs, time horizon and sensitivity analysis.

With respect to the sample, studies can be based on a representative national sample or enroll a specific group of patients. The epidemiological approach can take the form of a prevalence-based study, which measures costs attributable to a group of patients suffering from endometriosis during a given time interval. Alternatively, an incidence-based study quantifies lifetime costs of endometriosis from onset to death. As women may suffer from recurrent episodes of endometriosis, cost studies need to adopt an incidence-based approach.

Data can be collected prospectively/retrospectively from patient medical records, a survey, a claims database or the literature. Studies need to set up a prospective collection of primary data on healthcare resource use and costs. This type of analysis can be considered to be more reliable than retrospective analyses of patient medical records or claims databases. Alternatively, modeling approaches can be considered that are based on high-quality data, closely reflecting real-life practice and the evolution of endometriosis in patients.

Cost studies can be designed as a case series following up patients suffering from endometriosis, a case–control study comparing patients with/without endometriosis, or a cohort study contrasting options for diagnosis and treatment of endometriosis patients. For instance, a cost-of-illness analysis needs to distinguish between the disease endometriosis and the main symptoms (pain and subfertility) associated with endometriosis. To examine the costs associated with endometriosis itself, studies need to compare patients with endometriosis and pelvic pain to patients with a normal pelvis and

Endometriosis: Science and Practice, First Edition. Edited by Linda C. Giudice, Johannes L.H. Evers and David L. Healy.
© 2012 Blackwell Publishing Ltd. Published 2012 by Blackwell Publishing Ltd.

Table 3.1 Costs associated with endometriosis.

Direct healthcare costs					Direct non-healthcare costs	Indirect costs
Medication	**Diagnostic procedures**	**Surgical procedures**	**Healthcare providers**	**Other**		
Non-steroidal anti-inflammatory drugs	Ultrasound scan (transvaginal/abdominal/transrectal)	Laparoscopy	General practitioner	Accident and Emergency visit	Transportation to healthcare provider	Absence from work
Progestogen-only contraceptives	Ultrasound scan (kidney)	Laparotomy	Gynecologist	Hospitalization	Child care costs while in treatment	Reduced productivity while at work
Combined oral contraceptive pill	Magnetic resonance imaging	Colposcopy	Nurse	Alternative medicine (e.g. homeopathy, acupuncture, nutrition)		Reduced ability to carry out day-to-day activities
Danazol	Computed tomography	Cyst aspiration	Urologist	In vitro fertilization		
Gestrinone	Intravenous pelvography	Hysteroscopy	Gastroenterologist	Intrauterine insemination		
Gonadotropin-releasing hormone agonists	Barium enema	Hysterectomy	Anesthetist	Hormonal stimulation		
Add-back hormone replacement therapy	Sigmoidoscopy	Ovarian cystectomy	Radiologist			
Mirena coil	Biopsy and histological examination (vaginal endometriosis, peritoneal endometriosis, ovarian endometriosis, bowel endometriosis)	Adnectomy	Theater staff			
Clomiphene citrate	Serum markers (CA-125)	Ovariectomy	Hematologist			
Gonadotropins	Bacteriology/culture	Tubectomy	Counselor			
Antibiotics		Adhesiolysis	Physiotherapist			
Antidepressants		Resection endometriosis rectovaginal septum	Psychiatrist			
Aromatase inhibitors		Resection bladder endometriosis				
		Low anterior resection				
		Segmental bowel resection				
		Appendectomy				
		Resection cecum				
		Resection small bowel				
		Colostomy				
		Ureter reimplantation				
		Ureter-ureterostomy				
		Nephrectomy				
		Electrocoagulation peritoneal endometriosis				
		Laser coagulation peritoneal endometriosis				
		Laparoscopic uterosacral nerve ablation				
		Endometrial ablation				

pain or compare patients with endometriosis and infertility to patients with a normal pelvis and infertility. A case–control study design comparing patients with/without endometriosis seems to be suited for this purpose.

The economic impact of endometriosis on patients, the healthcare system and society is difficult to determine. Therefore, Table 3.1 identifies the major cost items that need to be considered when calculating the costs of endometriosis from a societal perspective. In addition to direct healthcare costs, studies need to focus on eliciting direct non-healthcare costs and indirect costs. With respect to the latter, attention needs to be paid to calculating the indirect costs of days lost to education and work and the costs of reduced ability to carry out normal everyday activities.

Estimates can be presented as charges based on official list prices or costs based on actual resource use. Studies need to move away from using charge data based on official list prices towards measuring costs based on actual resource use. This is because, for instance, charges for surgical treatment of endometriosis in hospital may not accurately reflect actual expenditure on administration, billing, capital depreciation, maintenance, laundry and other hospital services related to the surgical procedure. Alternatively, in studies that measure charges, these need to be converted into costs by means of cost-to-charge ratios. Such adjustment by cost-to-charge ratios is regularly used in cost studies set in the United States.

Evidence

Economic burden

The economic burden arising from endometriosis has been estimated for the US population in 2002. A study found annual direct healthcare costs of $2801 per patient (outpatient and hospital care amounted to 10% and 90% of costs, respectively) and annual indirect costs of $1023 per patient in 2002 values [1]. Extrapolating these findings to the US population, annual endometriosis costs amounted to about $22 billion assuming a prevalence of 10% in women of reproductive age [2].

In order to fully appreciate these costs, it is important to compare them with published cost estimates for other diseases in the United States in 2002. When comparing costs of diseases, caution need to be exercised as the methods used to derive cost estimates may differ between studies and diseases. Crohn's disease seems to be a good comparator as its treatment involves expensive medication and can draw on a medical or a surgical approach as is the case with endometriosis. Estimates of total annual costs of Crohn's disease were $865 million [3]. Migraine exhibits similarities to endometriosis in that it is a chronic condition, with a cyclic pattern, affecting individuals in a similar age group, and is more prevalent in women than in men. The annual economic burden of migraine was estimated at $13–17 billion [4].

In a retrospective review of administrative data for commercial payers of a US insurance company [5], the extrapolated cost of endometriosis per patient per month was $791, a cost that is higher than or similar to the cost for high-profile conditions such as hypertension ($500), diabetes ($916) and rheumatoid arthritis

($1121) in 2003 values. The costs of endometriosis could be explained by the high hospital admission rate and surgical procedures. Furthermore, due to the added cost related to comorbid conditions like interstitial cystitis, depression, migraine, irritable bowel syndrome, chronic fatigue syndrome, abdominal pain and infertility, women with endometriosis incurred total direct healthcare costs that were, on average, 63% higher than costs for an average woman in a commercially insured group.

Healthcare costs

Diagnosing endometriosis on the basis of symptoms is rendered difficult by the fact that the presentation of endometriosis is variable, each of the symptoms can have other causes (for example, irritable bowel syndrome or pelvic inflammatory disease), and a significant proportion of affected women are asymptomatic [6]. The ability to diagnose endometriosis by means of laparoscopy depends on the surgeon's skills and experience. As a result, 3–12 years may pass between symptom onset and definitive diagnosis [7,8]. During this time, unnecessary investigations and treatments are likely to be initiated, thus representing a cost of obtaining a diagnosis for women presenting with symptoms that may have several different causes. Better diagnostic methods would alleviate some of the distress felt between symptom onset and diagnosis and treatment, although the net effect on costs is unclear. As cost studies enrol patients who have been identified to suffer from endometriosis, they under-report the economic burden of endometriosis.

The costs of the most commonly used medical treatments of endometriosis have been evaluated in the United Kingdom [9]. The cost of 6 months of treatment amounted to $11–18 with progestogen-only contraceptives, $8 with the combined oral contraceptive pill, $225 with danazol, $945 with gestrinone, $1035 and $1145 with goserelin with and without add-back hormone replacement therapy, respectively, in 2002 values. Within the class of gonadotropin-releasing hormone agonists, a cost advantage of treatment with nafarelin acetate as compared with leuprolide acetate has been reported [10]. Direct healthcare costs of 6 months of treatment amounted to $2241 per patient with nafarelin acetate and $2623 with leuprolide acetate in 2002 values ($P < 0.05$). This cost difference arose from lower drug costs with nafarelin acetate ($P < 0.001$). There were no significant differences between medical treatments with nafarelin acetate and leuprolide acetate in terms of costs of outpatient drugs other than nafarelin and leuprolide acetate, outpatient services and inpatient admissions.

Hysterectomy, laparoscopy and laparotomy are commonly performed on patients with endometriosis. A US study showed that a total abdominal hysterectomy was the most commonly performed procedure, accounting for 55–60% of surgical procedures for women with endometriosis in the USA [11]. A total abdominal hysterectomy was associated with higher mean total costs when compared to laparotomy and to other uterus-related operations in 1991 and 1992 [11,12]. As compared with laparotomy, laparoscopy generally results in quicker recovery, decreased morbidity and lower costs [12]. Focusing on inpatient

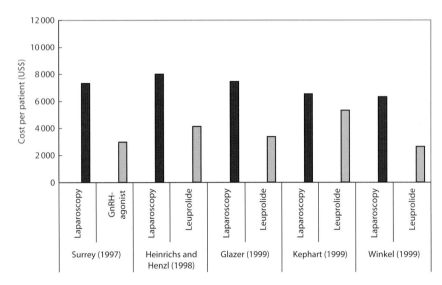

Figure 3.1 Healthcare costs of endometriosis diagnosis and treatment (2002 values).

costs, a cost analysis found that laparotomy ($9533) was nearly twice as expensive as laparoscopy ($5014) in 2002 values [13].

Is a surgical approach to diagnosis and treatment of endometriosis more or less expensive than a medical approach? Four cost analyses explored this question in endometriosis patients presenting with chronic pelvic pain [14–17]. The results suggested that medical treatment of endometriosis with gonadotropin-releasing hormone agonist therapy (with leuprolide acetate) was less expensive than laparoscopy [2] (Fig. 3.1). However, these studies did not take into account the fact that the lower costs of medical treatment may (or may not) be balanced by additional costs due to higher recurrence rates of endometriosis after medical treatment as compared with surgical treatment [18]. Therefore, the true cost difference between a surgical and medical approach remains unknown to date.

Indirect costs

Endometriosis is a chronic disease that targets the young, working-age population. Social, indirect, and intangible costs also contribute to the overall economic impact of endometriosis. These costs include, but are not limited to, time lost from education and work, the reduced ability to carry out normal everyday activities, loss in earned income, social withdrawal, and psychological disorders such as depression, which may manifest as a consequence of endometriosis.

Little is known about the productivity loss associated with endometriosis, although available estimates from cost-of-illness analyses suggest that endometriosis may impose considerable indirect costs. Estimates of the number of hours missed from work due to endometriosis ranged from 19.2 to 86.4 h per patient per year [1,19]. The productivity loss of 86.4 h translated into annual indirect costs of $1023 per patient in 2002 values. No studies are available quantifying the cost of adolescent endometriosis. Nevertheless, indirect costs associated with adolescent endometriosis are probably considerable due to school absences, behavioral and psychosocial consequences.

Cost-effectiveness

Theory

Information about the cost-effectiveness of diagnosis and treatment of endometriosis can be derived from economic evaluations. An economic evaluation is defined as a study contrasting at least two alternatives in terms of both costs and consequences [20]. With respect to endometriosis, this implies that economic evaluations compare different approaches to diagnosing and treating endometriosis in standard clinical practice. Three techniques can be used to conduct an economic evaluation of the diagnosis and treatment of endometriosis: cost-effectiveness analysis, cost-utility analysis and cost-benefit analysis.

Cost-effectiveness analysis denotes an economic evaluation where a single consequence is quantified in a natural unit, such as the number of patients who are symptom free at 1 year following treatment or the number of patients who need repeat treatment after 5 years. There are two specific types of cost-effectiveness analysis. In a cost-minimization analysis, only costs are analyzed and the least costly alternative is chosen provided that consequences are known to be equal between the intervention and the comparator. In a cost-consequence analysis, costs and more than one consequence are compared between the intervention and the comparator.

A study that measures consequences by specific health-related quality of life measures, such as quality-adjusted life-years, is referred to as a cost-utility analysis. The quality-adjusted life-year takes into account the quantity and quality of life. The quality of life associated with a health state is measured through the use of health utilities. A utility reflects the preference of the general public for the health state. Utilities are elicited on a scale of 0 (reflecting death) to 1 (reflecting perfect health) using techniques such as the visual analog scale, the standard gamble or the time trade-off. Quality of life data are then combined with estimates of the time period for which the outcomes last to generate quality-adjusted life-years.

Cost-benefit analysis refers to an economic evaluation where consequences are valued in monetary terms (a so-called "benefit"). A monetary value can be assigned to health benefits by means of, for instance, the willingness-to-pay technique. Assigning monetary values to consequences is, however, controversial and further work on methods to value consequences needs to be carried out. As both costs and benefits are expressed in monetary terms, benefits can be compared with costs of an approach to diagnose and treat endometriosis, and the net worth (benefits minus costs) of each of the approaches can be estimated.

Evidence

Diagnosis

A cost-effectiveness analysis evaluated the diagnostic performance of magnetic resonance imaging as compared with laparoscopy or laparotomy in patients with clinically suspected endometriosis [21]. Cost and consequence data originated from a single-center trial of 35 women. No sample size calculations were undertaken. Laparoscopy or laparotomy revealed a normal pelvis in six patients, surgically confirmed endometriosis in 26 patients, hematosalpingitis in one patient, benign cystic teratoma in one patient and ovarian cancer with internal hemorrhage in one patient. The overall sensitivity, specificity and accuracy of magnetic resonance imaging were 77%, 78% and 77%, respectively. The sensitivity of magnetic resonance imaging in combination with CA-125 assays was 85%. The laparoscopy cost per patient was $1845 and the abdominal surgery cost per patient was $7859 in 1996 values. The total cost for diagnosis and treatment per patient was $2294. When magnetic resonance imaging was performed, the magnetic resonance imaging cost per patient was $321 and the diagnostic laparoscopy cost per patient was $1845. The total cost for diagnosis and treatment per patient was not reported. The overall net savings were estimated to be $259 per patient. In conclusion, the authors stated that, in patients with suspected endometriosis, the use of pelvic magnetic resonance imaging in combination with serum CA-125 assay decreased the number of invasive surgical procedures and reduced healthcare costs.

A comparative study explored the diagnostic performance of transvaginal sonography and magnetic resonance imaging for the assessment of different locations of deep infiltrating endometriosis [22,23]. No statistically significant difference was found in accuracy between transvaginal sonography and magnetic resonance imaging as a result of the large overlap of 95% confidence intervals for all locations. In the absence of a difference in diagnostic performance, the authors carried out a cost-minimization analysis and argued that the use of magnetic resonance imaging to assess symptomatic women before surgery can increase the cost of preoperative evaluation. Therefore, transvaginal sonography was proposed as a cost-effective method for the assessment of different locations of deep infiltrating endometriosis.

Treatment

An economic evaluation compared surgical treatment with medical treatment with a gonadotropin-releasing hormone agonist [24]. Based on a review of studies, the author argued that surgical therapy offers no better results in terms of pain relief than a gonadotropin-releasing hormone agonist. Given the similar results obtained with surgical and medical treatment and the fact that medical treatment is less expensive, this cost-minimization analysis concluded that primary therapy with a gonadotropin-releasing hormone agonist appears to be a cost-effective approach to the management of endometriosis.

A cost-effectiveness analysis compared the costs and consequences of helium thermal coagulator treatment with medical treatment using gonadotropin-releasing hormone agonists in women with minimal-to-moderate endometriosis [25]. Although alternative medical and surgical treatments are available, the authors did not explicitly state why these two alternatives were chosen. The sample consisted of women presenting to a gynecology outpatient clinic with a history of pelvic pain, dysmenorrhea, dyspareunia, and dyschezia suggestive of endometriosis, or who had previously been diagnosed with the disease. Eighteen women received medical treatment and 17 received surgical treatment. In the medical group, three women (17%) were symptom free, 11 required surgical treatment of endometriosis, one had a laparoscopically assisted vaginal hysterectomy, and three became pregnant before their final reviews. In the surgical group, nine women (53%) were symptom free, four required Zoladex therapy, one required oral contraceptive pills, and three required repeat surgical treatment. Mean costs per patient amounted to £323.29 in the surgical group and £918.12 in the medical group in 2001 values ($P < 0.0001$). The authors reported that their cost results conflicted with those of some other studies, but suggested that this may originate from several patients in the medical group undergoing subsequent surgical treatment. It was concluded that surgical treatment with helium thermal coagulator therapy is a cheaper and more effective therapy.

Diagnosis and treatment

A cost-effectiveness analysis examined three approaches to endometriosis diagnosis and treatment in women with chronic pelvic pain: (a) laparoscopy to diagnose endometriosis followed, if necessary, by repeat laparoscopic surgery for persistent or recurrent symptoms; (b) minilaparoscopy for initial diagnosis and for repeat surgery; and (c) a 3-month course of a gonadotropin-releasing hormone agonist (if pain persisted, surgery by either laparoscopy or minilaparoscopy was performed) [26]. Consequence data were derived from multicenter placebo-controlled trials and authors' assumptions. Costs were based on average charges at Stanford University Hospital and clinics in 1997 values. With respect to consequences, 12% of patients had absent or mild pain at the start of treatment, 77% had absent or mild pain after 3 months of treatment and 82% had absent or mild pain after 6 months of treatment. Also, 88% of patients described their pain as moderate or severe at the start of treatment, 23% after 3 months of treatment and 18% after 6 months of treatment. Side-effects were significantly more severe after 6 months of treatment than after 3 months of treatment. Overall, 3 months of treatment were as effective in pain relief as 6 months and resulted in fewer severe side-effects. Total charges would be $725,635 for 100 patients using laparoscopy and $345,600 for 100 patients using minilaparoscopy. Total charges for 100 patients using gonadotropin-releasing hormone agonist would be $374,225 if 35 patients requiring further investigation were given laparoscopy and $275,700 if they were given minilaparoscopy. The authors concluded that administration of gonadotropin-releasing hormone agonist for 3 months would be a cost-effective means of presumptive diagnosis and treatment of endometriosis among women with chronic pelvic pain.

Conclusion

Endometriosis imposes a substantial economic burden on society. The high burden originates from the time delay between onset of symptoms and diagnosis, costly medical and surgical treatments, the chronic nature of endometriosis, and the indirect costs associated with reduced ability to work. Increasing awareness of the disease, cutting the time to diagnosis and providing centralized evidence-based specialized care are crucial steps in reducing the morbidity, healthcare expenditure and lost productivity associated with endometriosis.

The substantial economic burden underlines the need for further research into cost-effective approaches to diagnosing and treating endometriosis. To date, little is known about the cost-effectiveness of endometriosis diagnosis and treatment. The small number of economic evaluations and their methodological limitations preclude the recommendation of a specific approach to endometriosis diagnosis and treatment on economic grounds.

Acknowledgments

Professor D'Hooghe holds the Serono Chair for Reproductive Medicine at Leuven University Hospital Gasthuisberg. The authors have no conflicts of interest that are relevant to the content of this chapter.

References

1. Kunz K, Kuppermann M, Moynihan C et al. The cost of treatment of endometriosis in the California Medicaid population. Am J Managed Care 1995;1:25–29.

2. Simoens S, Hummelshoj L, D'Hooghe T. Endometriosis: cost estimates and methodological perspective. Hum Reprod Update 2007;13:395–404.

3. Sandler RS, Everhart JE, Donowitz M et al. The burden of selected digestive diseases in the United States. Gastroenterology 2002;122: 1500–1511.

4. Goldberg LD. The cost of migraine and its treatment. Am J Managed Care 2005;11:S62–S67.

5. Mirkin D, Murphy-Barron C, Iwasaki K. Actuarial analysis of private payer administrative claims data for women with endometriosis. J Managed Care Pharm 2007;13:262–272.

6. Kennedy S, Bergqvist A, Chapron C et al. ESHRE guideline for the diagnosis and treatment of endometriosis. Human Reproduction 2005;20:2698–2704.

7. Arruda MS, Petta CA, Abrao MS et al. Time elapsed from onset of symptoms to diagnosis of endometriosis in a cohort study of Brazilian women. Hum Reprod 2003;18:4–9.

8. Husby GK, Haugen R, Moen MH. Diagnostic delay in women with pain and endometriosis. Acta Obstet Gynecol Scand 2003;82:649–653.

9. Pearson S, Pickersgill A. The costs of endometriosis. Gynecol Forum 2004;9:23–27.

10. Zhao SZ, Arguelles LM, Wong JM et al. Cost comparisons between nafarelin and leuprolide in the treatment of endometriosis. Clin Therapeut 1998;20:592–602.

11. Zhao SZ, Wong JM, Davis MB et al. The cost of inpatient endometriosis treatment: an analysis based on the Healthcare Cost and Utilization Project Nationwide Inpatient Sample. Am J Managed Care 1998;4:1127–1134.

12. Gao X, Outley JK, Botteman M et al. The economic burden of endometriosis. Fertil Steril 2006;86:1561–1572.

13. Luciano AA, Lowney J, Jacobs SL. Endoscopic treatment of endometriosis-associated infertility. Therapeutic, economic and social benefits. J Reprod Med 1992;37:573–576.

14. Surrey E. An economically rational method of managing early-stage endometriosis. Med Interface 1997;10:119–124.

15. Glazer M. The clinical and economic benefits of GnRH agonist in treating endometriosis. Am J Managed Care 1999;5:S316–S325.

16. Kephart W. Evaluation of Lovelace Health Systems chronic pelvic pain protocol. Am J Managed Care 1999;5:S309–S315.

17. Winkel CA. Modeling of medical and surgical treatment costs of chronic pelvic pain: new paradigms for making clinical decisions. Am J Managed Care 1999;5:S276–S290.

18. Wellbery C. Diagnosis and treatment of endometriosis. Ame Fam Physician 1999;60:1753–1768.

19. Mathias SD, Kuppermann M, Liberman RF et al. Chronic pelvic pain: prevalence, health-related quality of life, and economic correlates. Obstet Gynecol 1996;87:321–327.

20. Drummond M, Sculpher MJ, Torrance GW et al. Methods for the Economic Evaluation of Health Care Programmes. Oxford: Oxford University Press, 2005.

21. Sugimura K, Imaoka I, Okizuka H. Pelvic endometriosis: impact of magnetic resonance imaging on treatment decisions and costs. Acad Radiol 1996;3:S66–S68.

22. Bazot M, Lafont C, Rouzier R et al. Diagnostic accuracy of physical examination, transvaginal sonography, rectal endoscopic sonography, and magnetic resonance imaging to diagnose deep infiltrating endometriosis. Fertil Steril 2009;92:1825–1833.

23. Guerriero S, Alcazar JL, Ajossa S et al. Modified ultrasound scanning is a cost-effective method for the detection of deep infiltrating endometriosis. Fertil Steril 2009;91:e38.

24. Winkel CA. A cost-effective approach to the management of endometriosis. Curr Opin Obstet Gynecol 2000;12:317–320.

25. Lalchandani S, Baxter A, Phillips K. Is helium thermal coagulator therapy for the treatment of women with minimal to moderate endometriosis cost-effective: a prospective randomised controlled trial. Gynecol Surg 2005;2:255–258.

26. Heinrichs WL, Henzl MR. Human issues and medical economics of endometriosis: three- vs. six-month GnRH-agonist therapy. J Reprod Infant Psychol 1998;43:S299–S308.

2 Pathogenesis

4

Pathogenesis: Development of the Female Genital Tract

Jolande A. Land[1] and Johannes L.H. Evers[2]

[1]Department of Obstetrics and Gynaecology, University Medical Center Groningen, Groningen, The Netherlands
[2]Department of Obstetrics and Gynaecology, and GROW, School of Oncology and Developmental Biology, Maastricht University Medical Centre, Maastricht, The Netherlands

Introduction

The most defining moment in life is fertilization, when the genotype or chromosomal sex of an individual is determined. If the fertilizing sperm provides an X chromosome, a 46XX zygote and a female genotype will result. Fertilization by a Y chromosome carrying sperm will give rise to a 46XY zygote and a male genotype. Embryonic development into male or female direction starts after the 7th week, after the bipotential gonads have differentiated into testes or ovaries. In the presence of a functioning testis, the female genital ducts (paramesonephric or müllerian ducts) regress, whereas the male genital ducts (mesonephric or wolffian ducts) differentiate into the male genital tract and the urogenital sinus develops into male external genitals. In the absence of a testis, the paramesonephric ducts differentiate into female internal genitals, and external female genitals are formed from the urogenital sinus. The phenotypic sex of an individual is determined by the aspect of the external genitals and the secondary sexual characteristics, which develop during fetal life and puberty.

In this chapter normal sexual differentiation will be discussed in chronological order. Unless stated otherwise, the timetable is given in weeks of menstrual age, calculated from the first day of the last menstrual period.

Undifferentiated phase

In a 5-week embryo, mesonephroi (midkidneys or interim kidneys) and genital ridges can be discerned. The middle part of the primitive gut (midgut) is continuous with the yolk sac via the vitelline duct, and the lower part of the primitive gut (hindgut) is continuous with the umbilical cord via the allantois. In the most caudal part of the embryo, the connection between the hindgut and the allantois

broadens to form the cloaca (Fig. 4.1). Between the 6th and 8th weeks, the cloaca is divided by the growth of the urorectal septum. The rectum is formed from the most caudal part and the upper part develops into the bladder and the urogenital sinus (Fig. 4.2).

The primordial germ cells are the precursors of spermatozoa and oocytes. In the 5th week primordial germ cells can be identified in the yolk sac. They migrate by amoeboid movements to the dorsal side of the embryo to form the genital ridges near the developing mesonephroi (Fig. 4.3). In the genital ridges the primordial germ cells induce the adjacent tissues (the mesonephroi and the coelomic epithelium) to proliferate and form the sex cords, which are considered as the primitive gonads (Fig. 4.4).

In the 4th week the mesonephric ducts are formed. They grow caudally and in a few days they connect with the urogenital sinus. Between the mesonephric ducts, at the level of the urogenital sinus a bulge is formed – the sinus tubercle. In the 6th week in male and female embryos, a new pair of ducts (paramesonephric ducts) begins to form just lateral to the mesonephric ducts. These

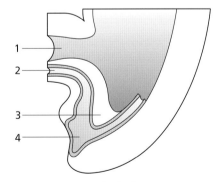

Figure 4.1 The urorectal septum divides the cloaca into two parts. 1, vitelline duct (connection with yolk sac); 2, allantois (connection with umbilical cord); 3, urorectal septum; 4, cloaca. Reproduced from Land [5] with permission from Elsevier.

Endometriosis: Science and Practice, First Edition. Edited by Linda C. Giudice, Johannes L.H. Evers and David L. Healy.
© 2012 Blackwell Publishing Ltd. Published 2012 by Blackwell Publishing Ltd.

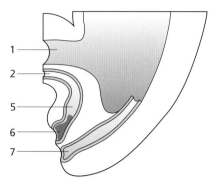

Figure 4.2 The caudal part of the cloaca forms the rectum, the cranial part the bladder and the urogenital sinus. 1, vitelline duct (connection with yolk sac); 2, allantois (connection with umbilical cord); 5, future bladder; 6, urogenital sinus; 7, rectum. Reproduced from Land [5] with permission from Elsevier.

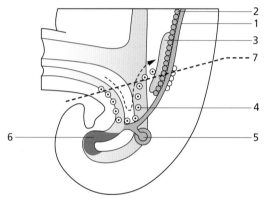

Figure 4.3 Migration of primordial germ cells from the yolk sac to the genital ridges. 1, mesonephric duct; 2, mesonephros (interim kidney); 3, genital ridge; 4, primordial germ cell; 5, ureteric bud and metanephros (permanent kidney); 6, urogenital sinus; 7, level of cross-section in Figure 4.4. Reproduced from Land [5] with permission from Elsevier.

ducts arise by the invagination of coelomic epithelium and grow caudally to the sinus tubercle. The two paramesonephric ducts proceed to fuse in the midline just before they reach the sinus tubercle (Fig. 4.5).

Up to the 7th week, in an undifferentiated embryo the external genitals consist of a cloacal membrane and a midline swelling (genital tubercle). At both sides of the cloacal membrane, urogenital folds and labioscrotal swellings can be distinguished.

In the 9th week, the cloacal membrane divides into a urogenital membrane and an anal membrane. Both membranes break down and the genital tubercle develops into a phallus. Although distinguishing sexual characteristics begin to appear during the 9th week, in male and female embryos the appearance of the external genitals is virtually similar up to the 14th week.

Differentiation of the gonads

For the development of a normal male phenotype, the presence of testis-determining factor (TDF) is mandatory. On the short arm of the Y chromosome, the sex-determining region (SRY) has been localized, containing TDF. In the presence of TDF, in the 8th week, sex cords start to differentiate into testes, in which Sertoli and Leydig cells develop. The Sertoli cells produce anti-müllerian hormone (AMH), which causes the paramesonephric ducts to regress (Fig. 4.6). Leydig cells produce testosterone, which is a prerequisite for development of the mesonephric ducts in the male direction. The primordial germ cells remain dormant in the testes until puberty. In the male, gametogenesis, the development of primordial germ cells into spermatozoa, takes place continuously from puberty until death.

In the female embryo, a Y chromosome with TDF is lacking. As a consequence, the sex cord cells do not differentiate into either Sertoli cells (producing AMH) or Leydig cells (producing testosterone). Therefore, in embryos lacking TDF male development is not stimulated and, as a default, female development ensues. In female embryos, the primitive sex cords degenerate and secondary sex cords are formed from the mesothelium of the genital ridge (Fig. 4.7). These secondary sex cords invest the primordial germ cells (oogonia), which multiply by mitotic division. The oogonia are surrounded by a single layer of granulosa cells, derived from the sex cord cells, and are subsequently called primordial follicles. Primordial follicles will be found in fetal ovaries from the 17th week onwards. As soon as oogonia are surrounded by granulosa cells, mitotic division stops and the primordial follicle will remain quiescent until follicular growth starts at puberty. The maximum number of primordial follicles, about 7 million, will be attained in a 20-week-old fetus. Thereafter atresia sets in: at birth about 1 million primordial follicles are left; at puberty only about 400,000 primordial

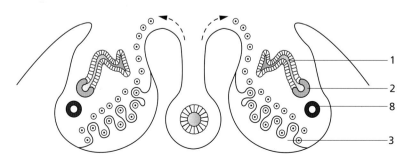

Figure 4.4 Sex cords are formed in the genital ridges. 1, mesonephric duct; 2, mesonephros (interim kidney); 3, genital ridge; 8, paramesonephric duct. Reproduced from Land [5] with permission from Elsevier.

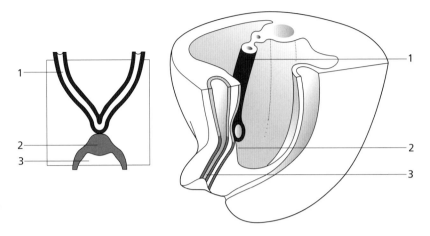

Figure 4.5 The mesonephric ducts end in the urogenital sinus. The paramesonephric ducts grow caudally to the sinus tubercle. 1, paramesonephric ducts; 2, sinus tubercle; 3, urogenital sinus. Reproduced from Land [5] with permission from Elsevier.

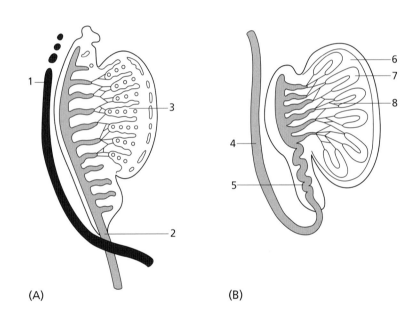

Figure 4.6 In the presence of testis-determining factor. (A) Development of the undifferentiated gonad into testis. (B) Development of the seminiferous tubules. 1, degenerating paramesonephric duct ; 2, mesonephric duct; 3, sex cord; 4, vas deferens; 5, epididymis ; 6, testis ; 7, seminiferous tubules ; 8, rete testis. Reproduced from Land [5] with permission from Elsevier.

(A)　　　　　　　　　　(B)

follicles are still available for reproduction. For the development of normal ovaries with a normal number of primordial follicles, two X chromosomes are mandatory.

Development of the internal genitals

In the male embryo, in the presence of TDF, the Sertoli cells in the testis will produce AMH. Between the 8th and 10th weeks, AMH induces a rapid regression of the paramesonephric ducts. Remnants of the paramesonephric ducts may be found in males after birth: the appendix of the testis and the prostatic utricle, which has occasionally given rise to endometrium-like tissue following the administration of high doses of estrogens in men with

prostatic carcinoma. After the 8th week, in addition to the Sertoli cells, Leydig cells develop in the fetal testis. Leydig cells produce testosterone, stimulated by placental human chorionic gonadotropin (hCG) initially, and by luteinizing hormone (LH) from the fetal pituitary later in pregnancy. Between the 8th and 10th weeks, testosterone induces the differentiation of the mesonephric ducts into the ductus deferens, epididymis and seminal vesicles. The prostate originates from the urogenital sinus.

In the female embryo, in the absence of TDF the gonads do not produce testosterone and consequently the mesonephric ducts degenerate. In the absence of TDF, no AMH is produced and the paramesonephric ducts will develop. In the undifferentiated phase, the paramesonephric ducts reach the sinus tubercle in the urogenital sinus, guided by the mesonephric ducts. Just above the

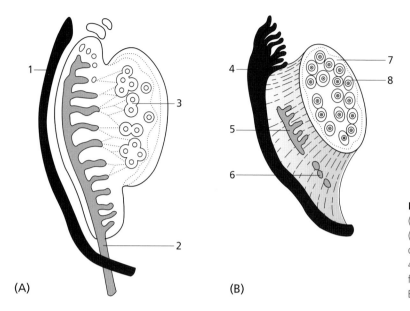

(A) (B)

Figure 4.7 In the absence of testis-determining factor. (A) Development of the undifferentiated gonad into ovary. (B) Development of primordial follicles. 1, paramesonephric duct; 2, degenerating mesonephric duct; 3, secondary sex cord; 4, tube; 5, epoophoron; 6, paroophoron; 7, ovary; 8, primordial follicle. Reproduced from Land [5] with permission from Elsevier.

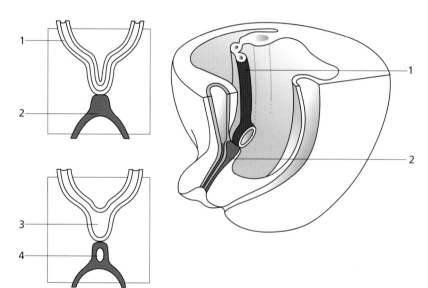

Figure 4.8 Paramesonephric ducts at the sinus tubercle. Formation of the genital canal and the vaginal plate. 1, paramesonephric duct; 2, sinovaginal bulb; 3, genital canal; 4, vaginal plate with lumen formation. Reproduced from Land [5] with permission from Elsevier.

sinus tubercle, the paramesonephric ducts fuse in the midline and the septum between the two ducts is resorbed, forming a tube with a single lumen. This tube, called the genital canal, becomes the uterus and the upper part of the vagina (Fig. 4.8). The unfused cranial parts of the paramesonephric ducts, above the genital canal, become the fallopian tubes.

In the 12th week tissue of the sinus tubercle thickens, forming a pair of swellings called the sinovaginal bulbs. These bulbs proliferate and form the vaginal plate which becomes canalized, creating the vaginal lumen. It still remains to be determined which part

of the vaginal plate is derived from the sinus tubercle, and which from the fused paramesonephric ducts. It is generally assumed that the lower one-third of the vagina has developed from the sinus tubercle (urogenital sinus) and the upper two-thirds from the paramesonephric ducts.

During the development of the vaginal plate, the urethra becomes separated from the vagina, with separated orificia in the vulva (Fig. 4.9). Finally, only in the 5th month of pregnancy, the membrane occluding the vaginal lumen degenerates and remnants persist as the vaginal hymen. Remnants of the mesonephric ducts

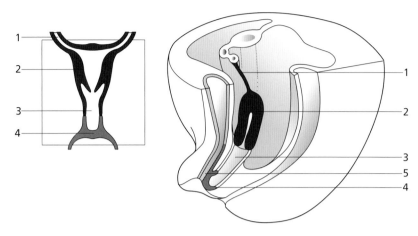

Figure 4.9 Development of the vagina from the vaginal plate, and of the uterus from the genital canal. 1, fallopian tube; 2, uterus; 3, vagina; 4, hymen; 5, urethra. Reproduced from Land [5] with permission from Elsevier.

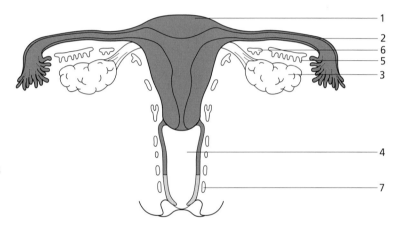

Figure 4.10 Development of the female internal genitals. Remnants of the mesonephric ducts. 1, uterus; 2, fallopian tube; 3, ovary; 4, vagina; 5, epoophoron; 6, paroophoron; 7, Gartner duct cyst. Reproduced from Land [5] with permission from Elsevier.

may persist in women in the form of epoophoron and paroophoron (parovarian cysts) and paravaginal Gartner duct cysts (Fig. 4.10).

Development of the external genitals

Fetal testes produce testosterone. In target tissue testosterone is converted by the enzyme 5α-reductase into dihydrotestosterone (DHT), which is a more potent androgen than testosterone. After the 10th week, the virilizing effect of DHT on the external genitals becomes apparent. In the male fetus, the perineal region separating the urogenital sinus from the anus begins to lengthen and labioscrotal swellings fuse in the midline to form the scrotum. By the 16th week the urogenital folds have fused and have enclosed the penile urethra completely.

In the absence of DHT in the female embryo, the perineum does not lengthen and the labioscrotal swellings and urogenital folds do not fuse. The urogenital folds become the labia minora, while the labia majora are formed from the labioscrotal swellings. The phallus bends caudally to become the clitoris. The urogenital sinus forms the vestibule of the vagina.

Sex-determining factor

Although it has been known since 1923 that males have an X and a Y chromosome and females have two X chromosomes, the role of the Y chromosome in sexual differentiation was only established in 1959. It was shown that the presence of a Y chromosome determines sexual differentiation in the male direction and that in the absence of a Y chromosome, differentiation is in the female direction.

Studies in individuals with sex chromosome anomalies revealed that the complete Y chromosome is not mandatory for the development of a normal male phenotype, but the presence of TDF is [1]. In 1990, the sex-determining region on the Y chromosome (SRY) was identified, and it became clear that the SRY gene activates several other genes located on the X chromosome and on autosomes. The prevailing view that for ovarian development no active genetic steps would be required seems incorrect. There is accumulating evidence that for the development of the undifferentiated gonad into an ovary, co-ordinated activity of a large number of genes is required [2].

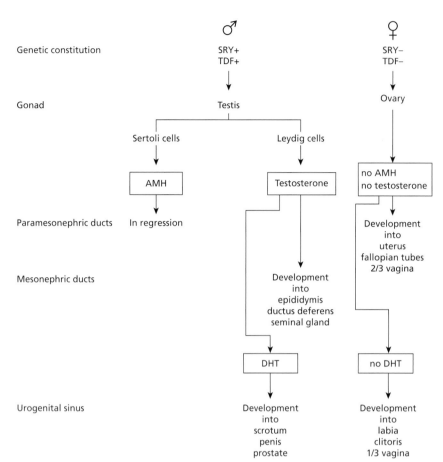

Figure 4.11 Summary of sexual differentiation. SRY, sex-determining region on the Y chromosome; TDF, testis-determining factor; AMH, anti-müllerian hormone; DHT, dihydrotestosterone. Reproduced from Land [5] with permission from Elsevier.

Embryonic origin of endometriosis

No consensus exists on whether endometriosis develops as a result of implantation of endometrial tissue or by metaplasia of coelomic epithelium or both. It has been suggested that peritoneal endometriosis and rectovaginal endometriosis are different disease entities that have separate etiologies. According to the metaplasia theory, endometriosis may be caused by aberrant differentiation or migration of the paramesonephric ducts, which could cause spreading of cells across the posterior pelvic floor. This could explain why peritoneal endometriosis is most commonly found in the pouch of Douglas and close to the posterior wall of the uterus. Environmental, genetic, and epigenetic factors may affect embryonic differentiation of the genital tract organs. These factors may alter the expression of critical genes in progenitor cells of pelvic tissues, which in turn may affect a woman's susceptibility to the development of endometriosis [3]. Deep infiltrating endometriotic nodules are most frequently seen in the rectovaginal septum, and are considered to arise from metaplasia in the remnants of the paramesonephric ducts. Some studies

have shown embryonic duct remnants with changes suggestive of gradual transformation to endometrial glands and estrogen receptor-positive stroma [4]. However there is no definitive proof of the embryonic remnant or müllerianosis theory, and the embryonic origin of endometriosis still remains speculative, as do the (epi) genetic and environmental factors affecting it.

Conclusion

The genetic sex of the embryo directs sexual differentiation in the male or female direction (Fig. 4.11). The SRY gene on the short arm of the Y chromosome has been shown to be the TDF. In an embryo in which TDF is expressed, the gonads will become testes, containing Sertoli and Leydig cells. Sertoli cells produce AMH, which in turn causes the paramesonephric ducts to regress. Leydig cells produce testosterone, which induces the mesonephric ducts to develop into male internal genitals (epididymis, ductus deferens, seminal glands). In target tissue, testosterone is converted into DHT which causes the urogenital sinus to differentiate into the male direction, and to form male external genitals (scrotum, penis) and the prostate.

In the absence of TDF, the undifferentiated gonad will develop into an ovary. The presence of a functional ovary, however, is not mandatory for normal female sexual differentiation. Since no AMH is produced, the paramesonephric ducts develop into female internal genitals (tubes, uterus, upper part of the vagina). The mesonephric ducts regress in the absence of testosterone, and in the absence of DHT the urogenital sinus develops into female external genitals (labia and clitoris) and the lower part of the vagina.

It has been speculated that environmental and (epi)genetic factors may affect embryonic and fetal genital differentiation and thus render a woman prone to endometriosis in adult life.

References

1. McLaren A. What makes a man a man? Nature 1990;346:216–217.
2. Wilhelm D, Palmer S, Koopman P. Sex determination and gonadal development in mammals. Physiol Rev 2007;87:1–283.
3. Bulun SE. Endometriosis: mechanisms of disease. N Engl J Med 2009;360:268–279.
4. Mai KT, Yazdi HM, Perkins DG, Parks W. Development of endometriosis from embryonic duct remnants. Hum Pathol 1998;29:319–322.
5. Land J. Geslachtelijke ontwikkeling. In: Heineman MJ, Evers JLH, Massuger LFAG, Steegers EAP (eds) Obstetrie en Gynaecologie, De Voortplanting van de Mens, 6th edn. Maarssen, The Netherlands: Elsevier, 2007.

5 Theories on the Pathogenesis of Endometriosis

Annemiek W. Nap

Department of Obstetrics and Gynaecology, Rijnstate Hospital, Arnhem, The Netherlands

Introduction

The first histological description of endometriosis was given by von Rokitansky in 1860 [1]. In 1896, Cullen suggested that endometriomas, or adenomyomas as he called them, resembled the mucous membrane of the uterus [2]. The term "endometriosis" was introduced by Sampson in 1921 [3]. Since the publication of his classic papers on the pathogenesis of endometriosis [3–5], extensive basic and clinical research concerning the pathogenesis of the disease has been carried out.

Despite this, the exact mechanisms of the development of endometriosis remain controversial. A growing body of evidence indicates that a combination of hormonal, immunological, anatomical, and genetic factors contribute to the development of endometriosis. In recent years, the notion of two distinct clinical entities, endometriosis as a phenomenon occurring intermittently in all women in their reproductive years, and endometriosis as a disabling disease occurring in a subset of women, regained support [6]. This concept, however, is not new: in 1953 the idea of intermittent occurrence of endometriosis was thus suggested by Scott: "If serial section of all pelvic tissue were feasible might not all 40 year old women with patent tubes and normal menstrual cycles regardless of parity reveal some endometriosis?" [7].

Because of the different locations, possible origins, appearances and hormone responsiveness, it has been suggested that peritoneal endometriosis, ovarian endometriosis, and adenomyotic nodules of the rectovaginal septum or deep invasive endometriosis are three different entities [8], each with a different pathogenesis.

Several hypotheses have been put forward to explain the pathogenesis of the disease. Three main concepts, some of which have historical interest only, can be distinguished as shown in Box 5.1. The concepts of *in situ* development, induction, transplantation, and retrograde menstruation are considered as the most important theories and will be described in this chapter.

The theories

In situ development

The oldest concept concerning the pathogenesis of endometriosis is based on the assumption that endometriosis develops *in situ* from local tissue. Development may occur from remnants of the wolffian or müllerian ducts, or from metaplasia of peritoneal or ovarian tissue. This view on the pathogenesis of endometriosis had wide support in the early part of the last century, and continues to be popular today. In particular, pathologists prefer this theory, and refer to it as the metaplastic theory.

Müllerian remnants

In the embryonic phase, the coelomic epithelium gives rise to the müllerian ducts which form the fallopian tubes, the uterine body, the cervix, and the upper part of the vagina. Aberrant differentiation or migration of the müllerian ducts could cause spreading of cells in the migratory pathway of fetal organogenesis across the posterior pelvic floor. This might explain the observation that endometriosis is often found in the cul-de-sac, uterosacral ligaments, and medial broad ligaments. Lauchlan introduced the term "secondary Müllerian system" by which he meant all mülllerian-type epithelium, including endometriotic lesions outside the cavities of the mülllerian ducts. Moreover, manifestations of mülllerian-directed metaplasia and non-neoplastic proliferations both epithelial and mesenchymal, which can be identified on or closely beneath the ovarian surface, the pelvic peritoneum and the omentum, and in retroperitoneal lymph nodes, are referred to as the secondary Müllerian system [9]. Others prefer to call this phenomenon "müllerianosis," as reviewed by Batt and co-workers [10]. The

Endometriosis: Science and Practice, First Edition. Edited by Linda C. Giudice, Johannes L.H. Evers and David L. Healy.
© 2012 Blackwell Publishing Ltd. Published 2012 by Blackwell Publishing Ltd.

finding of peritoneal pockets with and without endometriosis in adolescents and adults has been associated with congenital tract malformations. This suggests a possible link between embryological abnormalities and onset of the disease, explaining the higher incidence of endometriosis in women with müllerian anomalies [11], and even the presence of endometriosis in a young woman with Mayer–Rokitansky–Kuster–Hauser syndrome [12].

Furthermore, endometriosis diagnosed in adolescents before or shortly after menarche provides circumstancial evidence for an embryonic müllerian rest pathogenesis [13]. Even in human female fetuses, organoid structures outside the uterine cavity have been found resembling the structure of primitive endometrium and expressing both CA125 and estrogen receptor. This observation also sustains the müllerianosis hypothesis of an embryological origin for endometriosis, implicating alterations in the fine tuning of the female genital tract organogenesis [14].

Coelomic metaplasia

The theory of coelomic metaplasia suggests that the germinal epithelium of the ovary and the serosa of the peritoneum can be transformed into endometrium by metaplasia [2,15]. These metaplastic changes occur secondary to inflammatory processes [16] or hormonal influences [17]. The coelomic metaplasia hypothesis may explain the presence of endometriosis in parts of the body outside the pelvis. Endometriosis is rarely described in the chest, affecting diaphragm, pleura, and lungs. A small number of cases of histologically confirmed parenchymal pulmonary endometriosis have been reported [18].

The concept of *in situ* development is attractive since it can explain the occurrence of endometriosis in the absence of menstruation. Rarely, endometriosis has been reported in males. However, these were all older men suffering from prostate carcinoma, who were treated with long-term high doses of estrogens. In these cases, hypertrophy of remnants of the müllerian ducts in the prostate, the utricle, developed [18]. It should be questioned whether this should be defined as endometriosis.

Several points argue against the *in situ* development concept. First, if peritoneal cells can easily undergo metaplastic transformation, the disease should be observed more frequently in men. Second, if coelomic metaplasia resembles common metaplasia, the frequency of endometriosis should increase with advancing age. Third, ectopic endometrial implants are not uniformly distributed within the peritoneum. If metaplasia represents the pathophysiological process for development of the disease, one would have anticipated a more or less uniform distribution on peritoneal surfaces. Finally, endometriosis mainly affects the pelvic organs. Given that the coelomic membrane contributes to both the peritoneal cavity and the thoracic cavity, it should be expected that endometriosis would be present more often in the chest as well.

Induction

The theory of induction may be seen as an extension of the coelomic metaplasia theory, proposing that one or several endogenous, biochemical or immunological factors could induce endometrial differentiation in undifferentiated cells. The proponents of this theory assume that substances released by uterine endometrium and transported by blood and lymph streams induce the formation of endometriosis in different parts of the body.

In a rabbit model, Levander and Normann implanted fresh and denatured endometrium in the abdominal cavity of the rabbit and evaluated the tissue histologically for 7 days [19]. They observed degeneration of the endometrial implants during the first 4 days, with cyst formation and epithelial differentiation characteristic of endometrium in the surrounding connective tissue during the next 3 days. If the tissue was degraded before implantation, better results were obtained. From these observations, they concluded that dying endometrial tissue liberates specific substances activating undifferentiated mesenchyme to develop into endometrial tissue. Their findings were confirmed several years later by Merrill [20] who implanted viable and ischemic endometrial tissue within millipore filters intraperitoneally in the rabbit. Due to the small pore size, only chemical substances and no cells could pass. The presence of endometrium-like epithelium and glands was observed in the connective tissue adjacent to the implants, suggesting that cell-free endometrial products were capable of inducing endometrial metaplasia. However, these changes do not meet the criteria for endometriosis, since no endometrial stroma was found in the surrounding tissue.

Transplantation

The theory of transplantation implies that endometrium is replaced from the uterus to another location inside the body. Different routes of dissemination are involved in the concept of transplantation in the pathogenesis of endometriosis. Iatrogenic, lymphogenic, and hematogenic spread account for uncommon, extraperitoneal locations of endometriosis [21–24].

Retrograde menstruation

The most popular theory is Sampson's retrograde menstruation theory. Initially, Sampson assumed that endometriotic lesions are seedlings from diseased ovaries [3]. Later on, in 1927, he proposed that endometriosis is the result of the reflux of endometrial fragments through the fallopian tubes during menstruation, with subsequent implantation and growth on and into the peritoneum and the ovary [3–5].

The reflux implantation theory is based on the assumption that retrograde menstruation takes place and that viable endometrial tissue reaches the abdominal cavity and implants. These three conditions are the basic principles of the viability of Sampson's theory. They implicate that first, endometrial cells must enter the peritoneal cavity through the fallopian tubes. Second, cells within the menstrual effluent must be viable and be able to be transplanted onto the pelvic structures. Third, the anatomical distribution of endometriosis in the pelvic cavity must be correlated with the principles of transplantation for exfoliated cells. For a long time this theory was neglected, because menstrual effluent was considered to contain only non-viable endometrial tissue. Moreover, retrograde menstruation was thought to be a rare phenomenon. Sampson based his theory on clinical and anatomical observations. He realized that for his concept to be true, the viability of endometrial tissue retrogradely shed into the peritoneal cavity was crucial, and he stated: "If bits of Mullerian mucosa carried by menstrual blood escaping into the peritoneal cavity are always dead, the implantation theory, as presented by me, also is dead and should be buried and forgotten" [5]. Over the years experimental evidence has been provided supporting his hypothesis, and it is now the most widely accepted theory.

Arguments in favor of the retrograde menstruation theory

Several points argue in favor of the retrograde menstruation theory. Reflux of menstrual tissue is a common event in women with patent fallopian tubes. Halme and co-workers obtained peritoneal fluid by laparoscopy in the perimenstrual period [25]. Blood was found in 90% of the patients with patent tubes. If the fallopian tubes were occluded, only 15% had evidence of blood in the pelvis. Endometrial epithelial cells have been found in the peritoneal fluid of women during the early proliferative phase [26], suggesting that menstrual effluent contains endometrial cells. Shed menstrual tissue contains viable endometrium, single cells, and glandular structures [27].

The distribution of endometriotic lesions in the abdominal cavity corresponds to that of tubal reflux [28]. The peritoneal fluid flow in the abdomen is counter-clockwise, suggesting that refluxed endometrial cells in the peritoneal fluid are retained by the falciform ligament of the liver. Diaphragmatic endometriotic lesions have been found more frequently on the right side of the diaphragm than on the left [29]. Moreover, ovarian endometriomas are more frequently present in the left ovary than in the right, compatible with the anatomical differences in the left and right hemipelvis. These observations also support the tubal regurgitation theory [30].

Early endometriotic lesion formation

Assuming that shed menstrual endometrium is the basis for the development of endometriosis, stepwise endometriotic lesion formation can be investigated, in order to gain more information about the prerequisites for the development of endometriosis. An adequate model to study the phenomena involved in this process is the chicken chorio-allantoic membrane (CAM) [31]. This is an *ex vivo* model, using the covering membrane of the chicken embryo onto which tissue can be transplanted, and the behavior of the tissue can be observed. Moreover, interventions can be carried out and the consequences of these interventions can be studied.

In order to visualize the different steps in the process of endometriotic lesion formation, human menstrual endometrial fragments were collected by aspiration. These fragments consisted of endometrial glands and stroma, and they were transplanted onto the CAM (Plate 5.1). After 24, 48 and 72 h, cross-sections of the CAMs were cut and immunohistochemically stained. After 24 h, direct contact between the CAM mesenchyme and the menstrual tissue fragment was present. The endometrial tissue seemed to fall apart during migration towards the CAM mesenchyme. After 48 h, the menstrual endometrium was reorganizing inside the CAM mesenchyme, and after 72 h a complete endometrium fragment with glands and stroma was present in the CAM mesenchyme. Inside the endometrium fragment, blood vessels attracted from the CAM were present. This experiment showed that in order to form an endometriotic lesion, viable endometrium is necessary, as well as the ability to adhere to a matrix, the ability to degrade this matrix, and to attract new blood vessels in order to survive [32].

Endometrial cells express adhesive molecules. Biopsied proliferative and secretory endometrial fragments, as well as antegradely shed menstrual endometrial fragments, can adhere at locations where the mesothelial lining of the peritoneum is damaged, exposing the basement membrane or the extracellular matrix [33,34]. This suggests that an intact mesothelial lining serves as a barrier and prevents adhesion of menstrual endometrial fragments to the peritoneal lining, thus preventing the implantation of endometrial tissue [35]. However, the mesothelium is fragile and can easily be damaged by surgery, inflammatory cells or endometrium, thereby facilitating adhesion of endometrium. Analogous to tumor cells and tumor ascites, isolated cells from menstrual effluent as well as conditioned medium prepared from menstrual effluent are able to induce morphological alterations in mesothelial cells [36,37]. Therefore, menstrual endometrium is harmful to the mesothelium and may create its own adhesion sites at the mesothelial lining, thereby facilitating the development of endometriosis [37]. As a consequence of the contact with menstrual endometrium, the mesothelial lining undergoes morphological alterations: the menstrual endometrium initiates a reversible, energy-dependent transition process from an epithelial to a mesenchymal phenotype of the mesothelium [38].

Adhesive properties of endometrial cells determine the process of attachment of retrogradely shed endometrium to the peritoneal lining. Several cell adhesion molecules are expressed by endometrial cells, including integrins, cadherins, laminin-binding proteins, the immunoglobulin superfamily and CD44 [39]. They modulate cell–matrix and cell–cell attachments. In endometrium and endometriosis, integrins and cadherins have been studied extensively. The integrins belong to a large family of transmembrane glycoproteins that provide an anchorage for cells to the extracellular matrix and are involved in direct invasion and motility of cells [40]. The expression of integrins in the endometrium changes during the menstrual cycle [41–43]. Aberrant patterns of integrin expression have been associated with reproductive problems, including endometriosis [44,45].

Cadherins are transmembrane glycoproteins which mediate cell–cell adhesion. They can act as invasion suppressor molecules by inhibiting the ability of cells to escape from their primary site to initiate invasion. Immunohistochemical studies have demonstrated that epithelial cadherin (E-cadherin) is expressed in epithelial glandular cells derived from menstrual effluent, endometrium throughout the menstrual cycle, peritoneal fluid, peritoneum and endometriosis, indicating a role in the maintenance of the epithelial architecture in endometrium [42,46]. *In vitro*, E-cadherin-positive cells are retained in tumor tissue by cell–cell interaction, but when E-cadherin is absent or inactivated, these cells are no longer constrained and invasion can occur [47]. E-cadherin is therefore considered one of the central players in the establishment of metastasis in human carcinomas [45]. Endometriosis cells and carcinoma cells may share molecular mechanisms of invasion and metastasis that are related to the absence of E-cadherin [45,48].

Fragments of endometrium express matrix metalloproteinases (MMPs), molecules that are able to degrade the extracellular matrix (ECM). Endometriotic lesion formation is an invasive event, which requires ECM breakdown. The ECM consists of collagens, proteoglycans, and glycoproteins including fibronectin and laminin. In addition to its role in determining cell shape, the ECM is important in metabolic processes, influencing cellular proliferation, differentiation and apoptosis, and it serves as a repository for biologically active growth factors. Remodeling and breakdown of the ECM are mainly regulated by MMPs. MMPs are a family of structurally related, zinc-containing endoproteases that share structural domains but differ in substrate specificity, cellular sources, and inducibility. All MMPs share the following functional features: they are capable of degrading ECM components, they are secreted in a latent proform and require activation for proteolytic activity, they contain Zn^{2+} at their active site and need calcium for stability, they function at a neutral pH, and they are inhibited by specific tissue inhibitors of metalloproteinases (TIMPs) [49]. According to their substrate specificity and structure, members of the MMP family can be classified into subclasses: the collagenases, gelatinases, stromelysins, membrane-type MMPs, and other MMPs.

The activity of MMPs is controlled by the induction of gene expression and by the activation of latent proenzymes. Induction at the level of gene expression is mediated by growth factors, hormones, and inflammatory cytokines including interleukin-1 (IL-1), IL-6, tumor necrosis factor-α (TNF-α), epidermal growth factor (EGF), platelet-derived growth factor (PDGF) and basic fibroblast growth factor (bFGF) [50,51]. The activation of the latent proenzymes can be achieved by (1) stepwise activation in which plasmin is assumed to be the most potent physiological activator *in vivo*, (2) activation at the cell surface by membrane type (MT)-MMPs, and (3) intracellular activation [52,53]. In turn, the activity of MMPs in tissues is controlled by the antagonizing actions of their natural inhibitors, the TIMPs. TIMPs are present in the majority of tissues and body fluids, and are expressed by a variety of cells. TIMP-1, -2, -3, and -4 are structurally related and bind non-covalently to active MMPs. They have the ability to interact with the zinc-binding site within the catalytic domain of active MMPs.

In many reproductive processes, including menstruation, ovulation, and embryo implantation, MMPs are expressed in a highly regulated manner [54,55]. In the endometrium, MMP expression is most pronounced during menstruation. A limited number of MMPs is expressed at low levels during the proliferative phase, whereas expression generally declines during the early secretory phase and reappears in the late secretory phase. Endometrial MMP expression is regulated by hormones, cytokines, and growth factors. In particular, progesterone is a potent repressor both *in vitro* [56,57] and *in vivo* [58]. The mechanism through which progesterone modulates MMP and TIMP activity is not yet clear. It has been proposed that progesterone regulates MMP expression indirectly through controlling the plasminogen activator pathway. Progesterone can increase the levels of plasminogen activator inhibitor (PAI)-1 and thus reduce plasmin-mediated activation of latent MMPs [59]. Locally produced retinoic acid and transforming growth factor-β (TGF-β) were shown to act as mediators of the progesterone suppression of MMPs, while enhancing expression of TIMPs [60]. On the other hand, arguments against progesterone as the primary regulator of endometrial collagenase activity are that *in vivo* circulating progesterone levels decrease too early to explain the perimenstrual increase in MMP expression, and tissue degradation at menstruation occurs at focal points rather than throughout the entire endometrium [61].

The involvement of MMPs in the development of endometriosis was suspected after finding collagen breakdown products in the peritoneal fluid of patients with mild endometriosis [58]. Later, intervention studies in mice and in the CAM with experimentally induced endometriosis demonstrated that lesion formation can be prevented by inhibiting the production and activation of MMPs [62,63].

Ectopically implanted endometrium needs to trigger an angiogenic response, activating angiogenesis within and around the tissue, in order to survive in its new environment. Angiogenesis is the formation of new blood vessels from pre-existing capillaries. It involves the proteolytic degradation of the ECM, proliferation and migration of endothelial cells, and ultimately formation of a patent tubular network supplying the angiogenic stimulus [64]. Angiogenesis is essential in growth, wound healing, and in the female reproductive system, including processes in the menstrual cycle and pregnancy [65]. It occurs when the balance of local factors favoring vascular growth exceeds those factors inhibiting angiogenesis. Disruption of the balance between inhibitors and activators in favor of excessive angiogenesis may result in conditions such as cancer, atherosclerosis, chronic inflammation, and endometriosis [66]. Several factors of a peptide and non-peptide nature induce angiogenesis *in vivo*. Vascular endothelial growth factor (VEGF) is suggested to be the most important factor, based on its ability to induce endothelial cell proliferation and migration, induce vasodilation, and increase endothelial cell permeability [65].

Endometrial cells have angiogenic potential. In the endometrium, angiogenesis is regulated by many angiogenic factors, of which VEGF-A appears to be the most important. In the proliferative phase of the menstrual cycle, estradiol triggers VEGF-A expression in endometrial epithelial cells and stromal fibroblasts, which is increased in the secretory phase [67]. Prior to menstruation, the endometrium becomes hypoxic as a result of vasoconstriction, which enhances the production of VEGF-A in the endometrial tissue even more [68]. In eutopic endometrium of endometriosis patients, endothelial cell proliferation and VEGF-A contents are significantly higher than in the endometrium of disease-free women [69,70].

Clinical studies on the vascularization of endometriotic lesions are rare, despite the fact that at laparoscopy, active superficial endometriotic lesions are easily recognized by the abundant vasculature. When comparing the vascular density and luminal diameter in red, black, and white lesions as well as in endometriomas and lesions in the rectovaginal septum, red lesions are better vascularized. This is the result of a larger vessel diameter rather than the number of vessels, which is significantly higher in black lesions [69]. No differences in the numbers of vessels between the different types of lesions have been reported, but red lesions have more vessels with a small diameter (<10 μm), whereas black lesions have significantly more vessels with a larger diameter (>20 μm) [71]. The fact that endothelial cell proliferation and smooth muscle cell-negative blood vessels are observed in endometriotic lesions suggests that an active angiogenic process is ongoing here.

In an experimental environment, studies in the CAM model indicate that human endometrium is highly angiogenic, and therefore perfectly capable of attracting blood vessels from the surrounding tissue [72]. In early endometriotic lesion formation, VEGF-A and angiogenesis are of significant value. Antagonizing the actions of VEGF-A by administering the soluble VEGF receptor sflt-1 reduces the number of lesions formed in nude mice after intraperitoneal injection of minced endometrial tissue [73]. Therefore, antagonizing angiogenesis by applying antiangiogenic therapy may be effective in preventing the development of endometriosis. More support for this hypothesis has been provided in studies in the CAM model. Administration of the antiangiogenic factors anti-human VEGF, anginex, endostatin and TNP-470 to the CAM significantly decreases the vascular density of the CAM. If endometriosis was induced experimentally in this model by transplantation of human endometrium fragments onto the CAM, administration of these antiangiogenic agents prevented endometriosis-like lesion formation [74]. Moreover, after endometriosis had been provoked by transplanting human endometrium fragments intraperitoneally in nude mice, application of these antiangiogenic agents resulted in a significant decrease in the number of endometriotic lesions in the mice compared to control mice not treated with antiangiogenic agents. The reduction in the number of lesions was explained by a decline in the number of newly developed vessels, as only mature vessels remained [75].

Arguments against the retrograde menstruation theory

The most important argument against Sampson's theory is that it is unable to explain the presence of endometriosis in the absence of menstruation. As stated above, endometriosis has been reported in women without menses and even in males. The retrograde menstruation theory inadequately elucidates these presentations of endometriosis.

One can also question the retrograde menstruation theory because it assumes that endometriosis is a form of autotransplant. Redwine asked whether endometriosis fulfills the criteria for an autotransplant [76]. If not, the retrograde menstruation theory might be insufficient to explain the pathogenesis of the disease. An autotransplant is defined as tissue transplanted from one site to another site in the same organism, due to either a pathological process or surgical intervention. An autotransplant essentially remains unchanged in its new location, unaffected by factors that alter its immunohistochemistry or change the autotransplant morphologically, histologically or biochemically. Examples of autotransplants include strips of ovarian cortex that are transplanted to the forearm in women prior to undergoing pelvic radiotherapy, and aortic valve substitutes constructed out of pulmonary valves.

In experimental settings, autotransplants as well as human-to-mouse xenografts have been used to study endometriosis and its medical and surgical treatment. This creation of autotransplants as experimental models of endometriosis is the strongest manifestation of the belief that endometriosis is identical to eutopic endometrium. Redwine has extensively reviewed the literature concerning eutopic endometrium and endometriosis in which hormone receptor levels as well as histological, morphological, and biological factors are compared. He concludes that the differences between eutopic endometrium and endometriosis are numerous, and the similarities are only limited. The balance of evidence therefore may suggest that endometriosis is not simply displaced normal endometrium, as would be expected in an autotransplant disease. For this incongruence, there are two possible explanations. Either normal endometrium is severely damaged on the way from the uterus to its ectopic location, or endometriosis does not originate from native endometrium but has a different provenance. The first explanation is difficult to imagine. No putative mechanism seems to exist to explain this kind of damage occurring to the endometrium when it is shed retrogradely. Endometriosis should therefore not be considered to be merely displaced normal endometrium. As this is one of the mainstays of Sampson's theory, according to those doubting the retrograde menstruation theory this concept should be discarded [76].

The phenomenon and the disease

Examination by laparoscopy of the healthy peritoneum often reveals endometrial implants [77]. Microscopic or minimal peritoneal lesions, called subtle lesions, are present in up to 20% of cases of unexplained subfertility, and also in many healthy women undergoing laparoscopy for tubal ligation. These subtle endometriotic lesions as observed during laparoscopy are so frequent that they may not be seen as a disease, but rather as a physiological phenomenon. Most of these implants tend to resolve spontaneously, being invisible or visible as white scars or old black lesions.

However, some implants in certain women develop into the disease endometriosis, characterized by adhesions perturbing local physiology, endometriotic ovarian cysts, or profound endometriotic lesions presenting as rectovaginal nodules. Usually, they manifest with abdominal pain, dysmenorrhea, dyspareunia and/or subfertility. The most intriguing and essential question for clinicians and investigators remains: why do some women develop symptomatic endometriosis whereas others do not? Women with symptomatic endometriosis differ from women without the disease. Differences can be acknowledged at the level of the endometrium, the uterus and the peritoneal environment.

Alterations in endometrium

The eutopic endometrium of women with endometriosis shares some alterations with the ectopic lesions that are not found in the endometrium of women without the disease. This implies that the primary defect is rooted in the eutopic endometrium of endometriosis patients [78]. A relatively new concept holds that the basal endometrial layer, which contains stem cell characteristics, exhibits an enhanced potential for dislocation and proliferation in women with endometriosis [79]. As a result of microtraumata, a mechanism of tissue injury and repair (TIAR) is activated, resulting in local production of estrogen. Eventually, dislocation of fragments of basal endometrium into the peritoneal cavity and infiltration into the depth of the myometrial wall occur, followed by infiltrative growth and chronic inflammation, resulting in endometriosis or adenomyosis [80].

Endogenous hormone production in the endometrium

In benign as well as malignant diseases of the female reproductive tract, local production of estrogens is an important element in the pathogenesis. This is also the case in endometriosis. The conversion of estrogens from androgens is catalyzed by aromatase P450. Aromatase is normally expressed in a number of human tissues, including the ovary and the adipose tissue, but usually not in normal endometrium [81,82]. However, this enzyme has been found in endometriotic tissue and in the endometrium of women with endometriosis [82,83]. Moreover, endometriosis tissue is often deficient in 17β-hydroxysteroid dehydrogenase (17β-HSD) type 2, which normally converts the strong estrogenic 17β-estradiol into the weak estrogenic estrone. Consequently, this protective mechanism that lowers estradiol levels is lost in endometriosis tissue

[84]. The higher estradiol level of menstrual effluent in women with endometriosis as compared to controls confirms this hypothesis [85]. As a result of increased estrogen production in eutopic and ectopic endometrium, a positive feedback loop is initiated, which results in the continuous local production of estrogen [83,86]. Estrogen stimulates the production of cyclooxygenase type 2 (COX-2) enzyme. This results in elevated levels of prostaglandin E_2 (PGE_2), which is a potent stimulator of aromatase activity in endometriosis.

The clinical relevance of these findings has been exemplified by the successful treatment of an aggressive case of postmenopausal endometriosis using an aromatase inhibitor [87], and the beneficial effects of non-steroidal anti-inflammatory drugs (NSAIDs) for the treatment of pain symptoms [88].

Escape of the endometrium from immune surveillance

Menstrual effluent evokes an inflammatory response on arriving in the abdominal cavity [89]. It attracts large numbers of polymorphonuclear neutrophils (PMNs), and subsequently phagocytic and chemotactic leukocytes from the circulation [89,90]. Prior to the onset of menstruation, a marked influx of bone marrow-derived cells is observed. Of these cells, approximately 70% are CD56+ natural killer cells (NK cells), 20% CD14+ macrophages, and 10% CD3+ T-cells [91]. The physiological role of the inflammatory response is to clear the ectopic cells and tissue from the abdomen. In women with endometriosis, this system of cleansing is insufficient or overwhelmed.

Longer menstrual periods and heavier menstrual blood flow will result in larger amounts of endometrial tissue in the abdominal cavity, which enhances the risk of developing symptomatic endometriosis. Larger tissue fragments may have an increased capability to develop into endometriotic lesions. They have a higher chance of survival, since cells residing inside are protected from the proteolytic enzymes and phagocytic activity. These cells continue to produce angiogenic factors as a result of the continued hypoxic conditions.

Endometrial cells of women with endometriosis are more resistant to cytolysis by autologous peritoneal macrophages than endometrial cells of controls [92]. Their antigenicity seems to be altered in a way that could be protective against cytotoxicity of NK cells, due to overexpression of human leukocyte antigen (HLA) class I [93,94].

The soluble form of intercellular adhesion molecule-1 (sICAM-1) is released from endometrial stromal cells in culture, predominantly during the proliferative phase. sICAM-1 can modulate the cytotoxic activity of CD8+ and NK cells. It competes with ICAM-1 to bind leukocyte function antigen-1 (LFA-1), which is expressed by activated leukocytes. Binding of sICAM-1 to LFA-1 makes leukocytes less available for binding with cell surface ICAM-1 on target cells, preventing the activation of these leukocytes. The eutopic endometrial cells from women with endometriosis express higher levels of sICAM than those of women without endometriosis [95]. The expression of sICAM in ectopic endometrial cells is higher when compared to their eutopic endometrium [96].

Heat shock proteins (hsp) protect protein substrates against conformational damage to promote the function of proteins, prevent aggregation and prevent formation of toxic inclusion bodies. They protect cells against cytotoxic outcomes. A variety of physical and chemical stimuli including heat shock, steroids, and oxidative damage induce the synthesis of hsp. They serve as ligands for T-lymphocytes [97]. Throughout the menstrual cycle, the expression of different hsp may vary. Hsp 90 remains stable, whereas hsp27, hsp60, and hsp70 increase during the secretory phase [98]. Eutopic endometrium from women with endometriosis expresses higher levels of hsp27 and hsp70 as compared to controls. Their expression, however, is lower in ectopic lesions than in eutopic endometrium in these women. This suggests that hsp protect endometrial cells from apoptosis by reducing the cytotoxic effects of cytokines and leukocytes accumulated in the secretory phase [99].

Protection from apoptosis

Apoptosis, or programmed cell death, is one of the crucial factors regulating cell turnover in human endometrium. It eliminates senescent cells from the functional layer of the endometrium at the end of the secretory phase and during menses. Several genes regulate apoptosis. P53, bax and c-myc stimulate it, while B-cell lymphoma/leukemia-2 (Bcl-2), Bcl-xL, and sentrin inhibit it [100]. The expression of Bcl-2 varies during the endometrial cycle. Maximum expression occurs during the proliferative phase, and its expression correlates with the production of estrogens and the expression of hormonal receptors by glandular cells. The action of Bcl-2 depends on the expression and concentration of bax. The variation of apoptosis throughout the menstrual cycle suggests that ovarian steroids may control endometrial apoptosis by up- and downregulation of Bcl-2 and bax expression [101].

Eutopic endometrium from women with endometriosis shows significantly reduced apoptosis as compared to women without endometriosis, especially during the late secretory, menstrual, and early proliferative phases of the cycle.

After arrival in the peritoneal cavity, survival of endometrial tissue is a prerequisite for the development of endometriotic lesions. Normally, cells that do not adhere to the peritoneal mesothelium enter apoptosis as they receive different signals from their adhesion receptors. In women with endometriosis, the percentage of apoptosis in shed endometrial cells is reduced, implying that the number of surviving cells entering the peritoneal cavity is greater [102,103]. The resistance to apoptosis of endometrium in women with endometriosis could be due to (1) an environment which contains a constant source of TNF-α, a primary local signal initiating and modulating apoptosis during menses [98], (2) an inappropriate transduction of the signal for apoptosis or (3) a lack of endometrium able to express inhibitive proteins in endometriosis patients [104].

Potential of the endometrium to implant

Laminin and fibronectin are key role players in normal and tumor cell adhesion. They promote interactions between epithelial cells and the ECM and provide substrates for adhesion and migration [105]. During the menstrual cycle, endometrium develops into a well-differentiated tissue, susceptible to implantation of an embryo. In normal eutopic endometrium, integrins are hormonally regulated [106]. Endometriotic tissue, however, is able to express different integrins independently of the hormonal situation. Cyclical modifications in the expression of certain integrins are absent in endometriosis. The αvβ3molecule is normally present in the endometrium at the time of implantation, but might be absent in endometriotic lesions. Integrin expression in ectopic endometrial tissue seems highly variable and aberrant as compared with eutopic endometrium, with the exception of integrin β3, which is always absent in the endometrium from women with endometriosis [44]. This suggests that endometrium of patients with endometriosis lacks appropriate differentiation patterns. Fibronectin receptors are present in endometriotic glands but not in endometrial glands, indicating that fibronectin receptors could contribute to the attachment of endometriotic cells during menstruation [107].

Potential of the endometrium to invade

After initial attachment to the peritoneal mesothelial lining, invasion into the mesothelium has to take place in order to develop an endometriotic lesion. For invasion, ECM degradation is a prerequisite, and MMPs regulate this process. MMP expression and regulation may be different in women with and without endometriosis, as abnormal expression of specific MMPs and TIMPs and an increased MMP/TIMP ratio have been reported in women with endometriosis as compared to women without the disease [108–115]. MMP-3 and MMP-7 mRNA expression is elevated in the eutopic endometrium of women with endometriosis during the secretory phase of the cycle, corresponding with a failure to respond to the repressing action of progesterone *in vitro*. The enhanced expression of MMPs especially during the progesterone-dominated secretory phase in women with endometriosis, while their activity is suppressed in disease-free women, suggests that progesterone insensitivity may contribute to the development of endometriosis [116].

Besides the apparent pivotal role of MMP expression in the initial development of endometriotic lesions, the high expression of various MMPs in the endometriotic lesions suggests a function of MMPs in lesion survival as well. It is now becoming evident that MMPs cleave a variety of substrates that are not solely ECM components. MMPs may be implicated in the regulation of growth factors, cytokines, angiogenesis, tissue organization and cell survival as well as in invasion [117], thereby influencing endometriotic lesion development as well as its maintenance.

Excessive angiogenesis

At laparoscopy, endometriotic lesions usually are surrounded by peritoneal blood vessels. Endometriotic deposits derive their blood supply from the surrounding microvasculature. Larger endometriotic lesions have been observed in areas with a rich blood supply, and better vascularized endometriotic lesions are more active. Different angiogenic factors are involved in endometriosis, including bFGF, TGF-α and -β, hepatocyte growth factor (HGF), angiopoietin and VEGF, which is the most important factor in endometriosis [118,119].

Comparing endometrium from women with endometriosis to that from disease-free women, in women with endometriosis an increased endothelial cell proliferation has been observed. Moreover, there is a higher expression of angiopoietin-1 and -2 mRNA, an increased microvessel density and higher levels of VEGF-A [120,121]. These factors indicate a dysregulation of the angiogenic activity in the eutopic endometrium of women with endometriosis.

Genital tract abnormalities

The relative incapacity to clean the peritoneum of refluxed endometrium can be worsened by certain anatomical predispositions that increase menstrual reflux that are often found in women with endometriosis. These include uterine malformations preventing or disturbing normal antegrade menstrual flux [122], waves of retrograde contractions of the tubular and myometrial musculature [123], and hypertonia of the uterotubular junction [124]. Menstruations in women with endometriosis are often longer and heavier [125,126], and cycles have a tendency to be shorter.

Peritoneal fluid

Shed endometrial cells differ from eutopic endometrial cells. It is still not clear whether this phenomenon is a cause or a consequence of endometriosis. This finding may also be explained by the different environment of these cells. The eutopic endometrium is influenced by bloodstream factors, whereas shed endometrial cells after arrival in the peritoneal cavity are regulated by peritoneal fluid. Evidence is available to support the notion that factors present in the peritoneal fluid are able to affect processes in the peritoneal cavity. The peritoneal fluid is a specific microenvironment, mainly originating as an ovarian exudation product. It contains many different cells, including macrophages, red blood cells and endometrial cells which are able to secrete large amounts of growth factors, cytokines, angiogenic factors, glycodelins and hsp.

Macrophages constitute 85% of the cells in peritoneal fluid. Their role varies during the menstrual cycle. Their number and level of activity reach a maximum at the end of the menstrual phase for removal of endometrial debris, spermatozoa, and follicular cells from the peritoneal cavity. In endometriosis patients, peritoneal macrophages are more numerous and more active [127,128]. They are not destroyed after completing their work as in the physiological situation, but are protected from apoptosis by overexpression of the antiapoptotic protein Bcl-2, thus remaining present in the peritoneal fluid [129]. Moreover, the endometrium of patients with endometriosis liberates only small amounts of cytokines regulating the activation of macrophages (IL-10 and IL-13), in contrast to the endometrium of disease-free women [130]. The cytotoxic power of the peritoneal macrophages in the endometrium of women with endometriosis is reduced [131]. Thus, these macrophages are overworked and hyperactive. Being deficient in their phagocytic role,

they could aggravate and even initiate endometriosis in different ways. They liberate excessive amounts of cytokines, growth factors, and angiogenic molecules. The presence of these factors could induce metaplasia of coelomic epithelium already altered by an inflammatory environment [104].

Genetic predisposition

Genetic predisposition may play a role in endometriosis, as first-degree relatives of women with endometriosis have a higher risk of developing endometriosis compared to the general population [132]. Studies in monozygotic twins found a high concordance for endometriosis [133,134]. However, the reported familial aggregation may be debatable when examined closely. Although comprehensive lists of candidate genes and their polymorphisms involved in endometriosis have been published [135], little progress has been observed in the identification of genetic variants that predispose to endometriosis [136].

Conclusion

The exact mechanisms in the pathogenesis of endometriosis remain obscure. None of the theories described in this chapter is sufficient to satisfactorily explain the pathogenesis of this disease. *In situ* development and induction explain only a part of the endometriosis manifestations. Retrograde shedding of menstrual effluent seems to be a universal phenomenon, but is not enough to develop endometriosis. The presence of ectopic endometrium has to be accompanied by additional factors in order for the disease to develop. Biochemical and molecular aberrations in the eutopic endometrium, abnormal sex steroid responsiveness, an inadequate immune response, uterine malformations, a proinflammatory peritoneal fluid environment, and genetic predisposition are all factors that may ultimately be involved in the development of symptomatic endometriosis.

References

1. Von Rokitansky C. Ueber Uterusdrusen-Neubildung in Uterus- und Ovarial-Sarcomen. Ztschr KK Gesellsch Der Aerzte zu Wien 1860;37:577–581.

2. Cullen TS. Adeno-myoma uteri diffusum benignum. Johns Hopkins Hosp Bull 1896;6:133–137.

3. Sampson JA. Perforating hemorrhagic (chocolate) cysts of the ovary: their importance and especially their relation to pelvic adenomas of endometrial type (adenomyoma of the uterus, rectovaginal septum, sigmoid, etc). Arch Surg 1921;3:245–323.

4. Sampson JA. Peritoneal endometriosis due to menstrual dissemination of endometrial tissue into the peritoneal cavity. Am J Obstet Gynecol 1927;14:422–469.

5. Sampson JA. The development of the implantation theory for the origin of peritoneal endometriosis. Am J Obstet Gynecol 1940;40:549–557.

6. Koninckx PR. Is mild endometriosis a condition occurring intermittently in all women? Hum Reprod 1994;9:2202–2205.

7. Scott RB, Te Linde RW, Wharton LR Jr. Further studies on experimental endometriosis. Am J Obstet Gynecol 1953;66:1082–1099.

8. Nisolle M, Donnez J. Peritoneal endometriosis, ovarian endometriosis, and adenomyotic nodules of the rectovaginal septum are three different entities. Fertil Steril 1997;68:585–596.

9. Lauchlan SC. The secondary Mullerian system. Obstet Gynecol Surv 1972;27:133–146.

10. Batt RE, Smith RA, Buck Louis GM et al. Mullerianosis. Histol Histopathol 2007;22:1161–1166.

11. Nawroth F, Rahimi G, Nawroth C et al. Is there an association between septate uterus and endometriosis? Hum Reprod 2006;2:542–544.

12. Mok-Lin EY, Wolfberg A, Hollinquist H et al. Endometriosis in a patient with Mayer-Rokitansky-Kuster-Hauser syndrome and complete uterine agenesis: evidence to support the theory of coelomic metaplasia. J Pediatr Adolesc Gynecol 2010;23(1):e35–37.

13. Batt RE, Mitwally MFM. Endometriosis from thelarche to midteens: pathogenesis and prognosis, prevention and pedagogy. J Pediatr Adolesc Gynecol 2003;16:337–347.

14. Signorile PG, Baldi F, Bussani R et al. Ectopic endometrium in human foetuses is a common event and sustains the theory of mullerianosis in the pathogenesis of endometriosis, a disease that predisposes to cancer. J Exp Clin Cancer Res 2009;28:49.

15. Meyer R. Ueber eine adenomatose Wuchenrung der Serosa in einer Bauchnarbe. Z Geburtsh Gynakol 1903;49:32–41.

16. Meyer R. Ueber Stand der frage der Adenomyositis und Adenomyome im Allgemeinen und ins Besondere uber Adenomyositis seroepithelialis und Adenomyometritis sarcomatosa. Zentralbl Gynakol 1919;36:745–750.

17. Novak E. Pelvic endometriosis. Spontaneous rupture of endometrial cysts, with a report of three cases. Am J Obstet Gynecol 1931;22:826–837.

18. Suginami H. A reappraisal of the coelomic metaplasia theory by reviewing endometriosis occurring in unusual sites and instances. Am J Obstet Gynecol 1991;165:214–218.

19. Levander G, Normann P. The pathogenesis of endometriosis. An experimental study. Acta Obstet Gynecol Scand 1955;34:366–398.

20. Merrill JA. Endometrial induction of endometriosis across millipore filters. Am J Obstet Gynecol 1996;94:780–789.

21. Javert CT. Pathogenesis of endometriosis based on endometrial homeoplasia, direct extension, exfoliation and implantation, lymphatic and haematogenic metastasis. Cancer 1949;2:399–410.

22. Ridley JH. The histogenesis of endometriosis. A review of facts and fancies. Obstet Gynecol Surv 1968;23:1–35.

23. Victory R, Diamond MP, Johns DA. Villar's node: a case report and systematic review of endometriosis externa of the umbilicus. J Minim Invasive Gynecol 2007;14:23–32.

24. Teng CC, Yang HM, Chen KF et al. Abdominal wall endometriosis: an overlooked but possibly preventable complication. Taiwan J Obstet Gynecol 2008;47.42–48.

25. Halme J, Hammond MG, Hulka JF et al. Retrograde menstruation in healthy women and in patients with endometriosis. Obstet Gynecol 1984;64:151–154.

26. Kruitwagen RFPM, Poels LG, Willemsen WNP et al. Endometrial epithelial cells in peritoneal fluid during the early follicular phase. Fertil Steril 1991;55:297–303.

27. Koks CAM, Dunselman GAJ, de Goeij AFPM et al. Evaluation of a menstrual cup to collect shed endometrium for in vitro studies. Fertil Steril 1997;68:560–564.

28. Jenkins S, Olive DL, Haney AF. Endometriosis: pathogenetic implications of the anatomic distribution. Obstet Gynecol 1968;67:355–358.

29. Vercellini P, Abbiati A, Vigano P et al. Asymmetry in distribution of diaphragmatic endometriotis lesions : evidence in favour of the menstrual reflux theory. Hum Reprod 2007;22:2359–2367.

30. Vercellini P, Aimi G, de Giorgi O et al. Is cystic ovarian endometriosis an asymmetric disease? Br J Obstet Gynaecol 1998;105:1018–1021.

31. Maas JWM, Groothuis PG, Dunselman GAJ et al. Development of endometriosis-like lesions after transplantation of human endometrial fragments onto the chick embryo chorioallantoic membrane model. Hum Reprod 2001;16:627–631.

32. Nap AW, Groothuis PG, Demir AY et al. Tissue integrity is essential for ectopic implantation of human endometrium in the chicken chorioallantoic membrane. Hum Reprod 2003;18:30–34.

33. Groothuis PG, Koks CAM, de Goeij AFPM et al. Adhesion of human endometrial fragments to peritoneum in vitro. Fertil Steril 1999;71:1119–1124.

34. Koks CAM, Groothuis PG, Dunselman GAJ et al. Adhesion of shed menstrual tissue in an in-vitro model using amnion and peritoneum: a light and electron microscopic study. Hum Reprod 1999;14:816–822.

35. Dunselman GAJ, Groothuis PG, de Goeij AFPM et al. The mesothelium, Teflon or Velcro? Hum Reprod 2001;16:605–607.

36. Koks CAM, Demir-Weusten AY, Groothuis PG et al. Menstruum induces changes in mesothelial cell morphology. Gynaecol Obstet Invest 2000;50:13–18.

37. Demir-Weusten AY, Groothuis PG, Dunselman GAJ et al. Morphological changes in mesothelial cells induced by shed menstrual endometrium in vitro are not primarily due to apoptosis or necrosis. Hum Reprod 2000;15:1462–1468.

38. Demir AY, Groothuis PG, Nap AW et al. Menstrual effluent induces epithelial to mesenchymal transitions in mesothelial cells. Hum Reprod 2004;19:21–29.

39. Stetler-Stevenson WG, Liotta LA, Kleiner DE. Extracellular matrix 6: role of matrix metalloproteinases in tumour invasion and metastasis. FASEB J 1993;7:1434–1444.

40. Curran S, Murray GI. Matrix metalloproteinases: molecular aspects of their roles in tumour invasion and metastasis. Eur J Cancer 2000;36:1621–1630.

41. Tabibzadeh S. Patterns of expression of integrin molecules in human endometrium throughout the menstrual cycle. Hum Reprod 1992;7:876–882.

42. Van der Linden PJQ, de Goeij AFPM, Dunselman GAJ et al. Expression of cadherins and integrins in human endometrium throughout the menstrual cycle. Fertil Steril 1995;63:1210–1216.

43. Lessey BA. Endometrial integrins and the establishment of uterine receptivity. Hum Reprod 1998;13 suppl 3:247–258.

44. Lessey BA, Castelbaum AJ, Sawin SW et al. Aberrant integrin expression in the endometrium of women with endometriosis. J Clin Endocrinol Metab 1994;79:643–649.

45. Starzinski-Powitz A, Handrow-Metzmacher H, Kotzian S. The putative role of cell-adhesion molecules in endometriosis: can we learn from tumour metastasis? Molec Med Today 1999;5:304–309.

46. Van der Linden PJQ, de Goeij AFPM, Dunselman GAJ et al. Expression of integrins and E-cadherin in cells from menstrual effluent, endometrium, peritoneal fluid, peritoneum and endometriosis. Fertil Steril 1994;61:85–90.

47. Guilford P. E-cadherin downregulation in cancer: fuel on the fire? Molec Med Today 1999;5:172–177.

48. Gaetje R, Kotzian S, Hermann G et al. Nonmalignant epithelial cells, potentially invasive in human endometriosis, lack the tumour suppressor molecule E-cadherin. Am J Pathol 1997;150:461–467.

49. Creemers EEJM, Cleutjens JPM, Smits JFM et al. Matrix metalloproteinase inhibition after myocardial infarction. A new approach to prevent heart failure? Circ Res 2001;89:201–210.

50. Malik N, Greenfield BW, Wahl AF et al. Activation of human monocytes through CD40 induces matrix metalloproteinases. J Immunol 1996;156:3952–3960.

51. Schonbeck U, Mach F, Sukhova GK et al. Regulation of matrix metalloproteinase expression in human vascular smooth muscle cells by T lymphocytes: a role for CD40 signaling in plaque rupture? Circ Res 1997;81:448–454.

52. Murphy G, Willenbrock F, Crabbe T et al. Regulation of matrix metalloproteinase activity. Ann NY Acad Sci 1994;732:31–41.

53. Nagase H. Activation mechanisms of matrix metalloproteinases. Biol Chem 1997;378:151–160.

54. Marbaix E, Kokorine I, Henriet P et al. The expression of interstitial collagenase in human endometrium is controlled by progesterone and by oestradiol and is related to menstruation. Biochem J 1995;305:1027–1030.

55. Hulboy DL, Rudolph LA, Matrisian LM. Matrix metalloproteinases as mediators of reproductive function. Molec Hum Reprod 1997;3:27–45.

56. Rodgers WH, Matrisian LM, Giudice LC et al. Patterns of matrix metalloproteinase expression in cycling endometrium imply differential functions and regulation by steroid hormones. J Clin Invest 1994;94:946–953.

57. Bruner KL, Eisenberg E, Gorstein F et al. Progesterone and transforming growth factor-β co-ordinately regulate suppression of endometrial matrix metalloproteinases in a model of experimental endometriosis. Steroids 1999;64:648–653.

58. Spuijbroek MDEH, Dunselman GAJ, Menheere PPCA et al. Early endometriosis invades the extracellular matrix. Fertil Steril 1992;58:929–933.

59. Clark DA. Cytokines in uterine bleeding. In Alexander NJ, d'Arcangues C (eds) Steroid Hormones and Uterine Bleeding. Washington, DC: American Association for the Advancement of Science, 1992, pp. 263–275.

60. Osteen KG, Bruner-Tran KL, Keller NR et al. Progesterone-mediated endometrial maturation limits matrix metalloproteinase (MMP) expression in an inflammatory-like environment: a regulatory system altered in endometriosis. Ann NY Acad Sci 2002;955:37–47.

61. Salamonsen LA, Woolley DE. Matrix metalloproteinases in normal menstruation. Hum Reprod 1996;11(Suppl 2):124–133.

62. Bruner KL, Matrisian LM, Rodgers WH et al. Suppression of matrix metalloproteinases inhibits establishment of ectopic lesions by human endometrium in nude mice. J Clin Invest 1997;99:2851–2857.

63. Nap AW, Dunselman GAJ, de Goeij AFPM et al. Inhibiting MMP activity prevents the development of endometriosis in the chicken chorioallantoic membrane model. Hum Reprod 2004;19:2180–2187.

64. Folkman J. Tumor angiogenesis. Adv Cancer Res 1985;43:175–203.

65. Griffioen AW, Molema G. Angiogenesis: potentials for pharmacologic intervention in the treatment of cancer, cardiovascular diseases, and chronic inflammation. Pharm Rev 2000;52:237–268.

66. McLaren J. Vascular endothelial growth factor and endometriotic angiogenesis. Hum Reprod Update 2000;6:45–55.

67. Charnock-Jones DS, Sharkey AM, Rajput-Williams J et al. Identification and localization of alternately spliced mRNAs for vascular endothelial growth factor in human uterus and estrogen regulation in endometrial carcinoma cell lines. Biol Reprod 1993;48:1120–1128.

68. Smith SK. Regulation of angiogenesis in the endometrium. Trends Endocrinol Metab 2001;12:147–151.

69. Donnez J, Smoes P, Gillerot S et al. Vascular endothelial growth factor (VEGF) in endometriosis. Hum Reprod 1998;13:1686–1690.

70. Wingfield M, Macpherson A, Healy DL et al. Cell proliferation is increased in the endometrium of women with endometriosis. Fertil Steril 1995;64:340–346.

71. Matsuzaki S, Canis M, Murakami T et al. Immunohistochemical analysis of the role of angiogenic status in the vasculature of peritoneal endometriosis. Fertil Steril 2001;76:712–716.

72. Maas JWM, Le Noble FAC, Dunselman GAJ et al. The chick embryo chorioallantoic membrane as a model to investigate the angiogenic properties of human endometrium. Gynecol Obstet Invest 1999;48:108–112.

73. Hull ML, Charnock-Jones DS, Chan CLK et al. Antiangiogenic agents are effective against endometriosis. J Clin Endocrinol Metab 2003;88:2889–2899.

74. Nap AW, Dunselman GAJ, Griffioen AW et al. Angiostatic agents prevent the development of endometriosis-like lesions in the chicken chorioallantoic membrane. Fertil Steril 2005;83:793–795.

75. Nap AW, Griffioen AW, Dunselman GAJ et al. Anti-angiogenesis therapy for endometriosis. J Clin Endocrinol Metab 2004;89:1089–1095.

76. Redwine DB. Was Samspon wrong? Fertil Steril 2002;78:686–693.

77. Donnez J, Squifflet J, Casanas-Roux F et al. Typical and subtle atypical presentations of endometriosis. Obstet Gynecol Clin North Am 2003;30:83–93.

78. Garai J, Molnar V, Varga T et al. Endometriosis: harmful survival of an ectopic tissue. Front Biosci 2006;11:595–619.

79. Leyendecker G, Herbertz M, Kunz G et al. Endometriosis results from the dislocation of basal endometrium. Hum Reprod 2002;17:2725–2736.

80. Leyendecker G, Wildt L, Mall G. The pathophysiology of endometriosis and adenomyosis: tissue injury and repair. Arch Gynecol Obstet 2009;280:529–538.

81. Kitawaki J, Noguchi T, Amatsu T et al. Expression of aromatase cytochrome P450 protein and messenger ribonucleic acid in human

endometriotic and adenomyotic tissues but not in normal endometrium. Biol Reprod 1997;57:514–519.

82. Noble LS, Simpson ER, Johns A et al. Aromatase expression in endometriosis. J Clin Endocrinol Metab 1996;81:174–179.

83. Noble LS, Takayama K, Zeitoun KM et al. Prostaglandin E₂ stimulates aromatase expression in endometriosis-derived stromal cells. J Clin Endocrinol Metab 1997;82:600–606.

84. Zeitoun K, Takayama K, Sasano H et al. Deficient 17β-hydroxysteroid dehydrogenase type 2 expression in endometriosis: failure to metabolize 17β-estradiol. J Clin Endocrinol Metab 1998;83:4474–4480.

85. Takahashi K, Nagata H, Kitao M. Clinical usefulness of determination of estradiol level in the menstrual blood for patients with endometriosis. Nippon Sanka Fujinka Gakkai Zasshi 1989;41:1849–1850.

86. Bulun SE, Yang S, Fang Z et al. Role of aromatase in endometrial disease. J Ster Biochem Molec Biol 2001;79:19–25.

87. Takayama K, Zeitoun K, Gunby RT et al. Treatment of severe postmenopausal endometriosis with an aromatase inhibitor. Fertil Steril 1998;69:709–713.

88. Corson SL, Bolognese RJ. Ibuprofen therapy for dysmenorrhea. J Reprod Med 1978;20:246–252.

89. Haney AF, Muscato JJ, Weinberg JB. Peritoneal fluid cell populations in infertility patients. Fertil Steril 1981;35:696–698.

90. Hill JA, Faris HM, Schiff I et al. Characterization of leukocyte subpopulations in the peritoneal fluid of women with endometriosis. Fertil Steril 1988;50:216–222.

91. Jones RK, Bulmer JN, Searle RF. Phenotypic and functional studies of leukocytes in human endometrium and endometriosis. Hum Reprod Update 1998;4:702–709.

92. Oosterlynck DJ, Cornillie FJ, Waer M et al. Women with endometriosis show a defect in natural killer activity resulting in a decreased cytotoxicity to autologous endometrium. Fertil Steril 1991;56:45–51.

93. Ota H, Igarashi S. Expression of major histocompatibility complex class II antigen in endometriotic tissue in patients with endometriosis and adenomyosis. Fertil Steril 1993;60:834–838.

94. Semino C, Barocci A, Semino PL et al. Role of major histocompatibilty complex class-I expression and natural killer-like T-cells in the genetic control of endometriosis. Fertil Steril 1995;64:909–916.

95. Somigliana E, Vigano P, Gaffuri B et al. Human endometrial cells as a source of soluble intercellular adhesion molecule (ICAM)-1 molecules. Hum Reprod 1996;11:1190–1194.

96. Vigano P, Gaffuri B, Somogliana E et al. Expression of intercellular adhesion molecule (ICAM) mRNA and protein is enhanced in endometriosis versus endometrial stromal cells in culture. Mol Hum Reprod 1998;4:1150–1156.

97. Sharpe-Timms KL. Endometrial anomalies in women with endometriosis. Ann NY Acad Sci 2001;943:131–147.

98. Tabibzadeh S, Kong QF, Satyaswaroop PG et al. Heat shock proteins in human endometrium throughout the menstrual cycle. Hum Reprod 1996;11:633–640.

99. Jaattela M. Overexpression of major heat shock protein hsp70 inhibits tumour necrosis factor-induced activation of phospholipase A2. Immunology 1993;151:4286–4294.

100. Sattler M, Liang H, Nettesheim D et al. Structure of Bcl-xL-BaK peptide complex: recognition between regulators of endometriosis. Science 1997;225:983–986.

101. Tabibzadeh S, Zupi E, Babaknia A et al. Site and menstrual cycle-dependent expression of proteins of the tumour necrosis factor (TNF) receptor family, and Bcl-2 oncoprotein and phase-specific production of TNFα in human endometrium. Hum Reprod 1995;10:277–286.

102. Gebel HM, Braun DP, Tambur A et al. Spontaneous apoptosis of endometrial tissue is impaired in women with endometriosis. Fertil Steril 1998;69:1042–1047.

103. Beliard A, Noel A, Foidart JM. Reduction of apoptosis and proliferation in endometriosis. Fertil Steril 2004;82:80–85.

104. Vinatier D, Orazi G, Cosson M et al. Theories on endometriosis. Eur J Obstet Gynecol Reprod Med 2001;96:21–34.

105. Hunt G. The role of laminin in cancer invasion and metastasis. Exp Cell Biol 1989;57:165–176.

106. Lessey BA, Damjanovich L, Coutifaris C et al. Integrin adhesion molecules in the human endometrium. Correlation with the normal and abnormal menstrual cycle. J Clin Invest 1992;90:188–195.

107. Beliard A, Donnez J, Nisolle M et al. Localization of laminin, fibronectin, E-cadherin, and integrins in endometrium and endometriosis. Fertil Steril 1997;67:266–272.

108. Osteen KG, Bruner KL, Sharpe-Timms KL. Steroid and growth factor regulation of matrix metalloproteinase expression and endometriosis. Semin Reprod Endocrinol 1996;14:247–255.

109. Osteen KG, Keller NR, Feltus FA et al. Paracrine regulation of matrix metalloproteinase expression in the normal human endometrium. Gynecol Obstet Invest 1999;48 suppl 1:2–13.

110. Sillem M, Prifti S, Neher M et al. Extracellular matrix remodelling in the endometrium and its possible relevance to the pathogenesis of endometriosis. Steroids 1998;64:648–653.

111. Sharpe-Timms KL, Keisler LW, McIntush EW et al. Tissue inhibitor of metalloproteinase-1 concentrations are attenuated in peritoneal fluid and sera of women with endometriosis and restored in sera by gonadotrophin releasing hormone agonist therapy. Fertil Steril 1998;69:1128–1134.

112. Chung HW, Wen Y, Chun SH et al. Matrix metalloproteinase-9 and tissue inhibitor of metalloproteinase-3 mRNA expression in ectopic and eutopic endometrium in women with endometriosis: a rationale for endometriotic invasiveness. Fertil Steril 2001;75:152–159.

113. Cox KE, Piva M, Sharpe-Timms KL. Differential regulation of matrix metalloproteinase-3 gene expression in endometriotic lesions compared with endometrium. Biol Reprod 2001;65:1297–1303.

114. Sharpe-Timms KL, Cox KE. Paracrine regulation of matrix metalloproteinase expression in endometriosis. Ann NY Acad Sci 2002;955:147–156.

115. Pitsos M, Kanakas N. The role of matrix metalloproteinases in the pathogenesis of endometriosis. Reprod Sci 2009;16:717–726.

116. Osteen KG, Bruner-Tran KL, Eisenberg E. Reduced progesterone action during endometrial maturation: a potential risk factor for the development of endometriosis. Fertil Steril 2005;83:529–537.

117. Stamenkovic I. Extracellular matrix remodelling: the role of matrix metalloproteinases. J Pathol 2003;200:448–464.

118. May K, Becker CM. Endometriosis and angiogenesis. Minerva Ginecol 2009;60:245–254.

119. Taylor RN, Yu J, Torres PB et al. Mechanistic and therapeutic implications of angiogenesis in endometriosis. Reprod Sci 2009;16:140–146.

120. Bourlev V, Volkov N, Pavlovitch S et al. The relationship between microvessel density, proliferative activity and expression of vascular endothelial growth factor-A and its receptors in eutopic endometrium and endometriotic lesions. Reproduction 2006;132:501–509.

121. Di Carlo C, Bonifacio M, Tommaselli GA et al. Metalloproteinases, vascular endothelial growth factor, and angiopoietin 1 and 2 in eutopic and ectopic endometrium. Fertil Steril 2009;91:2315–2323.

122. Sanfilippo JS, Wakim NG, Schikler KN et al. Endometriosis in association with uterine anomaly. Am J Obstet Gynecol 1986;154:39–43.

123. Salamanca A, Beltran E. Subendothelial contractibility in menstrual phase visualized by transvaginal sonography in patients with endometriosis. Fertil Steril 1995;64:193–195.

124. Ayers JWT, Friedman AP. Utero-tubal hypotonia associated with pelvic endometriosis. American Fertility Society Annual Meeting, 1985, Abstract 131.

125. Darrow SL, Vena JE, Batt RE et al. Menstrual cycle characteristics and the risk of endometriosis. Epidemiology 1993;4:135–142.

126. Vercellini P, de Giorgi O, Aimi G et al. Menstrual characteristics in women with and without endometriosis. Obstet Gynecol 1997;90:264–268.

127. Martinez-Roman S, Balasch J, Creus M et al. Transferrin receptor (CD71) expression in peritoneal macrophages from fertile and infertile women with and without endometriosis. Am J Reprod Immunol 1997;38:413–417.

128. Raiter-Tenenbaum A, Baranao RI, Etchepareborda JJ et al. Functional and phenotypic alterations in peritoneal macrophages from patients with early and advanced endometriosis. Arch Gynecol Obstet 1998;261:147–157.

129. McLaren J, Prentice A, Charnock-Jones DS et al. Immunolocalization of the apoptosis regulating proteins Bcl-2 and bax in human endometrium and isolated peritoneal fluid macrophages in endometriosis. Hum Reprod 1997;12:146–152.

130. McLaren J, Dealtry G, Prentice A et al. decreased levels of the potent regulator of monocyte/macrophage activation, interleukin-13, in the peritoneal fluid of patients with endometriosis. Hum Reprod 1997;12:1307–1310.

131. Halme J, Becker S, Wing R. Accentuated cyclic activation of peritoneal macrophages in patients with endometriosis. Am J Obstet Gynecol 1984;148:85–90.

132. Simpson JL, Bischoff FZ, Kamat A et al. Genetics of endometriosis. Obstet Gynecol Clin North Am 2003;30:21–40.

133. Hadfield RM, Mardon HJ, Barlow DH et al. Endometriosis in monozygotic twins. Fertil Steril 1997;68:941–942.

134. Treloar SA, O'Connor DT, O'Connor VM et al. Genetic influences on endometriosis in an Australian twin sample. Fertil Steril 1997;71:701–710.

135. Zondervan K, Cardon L, Kennedy S. Development of a website for the genetic epidemiology of endometriosis. Fertil Steril 2002;78:777–781.

136. Guo SW. Epigenetics of endometriosis. Molec Hum Reprod 2009;15:587–607.

6 Understanding the Pathogenesis of Endometriosis: Gene Mapping Studies

Jodie N. Painter[1], Krina T. Zondervan[2] and Grant W. Montgomery[1]

[1]Molecular Epidemiology, Queensland Institute of Medical Research, Brisbane, Australia
[2]Wellcome Trust Centre for Human Genetics, University of Oxford, Oxford, UK

Introduction

Endometriosis affects 6–10% of women during their most productive years. The disease has a large impact on the lives of affected women and healthcare treatment costs are substantial. The causes of endometriosis are still largely unknown and current treatments rely on surgery and/or ovarian suppressive agents. A major objective for research in endometriosis is to understand mechanisms leading to implantation of lesions outside the uterus and subsequent progression of the disease [1]. There is good evidence for a genetic contribution to disease risk and recent advances in human genetics provide powerful approaches to mapping genetic variation contributing to risk for common complex diseases. Therefore, genetic studies offer an important approach to understanding the biology of endometriosis and in this chapter we review recent developments in human genetics and how they are being applied in the search for genes contributing to the risk of developing the disease.

Genetic contributions to endometriosis

Endometriosis is a complex condition, influenced by both genetic and environmental factors. Familial aggregation of endometriosis is firmly established in humans [2–6] and non-human primates [7]. Higher rates of endometriosis are found among the relatives of endometriosis cases compared to those of controls in both hospital [3,8] and population-based samples [4]. The relative recurrence risk to siblings, which is the increase in risk to an individual whose sibling is affected compared to the risk in the general population, has been estimated at 2.3 in an Australian sample of twins and their families [5]. It is difficult to obtain an accurate estimate of this recurrence risk because the population prevalence is unknown and there is inevitable bias in ascertaining endometriosis cases through surgery that will influence the estimated risk to siblings.

Most of the early studies – investigating the genetic influence on endometriosis by looking at prevalence rates among first-degree relatives of cases versus controls – considered only small sample sizes and many suffered from ascertainment bias. Increased opportunity for diagnosis among family members of cases compared with controls and familial aggregation of confounding risk factors such as early age at menarche have led to questions about the genetic contribution to endometriosis [9]. These are certainly important considerations, arising principally because of the nature of the disease and the lack of non-invasive diagnostic tools. The strongest evidence supporting a genetic background to endometriosis comes from the larger studies in twins [5,10–12] and in the Icelandic population [4]. Monozygotic (MZ) twins show greater concordance for endometriosis than dizygotic (DZ) twins [10,11], with intra-pair correlation rates of $r_{MZ} = 0.52$ versus $r_{DZ} = 0.19$ reported in a large study of >3000 Australian twins [12]. The same study concluded that genetic factors contribute about half of the variation in endometriosis risk with an estimate of heritability of 51% [12].

Further evidence supporting a genetic background for endometriosis comes from studies in the rhesus macaque, an ideal animal model for endometriosis. Females have monthly menstrual cycles, experience menarche and menopause, and develop spontaneous disease that is histologically and morphologically identical to that seen in humans [7]. A study in a pedigree of >1800 rhesus macaques at the University of Wisconsin-Madison showed familial aggregation of endometriosis, with a significantly higher average kinship coefficient among affected macaques compared with unaffected and a higher recurrence risk for full sibs (0.75) compared with maternal half-sibs (0.26) and paternal half-sibs (0.18).

We should continue to evaluate the contribution of genetic factors to endometriosis risk as new genetic data emerge and better diagnos-

Endometriosis: Science and Practice, First Edition. Edited by Linda C. Giudice, Johannes L.H. Evers and David L. Healy.
© 2012 Blackwell Publishing Ltd. Published 2012 by Blackwell Publishing Ltd.

tic tools are developed. However, despite difficulties in interpretation, current evidence provides substantial support for a genetic contribution to endometriosis risk. Consequently, genetic approaches can be used to map genes contributing to risk of endometriosis.

Candidate genes

General approaches to gene mapping include the study of specific candidate genes usually chosen from an understanding of the biological mechanisms thought to contribute to disease. Many of the published studies have been reviewed recently [13–17]. The choice of candidates for study in endometriosis is problematic because we have limited information on disease mechanisms and many gene pathways could be involved. Furthermore, within these pathways there are many genes that could be considered for investigation, and no candidate study to date has explored these in a systematic fashion. Lastly, most studies have genotyped only a small number of selected variants in relatively small samples from endometriosis cases and controls to test for association with disease.

Candidates tested include genes from detoxification pathways, sex steroid pathways, and cytokine signaling pathways, cell cycle regulation adhesion molecules and matrix enzymes [13,17]. Endometriosis is an estrogen-dependent disease and therefore genes from pathways of sex steroid biosynthesis and signaling have been investigated. Many reported positive findings of associations for cytochrome P450, family 17, subfamily A, polypeptide 1 (CYP17A1), cytochrome P450, family 19, subfamily A, polypeptide 1 (CYP19A1), androgen receptor (AR), progesterone receptor (PGR), and estrogen receptors (ESR1 and ESR2) have problems with study design and data analysis in the original reports. Meta-analysis of the studies provided limited support for association between endometriosis and either PGR or ESR1 [16]. A subsequent study in a large family-based sample failed to support any association between PGR and endometriosis [18]. Recently, a small study reported an association (P-value = 0.023, odds ratio (OR) = 3.12) between endometriosis and a variant causing a splice site defect that abrogates gene expression of cytochrome P450, family 2, subfamily C, polypeptide 19 (CYP2C19) [19], but a second small study could not replicate this finding [20].

Several studies have evaluated genes from detoxification pathways because of the postulated effects of environmental estrogens [21], although evidence supporting this has recently been called into question [22]. Glutathione S-transferase enzymes involved in the pathway for detoxification of a range of toxic compounds and carcinogens have been studied extensively. Polymorphisms in glutathione S-transferase M1 (GSTM1) on chromosome 1p13.3 and glutathione S-transferase theta 1 (GSTT1) on chromosome 22q11.23 have been evaluated in over 20 studies [14]. There is some evidence for increased risk of developing endometriosis associated with variants in both enzymes. However, there is significant heterogeneity between studies and suggestions of publication bias. Results should be viewed with caution, especially for GSTM1 [14]. Meta-analysis of multiple studies for the detoxification enzymes N-acetyltransferase 2 (arylamine N-acetyltransferase) (NAT2) on chromosome 8p22 and cytochrome P450, family 1, subfamily A, polypeptide 1 (CYP1A1) on chromosome 15q24.1 found no evidence for association between the NAT2 acetylation polymorphism and endometriosis [15]. There may be some evidence for a small increase in risk for alleles at the MspI polymorphism in CYP1A1, but the evidence is not strong and further studies are needed to confirm the result [15].

In general, candidate gene studies have not provided the new insights into the causes of endometriosis that were hoped for. It is standard practice to replicate any significant findings in at least one independent sample before accepting the results of association studies. Less than half of the reported associations with endometriosis have been investigated in a separate sample and many associations failed to replicate in subsequent studies [17]. A number of factors have contributed to this failure, including study power, experimental design, data analysis, publication bias, population differences, and technical issues.

Recent gene discoveries in complex disease studies clearly demonstrate that the effect size for the vast majority of common risk variants is low, with ORs for the risk allele in the range of 1.1–1.5 [23–25]. However, most candidate gene studies in endometriosis have tested small samples and lack the necessary power to detect the small effects we expect to contribute to the risk of the disease [17,26]. For a complex disease such as endometriosis, where etiology is likely to be due to many genes as well as environmental factors, large sample sizes of at least 1000 cases and 1000 controls are likely to be required to detect genetic effects [27]. Moreover, it is important to recognize the effect of publication bias, which means that results that appear significant are more likely to be published [28,29]. In addition, some studies do not take adequate account of statistical issues such as multiple testing or technical issues in genotyping [16]. This publication bias, together with problems in experimental design, suggests that many reported associations are false-positive results. Our review of the large number of studies conducted for association with endometriosis does not support any gene variants being robustly associated with increased risk of endometriosis [17].

Even if association results are "true" associations, the strength of the effect is often overestimated in the initial study, an effect referred to as the "winner's curse" [29]. This means that replication studies often need more samples and greater power than the original study to detect the effect. Some cases of failure to replicate findings from the original study might be due to replication studies being underpowered [29,30]. If we are to make progress in understanding genetic contributions to endometriosis risk, researchers must give proper consideration to study power and experimental design. To uncover genetic variants underlying endometriosis, much larger studies than typically conducted are required and can be achieved by combining samples from multiple sites. Experience has shown that the way to make progress in complex disease genetics is to combine sample collections in large consortia that do have the power to detect "true" associations.

Linkage studies

In the 1980s and 1990s, a popular alternative approach to candidate gene studies was the hypothesis-free linkage study. Having delivered great successes for gene mapping in diseases caused by a single gene mutation and clear mendelian segregation patterns (e.g. Huntington disease or cystic fibrosis), linkage studies were also applied to gene mapping in complex traits. The underlying principle of a linkage study – which is carried out in families with multiple cases – is to search for genomic regions shared more frequently between relatives carrying the disease than expected, and therefore likely to carry variants increasing disease risk. Highly variable (informative) genetic markers from across the genome are typed in families and the data analyzed to identify shared regions of the genome [31–33]. To conduct linkage studies, samples must be collected from close relatives with disease. For common diseases like endometriosis with a relatively low recurrence risk to sibs, the best design is to analyze pairs of sisters both carrying the disease [33]. Studying affected sisters is also more suitable for those diseases where it is difficult to determine "unaffected" status. This is important in the case of endometriosis where a laparoscopy would be required for definitive diagnosis of unaffected status.

Families of sisters with surgically confirmed endometriosis were recruited in studies in Australia and the UK over a period of 10 years. A genome scan with 1176 affected sister-pair families was completed in the combined Australian and UK families [34]. Power calculations suggested that the study sample had 80% power to detect a locus with a recurrence risk to sisters of 1.35 [5]. Microsatellite markers spaced about every 10 cM (approximately every 10 megabases (Mb)) across the genome were typed in DNA samples from the sisters and from other family members. The combined data identified one peak of significant linkage on chromosome 10 with a logarithm of odds (LOD) score of 3.09 (genome-wide P-value 0.047). A second peak on chromosome 20 showed suggestive evidence for linkage. The results were consistent for both datasets with evidence for linkage to chromosome 10 in both the Australian and the UK families. Fine-mapping with an additional four microsatellite markers on chromosome 10 resulted in a small increase in the evidence for linkage. The peak of maximum linkage was located at 148.75 cM (127.92 Mb).

A separate linkage analysis was conducted in a subset of families with three or more affected women (Oxford: n = 52; Australia: n = 196) to test whether the apparent concentration of cases in high-risk families might reflect the presence of a rare genetic variant with relatively large effect acting in this subset of families. This would be similar to the discovery of linkage to the breast cancer 1, early-onset (BRCA1) and breast cancer 2, early-onset (BRCA2) genes shown to carry mutations responsible for breast cancer in a small subset of patients with strong familial inheritance

patterns [35,36]. The analysis identified a significant linkage peak on chromosome 7p in this subset of families [37]. This suggests that there may be a high-penetrance susceptibility locus for endometriosis in this region in a small subset of high-risk families.

The inherent problem with linkage studies is that the genomic region linked to a condition is very large, typically involving 10–100 Mb and containing hundreds of genes. This means that although a linkage study can identify a region of interest, it is unable to pinpoint a specific gene or variant. A different study design – the association study – is required for this purpose. In an association study, specific genetic variants are examined for their association with disease, typically by comparing their frequency in cases versus controls, although family-based designs can also be used. Most of the common variants in the human genome are single base differences or single nucleotide polymorphisms (SNPs). Methods have been developed to easily genotype large numbers of SNPs and these are now the markers of choice for many applications, including both linkage and association studies. Moreover, in-depth studies of variation within populations across the human genome, utilizing data generated by the International HapMap Project (www.hapmap.org), have shown that the inheritance of common SNPs (with a population frequency > 0.01) located close together is not independent (also termed linkage disequilibrium or LD) [38]. This means that one SNP can act as a proxy or 'tag' for another, and it is this feature that allows investigators to capture most of the common variation in a particular genomic region by typing a selected number of tagSNPs.

Association studies have attempted to identify the genes or variants contributing to endometriosis risk under the chromosome 7 and 10 linkage peaks by analyzing candidate genes. Several genes on chromosome 10q have previously been implicated in endometriosis and endometrial cancer [39]. These include empty spiracles, homolog of Drosophila, 2 (EMX2), phosphatase and tensin homolog (PTEN) and the fibroblast growth factor receptor 2 gene (FGFR2). EMX2 is a transcription factor essential for reproductive tract development also expressed in the adult uterine endometrium with decreased expression during the luteal phase of the menstrual cycle [40,41]. PTEN promotes cell survival and proliferation and inactivation of PTEN is an early event in endometrial hyperplasia and the development of ovarian and endometrial cancers [42]. FGFR2 has been implicated in both endometrial and breast cancer [43,44].

To examine whether common variations in EMX2, PTEN or FGFR2 might contribute to the linkage signal on chromosome 10, sets of tagSNPs were selected to capture common variations across each of the three genes. Variants reported to contribute to risk of endometrial cancer or breast cancer were included in the SNP sets which were then typed in a large sample of endometriosis cases and matched controls. Using a case–control approach involving 958 cases from families contributing to the linkage study, there was no evidence for any association with endometriosis risk, suggesting that the linkage signal is not due to common variants in any of these genes [39,45]. However, these studies cannot completely exclude a role for variation in these genes and the pathology of endometriosis. Linkage studies identify regions of the genome that are shared in sisters with the disease more often than by chance. However, the mutations that segregate within families need not be the same between all families included in the analysis, as different families may have different mutations in the same gene or gene region. Indeed, the recent consensus is that linkage signals are caused by different variants across families that are rare in the general population. The association studies mentioned [39,45] assume that underlying variants are common in the general population. Consequently, rare family specific variants in any of the three genes could still contribute to endometriosis risk. Extensive DNA sequencing of candidate genes would be required to identify such rare variants.

Genome-wide association studies

Lack of progress in locating true risk variants from either candidate gene association studies or linkage mapping approaches is not confined to endometriosis. This has been a common problem in complex disease studies and much effort has been directed to developing better methods [24]. Spectacular advances in genotyping technology, greater understanding of the structure of common variations in the human genome, and continued advances in computing power and software tools have led to a powerful method for mapping disease genes known as genome-wide association (GWA) studies (Fig. 6.1). Genetic markers capturing most of the common variations across the genome can now be screened in a single experiment and provide the first effective approach to search for genetic variants contributing to the etiology of complex human diseases. There are 10–15 million common SNPs that segregate in human populations and genotyping them all remains a major task. However, the International HapMap Project [38] has characterized patterns of SNP variation in the human genome, and demonstrated that genotyping a representative set of 500,000 to 1 million tagSNPs could sample most of the common variations in the genome. Commercial genotyping platforms now routinely type up to 1 million SNPs on a single chip. Therefore, a typical GWA study would genotype ~500,000 tagSNPs in several thousand cases and controls and test for association with disease (see Fig. 6.1).

The design of a study is important and the best approach will depend on the characteristics of the disease or trait being studied [46]. In particular, the choice of population controls or controls screened for absence of disease can influence the outcome of the studies. Another important consideration is to ensure that cases and controls are well matched for ethnicity to reduce the chances of false-positive association signals caused by ethnic differences in allele frequency if one ethnic group is over-represented in either the case or control group.

Once genotyping is complete, the results are subjected to standard, rigorous, quality control procedures. These include removal of individuals or markers with missing genotypes because these suggest poor-quality DNA or poor-quality assays, respectively.

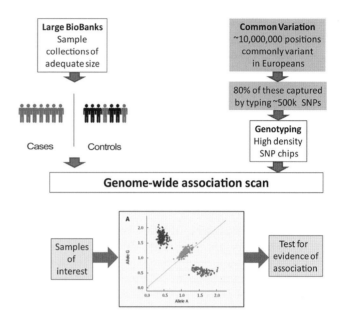

Figure 6.1 Schematic representation of typical genome-wide association studies. Large sample collections of disease cases and controls have been collected and stored in BioBanks. Greater understanding of the structure of variation in the human genome and developments in technology for massive parallel genotyping of single nucleotide polymorphisms (SNPs) has led to the development of commercial genotyping systems that can type over 1 million SNPs in a single experiment. These SNPs are chosen to "tag" common variations in the human genome. Case and control samples are genotyped with these commercial SNP chips and data analyzed to identify novel disease associations.

Tests are also conducted to remove outlier individuals that may come from different ethnic backgrounds than the target study population. Association results are generally presented in terms of significance values for all SNPs across the genome in a "Manhattan" plot (Plate 6.1). Significant association results are seen as points above a stringent threshold, determined by the probability of finding a false positive and allowing for the many statistical tests conducted.

Once genetic association with the disease has been identified in an initial discovery sample, it is essential to replicate the finding in independent samples. As GWA studies test association for hundreds of thousands of individual SNPs, despite setting a stringent significance threshold this nevertheless still presents an opportunity for false positives to occur due to multiple testing. Replication of the initial finding provides an important safeguard against the possibility of false-positive results. Another reason for replicating the results is to get an independent estimate for the size of the effect. Results identified in the initial discovery sample often overestimate the size of the effect because of the previously mentioned phenomenon of the winner's curse [47]. Replication in independent samples usually provides a better estimate of the size of the effect expected in other populations.

Once significant association has been detected, the region around the locus is examined to determine the location of association signals relative to genes in the region and the pattern of local variation (see Plate 6.1). One consequence of genotyping tagging variants in the discovery sample is that SNPs that are statistically associated with disease are unlikely to be the causal variant. The causal variant was probably not present on the SNP chip used to genotype the discovery sample and the true causal variant(s) will be correlated with one or more of the common variants typed on the chip. The causal variant is most likely to lie within a region of 50,000–200,000 bases from the "tag" SNP, but this will vary between chromosomal locations influenced by patterns of LD in the region. This in turn depends on the past history of selection in these regions in human populations [48], with regions containing genes subject to more recent selection showing stronger patterns of LD over longer distance.

Often there are many genes within the broad regions tagged by the risk variant first discovered in the GWA studies. Therefore, the next step is to try to identify the likely causal variant and the gene or genes causing disease risk. Alternatively, signals could map to areas of the genome without obvious genes (indeed, in a recent study of replicated GWA signals, 43% of these were found to be in large intergenic regions, previously termed "gene deserts") [23]. Such findings are likely to point to regulatory regions which affect the expression of genes further away, and which will need to be followed up with further functional studies of gene expression. Functional studies can be difficult, but are essential to define the genes and pathways contributing to disease for future development of improved diagnostic tests or novel therapies.

Genome-wide association studies have been very successful. In the last 3 years over 1000 variants have been detected that are associated with a range of human traits and common diseases [25]. These discoveries have provided new and exciting insights into the biology of many diseases. We can draw several general conclusions from the studies. Common variants in the population (with an allele frequency > 5%) have been found that are robustly associated with most diseases that have been analyzed. Many of these variants are in genes that contribute to biological pathways that were previously not known to be involved in disease or are located in regions that do not contain known protein-coding genes. However, the sizes of effects on disease risk are typically small, with odds ratios for the risk alleles in the range of ~1.1 to ~1.5. Even where risk alleles in several genes have been detected for a particular disease, adding the effects of the different SNPs associated with the disease usually explains only a small fraction of the familial risk (or heritability) [49]. This varies across diseases since some diseases and traits have different genetic architecture. For example, in age-related macular degeneration, approximately 50% of genetic variation has been accounted for by only six loci [50], whereas for adult height only 6% of genetic variation was accounted for by ~50 loci [49]. How to find the variants responsible for these "missing" heritabilities has become a key focus for many investigators, after the initial identification of robust associations [51].

Gene discovery in endometriosis cases: applying genome-wide screens

Conducting GWA studies in well-powered endometriosis case–control studies is a critical next step in finding genes for endometriosis risk, and several groups have recently published their first GWA results. A study by Juneau Biosciences [52] on 761 surgically confirmed cases and 1531 controls of European ancestry was published in abstract form. This study identified a number of signals with low P-values ($<1\times10^{-5}$) but no association signals reached genome-wide significance. The most significant result ($P = 3.09 \times 10^{-7}$) was for rs2286276 on chromosome 7 located in an intron of the transducin β-like 2 gene (TBL2). This SNP is located on a different chromosomal arm from the area of significant linkage found in the linkage study including ≥3 affected sisters described previously [46], and the results would therefore be unrelated. Further cases are being collected to increase the power of the study and the results will need to be replicated in an independent sample.

The first GWA study to be published as an article in a peer-reviewed scientific journal was by Uno *et al* [53], describing the results of a GWA in a Japanese sample. The most significant result for this study, which included a GWA analysis in a "discovery" set of 1423 cases and 1318 controls, was for rs10965235 located on chromosome 1 within the cyclin-dependent kinase inhibitor 2B antisense RNA (CDKN2BAS) gene ($P=1.52\times10^{-4}$, OR=1.31). Cases included a mixture of surgically confirmed and clinically diagnosed women. This SNP was replicated in an independent "replication" sample of 484 cases and 3974 controls ($P=6.79\times10^{-6}$, OR=1.56), resulting in a genome-wide significant P-value for the combined analysis (or meta-analysis) including both samples of $P=5.57\times10^{-12}$ (OR=1.44). The next most significant result was for rs16826658 on chromosome 1, located within an LD block close to the wingless-type MMTV integration site family 4 (WNT4) gene (meta-analysis $P=9.84\times10^{-6}$, OR=1.18). WNT4 is important for the development of the female reproductive tract, ovarian follicle development and steroidogenesis [54,55], making this gene an interesting biological candidate.

A smaller, independent study reporting a meta-analysis of two additional sets of Japanese samples [56], including a total of 696 cases and 825 controls, found evidence for association for SNPs around the interleukin-1, alpha proprotein (IL1A) gene on chromosome 2, where the most significant P-value was for rs3783525 of $P=1.4\times10^{-6}$ (OR=1.52). Most of the cases were surgically confirmed, although approximately a quarter had ultrasound evidence of endometrioma only. Levels of IF1A in both serum and peritoneal fluid have been shown to be elevated in infertile women with endometriosis compared to controls, particularly in cases with advanced disease [57]. The biological relevance highlights this gene as a potential functional candidate, but this association should be replicated in an independent sample for confirmation.

The largest GWA study conducted to date is that reported by the International ENDOGENE Consortium (IEC). The IEC followed on from a collaboration formed by researchers at the

Queensland Institute of Medical Research in Australia and at Oxford University in the UK [5] in 2000 to conduct the combined linkage scans of affected sister-pair families discussed above [34]. In addition to the affected sister-pair families, individual cases were also recruited in both Australia and the UK. More recently, researchers from the Nurses' Health Study in Boston, US, have joined the collaboration, culminating in the formation of the IEC in 2008. Collectively, the different sites have recruited ~5500 independent cases with clinically confirmed disease [58].

In addition to the analysis of SNP–disease associations, there has been considerable recent interest in applying GWA data to the analysis of genome-level genetic architecture underlying complex traits. Statistical methods have been developed that use GWA data to investigate, for instance, the proportion of variation in disease risk that is attributable to genetic variants (closely related to the estimation of the heritability of a trait) [59] and whether disease status in one sample (e.g. a GWA study discovery sample) can predict disease status in an independent sample (e.g. a GWA study replication sample) [60]. The discovery stage of the IEC GWA study was conducted in 3194 surgically confirmed endometriosis cases and 7060 controls from Australia and the UK. Prior to conducting our association analyses, we first investigated potential differences in the genetic contribution to stage B (moderate-to-severe disease, equivalent to the Revised American Fertility Society (rAFS) classification stages III–IV [61]) and stage A (equivalent to rAFS stages I–II) endometriosis [58]. Of the 3050 cases with stage information, 1686 (55%) were stage A while 1364 (45%) were stage B. Both analyses suggested a greater genetic loading for stage B endometriosis, with the proportion of phenotypic variation due to common variants estimated to be significantly higher for stage B (0.34) than for stage A cases (0.15; $P=1.8\times10^{-4}$). The prediction analyses confirmed the greater genetic loading for stage B disease: for example, SNP data from UK stage B cases predicted stage B disease status in Australian samples better (smallest $P=3.5\times10^{-7}$) than using data from all cases (smallest $P=8.4\times10^{-6}$), and the proportion of variation explained by the SNPs in stage B analysis was again higher than for all endometriosis. The results were similar when using Australian cases to predict disease status in the UK samples, indicating that our association analyses should be carried out separately using "all" and stage B endometriosis cases versus controls.

As expected from the proportion of variation and prediction analyses, the strongest signals of association in the IEC GWA study were observed following the analysis of stage B cases versus controls. In both analyses, the most significantly associated SNP was rs12700667, with a P-value of 2.6×10^{-7} (OR=1.22) when including all cases, and reaching genome-wide significance with $P=1.5\times10^{-9}$ (OR=1.38) when including only stage B cases. This SNP was replicated in our independent cohort of 2392 self-reported surgically confirmed cases and 2271 controls from the US ($P=1.2\times10^{-3}$, OR= 1.17). As stage information was not available for the US cases, the meta-analysis of the two datasets was conducted using all 5586 endometriosis cases and 9331 controls, reaching a genome-wide level of significance with $P=1.4\times10^{-9}$ (OR=1.20). The rs12700667

SNP is located within a large intergenic region spanning approximately 924 kilobases (Kb) on the short arm of chromosome 7, within a 48 Kb block of strong LD. Within this block sequence conservation across species and the presence of regulatory elements such as non-coding RNA, transcription factor binding sites and areas of open chromatin (which are indicative of transcriptional activity) suggest this region may regulate the activity of nearby genes. Plausible candidates include the closest gene, nuclear factor (erythroid-derived 2)-like 3 (NFE2L3), located 331 Kb away and highly expressed in placenta. Further away, located 1.35 Mb from rs12700667, are two functional candidate genes HOXA10 and HOXA11, members of the homeobox A family of transcription factors mentioned previously. Both of these genes have crucial roles in uterine development, and in adults, expression levels increase during the luteal phase of the menstrual cycle when implantation of a developing embryo may occur. Studies have shown that HOXA10 levels fail to increase in women with endometriosis, which may contribute to the infertility associated with this disease [62].

To determine the significance of the published GWA "hits" to endometriosis, we also performed a meta-analysis incorporating the data available to us at the time – our own GWA results for our "discovery" samples and those of the first Japanese GWA. Comparing both studies, results were available for 93 SNPs. Uno et al [53] did not report our top SNP (rs12700667) among the 100 SNPs they included in their replication analysis but given their smaller sample size, their study would only have had 13% power to detect its effect, assuming a similar effect size in the Japanese population. Likewise, we found no evidence of association for their top SNP rs10965235 on chromosome 9, as this SNP is monomorphic in individuals of European descent, nor for any SNPs in moderate-to-high LD with rs10965235 in the Japanese population. These results are likely to reflect the different ancestral genetic backgrounds of the populations investigated in each study. We did find evidence for replication for rs7521902, close to the WNT4 gene, again with a higher P-value for stage B cases ($P=7.5\times10^{-6}$, OR=1.25) than for all endometriosis cases ($P=9.0\times10^{-5}$, OR=1.16). Importantly, meta-analysis of the combined GWA results produced a genome-wide significant P-value $=4.2\times10^{-8}$ (OR=1.19), confirming the status of WNT4 as a plausible candidate gene for endometriosis.

Together, the current group of GWA studies have offered intriguing evidence pointing to chromosomal areas that may harbor novel candidate genes contributing to the risk of developing endometriosis. Much laboratory and statistical work remains to be done to locate the causal SNPs that are ultimately responsible for the increased disease risk, and how (and upon which genes) these genetic variants exert their effects.

Genetic contribution to common disease is largely unexplained

The focus of GWA studies has been to identify the top association signals that can be replicated in independent samples. However, as discussed above, the effect size for risk alleles identified in these studies is generally low. For most diseases, the combined effects of all genes explain only a small fraction of the variation thought to be due to genetic contributions to disease. For example, our GWA SNP rs12700667 is estimated to contribute only 0.69% to the estimated 51% heritability of endometriosis [12,58]. The most likely explanations for the "missing" heritability are that either there are many variants with small odds ratios that do not reach formal statistical significance despite large GWA studies or that causal variants are not tagged well by SNPs on the current commercial chips (e.g. because they occur at lower frequency or are in areas of the genome for which it is difficult to develop SNP assays).

Several lines of evidence from different disease studies suggest that many genes of small effect do contribute to disease risk. A recent analysis of genome-wide data in schizophrenia showed that the data were consistent with a substantial proportion of disease risk coming from many genes of small effect [60], suggesting that hundreds or even thousands of variants contribute to disease risk. The general trend in gene discovery is to combine results from many sites and conduct large meta-analyses of genome-wide data [63]. These combined studies have greater power and most discover additional loci exceeding the threshold for genome-wide significance and associated with disease risk. Larger studies are in progress, with some studies of complex traits conducting combined data analysis of over 100,000 individuals. Given that the variants with largest effects were mostly discovered in the initial "smaller" studies, effect sizes of the novel variants from the large meta-analyses decrease as studies get larger.

The second possible explanation for the "missing" heritability is that causal variants are not tagged well by SNPs on the current commercial chips. It is often stated that the current dense SNP chips capture approximately 90% of variation for Caucasians. However, this estimate is based on estimates from analysis with the ~3 million common SNPs typed in the HapMap Project and not an estimate from all common variations in the genome. Moreover, the SNP chips are unlikely to cover much of the rare variations in the genome. DNA sequencing is required to uncover this additional variation, and large-scale projects, such as the 1000 Genomes Project (www.1000genomes.org/) which will systematically search the genome for this variation are currently under way. In a recent example, the number of rare SNPs (defined as SNPs with minor allele frequencies of <3%) across 31 Kb of coding sequence was increased ~7-fold (from 23 to 179) through the resequencing of pools of type 1 diabetes cases and controls [64].

Resequencing of genomic regions is uncovering new variations and emerging evidence points to both common and rare variants contributing to disease risk. Rare functional variants may contribute substantially to susceptibility for some common diseases [65,66]. GWA studies were designed to target common variants. Current DNA databases survey variants from limited numbers of individuals and the small discovery panels used for previous SNP discovery fail to detect low-frequency alleles [67,68]. Full-sequence data on many individuals will be important to fully define genetic variation in any region of interest and insure that genotyping adequately tags all variants within the region.

Individual, rare functional variants will need to have large effects on disease risk if they are to explain much of the variation since the contribution to disease risk in the population is a function of the minor allele frequency and the effect size. However, multiple such variants in one particular gene could still account for a sizeable contribution to risk of that gene, even if the effects for each of the individual variants are small. For example, rare deletions and amino acid substitutions were discovered in GDF9 and shown to contribute to the risk for dizygotic twinning [69,70]. The proportion of mothers of dizygotic twins carrying any GDF9 variant (4.12%) was significantly higher ($P < 0.0001$) than the proportion of carriers in controls (2.29%). However, individual allele frequencies ranged from 0.002 to 0.012 in cases. Recently Nejentsev et al [64] resequenced a candidate gene for type 1 diabetes and detected four new variants at ~1% frequency that in total contributed more to variation in risk in the population than a single common variant in the same gene detected by a previous GWA study. Causal variants at lower frequencies must either have very large odds ratios to be detectable in population-based case–control studies, or statistical methods must be adopted to combine the evidence of multiple variants with small effects at a local level [71]. Nevertheless, the sample size of genotyping projects to detect such variants will need to be even larger than current GWA studies.

Beyond the top hits

Association results must pass stringent thresholds for significance and be replicated in independent studies before risk variants are accepted as contributing to disease. Only a few of the top signals meet these criteria in most genome-wide studies. However, it can be seen from the example in Plate 6.1 that many other variants lie just below the threshold. Some of these will be "truly" associated with disease, but cannot be distinguished from the other false-positive signals. Larger studies help to discover more of the risk variants, but the application of multivariate statistical approaches to the entire marker dataset can also be used in other important ways to understand the nature of genetic contributions to disease risk, as shown recently in the study of schizophrenia [60]. Analysis of the GWA data for schizophrenia and bipolar disorder revealed a strong overlap in genetic risk. This was specific for schizophrenia and bipolar disorder since applying the same analysis showed no evidence for shared genetic risk between schizophrenia and other diseases studied as part of the Wellcome Trust Case Control Consortium.

This approach can be used to further our knowledge of the genetic background of endometriosis by analysis with data from co-morbid conditions. Studies have shown increased numbers of cases of ovarian cancer, non-Hodgkin lymphoma and melanoma in patients with a history of endometriosis [72–74]. There is also evidence for genetic co-morbidity between endometriosis and migraine [75]. Epidemiological studies can be difficult to conduct because there may be problems with ascertainment and large

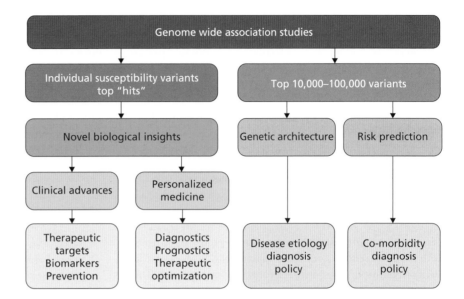

Figure 6.2 Schematic representation of pathways by which results from genome-wide association studies might be translated into relevant clinical outcomes.

cohorts must be recruited to have sufficient numbers of patients with both endometriosis and cancers to enable firm conclusions to be drawn. The advent of genome-wide marker data offers an alternative approach by evaluating shared genetic contributions to disease traits directly. Thus, analysis of GWA data across disease studies can lead to a better understanding of the shared genetic contributions to disease and to reassessment of diagnostic criteria.

Another application is to use the GWA data to estimate the genetic contributions to subclasses of disease. It is often difficult to determine the relationship between disease classes with strongly overlapping symptoms. The rAFS classification system is commonly used to stage disease severity in endometriosis and assigns patients to one of four stages (I–IV) on the basis of the extent of the disease and the associated adhesions present [61]. Other classification systems have been proposed, including ovarian versus peritoneal disease [61] and deep infiltrating versus superficial disease [76]. Whether these subclasses represent the natural history of one disorder or are in fact different disease subtypes altogether is an important consideration in endometriosis research, but as yet remains unclear. Analysis of genome-wide marker data can assess the genetic contribution to individual disease subclasses and also the shared genetic contribution to each subclass and provide new insights into the different disease presentations. Large samples with detailed phenotypic data on symptoms and disease classification will facilitate these studies and may provide important insights for future diagnosis and treatment.

Translation of genome-wide association study results to the clinic

Likely pathways for translation of results from GWA analyses into the clinic are summarized in Figure 6.2. Discoveries from GWA studies are important, but in most cases do not provide immediate results that can be translated directly into the clinic. As noted above, most novel variants have small effects. For most diseases, the known variants account for only a small proportion of population risk and so they have limited predictive value. A substantial proportion of genetic variation would have to be accounted for by genetic markers to construct risk predictors that are more informative than current predictors based upon family history. Nevertheless, GWA results have provided novel insights into the pathogenesis of many diseases. Variants that increase the risk of type 2 diabetes influence β-cell development and function and focus attention on insulin secretion in the development of disease [77]. Discoveries in inflammatory bowel disease have highlighted the importance of the autophagy pathway in disease development [78]. Better understanding of disease pathogenesis has already opened up new avenues for research likely to provide opportunities for drug discovery in the future (see Fig. 6.2). Many novel variants are located in regions with multiple genes or in intergenic regions with no genes in the immediate vicinity. Consequently, additional research will be necessary to identify the causal variant(s) or the gene(s) and pathway affected before these discoveries can be assessed.

Genetic profiles can be used to investigate genetic co-morbidity and to evaluate use of current diagnostic criteria in closely related disease conditions. This could be an important outcome of many of the current studies. Larger GWA studies will continue to identify novel genes and pathways and provide insight into the genetic architecture of complex diseases. However, these large GWA studies combine data across multiple sites. There may be important but subtle differences in disease definitions and ascertainment of cases between sites. Consequently, only common effects might be detected in these meta-analyses and some important genes will be missed, particularly if they contribute considerably more to disease etiology in one dataset than another. Investigating genetic co-morbidity and the relationships between disease subclasses is likely to lead to a better understanding of disease etiology and help with diagnosis and treatment decisions (see Fig. 6.2). In the future, results from these genetic studies can be used to inform new studies with more targeted recruitment of disease cases or collection of specific phenotypic information to better understand disease biology.

Conclusion

Genome-wide association studies provide a powerful approach to the discovery of genes or variants contributing to risk for development of complex diseases. In the last 3 years, novel genes and pathways for many diseases have been identified. The success has varied for different diseases. For age-related macular degeneration and Crohn's disease, a small number of variants with moderate effects contribute substantially to disease risk. Results for other diseases and traits have been less promising. The reasons for these differences relate to the biology and unknown genetic architecture of each disease and also to the accuracy of diagnosis and classification of disease.

Several groups have now formally published GWA studies for endometriosis. These have suggested promising novel candidate genes and regions that should be studied in the future, but as the effect sizes for the associated variants are small, the results also indicate that it will not be easy to identify high-risk genes for this disease. Several groups have substantial collections of cases suitable for genome-wide studies, but collectively the number of cases is far less than for many other diseases. Most studies have recruited women with an existing diagnosis of endometriosis. In some cases, studies rely on self-report diagnosis and in others medical records have been obtained to confirm the diagnosis. There are problems in accurately assessing stage of disease retrospectively using the clinical records alone, and consequent limitations in the information on stage of disease and other clinical data that could be used in the genetic studies. In addition, diagnosis of the disease has changed over time with developments in surgical methods, and a number of different disease classifications exist. Candidate gene studies have not identified any genes robustly associated with endometriosis, most likely due to a combination of poor study design and the intrinsic difficulty in selecting a gene of interest *a priori*. Linkage studies for the disease identified several linkage peaks, but the gene or genes contributing to these linkage signals have not yet been identified. However, these results are not good indicators of the likely success of genome-wide association studies in endometriosis and we await their outcome with considerable interest.

Access to large, well-characterized datasets still restricts progress in the genetics of endometriosis. Candidate gene studies in small samples with no power to detect the effects we expect for common variants contributing to disease risk add little to our understanding of endometriosis. Resources would be better spent on further collections of large, well-phenotyped cohorts suitable for discovery or replication samples. The goal is to understand pathways to disease and develop improved methods of prevention,

diagnosis, and treatment. Genetic approaches can now find genes or variants associated with disease and can help to achieve this goal. GWA studies to detect common variants in endometriosis are now being published and have indicated some interesting chromosomal regions for follow-up. The next step will be to perform sequencing studies to examine rare, possibly causal variants, but based on the examples from other disease projects, we will need to conduct larger studies in the future to identify a comprehensive set of the variants contributing most to endometriosis risk.

References

1. Rogers PA, D'Hooghe TM, Fazleabas A et al. Priorities for endometriosis research: recommendations from an international consensus workshop. Reprod Sci 2009;16:335–346.

2. Kennedy S. The genetics of endometriosis. J Reprod Med 1998;43:263–268.

3. Simpson JL, Bischoff FZ. Heritability and molecular genetic studies of endometriosis. Ann NY Acad Sci 2002;955:239–251.

4. Stefansson H, Geirsson RT, Steinthorsdottir V et al. Genetic factors contribute to the risk of developing endometriosis. Hum Reprod 2002;17:555–559.

5. Treloar S, Hadfield R, Montgomery G et al. The International Endogene Study: a collection of families for genetic research in endometriosis. Fertil Steril 2002;78:679–685.

6. Zondervan KT, Cardon LR, Kennedy SH. The genetic basis of endometriosis. Curr Opin Obstet Gynecol 2001;13:309–314.

7. Zondervan KT, Weeks DE, Colman R et al. Familial aggregation of endometriosis in a large pedigree of rhesus macaques. Hum Reprod 2004;19:448–455.

8. Kennedy S, Mardon H, Barlow D. Familial endometriosis. J Assist Reprod Genet 1995;12:32–34.

9. Di W, Guo SW. The search for genetic variants predisposing women to endometriosis. Curr Opin Obstet Gynecol 2007;19:395–401.

10. Hadfield RM, Mardon HJ, Barlow DH, Kennedy SH. Endometriosis in monozygotic twins. Fertil Steril 1997;68:941–942.

11. Moen MH. Endometriosis in monozygotic twins. Acta Obstet Gynecol Scand 1994;73:59–62.

12. Treloar SA, O'Connor DT, O'Connor VM, Martin NG. Genetic influences on endometriosis in an Australian twin sample. Fertil Steril 1997;17:701–710.

13. Falconer H, D'Hooghe T, Fried G. Endometriosis and genetic polymorphisms. Obstet Gynecol Surv 2007;62:616–628.

14. Guo SW. Glutathione S–transferases M1/T1 gene polymorphisms and endometriosis: a meta–analysis of genetic association studies. Molec Hum Reprod 2005;11:729–743.

15. Guo SW. The association of endometriosis risk and genetic polymorphisms involving dioxin detoxification enzymes: a systematic review. Eur J Obstet Gynecol Reprod Biol 2006;124:134–143.

16. Guo SW. Association of endometriosis risk and genetic polymorphisms involving sex steroid biosynthesis and their receptors: a meta-analysis. Gynecol Obstet Invest 2006;61:90–105.

17. Montgomery GW, Nyholt DR, Zhao ZZ et al. The search for genes contributing to endometriosis risk. Hum Reprod Update 2008;14:447–457.

18. Treloar SA, Zhen Zhao Z, Armitage T et al. Association between polymorphisms in the progesterone receptor gene and endometriosis. Molec Hum Reprod 22005;11:641–647.

19. Cayan F, Ayaz L, Aban M, Dilek S, Gumus LT. Role of CYP2C19 polymorphisms in patients with endometriosis. Gynecol Endocrinol 2009;25:530–535.

20. Bozdag G, Alp A, Saribas Z, Tuncer S, Aksu T, Gurgan T. CYP17 and CYP2C19 gene polymorphisms in patients with endometriosis. Reprod Biomed Online 2010;20:286–290.

21. Rier SE, Martin DC, Bowman RE, Becker JL. Immunoresponsiveness in endometriosis: implications of estrogenic toxicants. Environ Health Perspect 1995;103 Suppl 7:151–156.

22. Guo SW, Simsa P, Kyama CM et al. Reassessing the evidence for the link between dioxin and endometriosis: from molecular biology to clinical epidemiology. Molec Hum Reprod 2009;15:609–624.

23. Hindorff LA, Sethupathy P, Junkins HA. Potential etiologic and functional implications of genome-wide association loci for human diseases and traits. Proceedings of the National Academy of Science USA Proc Natl Acad Sci USA 2009;106:9362–9367.

24. McCarthy MI, Abecasis GR, Cardon LR et al. Genome-wide association studies for complex traits: consensus, uncertainty and challenges. Nat Rev Genet 2009;9:356–369.

25. Visscher PM, Montgomery GW. Genome-wide association studies and human disease: from trickle to flood. JAMA 2009;302:2028–2029.

26. Zondervan K, Cardon L, Desrosiers R et al. The genetic epidemiology of spontaneous endometriosis in the rhesus monkey. Ann NY Acad Sci 2002;955:233–238.

27. Zondervan KT, Cardon LR. The complex interplay among factors that influence allelic association. Nat Genet Rev 2004;5:89–100.

28. Hirschhorn JN, Lohmueller K, Byrne E, Hirschhorn K. A comprehensive review of genetic association studies. Genet Med 2002;4:45–61.

29. Ioannidis JP, Ntzani EE, Trikalinos TA, Contopoulos-Ioannidis DG. Replication validity of genetic association studies. Nat Genet 2001;29:306–309.

30. Lohmueller KE, Pearce CL, Pike M, Lander ES, Hirschhorn JN. Meta-analysis of genetic association studies supports a contribution of common variants to susceptibility to common disease. Nat Genet 2003;33:177–182.

31. Kruglyak L, Lander ES. Complete multipoint sib-pair analysis of qualitative and quantitative traits. Am J Hum Genet 1995;57:439–454.

32. Lander E, Kruglyak L. Genetic dissection of complex traits: guidelines for interpreting and reporting linkage results. Nat Genet 1995;11:241–247.

33. Risch N. Linkage strategies for genetically complex traits. II. The power of affected relative pairs. Am J Hum Genet 1990;46:229–241.

34. Treloar SA, Wicks J, Nyholt DR et al. Genomewide linkage study in 1,176 affected sister pair families identifies a significant susceptibility locus for endometriosis on chromosome 10q26. Am J Hum Genet 2005;77:365–376.

35. Miki Y, Swensen J, Shattuck-Eidens D et al. A strong candidate for the breast and ovarian cancer susceptibility gene BRCA1. Science 1994;266:66–71.

36. Wooster R, Bignell G, Lancaster J et al. Identification of the breast cancer susceptibility gene BRCA2. Nature 1995;378:789–792.

37. Zondervan KT, Treloar SA, Lin J et al. Significant evidence of one or more susceptibility loci for endometriosis with near-Mendelian autosomal inheritance on chromosome 7p13–15. Hum Reprod 2007;22:717–728.

38. Frazer KA, Ballinger DG, Cox DR et al. A second generation human haplotype map of over 3.1 million SNPs. Nature 2007;449:851–861.

39. Treloar SA, Zhao ZZ, Le L et al. Variants in EMX2 and PTEN do not contribute to risk of endometriosis. Molec Hum Reprod 2007;13:587–594.

40. Daftary GS, Taylor HS. EMX2 gene expression in the female reproductive tract and aberrant expression in the endometrium of patients with endometriosis. J Clin Endocrinol Metab 2004;89:2390–2396.

41. Troy PJ, Daftary GS, Bagot CN, Taylor HS. Transcriptional repression of peri-implantation EMX2 expression in mammalian reproduction by HOXA10. Molec Cell Biol 2003;23:1–13.

42. Maxwell GL, Risinger JI, Gumbs C et al. Mutation of the PTEN tumor suppressor gene in endometrial hyperplasias. Cancer Res 1998;58:2500–2503.

43. Easton DF, Pooley KA, Dunning AM et al. Genome-wide association study identifies novel breast cancer susceptibility loci. Nature 2007;447:1087–1093.

44. Pollock PM, Gartside MG, Dejeza LC et al. Frequent activating FGFR2 mutations in endometrial carcinomas parallel germline mutations associated with craniosynostosis and skeletal dysplasia syndromes. Oncogene 2007;26:7158–7162.

45. Zhao ZZ, Pollock PM, Thomas S et al. Common variation in the fibroblast growth factor receptor 2 gene is not associated with endometriosis risk. Hum Reprod 2008;23:1661–1668.

46. Zondervan KT, Cardon LR. Designing candidate gene and genome-wide case-control association studies. Nat Protocols 2007;2:2492–2501.

47. Zollner S, Pritchard JK. Overcoming the winner's curse: estimating penetrance parameters from case-control data. Am J Hum Genet 2007;80:605–615.

48. Sabeti PC, Varilly P, Fry B et al. Genome-wide detection and characterization of positive selection in human populations. Nature 2007;449:913–918.

49. Visscher PM. Sizing up human height variation. Nat Genet 2008;40:489–490.

50. Seddon JM, Reynolds R, Maller J et al. Prediction model for prevalence and incidence of advanced age-related macular degeneration based on genetic, demographic, and environmental variables. Invest Ophthalmol Vision Sci 2009;50:2044–2053.

51. Manolio TA, Collins FS, Cox NJ et al. Finding the missing heritability of complex diseases. Nature 2009;461:747–753.

52. Albertson H, Fech G, Dintelman S, Farrington P, Ward K. Genome-wide association study identifies novel loci associated with endometriosis in a Caucasian population. American Society of Human Genetics Meeting, Hawaii, 2009.

53. Uno S, Zembutsu H, Hirasawa A et al. A genome-wide association study identifies genetic variants in the CDKN2BAS locus associated with endometriosis in Japanese. Nat Genet 2010;42:707–710.

54. Naillat F, Prunskaite-Hyyrylainen R, Pietila I et al. Wnt4/5a signalling coordinates cell adhesion and entry into meiosis during presumptive ovarian follicle development. Hum Molec Genet 2010;19:1539–1550.

55. Boyer A, Lapointe E, Zheng X et al. WNT4 is required for normal ovarian follicle development and female fertility. FASEB J 2010;24:3010–3025.

56. Adachi S, Tajima A, Quan J et al. Meta-analysis of genome-wide association scans for genetic susceptibility to endometriosis in Japanese population. J Hum Genet 2010;55:816–821.

57. Kondera-Anasz Z, Sikora J, Mielczarek-Palacz A, Jonca M. Concentrations of interleukin (IL)-1alpha, IL-1 soluble receptor type II (IL-1 sRII) and IL-1 receptor antagonist (IL-1 Ra) in the peritoneal fluid and serum of infertile women with endometriosis. Eur J Obstet Gynecol Reprod Biol 2005;123:198–203.

58. Painter JN, Anderson CA, Nyholt DR et al. Genome-wide association study identifies a locus at 7p15.2 associated with endometriosis. Nat Genet 2011;43:51–54.

59. Yang J, Benyamin B, McEvoy BP et al. Common SNPs explain a large proportion of the heritability for human height. Nat Genet 2010;42:565–569.

60. Purcell SM, Wray NR, Stone JL et al. Common polygenic variation contributes to risk of schizophrenia and bipolar disorder. Nature 2009;460:748–752.

61. American Fertility Society. Revised American Fertility Society classification of endometriosis: 1985. Fertil Steril 1985;43:351–352.

62. Zanatta A, Rocha AM, Carvalho FM et al. The role of the Hoxa10/HOXA10 gene in the etiology of endometriosis and its related infertility: a review. J Assist Reprod Genet 2010;27:701–710.

63. Aulchenko YS, Ripatti S, Lindqvist I et al. Loci influencing lipid levels and coronary heart disease risk in 16 European population cohorts. Nat Genet 2009;41:47–55.

64. Nejentsev S, Walker N, Riches D, Egholm M, Todd JA. Rare variants of IFIH1, a gene implicated in antiviral responses, protect against type 1 diabetes. Science 2009;324:387–389.

65. Bodmer W, Bonilla C. Common and rare variants in multifactorial susceptibility to common diseases. Nat Genet 2008;40:695–701.

66. Gorlov IP, Gorlova OY, Sunyaev SR, Spitz MR, Amos CI. Shifting paradigm of association studies: value of rare single-nucleotide polymorphisms. Am J Hum Genet 2008;82:100–112.

67. Curtin K, Iles MM, Camp NJ. Identifying rarer genetic variants for common complex diseases: diseased versus neutral discovery panels. Ann Hum Genet 2009;73:54–60.

68. Iles MM. What can genome–wide association studies tell us about the genetics of common disease? PLoS Genet 2008;4:e33.

69. Montgomery GW, Zhao ZZ, Marsh AJ et al. A deletion mutation in GDF9 in sisters with spontaneous DZ twins. Twin Res 2004;7:548–555.

70. Palmer JS, Zhao ZZ, Hoekstra C et al. Novel variants in growth differentiation factor 9 in mothers of dizygotic twins. J Clin Endocrinol Metab 2006;91:4713–4716.

71. Morris AP, Lindgren CM, Zeggini E et al. A powerful approach to sub-phenotype analysis in population-based genetic association studies. Genet Epidemiol 2010;34(4):335–343.

72. Brinton L, Gridley G, Persson I, Baron J, Bergqvist A. Cancer risk after a hospital discharge diagnosis of endometriosis. Am J Obstet Gynecol 1997;176:572–579.

73. Kvaskoff M, Mesrine S, Fournier A, Boutron-Ruault MC, Clavel-Chapelon F. Personal history of endometriosis and risk of cutaneous melanoma in a large prospective cohort of French women. Arch Intern Med 2007;167:2061–2065.

74. Varma R, Rollason T, Gupta JK, Maher ER. Endometriosis and the neoplastic process. Reproduction 2004;127:293–304.

75. Nyholt DR, Gillespie NG, Merikangas KR et al. Common genetic influences underlie comorbidity of migraine and endometriosis. Genet Epidemiol 2009;33:105–113.

76. Koninckx PR, Barlow D, Kennedy S. Implantation versus infiltration: the Sampson versus the endometriotic disease theory. Gynecol Obstet Invest 1999;47:3–9.

77. Majithia AR, Florez JC. Clinical translation of genetic predictors for type 2 diabetes. Curr Opin Endocrinol Diabetes Obes 2009;16:100–106.

78. Shih DQ, Targan SR. Insights into IBD pathogenesis. Curr Gastroenterol Rep 2009;11:473–480.

7   Pathogenesis: Epigenetics

Sun-Wei Guo

Shanghai Obstetrics and Gynecology Hospital, Fudan University Shanghai College of Medicine, Shanghai, People's Republic of China

Introduction

Endometriosis, characterized by the presence and growth of functional endometrial-like tissues outside the uterus, is a major contributor to pelvic pain and subfertility in women of reproductive age [1]. While remarkable advances have been made in the molecular biology of endometriosis, its etiopathogenesis and pathophysiology are still poorly understood and remain an enigma [2]. As a result, there are many uncertainties in the management of endometriosis, such as the optimal therapy, non-invasive diagnostics, and mechanisms of endometriosis-related pain and subfertility [1].

Endometriosis is undisputedly a hormonal disease, owing much to its estrogen dependency and aberrations in estrogen production and metabolism [3,4]. It also has been viewed as an immunological disease due to immunological aberrations in endometriosis [5,6]. In addition, it has been thought of as a disease caused by exposure to dioxins [7,8] yet human data, even 17 years after the first report based on a small animal study was published, are still equivocal at best [9,10]. Finally, it has been regarded as a genetic disease [11,12], due, apparently, to its reported familial aggregation. But even the reported familial aggregation, when examined closely, may be debatable [13]. Despite well over 100 publications reporting linkage or association of endometriosis with various genetic polymorphisms, no gene has been consistently identified so far, let alone genes that have verifiable predictive power in identifying high-risk women who are susceptible to endometriosis [13–15].

Endometriosis is no doubt a hormonal disease and certainly entails an array of immunological aberrations. While so far there is no solid evidence linking dioxin exposure to endometriosis, it may still be plausible that dioxin exposure, at the right time and dosage, might precipitate the initiation or progression of endometriosis through interaction with estrogen receptors [16] or by suppressing expression of progesterone receptors [17].

In the last decade, numerous large-scale gene expression-profiling studies have demonstrated, unequivocally, that many genes are deregulated in endometriosis [18–35]. It also has been shown that a single focus of endometriotic lesion is mono-clonal [36]. During their development from single progenitor cells to endometriotic lesions leading to various symptoms, endometriotic cells presumably need to make a series of sequential, perhaps dichotomous, and irrevocable cell fate choices. These choices are likely to be made without any change in DNA sequences. This cellular lineage, or identity, inevitably requires that cells transcribe, or enable transcription of, specific sets of genes while at the same time repressing others. To maintain cellular identity, the gene expression program must be iterated through cell divisions in a heritable fashion by epigenetic processes. Thus, it is conceivable that the initiation of endometriosis as well as its progression is triggered by the accumulation of pathological gene dysregulation. Hence, the common denominator for a disease that is hormonal, immunological and possibly environmental and genetic is the stable gene dysregulation, possibly through epigenetic means.

Indeed, transcription is regulated, in part, by the assembly of a plethora of complexes of transcription factors on regulatory regions of genes, and can be regulated at various levels: DNA modifications (both chemical and structural), post-transcriptional modifications, and post-translational modifications. These involve chemical modification of DNA (methylation), histone modification, and various mechanisms, such as specific factors, repressors, activators, general transcriptional factors, enhancers, microRNAs (miRNAs) [37,38], and recently discovered, double-stranded, non-coding RNAs (ncRNAs) [39]. These levels are either part of the epigenetic regulation (DNA methylation, histone modifications, miRNA) or closely related. After the DNA

Endometriosis: Science and Practice, First Edition. Edited by Linda C. Giudice, Johannes L.H. Evers and David L. Healy.
© 2012 Blackwell Publishing Ltd. Published 2012 by Blackwell Publishing Ltd.

is transcribed and mRNA formed, there are extra levels of regulation on how much the mRNA is translated into proteins. Post-translational modifications of protein products, localization and higher order interactions with other transcription factors, co-activators or co-repressors are one set of mechanisms through which transcription can be controlled at another level.

In view of this, epigenetics is likely to be involved in maintaining cellular identity or gene expression programs in ectopic endometrial cells. Here, I shall present evidence for epigenetic aberrations in endometriosis, examine possible roles that epigenetics may play in the pathogenesis of endometriosis, and discuss implications for the diagnosis, therapeutics, and prognosis of endometriosis.

Epigenetics

The word epigenetics (*epi-* in Greek means "over" or "above" so epigenetics means "on top of" or "in addition to" genetics) was coined by Conrad H. Waddington in the 1950s [40], and its definition has evolved following our deeper understanding of genes and their functions and regulations. It is used to describe the study of phenotypic changes and then stable gene expression programs *without* changes in DNA sequence or DNA content. The latest definition of an epigenetic trait is "a stably heritable phenotype resulting from changes in a chromosome without alterations in the DNA sequence" [41]. Epigenetic processes are known to be essential in development and differentiation, but they are also involved in disease and aging, and are responsible for some known phenomena such as X chromosome inactivation and genomic imprinting [42,43].

One important way in which genes are regulated is through the remodeling of chromatin. The nucleosome, a basic unit of chromatin, consists of an octamer formed of two copies of each of the four core histones (H2A, H2B, H3, and H4), around which 147 base pair (bp) DNA are wrapped in 1.65 left-handed superhelical turns [44]. The neighboring nucleosomes are connected by a stretch of free DNA called "linker DNA." The nucleosomes and histones are organized into chromatin. Dynamic changes in chromatin structure influence gene expression and are affected by chemical modifications of histone proteins such as methylation (DNA and histone) and acetylation (histone), and by non-histone, DNA-binding proteins [45]. Enzymes involved in this process include DNA methyltransferases (DNMTs), histone deacetylases (HDACs), histone acetylases (HATs), histone methyltraqnsferases (HMTs), and the methyl-CpG-binding protein MeCP2.

DNA methylation

DNA methylation refers to the covalent modification of postreplicative DNA by adding a methyl group (–CH_3) to specific dinucleotide sites along the genome, i.e. cytosines 5′ of guanines, or at CpG sites [46], which are typically enriched in gene promoters and/or the first exon where they aggregate to form the so-called CpG island. Approximately 60% of protein-coding genes in mammals contain CpG islands in their promoter regions. Normally, transcriptionally active mammalian genes are unmethylated, whereas tissue-specific and developmental genes are mostly methylated and silenced in differentiated tissues.

DNA methylation is by far the most studied and best understood epigenetic modification, starting from a proposal in 1975 that DNA methylation may cause stable maintenance of a gene expression pattern through subsequent mitotic cell divisions [47,48]. The process of DNA methylation is catalyzed by three main DNMTs in mammals: DNMT1, which is a "maintainance" methyltransferase, and DNMT3A and DNMT3B, which are "*de novo*" methyltransferases acting on previously unmethylated sites [49]. These enzymes catalyze the transfer from the methyl group donor S-adenosyl methionine. In general, promoter hypo- and hypermethylation are associated with gene expression and silencing, respectively. The patterns of DNA methylation are initiated and maintained by DNMTs.

Histone modifications

Besides DNA methylation, covalent histone modifications such as acetylation, methylation, ubiquitination, SUMOylation and ADP-ribosylation can also orchestrate DNA organization and gene expression [50]. Both the type of modification as well as the affected amino acid residue determine the subsequent changes in chromatin structure, making it either accessible or inaccessible for transcription. DNA methylation typically works in concert with histone modifications, dynamically controlling the chromatin structure and gene expression [51].

The exact mechanisms by which DNA methylation works in concert with histone modification to regulate gene expression are an active research area. It is thought that DNA methylation is the initiating event demarcating certain genomic sites for the establishment of a transcriptionally repressive chromatin state [52]. But DNA methylation may also depend on prior histone modification (e.g. H3K9 methylation), followed by binding of methyl CpG-binding domain proteins (MBDs) which lead to gene repression by recruiting HDACs [53].

MicroRNA

MicroRNAs (miRNAs) are a large class of endogenous, single-stranded, short, non-coding RNA of 20–30 nucleotides in length that match perfectly the 3′ untranslated regions (3′UTR) of target mRNAs and play a key role in regulating gene expression through interaction with mRNA of protein-coding genes. Evolutionarily highly conserved, miRNAs account for 2–3% of the human genome and collectively regulate about 30% of the human genes [54]. MiRNAs may be located within introns of coding genes or in intergenic regions, but also can be found, albeit more rarely, in coding exons [55–57]. As with DNA methylation or histone modifications, they also regulate gene expression without any change in DNA sequences, which is achieved through either inhibiting mRNA translation or, less frequently, inducing mRNA degradation. Because of this, miRNAs are subsumed in the epigenetics realm.

Discovered at the turn of the century [58–60], miRNA's essential role in development and its significance in health and disease soon became evident and are now an active research field [61]. Growing evidence shows that miRNA expression is deregulated in cancer, and that aberrant miRNA expression correlates with aberrant expression of tumor suppressor genes and oncogenes, and thus can be of diagnostic and prognostic value [62–65]. More recent research indicates that miRNA is not merely a suppressor of gene expression; it also plays a more diverse role in gene regulation [66]. Ørom et al report that miR-10a, an miRNA, can interact with the 5′ UTR of mRNAs encoding ribosomal proteins and enhance their translation [67].

The dynamic change of epigenetic modifications

One notable feature in epigenetics is that all epigenetic modifications are reversible and dynamic. The epigenome, the collection of DNA methylation states and histone modifications, can be influenced and modified by environmental and lifestyle factors throughout the entire lifespan [52]. Aging, for example, is associated with changes in DNA methylation patterns [68]. In addition, it is associated with a decline in global CpG methylation [69].

Diet also can impact on gene expression through epigenetic modifications. Folate deficiency is linked with open neural tube defects [70], likely due to the essential role that folate plays in converting methionine to S-adenosylmethionine, the main methyl group donor in DNA methylation reactions. Folate therapy restores the normal state of DNA methylation, normalizing gene expression [71].

Epigenetic regulation in endometrium

During the menstrual cycle, the endometrium, driven by steroid sex hormones, undergoes programmed morphological and functional changes in order to prepare for pregnancy. These changes involve co-ordinated control of many genes, and some of them have recently been shown to be regulated epigenetically (for an excellent review, see [72]).

Perhaps the first clue that epigenetics plays a role in the cyclic change of endometrium is from a 2004 report that the global methylation level, as measured by 5-methyl cytidine level, in human endometrium changes with the menstrual cycle, being higher in proliferative phase than in secretory phase [73]. This hypermethylation during the proliferative phase appears to be supported by the report that DNMT1 expression level is found to be higher in the proliferative phase than in the secretory phase in normal endometrium [74]. A more recent study found that DNMT1 expression level is the lowest in midsecretory phase and higher in the proliferative and late secretory phases [75]. In addition, the same study also found that DNMT3A expression level is lower in the secretory phase than in the proliferative phase, and to some extent so is DNMT3B. Consistent with these findings, the gene expression levels of DNMT3A and DNMT3B, but not DNMT1, were found to be decreased by treatment with estrogen and progestin [75]. The authors of the study

attributed the difference in DNMT1 expression level between mRNA and protein results to the different sensitivities of RT-PCR (reverse transcription polymerase chain reaction) and immunohistochemistry. While this explanation may sound valid, a more plausible scenario could be that the effect of progesterone and estrogen on DNMT1 expression may not be manifested at the transcription level, but rather at the post-transcriptional level. That is, while the treatment of progesterone and estrogen does not change the DNMT1 gene *expression*, it may reduce the DNMT1 protein *stability*. Regardless, these data, taken together, indicate that DNMTs have regulatory functions in the cyclical changes of endometrium.

Another strong piece of evidence for an epigenetic role in endometrium comes from a study investigating the expression of class I HDACs and two HATs in human endometrium [76]. It shows that HDAC1 and HDAC3 protein expression is constitutive throughout the menstrual cycle while HDAC1 expression is reduced in secretory phase endometrium [76]. In addition, two HATs, PCAF and GCN5, are also constitutively expressed in endometrium [76]. Munro et al report that the global histone acetylation levels of H2AK5, H3K9, H4K8, and H3K14/18 are increased in the early proliferative phase, subsequently declining until ovulation [72]. These data suggest that histone modifications are involved in endometrial function and their aberrations may be involved in endometrial pathology.

As reviewed by Munro et al [72], epigenetics has been implicated in numerous aspects of endometrial development: regeneration, proliferation, angiogenesis, differentiation, and implantation. Of note is the role of histone modifications in the control of decidualization, reported first by Sakai et al in 2003 [77] and later by Uchida and colleagues [78–81]. Treatment with HDAC inhibitors (HDACIs) yields differentiation in endometrial cells, similar to the joint treatment of progesterone and estrogen, leading to morphological transformation and induction of differentiation marker genes such as glycodelin and leukemia inhibitory factor (LIF).

In the last 2–3 years, there has been a growing interest in characterizing the role of miRNAs in endometrium (reviewed in [82]). Starting with Pan et al [83] who identified 65 out of 287 miRNAs expressed in normal endometrium, eutopic and ectopic endometrium from women with endometriosis, the same group also found an inverse correlation between the expression of miR-23a, miR-23b, and miR542-3p and the expression of their respective target genes aromatase and cyclooxygenase (COX)-2. In addition, the expression of these miRNAs and genes is differentially regulated by estrogen, medroxyprogesterone acetate, ICI-182780 and RU-486, or their respective combinations, in endometrial stromal and glandular epithelial cells. These data indicate that miRNAs play a role in gene regulation in endometrial function.

A more recent study further characterizes this role. Using isolated endometrial glandular epithelial cells from the time windows of maximum proliferative (late proliferative phase) and maximum P4 action (midsecretory phase), and by profiling both mRNA and miRNA expression levels, Kuokkanen et al found an inverse relationship between the expression of certain miRNAs and the suppression of their putative target genes that are involved in cell cycling [84]. Thus, they were able to show that miRNAs may post-transcriptionally downregulate the expression of cell cycle genes, thereby suppressing cell cycle progression and cell proliferation in secretory-phase endometrial epithelium [84]. Their results also suggest that progesterone acts to oppose estrogen action by fine-tuning expression of genes involved in endometrial function [85].

With demonstrated involvement in endometrium, it is perhaps not surprising to see reports demonstrating that miRNAs have a role in postnatal development of the uterus and also in embryo implantation in the mouse [86–91]. These results add to our knowledge base on endometrial biology and provide a reference point for investigation of various endometrial pathologies, benign and malignant, such as endometrial cancer, uterine leiomyoma, infertility, endometriosis, and perhaps also contraception [82,92–96].

Epigenetic aberrations in endometriosis

While the first study on aberrant methylation at hMLH1, p16 and PTEN in endometriosis was published in 2002 in the context of possible malignant transformation of endometriosis, the first piece of evidence showing that endometriosis may be an epigenetic disease came from a study, published in 2005, reporting that the putative promoter of HOXA10 in endometrium from women with endometriosis is hypermethylated as compared with that from women without endometriosis [97]. HOXA10 is a member of a family of homeobox genes that serve as transcription factors during development and has been shown to be important for uterine function. It is expressed in human endometrium, and its expression is dramatically increased during the midsecretory phase of the menstrual cycle, corresponding to the time of implantation and increase in circulating progesterone [98]. This suggests that HOXA10 may have an important function in regulating endometrial development during the menstrual cycle and in establishing conditions necessary for implantation [99].

In endometrium of women with endometriosis, however, HOXA10 gene expression is significantly reduced, indicating some defects in uterine receptivity [100,101], which may be responsible for reduced fertility in women with endometriosis. As promoter hypermethylation is generally associated with gene silencing, the observed HOXA10 promoter hypermethylation provides a plausible explanation as why HOXA10 gene expression is reduced in endometrium of women with endometriosis [97]. The HOXA10 promoter hypermethylation also has been demonstrated in induced endometriosis in baboons, which coincides with reduced HOXA10 expression [102]. In mice with induced endometriosis, HOXA10 promoter hypermethylation in eutopic endometrium also was confirmed [103]. HOXA10 hypermethylation, accompanied by overexpression of DNMT1 and DNMT3B, also has been reported recently in mice prenatally exposed to diethylstilbestrol [104]. Interestingly, *in utero* exposure to bisphenol-A, another endocrine disrupting chemical (EDC), results in HOXA10

*hypo*methylation and no change in expression of DNMT1, DNMT3A, and DNMT3B [105]. These aberrant methylations seem to be a novel mechanism of altered developmental programming induced by *in utero* exposure to EDCs.

The second piece of evidence came from a study demonstrating that the promoter of PR-B is hypermethylated in endometriosis [106]. In addition, the PR-B promoter hypermethylation is concomitant with reduced PR-B expression, providing support for the role of epigenetic aberration in PR-B downregulation. It is well known that there is a general tendency of progesterone resistance in endometriosis [2]. It is also known that PR-B is downregulated in endometriosis [107] and may, at least in part, be responsible for progesterone resistance since progesterone is mediated through its receptors, including PR-B. Yet why there is a persistent PR-B downregulation is a mystery. PR-B promoter hypermethylation provides a plausible explanation as why PR-B is persistently downregulated in endometriosis. Silencing of progesterone target genes by methylation is an epigenetic mechanism that mediates progesterone resistance. The relatively permanent nature of methylation may explain the widespread failure of treatments for endometriosis-related infertility.

With the finding of HOXA10 and PR-B hypermethylation in endometriosis, one may wonder whether these findings are simply a matter of luck or merely the tip of a much bigger iceberg. Perhaps the most important piece of evidence showing that endometriosis is an epigenetic disease comes from a study demonstrating that DNMT1, DNMT3A, and DNMT3B, the three genes coding for DNA methyltransferases that are involved in genomic DNA methylation, are all overexpressed in endometriosis [108]. Since these genes are involved in *de novo* as well as maintenance methylation, their aberrant expression suggests that aberrant methylation may be widespread in endometriosis. As methylation is closely linked with chromatin remodeling, the aberrant expression of these genes may also signal that there are aberrant epigenetic changes, other than methylation, in endometriosis.

Consistent with this view, several very recent studies provide further evidence for epigenetic changes in endometriosis. Steroidogenic factor-1 (SF-1), a transcriptional factor essential for activation of multiple steroidogenic genes for estrogen biosynthesis, is usually undetectable in normal endometrial stromal cells but aberrantly expressed in endometriotic stromal cells. Xue *et al* show that SF-1 promoter has increased methylation in endometrial cells yet in endometriotic cells it is hypomethylated [109]. They also found that ERβ promoter is hypomethylated in endometriotic cells, which accounts for its overexpression [110]. Izawa *et al* also show that the treatment of endometrial stromal cells, which normally do not express aromatase, with a demethylation agent (DMA), 5-aza-deoxycytidine, dramatically increased the aromatase mRNA expression [111]. Very recently, the same group reported that in ectopic endometrium aromatase is hypomethylated while in normal endometrium it is hypermethylated, and the difference provides a convincing explanation as to why aromatase is expressed in ectopic but not in normal endometrium [112].

Table 7.1 Genes identified so far to have epigenetic aberrations in endometriosis/adenomyosis.

Year of the first report	Gene name	Major finding	Modulation by HDACI and/or DMA	Reference
2005	HOXA10	Hypermethylated in eutopic endometrium	ND	[97,102,103]
2006	PR-B	Hypermethylated in ectopic endometrium, with concomitant decreased expression	TSA, upregulation	[106]
2007	Aromatase	Endometriotic cells secreted more aromatase than endometrial cells with added testosterone, yet when treated with a demethylation agent, endometrial cells increased the secretion	ADC, upregulation	[111]
2007	ERβ	Hypomethylated in ectopic endometrium	ND	[110]
2007	SF-1	Hypomethylated in ectopic endometrium	ND	[109]
2007	E-cadherin	Methylated and inactivated in an endometriotic epithelial-like cell line, and can be demethylated and reactivated by the treatment of TSA	TSA, reactivation	[116]
2010	Aromatase	Aromatase is hypomethylated in ectopic, but not in normal endometrium		[112]
2010	PR-B	Hypermethylated in ectopic endometrium from women with adenomyosis, with concomitant decreased expression	TSA and/or ADC, upregulation	[113]

ADC, 5-aza-2′-deoxycytidine; DMA, demethylation agent; HDACI, histone deacetylase inhibitor; ND, not done; TSA, trichostatin A.

In adenomyosis, a disorder which used to be called endometriosis interna, it has recently been found that, as in endometriosis, PR-B promoter is hypermethylated in ectopic but not in normal endometrial stromal cells [113]. Treatment with both trichostatin A (TSA, an HDACI) and 5-aza-2′-deoxycytidine (ADC, a demethylation agent) elevated PR-B gene and protein expression in ectopic, but not in normal, endometrial stromal cells. Both TSA and ADC treatment dose dependently inhibited the proliferation of ectopic endometrial stromal cells. TSA and ADC treatment also suppressed the cell cycle progression in ectopic endometrial stromal cells. Thus, this study provides the first piece of evidence that adenomyosis has epigenetic aberration and may also be an epigenetic disease amenable to rectification by pharmacological means.

Table 7.1 provides a complete list of genes with various epigenetic aberrations in endometriosis and adenomyosis identified so far.

Endometriotic cells are found to lack the intercellular adhesion protein E-cadherin, a known metastasis suppressor protein in epithelial tumor cells whose deregulation also seems to be associated with invasiveness of endometriotic cells [114,115]. In two immortalized endometriotic cell lines, E-cadherin was found to be hypermethylated, and treatment with TSA resulted in its reactivated expression with concomitant attenuated invasion [116]. This seems to suggest that, at least in endometriotic cell lines, E-cadherin silenced by methylation is associated with invasiveness.

Our *in silico* study based on large-scale gene expression profiling of paired ectopic and eutopic endometrium also suggests a theme of post-translational modification and histone deacetylation [117], again supporting the role of epigenetics in endometriosis.

MicroRNA deregulation in endometriosis

The identification and characterization of miRNAs differentially expressed in endometriosis are a rapid expanding field. Pan *et al* report an miRNA expression profiling study that identified 48 out of 287 miRNAs that are differentially expressed with progressive decline in expression level in endometrium from women without endometriosis (EN), paired eutopic and ectopic endometrium (EU and EC), and ectopic endometrium from women with endometriosis (EE) [83] (Table 7.2). The target genes of these identified miRNAs include many genes known to be involved in endometriosis, such as ERα, ERβ, PR, and TGF-β, suggesting that miRNA deregulation may be involved in endometriosis.

A follow-up study conducted by the same group further evaluated the expression of four miRNAs (miR-17-5p, miR-23a, miR-23b, and miR-542-3p) that were previously identified to be differentially expressed in ectopic and eutopic endometrium, and their predicted target genes, steroidogenic acute regulatory protein (StAR), aromatase and COX-2, and further assessed the influence of ovarian steroids on their expression in endometrial cells [118]. An inverse correlation existed between the expression level of miR-23a, miR-23b, and miR542-3p and that of their respective target genes aromatase and COX-2, respectively, but not between miR17-5p and StAR expression, as suspected. Thus, by showing that the altered expression of specific miRNAs affects the stability of their target genes known to be involved in endometriosis, the role of these miRNAs in pathogenesis of endometriosis is demonstrated.

By using miRNA array and by comparing seven pairs of eutopic and ectopic endometrium from women with endometriosis, Hall and colleagues identified 22 miRNAs that are differentially expressed with a fold change ≥±1.5 in ectopic versus eutopic endometrium (see Table 7.2) [119]. Fourteen of them were found to be upregulated, and the other eight downregulated in ectopic endometrium as compared with eutopic endometrium.

Using a similar approach and based on three pairs of eutopic and ectopic endometrial tissue samples, Filigheddu *et al* recently reported the identification of 50 miRNAs that are differentially expressed with a fold change ≥±2.0 in ectopic versus eutopic endometrium (see Table 7.2) [120]. They also identified the predicted target genes for these aberrantly expressed miRNAs by

Table 7.2 Deregulated miRNAs in endometriosis identified by various studies.

Author	Direction of deregulation	miRNA names	Remarks
Pan *et al* (2007) [83]	Downregulated as compared with normal endometrium	miR-23a let-7b, miR-100, miR-125a, miR-143, miR-195, miR-199a, miR-199a-AS, miR-21, miR-214, mi-R22, miR-221, miR-222, miR-23b, miR-24, miR-26a, miR-29a let-7a, let-7c, let-7d, let-7f, let-7i, miR-10b, miR-125b, miR-145, miR-27b, miR-99a, miR-107, miR-146b, miR-191, miR-30a-5p, miR-30b, miR-30c, miR-30d, miR-451, miR-103, miR-126, miR-15b, miR-16, *miR-17-5p*, miR-193b, miR-19b, miR-29c, miR-30e-5p, miR-342, miR-423, miR-494, miR-92	Based on four normal endometrial tissue samples, four pairs of eutopic and ectopic endometrial tissue samples, and four ectopic endometrial tissue samples The upper panel is a list of miRNAs with fold change in ectopic versus (paired) eutopic endometrium expression < 2.0, the middle panel, < 1.5 but ≥ 2.0, and the lower panel, ≥ 1.5 The underscored miRNA names are those that are identified to be *upregulated* in [119] or [120] or both. The italicized miRNA is also identified to be differentially expressed in the same direction in [120]
Ohlsson Teague *et al* (2009) [119]	Upregulated	**miR-145, miR-143, miR-99a**, miR-99b, **miR-126, miR-100**, miR-125b, **miR-150**, miR-125a, miR-223, miR-194, **miR-365, miR-29c, miR-1**	Based on seven pairs of eutopic and ectopic endometrial tissue samples
	Downregulated	**miR-196b, miR-20a**, *miR-34c*, miR-424, miR-142-3p, **miR-200b**, miR-141, **miR-200a**	The bold miRNAs are also identified to be differentially expressed in the same direction in [120]. The italicized miRNA is also identified to be downregulated in [94]
Filigheddu *et al* (2010) [120]	Upregulated	**miR-1, miR-100**, miR-101, **miR-126**, miR-130a, **miR-143, miR-145**, miR-148a, **miR-150**, miR-186, miR-199a, miR-202, miR-221, miR-28, miR-299-5p, miR-29b, **miR-29c**, miR-30e-3p, miR-30e-5p, miR-34a, **miR-365**, miR-368, miR-376a, miR-379, miR-411, miR-493-5p, **miR-99a**	Based on three pairs of eutopic and ectopic endometrial tissue samples
	Downregulated	miR-106a, miR-106b, miR-130b, miR-132, *miR-17-5p*, miR-182, miR-183, **miR-196b, miR-200a, miR-200b**, miR-200c, **miR-20a**, miR-25, miR-375, miR-425-5p, miR-486, miR-503, miR-638, miR-663, miR-671, miR-768-3p, miR-768-5p, miR-93	The bold miRNAs are also identified to be differentially expressed in the same direction in [119]
			The italicized miRNA is also identified to be differentially expressed in the same direction in [83], but not in their ectopic versus eutopic comparison
Burney *et al* (2009) [94]	Downregulated (eutopic versus normal endometrium)	miR-9, miR-9*, miR-34b, miR-34c-5p, miR-34c-3p, miRPlus_42 780	Based on three normal endometrial tissue samples, four eutopic endometrial tissue samples

a bioinformatics approach, and found that several of them actually match the genes that are known to be differentially expressed in ectopic versus eutopic endometrium.

Burney *et al* carried out miRNA expression profiling of early secretory eutopic endometrium in women with and without endometriosis [94]. From 1488 + 151 = 1639 miRNAs, they identified six miRNAs that were downregulated in eutopic endometrium in women with endometriosis as compared with women without. The six miRNAs are listed in Table 7.2. Four of the identified miRNAs were further validated by qRT-PCR and three of them were found to be indeed significantly downregulated in eutopic endometrium from women with endometriosis. They further identified the predicted mRNA targets for each of the three validated miRNAs by a bioinformatics approach, and went further to cross-reference the targets against the 2488 genes found, by the same group, to be differentially expressed between eutopic endometrium in women with and without endometriosis. They found that the miRNA downegulation correlated with the upregulation of their target genes involved in cell cycle regulation, suggesting that the downregulation of the miRNAs may indeed be involved in cellular proliferation of endometrial cells in eutopic endometrium from women with endometriosis.

The studies by Ohlsson Teague *et al* [119] and by Filigheddu *et al* [120] were carried out using paired eutopic and ectopic endometrial tissue samples. In contrast, Pan *et al* used normal as well as ectopic endometrial tissue samples as well as additional paired eutopic and ectopic endometrial tissue samples. By comparing the lists of identified differentially expressed miRNAs, one can find some agreement and discrepancies (see Table 7.2). First, the two studies with the similar design came up with some identical miRNAs that either upregulated or downregulated in ectopic versus eutoipc endometrium, nine being upregulated and four being downregulated (see Table 7.2). No miRNAs were "misclassified" between the two studies. If we use the list of miRNAs that are consistently identified by both studies as the "correct" one, then the correct rate for the Ohlsson Teague study is 13/22 = 59.1% while that for Filigheddu *et al* is 13/50 = 26.0%. Interestingly, the difference is not due entirely to the use of different criteria (i.e. 1.5- versus 2.0-fold of changes).

Second, the choice of tissue samples makes a difference in results. In Pan *et al* [83], the correlation coefficient on the ratio of expression between paired ectopic versus eutopic endometrium and that of ectopic versus normal endometrium is 0.41 ($P = 0.003$, based on data presented in Table 1 in [83]). While the ratios of miRNA expression in ectopic versus normal endometrium were all less than 1, the counterpart in paired ectopic versus eutopic endometrium ranged from 0.48 to 1.3, and only 17/48 = 35.4% of the ratios were below 0.67, or a fold reduction >1.5.

Third, different studies can yield quite different lists of differentially expressed miRNAs. We can see that the list identified by Pan *et al* [83], which also includes miRNAs that were differentially expressed between eutopic endometrium from women with and without endometriosis, had no overlap with that of Burney *et al* [94]. In addition, the list of miRNAs identified by Pan *et al* [83] that were downregulated in paired ectopic versus eutopic endometrium actually contains five miRNAs that were identified to be *upregulated* either by Ohlsson Teague *et al* [119] or Filigheddu *et al* [120], or both (see Table 7.2). Such discrepancies presumably result from several conceivable sources, such as study design, heterogeneity in patients, types of miRNA microarrays, statistical analytical methods employed, and finally, chance events. Thus, discrepancy is a fact of life and will probably be always with us. Standardization should help to reduce the extent of discrepancy, but probably will not remove it completely.

Lastly, different study designs have their pros and cons, and their own strengths and weaknesses. For example, while studies comparing paired ectopic and eutopic endometrium such as Ohlsson Teague *et al* [119] or Filigheddu *et al* [120] and, to some extent, Pan *et al* [83] can identify miRNAs aberrantly expressed in ectopic endometrium that may be associated with the development of endometriosis, by design, they *cannot* identify miRNAs that are *both* aberrantly expressed in the *same* direction in eutopic and ectopic endometrium.

So far no report on methylation and miRNA in endometriosis has been published. It is interesting to note that miR-34c has been shown to be underexpressed in endometriosis [119], yet epigenetic silencing of miR-34c has also been shown to be associated with CpG island methylation and can be restored by treatment with a DMA in colorectal cancer [121]. Thus, an obvious question is whether miR-34c expression also could be restored by treatment with either HDACIs or DMAs, or both.

MicroRNAs have been shown to play important roles in modulating innate and adaptive immune responses, T-cell differentiation and activation, and B-cell differentiation [122,123]. Hence they may also be involved in immunological aspects of endometriosis, which has been characterized so far.

It should be noted that miRNAs are not merely unidirectional negative regulators of gene expression. Vasudevan *et al* demonstrate that miRNA can also increase translation [124]. Recent research also demonstrates that many miRNAs interact closely with transcription factors, often forming a network for gene regulation. Human granulocytic differentiation, for example, is shown to be controlled by a regulatory circuitry involving miR-223 and two transcription factors, NFI-A and C/EBPα [125]. The two factors compete for binding to the miR-223 promoter: NFI-A maintains miR-223 at low levels, whereas its replacement by C/EBPα, following retinoic acid-induced differentiation, upregulates miR-223 expression. The competition by C/EBPα and the granulocytic differentiation are favored by a negative feedback loop in which miR-223 represses NFI-A translation. The interactions between miRNA and transcription factors can yield either a negative feedback loop [126] or a feedforward loop [127]. This adds another layer of complexity in gene regulation.

As a new class of post-transcriptional regulators of gene expression, the importance of miRNAs in the pathogenesis of endometriosis is only beginning to be unveiled. Existing evidence, mostly from cancer research, has shown that miRNAs are involved in numerous cellular processes, including differentiation, cell cycle progression, apoptosis, embryogenesis, angiogenesis, oncogenesis, and immune responses [128–132]. MiRNAs also have been found to be both regulators and targets of methylation and acetylation processes. It is thus reasonable to expect that miRNAs may similarly be regulators and targets in endometriosis as well and are involved in endometriosis pathogenesis. Thus, in light of their potentially important roles in endometriosis, miRNAs may well become promising therapeutic targets as their roles and mode of actions are unraveled in future studies. This enthusiasm is buoyed, perhaps in no small part, by the recognition that there are far fewer miRNAs (predicted to be around 1000) than mRNAs (~24,000 genes, plus numerous splicing variants) and also by the recent reports of successful and well-tolerated use of anti-miRs in animal studies [133–136], as well as the news of a stage I human trial on the use of anti-miR-122 in treating hepatitis C infection (www.fiercebiotech.com/story/first-mirna-drug-enters-human-studies/2008-05-28).

However, this enthusiasm is not unguarded and certainly not unbounded. Aside from various technical hurdles inevitably encountered with new technology, the seemingly vast gulf between the exciting preclinical findings and somewhat disappointing clinical trials as seen recently in endometriosis serves as a sobering reminder of how challenging translational research is [137,138]. Indeed, anti-miRNAs may have global, non-specific effects, causing collateral damage and untoward side-effects. It has been reported that cardiac-specific knockout of Dicer, a gene encoding a RNase III endonuclease essential for miRNA processing, leads to postnatal lethality [139]. Therefore, more research will be needed.

Therapeutic implications

Unlike DNA mutations or copy number changes, DNA methylation, histone and protein modifications are reversible. Hence, enzymes that regulate the epigenetic changes could be ideal targets for intervention by pharmacological means. From the above discussion, it could be speculated that the use of HDACIs and/or DMAs could also rectify miRNA deregulation in endometriosis. Given the evidence that endometriosis may be an epigenetic disease, encouraging *in vitro* results on the use of HDACIs as a potential therapy for endometriosis have been reported. Treatment of an endometrial stromal cell line with TSA resulted in decreased proliferation [140] and cell cycle arrest [141]. The effect is likely through, perhaps in part, the upregulation of PR-B by TSA [140], possibly through increased acetylation of histones in chromatins. Treatment of TSA also inhibited interleukin (IL)-1β-induced COX-2 expression [142]. This is significant, since COX-2 overexpression has been observed in ectopic endometrium [143], found to correlate with endometriosis-associated pain [144,145], and reported to be a biomarker for recurrence [146]. TSA treatment upregulated PPARγ expression in endometrial stromal cells [147]. PPARγ agonists have been reported to inhibit vascular endothelial growth factor (VEGF) expression and angiogenesis in endometrial cells [148], inhibit tumor necrosis factor (TNF)-induced IL-8 production in endometriotic cells [149], and repress ectopic implants in animal models of endometriosis [150–152].

In two endometriotic cell lines, TSA treatment resulted in attenuated invasion and reactivated E-cadherin expression [116]. This appears to suggest that some cellular phenotypes of endometriotic cells, such as invasiveness, may be mediated epigenetically and, as such, could be tamed by epigenetic reprogramming through pharmaceutical means. A recent study also reports that romidepsin, an HDACI, inhibited HDAC activity, produced acetylation of the histone proteins, upregulated p21, and downregulated cyclins B1 and D1, resulting in proliferation inhibition and apoptosis activation in an immortalized epithelial-like endometriotic cell [153]. In a preliminary study, TSA has been found to inhibit the expression of SLIT2 (Zhao *et al*, unpublished data), a member of the SLIT family of secretory glycoproteins that have recently been found to attract vascular endothelial cells *in vitro* and promote tumor-induced angiogenesis [154], and, more recently, found to be a constituent biomarker for recurrence of endometriosis [155]. In adenomyosis, the administration of TSA and/or ADC, a demethylation agent, reactivated PR-B gene and protein expression that is silenced in ectopic, but not in normal endometrial stromal cells [156]. In addition, both TSA and ADC treatment dose-dependently reduced cell viability of ectopic endometrial stromal cells. TSA and ADC treatment also suppressed the cell cycle progression in ectopic endometrial stromal cells [156]. This study provides the first piece of evidence that adenomyosis may also be an epigenetic disease amenable to rectification by pharmacological means. These data, taken together, provide strong evidence that endometriotic cells are sensitive to the epigenetic effects of HDACIs and suggest that HDACIs may have therapeutic potential in treating endometriosis.

There are indications that HDACIs may be analgesic when treating endometriosis. The first such indication comes from a report that three HDACIs, TSA, suberic bishydroxamate and valproic acid (VPA), suppress spontaneous and oxytocin-induced uterine contractility [157]. It has been shown that women with endometriosis have aberrant uterine contractility during menses with increased frequency, amplitude, and basal pressure tone as compared with those without [158]. It is suggested that in uterus from women with dysmenorrhea there is a lack of synchronization in fundal-cervical contraction [159]. Incidentally, progesterone, a traditional drug for treating endometriosis-associated dysmenorrhea, can also inhibit myometrial contraction [160].

The *in vivo* data also appear to be encouraging. In mice with surgically induced endometriosis, treatment with TSA significantly reduced the average size of ectopic implants as compared with controls [161]. And this finding has been replicated in rats treated with VPA [162] (Liu *et al*, unpublished data). In addition, it was found that induced endometriosis resulted in hyperalgesia or "central sensitization" while TSA or VPA treatment significantly improved mice' or rats' perception of pain induced by noxious stimuli [161,162] (Liu *et al*, unpublished data). More remarkably, VPA treatment results in lowered immunoreactivity to all mediators involved in central sensitization such as ASIC3, c-Fos, N-methyl-D-aspartate (NMDA) receptor 1, and CGRP in dorsal root ganglia. The immunoreactivities to all these mediators are all increased in rats with induced endometriosis, along with reduced tolerance to noxious thermal stimulus. These data are consistent with the report that chronic administration of VPA reduces brain NMDA signaling [163], and clearly indicate that VPA treatment not only retards the growth of ectopic implants but also impacts positively on the central nervous system.

The observation that VPA treatment results in reduced amount of menses in women with adenomyosis complaining of dysmenorrhea may be attributable to the fact that HDACIs have been reported to suppress TNF-α-induced tissue factor expression [164] and also suppress VEGF receptor expression [165] and can serve as antiangiogenic factors altering VEGF signaling [166]. Both tissue factor and VEGF (and its receptors) are known to be key players involved in abnormal uterine bleeding resulting from prolonged use of progestin-only contraceptives [167] and tissue factor has been shown to be overexpressed in endometriosis [168]. Tissue factor is also found to be overexpressed in adenomyosis and its expression correlates with the amount of menses in women with adenomyosis [175].

Taking advantage of an existing drug, VPA, that is an HDACI with known pharmacology, and the advantage that adenomyosis, once called endometriosis interna, can be diagnosed quite accurately by non-invasive imaging techniques and shares many similarities with endometriosis, Liu and Guo tested VPA on three patients as a new therapy and found that it was well tolerated and, after 2 months of use, pain symptoms were dramatically reduced [169]. In addition, the uterus size was reduced by an average of one-third. Results from more patients show that VPA can effectively alleviate adenomyosis-associated pain, reduce uterus size, and reduce the amount of menses, at the expense of prolonging the menstrual cycle length by 2–4 days [170].

There is indication that HDACIs appear to synergize with DMAs, resulting in a more potent antiproliferative effect than either used alone and more robust re-expression of methylation-silenced genes [156], as in cancer cells [171]. Clearly, future research should illuminate this further.

Diagnostic and prognostic implications

Besides providing novel targets for drug therapy, epigenetic aberrations, once identified, may also provide promising prospects for diagnostic and/or prognostic purposes. One attractive approach is the identification of DNA methylation markers, which can be used for many specimens, such as menstrual blood.

Any biomarker, in order to be clinical useful, should ideally have high specificity and sensitivity. In addition, it should be easily detectable in specimens procured in a minimally invasive manner. DNA methylation biomarkers appear to fit the latter requirement quite well.

Since menstrual blood contains the same DNA (and thus methylation status) as that from endometrial cells, and since the endometrium from women with endometriosis is somewhat different from that of women without [172], menstrual blood could be a valuable, abundant, non-invasive, and convenient source for detection of methylation changes, as reported [173]. A recent preliminary study using menstrual blood provides evidence that the frequency of ERβ hypermethylation in women with endometriosis is significantly less than that in women without (Shen *et al*, unpublished data). This seems to echo the result of Xue *et al* that ERβ is hypomethylated in endometriosis [110].

Of course, it is currently unclear whether the DNA methylation markers based on menstrual blood are of any use for early diagnosis of endometriosis. It is also unclear whether they would be of value for differential diagnosis of endometriosis, which could be more challenging. Much more work is warranted.

DNA methylation markers may also prove to be useful for prognostic purposes. The preliminary results of Shen *et al* seem to suggest that PR-B promoter hypermethylation found in tissue samples harvested at the time of surgery may be a biomarker for recurrence, which is consistent with the published findings [106,174]. In any case, very little has been published in this area, even though it is an area that is likely to be clinically most useful and could bring tangible results to better patient care. The identification of patients at high risk of recurrence should suggest further intervention. On the other hand, patients with low risk of recurrence may be advised not to take any medication, which often has side-effects.

Conclusion

Many publications now provide credible evidence that endometriosis is an epigenetic disorder, in the sense that epigenetics plays a *definite* role in the pathogenesis and pathophysiology of endometriosis. This is characterized, at least in part, by aberrant methylation and very recently by deregulation of miRNA expression in eutopic as well as ectopic endometrium. Published data also have shown that HDACIs have great potential as therapy for endometriosis and/or adenomyosis. In addition, DNA methylation based on miRNA-based biomarkers may hold potential in diagnosis and/or predicting recurrence risks.

Yet the epigenetics of endometriosis is still in its infancy. We are still far from identifying and characterizing all aberrant methylations and/or miRNA expression in endometriosis, let alone understanding their underlying causes, interactions and precise roles in the pathogenesis of endometriosis, and possible ways of intervention. So far, few, if any, data exist regarding any aberration in histone modification in endometriosis. These will require research not only on ectopic endometrium, but also on epigenetic regulation in normal endometrium since this should serve as a reference point against which comparison can be made. In addition, the research on epigenetic regulation in normal endometrium is not only important to better understand endometrial biology, but also critical to help delineate endometrial pathobiologies, such as endometrial cancer, uterine leiomyoma, infertility, endometriosis, and perhaps also contraception.

Regardless, endometriosis epigenetics is a burgeoning field and may transform our understanding of the pathogenesis and pathophysiology of endometriosis, opening new avenues for diagnosis, treatment, and prognostic prediction. So far we have only scratched its surface. With more research, we may come closer to preventing or at least treating this unrelentingly painful disease that is endometriosis.

Acknowledgment

This research was supported in part by grant 30872759 from the National Science Foundation of China, grants 074119517, 09PJD015, and 10410700200 from the Shanghai Science and Technology Commission, and grant (09–11) from the State Key Laboratory of Medical Neurobiology of Fudan University.

References

1. Giudice LC. Clinical practice. Endometriosis. N Engl J Med 2010;362(25):2389–2398.

2. Giudice LC, Kao LC. Endometriosis. Lancet 2004;364(9447): 1789–1799.

3. Gurates B, Bulun SE. Endometriosis: the ultimate hormonal disease. Semin Reprod Med 2003;21(2):125–134.

4. Kitawaki J, Kado N, Ishihara H et al. Endometriosis: the pathophysiology as an estrogen-dependent disease. J Steroid Biochem Mol Biol 2002;83(1–5):149–155.

5. Paul Dmowski W, Braun DP. Immunology of endometriosis. Best Pract Res Clin Obstet Gynaecol 2004;18(2):245–263.

6. Ulukus M, Arici A. Immunology of endometriosis. Minerva Ginecol 2005;57(3):237–248.

7. Rier SE, Martin DC, Bowman RE et al. Endometriosis in rhesus monkeys (Macaca mulatta) following chronic exposure to 2,3,7,8-tetrachlorodibenzo-p-dioxin. Fundam Appl Toxicol 1993;21(4):433–441.

8. Rier SE. The potential role of exposure to environmental toxicants in the pathophysiology of endometriosis. Ann N Y Acad Sci 2002; 955:201–212; discussion 230–232, 396–406.

9. Guo SW. The link between exposure to dioxin and endometriosis: a critical reappraisal of primate data. Gynecol Obstet Invest 2004; 57(3):157–173.

10. Guo SW, Simsa P, Kyama CM et al. Reassessing the evidence for the link between dioxin and endometriosis: from molecular biology to clinical epidemiology. Mol Hum Reprod 2009;15(10):609–624.

11. Simpson JL, Bischoff FZ, Kamat A et al. Genetics of endometriosis. Obstet Gynecol Clin North Am 2003;30(1):21–40, vii.

12. Barlow DH, Kennedy S. Endometriosis: new genetic approaches and therapy. Annu Rev Med 2005;56:345–356.

13. Di W, Guo SW. The search for genetic variants predisposing women to endometriosis. Curr Opin Obstet Gynecol 2007;19(4):395–401.

14. Falconer H, D'Hooghe T, Fried G. Endometriosis and genetic polymorphisms. Obstet Gynecol Surv 2007;62(9):616–628.

15. Guo SW. The relevance of genetics in endometriosis. In: Garcia-Velasco JA, Rizk B (eds) Endometriosis: Current Management and Future Trends. New Delhi: Jaypee Medical Publishers, 2009.

16. Ohtake F, Takeyama K, Matsumoto T et al. Modulation of oestrogen receptor signalling by association with the activated dioxin receptor. Nature 2003;423(6939):545–550.

17. Igarashi TM, Bruner-Tran KL, Yeaman GR et al. Reduced expression of progesterone receptor-B in the endometrium of women with endometriosis and in cocultures of endometrial cells exposed to 2,3,7,8-tetrachlorodibenzo-p-dioxin. Fertil Steril 2005;84(1):67–74.

18. Carson DD, Lagow E, Thathiah A et al. Changes in gene expression during the early to mid-luteal (receptive phase) transition in human endometrium detected by high-density microarray screening. Mol Hum Reprod 2002;8(9):871–879.

19. Arimoto T, Katagiri T, Oda K et al. Genome-wide cDNA microarray analysis of gene-expression profiles involved in ovarian endometriosis. Int J Oncol 2003;22(3):551–560.

20. Kao LC, Germeyer A, Tulac S et al. Expression profiling of endometrium from women with endometriosis reveals candidate genes for disease-based implantation failure and infertility. Endocrinology 2003;144(7):2870–2881.

21. Matsuzaki S, Canis M, Vaurs-Barrière C et al. DNA microarray analysis of gene expression in eutopic endometrium from patients with deep endometriosis using laser capture microdissection. Fertil Steril 2005;84(Suppl 2):1180–1190.

22. Wu Y, Kajdacsy-Balla A, Strawn E et al. Transcriptional characterizations of differences between eutopic and ectopic endometrium. Endocrinology 2006;147(1):232–246.

23. Burney RO, Talbi S, Hamilton AE et al. Gene expression analysis of endometrium reveals progesterone resistance and candidate susceptibility genes in women with endometriosis. Endocrinology 2007;148(8):3814–3826.

24. Eyster KM, Klinkova O, Kennedy V et al. Whole genome deoxyribonucleic acid microarray analysis of gene expression in ectopic versus eutopic endometrium. Fertil Steril 2007;88(6):1505–1533.

25. Flores I, Rivera E, Ruiz LA et al. Molecular profiling of experimental endometriosis identified gene expression patterns in common with human disease. Fertil Steril 2007;87(5):1180–1199.

26. Hever A, Roth RB, Hevezi P et al. Human endometriosis is associated with plasma cells and overexpression of B lymphocyte stimulator. Proc Natl Acad Sci USA 2007;104(30):12451–12456.

27. Konno R, Fujiwara H, Netsu S et al. Gene expression profiling of the rat endometriosis model. Am J Reprod Immunol 2007;58(4):330–343.

28. Mettler L, Salmassi A, Schollmeyer T et al. Comparison of c-DNA microarray analysis of gene expression between eutopic endometrium and ectopic endometrium (endometriosis). J Assist Reprod Genet 2007;24(6):249–258.

29. Chand AL, Murray AS, Jones RL et al. Laser capture microdissection and cDNA array analysis of endometrium identify CCL16 and CCL21 as epithelial-derived inflammatory mediators associated with endometriosis. Reprod Biol Endocrinol 2007;5:18.

30. Van Langendonckt A, Punyadeera C, Kamps R et al. Identification of novel antigens in blood vessels in rectovaginal endometriosis. Mol Hum Reprod 2007;13(12):875–886.

31. Hull ML, Escareno CR, Godsland JM et al. Endometrial-peritoneal interactions during endometriotic lesion establishment. Am J Pathol 2008;173(3):700–715.

32. Sherwin JR, Sharkey AM, Mihalyi A et al. Global gene analysis of late secretory phase, eutopic endometrium does not provide the basis for a minimally invasive test of endometriosis. Hum Reprod 2008; 23(5):1063–1068.

33. Zafrakas M, Tarlatzis BC, Streichert T et al. Genome-wide microarray gene expression, array-CGH analysis, and telomerase activity in advanced ovarian endometriosis: a high degree of differentiation rather than malignant potential. Int J Mol Med 2008;21(3):335–344.

34. Pelch KE, Schroder AL, Kimball PA et al. Aberrant gene expression profile in a mouse model of endometriosis mirrors that observed in women. Fertil Steril 2010;93(5):1615–1627.

35. Umezawa M, Tanaka N, Tainaka H et al. Microarray analysis provides insight into the early steps of pathophysiology of mouse

endometriosis model induced by autotransplantation of endometrium. Life Sci 2009;84(23–24):832–837.

36. Wu Y, Basir Z, Kajdacsy-Balla A et al. Resolution of clonal origins for endometriotic lesions using laser capture microdissection and the human androgen receptor (HUMARA) assay. Fertil Steril 2003;79(Suppl 1):710–717.

37. Ambros V. The functions of animal microRNAs. Nature 2004;431(7006):350–355.

38. Bartel DP. MicroRNAs: genomics, biogenesis, mechanism, and function. Cell 2004;116(2):281–297.

39. Kurokawa R, Rosenfeld MG, Glass CK. Transcriptional regulation through noncoding RNAs and epigenetic modifications. RNA Biol 2009;6(3):233–236.

40. Waddington CH. The Strategy of the Genes. London: Allen & Unwin, 1957.

41. Berger SL, Kouzarids T, Shiekhattar R et al. An operational definition of epigenetics. Genes Dev 2009;23(7):781–783.

42. Robertson KD, Wolffe AP. DNA methylation in health and disease. Nat Rev Genet 2000;1(1):11–19.

43. Rodenhiser D, Mann M. Epigenetics and human disease: translating basic biology into clinical applications. CMAJ 2006;174(3):341–348.

44. Luger K, Mäder AW, Richmond RK et al. Crystal structure of the nucleosome core particle at 2.8 A resolution. Nature 1997;389(6648): 251–260.

45. Li E. Chromatin modification and epigenetic reprogramming in mammalian development. Nat Rev Genet 2002;3(9):662–673.

46. Laird PW, Jaenisch R. The role of DNA methylation in cancer genetic and epigenetics. Annu Rev Genet 1996;30:441–464.

47. Holliday R, Pugh JE. DNA modification mechanisms and gene activity during development. Science 1975;187(4173):226–232.

48. Riggs AD. X inactivation, differentiation, and DNA methylation. Cytogenet Cell Genet 1975;14(1):9–25.

49. Brero A, Leonhardt H, Cardoso MC. Replication and translation of epigenetic information. Curr Top Microbiol Immunol 2006;301:21–44.

50. Peterson CL, Laniel MA. Histones and histone modifications. Curr Biol 2004;14(14):R546–551.

51. Vaissière T, Sawan C, Herceg Z. Epigenetic interplay between histone modifications and DNA methylation in gene silencing. Mutat Res 2008;659(1–2):40–48.

52. Jaenisch R, Bird A. Epigenetic regulation of gene expression: how the genome integrates intrinsic and environmental signals. Nat Genet 2003;33(Suppl):245–254.

53. Tamaru H, Selker EU. A histone H3 methyltransferase controls DNA methylation in Neurospora crassa. Nature 2001;414(6861):277–283.

54. Lewis BP, Shih IH, Jones-Rhoades MW et al. Prediction of mammalian microRNA targets. Cell 2003;115(7):787–798.

55. Lai EC, Tomancak P, Williams RW et al. Computational identification of Drosophila microRNA genes. Genome Biol 2003;4(7):R42.

56. Lim LP, Lau NC, Weinstein EG et al. The microRNAs of Caenorhabditis elegans. Genes Dev 2003;17(8):991–1008.

57. Rodriguez A, Griffiths-Jones S, Ashurst JL et al. Identification of mammalian microRNA host genes and transcription units. Genome Res 2004;14(10A):1902–1910.

58. Reinhart BJ, Slack FJ, Basson M et al. The 21-nucleotide let-7 RNA regulates developmental timing in Caenorhabditis elegans. Nature 2000;403(6772):901–906.

59. Lee RC, Ambros V. An extensive class of small RNAs in Caenorhabditis elegans. Science 2001;294(5543):862–864.

60. Lau NC, Lim LP, Weinstein EG et al. An abundant class of tiny RNAs with probable regulatory roles in Caenorhabditis elegans. Science 2001;294(5543):858–862.

61. He L, Hannon GJ. MicroRNAs: small RNAs with a big role in gene regulation. Nat Rev Genet 2004;5(7):522–531.

62. Calin GA, Ferracin M, Cimmino A et al. A MicroRNA signature associated with prognosis and progression in chronic lymphocytic leukemia. N Engl J Med 2005;353(17):1793–1801.

63. Croce CM, Calin GA. miRNAs, cancer, and stem cell division. Cell 2005;122(1):6–7.

64. Lu J, Getz G, Miska EA et al. MicroRNA expression profiles classify human cancers. Nature 2005;435(7043):834–838.

65. Lujambio A, Calin GA, Villanueva A et al. A microRNA DNA methylation signature for human cancer metastasis. Proc Natl Acad Sci USA 2008;105(36):13556–13561.

66. Takamizawa J, Konishi H, Yanagisawa K et al. Reduced expression of the let-7 microRNAs in human lung cancers in association with shortened postoperative survival. Cancer Res 2004;64(11): 3753–3756.

67. Ørom UA, Nielsen FC, Lund AH. MicroRNA-10a binds the 5′UTR of ribosomal protein mRNAs and enhances their translation. Mol Cell 2008;30(4):460–471.

68. Issa JP. Age-related epigenetic changes and the immune system. Clin Immunol 2003;109(1):103–108.

69. Fraga MF, Esteller M. Epigenetics and aging: the targets and the marks. Trends Genet 2007;23(8):413–418.

70. Tamura T, Picciano MF. Folate and human reproduction. Am J Clin Nutr 2006;83(5):993–1016.

71. Ingrosso D, Cimmino A, Perna AF et al. Folate treatment and unbalanced methylation and changes of allelic expression induced by hyperhomocysteinaemia in patients with uraemia. Lancet 2003;361(9370):1693–1699.

72. Munro SK, Farquhar CM, Mitchell MD et al. Epigenetic regulation of endometrium during the menstrual cycle. Mol Hum Reprod 2010;16(5):297–310.

73. Ghabreau L, Roux JP, Niveleau A et al. Correlation between the DNA global methylation status and progesterone receptor expression in normal endometrium, endometrioid adenocarcinoma and precursors. Virchows Arch 2004;445(2):129–134.

74. Liao X, Siu MK, Chan KY et al. Hypermethylation of RAS effector related genes and DNA methyltransferase 1 expression in endometrial carcinogenesis. Int J Cancer 2008;123(2):296–302.

75. Yamagata Y, Asada H, Tamura I et al. DNA methyltransferase expression in the human endometrium: down-regulation by progesterone and estrogen. Hum Reprod 2009;24(5):1126–1132.

76. Krusche CA, Vloet AJ, Classen-Linke I et al. Class I histone deacetylase expression in the human cyclic endometrium and endometrial adenocarcinomas. Hum Reprod 2007;22(11):2956–2966.

77. Sakai N, Maruyama T, Sakurai R et al. Involvement of histone acetylation in ovarian steroid-induced decidualization of human endometrial stromal cells. J Biol Chem 2003;278(19):16675–16682.

78. Uchida H, Maruyama T, Nagashima T et al. Histone deacetylase inhibitors induce differentiation of human endometrial adenocarcinoma cells through up-regulation of glycodelin. Endocrinology 2005;146(12):5365–5373.

79. Uchida H, Maruyama T, Nagashima T et al. Human endometrial cytodifferentiation by histone deacetylase inhibitors. Hum Cell 2006; 19(1):38–42.

80. Uchida H, Maruyama T, Ohta K et al. Histone deacetylase inhibitor-induced glycodelin enhances the initial step of implantation. Hum Reprod 2007;22(10):2615–2622.

81. Uchida H, Maruyama T, Ono M et al. Histone deacetylase inhibitors stimulate cell migration in human endometrial adenocarcinoma cells through up-regulation of glycodelin. Endocrinology 2007;148(2): 896–902.

82. Pan Q, Chegini N. MicroRNA signature and regulatory functions in the endometrium during normal and disease states. Semin Reprod Med 2008;26(6):479–493.

83. Pan Q, Luo X, Toloubeydokhti T et al. The expression profile of micro-RNA in endometrium and endometriosis and the influence of ovarian steroids on their expression. Mol Hum Reprod 2007;13(11): 797–806.

84. Kuokkanen S, Chen B, Ojalvo L et al. Genomic profiling of microRNAs and messenger RNAs reveals hormonal regulation in microRNA expression in human endometrium. Biol Reprod 2010;82(4):791–801.

85. Lessey BA. Fine tuning of endometrial function by estrogen and progesterone through microRNAs. Biol Reprod 2010;82(4):653–655.

86. Gonzalez G, Behringer RR. Dicer is required for female reproductive tract development and fertility in the mouse. Mol Reprod Dev 2009;76(7):678–688.

87. Nagaraja AK, Andreu-Vieyra C, Franco HL et al. Deletion of Dicer in somatic cells of the female reproductive tract causes sterility. Mol Endocrinol 2008;22(10):2336–2352.

88. Hu SJ, Ren G, Liu JL et al. MicroRNA expression and regulation in mouse uterus during embryo implantation. J Biol Chem 2008;283(34):23473–23484.

89. Hong X, Luense LJ, McGinnis LK et al. Dicer1 is essential for female fertility and normal development of the female reproductive system. Endocrinology 2008;149(12):6207–6212.

90. Xia HF, Jin XH, Song PP et al. Temporal and spatial regulation of miR-320 in the uterus during embryo implantation in the rat. Int J Mol Sci 2010;11(2):719–730.

91. Chakrabarty A, Tranguch S, Daikoku T et al. MicroRNA regulation of cyclooxygenase-2 during embryo implantation. Proc Natl Acad Sci USA 2007;104(38):15144–15149.

92. Boren T, Xiong Y, Hakam A et al. MicroRNAs and their target messenger RNAs associated with endometrial carcinogenesis. Gynecol Oncol 2008;110(2):206–215.

93. Wu W, Lin Z, Zhuang Z et al. Expression profile of mammalian microRNAs in endometrioid adenocarcinoma. Eur J Cancer Prev 2009;18(1):50–55.

94. Burney RO, Hamilton AE, Aghajanova L et al. MicroRNA expression profiling of eutopic secretory endometrium in women with versus without endometriosis. Mol Hum Reprod 2009;15(10): 625–631.

95. Cohn DE, Fabbri M, Valeri N et al. Comprehensive miRNA profiling of surgically staged endometrial cancer. Am J Obstet Gynecol 2010;202(6):656.

96. Wang T, Zhang X, Obijuru L et al. A micro-RNA signature associated with race, tumor size, and target gene activity in human uterine leiomyomas. Genes Chromosomes Cancer 2007;46(4):336–347.

97. Wu Y, Halverson G, Basir Z et al. Aberrant methylation at HOXA10 may be responsible for its aberrant expression in the endometrium of patients with endometriosis. Am J Obstet Gynecol 2005;193(2): 371–380.

98. Troiano RN, Taylor KJ. Sonographically guided therapeutic aspiration of benign-appearing ovarian cysts and endometriomas. Am J Roentgenol 1998;171(6):1601–1605.

99. Taylor HS, Arici A, Olive D et al. HOXA10 is expressed in response to sex steroids at the time of implantation in the human endometrium. J Clin Invest 1998;101(7):1379–1384.

100. Taylor HS, Bagot C, Kardana A et al. HOX gene expression is altered in the endometrium of women with endometriosis. Hum Reprod 1999;14(5):1328–1331.

101. Gui Y, Zhang J, Yuan L et al. Regulation of HOXA-10 and its expression in normal and abnormal endometrium. Mol Hum Reprod 1999;5(9):866–873.

102. Kim JJ, Taylor HS, Lu Z et al. Altered expression of HOXA10 in endometriosis: potential role in decidualization. Mol Hum Reprod 2007;13(5):323–332.

103. Lee B, Du H, Taylor HS. Experimental murine endometriosis induces DNA methylation and altered gene expression in eutopic endometrium. Biol Reprod 2009;80(1):79–85.

104. Bromer JG, Wu J, Zhou Y et al. Hypermethylation of HOXA10 by in utero diethylstilbestrol exposure: an epigenetic mechanism for altered developmental programming. Endocrinology 2009;150(7): 3376–3382.

105. Bromer JG, Zhou Y, Taylor MB et al. Bisphenol-A exposure in utero leads to epigenetic alterations in the developmental programming of uterine estrogen response. FASEB J 2010;24(7):2273–2280.

106. Wu Y, Strawn E, Basir Z et al. Promoter hypermethylation of progesterone receptor isoform B (PR-B) in endometriosis. Epigenetics 2006;1(2):106–111.

107. Attia GR, Zeitoun K, Edwards D et al. Progesterone receptor isoform A but not B is expressed in endometriosis. J Clin Endocrinol Metab 2000;85(8):2897–2902.

108. Wu Y, Strawn E, Basir Z et al. Aberrant expression of deoxyribonucleic acid methyltransferases DNMT1, DNMT3A, and DNMT3B in women with endometriosis. Fertil Steril 2007;87(1):24–32.

109. Xue Q, Lin Z, Yin P et al. Transcriptional activation of steroidogenic factor-1 by hypomethylation of the 5′ CpG island in endometriosis. J Clin Endocrinol Metab 2007;92(8):3261–3267.

110. Xue Q, Lin Z, Cheng YH et al. Promoter methylation regulates estrogen receptor 2 in human endometrium and endometriosis. Biol Reprod 2007;77(4):681–687.

111. Izawa M, Harada T, Taniguchi F et al. An epigenetic disorder may cause aberrant expression of aromatase gene in endometriotic stromal cells. Fertil Steril 2008;89(5 Suppl):1390–1396.

112. Izawa M, Taniguchi F, Uegaki T et al. Demethylation of a nonpromoter cytosine–phosphate-guanine island in the aromatase gene may cause the aberrant up-regulation in endometriotic tissues. Fertil Steril 2011;95(1):33–39.

113. Nie J, Liu XS, Guo SW. Promoter hypermethylation of progesterone receptor isoform B (PR-B) in adenomyosis and its rectification by a histone deacetylase inhibitor and a demethylation agent. Reprod Sci 2010;17(11):995–1005.

114. Starzinski-Powitz A, Gaetje R, Zeitvogel A et al. Tracing cellular and molecular mechanisms involved in endometriosis. Hum Reprod Update 1998;4(5):724–729.

115. Starzinski-Powitz A et al. In search of pathogenic mechanisms in endometriosis: the challenge for molecular cell biology. Curr Mol Med 2001;1(6):655–664.

116. Wu Y, Starzinski-Powitz A, Guo SW. Trichostatin A, a histone deacetylase inhibitor, attenuates invasiveness and reactivates E-cadherin expression in immortalized endometriotic cells. Reprod Sci 2007;14(4):374–382.

117. Wren JD, Wu Y, Guo SW. A system-wide analysis of differentially expressed genes in ectopic and eutopic endometrium. Hum Reprod 2007;22(8):2093–2102.

118. Toloubeydokhti T, Pan Q, Luo X et al. The expression and ovarian steroid regulation of endometrial micro-RNAs. Reprod Sci 2008;15(10):993–1001.

119. Ohlsson Teague EM, van der Hoek KH, van der Hoek MB et al. MicroRNA-regulated pathways associated with endometriosis. Mol Endocrinol 2009;23(2):265–275.

120. Filigheddu N, Gregnanin I, Porporato PE et al. Differential expression of microRNAs between eutopic and ectopic endometrium in ovarian endometriosis. J Biomed Biotechnol 2010;2010:369549.

121. Toyota M, Suzuki H, Sasaki Y et al. Epigenetic silencing of microRNA-34b/c and B-cell translocation gene 4 is associated with CpG island methylation in colorectal cancer. Cancer Res 2008;68(11):4123–4132.

122. Baltimore D, Boldin MP, O'Connell et al. MicroRNAs: new regulators of immune cell development and function. Nat Immunol 2008;9(8):839–845.

123. Bi Y, Liu G, Yang R. MicroRNAs: novel regulators during the immune response. J Cell Physiol 2009;218(3):467–472.

124. Vasudevan S, Tong Y, Steitz JA. Switching from repression to activation: microRNAs can up-regulate translation. Science 2007;318(5858):1931–1934.

125. Fazi F, Rosa A, Fatica A et al. A minicircuitry comprised of microRNA-223 and transcription factors NFI-A and C/EBPalpha regulates human granulopoiesis. Cell 2005;123(5):819–831.

126. Burk U, Schubert J, Wellner U et al. A reciprocal repression between ZEB1 and members of the miR-200 family promotes EMT and invasion in cancer cells. EMBO Rep 2008;9(6):582–589.

127. Sylvestre Y, de Guire V, Querido E et al. An E2F/miR-20a autoregulatory feedback loop. J Biol Chem 2007;282(4):2135–2143.

128. Kuehbacher A, Urbich C, Dimmeler S. Targeting microRNA expression to regulate angiogenesis. Trends Pharmacol Sci 2008;29(1):12–15.

129. Song L, Tuan RS. MicroRNAs and cell differentiation in mammalian development. Birth Defects Res C Embryo Today 2006;78(2):140–149.

130. Dykxhoorn DM, Chowdhury D, Lieberman J. RNA interference and cancer: endogenous pathways and therapeutic approaches. Adv Exp Med Biol 2008;615:299–329.

131. Rodriguez A et al. Requirement of bic/microRNA-155 for normal immune function. Science 2007;316(5824):608–611.

132. Cobb BS, Hertweck A, Smith J et al. A role for Dicer in immune regulation. J Exp Med 2006;203(11):2519–2527.

133. Esau C, Davis S, Murray SF et al. miR-122 regulation of lipid metabolism revealed by in vivo antisense targeting. Cell Metab 2006;3(2):87–98.

134. Elmén J, Lindow M, Schütz S et al. LNA-mediated microRNA silencing in non-human primates. Nature 2008;452(7189):896–899.

135. Elmén J, Lindow M, Silahtaroglu A et al. Antagonism of microRNA-122 in mice by systemically administered LNA-antimiR leads to up-regulation of a large set of predicted target mRNAs in the liver. Nucleic Acids Res 2008;36(4):1153–1162.

136. Stenvang J, Silahtaroglu A, Lindow M et al. The utility of LNA in microRNA-based cancer diagnostics and therapeutics. Semin Cancer Biol 2008;18(2):89–102.

137. Guo SW, Hummelshoj L, Olive DL et al. A call for more transparency of registered clinical trials on endometriosis. Hum Reprod 2009;24(6):1247–1254.

138. Guo SW, Olive DL. Two unsuccessful clinical trials on endometriosis and a few lessons learned. Gynecol Obstet Invest 2007;64(1):24–35.

139. Chen JF, Murchison EP, Tang R et al. Targeted deletion of Dicer in the heart leads to dilated cardiomyopathy and heart failure. Proc Natl Acad Sci USA 2008;105(6):2111–2116.

140. Wu Y, Guo SW. Inhibition of proliferation of endometrial stromal cells by trichostatin A, RU486, CDB-2914, N-acetylcysteine, and ICI 182780. Gynecol Obstet Invest 2006;62(4):193–205.

141. Wu Y, Guo SW. Histone deacetylase inhibitors trichostatin A and valproic acid induce cell cycle arrest and p21 expression in immortalized human endometrial stromal cells. Eur J Obstet Gynecol Reprod Biol 2008;137(2):198–203.

142. Wu Y, Guo SW. Suppression of IL-1beta-induced COX-2 expression by trichostatin A (TSA) in human endometrial stromal cells. Eur J Obstet Gynecol Reprod Biol 2007;135(1):88–93.

143. Ota H, Igarashi S, Sasaki M et al. Distribution of cyclooxygenase-2 in eutopic and ectopic endometrium in endometriosis and adenomyosis. Hum Reprod 2001;16(3):561–566.

144. Matsuzaki S, Canis M, Pouly JL et al. Cyclooxygenase-2 expression in deep endometriosis and matched eutopic endometrium. Fertil Steril 2004;82(5):1309–1315.

145. Buchweitz O, Staebler A, Wülfing P et al. COX-2 overexpression in peritoneal lesions is correlated with nonmenstrual chronic pelvic pain. Eur J Obstet Gynecol Reprod Biol 2006;124(2):216–221.

146. Yuan L, Shen F, Lu Y et al. Cyclooxygenase-2 overexpression in ovarian endometriomas is associated with higher risk of recurrence. Fertil Steril 2009;91(4 Suppl):1303–1306.

147. Wu Y, Guo SW. Peroxisome proliferator-activated receptor-gamma and retinoid X receptor agonists synergistically suppress proliferation of immortalized endometrial stromal cells. Fertil Steril 2009; 91(5 Suppl):2142–2147.

148. Peeters LL, Vigne JL, Tee MK et al. PPARgamma represses VEGF expression in human endometrial cells: implications for uterine angiogenesis. Angiogenesis 2005;8(4):373–379.

149. Ohama Y, Harada T, Iwabe T et al. Peroxisome proliferator-activated receptor-gamma ligand reduced tumor necrosis factor-alpha-induced interleukin-8 production and growth in endometriotic stromal cells. Fertil Steril 2008;89(2):311–317.

150. Aytan H, Caliskan AC, Demirturk F et al. Peroxisome proliferator-activated receptor-gamma agonist rosiglitazone reduces the size of experimental endometriosis in the rat model. Aust N Z J Obstet Gynaecol 2007;47(4):321–325.

151. Lebovic DI, Kir M, Casey CL. Peroxisome proliferator-activated receptor-gamma induces regression of endometrial explants in a rat model of endometriosis. Fertil Steril 2004;82(Suppl 3):1008–1013.

152. Lebovic DI, Mwenda JM, Chai DC et al. PPAR-gamma receptor ligand induces regression of endometrial explants in baboons: a prospective, randomized, placebo- and drug-controlled study. Fertil Steril 2007;88(4 Suppl):1108–1119.

153. Imesch P, Fink D, Fedier A. Romidepsin reduces histone deacetylase activity, induces acetylation of histones, inhibits proliferation, and activates apoptosis in immortalized epithelial endometriotic cells. Fertil Steril 2010;94(7):2838–2842.

154. Wang B, Xiao Y, Ding BB et al. Induction of tumor angiogenesis by Slit-Robo signaling and inhibition of cancer growth by blocking Robo activity. Cancer Cell 2003;4(1):19–29.

155. Shen FH, Liu X, Geng JG et al. Increased immunoreactivity to SLIT/ROBO1 in ovarian endometriomas and as a likely constituent biomarker for recurrence. Am J Pathol 2009;175(2):479–488.

156. Nie J, Liu XS, Guo SW. Promoter hypermethylation of progesterone receptor isoform B (PR-B) in adenomyosis and its rectification by a histone deacetylase inhibitor and a demethylation agent. Reprod Sci 2010;17(11):995–1005.

157. Moynihan AT, Hehir MP, Sharkey AM et al. Histone deacetylase inhibitors and a functional potent inhibitory effect on human uterine contractility. Am J Obstet Gynecol 2008;199(2):167.

158. Bulletti C, De Ziegler D, Setti PL et al. The patterns of uterine contractility in normal menstruating women: from physiology to pathology. Ann N Y Acad Sci 2004;1034:64–83.

159. Kitlas A, Oczeretko E, Swiatecka J et al. Uterine contraction signals – application of the linear synchronization measures. Eur J Obstet Gynecol Reprod Biol 2009;144(Suppl 1):S61–64.

160. Ruddock NK, Shi SQ, Jain S et al. Progesterone, but not 17-alpha-hydroxyprogesterone caproate, inhibits human myometrial contractions. Am J Obstet Gynecol 2008;199(4):391.

161. Lu Y, Nie J, Liu X et al. Trichostatin A, a histone deacetylase inhibitor, reduces lesion growth and hyperalgesia in experimentally induced endometriosis in mice. Hum Reprod 2010;25(4):1014–1025.

162. Zhao T, Liu X, Zhen X et al. Levo-tetrahydropalmatine (l-THP) retards the growth of ectopic endometrial implants and alleviates generalized hyperalgesia in experimentally induced endometriosis in rats. Reprod Sci 2011;18(1):28–45.

163. Basselin M, Chang L, Chen M et al. Chronic administration of valproic acid reduces brain NMDA signaling via arachidonic acid in unanesthetized rats. Neurochem Res 2008;33(11):2229–2240.

164. Wang J, Mahmud SA, Bitterman PB et al. Histone deacetylase inhibitors suppress TF-kappaB-dependent agonist-driven tissue factor expression in endothelial cells and monocytes. J Biol Chem 2007;282(39):28408–28418.

165. Dong XF, Song W, Li LZ et al. Histone deacetylase inhibitor valproic acid inhibits proliferation and induces apoptosis in KM3 cells via downregulating VEGF receptor. Neuro Endocrinol Lett 2007;28(6):775–780.

166. Deroanne CF, Bonjean K, Servotte S et al. Histone deacetylases inhibitors as anti-angiogenic agents altering vascular endothelial growth factor signaling. Oncogene 2002;21(3):427–436.

167. Lockwood CJ, Krikun G, Hickey M et al. Decidualized human endometrial stromal cells mediate hemostasis, angiogenesis, and abnormal uterine bleeding. Reprod Sci 2009;16(2):162–170.

168. Krikun G, Schatz F, Taylor H et al. Endometriosis and tissue factor. Ann N Y Acad Sci 2008;1127:101–105.

169. Liu X, Guo SW. A pilot study on the off-label use of valproic acid to treat adenomyosis. Fertil Steril 2008;89(1):246–250.

170. Liu X, Yuan L, Guo SW. Valproic acid as a therapy for adenomyosis: a comparative case series. Reprod Sci 2010;17(10):904–912.

171. Cameron EE, Bachman KE, Myöhänen S et al. Synergy of demethylation and histone deacetylase inhibition in the re-expression of genes silenced in cancer. Nat Genet 1999;21(1):103–107.

172. Vinatier D, Cosson M, Dufour P. Is endometriosis an endometrial disease? Eur J Obstet Gynecol Reprod Biol 2000;91(2):113–125.

173. Fiegl H, Gattringer C, Widschwendter A et al. Methylated DNA collected by tampons – a new tool to detect endometrial cancer. Cancer Epidemiol Biomarkers Prev 2004;13(5):882–888.

174. Shen F, Wang Y, Lu Y et al. Immunoreactivity of progesterone receptor isoform B and nuclear factor kappa-B as biomarkers for recurrence of ovarian endometriomas. Am J Obstet Gynecol 2008;199(5):486.

175. Liu XS, Nie J, Guo SW. Elevated immunoreactivity to tissue factor and its association with dysmenorrhea severity and the amount of menses in adenomyosis. Hum Reprod 2011;26:337–45.

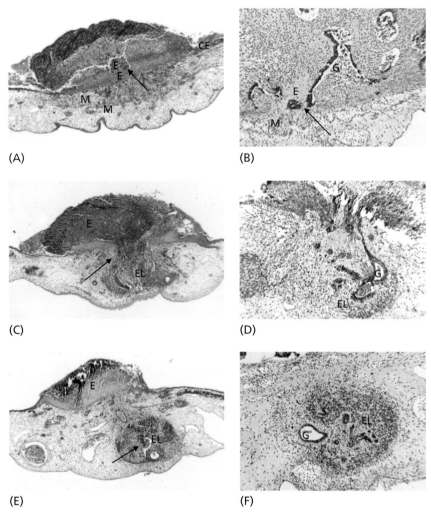

Plate 5.1 Development of endometriotic lesion after transplantation of biopsied menstrual endometrium onto the chorio-allantoic membrane (CAM). *Twenty-four hours after transplantation of menstrual endometrium onto the CAM.* (A) Direct contact (*arrow*) of endometrium (E) and CAM mesenchyme (M). CE, chorionic epithelium. (B) Detail. Direct contact (*arrow*) of endometrium (E) and CAM mesenchyme (M). Note the reorganizing cytokeratin positive glandular epithelial tissue (G) in the menstrual endometrium. *Forty-eight hours after transplantation of menstrual endometrium onto the CAM.* (C) Infiltration (*arrow*) of endometrial tissue (E). An endometriotic lesion (EL) is formed. (D) Detail. Note the reorganizing glandular tissue (G) in the endometriotic lesion (EL). *Seventy-two hours after transplantation of menstrual endometrium onto the CAM.* (E) Organized endometriotic lesion (EL), with enlarged vessels in the CAM (*arrow*). (F) Detail. Note the intact glands (G) and the surrounding endometrial stroma (S) in the endometriotic lesion (EL). A,C,E: hematoxylin and eosin staining; B,D,F: cytokeratin staining.

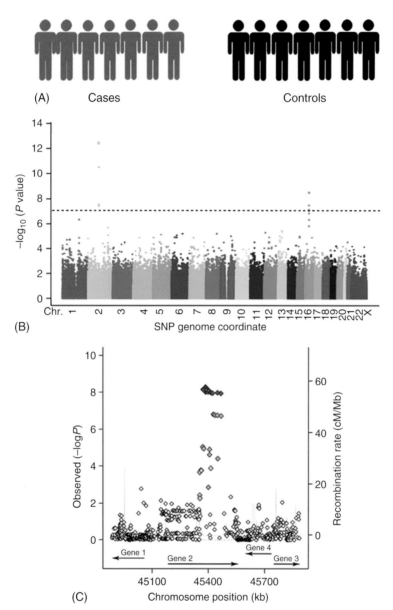

Plate 6.1 Schematic representation of typical results from a genome-wide association study. (A) Case and control samples are genotyped for 500,000 to 1,000,000 SNPs. (B) Following data cleaning and quality control of the data, individual SNP association results are plotted as −log10 (P-values) against position along the genome in a typical "Manhattan" plot. SNPs in different chromosomes are plotted in different colors to distinguish each chromosome plotted on the x axis. The dotted line represents the stringent threshold for genome-wide significance to account for the large number of association tests. Dots above the line represent individual variants showing genome-wide association with the disease. In many cases, multiple variants in the same gene or region will be associated with the disease. (C) A plot of association results in a specific region showing results for individual SNPs on a background of the estimated recombination rate (blue line) estimated from HapMap. Colors for the SNP results show the degree of linkage disequilibrium with SNP showing the strongest association result.

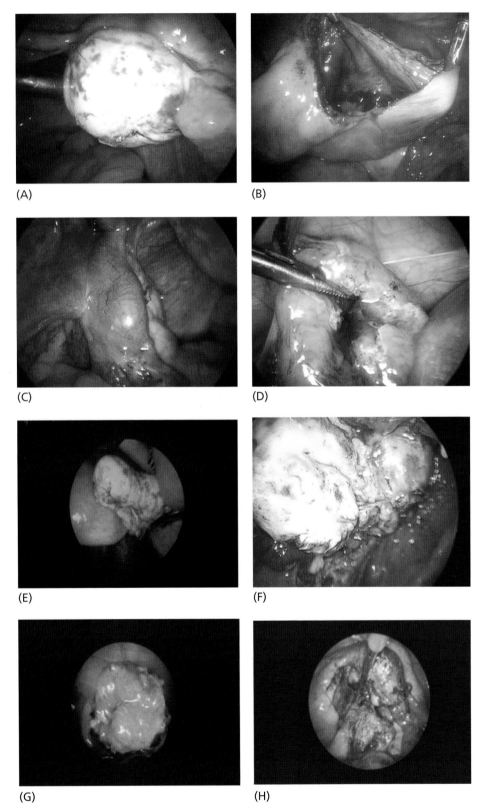

Plate 8.1 Least function scores. (A) Ovary = 3: not normal, but only minor trauma to the surface. Fimbria = 3: slight blunting. (B) Ovary = 2 (high): large endometrioma cleanly resected, good volume of ovary remaining, but more than minor damage. (C) Tube = 2 (high): distal tubal endometriosis moderately significant, cleanly vaporized by CO_2 laser. Could be associated with postoperative adhesions and loss of function. (D) Fimbria = 2 (high): clear intrafimbrial adhesions, treated with some damage to fimbria, still some reasonable architecture and function, but more than minor damage. (E) Ovary = 2 (low): large endometrioma has been removed, suture required for ovarian reconstruction, some damage to ovarian surface, and relatively small ovarian volume. (F) Tube = 2 (low): extensive resection and vaporization of tubal endometriosis seen in tube at 12 o'clock with resultant reduction in tubal function. Ovary = 2 (low): Small endometrioma removed with loss of ovarian volume, and extensive invasive ovarian surface endometriosis vaporized, with postoperative high risk of adhesions. (G) Fimbria = 2 (low): fimbrioplasty has been performed in obviously damaged tube, but with good patency expected. Very close to a score of 1. (H) Tube = 1: both tubes have extensive salpingitis isthmica nodosa.

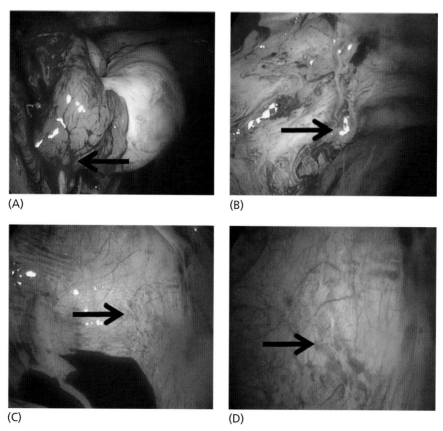

(A)

(B)

(C)

(D)

Plate 9.1 Retrograde menstruation, active and subtle endometriotic lesions. (A) Retrograde menstruation through the fallopian tubes during laparoscopy. (B) "Fresh" and active endometriotic lesion that recently adhered to peritoneum. (C,D) Diffuse and transient hemosiderin deposits on the peritoneum.

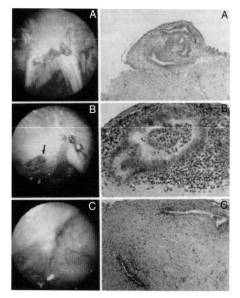

Plate 9.2 Peritoneal endometriosis subtypes (see Fig. 9.2 also). (A) Red endometriotic lesion at laparoscopy: numerous glands with active epithelium and abundant stroma on the peritoneal surface. (B) Typical black endometriotic lesion: combination of glands, stroma, and intraluminal debris. (C) White endometriotic lesion: occasional retroperitoneal glandular structures and scanty stroma. Reproduced from Nisolle and Donnez [3] with permission from Elsevier.

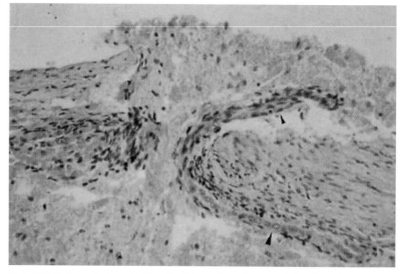

Plate 9.3 Continuum between the flat cells of the ovarian surface mesothelium (M) and the endometrioma-type epithelium (E) of the endometrioma (stain, Gomori's trichrome, original magnification, ×410). Reproduced from Nisolle and Donnez [3] with permission from Elsevier.

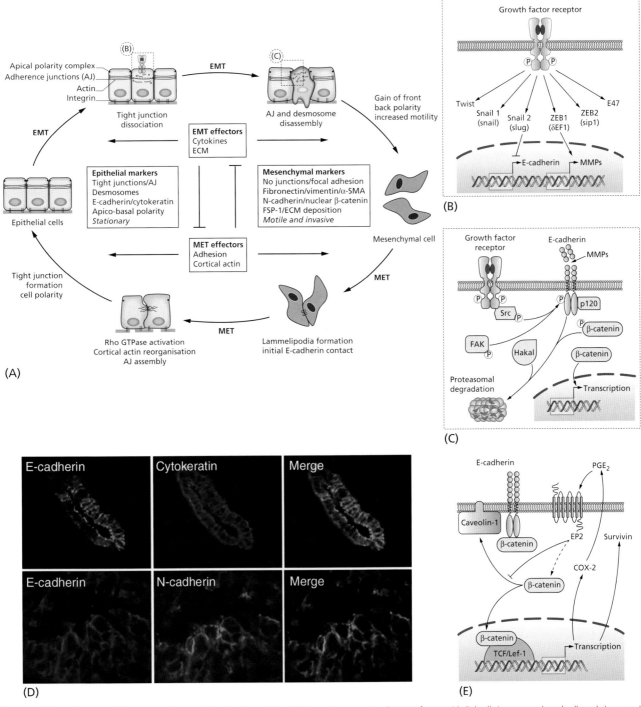

Plate 11.1 Signaling events in the onset and progression of endometriosis. (A) The cyclic progression that transforms epithelial cells into mesenchymal cells and vice versa in different contexts of development and pathology. The different stages during EMT (epithelial-mesenchymal transition) and the reverse process MET (mesenchymal-epithelial transition) are regulated by effectors of EMT and MET, which influence each other. Important events during the progression of EMT and MET are the regulation of tight junctions and adherence junctions. (B) A variety of transcription factors are activated through growth factor receptor stimulation leading to E-cadherin repression and induction of proinvasive genes like MMPs. (C) Destabilization of the E-cadherin/β-catenin complex by either phosphorylation of E-cadherin or β-catenin through Src and/or FAK targets phospho-E-cadherin or phospho-β-catenin to proteasomal degradation mediated by Hakai. In the absence of β-catenin phosphorylation, the cytoplasmic β-catenin is stabilized and modulates the transcription of proinvasive genes. α-SMA, α-smooth muscle actin; FSP-1, fibroblast-specific protein 1. Adapted from [95,173,174]. (D) Loss of E-cadherin expression and gain of N-cadherin expression, markers indicative of EMT, in deep infiltrating endometriotic lesions. The E-cadherin-negative but N-cadherin- and cytokeratin-positive endometriotic cells represent the subpopulation of endometriotic cells with an invasive phenotype in vitro [71]. (E) The role of PGE$_2$ in the stabilization of nuclear β-catenin activity by an EP2 receptor-dependent mechanism. Cytoplasmic β-catenin is sequestered to the plasma membrane in a complex with E-cadherin in the presence of caveolin-1, thereby suppressing nuclear β-catenin/TCF/Lef-1 activity. PGE$_2$ signaling through its receptor EP2 suppresses the ability of caveolin-1 to sequester β-catenin to the plasma membrane and induces the expression of β-catenin/TCF/Lef-1 target genes, including COX-2 and survivin. The resulting COX-2-PGE$_2$ feedback amplification loop might play an important role in endometriosis progression. Adapted from Rodriguez et al [105] with permission from the American Society for Microbiology.

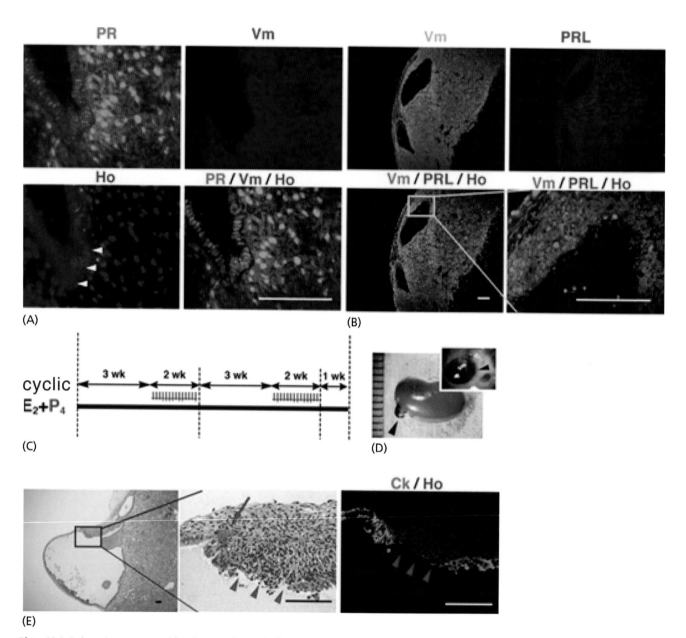

Plate 12.1 Endometrium reconstructed from human endometrial cells transplanted beneath the kidney capsule resembles endometriosis lesions and responds to hormones and hormone withdrawal. (A) Estrogen-treated NOG mice show upregulation of progesterone receptor (PR) in glands and vimentin-positive (Vm) stroma. (B) Estrogen + progesterone-treated mice show production of the decidual marker prolactin (PRL). (C) Hormonal treatment regime for induction of menstruation-like tissue breakdown and shedding shown (D) macroscopically and (E) microscopically in H&E and by immunofluorescence. The arrow shows hemorrhage in the stroma, the arrowheads, loss of epithelial layer. Reproduced from Masuda *et al* [35] with permission from National Academy of Sciences.

miRNA Regulatory Functions During Endometriosis Lesion Development

1: Adhesion and Wounding

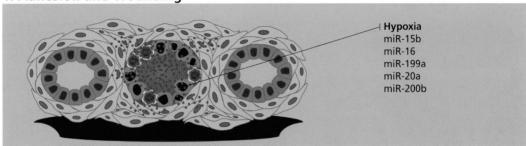

Hypoxia
miR-15b
miR-16
miR-199a
miR-20a
miR-200b

2: Inflammation

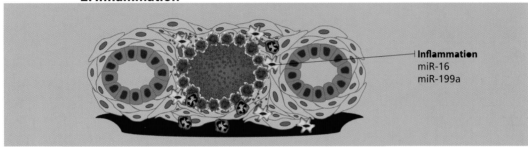

Inflammation
miR-16
miR-199a

3: Tissue Remodelling

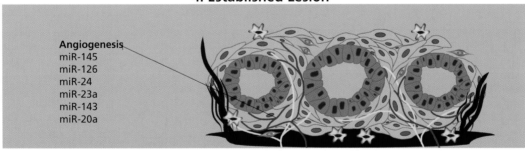

Cell Proliferation
miR-125a, miR-125b,
miR-143, miR-126,
miR-145, miR-20a,
miR-221, miR-222,
miR- 26a

Extracellular Matrix
Remodelling
miR-29c

Tissue Repair
miR-200b
miR-200c
miR -141
miR-21
miR-1
miR-194

4: Established Lesion

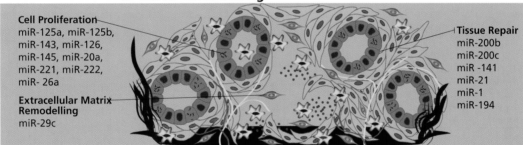

Angiogenesis
miR-145
miR-126
miR-24
miR-23a
miR-143
miR-20a

Legend

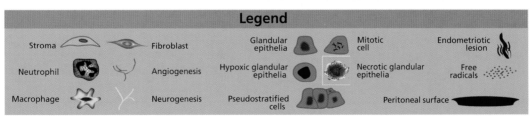

Stroma — Fibroblast — Glandular epithelia — Mitotic cell — Endometriotic lesion

Neutrophil — Angiogenesis — Hypoxic glandular epithelia — Necrotic glandular epithelia — Free radicals

Macrophage — Neurogenesis — Pseudostratified cells — Peritoneal surface

Plate 17.1 A model of miRNA regulation during endometriotic lesion development. In our proposed model for endometriotic lesion development at an ectopic site, displaced endometrial tissue in retrograde menstrual fluid progresses through a process of attachment and wounding, inflammation, tissue remodeling and lesion establishment. miRNA expression may play a role in these processes, regulating transcripts involved in hypoxia, inflammation, tissue repair, cellular proliferation, extracellular matrix remodeling and angiogenesis.

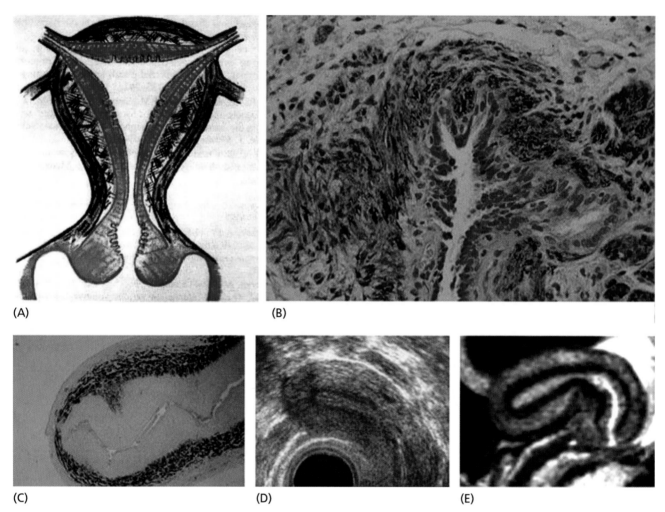

(A)   (B)

(C)   (D)   (E)

Plate 20.1 (A) A schematic representation of the endometrial-subendometrial unit ("archimetra") within the human uterus based on immunocytochemical results and the morphological and ontogenetic data. The endometrial-subendometrial unit is composed of the glandular (*green*), stromal part of the endometrium and the stratum subvasculare of the myometrium with predominantly circular muscular fibers (*orange*). Ontogenetically, the unit is derived from the paramesonephric ducts (*green*) and their surrounding mesenchyme (*orange*). The bulk of the human myometrium does not originate from the paramesonephric ducts (*blue*). It consists of the stratum vasculare with a three-dimensional meshwork of short muscular bundles and the stratum supravasculare with predominantly longitudinal muscular fibers. The stratum vasculare is the phylogenetically most recent acquisition and, in contrast to the endometrial-subendometrial unit, both the stratum vasculare and supravasculare develop late during ontogeny. The stratum vasculare and supravasculare surround the uterine corpus and extend caudally only to the uterine isthmus. There is a transitory zone within the stratum vasculare adjacent to the stratum subvasculare where muscular fibers of the two layers blend (light orange margin of the stratum vasculare). The endocervical mucoasa is the most caudal structure derived from the paramesonephric ducts. The underlying circular muscular fibers, which progressively diminish in the caudal direction, and the accompanying connective tissue blend with vaginal tissue elements (*red*) to form the vaginal portion of the cervix. (B) A peritoneal endometriotic lesion (×400) as an ectopic "microarchimetra." With endometrial glands, endometrial stroma and peristromal muscular tissue, the lesion is composed of all elements of the archimetra. (C) The primordial uterus in the 23rd week of pregnancy (×50) is composed of the elements of the archimetra, such as endometrium and archimyometrium (specific actin staining) . The archimetra is essentially the adult representation of the primordial uterus. (D) The "halo" in transvaginal sonography represents the archimyometrium, as does the "junctional zone" in MR imaging (E). Transvaginal sonography (TVS) and magnetic resonance imaging (MRI) of the uterus of a 29-year-old woman unaffected with endometriosis and adenomyosis. Sagittal scans of the uterine midline are shown. The myometrial-endometrial lining is sharp and smooth; the "halo" in TVS and the "junctional zone" in MRI are unaltered; there is symmetry with respect to the anterior and posterior myometrial walls and the texture of the myometrium in TVS appears to be homogenous. Modfied from Leyendecker *et al* [25] with permission from Wiley-Blackwell.

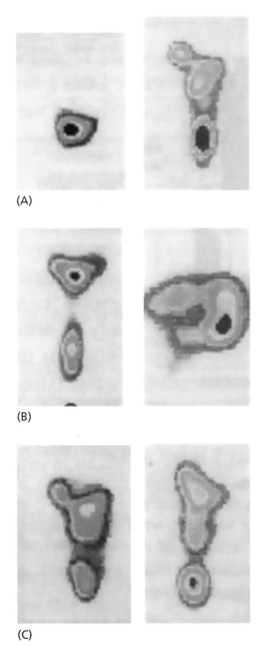

(A)

(B)

(C)

Plate 20.2 Representative scans obtained from hysterosalpingiscintigraphy in women without (*left panel*) and with (*right panel*) endometriosis 32 min following application of technetium-labeled macrospheres of sperm size in the posterior fornix of the vagina in six different women in the (A) early follicular, (B) midfollicular and (C) late follicular phases of the menstrual cycle. In normal women with normoperistalsis, the particles usually remain at the site of application during the early follicular phase (A, *left panel*). In women with endometriosis and hyperperistalsis, there is in this phase a massive transport of the particles through the uterine cavity in one of the tubes (A, *right panel*). In the midfollicular phase, normal women show only ascendance of the particles into the uterine cavity and sometimes a trend of ascendance into the tube ispsilateral to the dominant follicle (B, *left panel*). In women with endometriosis, the ascendance dramatically increases and in this example the particles are transported through the tube into the peritoneal cavity. This was, however, the contralateral tube to the dominant follicle (B, *right panel*). During the preovulatory phase in healthy women, the particles are rapidly transported into the "dominant" tube (C, *left panel*) while, due to dysperistalsis, there is a breakdown of directed sperm transport in women with endometriosis (C, *right panel*). These scans show the enormous power of the uterine peristaltic pump during the early and midfollicular phases of the cycle in women with hyperperistalsis and endometriosis. Continuous hyperperistalsis results in autotraumatization of the uterus. Modified from Kunz *et al* [8] and Leyendecker *et al* [20] with permission from Oxford University Press.

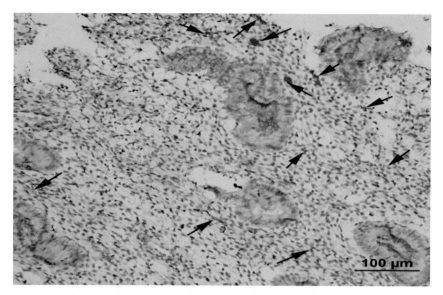

Plate 21.1 Nerve fibers stained for PGP9.5 in the functional layer of endometrium from a woman with endometriosis.

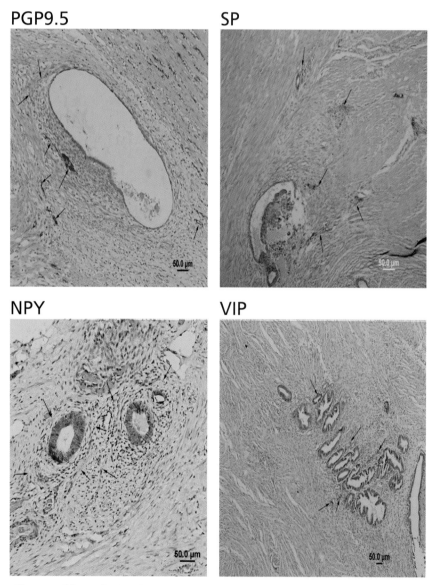

PGP9.5

SP

NPY

VIP

Plate 21.2 Nerve fibers stained for PGP9.5 (all nerve fibers), SP (sensory fibers), NPY (mainly sympathetic fibers) and VIP (mainly parasympathetic fibers) in peritoneal endometriosis (×200). Nerve fibers, stained with Fast Red, indicated by arrows.

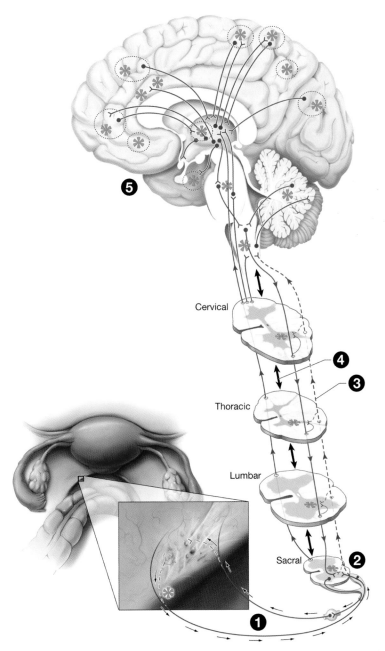

Plate 22.1 This figure illustrates how endometrial lesions can engage the nervous system to give rise to different types of pain associated with endometriosis and co-morbid conditions. **Part 1:** This part of the diagram depicts the laparoscopic view of pelvic organs in which a deeply infiltrating lesion on the left uterosacral ligament is expanded in the inset. Both peptidergic sensory (*blue*) and sympathetic nerve fibers (*green*) sprout axon branches (*red dashed lines*) from nerve fibers that innervate nearby blood vessels to innervate this lesion. Sensory fibers that sprouted new axons become sensitized (*red asterisk*). The extent of sensitization is dynamically modulated by estradiol and sympathetic-sensory coupling. **Part 2:** Two-way connection between innervated lesions and spinal cord is concentrated within sacral segments of the pelvic region. Sensitized peripheral nerve fibers, in turn, sensitize spinal sacral segment neurons. This "central sensitization," shown by the red asterisk in the sacral segment, can become independent of and is modulated differently from peripheral sensitization, described in the text. **Part 3:** Although input from peripheral afferent fibers to the spinal cord via their dorsal roots is concentrated in the segment associated with the body part the fibers innervate (sacral segments, branches of the fibers extend to other segments (*blue dashed lines*). Normally, these dorsal root branches have minimal impact on neurons in other segments unless the fibers become sensitized. Such remote actions are depicted by red dashed branches into the lumbar, thoracic and cervical spinal cord dorsal horn and the red asterisks at those levels. **Part 4:** Normally, multiple intersegmental spinal connections exist to co-ordinate healthy bodily functions via excitatory and inhibitory synaptic connections, shown by double-arrowed black lines. This intersegmental communication can influence how central sensitization modifies how neurons in remote segments process nociceptive and non-nociceptive sensory information ("remote central sensitization"), shown as red asterisks. Together, actions in Parts 3 and 4 can lead to increased nociception not only at sacral entry segments but also in any other segment. **Part 5:** Multiple connections exist that ascend from every level of the spinal cord to the brain (*blue lines*) and descend from the brain to the spinal cord (*green lines*). Thus, in health, input from the spinal cord engages neurons throughout the brain that themselves are interconnected via complex ascending and descending inhibitory/excitatory synapses. Input from sensitized spinal neurons can affect activity throughout the neuroaxis, altering normal processing of nociceptive and non-nociceptive information. Some regions that can be influenced are depicted by red asterisks. Although asterisks are shown on the medial surface of the cortex, some influenced areas extend to parts of the lateral prefrontal, frontal, parietal lobes and within the temporal lobe (*dotted black ellipses*). These influences can become independent of peripheral sensitization associated with lesions' innervation (Part 1). Such actions provide mechanisms for different types of endometriosis-associated and co-morbid pain, not only in the pelvis but also elsewhere. Reproduced from Stratton and Berkley [7] with permission from Oxford University Press.

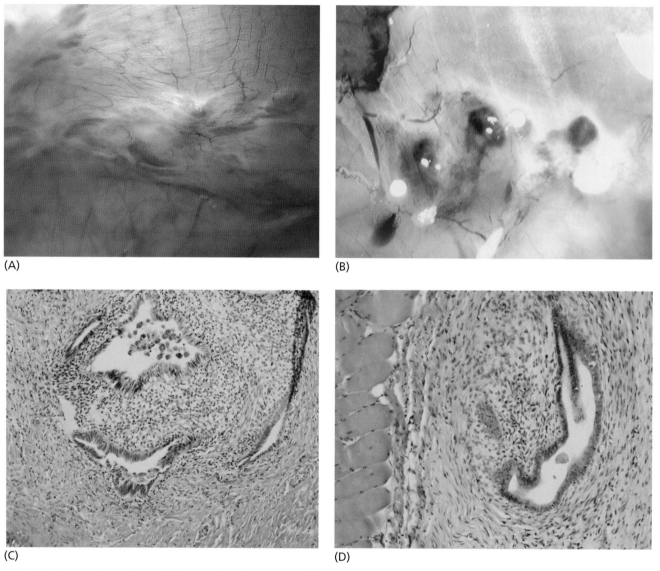

Plate 26.1 Gross morphology of human (A) (courtesy of Dr John A. Lucas, Vanderbilt University School of Medicine) and experimental endometriosis established by proliferative phase human endometrium in nude mice (B). Hematoxylin and eosin stains of human (C) and experimental endometriosis (D). Original magnification: ×15 (gross) and ×200 (microscopic).

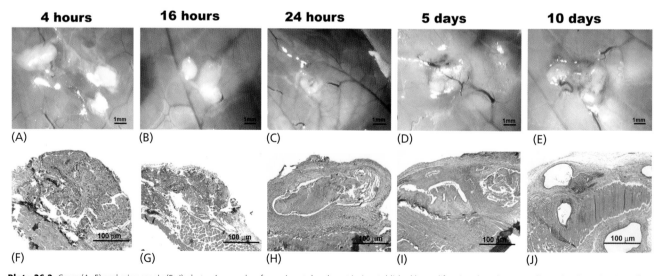

Plate 26.2 Gross (A–E) and microscopic (F–J) photomicrographs of experimental endometriosis established by proliferative phase human endometrium in nude mice. All mice were implanted with a slow-release estradiol capsule prior to introduction of human tissues. Mice were sacrificed 4 h to 10 days after human tissue injection. Original magnification: ×15 (gross) and ×40 (microscopic) (hematoxylin and eosin staining). Reproduced from Bruner-Tran et al [63] with permission from *The Endocrine Society*.

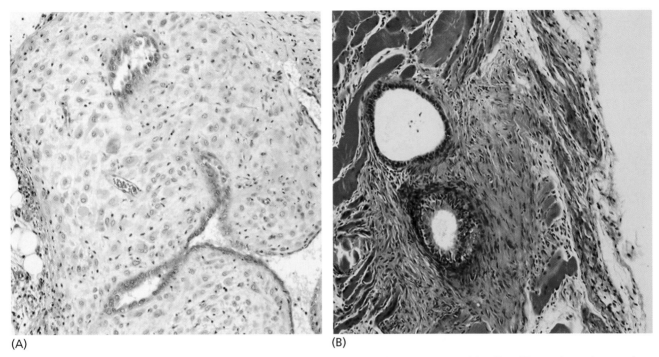

(A)

(B)

Plate 26.3 Hematoxylin and eosin stains of experimental endometriosis established by normal proliferative endometrium (A) and by proliferative phase endometrium from a patient with endometriosis (B). Ovariectomized mice were treated with estradiol (1 nM) and medroxyprogesterone acetate (100 mg/kg). Mice were sacrificed 10 days after human tissue injection.Original magnification, ×200.

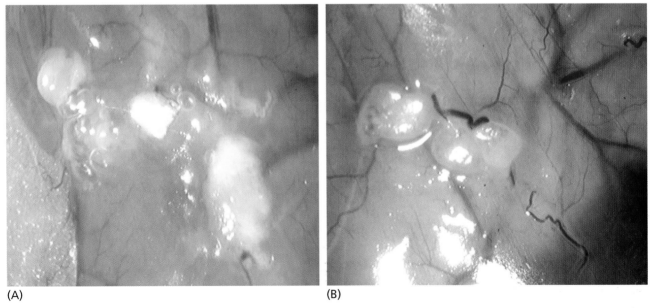

(A)

(B)

Plate 26.4 Gross morphology of experimental endometriosis established by proliferative phase normal endometrium (A) and proliferative phase eutopic endometrium from a patient with endometriosis (B). Mice were sacrificed 4 h after human tissue injection. Original magnification,×15.

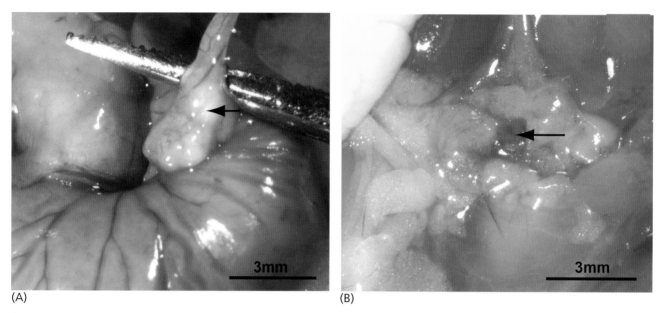

(A)   (B)

Plate 26.5 Gross morphology of experimental endometriosis established by proliferative phase normal endometrium. Tissues were injected into mice 5 days post ovariectomy (A) or less than 24 h post surgery (B). Note that lesion in (A) is well circumscribed and did not track to the site of surgical injury. The star-shaped lesion shown in (B) is much larger (6 mm × 6mm) and at the surgical site. Mice were sacrificed 5 days after human tissue injection. Original magnification,×15.

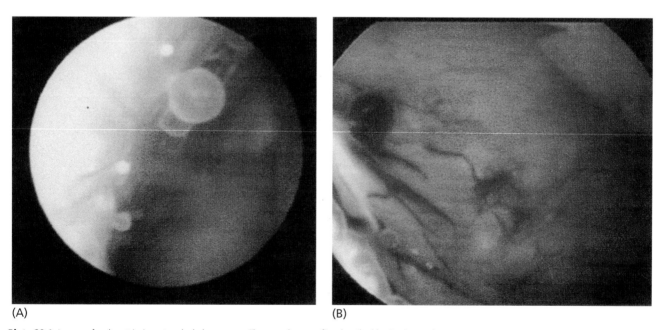

(A)   (B)

Plate 28.1 Images of endometriosis on transhydrolaparoscopy. The procedure was first described by Gordts *et al*.

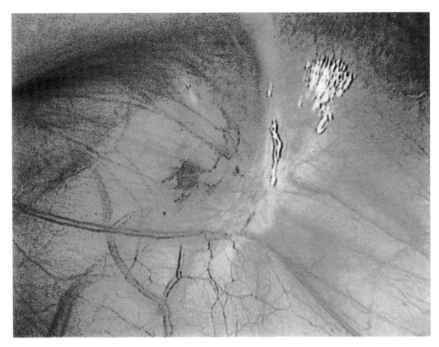

Plate 28.2 Laparoscopic view of non-typical endometriosis lesion.

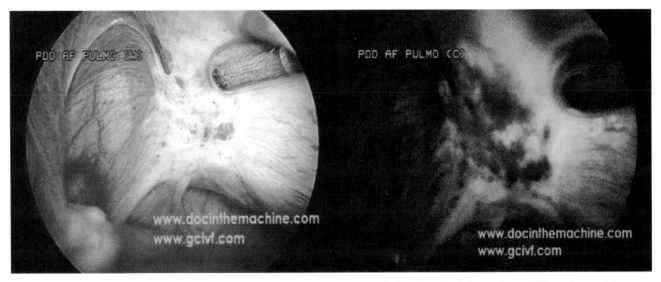

Plate 28.3 Differentiation between normal peritoneum and tissue harboring endometriosis can be further achieved with the use of a special filter to decrease light illuminating the tissue.

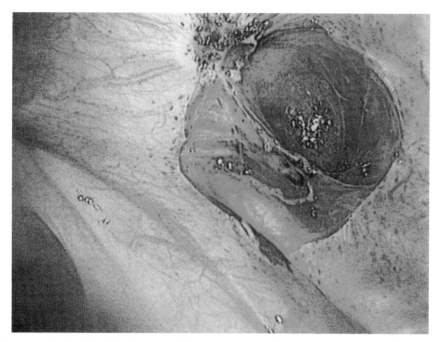

Plate 28.4 Deep endometriosis on the lateral pelvic wall has been excised. The tubular structure at the base of the excised peritoneum is the ureter.

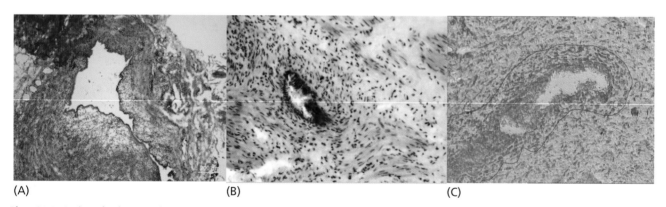

(A)   (B)   (C)

Plate 31.1 Histology of endometriotic lesions containing (A) sufficient or (B) insufficient endometrial tissue for laser capture. (C) A lesion undergoing laser capture in which the drawn line defines the area for capture. Photomicrographs were taken at different magnifications to best represent the images.

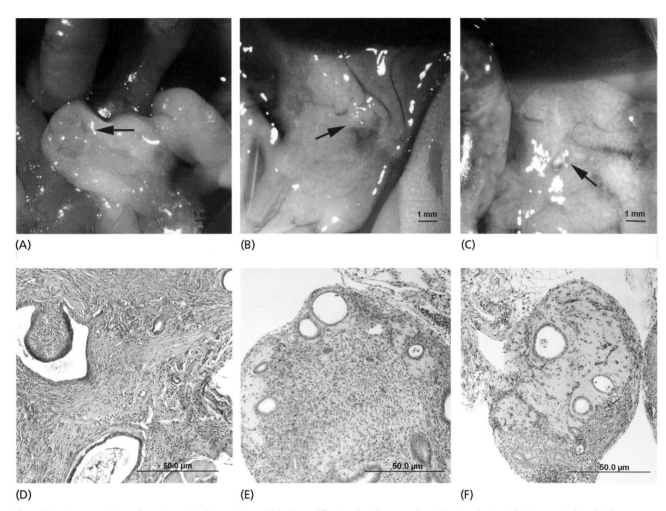

Plate 36.1 Gross morphology of experimental endometriosis established by proliferative phase human endometrium in nude mice. All mice were implanted with a slow-release estradiol capsule before introduction of human tissues. Mice were treated by gavage with vehicle (A), 5 mg/kg simvastatin (B), or 25 mg/kg simvastatin (C). (D–F) Hematoxylin and eosin stains of tissues from each treatment group (D, vehicle; E, 5 mg/kg simvastatin; F, 25 mg/kg simvastatin). Results are representative of three separate experiments using three different human biopsies. Original magnification: ✕100. *Arrows* point to endometrial implants. Reproduced from Bruner-Tran *et al* [71] with permission from the Endocrine Society.

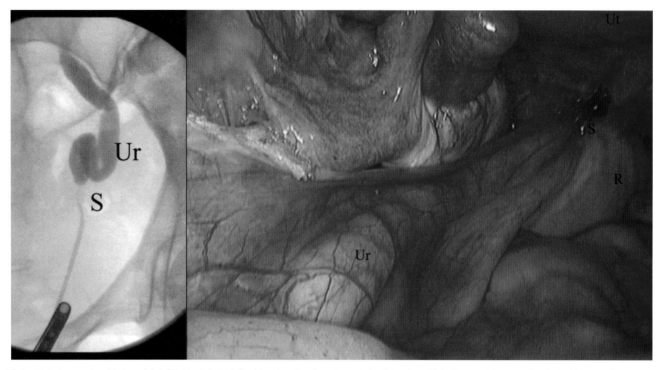

Plate 37.1 Deep endometriotic nodule infiltrating into the left pelvic sidewall and causing ureteric obstruction with hydroureter. Ur, ureter; S, stricture;Ut, uterus; R, rectum.

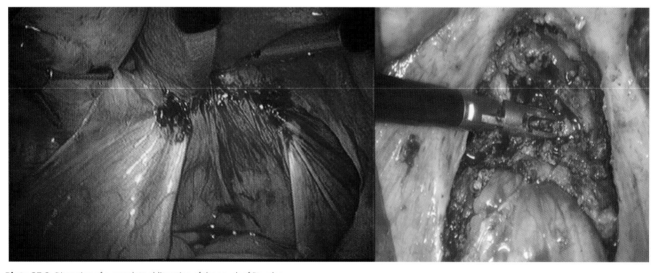

Plate 37.2 Dissection of a complete obliteration of the pouch of Douglas.

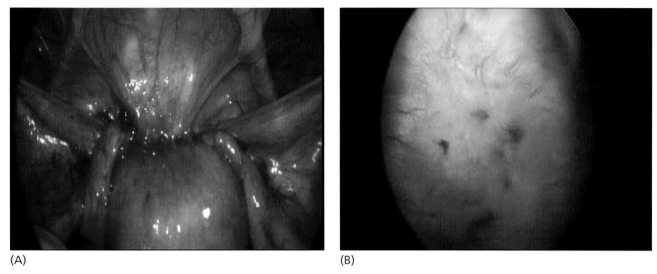

(A)   (B)

Plate 42.1 Bladder endometriotic nodule. (A) Laparoscopic view. (B) Cystoscopic view.

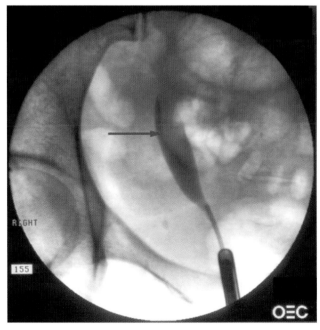

Plate 42.2 Retrograde uretogogram showing intrinsic ureteric lesion. Courtesy of Mr Dinesh Agarwal.

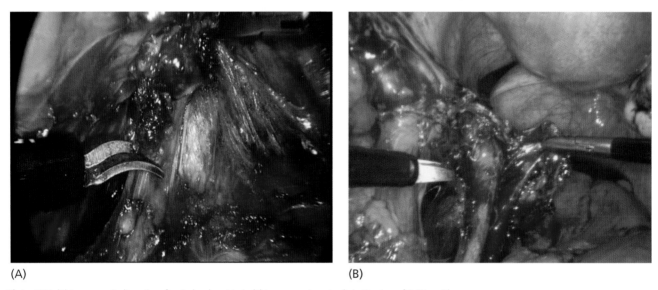

(A) (B)

Plate 42.3 (A) Laparoscopic dissection of vesical endometriosis. (B) Laparoscopic ureterolysis. Courtesy of Dr Weng Chan.

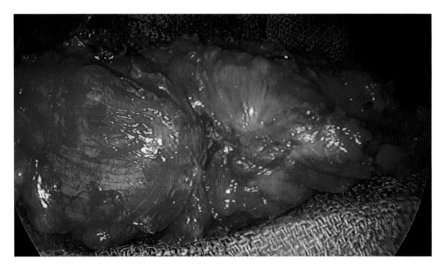

Plate 43.1 Segment of resected sigmoid colon with site of stricture due to endometriosis clearly visible.

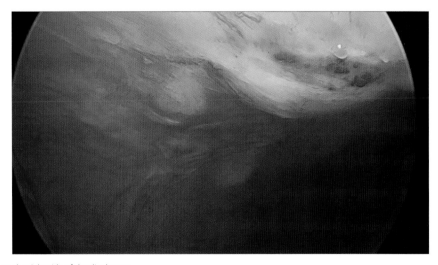

Plate 43.2 Endometriosis on the right side of the diaphragm.

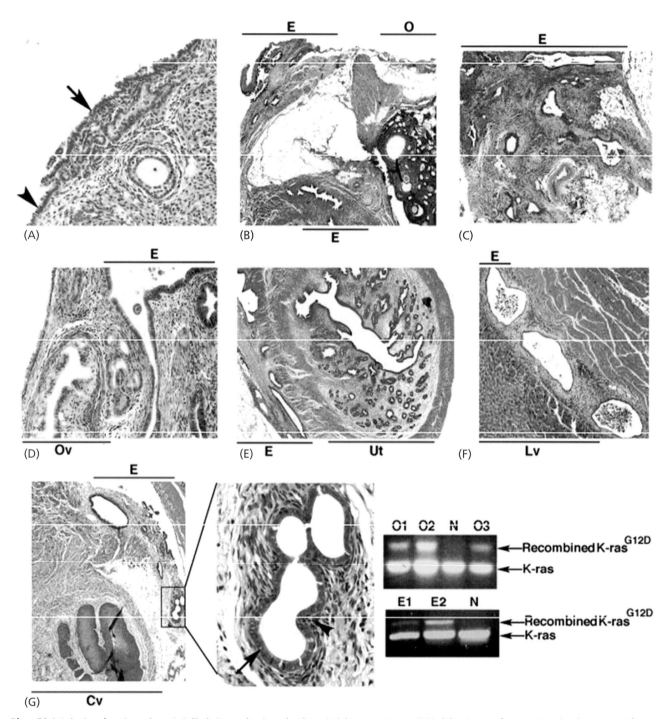

Plate 50.1 Induction of ovarian endometriotic-like lesions and peritoneal endometriosis by oncogenic K-rasG12D. (A) Activation of K-rasG12D within the ovarian surface epithelium (OSE) results in endometrioid glandular lesions (arrow); normal OSE is seen nearby (arrowhead). (B–G) Peritoneal endometriosis (E) in the soft tissue surrounding the ovary (O) (B), fat (C), on the surface of the oviduct (Ov) (D), uterus (Ut) (E), liver (Lv) (F), and cervix (Cv) (G). A higher magnification picture (G) shows the presence of both endometriotic epithelial glands (arrow) and stroma (arrowhead). (H) Cre-mediated recombination of K-rasG12D in ovarian endometriotic-like lesions (O1-O3), peritoneal endometriotic lesions (E1, E2), but not in control OSE (N) [19].

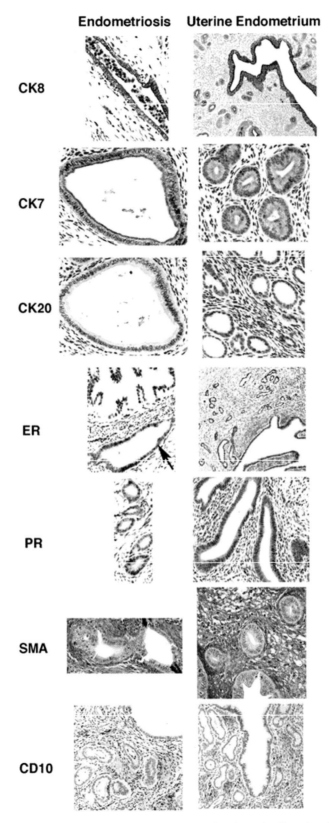

Endometriosis   Uterine Endometrium

CK8

CK7

CK20

ER

PR

SMA

CD10

Plate 50.2 Peritoneal endometriotic lesions and the uterine endometrium have a similar immunohistochemical profile. Both endometriotic and endometrial glands are positive for CK8, CK7, ER, PR, but not for CK20. Endometriotic stroma stains positively with endometrial-type stroma markers, SMA and CD10 [19].

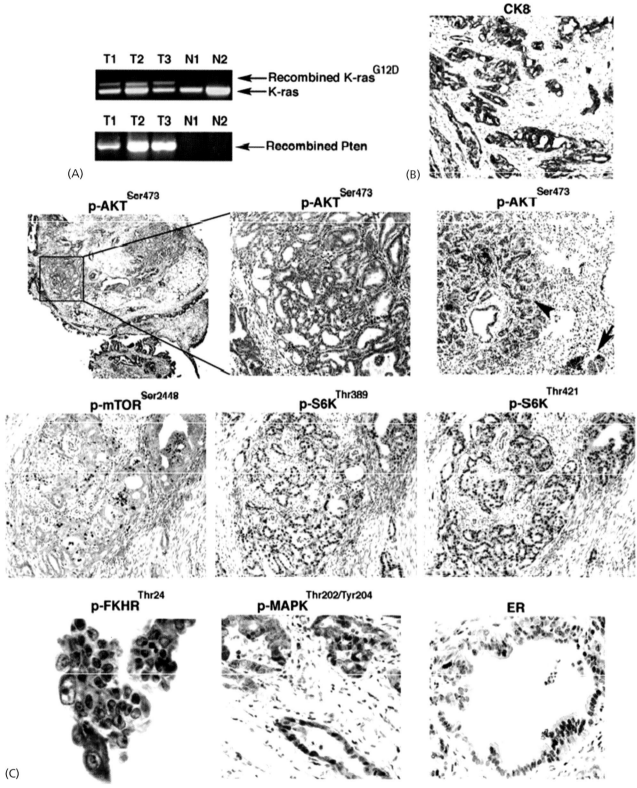

Plate 50.3 (A) Cre-mediated recombination of K-rasG12D and conditional deletion of Pten in tumors (T1-T3) isolated from AdCre-infected LSL-K-rasG12D/+; Ptenloxp/loxp (K-ras/Pten) mice; controls (N1, N2). (B,C) Immunohistochemical profile (CK8, PI3K/AKT/mTOR/FKHR and MAPK pathways, and ER) of primary ovarian tumors, peritoneal implants, and lung metastases in Cre-induced K-ras/Pten mice [19].

3   Disease Characterization

8

Endometriosis: Disease Classification and Behavior

G. David Adamson

Fertility Physicians of Northern California and Stanford University, Palo Alto, CA, USA

Introduction

Endometriosis remains an enigmatic disease. Our continued frustration in staging its clinical presentation and impact on associated pain and infertility reduces our ability to ameliorate its effect on millions of women. There are important reasons for staging endometriosis, or any other disease: to create a common language, to enable specificity of diagnosis, to standardize comparisons, and to facilitate research applications. The requirements of an ideal endometriosis classification system are that it: (1) be empirically and scientifically based, (2) enjoy general consensus, (3) have unambiguous definition of terms, (4) be comprehensive for all cases, (5) have a simple translation from anatomical feature to verbal description, (6) reflect disease, (7) predict fertility, (8) predict pain relief, (9) be useful to guide treatment, (10) indicate risk of recurrence, (11) identify clinical situations in which it does not apply, (12) be simple to calculate, and (13) be easy to communicate to patients. No such staging system has yet been developed for endometriosis. This chapter will address the behavior and symptoms of endometriosis and review some of the attempts at classifying endometriosis.

Classification systems of historical interest

In 1921 Sampson first classified endometriosis when he categorized hemorrhagic cysts and noted adhesions [1]. In 1927 he proposed his theory of retrograde menstruation. Subsequent classifications were based on histological criteria, anatomical presentation, histopathology and pain, clinical, anatomical and histopathological presentation, structure involvement or physical exam and surgical findings [2–6].

In 1973 Acosta proposed a system based on the site and distribution of lesions on the premise that severity determined the success of surgery [7]. There was more emphasis on adnexal adhesions as a fertility factor and recognition of the risk of the ovaries forming adhesions. Others proposed systems based on malignancy, lesions, site and distribution of lesions, laparoscopic findings, and therapy [8–13]. These systems were all criticized for multiple reasons, including their inability to predict clinical outcomes, especially pregnancy rates, in infertile patients.

American Fertility Society classification

In 1979 the American Fertility Society (AFS) first proposed a classification system which was flexible enough to describe any case, had an associated paper form to ensure complete documentation, was quantitative and so allowed for analysis, and had assigned cut-off points [14]. The AFS system was subsequently subjected to evaluation and critique by various authors, some of whom made suggestions for its improvement [15–18]. In 1982 Guzick used dose-response methodology to demonstrate that there was no correlation of pregnancy rates with severity following surgery and recommended a non-parametric monotonic estimate [19]. In 1982 Adamson utilized clustering techniques in an attempt to identify anatomical factors which predict pregnancy rates, but none were found [20]. Further recommendations were subsequently made to modify the AFS classification [21,22].

In 1985 the AFS revised the 1979 classification [23]. The new rAFS classification eliminated extensive disease stage, removed tubal endometriosis as a separate category, created a category for minimal disease, differentiated superficial and deep lesions of peritoneum and ovaries, required more detail for the adnexal adhesions, quantified filmy versus dense adhesions, considered posterior cul-de-sac obliteration to be severe disease, doubled the solitary adnexa score, and recorded additional pathology.

Endometriosis: Science and Practice, First Edition. Edited by Linda C. Giudice, Johannes L.H. Evers and David L. Healy.
© 2012 Blackwell Publishing Ltd. Published 2012 by Blackwell Publishing Ltd.

Limitations of the revised AFS system

Despite these revisions, the current rAFS system has serious limitations. First, it has an arbitrary scoring system in which the point scores do not reflect empirically derived relative weights, and the stage demarcation by point score is arbitrary with wide score ranges within the categories.

Second, there is potential for observer error. Endometriosis has many morphological presentations, including subtle and microscopic lesions [24–31]. Accuracy of documentation and identification of endometriomas can be problematic [32–33]. Staging can be affected by timing of laparoscopy and whether the staging is performed at laparoscopy or laparotomy [34,35].

Third, there is limited reproducibility of the staging. The correlation of intraobserver restaging has been reported to be only 0.38 and interobserver 0.52, with the greatest variation occurring in documenting the ovary and posterior cul-de-sac [36]. Only fair-to-good agreement has been reported and multiple lesion types in the same patient complicate staging [34,37].

Fourth, the rAFS system does not consider morphological lesion type or age-related evolution [38,39]. The association between gross and histopathological appearance as it relates to prostaglandin F production is not considered [30], nor is the association of morphology and pain [40], the three-dimensional aspect of lesions [26], and the possible appearance and disappearance of lesions [41].

Fifth, there is poor correlation between the extent of disease and pelvic pain. Some found no relationship between rAFS stage and pain [40,42,43]. Pelvic pain and dyspareunia have been associated with deeply invasive nodules, and pelvic pain has been correlated with penetration depth of lesions [43–46]. Pelvic pain and dyspareunia have also been correlated with severe dysmenorrhea in stage III and IV disease [47–49].

Sixth, the rAFS stages correlate poorly with infertility, except for extensive disease [50]. Lesion site and type do not predict pregnancy outcome and pregnancy rates have been determined not to differ according to stage [51–53]. Therefore, the current staging system does not effectively predict outcome of treatment [50].

Behavior and symptoms

Lesions

Endometriosis implants are peritoneal surface lesions of a few millimeters to 20 mm in diameter and are encapsulated by adhesions or fibrotic tissue, which pucker the typically bluish gray, dark brown or black "powder burn" lesions. In addition to their varying colors, which result from hemolyzed blood from ectopic endometrium, they vary considerably in their gross organic presentation. Small, new lesions may occur as clusters of nodules resembling hemorrhagic vesicles. Other implants may appear as clear, non-pigmented or light brown vesicles or as reddish polyps, white scar tissue or plaques, petechiae, or flame-like lesions – and all types may occur in the same patient. White, scarred peritoneum or pigmented lesions characterize late-stage endometriosis. Endometriosis foci may appear at the base of adhesions that result from chronic peritoneal surface irritation by the implants. Two-thirds of peritoneal pockets contain endometriosis around the rim or inside the defect [54,55]. Inexperienced laparoscopists may overlook or miss subtle lesions [31].

Implants may infiltrate the broad ligament, giving rise to endometriosis and red adhesions from the uterosacral ligaments to the ovary and fallopian tube. Black and red disease, sometimes associated with scarring, are easily seen. Disease may become deeply invasive and nodular, producing a reactive, inflammatory response in surrounding tissues and, consequently, more extensive and dense adhesions with potential cul-de-sac obliteration.

Endometriotic cysts usually are in the ovary. Superficial ovarian implants are irregularly shaped and variously pigmented and occur on the lateral and inferior surfaces. Upon cyst formation, cyclic hemorrhage within causes cyst growth because of slow reabsorption of the old blood content. Such "chocolate cysts" contain thick, tarry, dark brown fluid. With increase of intracystic pressure, endometriomas tend to rupture and leak irritating, hemosiderin macrophage content. Dense adhesion formation typically occurs at the rupture site, extending to adjacent organs and rendering surgical removal of the cyst difficult.

Histopathological analysis of endometrial tissue reveals endometrial glands and endometrial stroma as well as fibrosis and hemorrhage. Most endometriosis implants do not exhibit the typical cyclic histology seen in normal endometrium [56]. Endometriotic cyst walls are often lined with fibrous tissue of cuboidal epithelium, they vary in thickness, and exhibit little or no menstrual cyclicity. Hemorrhage to surrounding tissues may result in fibrosis as well as deposits of hemosiderin macrophages or pseudoxanthoma cells. Because some hemorrhaging is typical in surgical excision, histological detail and, thus, histological confirmation of endometriosis is lost.

Endometriosis can cause various symptoms; however, none is pathognomonic for the disease. Although many affected patients are asymptomatic, those patients who are symptomatic complain most commonly of pelvic pain, infertility, and dysfunctional uterine bleeding. Other, less common symptoms may occur from endometriosis implants in atypical sites.

Pelvic pain

Pelvic pain is the most common presenting symptom of endometriosis, occurring in approximately 80% of patients [57]. It may occur at any time in the menstrual cycle and is variously described as backache, rectal pressure, constant lower abdominal ache, and severe cramping. Pain most probably results from anatomical distortion and fixation of pelvic structures caused by fibrosis. Prostaglandin and histamine release may exacerbate pain symptoms, and in the absence of anatomical distortion, irritation from small implants in critical locations or deeply infiltrating implants [44] may cause disabling pain. In contrast, large endometriomas can be asymptomatic.

Dysmenorrhea is a classic symptom of endometriosis. Pain may radiate into the vagina, thighs or perineum. The onset usually occurs before the onset of menstruation and gradually improves over several days after initiation of flow. The severity and duration of the pain can vary from cycle to cycle. Antiprostaglandin therapy may reduce dysmenorrhea symptoms although the role of prostaglandins is uncertain.

Dyspareunia is also common in endometriosis patients. It is usually associated with implants of the uterosacral ligament, rectovaginal septum, upper vagina or posterior cul-de-sac and is worse during menstruation. A patient with a fixed, retroverted uterus and notable pelvic adhesions may experience pain with deep penetration. Vercellini *et al*, however, reported the severity of deep dyspareunia as inversely related to the stage of endometriosis [43].

The generally diffuse pelvic pain of dyschezia, which may result from endometriosis on or near the rectum or from adhesions, might be overlooked by a patient. The physician should inquire about the cyclic occurrence of painful bowel movements.

Infertility

The incidence of endometriosis in infertile women ranges from 4.5% to 33% (mean 14%) [58]. In comparison, the prevalence of endometriosis in women undergoing tubal ligation is 4.1% [59]. In one study, the reported incidence of endometriosis in infertile women and in fertile controls was 21% and 2%, respectively [60].

In the presence of adhesions or significant anatomical distortion, infertility may be caused by mechanical interference of oocyte pick-up and transport and altered tubal peristalsis. In the absence of anatomical distortion, the mechanism of subfertility associated with endometriosis implants alone is poorly understood. Several theories have been proposed: altered folliculogenesis, ovulatory dysfunction, sperm phagocytosis, impaired fertilization, defective implantation, inhibition of early embryo development, luteal-phase defects, and immunological alterations [61–71]. Chronic inflammatory peritoneal cavity changes are associated with increased peritoneal fluid volume and increased number, concentration and activity of macrophages [72–75]. The peritoneal fluid leukocytes may compromise fertility by exerting direct cytotoxic effects or by releasing cytokines and proteolytic enzymes into the pelvic milieu that affect gamete function or embryo growth.

Endometriosis implants alone may not cause infertility, and its association alone with subfertility is debated. Transplanted endometrium in laboratory animals reduced fertility only in the presence of adhesions [75–78]. Fertility was not adversely affected in the absence of pelvic distortion [79]. In women undergoing donor insemination, there was no difference in fecundity between those with endometriosis and those without [80]. Other investigators, however, have found lower fecundity in women with endometriosis undergoing donor insemination [81]. A multivariate study of potential infertility factors in a large cohort of infertile women revealed no change in the cumulative conception rate from endometriosis in the absence of adhesions [82].

Dysfunctional uterine bleeding

Abnormal uterine bleeding has frequently been associated with endometriosis [83]. However, many cases of bleeding can be attributed to co-existent pathology rather than true dysfunctional uterine bleeding (DUB). The available data are insufficient to conclude that endometriosis causes DUB [15,84].

Other symptoms

In addition to bowel implants that can cause rectal bleeding or obstruction, endometriosis can be located in the bladder, causing suprapubic pain, frequency, urgency, dysuria, and hematuria. Ureteral involvement may cause upper urinary tract symptoms such as flank pain or backaches. Pulmonary involvement can result in pleuritic pain, pleural effusion, cough, hemoptysis, or pneumothorax [85]. In patients with upper abdominal or shoulder pain, diaphragmatic endometriosis should be considered [86]. Cyclic headaches or seizures may indicate brain lesions [87]. Sciatica has been reported from endometriosis in the retroperitoneal space [88]. Some symptoms, such as pain or bowel obstruction, may persist (despite castration or menopause), usually from scarring or adhesions.

Potential synergies in the development of an improved classification system

Many potential modifications to the current rAFS classification system have been suggested (Table 8.1) [25,26,34,41,46,50,53,89–125]. The most significant improvement would probably result from a basic research breakthrough in endometriosis or in some aspect of general medicine that affects endometriosis, for example the role of genetics, angiogenesis, immunology and/or endocrinology in endometriosis. Imaging enhancements such as visual quantification of graphic pelvic mapping, computer technology for image storage, and three-dimensional endoscopic visualization might also result in an improved system. Furthermore, there is some hope that biological markers might some day enhance the ability of classification systems to be of clinical value [126].

It is likely that some complex combination of modifications is necessary to develop the ideal endometriosis classification system. Since such a classification system has eluded both basic and clinical scientists for decades, we report in this chapter a different approach to developing a system for fertility patients that has just been published: collect clinical data prospectively, utilize outcomes assessment for infertility, do comprehensive statistical analysis of the data and derive a new staging system from the data rather than from *a priori* assumptions. This new staging system has been validated prospectively and modified to optimize the staging system [127].

The purpose of our study was to develop a useful clinical tool (the Endometriosis Fertility Index or EFI) that predicts pregnancy rates in patients with surgically documented endometriosis who attempt non-*in vitro* fertilization (IVF) conception. The following methods were used. Data were prospectively collected at the time of surgery on a standardized form. The prospectively collected detailed clinical and surgical data on 579 consecutive infertile endometriosis patients were used to create a database with hundreds of variables [50]. The data

Table 8.1 Potential modifications to the rAFS (1985) staging system.

Classification	Reference(s)	Classification	Reference(s)
Anatomical factors		**Histological factors**	
Stage V for extensive (≥71) disease	[50,89]	Histological evaluation	[25,26,94–97]
Size, type, location, presentation	[52,90,91]		
Increase endometrioma score, omit adhesions	[46]		
Red versus black endometriomas	[90]		
Internal size of endometriomas	[91]		
Peritoneal fluid volume	[92]		
Type of active lesion	[41]		
Ovarian adhesions	[93]		
Tubal status	[94,95]		
Biomarkers		**Imaging findings**	
CA-125 levels	[97–100]	MR imaging	[110–114]
Prostaglandin $F_2\alpha$, PGE_2, C3c, C4 cytokines, TNF-2	[101]	Ultrasound findings	[115]
Interleukins	[93]	Radiological, ultrasound, pathological correlation	[116]
C-myc protooncogene polypeptide	[102]		
β3 Integrin	[103]	**Other**	
Immune markers	[104–108]	Pain classification system	[118]
Angiogenesis markers	[107]	Research classification	[34]
Peritoneal fluid evaluation	[92,101,109]	Premenstrual spotting	[119]
Other biomarkers	[126]	Additional confounding variables	[50,120]
Genes		Effectiveness of IVF	[121]
Genetic markers	[117]	Response to treatment	[122]
		Revised classification systems	[53,123–125]

IVF, *in vitro* fertilization; MR, magnetic resonance; PGE, prostaglandin E; TNF, tumor necrosis factor.

were then analyzed by sophisticated statistical analysis including life table survival and Cox proportional hazards regression analysis to identify those factors most predictive of pregnancy. Patients were censored from the study when they were lost to follow-up, became pregnant, had subsequent surgery for endometriosis, ovarian suppression medications or underwent assisted reproductive technologies. Preliminary analyses addressed the importance of groups of variables for predicting pregnancy and then evaluated alternative ways of combining the variables within groups. The main groups of variables were historical factors, results of hysteroscopy, and results of abdominal surgery. Subsequent analyses combined the most predictive variables and established a simple scoring system, the EFI. After developing the EFI, the same data were prospectively collected on 222 additional consecutive patients, the EFI calculated on each patient, and pregnancy rates predicted prospectively.

The historical factors evaluated in preliminary analyses included age, duration of infertility, and pregnancy history, which have repeatedly been shown to be predictive of subsequent pregnancy [50]. Many additional historical factors were

evaluated, including factors relating to the male partner, previous endometriosis treatment, and results of diagnostic tests.

The results of abdominal surgery were recorded in substantial detail, allowing for the comparison of three prospective operative coding systems: (1) rAFS total, lesion, adhesion, and cul-de-sac scores, (2) percentage of filmy and dense adhesions on the ovaries and tubes bilaterally, and (3) intraoperative pre- and post-treatment functional score. The functional score was determined by the surgeon for each tube, fimbria and ovary bilaterally where 0 = absent or non-functional; 1, 2, and 3 = severe, moderate, and mild dysfunction, respectively; and 4 = normal with respect to the capacity of the organ/structure to effect its purpose in the reproductive process (Plate 8.1). This means the ability of the tube to move over the ovary, to be the passage for the sperm from the uterus, to provide the early environment for the egg and embryo, and to enable transport of the embryo to the uterus; the fimbria to move over the ovary and to pick up an egg; and the ovary to house eggs, develop follicles, ovulate eggs, and allow them to be picked up by the fimbria. These three intraoperative scoring systems were considered supplements to the historical factors that were found to predict pregnancy rates: age, duration of infertility, and pregnancy history. It should be emphasized that the least function (LF) score is determined at the completion of the surgical intervention, not before. It therefore represents an estimate of functionality after the surgical intervention. Two-tailed *P*-values less than 0.05 were considered statistically significant.

The LF score determined intraoperatively following surgical intervention was a statistically significant predictor of fertility even after controlling for AFS total score and years infertile. The predictive power of the LF score after controlling for the AFS total score and years infertile demonstrates that the LF score measures something different from the AFS total score, presumably the postoperative functionality of the reproductive organs. There was high correlation between both adhesions and tubes and the LF score, and moderate correlation between filmy adhesions alone and the LF score.

The only variables that achieved statistical significance were duration of infertility, prior pregnancy with partner, LF score and uterine abnormality, the last being the least significant with a *P*-value of 0.04. These variables, together with alternative pregnancy history variables and various AFS scores, were considered for creation of the numerically simple EFI. Details are given in Plate 8.1. The EFI score ranges from 0 to 10 with 0 representing the poorest prognosis and 10 the best prognosis. Half of the points come from the historical factors and half from the surgical factors. The prospective testing of the EFI on 222 additional patients produced excellent results, showing a good correlation of predicted and actual outcomes for all stages of endometriosis. The estimated cumulative percent pregnant by value of the EFI score, based on all 801 patients, is presented graphically in Figure 8.1.

To assess the effect on the EFI of potential differences in the assignment of the LF scores by different surgeons, a sensitivity analysis was performed. The EFI, which changes only when the LF score category changes, only changed a little over 15% of the time: 4.2% of the time higher and 11.2% of the time lower. In only 5.4% of the cases was the EFI changed by more than 1 point. In practice, changes in the EFI are material only for the middle values, and knowing that the tendency is for the EFI to change downward, and only slightly, in the presence of uncertainty in the LF scores allows that to be taken into account clinically.

The EFI is useful only for infertility patients who have had surgical staging of their disease. It is not intended to predict any aspect of endometriosis-associated pain. It is required that the male and female gametes are sufficiently functional to enable attempts at non-IVF conception. One factor found to predict pregnancy that is not included in the EFI is uterine abnormality. Severe uterine abnormality that is clinically significant is so uncommon in infertile endometriosis patients that it is not included in the EFI. However, when this condition is found, it does need to be taken into account in predicting pregnancy rates. Deficiencies in the reproductive function of the gametes or uterus will obviously affect the prognosis and must be considered separately as fertility factors, just as they would with any patient with any other type of disease.

The LF score is central to the EFI. Its incorporation is justified in part because it has predictive power even after controlling for the AFS total score and years infertile. There is an association between AFS scores and the LF score. This finding occurred because adhesions and lesions provide most of the points in the AFS scoring system and are consistent with the perspective that dense adhesions, especially ovarian, cul-de-sac obliteration and endometriomas, contribute to infertility. There was also high correlation between both adhesions and tubes and LF score, and moderate correlation between filmy adhesions alone and LF score. This quantifies and is consistent with the surgical perspective that adhesions, especially dense adhesions, reduce the ability of the fallopian tubes to function normally, thereby reducing pregnancy rates. This relationship persists even though the LF score is determined after surgical treatment is completed because it is more difficult to achieve a good surgical result when initially there is more severe disease.

A legitimate criticism can be made that the LF score is subjective for any given surgeon, and even more subjective among different surgeons. The LF score in fact is an extremely robust measure of pelvic reproductive potential with much less variability than one might think. The score is easy for most surgeons with any degree of experience to determine for each structure. A normal tube, fimbria or ovary is usually easy to distinguish and score. An absent or completely non-functional structure is similarly relatively easy to distinguish for the tube, fimbria or ovary. Therefore, even though the scoring system provides discrimination over five numbers, only three have much subjectivity to them. The ability for most surgeons to discriminate between these choices in most cases should be quite high because surgically these choices are relatively easy. Furthermore, since only the lowest score of the tube, fimbria or ovary is used in calculating the LF score, any variability in choosing the correct function score for each structure is in a sense averaged out over the three choices. Also, the least score from each side is added with the least score from the other side, again buffering total score from any variability in choosing the LF score for a particular structure. When the LF score is added in to the EFI as one component of it, any variability or error is further buffered. This is demonstrated by the sensitivity analysis, which showed that even with substantial variation in the assignment of functional scores, the EFI varies very little. Therefore, even though the LF score is the largest component of the EFI, and is associated with some subjectivity, it remains a very robust measure of future reproductive potential.

The absence of male factors in the EFI mandates that the male's ability to reproduce must be evaluated independently from the female and treated appropriately, if necessary. Pregnancy history is included in the EFI as any prior pregnancy with any partner, in part because it is simpler than the other choices (e.g. pregnancy with current partner, total pregnancies, elective pregnancy termination). Age cut-offs are consistent with pregnancy rate seen in IVF and non-IVF populations, supporting the general application of our population of patients. The influence of duration of infertility is also consistent with that found in other populations [127,128].

ENDOMETRIOSIS FERTILITY INDEX (EFI) SURGERY FORM

LEAST FUNCTION (LF) SCORE AT <u>CONCLUSION</u> OF SURGERY

Score		Description			Left	Right
4	=	Normal		Fallopian Tube	☐	☐
3	=	Mild Dysfunction				
2	=	Moderate Dysfunction		Fimbria	☐	☐
1	=	Severe Dysfunction				
0	=	Absent or Nonfunctional		Ovary	☐	☐

To calculate the LF score, add together the lowest score for the left side and the lowest score for the right side. If an ovary is absent on one side, the LF score is obtained by doubling the lowest score on the side with the ovary.

	Left		Right		LF Score
Lowest Score	☐	+	☐	=	☐

ENDOMETRIOSIS FERTILITY INDEX (EFI)

Historical Factors			Surgical Factors		
Factor	**Description**	**Points**	**Factor**	**Description**	**Points**
Age			**LF Score** ☐		
	If age is ≤ 35 years	2		If LF Score = 7 to 8 (high score)	3
	If age is 36 to 39 years	1		If LF Score = 4 to 6 (moderate score)	2
	If age is ≥ 40 years	0		If LF Score = 1 to 3 (low score)	0
Years Infertile			**AFS Endometriosis Score**		
	If years infertile is ≤ 3	2		If AFS Endometriosis Lesion Score is < 16	1
	If years infertile is > 3	0		If AFS Endometriosis Lesion Score is ≥ 16	0
Prior Pregnancy			**AFS Total Score**		
	If there is a history of a prior pregnancy	1		If AFS total score is < 71	1
	If there is no history of prior pregnancy	0		If AFS total score is ≥ 71	0
Total Historical Factors			**Total Surgical Factors**		

EFI = TOTAL HISTORICAL FACTORS + TOTAL SURGICAL FACTORS:

Historical		Surgical		EFI Score
☐	+	☐	=	☐

ESTIMATED PERCENT PREGNANT BY EFI SCORE

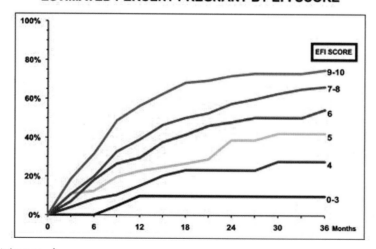

Figure 8.1 Endometriosis Fertility Index surgery form.

The EFI can be used to decide what type of treatment patients should undergo, for how long and at what cost before considering the assisted reproductive technologies (ART) following endometriosis surgery. It can be used to provide reassurance for many who have a good prognosis and to avoid wasted time and treatment for those with a poor prognosis. Since very few patients overall actually engage ART procedures, the EFI can bring major benefits to the vast majority of endometriosis patients who wish to have children.

American Association of Gynecologic Laparoscopists proposed endometriosis tabulation system

Previous endometriosis classification systems have failed to yield very useful insights about the disease, partly because they have had arbitrary divisions and scores which it was hoped might correlate with clinical management or prediction of treatment outcomes. For example, the rAFS classification system devotes most of its available points to adhesions, not endometriosis, and although peritoneal disease is the most common manifestation, only 10 points out of over 130 points are available for scoring peritoneal involvement.

The American Association of Gynecologic Laparoscopists (AAGL) proposed tabulation system is not a classification system but a new tabulation system that researchers and interested clinicians can use to document the morphology of endometriosis seen at surgery in their patients [128]. If the disease can be described accurately, then a clinically useful classification system may eventually be developed. If not, at least this tabulation system can more accurately gauge disease extent, which is important in evaluating results of treatment. This system is being developed with input from the world's leading experts in the research and surgical management of endometriosis. It contains the all the basic information thought to be important in quantifying the extent of disease in a patient. It is based on Excel, a commonly used spreadsheet with both Macintosh and PC versions, and can be expanded or simplified by end-users with facility in using Excel.

The interactive spreadsheet contained in "AAGLEndoTab" allows entry of administrative and clinical data on almost 1000 patients. As each patient is entered, the program automatically computes totals for each patient row as well as grand totals for all patient columns. Basic statistical calculations are offered, including ranges, sums, averages, and standard deviations. The data can be exported to a more robust statistical package for more in-depth analysis. This system is under development.

The AAGL system is quite comprehensive and the surgical data entry is intuitive. Operative laparoscopy is not required. Meticulous surgeons might actually use a measuring device, while others may make a snap clinical judgment. As long as the method of determination is consistent for each surgeon, qualified interpretations can be made with either method. Similarly, judgment on what constitutes "thick" or "filmy" adhesions is left to the surgeon's judgment.

ENZIAN classification system

European endometriosis experts have recently proposed a system based on clinical presentation, histology, localization, and extent of disease [129,130]. This system's future role and relationship to other classification systems are yet to be determined.

Conclusion

Multiple systems have been proposed for classifying endometriosis. Unfortunately, none has met with much success because of their inability to meet recognized clinical needs. However, the Endometriosis Fertility Index (EFI) is a simple, robust, and validated clinical tool that predicts pregnancy rates for patients following surgical staging of endometriosis. The EFI should be very useful in developing treatment plans in infertile endometriosis patients. It is hoped that further prospective validation by other clinical investigators will encourage widespread application of the EFI to the benefit of their patients. Further efforts by the AAGL and other investigators to develop tabulation and staging systems that will help predict outcomes for endometriosis patients with pelvic pain for both surgical and non-surgical treatment will hopefully bring additional value to the management of our patients.

References

1. Sampson JA. Perforating hemorrhagic (chocolate) cysts of ovary: their importance and especially their relation to pelvic adenomas of endometriotic type ("adenomyoma" of the uterus, rectovaginal septum, sigmoid, etc.). Arch Surg 1921;3:245–261.
2. Wicks MJ, Larsen CP. Histologic criteria for evaluating endometriosis. Nortwest Med 1949;48:611–614.
3. Huffman JW. External endometriosis. Am J Obstet Gynecol 1951;62:1243–1252.
4. Norwood GE. Sterility and fertility in women with pelvic endometriosis. Clin Obstet Gynecol 1960;3:456–471.
5. Riva HL, Kawasaki DM, Messinger AJ. Further experience with norethynodrel in treatment of endometriosis. Obstet Gynecol 1962;19:111–117.
6. Beecham CT. Classification of endometriosis. Obstet Gynecol 1966;28:437.
7. Acosta AA, Buttram VC Jr, Besch PK et al. A proposed classification of pelvic endometriosis. Obstet Gynecol 1973;42:19–25.
8. Mitchell GW, Farber M. Medical versus surgical management of endometriosis. In: Reid DE, Christian CD (eds) Controversy in Obstetrics and Gynecology. Philadelphia: WB Saunders, 1974, p. 69.
9. Dmowski WP, Cohen MR. Treatment of endometriosis with an antigonadotropin, Danazol: a laparoscopic and histologic evaluation. Obstet Gynecol 1975;46:147–154.

10. Kistner RW, Siegler AM, Behrman SJ. Suggested classification for endometriosis: relationship to infertility. Fertil Steril 1977;28:1008–1010.

11. Ingersoll FM. Selection of medical or surgical treatment of endometriosis. Clin Obstet Gynecol 1977;20:849–864.

12. Buttram VC Jr. An expanded classification of endometriosis. Fertil Steril 1978;30:240–242.

13. Cohen MR. Laparoscopy and the management of endometriosis. J Reprod Med 1979;23:81–84.

14. American Fertility Society. Classification of endometriosis. Fertil Steril 1979;32:633–634.

15. Buttram VC Jr. Conservative surgery for endometriosis in the infertile female: a study of 206 patients with implications for both medical and surgical therapy. Fertil Steril 1979;31:117–123.

16. Hasson HM. Classification for endometriosis. Fertil Steril 1981;35:368–369.

17. Andrews WC. Classification of endometriosis. Fertil Steril 1981;35:124–125.

18. Rock JA, Guzick DS, Sengos C et al. The conservative surgical treatment of endometriosis: evaluation of pregnancy success with respect to the extent of disease as categorized using contemporary classification systems. Fertil Steril 1981;35:131–137.

19. Guzick DS, Bross DS, Rock JA. Assessing the efficacy of the American Fertility Society's classification of endometriosis: application of a dose-response methodology. Fertil Steril 1982;38:171–176.

20. Adamson GD, Frison L, Lamb EJ. Endometriosis: studies of a method for the design of a surgical staging system. Fertil Steril 1982;38:659–666.

21. Buttram VC Jr. Evolution of the revised American Fertility Society classification of endometriosis. Fertil Steril 1985;43:347–350.

22. Candiani GB. The classification of endometriosis: historical evolution, critical review and present state of the art. Acta Eur Fertil 1986;17:85–92.

23. American Fertility Society. Revised American Fertility Society classification of endometriosis. Fertil Steril 1985;43:351–352.

24. Martin DC, Hubert GD, Vander Zwaag R et al. Laparoscopic appearances of peritoneal endometriosis. Fertil Steril 1989;51:63–67.

25. Nisolle M, Paindaveine B, Bourdon A et al. Histologic study of peritoneal endometriosis in infertile women. Fertil Steril 1990;53:984–988.

26. Donnez J, Nisolle M, Casanas-Roux F. Three-dimensional architectures of peritoneal endometriosis. Fertil Steril 1992;57:980–983.

27. Vasquez G, Cornillie F, Brosens IA. Peritoneal endometriosis: scanning electron microscopy and histology of minimal pelvic endometriotic lesions. Fertil Steril 1984;42:696–703.

28. Murphy AA, Green WR, Bobbie D et al. Unsuspected endometriosis documented by scanning electron microscopy in visually normal peritoneum. Fertil Steril 1986;46:522–524.

29. Jansen RP, Russell P. Nonpigmented endometriosis: clinical, laparoscopic, and pathologic definition. Am J Obstet Gynecol 1986;155:1154–1159.

30. Vernon MW, Beard JS, Graves K et al. Classification of endometriotic implants by morphologic appearance and capacity to synthesize prostaglandin F. Fertil Steril 1986;46:801–806.

31. Stripling MC, Martin DC, Chatman DL et al. Subtle appearance of pelvic endometriosis. Fertil Steril 1988;49:427–431.

32. Candiani GB, Vercellini P, Fedele L. Laparoscopic ovarian puncture for correct staging of endometriosis. Fertil Steril 1990;53:994–997.

33. Vercellini P, Vendola N, Boccioline L et al. Reliability of the visual diagnosis of ovarian endometriosis. Fertil Steril 1991;56:1198–1200. Comment in: Fertil Steril 1992;58:221–222; discussion 223–224.

34. Canis M, Bouquet de Jolinieres J, Wattiez A et al. Classification of endometriosis. Baillière's Clin Obstet Gynaecol 1993;7:759–774.

35. Lin SY, Lee RK, Hwu YM et al. Reproducibility of the revised American Fertility Society classification of endometriosis using laparoscopy or laparotomy. Int J Gynaecol Obstet 1998;60:265–269.

36. Hornstein MD, Gleason RE, Orav J et al. The reproducibility of the revised American Fertility Society classification of endometriosis. Fertil Steril 1993;59:1015–1021.

37. Rock JA. The revised American Fertility Society classification of endometriosis: reproducibility of scoring. ZOLADEX Endometriosis Study Group. Fertil Steril 1995;63:1108–1110.

38. Redwine DB. The distribution of endometriosis in the pelvis by age groups and fertility. Fertil Steril 1987;47:173–175.

39. Redwine DB. Age-related evolution in color appearance of endometriosis. Fertil Steril 1987;48:1062–1063.

40. Vercellini P, Boccioline L, Vendola N et al. Peritoneal endometriosis. Morphologic appearance in women with chronic pelvic pain. J Reprod Med 1991;36:533–536.

41. Wiegerinck MA, van Dop PA, Brosens IA. The staging of peritoneal endometriosis by the type of active lesion in addition to the revised American Fertility Society classification. Fertil Steril 1993;60:461–464.

42. Fedele L, Parazzini F, Bianchi S et al. Stage and localization of pelvic endometriosis and pain. Fertil Steril 1990;53:155–158. Comment in: Fertil Steril 1990;54:180–181.

43. Vercellini P, Trespidi L, de Giorgi O et al. Endometriosis and pelvic pain: relation to disease stage and localization. Fertil Steril 1996;65:299–304.

44. Cornillie FJ, Oosterlynck D, Lauwerysn JM et al. Deeply infiltrating pelvic endometriosis: histology and clinical significance. Fertil Steril 1990;53:978–983.

45. Ripps BA, Martin DC. Correlation of focal pelvic tenderness with implant dimension and stage of endometriosis. J Reprod Med 1992;37:620–624.

46. Koninckx PR, Meuleman C, Demeyere S et al. Suggestive evidence that pelvic endometriosis is a progressive disease, whereas deeply infiltrating endometriosis is associated with pelvic pain. Fertil Steril 1991;55:759–765.

47. Fedele L, Bianchi S, Boccioline L et al. Pain symptoms associated with endometriosis. Obstet Gynecol 1992;79:767–769.

48. Muzii L, Marana R, Pedulla S et al. Correlation between endometriosis-associated dysmenorrhea and the presence of typical or atypical lesions. Fertil Steril 1997;68:19–22.

49. Stovall DW, Bowser LM, Archer DF et al. Endometriosis–associated pelvic pain: evidence for an association between the stage of disease and a history of chronic pelvic pain. Fertil Steril 1997;68:13–18.

50. Adamson GD, Hurd SJ, Pasta DJ et al. Laparoscopic endometriosis treatment: is it better? Fertil Steril 1993;59:35–44.

51. Kurata S, Ishimaru T, Masuzaki H et al. Relationship between the prognosis of conception and the location of pelvic involvement in the endometriosis: significance of the TOP (tube, ovary, peritoneum) classification. Asia Oceania J Obstet Gynaecol 1993;19:391–399.

52. Palmisano GP, Adamson GD, Lamb EJ. Can staging systems for endometriosis based on anatomic location and lesion type predict pregnancy rates? Int J Fertil Menopausal Stud 1993;38:241–249.

53. Guzick DS, Silliman NP, Adamson GD et al. Prediction of pregnancy in infertile women based on the American Society of Reproductive Medicine's revised classification of endometriosis. Fertil Steril 1997;67:822–829.

54. Chatman DL, Zbella EA. Pelvic peritoneal defects and endometriosis: further observations. Fertil Steril 1986;46:711–714.

55. Redwine DB. Peritoneal pockets and endometriosis: confirmation of an important relationship, with further observations. J Reprod Med 1989;34:270–272.

56. Metzger DA, Olive DL, Haney AF. Limited hormonal responsiveness of ectopic endometrium: histologic correlation with intrauterine endometrium. Hum Pathol 1988;19:1417–1424.

57. Pittaway DE. Diagnosis of endometriosis. Infertil Reprod Med Clin North Am 1992;3:619.

58. Pauerstein C. Clinical presentation and diagnosis. In: Schenken RS (ed) Endometriosis: Contemporary Concepts in Clinical Management. Philadelphia: JB Lippincott, 1989.

59. Eskenazi B, Warner ML. Epidemiology of endometriosis. Obstet Gynecol Clin North Am 1997;24:235–258.

60. Strathy JH, Molgaard CA, Coulam CB et al. Endometriosis and infertility: a laparoscopic study of endometriosis among fertile and infertile women. Fertil Steril 1982;38:667–672.

61. Fakih H, Baggett B, Holtz G et al. Interleukin-1: a possible role in the infertility associated with endometriosis. Fertil Steril 1987;47:213–217.

62. Dmowski WP, Radwanska E, Binor Z et al. Mild endometriosis and ovulatory dysfunction: effect of danazol treatment on success of ovulation induction. Fertil Steril 1986;46:784–789.

63. Tummon IS, Maclin VM, Radwanska E et al. Occult ovulatory dysfunction in women with minimal endometriosis or unexplained infertility. Fertil Steril 1988;50:716–720.

64. Muscato JJ, Haney AJ, Weinberg JB. Sperm phagocytosis by human peritoneal macrophages: a possible cause of infertility in endometriosis. Am J Obstet Gynecol 1982;144:503–510.

65. Mahadevan MM, Trounson AO, Leeton JF. The relationship of tubal blockage, infertility of unknown cause, suspected male infertility, and endometriosis to success of in vitro fertilization and embryo transfer. Fertil Steril 1983;40:755–762.

66. Yovich JL, Yovich JM, Tuvik AI et al. In vitro fertilization for endometriosis. Lancet 1985;ii:552.

67. Grant A. Additional sterility factors in endometriosis. Fertil Steril 1966;17:514–519.

68. Damewood MD, Hesla JS, Schlaff WD et al. Effect of serum from patients with minimal to mild endometriosis on mouse embryo development in vitro. Fertil Steril 1990;54:917–920.

69. Taketani Y, Kuo T-M, Mizuno M. Tumor necrosis factor inhibits the development of mouse embryos co-cultured with oviducts: possible relevance to infertility associated with endometriosis. J Mamm Ovar Res 1991;8:175.

70. Pittaway DE, Maxson W, Daniell J et al. Luteal phase defects in infertility patients with endometriosis. Fertil Steril 1983;39:712–713.

71. Gilmore SM, Aksel S, Hoff C et al. In vitro lymphocyte activity in women with endometriosis – an altered immune response? Fertil Steril 1992;58:1148–1152.

72. Drake TS, Metz SA, Grunert GM et al. Peritoneal fluid volume in endometriosis. Fertil Steril 1980;34:280–281.

73. Dunselman G, Hendrix M, Bouckaert P et al. Functional aspects of peritoneal macrophages in endometriosis of women. J Reprod Fertil 1988;82:707–710.

74. Haney A, Muscato J, Weinberg J. Peritoneal fluid cell populations in infertility patients. Fertil Steril 1981;35:696–698.

75. Halme J, Becker S, Hammond M et al. Pelvic macrophages in normal and infertile women: the role of patent tubes. Am J Obstet Gynecol 1982;142:890–895.

76. Schenken RS, Asch RH, Williams RF et al. Etiology of infertility in monkeys with endometriosis: luteinized unruptured follicles, luteal phase defects, pelvic adhesions, and spontaneous abortions. Fertil Steril 1984;41:122–130.

77. Schenken RS, Asch RH. Surgical induction of endometriosis in the rabbit: effects on fertility and concentrations of peritoneal fluid prostaglandins. Fertil Steril 1980;34:581–587.

78. Kaplan CR, Eddy CA, Olive DL et al. Effects of ovarian endometriosis on ovulation in rabbits. Am J Obstet Gynecol 1989;160:40–44.

79. Dunselman GAJ, Dumoulin JCM, Land JA et al. Lack of effect of peritoneal endometriosis on fertility in the rabbit model. Fertil Steril 1991;56:340–342.

80. Chauhan M, Barratt CLR, Cooke SMS et al. Differences in the fertility of donor insemination recipients – a study to provide prognostic guidelines as to its success and outcome. Fertil Steril 1989;51:815–819.

81. Jansen RPS. Minimal endometriosis and reduced fecundability; prospective evidence from an artificial insemination by donor program. Fertil Steril 1986;46:141–143.

82. Dunphy BC, Kay R, Barratt CLR et al. Female age and the length of involuntary infertility prior to investigation and fertility outcome. Hum Reprod 1989;4:527–530.

83. Scott RB, te Linde RW. External endometriosis – the scourge of the private patient. Ann Surg 1950;131:697.

84. Soules MR, Malinak LR, Bury R et al. Endometriosis and anovulation: a coexisting problem in the infertile female. Am J Obstet Gynecol 1976;125:412–417.

85. Foster DC, Stern JL, Buscema J et al. Pleural and parenchymal pulmonary endometriosis. Obstet Gynecol 1981;58:552–556.

86. Nezhat C, Seidman D, Nezhat F et al. Laparoscopic surgical management of diaphragmatic endometriosis. Fertil Steril 1998;69:1048–1055.

87. Thibodeau LL, Prioleau GR, Manuelidis EE et al. Cerebral endometriosis: case report. J Neurosurg 1987;66:609–610.

88. Denton RO, Sherrill JD. Sciatic syndrome due to endometriosis of sciatic nerve. South Med J 1955;48:1027–1031.

89. Canis M, Pouly JL, Wattiez A et al. Incidence of bilateral adnexal disease in severe endometriosis (revised American Fertility Society [AFS], stage IV): should a stage V be included in the AFS classification? Fertil Steril 1992;57:691–692.

90. Brosens I, Donnez J, Benagiano G. Improving the classification of endometriosis. Hum Reprod 1993;8:1792–1795.

91. Brosens IA. Endoscopic exploration and classification of the chocolate cysts. Hum Reprod 1994;9:2213–2214.

92. Syrop CH, Halme J. A comparison of peritoneal fluid parameters of infertile patients and the subsequent occurrence of pregnancy. Fertil Steril 1986;46:631–635.

93. Murakami T, Okamura C, Matsuzaki S et al. Prediction of pregnancy in infertile women with endometriosis. Gynecol Obstet Invest 2002;5:26–32.

94. Fujishita A, Khan KN, Masuzaki H et al. Influence of pelvic endometriosis and ovarian endometrioma on fertility. Gynecol Obstet Invest 2002;53 Suppl 1:40–45.

95. Brosens I. Pelvic endometriosis: some pathophysiological and clinical conditions. Rev Med Suisse Romande 1992;112:787–792.

96. Mettler L, Schollmeyer T, Lehmann-Willenbrock E et al. Accuracy of laparoscopic diagnosis of endometriosis. JSLS 2003;7:15–18.

97. Barbieri RL, Niloff JM, Bast RC Jr et al. Elevated serum concentrations of CA-125 in patients with advanced endometriosis. Fertil Steril 1986;45:630–634.

98. Pittaway DE, Rondinone D, Miller KA et al. Clinical evaluation of CA-125 concentrations as a prognostic factor for pregnancy in infertile women with surgically treated endometriosis. Fertil Steril 1995;64:321–324.

99. Lanzone A, Marana R, Muscatello R et al. Serum CA-125 levels in the diagnosis and management of endometriosis. Gynecol Endocrinol 1992;6:265–269.

100. Fedele L, Arcaini L, Vercellini P et al. Serum CA 125 measurements in the diagnosis of endometriosis recurrence. Obstet Gynecol 1988;72:19–22.

101. Badawy SZ, Cuenca V, Marshall L et al. Cellular components in peritoneal fluid in infertile patients with and without endometriosis. Fertil Steril 1984;42:704–708.

102. Schenken RS, Johnson JV, Riehl RM. c-myc protooncogene polypeptide expression in endometriosis. Am J Obstet Gynecol 1991;164:1031–1036; discussion 1036–1037.

103. Lessey BA, Castelbaum AJ, Sawin SW et al. Aberrant integrin expression in the endometrium of women with endometriosis. J Clin Endocrinol Metab 1994;79:643–649.

104. Rier SE, Yeaman GR. Immune aspects of endometriosis: relevance of the uterine mucosal immune system. Semin Reprod Endocrinol 1997;15:209–220.

105. Olive DL, Montoya I, Riehl RM et al. Macrophage-conditioned media enhance endometrial stromal cell proliferation in vitro. Am J Obstet Gynecol 1991;164:953–958.

106. Surrey ES, Halme J. Effect of platelet-derived growth factor on endometrial stromal cell proliferation in vitro: a model for endometriosis? Fertil Steril 1991;56:672–679.

107. Smith SK. Vascular endothelial growth factor and the endometrium. Hum Reprod 1996;11 Suppl 2:56–61.

108. Halme J, Mathur S. Local autoimmunity in mild endometriosis. Int J Fertil 1987;32:309–311.

109. Spuijbroek MD, Dunselman GA, Menheere PP et al. Early endometriosis invades the extracellular matrix. Fertil Steril 1992;58:929–933.

110. Zawin M, McCarthy S, Scoutt L et al. Endometriosis: appearance and detection at MR imaging. Radiology 1989;171:693–696.

111. Sugimura K, Takemori M, Sugiura M et al. The value of magnetic resonance relaxation time in staging ovarian endometrial cyst. Br J Radiol 1992;65:502–506.

112. Tanaka YO, Itai Y, Anno I et al. MR staging of pelvic endometriosis: role of fat-suppression T1-weighted images. Radiat Med 1996;14:111–116.

113. Thomassin I, Bazot M, Detchev R et al. Symptoms before and after surgical removal of colorectal endometriosis that are assessed by magnetic resonance imaging and rectal endoscopic sonography. Am J Obstet Gynecol 2004;190:1264–1271.

114. Zanardi R, del Frate C, Zuiani C et al. Staging of pelvic endometriosis based on MRI findings versus laparoscopic classification according to the American Fertility Society. Abdom Imaging 2003;28:733–742.

115. Roseau G, Dumontier I, Palazzo L et al. Rectosigmoid endometriosis: endoscopic ultrasound features and clinical implications. Endoscopy 2000;32:525–530.

116. Woodward PJ, Sohaey R, Mezzetti TP Jr. Endometriosis: radiologic-pathologic correlation. Radiographics 2001;21:193–216; questionnaire 288–294.

117. Kennedy S. The genetics of endometriosis. J Reprod Med 1998;43 (3 Suppl):263–268.

118. American Society for Reproductive Medicine. Management of endometriosis in the presence of pelvic pain. Fertil Steril 1993;60:950–951.

119. Jansen RP. Endometriosis symptoms and the limitations of pathology-based classification of severity. Int J Gynaecol Obstet 1993;40 Suppl:S3–S7.

120. Forman RG, Robinson JN, Mehta Z et al. Patient history as a simple predictor of pelvic pathology in subfertile women. Hum Reprod 1993;8:53–55.

121. Olivennes F, Feldberg D, Liu HC et al. Endometriosis: a stage-by-stage analysis – the role of in vitro fertilization. Fertil Steril 1995;64:392–398.

122. Lockhat FB, Emembolu JO, Konje JC. The evaluation of the effectiveness of an intrauterine–administered progestogen (levonorgestrel) in the symptomatic treatment of endometriosis and in the staging of the disease. Hum Reprod 2004;19:179–184.

123. Schenken RS, Guzick DS. Revised endometriosis classification: 1996. Fertil Steril 1997;67:815–816.

124. Roberts CP, Rock JA. The current staging system for endometriosis: does it help? Obstet Gynecol Clin North Am 2003;30:115–132.

125. Hunault CC, Habbema JDF, Eijkemans MJC et al. Two new prediction rules for spontaneous pregnancy leading to live birth

among subfertile couples, based on the synthesis of three previous models. Hum Reprod 2004;19(9):2019–2026.

126. Giudice LC, Telles TL, Lobo S et al. The molecular basis for implantation failure in endometriosis: on the road to discovery. Ann NY Acad Sci 2002;955:252–264.

127. Adamson GD, Pasta DJ. Endometriosis Fertility Index: the new, validated endometriosis staging system. Fertil Steril 2010;94(5):1609–1615.

128. Endometriosis Classification Committee, Ad Hoc Committee of the AAGL. AAGL Endometriosis Tabulation System. 2007. AAGL. Cypress, California, USA.

129. Tuttlies F, Keckstein J, Ulrich U et al. ENZIAN-score, a classification of deep infiltrating endometriosis. Zentralbl Gynakol 2005;127:275–281.

130. Tuttlies F. ENZIAN-Klassifikation zur kiskussion gestellt: eine neue differnezierte klassifikation der tief infiltrierenden endo-metriose. J Gynakol Endokrinol 2008;2:6–13.

9 Peritoneal, Ovarian, and Rectovaginal Endometriosis are Three Different Entities

Jacques Donnez, Olivier Donnez, Jean-Christophe Lousse and Jean Squifflet

Department of Gynecology, Université Catholique de Louvain, Institut de Recherche Expérimentale et Clinique, Brussels, Belgium

Introduction

Because of the difference in site, possible origin, pathogenesis, appearance and hormone responsiveness, we have suggested since 1996 that peritoneal, ovarian, and rectovaginal endometriosis are three distinct entities [1–3]. Peritoneal endometriosis can be explained by the transplantation theory. Coelomic metaplasia of invaginated epithelial inclusions may be responsible for the development of ovarian endometriosis. The rectovaginal endometriotic lesion is an adenomyotic nodule whose histopathogenesis is not related to implantation of regurgitated endometrial cells, but to either metaplasia of müllerian remnants located in the rectovaginal septum or metaplasia of the retrocervical area.

The goal of this chapter is to describe the "three entities" theory and share with readers our arguments supporting this hypothesis.

Peritoneal endometriosis

Pathogenesis

Retrograde menstruation

Several theories relating to the pathogenesis of endometriosis have been proposed since its first detailed description in 1860 by von Rokitansky [4]. The most widely accepted theory, the transplantation theory, was proposed in 1927 by Sampson [5], who observed that endometrial cells regurgitated through the fallopian tubes during menstruation, with subsequent implantation and growth on the peritoneum (Fig. 9.1).

The transplantation theory hinges upon the assumption that retrograde menstruation takes place and that viable endometrial cells reach the abdominal cavity and implant. Although Sampson based his theory essentially on clinical and anatomical observations rather than experimental data, a large body of evidence has grown up over the years to make this a very plausible explanation. It has been demonstrated that retrograde menstruation is a common event in women with patent fallopian tubes. Halme *et al* [6] obtained peritoneal fluid (PF) by laparoscopy during the perimenstrual period, and blood was found in 90% of patients with patent tubes. Sampson's transplantation theory is also substantiated by the distribution of lesions in the peritoneal cavity [7] and demonstration of the viability of shed menstrual endometrium in tissue culture [6,8,9]. This theory is further corroborated by the high prevalence of pelvic endometriosis in girls with müllerian anomalies and subsequent menstrual outflow obstruction [10]. Moreover, menstrual periods are often longer and heavier in women with endometriosis [10–12] and cycles tend to be shorter [13].

Although retrograde menstruation occurs in most cycling women with patent tubes [6], clinical endometriosis develops in only 10–15% of women during their reproductive life. Additional factors that increase susceptibility to endometriosis must therefore exist and remain to be identified. The development of peritoneal endometriotic lesions involves a whole series of events, starting with the survival of refluxed endometrial cells and evasion of the immune surveillance system, adhesion of these cells to the peritoneum, invasion of the mesothelial lining and degradation of the underlying extracellular matrix (ECM), proliferation, resistance to apoptosis and, finally, generation of neovascularization [14–16] (see Fig. 9.1).

Evading the immune surveillance system

Menstrual effluent in the pelvic cavity could spur an inflammatory response that may result in the release of diverse chemoattractants, such as MCP-1 and regulated on activation, normal T-cell expressed and secreted (RANTES) chemokine, that recruit large numbers of polymorphonuclear neutrophils and, subsequently, phagocytic and

Endometriosis: Science and Practice, First Edition. Edited by Linda C. Giudice, Johannes L.H. Evers and David L. Healy.
© 2012 Blackwell Publishing Ltd. Published 2012 by Blackwell Publishing Ltd.

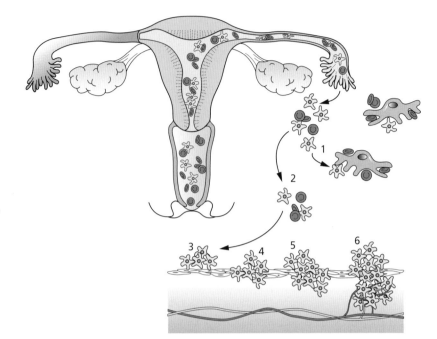

Figure 9.1 The retrograde transplantation theory. During menses, endometrial tissue and erythrocytes are retrogradely shed through the fallopian tubes into the peritoneal cavity. (1), Endometrial tissue fragments evade the immune surveillance system (peritoneal macrophages particularly) (2), adhere to the peritoneum (3), invade the peritoneal mesothelial lining (4), proliferate (5) and acquire a blood supply (6), leading to macroscopic peritoneal endometriotic lesion development. Reproduced from Lousse *et al* [15] with permission from Elsevier.

chemotactic leukocytes from the circulation [17–20]. The physiological role of the inflammatory response is to clear ectopic cells and tissue from the abdomen. This system appears to be effective in most women, although microscopic or minimal peritoneal lesions, termed "subtle lesions," are probably intermittently present in all women with patent fallopian tubes and menstrual cycles (Plate 9.1) [21].

In women who develop endometriosis, this "cleaning" system may be overwhelmed or simply inefficient. Anomalies in the peritoneal environment that alter the cellular and humoral immune system, natural killer (NK) cells, macrophages, peritoneum or local hormone concentrations may indeed result in deficient defense processes [15,16,22].

The eutopic endometrium of women with endometriosis has been shown to be more resistant to lysis by NK cells than the eutopic endometrium of controls [23]. It has been postulated that lymphocytes can adhere to endometrial cells through the lymphocyte function-associated antigen-1 (LFA-1)–intercellular adhesion molecule-1 (ICAM-1)-dependent pathway and make them a target for NK cells. Soluble forms of ICAM-1 secreted by PF endometrial and endometriotic cells can also bind to LFA-1-presenting lymphocytes and possibly prevent recognition of endometrial cells by these lymphocytes and subsequent NK cell-mediated cytotoxicity [24].

Endometrial cell adhesion to the peritoneum

The exact mechanism of endometrial cell adhesion to peritoneum is not known and cannot be studied *in vivo* in women. Therefore, interaction between human endometrium and peritoneum has essentially been studied in various *in vitro* models using amniotic membranes [25,26], autologous peritoneum [27–30] or autologous monolayered mesothelial cell cultures [31–34] as a model for pelvic peritoneum.

It has been reported that peritoneal mesothelium acts as a barrier preventing attachment of ectopic endometrium, and it has

been suggested that peritoneal damage is required for adhesion of endometrial fragments [25,26]. However, other investigators have observed that endometrium can attach to the intact mesothelial surface of the peritoneum in *in vitro* and experimental models [28,29,35]. Endometrial cell adhesion to mesothelial cells is a rapid process, occurring within 1 h of co-culture [29], and proliferative, secretory, and menstrual endometrium all attach to peritoneum in a similar manner [30]. Although both endometrial epithelial cells (EECs) and endometrial stromal cells (ESCs) were found to adhere to peritoneal mesothelial cells (PMCs) in monolayer culture [36], previous studies have demonstrated that ESCs in particular are involved in the initial attachment process [29,30,33,35].

Cell adhesion molecules (CAMs) are transmembrane receptors that facilitate intercellular binding and interactions with the ECM. They are important mediators of cell–cell and cell–matrix adhesion, and are members of a number of families including integrins, the immunoglobulin superfamily, cadherins, and selectins. CAMs have been detected in eutopic endometrium, menstrual effluent and endometriotic tissue samples of patients [37–42], and specific alterations in their expression could facilitate binding of refluxed menstrual endometrium in ectopic sites. CD44, the principal receptor for hyaluronic acid (HA), is expressed by ESCs and EECs *in vivo* and in cell culture [43,44]. In addition, the CD44 ligand, HA, is synthesized by mesothelial cells [45], and *in vitro* studies demonstrate that disruption of HA at the surface of mesothelial cells inhibits binding of ESCs and EECs to mesothelium [44]. The potential role for integrins in the initial attachment of endometrial cells to peritoneum has also been evaluated. Integrins are heterodimeric transmembrane cell adhesion receptors composed of an α and a β subunit. Witz *et al* [36] demonstrated that the $\alpha2\beta1$ and $\alpha3\beta1$ integrins are present on the apical surface of mesothelial cells. However, function blocking anti-integrin antibodies did not inhibit adhesion of endometrial cells to mesothelial cells, suggesting that integrins may not be involved in the initial adhesion process [36].

Invasion of the mesothelium

The establishment of endometriotic lesions requires ECM breakdown. The peritoneal ECM consists of collagens, proteoglycans, and glycoproteins, including fibronectin and laminin [42]. In addition to its role in determining cell shape, the ECM is important in metabolic processes, influencing cellular proliferation, differentiation and apoptosis, and angiogenesis.

Two families of proteolytic enzymes may be involved in ECM breakdown: matrix metalloproteinases (MMPs) and the plasminogen/plasmin activation system [46]. Once endometrial tissue adheres to the ECM, endometrial metalloproteinases begin active remodeling of the ECM, leading to endometrial invasion of the submesothelial space of the peritoneum [35,47–49]. MMPs have been shown to play a key role in the initiation of menstruation and contribute to the implantation and further invasion of seeded endometriotic explants [50–52]. The activity of MMPs is usually controlled by the induction of gene expression and activation of latent proenzymes. Induction of gene expression is mediated by growth factors, hormones, and inflammatory cytokines [53,54]. In turn, the activity of MMPs in tissues is controlled by the antagonizing actions of their natural inhibitors. Expression of various MMPs and a number of their tissue inhibitors was altered in endometriosis and in the endometrium and PF of patients with endometriosis [6,55–57]. A direct correlation between MMP-1 expression and the activity of endometriotic foci has also been reported [58]. Moreover, suppressing MMP secretion by progesterone treatment or blocking enzyme activity with the tissue inhibitor of metalloproteinase-1 was found to prevent formation of ectopic lesions in a nude mouse model of endometriosis [59].

The second family of proteases that may be involved in peritoneal invasion of endometrial tissue is the plasminogen/plasmin system. Indeed, plasminogen and urokinase-type plasminogen activator (uPA) have been detected at higher concentrations in ectopic than eutopic endometrium [56].

Endometriotic lesion survival

Cell proliferation is a fundamental process in the development of endometriotic lesions. In a nude mouse model of endometriosis, Nisolle *et al* [60] demonstrated that shortly after attachment of ESCs, rearrangement of epithelial and stromal cells occurs, leading to the development of endometriotic lesions and cystic glands within just 5 days. Extensive proliferation was observed in glandular cells as early as 3 days after transplantation.

Growth of endometriotic tissue can be regulated by ovarian steroid hormones (estrogen) and a number of cytokines and growth factors such as interleukin (IL)-6, IL-8, tumor necrosis factor (TNF)-α and hepatocyte growth factor (HGF) [61,62]. Ectopic and regurgitated endometrial cells also show resistance to apoptosis, contributing to the development of endometriotic lesions [63,64].

Establishment of a blood supply

In any autotransplanted tissue or organ, development of an adequate blood supply is critical for survival of the tissue and supply of oxygen and nutrients, as well as removal of waste products; this is also the case for shed menstrual endometrial tissue that has reached the abdominal cavity and implanted in the peritoneum [65,66]. Angiogenesis involves proliferation, migration, and extension of endothelial cells, adherence of these cells to the ECM, remodeling of the ECM, and formation of a new lumen [65,67].

Menstrual effluent contains high concentrations of vascular endothelial growth factor (VEGF), one of the main factors stimulating angiogenesis. Increased levels of angiogenic factors and angiogenic activity have been detected in the PF of women with endometriosis [68–70]. The presence of VEGF has been confirmed in epithelial glands, stromal cells, and macrophages from ectopic endometrium. High VEGF levels found in endometriotic lesions could result in an increase in the subperitoneal vascular network and facilitate the initial development and maintenance of endometriotic lesions [65,71,72].

The fact that angiostatic treatment was shown to reduce the number of lesions in several studies [73–75] confirms that, after implantation of endometrial tissue, an ongoing angiogenic process is required for its survival. These reports suggest that antiangiogenic therapy could be considered a new clinical approach to endometriosis, as recently reviewed by van Langendonckt *et al* [76].

Evolution, activity, and appearance of peritoneal endometriotic lesions

Peritoneal lesions go through various stages and have a range of aspects, appearing as red, black or white lesions (Fig. 9.2 and Plate 9.2), red lesions being the most active in terms of cell proliferation, inflammatory response, and vascularization [3,65,77,78].

Red lesions

There is an obvious similarity between eutopic endometrium and red peritoneal lesions [2,3,79]. Morphologically, red lesions are systematically located on the peritoneal surface. The glandular proliferation status of red lesions is similar to that of eutopic endometrium, revealing a comparable degree of activity. An extensive vascular network is observed between the stroma recently implanted onto the peritoneal surface and peritoneal and subperitoneal layers, demonstrating the importance of angiogenesis in the early stages of development after implantation [2].

These morphological and histological similarities between peritoneal lesions and eutopic endometrium suggest that eutopic endometrium and red lesions are similar tissues, red lesions being recently implanted regurgitated endometrial cells [3]. This observation constitutes an additional argument supporting the transplantation theory for peritoneal endometriosis. Detachment of glands from viable red endometrial implants, explained by the presence of MMPs, could initiate their implantation in other peritoneal sites, as in a "metastatic" process [58].

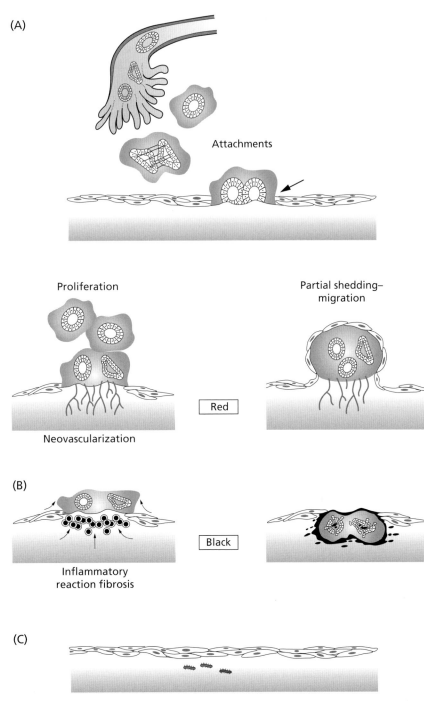

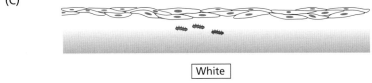

Figure 9.2 Peritoneal endometriosis subtypes (see also color Plate 9.2). (A) Red endometriotic lesion at laparoscopy: numerous glands with active epithelium and abundant stroma on the peritoneal surface. (B) Typical black endometriotic lesion: combination of glands, stroma, and intraluminal debris. (C) White endometriotic lesion: occasional retroperitoneal glandular structures and scanty stroma. Reproduced from Nisolle and Donnez [3] with permission from Elsevier.

Black lesions

After partial shedding, red lesions regrow constantly until the next shedding, but this finally induces a fibromuscular reaction, provoking a scarification process that encloses the implant. The embedded implant becomes a "black" lesion because of the presence of intraluminal debris (see Plate 9.3). This scarification process is probably responsible for the reduction in vascularization,

as proved by the significant decrease in relative surface areas of the capillaries and stroma [2,3,79].

White lesions

In some cases, the scarification process totally devascularizes the endometriotic foci, and white plaques of old collagen are all that remain of the ectopic implant [3]. White opacification and yellow-brown lesions are latent stages of endometriosis. They are probably inactive lesions that could be quiescent for a long time.

Other theories on the pathogenesis of peritoneal endometriosis
Metaplasia
This theory proposes that endometriosis develops from metaplasia of cells lining the visceral and abdominal peritoneum [80]. Some undetermined stimulus, hormonal, infectious or environmental, is believed to induce metaplastic changes in the peritoneal lining, resulting in endometrial implants. Support for this hypothesis lies in several lines of evidence. Embryologically, the thoracic, abdominal and pelvic peritoneum and the müllerian ducts are derived from the same lineage – the coelomic wall of the developing embryo. Clinically, this hypothesis would account for the rare occurrence of endometriosis in men [81,82], prepubescent and adolescent girls [83], distant ectopic sites, such as catamenial endometriosis in the thoracic cavity [84], and women with a congenital absence of müllerian structures [85]. Conclusive proof of the coelomic metaplasia theory remains elusive despite such intriguing observations. Furthermore, if this were the primary etiology of endometriosis, increased incidence would be expected with aging, similar to metaplasia in other organs.

Embryonic rests
This theory claims that cells of müllerian origin within the peritoneal cavity may be induced to form endometrial tissue when subjected to the appropriate stimuli [86]. This hypothesis could account for some cases of rectovaginal endometriosis, as well as in any site along the migration pathway of the embryonic müllerian system. This theory remains speculative, however, as it based on the assumption that these embryonic rests persist into adulthood.

Lymphatic or vascular metastasis
Sampson [5,87] suggested that endometrial cells could extend to ectopic sites via lymphatic and hematogenous spread, accounting for the presence of endometriosis in distant sites outside the pelvis, including the brain, lung, lymph nodes, knee, extremities, and abdominal wall. Clinically, this hypothesis is supported by the presence of endometrial tissue in the uterine vasculature, which has been documented in patients with adenomyosis [5]. In addition, intravenous injection of endometrial tissue has been demonstrated to result in pulmonary endometriosis in rabbits [88]. Although it is possible that some lymphovascular trafficking of endometrial cells contributes to the pathogenesis of endometriosis, this is not likely to be the primary mechanism of disease spread, because the incidence of hepatic, pulmonary, and thoracic endometriosis is rare.

Stem cell involvement
There is increasing interest in the concept that endometrial stem/progenitor cells may be responsible for the highly regenerative capacity of human endometrium. Initial evidence from cell

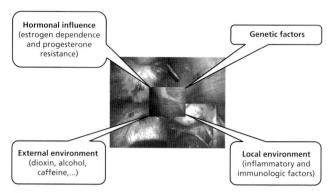

Figure 9.3 Endometriosis: a multifactorial disease.

cloning studies suggests that adult stem cells are probably present in human endometrium [89,90]. Although stem/progenitor cells are speculated to persist in adult endometrium to replace glandular epithelium and stroma that are shed with each menstrual cycle, recent studies indicate that bone marrow may be another source of endometrial stem cells [91,92]. This new stem cell theory suggests that endometriosis arises from retrograde menstruation of endometrial stem/progenitor cells [93,94]. In line with this hypothesis, a previous study reported that women with endometriosis shed more of the basalis layer, suspected to contain endometrial stem/progenitor cells [93], than control patients [95].

Endometriosis: a multifactorial disease
Endometriosis is nowadays considered to be a multifactorial disease [96]. In addition to the etiopathogenic factors previously mentioned, genetic, environmental, and hormonal factors have also been implicated in the establishment, development, maintenance, and progression of endometriotic lesions (Fig. 9.3).

Endometriosis is a condition showing hereditary tendencies, and a polygenic/multifactorial etiology has been suggested. A number of candidate genes have been identified with potential biological plausibility [97]. Some of these genes point to abnormalities in detoxification enzymes, which could lead to vulnerability to environmental stimuli, while others (tumor suppressor genes) are associated with malignant transformation [96,98]. There is evidence of genetic linkage to chromosomes 7 and 10, but genes (or variants) in these regions contributing to disease risk have yet to be determined [97]. In recent years, evidence has also emerged that endometriosis may be an epigenetic disease, as various epigenetic aberrations have been demonstrated in patients [99], which could constitute a common denominator for hormonal and immunological aberrations in endometriosis.

Endocrine-disrupting compounds, such as dioxins or dioxin-like polychlorinated biphenyls (PCBs), could play a role in the establishment or development of endometriosis. Experimental data in monkeys exposed to dioxin show development of endometriosis in a dose-dependent manner [100]. Heilier *et al* [101] have provided the first epidemiological evidence of a clear association between increased dioxin and dioxin-like PCBs impregnation and the risk of endometriosis.

Endometriosis is also known to be an estrogen-dependent disease, but progesterone resistance has also been postulated to be a mechanism of disease progression [102]. It has been documented that endometriotic lesions show high estradiol biosynthesis and low estradiol inactivation compared to endometrium from unaffected women [102]. Aromatase, which is the central enzyme in the biosynthesis of estradiol, has been reported to be involved in estrogen production and expressed in eutopic and ectopic endometrium of endometriosis patients [102,103]. However, in a recent study, we failed to confirm previously published studies on aromatase expression in human endometriotic lesions. Indeed, we observed no aromatase protein in the glandular or stromal compartments of ectopic endometrial tissue, and barely detectable aromatase mRNA expression [104,105], suggesting that locally produced aromatase (within endometriotic lesions) could be less implicated than previously postulated [106].

Summary

We regard red lesions as early endometriosis and black lesions as advanced endometriosis [107]. White lesions are believed to be healed endometriosis or quiescent or latent lesions. This hypothesis corroborates the clinical findings of Redwine [108] and of Goldstein et al [109] that red lesions precede the others and that with time, their presence decreases, being replaced by black and ultimately white lesions. Red petechial lesions are found in adolescents [109].

The exact reason why some implants or cells do not respond to hormonal therapy is not known, but at least four hypotheses have been proposed:

• that the drug does not gain access to the endometriotic foci because fibrosis surrounding the foci prevents access locally

• that endometriotic cells may have their own genetic programming, whereas endocrine influence appears to be only secondary and dependent on the degree of differentiation of the individual cell

• that fewer estrogen receptors (ERs) are present in ectopic peritoneal endometrium when compared with eutopic endometrium

• that the different regulatory mechanisms of endometriotic steroid receptors may result in deficient endocrine dependency because the receptors, although present, are biologically inactive.

Ovarian endometriosis

Pathogenesis

The pathogenesis of typical ovarian endometriosis is a source of controversy [110–112]. The original article by Sampson [113] on this condition indicated that perforation of the so-called chocolate cyst led to spillage of adhesions and the spread of peritoneal endometriosis. The findings of Hughesdon [114] contradicted Sampson's [113] hypothesis and suggested that adhesions are not the consequence, but rather the cause, of endometrioma formation. Hughesdon demonstrated, by serial section of ovaries

containing an endometrioma, that 90% of typical endometriomas are formed by invagination of the cortex after the accumulation of menstrual debris from bleeding of endometrial implants, which are located on the ovarian surface and adherent to the peritoneum.

The site of perforation, as described by Sampson [113], could represent the stigma of invagination. The observations of Brosens et al [115], based on ovarioscopy and in situ biopsies, were in agreement with the hypothesis of Hughesdon [114]. In 93% of typical endometriomas, the pseudocyst is formed by an accumulation of menstrual debris from the shedding and bleeding of active implants located by ovarioscopy at the site of inversion, resulting in a progressive invagination of the ovarian cortex [114].

Other investigators have suggested that large endometriomas may develop as a result of the secondary involvement of functional ovarian cysts in the process of endometriosis [116]. We recently published a different hypothesis on the development of ovarian endometriosis [110,117]. Coelomic metaplasia of invaginated epithelial inclusions could be responsible for this pathogenesis (Fig. 9.4). This hypothesis, based on the metaplastic potential of the pelvic mesothelium, is already a widely accepted theory on the pathogenesis of common epithelial ovarian tumors [118].

Although recent papers and debates have tried to classify endometriomas, there is still considerable uncertainty. We believe that ovarian endometriosis is caused by metaplasia of the invaginated coelomic epithelium [112–117]. Our arguments for this are as follows.

• In our series, we found that 12% of endometriomas were not fixed to the broad ligament and that Hughesdon's [114] theory cannot explain the formation of the endometriomas in these cases.

• It was not unusual to find multilocular endometriomas that could not be explained by the theory of adhesions and by bleeding of active superficial implants adherent to the peritoneum.

• The epithelium covering the ovary, which is the mesothelium, can invaginate into the ovarian cortex. Invaginations of the mesothelial layer covering the ovarian tissue were described by Motta et al [119] in animal and human fetal ovaries and also were visualized in human adult ovaries [3,117]. In our serial sections of the ovary, we frequently observed mesothelial inclusions. Under the influence of unknown growth factors, these inclusions could be transformed into intraovarian endometriosis by metaplasia.

• The fact that primordial follicles were found surrounding the endometriotic cyst also is in agreement with our hypothesis. When the mesothelium invaginates deep into the ovary, the follicles located at the invagination site are pushed concomitantly with the mesothelium.

• Our main argument is based upon the presence of epithelial invaginations in continuum with endometrial tissue, proving the metaplasia theory [3,117] (Plate 9.3).

• Another major argument is related to the demonstration of the capacity of the endometrioma wall to invaginate secondarily into the ovarian cortex [117]. Such secondary invaginations were observed in 33% of our cases and represent the so-called deep ovarian endometriosis that actually is just an extension of the endometrioma wall.

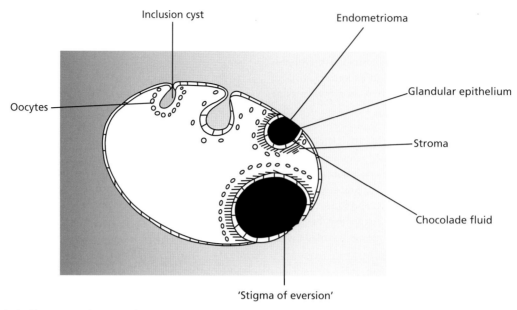

Oocytes

Inclusion cyst

Endometrioma

Glandular epithelium

Stroma

Chocolade fluid

'Stigma of eversion'

Figure 9.4 Hypothesis of histogenesis of ovarian endometriomas.

• Arguments to support our hypothesis can also be found in the literature. First, endometriomas have been described in patients with Rokitansky–Küster–Hauser syndrome, who do not have a uterus and therefore do not have retrograde menstruation [120]. Second, common epithelial tumors of the ovary are considered to be derived from the surface epithelium covering the ovary and from the underlying stroma [118].

Thus, our theory differs from the theories of Hughesdon [114] and of Brosens *et al* [115], who consider that the pathogenesis of the typical ovarian endometrioma now has been clarified as a process originating from a free superficial implant that is in contact with the ovarian surface and is sealed off by adhesions, with the menstrual shedding and bleeding of this small implant resulting in progressive invagination of the ovarian cortex and formation of the pseudocyst.

In our opinion, the endometrioma must be considered as an invagination but not as the result of the bleeding of a superficial implant. Metaplasia of the coelomic epithelium invaginated into the ovarian cortex was proved and explains the formation of the endometrioma [117]. The deep-infiltrating ovarian endometriosis described by our group is only the consequence of the invagination of endometriotic tissue into the ovary and probably is responsible for the recurrence of ovarian endometriosis after cyst excision or vaporization [121–125]. These findings give us supplementary arguments favoring the surgical technique already proposed in 1987, which consists of vaporization of the internal wall of the cyst [122].

Ovarian endometriomas pathogenesis and ovarian reserve

In a recent Cochrane review, Hart *et al* [125] concluded that excisional surgery of endometriomas results in a more favorable outcome than drainage and ablation in terms of recurrence, pain symptoms, subsequent spontaneous pregnancy in previously subfertile women, and ovarian response to stimulation. This review was based on three randomized studies comparing the two approaches of cystectomy and ablation by bipolar coagulation [126–128]. Unfortunately, all three studies failed to prospectively analyze the ovarian reserve after surgery.

When we attempt to address the question of ovarian function after surgery, data in the literature are contradictory, but in Geber's group, patients <35 years of age with previous ovarian surgery had fewer retrieved oocytes than patients in the control group [129]. Exacoustos *et al* [130] showed that ovarian stripping of endometriomas, but not ovarian dermoids, is associated with a significant decrease in residual ovarian volume, which may result in diminished ovarian reserve and function. Histological studies have demonstrated the presence of follicles in excised tissue. One or more primordial follicles were found in 68.9% of endometrioma capsules removed by cystectomy in a study by Hachisuga and Kawarabayashi [131]. Compared with cystectomy for dermoid cysts, cystectomy for endometriomas was much more frequently associated with ablation of follicles [132]. Close to the ovarian hilus, ovarian tissue removed along the endometrioma wall contained primordial, primary, and secondary follicles in 69% of cases [133].

In a very recent study [110,112], we demonstrated that preservation of the vascular blood supply to the ovary is of major importance, as it is vital for the maintenance of ovarian volume and antral follicle count (AFC). We showed that a combined (partial cystectomy and vaporization) approach allows preservation of normal ovarian volume, as well as a normal AFC (Table 9.1).

Table 9.1 Ovarian volume and AFC 6 months after surgery in women treated for endometriomas by the combined technique and in women of similar age with normal ovaries and regular ovulatory cycles presenting for IVF because of male factor infertility.

	Ovarian volume (cm³)	Antral follicle count
Combined technique (n = 31)	7.64 ± 2.95	6.1 ± 3.2
Women without endometriosis (n = 20)	7.99 ± 5.33	6.2 ± 4.8

Ovarian volume and AFC 1 year after surgery in women with unilateral endometriomas and contralateral normal ovaries serving as controls

	Ovarian volume (cm³)	Antral follicle count
Combined technique (n = 20)	7.45 ± 2.93	5.5 ± 2.4
Contralateral normal ovaries (n = 20)	7.82 ± 3.91	5.7 ± 1.6

The so-called rectovaginal or deep endometriosis

Another form of the disease is deep-infiltrating endometriosis of the rectovaginal septum. In 1922, Sampson [134] defined cul-de-sac obliteration as "extensive adhesions in the cul-de-sac, obliterating its lower portion and uniting the cervix or the lower portion of the uterus to the rectum; with adenoma of the endometrial type invading the cervical and the uterine tissue and probably also (but to a lesser degree) the anterior wall of the rectum."

Pathogenesis

This form of the disease (third entity in our theory) has been defined as deep endometriosis, rectovaginal endometriosis or adenomyosis of the rectovaginal septum [135–140]. In the literature, it is also called deep-infiltrating endometriosis or posterior deep-infiltrating endometriosis. The term "deep-infiltrating endometriosis" was coined by Koninckx and Martin and first published in 1995 [141]. In their classification, this form was described as a lesion deeply infiltrating the rectovaginal septum from the peritoneal pouch [142]. However, Koninckx himself now considers the concept of deep-infiltrating endometriosis no longer valid as an explanation for deep nodular "rectovaginal" lesions [143,144]. In fact, he has gone full circle, returning to his original question published in 1992 [144]: "Deep endometriosis: a consequence of infiltration or retraction or possible adenomyosis externa?".

On the other hand, the notion that peritoneal endometriosis and rectovaginal endometriosis are two distinct entities was already proposed back in 1996 [2], and the concept of essentially retroperitoneal or retrocervical disease was reported in 2001

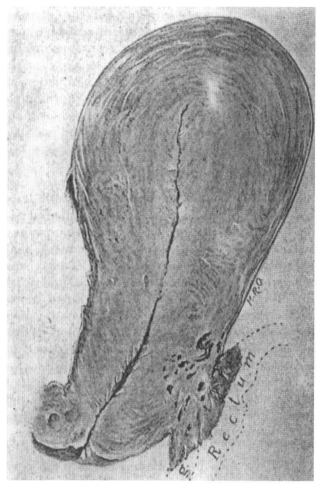

Figure 9.5 Drawing from Sampson's manuscript, clearly demonstrating the cervical origin of the nodular lesion described as "an adenoma of the endometrial type" invading the cervical and the uterine tissue and probably also (but at a lesser degree) the anterior wall of the rectum. Reproduced from Sampson [134] with permission from the American Medical Association.

[145]. The hypothesis is that these lesions are retroperitoneal and may result, in some cases (<10%), from metaplasia of müllerian rests. In other cases (>90%), the origin of the lesion is the posterior part of the cervix, where the vagina is attached [145,146].

Surprisingly, this concept of "retrocervical disease" appears to have already been suggested by Sampson in one of his drawings and manuscripts. Indeed, as early as 1927, Sampson [5] suggested a link between the cervix and the rectum. He defined cul-de-sac obliteration as "extensive adhesions in the cul-de-sac, obliterating its lower portion and uniting the cervix or the lower portion of the uterus to the rectum, with adenoma of the endometrial type invading the cervical and the uterine tissue and probably also (but to a lesser degree) the anterior wall of the rectum" (Fig. 9.5). It therefore looks increasingly likely that the correct description of deep nodular lesions was actually given over 80 years ago.

Although Chapron *et al* [147,148] and Abrao *et al* [149] continue to favor a peritoneal origin, it is highly unlikely that

	1989–1992	1993–1996	1997–2000	2000–2004	2004–2008
Endometriosis	1107	1389	1513	1980	2244
Peritoneal and ovarian endometriosis	1058 (95.5%)	1077 (78.8%)	931 (61.6%)	1168 (58.9%)	1152 (51.4)
Adenomyotic nodules	49 (4.5%)	312 (22.4%)	582 (38.4%)	812 (41.1%)	1092 (48.6%)

Table 9.2 Increasing prevalence of adenomyotic nodules among endometriosis sufferers.

retroperitoneal lesions of a few millimeters in size could induce retroperitoneal lesions of more than 3 cm in size. The nodular aspect of these lesions located in the rectovaginal septum or behind the cervix is due to smooth muscle proliferation. These deep lesions are retroperitoneal and may extend laterally or to the anterior rectal wall [144,146,150].

Do we have arguments to support a retrocervical origin?

Arguments in favor of retrocervical and retroperitoneal disease are numerous.

• The marked increase in the prevalence of rectovaginal nodules compared to peritoneal and ovarian endometriosis during these last 15 years (Table 9.2) could be due to environmental factors.

• Heilier et al [101] were recently able to determine that dioxin-like PCDDs (polychlorinated-dibenzo-dioxins) and PCBs were significantly higher in the serum of women suffering from deep nodular lesions than women with peritoneal endometriosis or controls. It has been suggested that these compounds, which act as endocrine disruptors, could be related to the increased prevalence of deep endometriosis observed in recent decades.

• In Belgium, where the highest dioxin levels have been described (elevated population and industrial concentrations) [151], the prevalence of deep lesions is among the highest in the world.

• Laparoscopic visualization reveals only the tip of the iceberg, with more than 90% of the lesion being retroperitoneal [3,138,139].

• Magnetic resonance images demonstrate that the majority of deep endometriotic lesions (>90%) originate from the retrocervical space [139].

• These lesions originate from the tissue of the rectovaginal septum or the posterior part of the cervix, and consist essentially of smooth muscle (90% of the content) with active glandular epithelium and scanty stroma [3]. The considerable fibromuscular content of nodules was also recently demonstrated by van Kaam et al [152]. Smooth muscle proliferation and fibrosis, consistently observed, are responsible for the nodular aspect of endometriosis. Histologically, this entity is completely different from peritoneal endometriosis, which can infiltrate the peritoneal surface and beneath the peritoneum. Even if peritoneal lesions may sometimes be found penetrating the subperitoneal layers by more than 5 mm, the claim that these lesions could induce the formation of deep nodular lesions (often more than 2 cm in size) is not borne out [2,3,145].

• The key argument proving that deep lesions and endometrial lesions are distinct entities is their differential expression of HOXA-10 and HOXA-13. HOX genes are highly evolutionary and act as regulators of embryonic morphogenesis and differentiation. Genes from the HOXA cluster are involved in the development of the paramesonephrotic duct and its differentiation into the female reproductive tract, and show a differential pattern of HOX gene expression along the anteroposterior axis [91]. HOXA-9 is expressed in the area destined to become the fallopian tube, HOXA-10 in the primordial uterus, HOXA-11 in the primordia of the lower uterine segment and cervix, while HOXA-13 is expressed in the upper vagina. This provides clear biological evidence that deep endometriotic nodules do not originate from infiltrating peritoneal endometriosis [153].

• Hyperplasia of smooth muscle present in the nodule often provokes perivisceritis, visible on barium enema, because of the inflammatory process and secondary retraction of the rectal serosa and muscularis. The absence of evolution of the rectal lesion after removal of the nodule supports our hypothesis concerning its purely retrocervical or rectovaginal septum origin [3,135–140]. Indeed, lateral and posterior extension occurs retroperitoneally via the lymphatics or nerves [3,135,140,153–155]. The mode of propagation is very similar to the propagation of cervical cancer.

In 28% of cases, the rectovaginal adenomyotic nodule is not associated with peritoneal endometriosis [138,154,156]. In such cases, the hypothesis of deep invasion by a peritoneal lesion, with subsequent formation of a retroperitoneal nodular lesion as suggested by some authors [147,149], is obsolete. Finally, literature on the subject reveals strong arguments from the original pioneers. As early as 1896, Cullen reported that deep lesions were the consequence of direct extension of lower uterine adenomyosis [157]. Sampson, in 1922 (see Fig. 9.5), confirmed this description by asserting that adenoma of the endometrial type invades the cervical and uterine tissue and unites the cervix and rectum [158]. One of the drawings in the series by Renish [159], recently reported by Hudelist et al [160], clearly demonstrates extension from the posterior part of the cervix where the vagina is attached [160]. A drawing by Lockyer from 1918 is similar [161]. It should be noted that Lockyer removed a large part of the anterior wall of the rectum, demonstrating that an overly aggressive approach was already being implemented as far back as 1912.

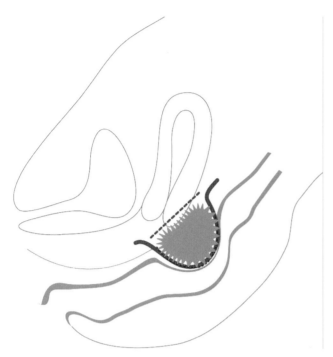

Figure 9.6 Shaving technique.

Table 9.3 Complication rate after surgery for deep rectovaginal endometriotic nodules using the shaving technique compared to bowel resection (selected systematic review).

	Shaving technique (data from present study) n = 500	Rectal resection (selected systematic review)*
Laparoconversion	0%	5–11%
Repeat surgery	<0.1%	10%
Urinary retention	0.8% (n = 4)	3–5%
Ureteral lesions (uroperitoneum)	0.8% (n = 4)	2–4%
Fecal peritonitis, anastomotic leakage	0%	3–5%
Severe anastomotic stenosis	–	3%
Occlusion	0%	1%
Sepsis (pelvic abscess)	0%	2–4%
Rectovaginal fistula	0%	6–9%
Rectal perforation upon shaving (diagnosed and repaired during surgery, no further complications)	1.4% (n = 7)	–

*Source: Donnez and Squifflet [171].

Are deep endometriotic nodules like non-hormone-dependent adenomyomas?

A deep endometriotic nodule exhibits a varied functional response [2,3,162] to ovarian hormones and does not respond to physiological levels of progesterone (P). Secretory changes are always absent during the second half of the menstrual cycle, indicating that endometrium in nodules does not have the same characteristics as eutopic endometrium [2,3].

Like an adenomyoma, this lesion is a circumscribed nodular aggregate of smooth muscle, endometrial glands and, usually, endometrial stroma [2,3,116,162,163]. The similarity in the histological descriptions of uterine adenomyosis and deep endometriotic nodules has led us to suggest that the so-called endometriotic nodule of the rectovaginal septum is the same as an adenomyoma or an "adenomyotic nodule."

The presence of smooth muscle-like cells in deep nodular lesions may be explained by several hypotheses.

• Fibromuscular cells may develop in some cases from remnants of the müllerian duct, as suggested by Donnez *et al* in 1996 [2] and Nisolle and Donnez in 1997 [3]. This is probably the case for lesions that are clearly situated in the rectovaginal septum and separated from the cervix (type I in Squifflet and Donnez's classification) [156].

• Smooth muscle-like cells may be the consequence of extension of fibromuscular cells from the cervix [140,145,153]. Ninety percent of deep lesions clearly originate from the cervix or are at least strongly connected to it.

• These smooth muscle-like cells may result from smooth muscle metaplasia or endometrial stromal fibroblasts [3,114].

• They may also originate from differentiation of local tissue fibroblasts, as a result of a reaction of the local environment to the presence of ectopic endometrium in the rectovaginal septum, as recently suggested by van Kaam *et al* [152].

Steroid receptor content of nodules throughout the cycle suggests that they are probably not regulated by steroids [3,163–165]. A low ER content could be the key factor in explaining the out-of-phase endometrium, despite normal P levels, but a reduction in progesterone receptor (PR) content could also cause resistance to P action and result in inadequate secretory transformation [3,163]. The absence of response to P levels suggests that the different regulatory mechanisms of endometriotic steroid receptors result in deficient endocrine dependency or that the receptors are present but biologically inactive [3,166–168]. This explains the poor response of nodules to hormonal therapy.

The low mitotic activity observed in this pathology could account for the relatively slow evolution of deep endometriotic nodules and the weak response to medical therapy, necessitating surgical excision [135–140].

Surgery: to shave or not to shave?

There is no doubt that we should operate in cases of symptomatic deep nodular lesions, but surgical techniques have taken some considerable time to evolve. However, all of them involve (i) separation of the anterior rectum from the posterior vagina and (ii) excision or ablation of deep endometriosis after complete dissection of the nodule from the posterior part of the cervix.

Surgery for deep rectovaginal endometriosis was first described by Reich *et al* [169] and Donnez in 1991 [170], and the first two large series including 231 and 500 women respectively were published in 1995 and 1997 [137,138]. Two further large series including 1942 and 2147 patients respectively were subsequently published [138,140].

In a very recent paper, Donnez and Squifflet [171] demonstrated that the shaving technique (Fig. 9.6) has a lower complication rate (3%) and similar recurrence rate (7%) compared to bowel resection. Moreover, the pregnancy rate is high (Table 9.3).

Although these papers concluded that it is prudent to curtail rather than encourage the widespread use of an aggressive and potentially morbid procedure, increasingly aggressive surgery, including bowel resection, is still systematically proposed in cases of deep endometriosis with muscularis involvement, even in the absence of mucosal involvement [147–149,172–178]. All these studies are retrospective and non-randomized, however, and do not evaluate the long-term outcome of this surgery compared to shaving surgery (see Fig. 9.6). The lack of evidence of better improvement in cases of bowel resection was recently underlined by Vercellini *et al* [179].

The debate is not new. In a recent paper by Hudelist *et al* [160], different past series and theories on the etiology of adenomyosis and endometriosis are described, and we are shown a specimen of deep endometriosis involving the rectum (a typical hourglass-shaped nodule). Back in 1912, Renish [159] performed resection of the anterior rectal wall (the first "disk resection") together with hysterectomy, while Lockyer performed hysterectomy and bowel resection over a length of 20 cm for the same type of lesion (drawing by Lockyer from 1918) [161]. Ninety years later, the debate rages on, not only rearing its head during the World Congress on Endometriosis [180], but also in the literature, with two conflicting articles recently appearing in the same journal: "Should we operate for deep-infiltrating endometriosis? No. Choose realism instead of idealism!" by Fernandez *et al* [181] and: "Yes, patients with deep-infiltrating endometriosis should be operated! Prefer optimistic will to pessimistic intelligence!" by Canis *et al* [182].

Conclusion

Peritoneal endometriosis, the different aspects (black, red, and white) of which represent distinctive steps in the evolutionary process, can be explained by the transplantation theory. Red lesions are the most active and most highly vascularized lesions and are considered to be the first stage of peritoneal endometriosis. According to our histological findings, coelomic metaplasia of invaginated epithelial inclusions could be responsible for the development of ovarian endometriosis. The epithelium covering the ovary, which originally derives from the coelomic epithelium, has great metaplastic potential and provokes epithelial inclusion cysts by invagination. Under the influence of unknown growth factors, these inclusions could be transformed into intraovarian

endometriosis by metaplasia. The rectovaginal endometriotic nodule is an adenomyotic nodule whose histopathogenesis is not related to the implantation of regurgitated endometrial cells. Metaplastic changes either from müllerian rests or from a retrocervical area into endometriotic glands involving the rectovaginal septum are responsible for the striking proliferation of the smooth muscle, creating an adenomyomatous appearance similar to that of adenomyosis in the endometrium.

References

1. Donnez J, Nisolle M, Casanas-Roux F. Three-dimensional architecture of peritoneal endometriosis. Fertil Steril 1992;57:980–983.

2. Donnez J, Nisolle M, Smoes P, Gillet N, Beguin S, Casanas-Roux F. Peritoneal endometriosis and "endometriotic" nodules of the rectovaginal septum are two different entities. Fertil Steril 1996;66:362–368.

3. Nisolle M, Donnez J. Peritoneal endometriosis, ovarian endometriosis, and adenomyotic nodules of the rectovaginal septum are three different entities. Fertil Steril 1997;68:585–596.

4. Von Rokitansky C. Ueber Uterusdursen-Neubildung in Uterus and Ovarialsarcomen (Uterine gland proliferation in uterine and ovarian sarcomas). Zeitschr Gesellsch Aerzte Wien 1860;37:577.

5. Sampson JA. Peritoneal endometriosis due to menstrual dissemination of endometrial tissue into the peritoneal cavity. Am J Obstet Gynecol 1927;14:422–469.

6. Halme J, Hammond MG, Hulka JF, Raj SG, Talbert LM. Retrograde menstruation in healthy women and in patients with endometriosis. Obstet Gynecol 1984;64:151–154.

7. Jenkins S, Olive DL, Haney AF. Endometriosis: pathogenetic implications of the anatomic distribution. Obstet Gynecol 1986;67:335–338.

8. Kruitwagen RF, Poels LG, Willemsen WN, Jap PH, Thomas CM, Rolland R. Retrograde seeding of endometrial epithelial cells by uterine-tubal flushing. Fertil Steril 1991;56:414–420.

9. Koks CA, Dunselman GA, de Goeij AF, Arends JW, Evers JL. Evaluation of a menstrual cup to collect shed endometrium for in vitro studies. Fertil Steril 1997;68:560–564.

10. Sanfilippo JS, Wakim NG, Schikler KN, Yussman MA. Endometriosis in association with uterine anomaly. Am J Obstet Gynecol 1986;154:39–43.

11. Darrow SL, Vena JE, Batt RE, Zielezny MA, Michalek AM, Selman S. Menstrual cycle characteristics and the risk of endometriosis. Epidemiology 1993;4:135–142.

12. Vercellini P, de Giorgi O, Aimi G, Panazza S, Uglietti A, Crosignani PG. Menstrual characteristics in women with and without endometriosis. Obstet Gynecol 1997;90:264–268.

13. Arumugam K, Lim JM. Menstrual characteristics associated with endometriosis. Br J Obstet Gynaecol 1997;104:948–950.

14. Spuijbroek MD, Dunselman GA, Menheere PP, Evers JL. Early endometriosis invades the extracellular matrix. Fertil Steril 1992;58:929–933.

15. Lousse JC, Defrère S, van Langendonckt A et al. Iron storage is significantly increased in peritoneal macrophages of endometriosis patients

and correlates with iron overload in peritoneal fluid. Fertil Steril 2009;91:1668–1675.

16. Lousse JC, Defrère S, González Ramos R, van Langendonckt A, Colette S, Donnez J. Involvement of iron, nuclear factor-kappa B (NF-κB) and prostaglandins in the pathogenesis of peritoneal endometriosis-associated inflammation: a review. J Endometr 2009;1:19–29.

17. Haney AF, Muscato JJ, Weinberg JB. Haney AF, Muscato JJ, Weinberg JB. Peritoneal fluid cell populations in infertility patients. Fertil Steril 1981;35:696–698.

18. Hill JA, Faris HM, Schiff I, Anderson DJ. Characterization of leukocyte subpopulations in the peritoneal fluid of women with endometriosis. Fertil Steril 1988;50:216–222.

19. Song M, Karabina SA, Kavtaradze N, Murphy AA, Parthasarathy S. Presence of endometrial epithelial cells in the peritoneal cavity and the mesothelial inflammatory response. Fertil Steril 2003;79:789–794.

20. Cao X, Yang D, Song M, Murphy A, Parthasarathy S. The presence of endometrial cells in the peritoneal cavity enhances monocyte recruitment and induces inflammatory cytokines in mice: implications for endometriosis. Fertil Steril 2004;82:999–1007.

21. Donnez J, van Langendonckt A. Typical and subtle atypical presentations of endometriosis. Curr Opin Obstet Gynecol 2004;16:431–437.

22. Vinatier D, Orzi G, Cosson M, Dufour P. Theories of endometriosis. Eur J Obstet Gynecol Reprod Biol 2001;96:21–34.

23. Oosterlynck DJ, Cornillie FJ, Waer M, Vandeputte M, Koninckx PR. Women with endometriosis show a defect in natural killer activity resulting in a decreased cytotoxicity to autologous endometrium. Fertil Steril 1991;56:45–51.

24. Viganò P, Gaffuri B, Somigliana E, Busacca M, Di Blasio AM, Vignali M. Expression of intercellular adhesion molecule (ICAM)-1 mRNA and protein is enhanced in endometriosis versus endometrial stromal cells in culture. Mol Hum Reprod 1998;4:1150–1156.

25. Van der Linden PJ, de Goeij AF, Dunselman GA, Erkens HW, Evers JL. Endometrial cell adhesion in an in vitro model using intact amniotic membranes. Fertil Steril 1996;5:76–80.

26. Groothuis PG, Koks CA, de Goeij AF, Dunselman GA, Arends JW, Evers JL. Adhesion of human endometrium to the epithelial lining and extracellular matrix of amnion in vitro: an electron microscopic study. Hum Reprod 1998;13:2275–2281.

27. Groothuis PG, Koks CA, de Goeij AF, Dunselman GA, Arends JW, Evers JL. Adhesion of human endometrial fragments to peritoneum in vitro. Fertil Steril 1999;71:1119–1124.

28. Witz CA, Montoya-Rodriguez AI, Schenken RS. Whole peritoneal explants: a novel model of the early endometriosis lesion. Fertil Steril 1999;71:56–60.

29. Witz CA, Thomas MR, Montoya-Rodriguez IA, Nair AS, Centonze VE, Schenken RS. Short-term culture of peritoneum explants confirms attachment of endometrium to intact peritoneal mesothelium. Fertil Steril 2001;75:385–390.

30. Debrock S, Vander Perre S, Meuleman C, Moerman P, Hill JA, D'Hooghe TM. In vitro adhesion of endometrium to autologous peritoneal membranes: effect of the cycle phase and the stage of endometriosis. Hum Reprod 2002;17:2523–2528.

31. Zhang R, Wild RA, Ojago JM. Effect of tumor necrosis factor-α on adhesion of human endometrial stromal cells to peritoneal mesothelial cells: an in vitro system. Fertil Steril 1993;59:1196–1201.

32. Wild RA, Zhang R, Medders D. Whole endometrial fragments form characteristics of in vivo endometriosis in a mesothelial cell co-culture system: an in vitro model of the histogenesis of endometriosis. J Soc Gynecol Invent 1994;1:165–168.

33. Lucidi RS, Witz CA, Chrisco M, Binkley PA, Shain SA, Schenken RS. A novel in vitro model of the early endometriotic lesion demonstrates that attachment of endometrial cells to mesothelial cells is dependent on the source of endometrial cells. Fertil Steril 2005;84:16–21.

34. Debrock S, de Strooper B, Vander Perre S, Hill JA, D'Hooghe TM. Tumour necrosis factor-α, interleukin-6 and interleukin-8 do not promote adhesion of human endometrial epithelial cells to mesothelial cells in a quantitative in vitro model. Hum Reprod 2006;21:605–609.

35. Nisolle M, Casanas-Roux F, Donnez J. Early-stage endometriosis: adhesion and growth of human menstrual endometrium. Fertil Steril 2000;74:306–312.

36. Witz CA, Dechad H, Montoya-Rodriguez IA et al. An in vitro model to study the pathogenesis of the early endometriosis lesion. Ann NY Acad Sci 2002;955:296–307.

37. Van der Linden PJ, de Goeij AF, Dunselman GA, Arends JW, Evers JL. P-cadherin expression in human endometrium and endometriosis. Gynecol Obstet Invest 1994;38:183–185.

38. Van der Linden PJ, de Goeij AF, Dunselman GA, Erkens HW, Evers JL. Expression of cadherins and integrins in human endometrium throughout the menstrual cycle. Fertil Steril 1995;63:1210–1216.

39. Bridges JE, Prentice A, Roche W, Englefield P, Thomas EJ. Expression of integrin adhesion molecules in endometrium and endometriosis. Br J. Obstet Gynaecol 1994;101:696–700.

40. Kim LT, Yamada KM. Evidence that beta1 integrins in keratinocyte cell-cell junctions are not in the ligand-occupied conformation. J Invest Dermatol 1997;108:876–880.

41. Regidor PA, Vogel C, Regidor M, Schindler AE, Winterhager E. Expression patter of integrin adhesion molecules in endometriosis and human endometrium. Hum Reprod Update 1998;4:710–718.

42. Witz CA. Cell adhesion molecules and endometriosis. Semin Reprod Med 2003;21:173–182.

43. Yaegashi N, Fujita N, Yajima A, Nakamura M. Menstrual cycle dependent expression of CD44 in normal human endometrium. Hum Pathol 1995;26:862–865.

44. Dechaud H, Witz CA, Montoya-Rodriguez IA, Degraffenried L, Schenken RS. Mesothelial cell-associated hyaluronic acid facilitates endometrial stromal and epithelial cell binding to mesothelium. Fertil Steril 2001;76:1012–1018.

45. Yung S, Thomas GJ, Stylianou E, Williams JD, Coles GA, Davies M. Source of peritoneal proteoglycans. Human peritoneal mesothelial cells synthesize and secrete mainly small dermatan sulfate proteoglycans. Am J Pathol 1995;146:520–529.

46. Rodgers WH, Matrisian LM, Giudice LC et al. Patterns of matrix metalloproteinase expression in cycling endometrium imply differential functions and regulation by steroid hormones. J Clin Invest 1994;94:946–953.

47. Witz CA, Sook C, Montoya-Rodriguez IA, Schenken RS. The α1β2 and α3β1 integrins do not mediate attachment of endometrial cells to peritoneal mesothelium. Fertil Steril 2002;78:796–803.

48. Witz CA, Cho S, Centonze VE, Montoya-Rodriguez IA, Schenken RS. Time series analysis of transmesothelial invasion by endometrial stromal and epithelial cells using three-dimensional confocal microscopy. Fertil Steril 2003;79:770–778.

49. Dunselman GA, Groothuis PG, de Goeij AF, Evers JL. The mesothelium, Teflon or Velcro? Mesothelium in endometriosis pathogenesis. Hum Reprod 2001;16:605–607.

50. Marbaix E, Kokorine I, Moulin P, Donnez J, Eeckhout Y, Courtoy PJ. Menstrual breakdown of human endometrium can be mimicked in vitro and is selectively and reversibly blocked by inhibitors of matrix metalloproteinases. Proc Natl Acad Sci USA 1996;93:9120–9125.

51. Singer CF, Marbaix E, Kokorine I et al. Paracrine stimulation of interstitial collagenase (MMP-1) in the human endometrium by interleukin 1alpha and its dual block by ovarian steroids. Proc Natl Acad Sci USA 1997;94:10341–10345.

52. Henriet P, Cornet PB, Lemoine P et al. Circulating ovarian steroids and endometrial matrix metalloproteinases (MMPs). Ann NY Acad Sci 2002;955:119–138.

53. Malik N, Greenfield BW, Wahl AF, Kiener PA. Activation of human monocytes through CD40 induces matrix metalloproteinases. J Immunol 1996;156:3952–3960.

54. Schonbeck U, Mach F, Sukhova GK et al. Regulation of matrix metalloproteinase expression in human vascular smooth muscle cells by T lymphocytes: a role for CD40 signaling in plaque rupture? Circ Res 1997;81:448–454.

55. Osteen KG, Bruner KL, Sharpe-Timms KL. Steroid and growth factor regulation of matrix metalloproteinase expression and endometriosis. Semin Reprod Endocrinol 1996;14:247–255.

56. Sillem M, Prifti S, Neher M, Runnebaum B. Extracellular matrix remodelling in the endometrium and its possible relevance to the pathogenesis of endometriosis. Hum Reprod Update 1998;4:730–735.

57. Sharpe-Timms KL, Cox KE. Paracrine regulation of matrix metalloproteinase expression in endometriosis. Ann NY Acad Sci 2002;955:147–156.

58. Kokorine I, Nisolle M, Donnez J, Eeckhout Y, Courtoy PJ, Marbaix E. Expression of interstitial collagenase (matrix metalloproteinase-1) is related to the activity of human endometriotic lesions. Fertil Steril 1997;68:246–251.

59. Bruner KL, Matrisian LM, Rodgers WH, Gorstein F, Osteen KG. Suppression of matrix metalloproteinases inhibits establishment of ectopic lesions by human endometrium in nude mice. J Clin Invest 1997;99:2851–2857.

60. Nisolle M, Casanas-Roux F, Marbaix E, Jadoul P, Donnez J. Transplantation of cultured explants of human endometrium into nude mice. Hum Reprod 2000;15:101–106.

61. Harada T, Iwabe T, Terakawa N. Role of cytokines in endometriosis. Fertil Steril 2001;76:1–10.

62. Khan KN, Masuzaki H, Fujishita A, Kitajima M, Sekine I, Ishimaru T. Immunoexpression of hepatocyte growth factor and c-Met receptor in the eutopic endometrium predicts the activity of ectopic endometrium. Fertil Steril 2003;79:173–181.

63. Garcia-Velasco JA, Arici A. Apoptosis and the pathogenesis of endometriosis. Semin Reprod Med 2003;21:165–172.

64. Beliard A, Noel A, Foidart JM. Reduction of apoptosis and proliferation in endometriosis. Fertil Steril 2004;82:80–85.

65. Donnez J, Smoes P, Gillerot S, Casanas-Roux F, Nisolle M. Vascular endothelial growth factor (VEGF) in endometriosis. Hum Reprod v1998;13:1686–1690.

66. Groothuis PG, Nap AW, Winterhager E, Grummer R. Vascular development in endometriosis. Angiogenesis 2005;8:147–156.

67. Folkman J, Shing Y. Angiogenesis. J Biol Chem 1992;267:10931–10934.

68. Oosterlynck DJ, Meuleman C, Sobis H, Vandeputte M, Koninckx PR. Angiogenic activity of peritoneal fluid from women with endometriosis. Fertil Steril 1993;59:778–782.

69. Koninckx PR, Kennedy SH, Barlow DH. Endometriotic disease: the role of peritoneal fluid. Hum Reprod Update 1998;4:741–751.

70. McLaren J. Vascular endothelial growth factor and endometriotic angiogenesis. Hum Reprod Update 2000;6:45–55.

71. McLaren J, Prentice A, Charnock-Jones DS, Smith SK. Vascular endothelial growth factor (VEGF) concentrations are elevated in peritoneal fluid of women with endometriosis. Hum Reprod 1996;11:220–223.

72. Shifren JL, Tseng JF, Zaloudek CJ et al. Ovarian steroid regulation of vascular endothelial growth factor in the human endometrium: implications for angiogenesis during the menstrual cycle and in the pathogenesis of endometriosis. J Clin Endocrinol Metab 1996;81:3112–3118.

73. Dabrosin C, Gyorffy S, Margetts P, Ross C, Gauldie J. Therapeutic effect of angiostatin gene transfer in a murine model of endometriosis. Am J Pathol 2002;161:909–918.

74. Hull ML, Charnock-Jones DS, Chan CL et al. Antiangiogenic agents are effective inhibitors of endometriosis. J Clin Endocrinol Metab 2003;88:2889–2899.

75. Nap AW, Griffioen AW, Dunselman GA et al. Antiangiogenesis therapy for endometriosis. J Clin Endocrinol Metab 2004;89:1089–1095.

76. Van Langendonckt A, Donnez J, Defrère S, Dunselman GA, Groothuis PG. Antiangiogenic and vascular-disrupting agents in endometriosis: pitfalls and promises. Mol Hum Reprod 2008;14:259–268.

77. Van Langendonckt A, Casanas-Roux F, Eggermont J, Donnez J. Characterization of iron deposition in endometriotic lesions induced in the nude mouse model. Hum Reprod 2004; 19:1265–1271.

78. González Ramos R, Donnez J, Defrère S et al. Nuclear factor-kappa B is constitutively activated in peritoneal endometriosis. Mol Hum Reprod 2007;13:503–509.

79. Nisolle M, Casanas-Roux F, Anaf V, Mine JM, Donnez J. Morphometric study of the stromal vascularization in peritoneal endometriosis. Fertil Steril 1993;59:681–684.

80. Ridley JH, Edwards IK. Experimental endometriosis in the human. Am J Obstet Gynecol 1958;76:783–790.

81. Oliker AJ, Harris AE. Endometriosis of the bladder in a male patient. J Urol 1971;106:858–859.

82. Schrodt GR, Alcorn MO, Ibanez J. Endometriosis of the male urinary system: a case report. J Urol 1980;124:722–723.

83. Schifrin BS, Erez S, Moore JG. Teen-age endometriosis. Am J Obstet Gynecol 1973;116:973–980.

84. Cassina PC, Hauser M, Kacl G, Imthurn B, Schröder S, Weder W. Catamenial hemoptysis. Diagnosis with MRI. Chest 1997;111:1447–1450.

85. Olive DL, Henderson DY. Endometriosis and mullerian anomalies. Obstet Gynecol 1987;69:412–415.

86. Von Recklinghausen F. Adenomyomas and cystadenomas of the wall of the uterus and tube: their origin as remnants of the wolffian body. Wien Klin Wochenschr 1896;8:530.

87. Sampson JA. Heterotopic or misplaced endometrial tissue. Am J Obstet Gynecol 1925;10:649–664.

88. Hobbs JE, Bortnick AR. Endometriosis of the lung: an experimental and clinical study. Am J Obstet Gynecol 1940;40:832–843.

89. Chan RW, Schwab KE, Gargett CE. Clonogenicity of human endometrial epithelial and stromal cells. Biol Reprod 2004;70:1738–1750.

90. Schwab KE, Chan RW, Gargett CE. Putative stem cell activity of human endometrial epithelial and stromal cells during the menstrual cycle. Fertil Steril 2005;84:1124–1130.

91. Taylor HS, Vanden Heuvel GB, Igarashi P. A conserved Hox axis in the mouse and human reproductive system: late establishment and persistent adult expression of the Hoxa cluster genes. Biol Reprod 1997;57:1338–1345.

92. Du H, Taylor HS. Contribution of bone marrow-derived stem cells to endometrium and endometriosis. Stem Cells 2007;25:2082–2086.

93. Gargett CE. Uterine stem cells: what is the evidence? Hum Reprod Update 2007;13:87–101.

94. Sasson IE, Taylor HS. Stem cells and the pathogenesis of endometriosis. Ann NY Acad Sci 2008;1127:106–115.

95. Leyendecker G, Herbertz M, Kunz G, Mall G. Endometriosis results from the dislocation of basal endometrium. Hum Reprod 2002;17:2725–2736.

96. Giudice LC, Kao LC. Endometriosis. Lancet 2004;364:1789–1799.

97. Montgomery GW, Nyholt DR, Zhao ZZ et al. The search for genes contributing to endometriosis risk. Hum Reprod Update 2008;14:447–457.

98. Simpson JL, Bischoff FZ. Heritability and molecular genetic studies of endometriosis. Ann NY Acad Sci 2002;955:239–251.

99. Guo SW. Epigenetics of endometriosis. Mol Hum Reprod 2009;15:587–607.

100. Rier SE, Martin DC, Bowman RE, Dmowski WP, Becker JL. Endometriosis in rhesus monkey s (Macaca mulatta) following chronic exposure to 2,3,7,8-tetrachlorodibenzo-p-dioxin. Fundam Appl Toxicol 1993;21:433–441.

101. Heilier JF, Nackers F, Verougstraete V, Tonglet R, Lison D, Donnez J. Increased dioxin-like compounds in the serum of women with peritoneal endometriosis and deep endometriotic (adenomyotic) nodules. Fertil Steril 2005;84:305–312.

102. Bulun SE. Endometriosis. N Engl J Med 2009;360:268–279.

103. Attar E, Bulun SE. Aromatase and other steroidogenic genes in endometriosis: translational aspects. Hum Reprod Update 2006;12:49–56.

104. Colette S, Lousse JC, Defrère S et al. Absence of aromatase protein and mRNA expression in endometriosis. Hum Reprod 2009;24:2133–2141.

105. ColetteS, Donnez J. Endometriosis. N Engl J Med 2009;306:1911–1912.

106. Colette S, Donnez J. Aromatase et endométriose: mythe ou réalité? Editorial. Gynécol Obstet Fertil 2010; 38:305–306.

107. Nisolle M, Casanas-Roux F, Anaf V, Mine JM, Donnez J. Morphometric study of the stromal vascularization in peritoneal endometriosis. Fertil Steril 1993;59:681–684.

108. Redwine DB. Age-related evolution in color appearance of endometriosis. Fertil Steril 1987;48:1062–1063.

109. Goldstein MP, de Cholnoky C, Emans SJ, Leventhal JM. Laparoscopy in the diagnosis and management of pelvic pain in adolescents. J Reprod Med 1980;44:251–258.

110. Donnez J, Lousse JC, Jadoul P, Donnez O, Squifflet J. Laparoscopic management of endometriomas using a combined technique of excisional (cystectomy) and ablative surgery. Fertil Steril 2009;94:28–32.

111. Brosens I. The typical ovarian endometrioma has a surface origin. Letter to the Editor. Fertil Steril 2010;94(5):e73.

112. Donnez J. Letter to the Editor. Reply of the authors (The typical ovarian endometrioma has a surface origin, Brosens I). Fertil Steril 2010;94(5):e74.

113. Sampson JA. Perforating haemorrhagic (chocolate) cysts of the ovary. Arch Surg 1921;3:245–323.

114. Hughesdon PE. The structure of endometrial cysts of the ovary. J Obstet Gynaecol Br Emp 1957;44:69–84.

115. Brosens IA, Puttemans PJ, Deprest J. The endoscopic localizationof endometrial implants in the ovarian chocolate cyst. Fertil Steril 1994;61:1034–1038.

116. Nezhat F, Nezhat C, Allan CJ, Metzger DA, Sears DL. Aclinical and histological classification of endometriomas: implications for a mechanism of pathogenesis. J Reprod Med 1992;37:771–776.

117. Donnez J, Nisolle M, Gillet N, Smets M, Bassil S, Casanas-Roux F. Large ovarian endometriomas. Hum Reprod 1996;11:641–646.

118. Serov SF, Scully RE, Sobin LH. Histological Typing of Ovarian Tumors. International Histological Classification of Tumors, No 9. Geneva: World Health Organization, 1973, pp.17–21.

119. Motta PM, van Blerkom J, Mekabe S. Changes in the surface morphology of ovarian germinal epithelium during the reproductive life and in some pathological conditions. Submicrosc Cytol 1992;99:664–667.

120. Rosenfeld DL, Lecher BD. Endometriosis in a patient with Rokitansky–Kuster–Hauser syndrome. Am J Obstet Gynecol 1981; 139:105–107.

121. Canis M, Wattiez A, Pouly JL et al. Laparoscopic treatment of endometriosis. In: Brosens IA, Donnez J (eds) The Current Status of Endometriosis. Research and Management. Carnforth: Parthenon Publishing, 1993, pp.407–417.

122. Donnez J. CO2 laser laparoscopy in infertile women with endometriosis and women with adnexal adhesions. Fertil Steril 1987;48:390–394.

123. Donnez J, Nisolle M, Casanas-Roux F. Classification and endoscopic treatment of ovarian endometriosis. In: Popkin E (ed) Woman's Health Today. Carnforth: Parthenon Publishing, 1994, pp.112–115.

124. Nisolle M, Donnez J. Conservative laparoscopic treatment of ovarian endometriosis. In: Shaw RW (ed) Endometriosis: Current Understanding and Management. London: Blackwell Science, 1995, pp.237–247.

125. Hart R, Hickey M, Maouris P, Buckett W. Excisional surgery versus ablative surgery for ovarian endometriomata. Cochrane Database Syst Rev 2008;16:CD004992.

126. Beretta P, Franchi M, Ghezzi F, Busacca M, Zupi E, Bolis P. Randomized clinical trial of two laparoscopic treatments of endometriomas: cystectomy versus drainage and coagulation. Fertil Steril 1998;70:1176–1180.

127. Alborzi S, Momtahan M, Parsanezhad M, Dehbashi S, Zolghadri J, Alborzi S. A prospective, randomized study comparing laparoscopic ovarian cystectomy versus fenestration and coagulation in patients with endometriomas. Fertil Steril 2004;82:1633–1637.

128. Alborzi S, Ravanbakhsh R, Parsanezhad M, Alborzi M, Alborzi S, Dehbashi S. A comparison of follicular response of ovaries to ovulation induction after laparoscopic ovarian cystectomy or fenestration and coagulation versus normal ovaries in patients with endometrioma. Fertil Steril 2007;88:507–509.

129. Geber S, Ferreira D, Spyer Prates L, Sales L, Samaio M. Effects of previous ovarian surgery for endometriosis on the outcome of assisted reproduction treatment. Reprod Biomed Online 2002;5:162–166.

130. Exacoustos C, Zupi E, Amadio A et al. Laparoscopic removal of endometriomas: sonographic evaluation of residual functioning ovarian tissue. Am J Obstet Gynecol 2004;191:68–72.

131. Somigliana E, Ragni G, Benedetti F, Borroni R, Vegetti W, Crosignani P. Does laparoscopic excision of endometriotic ovarian cysts significantly affect ovarian reserve? Insights from IVF cycles. Hum Reprod 2003;18:2450–2453.

132. Hachisuga T, Kawarabayashi T. Histopathological analysis of laparoscopically treated ovarian endometriotic cysts with special reference to loss of follicles. Hum Reprod 2002;17:432–435.

133. Muzii L, Bellati F, Bianchi A et al. Laparoscopic stripping of endometriomas: a randomized trial on different surgical techniques. Part II: pathological results. Hum Reprod 2005;20:1987–1992.

134. Sampson JA. Intestinal adenomas of endometrial type. Arch Surg 1922;5:21–27.

135. Donnez J, Nisolle M, Squifflet J, Smets M. Laparoscopic treatment of rectovaginal septum adenomyosis. In: Donnez J, Nisolle M (eds) An Atlas of Laser Operative Laparoscopy and Hysteroscopy. Carnforth, UK: Parthenon Publishing, 2001, pp.83–93.

136. Donnez J, Nisolle M. Advanced laparoscopic surgery for the removal of rectovaginal septum endometriotic and adenomyotic nodules. Baillière's Clin Obstet Gynecol 1995;9:769–774.

137. Donnez J, Nisolle M, Casanas-Roux F, Bassil S, Anaf V. Rectovaginal septum endometriosis or adenomyosis: laparoscopic management in a series of 231 patients. Hum Reprod 1995;10:630–635.

138. Donnez J, Nisolle M, Gillerot S, Smets M, Bassil S, Casanas-Roux F. Rectovaginal septum adenomyotic nodules: a series of 500 cases. Br J Obstet Gynaecol 1997;104:1014–1018.

139. Donnez J, Squifflet J. Laparoscopic excision of deep endometriosis. Obstet Gynecol Clin North Am 2004;31:567–580.

140. Donnez J, Jadoul P, Donnez O, Squifflet J. Laparoscopic excision of rectovaginal and retrocervical endometriotric lesions. In: Donnez J (ed) Atlas of Operative Laparoscopy and Hysteroscopy. Oxford: Informa Healthcare, 2007, pp. 63–75.

141. Koninckx PR, Martin DC. Surgical treatment of deeply infiltrating endometriosis. In: Shaw RW (ed) Endometriosis: Current Understanding and Management. London: Blackwell Scientific, 1995, pp.264–281.

142. Cornillie FJ, Oosterlynck D, Lauweryns JM, Koninckx PR. Deeply infiltrating pelvic endometriosis: histology and clinical significance. Fertil Steril 1990;53:978–983.

143. Koninckx PR, de Cicco C, Schonmann R, Corona R, Betsas G, Ussia A. Endometriosis lesions that compromise the rectum deeper than the inner muscularis layer have more than 40% of the circumference of the rectum affected by the disease. J Min Inv Gynecol 2008;15:774–775; author reply 775–776.

144. Koninckx PR, Martin D. Deep endometriosis: a consequence of infiltration or retraction or possible adenomyosis externa? Fertil Steril 1992;58:924–928.

145. Donnez J, Donnez O, Squifflet J, Nisolle M. The concept of "adenomyotic disease of the retroperitoneal space" is born. Gynaecol End 2001;10:91–94.

146. Squifflet J, Donnez J. Endometriosis is not only a gynecologic disease. Acta Gastro-enterol Belg 2004;67:272–277.

147. Chapron C, Chopin N, Borghese B et al. Deeply infiltrating endometriosis: pathogenetic implications of the anatomical distribution. Hum Reprod 2006;21:1839–1845.

148. Chapron C, Liaras E, Fayet P et al. Magnetic resonance imaging and endometriosis: deeply infiltrating endometriosis does not originate from the rectovaginal septum. Gynecol Obstet Invest 2002;53:204–208.

149. Abrao MS, Gonçalves MO, Dias JA Jr, Podgaec S, Chamie LP, Blasbalg R. Comparison between clinical examination, transvaginal sonography and magnetic resonance imaging for the diagnosis of deep endometriosis. Hum Reprod 2007;22:3092–3097.

150. Donnez J, Nisolle M, Squifflet J. Ureteral endometriosis: a complication of rectovaginal endometriotic (adenomyotic) nodules. Fertil Steril 2002;77:32–37.

151. Koninckx PR, Braet P, Kennedy SH, Barlow DH. Dioxin pollution and endometriosis in Belgium. Hum Reprod 1994;9:1001–1002.

152. Van Kaam KJAF, Schouten JP, Nap AW, Dunselman GAJ, Groothuis PG. Fibromuscular differentiation in deeply infiltrating endometriosis is a reaction of resident fibroblasts to the presence of ectopic endometrium. Hum Reprod 2008;23:2692–2700.

153. Van Langendonckt A, Marques de Safe G, Gonzalez D, Squifflet J, Donnez J. HOXA-10 and HOXA-13 gene expression in endometriotic nodules of the vaginal septum. Eur J Obstet Gynaecol Reprod Biol 2005;123 Suppl 1:S35.

154. Donnez J, Nisolle M, Casanas-Roux F, Brion P, da Costa Ferreira N. Stereometric evaluation of peritoneal endometriosis and endometriotic nodules of the rectovaginal septum. Hum Reprod 1995;11:224–228.

155. Anaf V, Simon P, El Nakadi I et al. Hyperalgesia, nerve infiltration and nerve growth factor expression in deep adenomyotic nodules, peritoneal and ovarian endometriosis. Hum Reprod 2002;17:1895–1900.

156. Squifflet J, Feger C, Donnez J. Diagnosis and imaging of adenomyotic disease of the retroperitoneal space. Gynecol Obstet Invest 2002;54:43–51.

157. Cullen T. Adeno–myoma uteri diffusum benignum. Johns Hopkins Hosp Rep 1896;133.

158. Sampson J. Ovarian hematomas of endometrial type (perforating hemorrhagic cysts of the ovary) and implantation adenomas of endometrial type. Boston Med Surg J 1922;180:445–456.

159. Renish N. Ein Beitrag zur Adenomyositis uteri et recti. Zeischr Geburtshilfe Gynaekol 1912;70:585.

160. Hudelist G, Keckstein J, Wright JT. The migrating adenomyoma: past views on the etiology of adenomyosis and endometriosis. Fertil Steril 2009;92(5):1536–1543.

161. Lockyer C. Fibroids and Allied Tumours (Myoma and Adenomyoma). London: Macmillan, 1918.

162. Vercellini P, Frontino G, Pietropaolo G, Gattei U, Daguati R, Crosignani PG. Deep endometriosis: definition, pathogenesis, and clinical management. J Am Assoc Gynecol Laparosc 2004;11: 153–161.

163. Nakamura M, Katabuchi H, Tohya TR, Fukumatsu Y, Matsuura K, Okamura H. Scanning electron microscopic and immunohisto-chemical studies of pelvic endometriosis. Hum Reprod 1993;8:2218–2226.

164. Kim MR, Park DW, Lee JH et al. Progesterone-dependent release of transforming growth factor-beta1 from epithelial cells enhances the endometrial decidualization by turning on the Smad signalling in stromal cells. Mol Hum Reprod 2005;11:801–808.

165. Haining RE, Cameron IT, van Papendorp C et al. Epidermal growth factor in human endometrium: proliferative effects in culture and immunocytochemical localization in normal and endometriotic tissues. Hum Reprod 1991;6:1200–1205.

166. Hirama Y, Ochiai K. Estrogen and progesterone receptors of the out-of-phase endometrium in female infertile patients. Fertil Steril 1995;63:984–988.

167. Laatikainen T, Andersson B, Karkkainen J, Wahlström T. Progestin receptor levels in endometriomas with delayed or incomplete changes. Obstet Gynecol 1983;62:592–595.

168. Spirtos NJ, Yurewicz EC, Moghissi KS, Magyar DM, Sundareson AS, Bottoms SF. Pseudocorpus luteum insufficiency: a study of cytosol progesterone receptors in human endometrium. Obstet Gynecol 1985;65:535–540.

169. Reich H, McGlynn F, Salvat J. Laparoscopic treatment of cul-de-sac obliteration secondary to retrocervical deep fibrotic endometriosis. J Reprod Med 1991;36:516–522.

170. Donnez J. Excision of deep endometriotic nodules by laparoscopy. In: Donnez J (ed) Laser Surgery. Leuven: Nauwelaerts Printing, 1991, p.148.

171. Donnez J, Squifflet J. Complications, pregnancy and recurrence in a prospective series of 500 patients operated on by the shaving technique for deep rectovaginal endometriotic nodules. Hum Reprod 2010;25(8):1949–1958.

172. Fleisch MC, Xafis D, Bruyne FD, Hucke J, Bender HG, Dall P. Radical resection of invasive endometriosis with bowel or bladder involvement – long-term results. Eur J Obstet Gynecol Reprod Biol 2005;123(2):224–229.

173. Chapron C, Chopin N, Borghese B, Malartic C, Decuypere F, Foulot H. Surgical management of deeply infiltrating endometriosis: an update. Ann NY Acad Sci 2004;1034:326–337.

174. Emmanuel KR, Davis C. Outcomes and treatment options in rectovaginal endometriosis. Curr Opin Obstet Gynecol 2005;17:399–402.

175. Ford J, English J, Miles WF, Giannopoulos T. A new technique for laparoscopic anterior resection for rectal endometriosis. JSLS 2005;9:73–77.

176. Daraï E, Marpeau O, Thomassin I, Dubernard G, Barranger E, Bazot M. Fertility after laparoscopic colorectal resection for endometriosis: preliminary results. Fertil Steril 2005;84:945–950.

177. Redwine DB, Wright JT. Laparoscopic treatment of complete obliteration of the cul-de-sac associated with endometriosis: long-term follow-up of en bloc resection. Feril Steril 2001;76:358–365.

178. Meuleman C, D'Hoore A, van Cleynenbreugel B, Beks N, D'Hooghe T. Outcome after multidisciplinary CO2 laser laparoscopic excision of deep infiltrating colorectal endometriosis. Reprod Biomed Online 2009;18:282–289.

179. Vercellini P, Crosignani PG, Abbiati A, Somigliani E, Viagano P, Fedele L. The effect of surgery for symptomatic endometriosis: the other side of the story. Hum Reprod Update 2009;15:177–178.

180. Donnez J. Is accreditation for surgery necessary? World Endometriosis Society e-journal 2008;10:6–7.

181. Fernandez H, Deffieux X, Faivre E, Gervaise A. Should we operate deep infiltrating endometriosis? No. "Choose realism instead of idealism". Gynécol Obstet Fertil 2008;36:214–217.

182. Canis M, Matsuzaki S, Jardon K et al. Yes, patients with deep infiltrating endometriosis should be operated! "Prefer optimistic will to pessimistic intelligence!" Gynécol Obstet Fertil 2008;36:218–221.

10 Extra-abdominal Endometriosis

Antonio Bobbio[1], Diane Damotte[2], Anne Gompel[3] and Marco Alifano[1]

[1]Department of Thoracic Surgery, Cochin-Hôtel-Dieu Hospital, Paris V University, Paris, France
[2]Department of Pathology, Cochin-Hôtel-Dieu Hospital, Paris V University, Paris, France
[3]Department of Medical Gynecology, Cochin-Hôtel-Dieu Hospital, Paris V University, Paris, France

Introduction

Endometriosis is a disease characterized by the growth of endometrium outside the uterine cavity or myometrium. It occurs more frequently in the pelvis and in the rest of the peritoneal cavity, but endometriosis of virtually all the body compartments has been reported. A classification of extragenital endometriosis was formulated by Markham *et al* in 1989, which distinguishes digestive, urinary, thoracic, and other site implants [1]. In this chapter, we will summarize the current knowledge on thoracic endometriosis and briefly present some other less frequent sites of extragenital endometriosis such as skin, muscular and nerve tissue implants.

Thoracic endometriosis

Thoracic endometriosis is nowadays recognized as a common condition. The thoracic endometriosis syndrome (TES) includes five well-recognized clinical entities: catamenial pneumothorax, catamenial hemothorax, catamenial hemoptysis, catamenial chest pain, and lung nodules, but less frequent presentations are possible [2]. Although TES is defined as the clinical manifestations related to the intrathoracic growth of endometrial tissue, it has been suggested to classify within this term cases with catamenial manifestations (pneumothorax, hemoptysis), also in the absence of histological documentation of endometriosis, but this is not fully accepted [2]. On the other hand, some manifestations (especially pneumothorax) that are generally catamenial if endometriosis-related, may be non-catamenial but endometriosis-related. In any case, the exact time relationship with menses is variable and presentations in the immediate pre- or postmenstrual period are often called catamenial, although they should not be classified accordingly. Overall, a large degree of overlap in definitions exists.

Epidemiology

Unlike pelvic endometriosis, which is thought to affect 5–15% of women of reproductive age [3], thoracic endometriosis has been considered an extremely rare condition until recent years. In a review paper published in 1996, Joseph and Sahan found 110 cases published in the previous 50 years; 73% of them were catamenial pneumothoraces, the remaining being represented by the other manifestations of the TES [4]. Since this publication, an increasing number of case reports and some surgical series have been published, probably because of an increased recognition of the condition. Retrospective analysis of all pneumothoraces operated on in our surgical department in a 6-year period showed that catamenial pneumothorax accounted for 24.6% (28/114) of cases of female patients referred for a pneumothorax initially considered idiopathic [5]. Interestingly thoracic endometriosis was found in 18/28 of these cases, whereas among patients with non-catamenial pneumothorax, thoracic endometriosis was finally histologically diagnosed in 11/86 cases. Thus, only 55 out of the 114 female patients had a pneumothorax, which was neither catamenial nor endometriosis related. Some other recent surgical series have confirmed the high incidence of catamenial pneumothorax or endometriosis-related non-catamenial pneumothorax among women referred for surgery [6–8]. If catamenial pneumothorax, endometriosis related or not and non-catamenial but endometriosis-related pneumothorax is now considered as a relatively common condition, the remaining manifestations of thoracic endometriosis syndrome remain rare.

Etiological mechanisms

The etiological mechanisms of endometriosis are described in detail in other chapters of this book; herein we will briefly analyze the specific aspects of the etiology of thoracic endometriosis.

Among the three etiological theories of endometriosis (coelomic metaplasia, lymphatic or hematogenous embolization from uterus or pelvis, and retrograde menstruation with subsequent transperitoneal-transdiaphragmatic migration of endometrial tissue), none may explain all the clinical manifestations of thoracic endometriosis. In particular, neither the theory of coelomic metaplasia nor that of lymphatic or vascular embolization is able to reliably explain the right-sided predominance of the disease, whereas the theory of transperitoneal-transdiaphragmatic migration of endometrial tissue cannot explain the occurrence of intrapulmonary localization. Thus, it is nowadays suggested that the disease has probably a multifactorial etiology, with some mechanism being dominant [4,9].

We suggest that the Sampson theory is probably the most appropriate to explain most of the manifestations of thoracic endometriosis: after retrograde menstruation, endometrial tissue may undergo either lymphatic or vascular embolization with possible pulmonary embolization (responsible for catamenial hemoptysis, endometriotic lung nodules, and some rare cases of catamenial pneumothorax due to visceral pleura endometriosis) or transperitoneal-transdiaphragmatic migration, responsible, as described below, for catamenial or endometriosis-related pneumothorax or hemothorax [10]. This theory would explain the right-sided predominance of both diaphragmatic and intrathoracic involvement of the disease. In fact, movement of fluids in the peritoneal cavity ("peritoneal circulation") follows predictable patterns: a preferential flow of fluids (air, cell aggregates, pus) exists from the pelvis to the right subdiaphragmatic area through the right paracolic gutter. Subsequently, the transdiaphragmatic passage of endometrial tissue could occur through either congenital or, more frequently, acquired diaphragmatic defects. In fact, the endometrial implants in the abdominal aspect of the diaphragm undergo cyclical necrosis and subsequent cycles may lead to the production of holes. Once into the pleural space, the viable endometrial tissue may colonize either the diaphragm and/or the rest of the pleural space. Although isolated diaphragmatic endometriosis is a frequent feature, the association of diaphragmatic and pleural endometriosis is possible [5–8].

Pathogenic mechanisms of pneumothorax

For pneumothorax occurring during the menstrual period, it should be remembered that air may be forced to enter the peritoneum thanks to the absence of mucus plug, by uterine contractions, physical efforts, or sexual intercourse and then it may reach the pleural space, through diaphragmatic defects, because of the negative intrathoracic pressure [2,3,11]. In our recently published experience [5], diaphragmatic abnormalities in terms of nodules and/or fenestrations were found in 22 out of 28 cases of catamenial pneumothorax (endometriosis was found in 18/28 of these cases), and in 11/11 cases of non-catamenial but endometriosis-related pneumothorax. The transdiaphragmatic passage of air implies the occurrence of a pneumoperitoneum as an intermediate step. Pneumoperitoneum has been described to occur during pelvic examination, postpartum knee-to-chest exercise, bending over, vaginal douching, and post coitus. We reported on four cases of associated pneumoperitoneum and

pneumothorax, and in one of them we had the opportunity to photograph the transdiaphragmatic passage of air [12,13]. Furthermore, we have reported a case of successful tubal ligature in the treatment of recurrent pneumothorax after failure of previous surgical therapy. In cases of non-catamenial but endometriosis-related pneumothorax, we suggested that the same factors responsible for pneumothorax during menses may also cause it in other periods, if the causative factor is sufficient to overcome the resistance of the mucus plug or if it is more permeable than usual.

The mechanism of transdiaphragmatic passage of air cannot explain the pathogenesis of all the reported cases of catamenial pneumothorax: alveolar leak secondary to sloughing of endometrial tissue from the visceral pleura may be another mechanism, advocated in approximately 30% of cases in the review by Korom *et al* [6]. In our recent report we found visceral pleural endometriosis (which was often associated with diaphragmatic endometriosis) in 11/28 cases of catamenial pneumothorax and in 3/11 cases of non-catamenial but endometriosis-related pneumothorax [5]. Some authors, especially in the past, did not find diaphragmatic defects or pleural endometriosis in patients with catamenial pneumothorax. Thus catamenial pneumothorax has been sometimes considered as a consequence of hormonal changes typical of the menstrual period: increased local or circulating levels of prostaglandin $F_2\alpha$, a potent vascular and bronchiolar constrictor, might be responsible for alveolar rupture and pneumothorax. Finally, it has been suggested that pulmonary endometrial implants may swell during the menstrual period inside terminal bronchioles, thus causing localized hyperinflation by a check-valve mechanism which, in turn, might cause pneumothorax [14].

Clinical presentations
Catamenial pneumothorax
Catamenial pneumothorax (CP) takes its name from its temporal relationship with menses: CP is generally defined as a recurrent pneumothorax occurring within 72 h from the onset of menstruation, but somewhat different time frames have been adopted [2]. For simple statistical considerations, the recurrent character of the pneumothorax during the menstrual period is essential to classify a pneumothorax as catamenial and not just as a mere temporal coincidence [2]. The strict relationship with menses is a typical manifestation of the disease; this relationship is confirmed by the majority of reports and outlined in review papers [6–8]. However, a recurrent endometriosis-related pneumothorax may also be observed in the intermenstrual period [5]. There are no specific eliciting factors in most cases of catamenial pneumothorax, but it has been suggested that physical efforts or sexual intercourse may be causative factors [15]. Though, by definition, catamenial pneumothorax occurs in the menstrual period, it may not occur with every menstrual cycle. In our recent prospective study, 1–4 episodes had occurred in the studied population prior to video-thoracoscopic examination [5], but several reports describe patients who experienced more than 10 episodes before receiving treatment with curative intent.

Age at presentation of catamenial pneumothorax or of non-catamenial but endometriosis-related pneumothorax seems to be higher than in non-catamenial pneumothorax. These patients frequently also have a history of known pelvic endometriosis and/or infertility. Catamenial pneumothorax is unilateral and right-sided in almost all instances, but left-sided pneumotoraces have much more rarely been reported. Bilateral occurrence is also possible, but it is also extremely infrequent.

The presentation of catamenial pneumothorax is the same as other kinds of pneumothorax: cough, chest pain, and shortness of breath are the most common symptoms. Chest pain may present as usually seen in patients with spontaneous pneumothorax or as periscapular or neck-radiated pain ("diaphragmatic pain"). Symptoms may be either discrete or very severe but in most instances, they are of mild intensity. In the review by Joseph and Sahn [4], among 80 patients with catamenial pneumothorax, the size of pneumothorax was small in 42 cases, medium in 19, large in four, and unspecified in 15. CP may be associated with the other manifestations of TES, but this kind of occurrence is unusual. As a general rule in TES, catamenial pneumothorax may occur only in the presence of a cyclic hormonal activity and, in most instances, of an intact genital apparatus. However, occurrence after hysterectomy with bilateral oophorectomy in cases of hormonal replacement therapy has been reported [15]. Similarly, a case has been published describing recurrent pneumothorax during pregnancy in a patient who had catamenial pneumothorax diagnosed before becoming pregnant [16]. Laboratory investigations may show increased levels of cancer antigen CA-125 in endometriosis-related catamenial pneumothorax [7].

Catamenial hemothorax

In the review by Joseph and Sahn, catamenial hemothorax accounted for 14% of manifestations of the TES [4]. Pelvic endometriosis was present in 100% of cases, whereas a history of pelvic surgery was reported in four out of 15 patients. Catamenial hemothorax may present in association with catamenial pneumothorax, but this occurrence is uncommon [2,4]. The right side is involved in almost all cases, although a case has been reported of associated right pneumothorax and left hemothorax [17]. The most common presenting symptoms are non-specific and include cough, chest pain, and shortness of breath [2]. In some instances signs can mimic those of pulmonary embolism [18]. The amount of bloody effusion is variable: in the review by Joseph and Sahn [4], it was large, moderate and small in two, three, and 10 cases, respectively. Catamenial hemothorax has been reported as being responsible for anaemia and collections of 7 L over 2 weeks [18]. At thoracocentesis, grossly bloody fluid is retrieved and laboratory examination can show high protein and lactate dehydrogenase levels [18]. Cytological examination may show endometrial cells. In almost all cases, chest x-ray shows the presence of pleural effusion without specific characteristics. Computed tomography (CT) scan confirms the presence of the effusion and may show additional features such as nodular lesions of pleura, multiloculated effusions, or bulky pleural masses.

Catamenial hemoptysis

Cyclical hemoptysis occurring during menses is an extremely rare condition; in the review by Joseph and Sahn, catamenial hemoptysis was the clinical presentation in eight out of 110 patients (7%) [4]. The amount of bleeding is quite variable (5–15 mL of blood per episode in those reports in which quantitative values are available) but neither cases of massive hemoptysis nor deaths have been described. The source of bleeding is an endometrial implant located in the pulmonary parenchyma or in the large airways in the vast majority of cases, this having represented an important obstacle to histological confirmation. The diagnostic work-up is still a matter of debate, but the key is undoubtedly careful history taking and clinical examination. A temporal association of symptoms with menses may not be recognized or appreciated and diagnostic delays up to 4 years from the onset of symptoms have been reported [19]. The exclusion of alternative causes of recurrent hemoptysis such as tuberculosis, opportunistic infections, bronchiectasis, pulmonary infarction, bronchial neoplasms, arteriovenous malformations, and anomalous vessels should always be pursued [20].

Several imaging methods have been employed in patients with suspected catamenial hemoptysis. Chest x-ray may display pulmonary densities or nodular infiltrates, but it shows normal findings even in a significant number of patients with current bleeding. Chest CT is probably the most sensitive tool, provided that it is performed during the menses [21]. CT findings of pulmonary endometriosis include ill-defined or well-defined opacities, nodules, thin-walled cavities, bullous formations, and ground-glass opacities. All these lesions, which are expressions of either endometrial implants or/and secondary hemorrhage, may change in size during the menstrual cycle. Unfortunately, CT scan may have a low diagnostic yield in tracheobronchial endometriosis without parenchymal involvement [22]. Descriptions of bronchoscopic findings in patients with tracheobronchial endometriosis are extremely rare. The presence of multiple, bilateral purplish-red submucosal lesions with easy touch oozing has been observed in most cases and seems the most common feature, but the spectrum of tracheobronchial abnormalities may also include a striking diffuse hyperemia with pronounced mucosal oozing, and a single, tiny red mucosal spot. Curiously, bronchial biopsy almost constantly fails to provide a tissue diagnosis regardless of the bronchoscopic findings, whereas brush cytology frequently shows distinctive features of endometrial cells. Even when all the bronchoscopic sampling procedures do not yield a diagnosis of endometriosis, follow-up bronchoscopic examination in the middle of the menstrual cycle may typically show disappearance of the previously reported findings [23].

Lung nodules

Lung nodules in the setting of TES are not infrequent radiological features, but they are associated in most cases with clinical symptoms such as chest pain (in the subpleural location) or, mainly, catamenial hemoptysis [2,21]. In extremely rare instances, however, single or multiple nodules can be the presentation of

TES in the absence of any other clinical or radiological manifestation, such an event having been registered in only seven out of 110 patients (6%) in the series by Joseph and Sahn [4]. Isolated lung nodules tend to be observed at an older age than any other clinical presentation of TES, a decreased hormonal support for the endometrial tissue in the older ages having been claimed as the likely explanation for the less common and pronounced clinical manifestations associated with these nodules. Finally, lung nodules have a less frequent, although evident, right-sided preferential location as compared to the other manifestations of TES [2].

Exceptional presentations

In the setting of TES, catamenial chest pain is related in almost all instances to catamenial pneumothorax or hemothorax. Two gynecological series have reported on cases of diaphragmatic endometriosis diagnosed at laparoscopy in which chest pain without pneumothorax or hemothorax was the only clinical complaint [24,25]. Shoulder pain was frequently associated and it sometimes radiated up to the neck or the arm [25]. In other instances, epigastric or right upper quadrant pain was reported. In most patients it was a pure catamenial pain, whereas in others it began several days before menstruation. The possibility of persistent pain with exacerbation during menses has also been reported [24]. Seeliger et al recently reported on a patient who had an extraordinarily large jelly-like paracardiac and abdominal mass which protruded through an intercostal space, causing a pulsating subcutaneous tumor [26]. Also, a single case of endometriosis in the thoracic aorta has been reported. It involved the area of an old repair of a coarctation and presented as intractable hypertension after elective cesarean section [27]. Finally, a unique case of catamenial chest pain with pneumomediastinum without pneumothorax is known. Tissue diagnosis was not obtained, but a favorable outcome was observed with danazol therapy [28].

Management

Operative treatment

Management of thoracic endometriosis should be multidisciplinary and include bronchoscopy, surgery, if possible by video-assisted technology, and hormonal treatment. Operative bronchoscopy with Nd:YAG laser has been rarely employed to treat endobronchial localizations of endometriosis, responsible for cyclic hemoptysis; experience with video-assisted thoracoscopy in the management of catamenial pneumothorax or hemothorax is, on the other hand, nowadays more widespread. At video-assisted thoracoscopy, once the pathogenic mechanism is identified at exploration, a targeted treatment may be carried out in most instances. Diaphragmatic involvement by either Sendometrial tissue or perforations is probably best managed by diaphragmatic resection. Simple suture of holes has been reported to be followed by recurrence, and it does not provide tissue for diagnosis. Diaphragmatic resection and suture may be achieved by endoscopic stapler devices [5,29], provided that the resected surface is smaller than 3 cm of long axis. If more extended

resection is necessary, as in the majority of cases, we suggest the use of a utility mini-thoracotomy to allow diaphragmatic resection and repair with X-shaped stitches. The insertion of a polyglactin mesh to cover the tendinous part of the diaphragm, to avoid leaving occult defects, has also been proposed [7]. Treatment of other lesions possibly involved in the pathogenesis of pneumothorax may be generally carried out by video-assisted thoracoscopy. In particular, bullous dystrophy can be resected as usual in the treatment of pneumothorax, and care should be taken to identify visceral or parietal pleura endometriosis, whose treatment by small wedge resection or limited pleurectomy we strongly suggest. We advocate associated talc pleurodesis instead of pleural abrasion because of the higher recurrence rate observed with this last method of pleural symphysis [5].

With regard to the treatment of catamenial hemothorax, pleurectomy, carried out by either thoracoscopy or thoracotomy, has been recently used [17], but none of the reports on the topic gives information on the extent of pleural resection. We suggest that at least the portions macroscopically involved by the disease be resected in order to remove active endometrial foci, to prevent further spread of the disease, and to produce a permanent symphysis (if the extent of pleurectomy is important). Wedge resection of implants in lung parenchyma may also be achieved by video-assisted thoracoscopy [30].

In the case of catamenial hemoptysis, surgery has been advocated in cases of failure of medical treatment [31], intolerable drug-related side-effects or symptom recurrence after the cessation of hormonal therapy. Surgery has also been proposed as an alternative to medical treatment. Open surgery may be employed in the treatment of catamenial hemoptysis when video-assisted thoracoscopy or video-assisted thoracic surgery is not adequate. Parenchymal sparing procedures should be employed whenever possible (wedge resections, subsegmentectomy, segmentectomy), but lobectomy may be seldom necessary [31].

Hysterectomy with bilateral salpingo-oophorectomy obviously represents the definitive treatment of endometriosis, but it should be considered only in cases of failure of other treatment modalities; remarkably, if hormonal replacement therapy is undertaken in this setting, thoracic endometriosis manifestations may recur [4].

Medical treatment

The aim of medical treatment is to block hormonal support to existing endometrial implants and to prevent further seeding. Reports on the use of oral contraceptives, progestatives, danazol, and gonadotropin-releasing hormone (GnRH) agonists are all available in the literature, but no controlled trial on the efficacy of these drugs in the setting of catamenial pneumothorax is available [2–4]. Furthermore, there is no definitive argument to suggest that a specific drug is superior to the others. Thus, the choice of drug is based on the team's specific experience, as well as on considerations about costs, side-effects, and pregnancy wishes [3].

The majority of experience in the last decade has been obtained with GnRH agonists and the antigonadotropic progestin ciproterone acetate [32]. In a comprehensive series, medical treatment alone was unfortunately associated with an unacceptably high recurrence rate of more than 50%, regardless of the drug(s) used [4]; in a more recent series, failure rate as high as 100% [33] has been observed. Regression of endometrial implants with hormonal therapy is not complete and/or recurrent embolization from pelvic foci is a continuous process in a large percentage of cases. Interestingly, in the retrospective analysis by Joseph and Sahn, surgical treatment of catamenial pneumothorax resulted in a far lower recurrence rate than hormonal therapy: the 6- and 12-month recurrence rates of catamenial pneumothorax were 50% and 60% respectively for medical treatment, and 5% and 25% respectively for surgical management [4]. On the basis of these considerations, we proposed, in the setting of catamenial pneumothorax, a treatment strategy based on a sequential approach of surgery followed by a 6-month period of hormonal treatment by GnRH agonists (or ciproterone acetate in case of contraindications or poor tolerance), in order to achieve complete ovarian rest during the time necessary for complete pleural symphysis [2,5].

Pathology

Thoracic endometriosis consists of the presence of endometrial tissue within the thoracic cavity. Regardless of the site, endometriotic foci consist of endometrial stroma and glands in different states, often with ectatic glands, mostly lined by pseudostratified cuboidal to cylindrical epithelium and sometimes filled with hemosiderin-laden macrophages [21] (Fig. 10.1). It is not clear if the presence of both stroma and glands is mandatory to affirm the diagnosis of extrapelvic endometriosis; we suggested that thoracic endometriosis may be considered histologically proven when both glands and stroma are present, whereas when only endometrial stroma staining positively with CD10 antigen and with estrogen/progesterone receptors are observed, endometriosis can be considered probable [4].

Macroscopically brown nodules in either pleura or diaphragm may correspond to hemorrhagic foci with hemosiderin-laden macrophages. Although this aspect may suggest endometriosis, this diagnosis cannot be definitively affirmed in the absence of the criteria described above [4].

Outcome

As discussed above, catamenial pneumothorax has a high recurrence rate. The exact figures are incompletely known, as few studies have addressed the issue of middle- and long-term outcomes. In the retrospective series by Bagan et al [7], reporting on 10 cases seen in the same institution, the recurrence rate (with a mean follow-up of 55.7 months) was high (3/5) among patients treated by simple thoracoscopic pleurodesis, and all of them (5/5) had persistent catamenial chest pain. In contrast, none of the patients who had diaphragmatic abnormalities identified and treated experienced recurrence of catamenial pneumothorax or chest pain.

In our retrospective series on spontaneous pneumothorax in women, the overall postsurgery recurrence rate was 14%, with a mean follow-up of 32.7 months [5]. Recurrence rates for

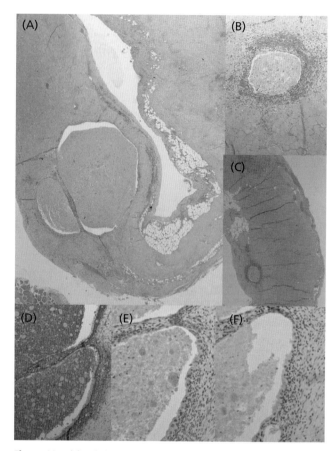

Figure 10.1 (A) Pathological examination of a resected diaphragmatic specimen. Two cystic endometrial glands filled with cell debris and iron-loaded macrophages are evident. Hematoxylin and eosin stain, initial magnification ×20. (B) Histopathological view at higher magnification of cystic endometrial glands. Endometrial stroma with blood is also evident. Hematoxylin and eosin stain, initial magnification ×100. (C) Histopathological view at lower magnification of cystic endometrium inside the resected diaphragm. Hematoxylin and eosin stain, initial magnification, ×4. (D) Immunohistochemistry with anti-CD10 antibody of a resected diaphragmatic specimen containing an endometrial implant: note the positive staining of endometrial stroma. Initial magnification ×100. (E) Immunohistochemistry with antibody against estrogen receptor of a resected diaphragmatic specimen containing an endometrial implant: note the positive staining of both endometrial gland and stroma. Initial magnification ×100. (F) Immunohistochemistry with antiFbody against progesterone receptor of a resected diaphragmatic specimen containing an endometrial implant: note the positive staining of both endometrial gland and stroma. Initial magnification ×100

catamenial pneumothorax, non-catamenial but endometriosis-related, and non-catamenial/non-endometriosis-related pneumothorax were 32%, 27%, and 5.3%, respectively. These globally mediocre results in catamenial pneumothorax and endometriosis-related pneumothorax prompted us to switch our technique of pleurodesis from pleural abrasion to talc insufflations. With an aggressive approach based on video-assisted thoracic surgery (with resection of all diseased areas and talc pleurodesis) and a 6-month hormonal treatment, the recurrence rate dropped to 0% [5]. Since the time when the study was published, two recurrences have occurred in spite of this approach and required iterative surgery and hormonal treatment (unpublished observations).

Information about the long-term outcome of the other manifestations of the thoracic endometriosis is inconsistent.

Other sites of extragenital endometriosis

Cutaneous and incisional endometriosis

Cutaneous endometriosis is reported as being a common site of extrapelvic endometriosis with a prevalence among women with endometriosis ranging between 1% and 5%. Among all cutaneous forms, scar endometriosis is the most frequent and its occurrence in the Pfannenstiel surgical incision is widely documented [34]. Endometriosis has also been observed in abdominal scar after myomectomy or hysterectomy and in a trocar incision site following laparoscopic treatment of endometriosis. Spontaneous cutaneous endometrosis is much more rare and is frequently observed in association with severe pelvic disease. Direct extension through the round ligament or through the omphalomesenteric duct is responsible for inguinal or umbilical implants, respectively. Of note, the right inguinal side is more likely to be affected than the left side.

Intramedullary and sciatic endometriosis

Six cases of intraspinal endometriosis were collected in a literature review published in 2006 [35]. Symptoms, which have often a menstrual occurrence, encompass meningeal irritation, nerve compression and even paraplegia. Intramedullary implants have been advocated to originate from reverse transport via the venous plexus of Betson. Diagnosis is generally established at time of surgery which is scheduled for medullary decompression. Radical resection is rarely achieved and medical therapy is mandatory.

Cyclical sciatica is a clinical syndrome defined by Head in 1962 which refers to endometriosis implants contiguous to nerve sciatic roots [36]. Typically nerve compression is intrapelvic but compression distally in the right sciatic notch has also been described.

Muscular endometriosis

Few cases of muscular implants have been reported. Gastrocnemius, trapezius deltoid and vastus lateralis muscular implants have been described [37]. Localized pain is the most common symptom and a swelling mass is present at physical examination. Diagnosis is established at the time of surgical excision, but without medical treatment local recurrence is to be expected.

Conclusion

Extra-abdominal and extrathoracic endometriosis are rarely seen in clinical practice. On the other hand, catamenial pneumothorax and endometriosis-related non-catamenial pneumothorax account for a significant proportion of spontaneous pneumothoraces in women. Pathogenic mechanisms are now sufficiently elucidated. Multimodality treatment, including aggressive surgery, hormonal treatment and close follow-up, is mandatory to best manage these patients. In spite of this approach, the problem of recurrence is not completely solved, suggesting that research should continue to further improve the management of these patients.

References

1. Markham SM, Carpenter SE, Rock JA. Extrapelvic endometriosis. Obstet Gynecol Clin North Am 1989;16:193–194.

2. Alifano M, Trisolini R, Cancellieri A, Regnard JF. Thoracic endometriosis: current knowledge. Ann Thorac Surg 2006;81:761–769.

3. Olive DL, Schwartz LB. Endometriosis. N Engl J Med 1993; 328:1759–1769.

4. Joseph J, Sahn S. Thoracic endometriosis syndrome: new observations from an analysis of 110 cases. Am J Med 1996;100:164–169.

5. Alifano M, Jablonski C, Kadiri H et al. Catamenial and noncatamenial, endometriosis-related or nonendometriosis-related pneumothorax referred for surgery. Am J Respir Crit Care Med 2007; 176:1048–1053.

6. Korom S, Canyurt H, Missbach A et al. Catamenial pneumothorax revisited: clinical approach and systematic review of the literature. J Thorac Cardiovasc Surg 2004;128:502–508.

7. Bagan P, Berna P, Assouad J et al. Value of cancer antigen 125 for diagnosis of pleural endometriosis in females with recurrent pneumothorax. Eur Respir J 2008;31:140–142.

8. Ciriaco P, Negri G, Libretti L et al. Surgical treatment of catamenial pneumothorax: a single centre experience. Interact Cardiovasc Thorac Surg 2009;8:349–352.

9. Morcos M, Alifano M, Gompel A, Regnard JF. Life-threatening endometriosis-related hemopneumothorax. Ann Thorac Surg 2006; 82:726–729.

10. Sampson JA. Peritoneal endometriosis due to the menstrual dissemination of endometrial tissue into the peritoneal cavity. Am J Obstet Gynecol 1927;14:422–469.

11. Kirschner PA. Porous diaphragm syndromes. Chest Surg Clin North Am 1998;8:449–472.

12. Roth T, Alifano M, Schussler O, Magdeleinat P, Regnard JF. Catamenial pneumothorax: an original chest x-ray sign and thoracoscopic treatment. Ann Thorac Surg 2002;74:563–565.

13. Jablonski C, Alifano M, Regnard JF, Gompel A. Pneumoperitoneum associated with catamenial pneumothorax in women with thoracic endometriosis. Fertil Steril 2009;91:930.

14. Lillington GA, Mitchell SP, Wood GA. Catamenial pneumothorax. JAMA 1972;219:1328–1332.

15. Muller NL, Nelems B. Postcoital catamenial pneumothorax. Report of a case not associated with endometriosis and successfully treated with tubal ligation. Am Rev Respir Dis 1986;134:803–804.

16. Schoenfeld A, Ziv E, Zeelel Y, Ovadia J. Catamenial pneumothorax: a literature review and report of an unusual case. Obstet Gynecol Surv 1986;41:20–24.

17. Ziedalski TM, Sankaranarayanan V, Chitkara RK. Thoracic endometriosis: a case report and literature review. J Thorac Cardiovasc Surg 2004;127:1513–1514.

18. Shepard MK, Mancini MC, Campbell GD, George R. Right-sided hemothorax and recurrent abdominal pain in a 34-year-old woman. Chest 1993;103:1239–1240.

19. Cassina PC, Hauser M, Kacl G, Imthurn B, Schroder S, Weder W. Catamenial hemoptysis. Diagnosis with MRI. Chest 1997;111:1447–1450.

20. Guidry CG, George RB. Diagnostic studies in catamenial hemoptysis. Chest 1990;98:260–261.

21. Elliot DL, Barker AF, Dixon LM. Catamenial hemoptysis. New methods of diagnosis and therapy. Chest 1985;87:687–688.

22. Wang HC, Kuo PH, Kuo SH, Luh KT. Catamenial hemoptysis from tracheobronchial endometriosis: reappraisal of diagnostic value of bronchoscopy and bronchial brush cytology. Chest 2000;118:1205–1208.

23. Hope-Gill B, Prathibha BV. Catamenial haemoptysis and clomiphene citrate therapy. Thorax 2003;58:89–90.

24. Mouroux J, Perrin C, Venissac N, Blaive B, Richelme H. Management of pleural effusion of cirrhotic origin. Chest 1996;109:1093–1096.

25. Redwine DB. Diaphragmatic endometriosis: diagnosis, surgical management, and long-term results of treatment. Fertil Steril 2002;77:288–296.

26. Seeliger T, Voigt JU, Singer H, Daniel WG, Rupprecht H. Pulsating thoracic tumor caused by extragenital endometriosis in a patient with Noonan syndrome. Ann Thorac Surg 2004;77:2204–2206.

27. Notzold A, Moubayed P, Sievers HH. Endometriosis in the thoracic aorta. N Engl J Med 1998;339:1002–1003.

28. Shahar J, Angelillo VA. Catamenial pneumomediastinum. Chest 1986;90:776–777.

29. Alifano M, Roth T, Camilleri Broet S, Schussler O, Magdeleinat P, Regnard JF. Catamenial pneumothorax. A prospective study. Chest 2003;124:1004–1008.

30. Inoue T, Kurokawa Y, Kaiwa Y et al. Video-assisted thoracoscopic surgery for catamenial hemoptysis. Chest 2001;120:655–658.

31. Kristianen K, Fjeld NB. Pulmonary endometriosis causing haemoptysis. Report of a case treated with lobectomy. Scand J Thorac Cardiovasc Surg 1993;27:113–115.

32. Slabbynck H, Laureys M, Impens N, de Vroey P, Schandevyl W. Recurring catamenial pneumothorax treated with a Gn-RH analogue. Chest 1991;100:851.

33. Tripp HF Thomas LP, Obney JA. Current therapy of catamenial pneumothorax. Heart Surg Forum 1998;1:146–149.

34. Douglas C, Rotimi O. Extragenital endometriosis – a clinicopathological review of a Glasgow hospital experience with case illustrations. J Obstet Gynaecol 2004;24:804–808.

35. Agrawal A, Shetty BJ, Makannavar JH, Shetty L, Shetty J, Shetty V. Intramedullary endometriosis of the conus medullaris: case report. Neurosurgery 2006;59(2):E428.

36. Papapietro N, Gulino G, Zobel BB, di Martino A, Denaro V. Cyclic sciatica related to an extrapelvic endometriosis of the sciatic nerve: new concepts in surgical therapy J Spinal Disord Tech 2002;15:436–439.

37. Poli-Neto OB, Rosa-E-Silva JC, Barbosa HF, Candido-Dos-Reis FJ, Nogueira AA. Endometriosis of the soleus and gastrocnemius muscles. Fertil Steril 2009;91:1294.

4 Biological Basis and Pathophysiology of Endometriosis

11 Biology of Eutopic and Ectopic Endometrium in Women with Endometriosis

Petra A.B. Klemmt and Anna Starzinski-Powitz

Institute for Cell Biology and Neuroscience, Johann Wolfgang Goethe University, Frankfurt, Germany

Introduction

In this chapter we will address the cell biology of eutopic and ectopic endometrium in the context of cell differentiation, escape mechanisms and the influence of the pelvic microenvironment on the development of endometriotic lesions. We revisited experimental and descriptive observations regarding the presumed changes in eutopic endometrial phenotype in affected women and the emergence and differential expression of molecules in endometriotic foci. Here we focus on the molecular mechanisms of cell–cell adhesion, particularly the role of cadherin expression and the integrin/extracellular matrix (ECM) expression profile and their putative modulation by growth factors, prostaglandins and interleukins increased in the pelvic fluid of affected women.

(Patho)biology of eutopic and ectopic endometrium

Endometrium is composed of a lining surface epithelium and associated glands with a connective tissue stroma in which spiral arteries are embedded. Within the endometrium, two distinct areas can be distinguished. The lamina basalis, a germinal layer, contains undifferentiated glands embedded in stroma which persists from cycle to cycle, and the transient superficial lamina functionalis, which consists of loose stroma and differentiating glands. The lamina functionalis responds to ovarian steroids during the menstrual cycle and is shed during menstruation. The morphological changes in endometrial structure have been well described and are coincident with the cyclic changes in the ovary [1,2]. In addition to histological profiling, the changes in gene expression across the menstrual cycle have also been evaluated and can be used to distinguish the different phases [3].

The regular (28-day) menstrual cycle can be divided into three phases: the proliferative phase (cycle days 5–14), the secretory phase (early, mid and late luteal phase, cycle days 15–28) and shedding/menstruation (cycle days 1–4) if no implantation occurs. The proliferative phase is characterized by re-epithelialization of the luminal edge and growth of the stromal and glandular elements in response to ovarian estrogen, the dominant hormone during this phase. Estrogen is dependent on follicle-stimulating hormone (FSH) produced by the adenohypophysis. Ovulation usually occurs after a surge in circulating luteinizing hormone (LH). The postovulatory rise in ovarian progesterone in the secretory phase induces profound remodeling of the estrogen-primed endometrium, characterized initially by growth and coiling of the spiral arteries, secretory transformation of the glands, influx of distinct immune cells, and subsequently by predecidualization of the stromal compartments independent of the presence of an implanting blastocyst. The decidual transformation represents a process of morphological and biochemical differentiation and involves extensive reprogramming at the molecular level. In this context, altered steroid hormone receptor expression and steroid metabolism, remodeling of the ECM and cytoskeleton, altered expression of intracellular enzymes, growth factors and cytokines and their receptors, and induction of apoptosis modulators and decidua-specific transcription factors have been reported [37]. A recent study compared the gene expression profile of the lamina functionalis with the lamina basalis and the intermediate area between those two endometrial layers confirmed the upregulation of genes necessary for ECM remodeling and apoptosis markers in the menstrual lysed superficial layer but not in the lamina basalis [8].

The naturally occurring myometrial contraction waves transport the menstrual effluent to a certain extent retrograde through the fallopian tubes into the peritoneal cavity [9,10]. Due to this physiological phenomenon, shed endometrial fragments can be detected in the peritoneal fluid in up to 59% of women

Endometriosis: Science and Practice, First Edition. Edited by Linda C. Giudice, Johannes L.H. Evers and David L. Healy.
© 2012 Blackwell Publishing Ltd. Published 2012 by Blackwell Publishing Ltd.

with and without endometriosis [11–19]. Further studies confirmed that the retrogradely refluxed menstrual efflux contains viable endometrial cells [20,21] which have been shown to express cell adhesion molecules [22–24]. Interestingly in this context, *de novo* increase in ECM deposition and cell adhesion molecules in menstrual endometrium has been suggested to facilitate ectopic implantation [8]. Furthermore, endometrium and shed menstrual fragments from women with endometriosis express haptoglobin [16] which is implicated in facilitating escape from immune destruction by reducing the phagocytotic activity of peritoneal macrophages and altering their cytokine expression profile [25].

The successive cycles of proliferation, differentiation, and shedding/menstruation of the endometrium during the reproductive lifespan of a woman indicate the presence of cells with stem cell characteristics [26,27]. This notion is supported by emerging evidence of stem cell marker expression in the lamina basalis and the presence of colony-forming cells [28–31]. In line with this, it has been debated whether endometriosis is actually a stem cell-driven disease [32–34] and might be caused by retrograde transported endometrial fragments containing dislocated basal endometrium [35,36]. Indeed, alongside shed endometrial fragments, menstrual blood contains cells with adult stem cell characteristics. Endometrial mesenchymal stem cells were identified which were able to differentiate *in vitro* into various lineages and exhibited matrix metalloproteinase (MMP) expression [37–39]. Interestingly, a histological study showed that bone marrow-derived mesenchymal stem cells (BM-MSC) participate in endometrial regeneration [40]. Based on this observation, another study showed that BM-MSC have the potential to differentiate down the stromal fibroblast lineage and were able to secrete biochemical markers of decidualization, namely prolactin (PRL) and insulin-like growth factor binding protein-1 (IGFBP-1) [41].

Women with endometriosis display a more prolonged and heavier menstrual flow than women without endometriosis [42], which is flushed into the peritoneal cavity more frequently and to a greater extent in women with proven endometriosis than in women with patent tubes unaffected by the condition [9,13,16,18]. Accumulating evidence also suggests that endometrium from women with endometriosis displays morphologically normal but structurally and biochemically abnormal responses [43–46]. In this context abnormal remodeling of ECM of endometrial stroma [47–50] and aberrant integrin expression have been associated with implantation defects [51]. Transcriptome analysis also revealed altered gene expression in the eutopic endometrium from women with endometriosis linked to implantation failure [52] and in ectopic endometrium [53]. The ability to contract ECM is upregulated in eutopic and even higher in ectopic endometrium from women with endometriosis and is attenuated if decidualization is induced [54]. Furthermore, endometrial stroma from women with endometriosis exhibits an impaired and/or reduced differentiation into decidual cells [46,55] and endometriotic stroma cells from peritoneal, ovarian or deeply infiltrating lesions show markedly reduced differentiation capacity [46].

Normally, endometrial stroma controls epithelial cell proliferation and survival. In endometriotic lesions, however, the epithelium exhibits increased proliferation and survival. A recent study demonstrated that this observation is linked to an increase in survivin expression in both eutopic and ectopic epithelium from women with endometriosis [56]. In this context, the endometriotic stromal cells lose the ability to regulate the epithelial survivin expression through the PI3 kinase/Akt pathway in both eutopic and ectopic epithelium, leading to increased cell proliferation and survival. These observations suggest that eutopic and to a greater extent ectopic endometrium from women with endometriosis contain less differentiated cells. Due to their reduced differentiation, they might be less likely to undergo apoptosis and remain able to respond to factors present in a novel environment.

Peritoneal cavity: role of peritoneal fluid in endometriosis

Peritoneal fluid (PF) is an important constituent of the peritoneal environment and is composed from different sources: plasma transudate, ovarian exudate, tubal fluid, retrograde menstruation, and macrophage secretions [57]. Depending on their location and depth of infiltration, early endometriotic foci are under the influence of various factors such as hormones, cytokines, growth factors and other factors present in peritoneal or ovarian fluid or the bloodstream [58]. Many investigators have shown that PF and follicular fluid from women with endometriosis enhance eutopic and ectopic endometrial cell proliferation [57,59–61]. It has been shown that this increased proliferation can depend on growth factors such as tumor necrosis factor-α (TNF-α) circulating in the PF from women with endometriosis [61–64]. Furthermore, the effect of steroid hormones and other cytokines on the proliferation potential of endometrial and endometriotic cells has also been reported [63,65–68]. Apart from stimulating the proliferative potential, the invasive phenotype of peritoneal lesion cells [69–71] is increased even further in the presence of peritoneal fluid [72], a process likely to be accompanied by a loss or downregulation of E-cadherin. The PF also contains soluble ECM proteins, e.g. laminin, collagen type IV, versican and hyaluronan, which on one hand could be released from the follicular fluid during ovulation [73] and/or on the other hand be brought along by lysed menstrual endometrial cells [8]. Thus PF contains factors which enable the endometrial cells to escape from their tissue organization and infiltrate into the underlying tissue of neighboring organs.

Evidence in the literature indicates that the development and maintenance of an endometriotic lesion could be regarded as a local pelvic inflammatory process with altered function of immune-related cells in the peritoneal environment. In this context, the quantity and quality of menstrual endometrium, impaired immune recognition and clearance of ectopic endometrial cells as well as the formation of endometrial autoantibodies may influence lesion progression [74]. Peritoneal macrophages from women with endometriosis display a reduced capacity to mediate the destruction of endometrial cells and fail to destroy matched endometriotic cells [75]. Thus it was proposed that this increased resistance of ectopic endometrial cells to macrophage-mediated cytolysis might facilitate the survival of these cells within the peritoneal cavity of women with endometriosis. Recent studies support this notion by showing that the CD36-dependent phagocytosis of endometriotic cells by peritoneal macrophages is inhibited by prostaglandin E_2 (PGE_2) [76]. Consistent with this, an increased level of PGE_2 in PF from women with endometriosis has been reported [77,78].

One likely source of the increased levels of PGE_2 in PF are the endometriotic cells themselves as they have been shown to produce high amounts of PGE_2 *in vitro* [79]. As Banu *et al* [79] have demonstrated, inhibition of PGE_2 or its receptor EP2 affects proliferation of cultured endometriotic cells but not of eutopic endometrial cells. This suggests that prostaglandins are one type of effector of the pathogenesis of endometriosis. In line with this, altered leukocyte populations within endometriotic lesions have also been linked with the progression of endometriosis. These leukocytes may secrete abnormal levels of cytokines and growth factors with growth-promoting and angiogenic properties [12,80,81]. An overview of the effect of immunological and endocrine factors has been given by several authors [74,82–86].

Cell adhesion molecules in eutopic endometrium and endometriosis: general remarks

An important property of cells that allows them to form tissues is their intrinsic adhesiveness mediated by cell adhesion molecules (CAM). CAMs are a heterogeneous group of membrane-bound surface molecules that are subdivided into various families, due to structural and biochemical features as well as sequence homologies. These families include, among others, cadherins, integrins, selectins, the immunoglobulin superfamily, and CD44 and its isoforms [87–89]. Of these, two major classes of adhesions can be distinguished: cell–cell and cell–ECM adhesion. Cadherins, a focus in this chapter, belong to a group of calcium-dependent transmembrane glycoproteins mediating cell–cell interactions [90]. Cadherins are important constituents of adherence junctions (zonula adherence) of epithelial cells where they are responsible for cytoskeletal organization and cell polarization [91]. Integrins are implicated in the assembly of ECM proteins, cell adhesion and migration on ECM proteins, in supporting cell survival and proliferation and influencing the expression of differentiation-related genes [92].

In the following two sections we will mainly deal with two classes of CAMs: cadherins and integrins with their ligands, the ECM proteins.

Cadherin-mediated cell–cell adhesion and regulatory circuits: impact on the pathogenesis of endometriosis

Major actions of tissue formation, regardless of physiological or pathological tissue, require the presence and tight regulation of cell–cell adhesion proteins. There are a number of different types of cell–cell adhesion proteins such as cadherins, L1, NCAM, CD44 and so on [89,93]. Some of these have been claimed to contribute to tumor formation and metastasis when deregulated [94–98]. Of those, cadherins are postulated to be targets and/or effectors in the pathogenesis of endometriosis. Here we would like to provide some background knowledge on cadherins, particularly E-cadherin and to some extent N-cadherin in normal tissue, tumors and endometriosis to suggest how these proteins might influence endometriosis as pathological effectors.

The calcium-dependent transmembrane protein family cadherin is an important class of cell–cell adhesion proteins. The best investigated members of the cadherin family are the so-called classic cadherins which exhibit a similar gene and protein domain organization as well as substantial amino acid sequence homologies. The classic cadherins are E-cadherin, N-cadherin, P-cadherin and M-cadherin [99]. Normally, the cadherins of two adjacent cells interact in a homophilic manner, i.e. E-cadherin interacts with E-cadherin, N-cadherin with N-cadherin, and so on. The first discovered and best characterized cadherin is certainly E-cadherin, which is present in and a marker of differentiated epithelial tissues (for example, of endometrium, ovary, mammary gland, colon, lung, skin, etc.). Many studies have indicated that E-cadherin is a suppressor protein of metastasis of carcinomas and possibly also of tumor progression [99]. N-cadherin, regarded as a mesenchymal cadherin, was first identified in neuronal cells where it stabilizes the synapses. In addition, it is a central component of intercalating disks in the heart.

The classic cadherins show basically the same sort of interactions with associated proteins, the catenins. While β-catenin binds to the most C-terminal amino acids of those, p120catenin interacts with their juxtamembrane region. It is supposed that the cadherin–catenin complex interacts with the actin cytoskeleton involving α-catenin and other proteins, thereby regulating cellular morphology [100]. Upon specific stimuli, for example by certain cytokines, β-catenin and p120catenin may eventually dissociate from the cadherins, and, instead of undergoing degradation, travel to the nucleus and interact with transcription factors to regulate gene expression. Thus, influencing cadherins by, for example, receptor tyrosine kinase (RTK) or WNT signaling pathways can initiate changes of the protein expression profile of a given cell or a group of cells, both in physiological (e.g. developmental) and pathophysiological (e.g. tumorigenic) processes (Plate 11.1). Noteworthy here are the many experiments demonstrating that functional inactivation or absence of E-cadherin induced by DNA mutations or epimutations (influencing the expression status of the E-cadherin gene) is a basis for the migratory potential of epithelial cells and carcinomas to metastasize (for explanation see below).

An important feature of cadherins possibly important for the pathogenesis of endometriosis is that their spatial and temporal expression is controlled by cytokines such as epithelial growth factor (EGF), hepatocyte growth factor (HGF) and others. Activation of the EGF and HGF receptors or other RTKs promote the transition of the epithelial to a mesenchymal cell morphology,

Table 11.1 Analysis of the cadherin expression profile in endometriotic lesions. Biopsies of deep infiltrating and peritoneal lesions were obtained during laparotomy or laparoscopy and the presence of N-cadherin and E-cadherin in the lesions was scored by performing double immunostaining on methanol-fixed cryosections.

Deep infiltrating endometriosis			Peritoneal endometriosis		
Biopsy no	N-cadherin	E-cadherin	Biopsy no	N-cadherin	E-cadherin
2	+	−	72	+	−
4	+	+	76	−	−
9	−	+	88	+	−
10	+	+	93	+	−
14	−	+	96	−	+
27	−	−	98	−	+
28	+	−	100	−	−
33	−	−	101	−	−
45	+	−			
48	−	+			
56	−	+			

a phenomenon called epithelial-mesenchymal transition (EMT). Downregulation of E-cadherin and upregulation of N-cadherin or other mesenchymal cadherins is one of the key events of EMT which is important in developmental processes and eventually in the progression of carcinomas. Along with EMT, a whole set of mesenchymal proteins including MMPs are upregulated as well and the migratory and invasive behavior of the cells increases. This process can be reversed and then it is called mesenchymal-epithelial transition (MET). For further explanations see Plate 11.1A–C.

Cadherins in eutopic and ectopic endometrium

As described above, eutopic and ectopic endometrium are composed of epithelial glands and stroma. Just as in other epithelial tissues, eutopic as well as ectopic epithelial glands are characterized by the expression of cytokeratins, the epithelial specific intermediate filament proteins, and E-cadherin. While in all glandular cells of the eutopic endometrium E-cadherin protein can be detected, this is not the case for glands in endometriosis lesions. Although histologically not distinguishable from glands of the eutopic endometrium, those of deep infiltrating and peritoneal endometriosis lesions have been shown to contain E-cadherin-negative cells of epithelial character as indicated by the presence of the epithelial-specific intermediate filaments (see Plate 11.1D; Table 11.1) [69–71]. Some of the endometriotic gland cells express N-cadherin (see Plate 11.1D; Table 11.1) which a terminally differentiated epithelial cell would normally not do. Consistent with these observations is that primary epithelial cells from endometriotic lesions but not those of eutopic endometrium are able to invade collagen gel or Matrigel [69]. In addition, only E-cadherin-negative immortalized epithelial cell lines could be generated from endometriotic lesions. These cell lines were shown to express N-cadherin and are able to invade Matrigel which

is in agreement with the results obtained with primary cells [71]. A possible conclusion of these findings could be that E-cadherin-negative/N-cadherin-positive cells still exhibit developmental plasticity and invasive potential, promoting the relatively high recurrence rate of endometriosis.

Why endometriosis lesions do contain E-cadherin-negative cells is not quite clear yet. But a reasonable explanation could be the activation of regulatory circuits in epithelial cells by factors which are present in the pelvic fluid at high concentrations and that may induce a change in the cadherin outfit and thus of the functional status of cells in the endometriotic lesions (see below).

Cadherins and regulatory circuits potentially relevant for the pathogenesis of endometriosis

Here we would like to highlight some regulatory loops which are possibly relevant for the pathogenesis of endometriosis and clearly have been shown to have an impact on E-cadherin and associated proteins as well as N-cadherin, thus changing important functional features of cells.

As already mentioned, numerous reports in the past two decades have indicated that the pelvic fluid of endometriosis patients contains different types of cytokines and other factors which are elevated when compared to control women. Many of those are ligands of receptors which are present in endometriotic cells and possibly induce EMT when activated (for example, EGF or HGF receptors; see Plate 11.1 and above). EMT renders the cells more motile and invasive by downregulation of E-cadherin and upregulation of N-cadherin. Thus, EMT, partially or completely, might be a realistic scenario to occur during the pathogenesis of endometriosis as we have detected E-cadherin-negative/N-cadherin-positive epithelial cells in endometriotic lesions.

In addition to the elevated levels of ligands of RTKs (e.g. HGF, TGF-β) or the inflammatory interleukin (IL)-6 [101–104], PGE_2 is a major substance elevated in the pelvic fluid of endometriosis patients. It is (also) produced by endometriotic cells themselves in culture [79] and presumably also *in vivo*. PGE_2 is a ligand of the G-protein-coupled receptor EP2 which is also expressed by endometriotic cells, thus allowing autocrine regulatory loops to occur. Recently, it has been described that PGE_2 and its receptor EP2 are involved in controlling β-catenin-mediated transcriptional activity (explained in Plate 11.1C and E) [105]. In this, membrane protein caveolin-1 is sequestering β-catenin at the membrane in a complex with E-cadherin, thus preventing transcription of β-catenin-dependent genes such as cell cycle activating genes. In addition, this mechanism also inhibits the transcription of the cyclo-oxygenase (COX)-2 gene (which produces PGE_2 in response to inflammatory cytokines and cytokines [106]) and the survivin gene whose gene product is an inhibitor of apoptosis and has been implicated in the survival of endometriotic cells [56,107,108]. Although not formally proven, PGE_2 might enhance β-catenin stability through an EP2 receptor-mediated mechanism [105] (Plate 11.1E) This is an interesting observation since β-catenin is one of the essential players in the regulation of developmental processes (e.g. stem cell renewal in different tissues, control of differentiation in mammary glands, development of carcinomas, etc.).

The enzymes COX-1 and COX-2 produce PGE_2 from arachidonic acid. Possibly important are suggestions from cancer studies that there is a connection between COX-2 and the expression of E-cadherin protein. First evidence has come from experiments showing that COX-2 inhibition by the selective inhibitor celecoxib led to upregulation of E-cadherin. In agreement with this, PGE_2 induces the transcriptional repressors ZEB1 and snail which are involved in blocking expression of E-cadherin during EMT [109].

Altogether, it seems that various regulatory loops exist which at some point do influence the expression of the tumor and metastasis suppressor protein E-cadherin. This in turn can have an impact on the stability of β-catenin which, when stabilized, drives the transcription of cell cycle genes and those important for the mesenchymal phenotype of cells (see Plate 11.1).

Extracellular matrix remodelling and integrin expression in endometriotic foci

Integrins are a family of structurally and functionally related cell membrane glycoproteins consisting of a α- and a β-subunit that mediate cell–matrix adhesion, thus linking the ECM with the intracellular cytoskeleton [87,110]. Binding of integrins to ECM components promotes the formation of focal contacts in which integrins associate with the termini of F-actin filaments through talin, α-actinin and vinculin. Formation of focal contacts is regulated by intracellular signals, which promote or inhibit integrin clustering and cytoskeletal association (inside-out signaling) [111,112]. Integrins bind virtually all major components of the ECM including several types of collagen, fibronectin, laminin, osteopontin, tenascin, thrombospondin, vitronectin, von Willebrand factor, and fibrinogen. Integrins are implicated in assembly of extracellular matrices, cell adhesion and migration on ECMs and can modulate many different signal transduction cascades, support cell survival and proliferation, and influence the expression of differentiation-related genes (outside-in signaling).

The ECM has an active and complex role in regulating the behavior of cells that contact it by providing order in the extracellular space, offering ligands that activate intracellular signaling pathways and serving as a reservoir for growth factors, cytokines, and other soluble factors. The ECM is an extremely dynamic structure and its remodeling requires the synthesis and deposition of new ECM components and the proteolytic breakdown of existing components [50,113], thereby influencing cell adhesion, survival, development, migration, proliferation, differentiation, shape, and function [114,115].

Components of the ECM in tissues are mainly produced locally by cells situated within it, and spatial and temporal expression patterns within tissues have been reported. Of the 20 different collagen types known at present [116], type I, II, IV, V, and VI collagens have been detected in human endometrium [49,117–121]. Collagen type I is localized in the ECM of endometrial stromal

cells throughout the menstrual cycle [119]. The basement membrane of glandular epithelium contains collagen type IV during the proliferative and secretory stages with increased deposition in the ECM of endometrial stromal cells during the secretory stage of the cycle [118,119,121]. Fibronectin is constitutively expressed in the ECM of stromal cells during the menstrual cycle [118,122] and has also been detected occasionally in the epithelial basement membrane [123]. Laminin is localized constitutively in the basement membrane of glandular epithelium and in the ECM of stromal cells in the secretory stage of the cycle [119,122,124] but has also been detected in the ECM of endometrial stromal cells throughout the cycle [123]. A recent study indicates that certain laminin isoforms are differentially expressed in the endometrial basement membrane. Laminin-1 was constitutively present throughout the menstrual cycle in contrast to laminin-5 which switched from an even distribution to a patchy expression during the secretory phase [121]. Vitronectin appears to be expressed predominantly in the proliferative stage in the ECM of endometrial stromal cells with an increase in deposition beneath the glandular epithelium [118]. Interestingly, tenascin-C exhibits a spatial expression pattern during the menstrual cycle. It is expressed abundantly in the stromal compartment during the proliferative phase and shifts to a strong periglandular expression in secretory endometrium [123,125].

As mentioned above, endometrial integrin expression is modulated by the deposition and remodeling of ECM proteins. Thus, constitutive and cycle-dependent patterns of endometrial integrin expression have been reported in the epithelial or stromal compartment [24,126,127]. The integrins α1β1, α4β1, and αvβ3 are expressed on glandular epithelium in the secretory stage of the menstrual cycle, coinciding with the window of implantation (cycle days 20–24) in endometrium of fertile women [126]. Constitutive expression in endometrial glandular epithelium is observed for integrins α2β1, α3β1 and α6β1 [128] and α2β1, α3β1, α4β1, α5β1 and α6β1 in the ECM of stromal cells [121,122]. Additionally, endometrial stromal cells express αvβ3 in the proliferative stage and α1β1 in the secretory stage of the menstrual cycle [128,129].

How could extracellular matrix components and integrins be involved in the pathogenesis of endometriosis?

It is known from other tissues that ECM components such as collagens, fibronectin, laminin, vitronectin and tenascin-C promote cell adhesion, migration, proliferation, protease activity, tumor growth, angiogenesis, and metastasis and are thus involved in fundamental processes such as embryogenesis, malignancy, homeostasis, wound healing, host defense, and maintenance of tissue integrity [130–133]. In line with this, cell adhesion molecules and ECM-degrading enzymes are important for the attachment and invasion of endometriotic cells through host tissue [134–136]. The expression profile of MMPs and their inhibitors, tissue inhibitor of metalloproteinases (TIMP) in eutopic and ectopic endometrium and their importance in the onset and maintenance of endometriotic lesions have been reviewed [50]. Important to note, however, is the fact that the expression of MMPs is upregulated in shed menstrual endometrium and in endometriotic lesions. As mentioned earlier, menstrual endometrium shows signs of de novo ECM protein synthesis and mesenchymal stem cells (MSC) in PF were shown to secrete MMPs. Furthermore, the presence of integrins was demonstrated in menstrual effluent, shed endometrial cells in peritoneal fluid and endometriotic lesions [24], suggesting that the development and maintenance of endometriotic lesions might involve complex interactions between the ECM and integrins.

At first glance, the spatial and temporal expression patterns of the ECM components collagen type I and type IV, laminin-1, vitronectin, and fibronectin are comparable in eutopic and ectopic endometrium from women with endometriosis and healthy fertile women [117,122,123]. To date, the only reported ECM component displaying a different expression profile is tenascin-C. Its expression levels are higher in endometriotic tissues than in endometrium and no cycle stage-dependent expression has been observed [123,125]. This is in contrast to endometrium where it is expressed in stromal ECM in proliferative endometrium and is remodeled during the secretory phase of the cycle where it displays an increase in deposition beneath the glandular epithelium. Thus tenascin-C, an adhesion-modulating ECM protein, has an important function in the regeneration of the endometrial stroma. It has been shown to modulate the adhesion of cells to fibronectin [137–139] and might regulate human endometrial development by interaction with mitotic cells [140]. In cells strictly anchorage dependent for growth, tenascin-C might delay proliferation whereas cancer cells are stimulated to divide [141,142]. It has been reported that tenascin-C appears during tumor development as a result of interactions between neoplastic epithelium and stroma and thus could be a stromal marker for the invading capacity of human endometrial malignancies [143]. Fibronectin splice variants have been shown to enhance motility and invasion of breast cancer stromal cells [144] which might be linked to an increase in tenascin-C in those tissues [145]. Laminin-5 was also reported to be altered in endometriotic foci where it appeared patchy and discontinuous in the basement membrane [121] and is also downregulated in eutopic endometrium from women with endometriosis [52]. An aberrant laminin-5 expression is associated with endometrial malignancies [146] and is implicated in epithelial tumor invasion [147,148]. The motile phenotype of breast epithelium was shown to be modulated by MMP-2-driven laminin-5 remodeling [149] and is linked to EMT in hepatocellular carcinoma [150] and Madin-Darby canine kidney (MDCK) cells [151].

As mentioned above, ECM proteins play an important role in tissue homeostasis and an aberrant ECM deposition might be crucial for ectopic lesion formation. In line with this notion, cell–cell and cell–matrix interactions were reported to be involved in the attachment of shed menstrual endometrium to the peritoneal lining and in the onset of early endometriotic lesions [22,24,152,153]. The peritoneal ECM contains collagens type I and type IV, fibronectin and laminin, and in this respect is very

similar to the endometrium [154]. The adhering endometrial cells cause local destruction of the underlying surface layer, including retraction and shrinking, thereby exposing adhesion sites [21]. Menstrual and cultured endometrial stromal cells preferentially adhere to collagen type IV and type I [22,155]. The adhesion-promoting effect of ECM components has been shown for endometrial and endometriotic stromal cells [22,156,157]. Notably, stromal cells derived from peritoneal and ovarian lesions and eutopic endometrial stromal cells from women with endometriosis display greater adhesive capacity on ECM proteins than those from healthy controls or deeply infiltrating lesions [157]. Furthermore, the presence of exposed or soluble ECM proteins in the peritoneal cavity not only promotes cell–matrix adhesion but facilitates and modulates the proliferative phenotype of ectopic endometrial stromal cells [157]. In line with this, it was shown that menstrual endometrium supplies its own de novo ECM deposition which has been suggested to facilitate ectopic implantation [8].

Both ectopic and eutopic endometrium express the ECM components collagen type IV, laminin-1, vitronectin, and fibronectin with a similar pattern throughout the menstrual cycle [122]. In line with the ECM expression pattern, cycle stage-dependent expression of the integrin $\alpha 1\beta 1$ [122,129], aberrant expression or the lack of $\alpha v\beta 3$ [51,157], constitutive expression of $\alpha 2\beta 1$, $\alpha 3\beta 1$ and $\alpha 6\beta 1$ in glandular epithelium [129] and $\alpha 2\beta 1$, $\alpha 3\beta 1$, $\alpha 4\beta 1$, $\alpha 5\beta 1$ and $\alpha 6\beta 1$ in the ECM of stromal cells [121,122,129], reduced expression of integrin subunits $\alpha 2$ and $\alpha 3$ [52] and a depolarized expression of the integrin subunit $\alpha 6$ [158] in eutopic endometrium from women with endometriosis have been documented. In contrast, $\alpha 4\beta 1$, $\alpha 5\beta 1$ and $\alpha v\beta 3$ are expressed throughout the cycle on glandular epithelium in endometriosis [122,159], with increased levels of the integrin $\alpha 3\beta 1$ and decreased levels of $\alpha 6\beta 1$ in the stromal component [159], indicating that integrins are aberrantly expressed in endometriosis [126,128].

Notably, the appearance of the integrin $\alpha 5\beta 1$, the classic fibronetin receptor, in glandular epithelium in endometriotic lesions is very interesting. As mentioned earlier, fibronectin, normally expressed in interstitial ECM, can be occasionally detected in basement membranes. Integrins not only link the ECM with cytoplasmic structures, but also trigger signal cascades and thus alter the cellular phenotype. It has been shown that snail, a transcription factor mediating EMT, is able to upregulate mesenchymal gene expression including fibronectin, vimentin, and N-cadherin [160–162]. Furthermore, snail was shown to regulate the expression of basement membrane proteins and the upregulation of the corresponding integrin, and thereby cell–matrix interaction [163]. This could explain the presence of fibronectin in the basement membrane and $\alpha 5\beta 1$ in glandular epithelium in endometriosis. In addition, altered deposition of tenascin-C [123,125], aberrant laminin-5 distribution [121] and increased proteolytic activity and tissue remodeling have been observed in endometriotic lesions [136,164,165]. Despite the constitutive expression of the laminin-5 receptor $\alpha 3\beta 1$ in endometriotic glandular epithelium, it displays altered cellular

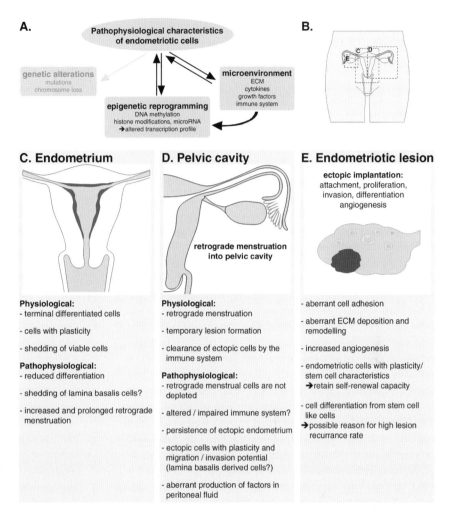

Figure 11.1 Model for events in endometriotic lesion formation. (A) The possible underlying mechanisms in endometriosis progression are not genetic alterations but epigenetic changes as a response to a different microenvironment for the misplaced endometrial cells. (B) The female pelvic cavity. The insets (C–E) indicate the different prerequisites in the development of endometriosis.

localization [121], indicating that these cells might undergo EMT. This could link the upregulation of α5β1 and fibronectin and the mosaic formation of E-cadherin-negative and N-cadherin-positive cells in endometriotic epithelium with the proteolytic degradation of laminin-5.

Reflection on current knowledge and perspectives

It is widely accepted in the field that during menstruation, retrograde transport of shed endometrial cells or fragments into the pelvic cavity is a normal phenomenon in healthy women [13,14,16,19,166]. In most cases (80–90% of women) the displaced menstrual components are removed by the immune system [74,83]. In the remaining cases, however, the menstrual components escape this clearing process and can adhere to the mesothelial lining [22,152,167], proliferate [157] and eventually invade the underlying tissue [168]. Along with these processes, angiogenesis is a prerequisite for progression and maintenance of the disease [169].

A central question arising in this context is why in some women endometriosis is established as disease while in others it appears to be a normal and temporary phenomenon. Several views exist on whether or not the disease process is mainly driven by intrinsic changes of the eutopic endometrium or regulated by the pelvic microenvironment in which the shed menstrual cells and tissue fragments are present and confronted with a variety of biological factors.

The menstrual effluent is composed of a variety of cells which differ in their responsiveness to environmental cues. As remodeling and regeneration of the endometrium begins with menstruation, the menstrual fluid contains fully differentiated cells which are prone to apoptosis but also cells which have only just embarked on the differentiation process. This suggests that the less differentiated cells misplaced in an ectopic environment represent the candidate cell population causing the disorder and not those already marked for apoptosis. These aspects are put into context in Figure 11.1.

Once the candidate cell population enters the pelvic cavity, its fate presumably depends on the presence of factors and immune cells [81,84]. Only the cells with differentiation capacity may be able to respond to factors such as prostaglandins, interleukins, cytokines and growth factors, leading to the pathophysiological characteristics of endometriotic cells [82,84,170]. In fact, many observations indicate that genetic alterations such as DNA mutations including substitution or chromosomal loss are not the major cause of endometriosis. It rather appears that the environmental influence supports epigenetic reprogramming (changes in DNA methylation, histone modifications and microRNA expression patterns) which finally leads to an aberrant expression profile of genes (see Fig. 11.1A) [171].

Based on these observations, several logical consequences arise which underlie these arguments. These comprise the differential expression pattern of proteins, e.g. down- or upregulation, altered cellular location, modification and/or activity. The gene expression profile and differentiation capacity strongly depend on the local microenvironment. One could postulate that endometriosis is a stem cell-driven disease arising from less differentiated cells or endometrial stem cells/mesenchymal stem cells present in menstrual effluent. One scenario could be that peritoneal lesions are established from shed endometrial cells/fragments originating from the lamina basalis which contains the stem cell reservoir. Under the influence of the new microenvironment, these misplaced stem cells undergo an aberrant differentiation program giving rise to endometriotic foci. The developing lesions in turn secrete factors which have an impact on eutopic gene expression profiles. In parallel to differentiation, the misplaced stem cells also might undergo self-renewal (an intrinsic feature of stem cells), thereby keeping the cell reservoir for recurrence of endometriotic lesions. The uterine lumen is connected via the patent fallopian tubes with the peritoneal cavity, allowing for an exchange of factors and changing fluid volumes depending on the menstrual cycle, suggesting a possible contribution of PF to uterine fluid volume [172]. Another scenario could be that the eutopic endometrium of endometriosis patients is intrinsically different in its gene expression profile, for whatever reason, leading to endometriosis development at ectopic sites. The current studies, however, do not allow us to separate these two possible scenarios as they might actually be two sides of the same coin.

Acknowledgments

We are most grateful to and dedicate this chapter to our former collaborator Prof. Dr Rolf Bauman MD, who is now retired. He generously shared with us his enormous knowledge of clinical work and therapeutical options of endometriosis. Based on his support with endometriotic tissue, we were able to generate our results and, most importantly, the immortalized endometriotic cell lines which are now a valuable tool for many groups all over the globe. Special gratitude also goes to Prof. Dr Helen Mardon for her vast contribution to the scientific education of one of us (PK) and her continued willingness to discuss the issues of endometriosis and reproduction.

References

1. Wynn R. The human endometrium: cyclic and gestational changes. In: Wynn R, Jollie W (eds) Biology of the Uterus. New York: Plenum, 1989, pp. 289–332.

2. Noyes R. Dating the endometrial biopsy. Fertil Steril 1950;1:2–25.

3. Talbi S, Hamilton AE, Vo KC et al. Molecular phenotyping of human endometrium distinguishes menstrual cycle phases and underlying biological processes in normo-ovulatory women. Endocrinology 2006;147(3):1097–1121.

4. Popovici RM, Kao LC, Giudice LC. Discovery of new inducible genes in in vitro decidualized human endometrial stromal cells using microarray technology. Endocrinology 2000;141(9):3510–3513.

5. Oliver C, Cowdrey N, Abadia-Molina AC et al. Antigen phenotype of cultured decidual stromal cells of human term decidua. J Reprod Immunol 1999;45(1):19–30.

6. Brar AK, Handwerger S, Kessler CA et al. Gene induction and categorical reprogramming during in vitro human endometrial fibroblast decidualization. Physiol Genom 2001;7(2):135–148.

7. Salamonsen LA. Current concepts of the mechanisms of menstruation: a normal process of tissue destruction. Trends Endocrinol Metab 1998;9(8):305–309.

8. Gaide Chevronnay HP, Galant C, Lemoine P et al. Spatiotemporal coupling of focal extracellular matrix degradation and reconstruction in the menstrual human endometrium. Endocrinology 2009; 150(11):5094–5105.

9. Bulletti C, de Ziegler D, Polli V et al. Characteristics of uterine contractility during menses in women with mild to moderate endometriosis. Fertil Steril 2002;77(6):1156–1161.

10. Van Gestel I, Ijland MM IJ, Hoogland HJ et al. Endometrial wave-like activity in the non-pregnant uterus. Hum Reprod Update 2003; 9(2):131–138.

11. Koninckx PR, Ide P, Vandenbroucke W et al. New aspects of the pathophysiology of endometriosis and associated infertility. J Reprod Med 1980;24(6):257–260.

12. Badawy SZ, Cuenca V, Marshall L et al. Cellular components in peritoneal fluid in infertile patients with and without endometriosis. Fertil Steril 1984;42(5):704–708.

13. Bartosik D, Jacobs SL, Kelly LJ. Endometrial tissue in peritoneal fluid. Fertil Steril 1986;46(5):796–800.

14. Kulenthran A, Jeyalakshmi N. Dissemination of endometrial cells at laparoscopy and chromotubation – a preliminary report. Int J Fertil 1989;34(4):256–258.

15. Beyth Y, Yaffe H, Levij S et al. Retrograde seeding of endometrium: a sequela of tubal flushing. Fertil Steril 1975;26(11):1094–1097.

16. Sharpe-Timms KL. Haptoglobin expression by shed endometrial tissue fragments found in peritoneal fluid. Fertil Steril 2005;84(1):22–30.

17. Kruitwagen RF, Poels LG, Willemsen WN et al. Endometrial epithelial cells in peritoneal fluid during the early follicular phase. Fertil Steril 1991;55(2):297–303.

18. Kruitwagen RF, Poels LG, Willemsen WN et al. Retrograde seeding of endometrial epithelial cells by uterine-tubal flushing. Fertil Steril 1991;56(3):414–420.

19. Halme J, Hammond MG, Hulka JF et al. Retrograde menstruation in healthy women and in patients with endometriosis. Obstet Gynecol 1984;64(2):151–154.

20. Keettel WC, Stein RJ. The viability of the cast-off menstrual endometrium. Am J Obstet Gynecol 1951;61(2):440–442.

21. Koks CA, Demir Weusten AY, Groothuis PG et al. Menstruum induces changes in mesothelial cell morphology. Gynecol Obstet Invest 2000;50(1):13–18.

22. Koks CA, Groothuis PG, Dunselman GA et al. Adhesion of menstrual endometrium to extracellular matrix: the possible role of integrin alpha(6)beta(1) and laminin interaction. Mol Hum Reprod 2000;6(2):170–177.

23. Griffith JS, Liu YG, Tekmal RR et al. Menstrual endometrial cells from women with endometriosis demonstrate increased adherence to peritoneal cells and increased expression of CD44 splice variants. Fertil Steril 2010;93(6):1745–1749.

24. Van der Linden PJ, de Goeij AF, Dunselman GA et al. Expression of integrins and E-cadherin in cells from menstrual effluent, endometrium, peritoneal fluid, peritoneum, and endometriosis. Fertil Steril 1994;61(1):85–90.

25. Sharpe-Timms KL, Zimmer RL, Ricke EA et al. Endometriotic haptoglobin binds to peritoneal macrophages and alters their function in women with endometriosis. Fertil Steril 2002;78(4):810–819.

26. Prianishnikov VA. On the concept of stem cell and a model of functional-morphological structure of the endometrium. Contraception 1978;18(3):213–223.

27. Bonatz G, Klapper W, Barthe A et al. Analysis of telomerase expression and proliferative activity in the different layers of cyclic endometrium. Biochem Biophys Res Commun 1998;253(2):214–221.

28. Gargett CE, Chan RW, Schwab KE. Endometrial stem cells. Curr Opin Obstet Gynecol 2007;19(4):377–383.

29. Schwab KE, Chan RW, Gargett CE. Putative stem cell activity of human endometrial epithelial and stromal cells during the menstrual cycle. Fertil Steril 2005;84 Suppl 2:1124–1130.

30. Chan RW, Schwab KE, Gargett CE. Clonogenicity of human endometrial epithelial and stromal cells. Biol Reprod 2004;70(6):1738–1750.

31. Gargett CE, Schwab KE, Zillwood RM et al. Isolation and culture of epithelial progenitors and mesenchymal stem cells from human endometrium. Biol Reprod 2009;80(6):1136–1145.

32. Starzinski-Powitz A, Zeitvogel A, Schreiner A et al. [Endometriosis – a stem cell disease?] Zentralbl Gynakol 2003;125(7–8):235–238.

33. Gargett CE, Chan RWS, Schwab KE. Hormone and growth factor signaling in endometrial renewal: role of stem/progenitor cells. Molec Cell Endocrinol 2008;288(1–2):22–29.

34. Sasson IE, Taylor HS. Stem cells and the pathogenesis of endometriosis. Ann NY Acad Sci 2008;1127:106–115.

35. Leyendecker G, Herbertz M, Kunz G et al. Endometriosis results from the dislocation of basal endometrium. Hum Reprod 2002;17(10):2725–2736.

36. Leyendecker G. Evidence that endometriosis results from the dislocation of basal endometrium? Hum Reprod 2003;18(5):1130-a-1.

37. Meng X, Ichim TE, Zhong J et al. Endometrial regenerative cells: a novel stem cell population. J Transl Med 2007;5:57.

38. Musina RA, Belyavski AV, Tarusova OV et al. Endometrial mesenchymal stem cells isolated from the menstrual blood. Bull Exp Biol Med 2008;145(4):539–543.

39. Toyoda M, Cui C, Umezawa A. Myogenic transdifferentiation of menstrual blood-derived cells. Acta Myol 2007;26(3):176–178.

40. Taylor HS. Endometrial cells derived from donor stem cells in bone marrow transplant recipients. JAMA 2004;292(1):81–85.

41. Aghajanova L, Horcajadas JA, Esteban FJ et al. The bone marrow-derived human mesenchymal stem cell: potential progenitor of the endometrial stromal fibroblast. Biol Reprod 2010;82(6):1076–1087.

42. Vercellini P, de Giorgi O, Aimi G et al. Menstrual characteristics in women with and without endometriosis. Obstet Gynecol 1997;90(2):264–268.

43. Giudice LC, Telles TL, Lobo S et al. The molecular basis for implantation failure in endometriosis: on the road to discovery. Ann NY Acad Sci 2002;955:252–264; discussion 93–95, 396–406.

44. Lessey BA. Implantation defects in infertile women with endometriosis. Ann NY Acad Sci 2002;955:265–280; discussion 93–95, 396–406.

45. Sharpe-Timms KL. Endometrial anomalies in women with endometriosis. Ann NY Acad Sci 2001;943:131–147.

46. Klemmt PA, Carver JG, Kennedy SH et al. Stromal cells from endometriotic lesions and endometrium from women with endometriosis have reduced decidualization capacity. Fertil Steril 2006;85(3):564–572.

47. Skinner JL, Riley SC, Gebbie AE et al. Regulation of matrix metalloproteinase-9 in endometrium during the menstrual cycle and following administration of intrauterine levonorgestrel. Hum Reprod 1999;14(3):793–799.

48. Bilalis DA, Klentzeris LD, Fleming S. Immunohistochemical localization of extracellular matrix proteins in luteal phase endometrium of fertile and infertile patients. Hum Reprod 1996;11(12):2713–2718.

49. Jokimaa V, Oksjoki S, Kujari H et al. Altered expression of genes involved in the production and degradation of endometrial extracellular matrix in patients with unexplained infertility and recurrent miscarriages. Mol Hum Reprod 2002;8(12):1111–1116.

50. Pitsos M, Kanakas N. The role of matrix metalloproteinases in the pathogenesis of endometriosis. Reprod Sci 2009;16(8):717–726.

51. Lessey BA, Castelbaum AJ, Sawin SW et al. Aberrant integrin expression in the endometrium of women with endometriosis. J Clin Endocrinol Metab 1994;79(2):643–649.

52. Kao LC, Germeyer A, Tulac S et al. Expression profiling of endometrium from women with endometriosis reveals candidate genes for disease-based implantation failure and infertility. Endocrinology 2003;144(7):2870–2881.

53. Meola J, Rosa ESJC, Dentillo DB et al. Differentially expressed genes in eutopic and ectopic endometrium of women with endometriosis. Fertil Steril 2010;93(6):1750–1773.

54. Tsuno A, Nasu K, Yuge A et al. Decidualization attenuates the contractility of eutopic and ectopic endometrial stromal cells: implications for hormone therapy of endometriosis. J Clin Endocrinol Metab 2009;94(7):2516–2523.

55. Aghajanova L, Horcajadas JA, Weeks JL et al. The protein kinase A pathway-regulated transcriptome of endometrial stromal fibroblasts reveals compromised differentiation and persistent proliferative potential in endometriosis. Endocrinology 2010;151(3):1341–1355.

56. Zhang H, Li M, Zheng X et al. Endometriotic stromal cells lose the ability to regulate cell-survival signaling in endometrial epithelial cells in vitro. Mol Hum Reprod 2009;15(10):653–663.

57. Bahtiyar MO, Seli E, Oral E et al. Follicular fluid of women with endometriosis stimulates the proliferation of endometrial stromal cells. Hum Reprod 1998;13(12):3492–3495.

58. Koninckx PR, Kennedy SH, Barlow DH. Pathogenesis of endometriosis: the role of peritoneal fluid. Gynecol Obstet Invest 1999;47 Suppl 1:23–33.

59. Surrey ES, Halme J. Effect of peritoneal fluid from endometriosis patients on endometrial stromal cell proliferation in vitro. Obstet Gynecol 1990;76(5 Pt 1):792–797.

60. Overton CE, Fernandez-Shaw S, Hicks B et al. In vitro culture of endometrial stromal and gland cells as a model for endometriosis: the effect of peritoneal fluid on proliferation. Fertil Steril 1997;67(1):51–56.

61. Braun DP, Ding J, Dmowski WP. Peritoneal fluid-mediated enhancement of eutopic and ectopic endometrial cell proliferation is dependent on tumor necrosis factor-alpha in women with endometriosis. Fertil Steril 2002;78(4):727–732.

62. Iwabe T, Harada T, Tsudo T et al. Tumor necrosis factor-alpha promotes proliferation of endometriotic stromal cells by inducing interleukin-8 gene and protein expression. J Clin Endocrinol Metab 2000;85(2):824–829.

63. Badawy SZ, Holland J, Landas S et al. The role of estradiol, progesterone, and transforming growth factor on human endometrioma cell culture. Am J Reprod Immunol 1996;36(1):58–63.

64. Hammond MG, Oh ST, Anners J et al. The effect of growth factors on the proliferation of human endometrial stromal cells in culture. Am J Obstet Gynecol 1993;168(4):1131–1136; discussion 6–8.

65. Holinka CF. Growth and hormonal responsiveness of human endometrial stromal cells in culture. Hum Cell 1998;1(2):207–217.

66. Yoshioka H, Harada T, Iwabe T et al. Menstrual cycle-specific inhibition of the proliferation of endometrial stromal cells by interleukin 6 and its soluble receptor. Am J Obstet Gynecol 1999;180(5):1088–1094.

67. Irwin JC, Utian WH, Eckert RL. Sex steroids and growth factors differentially regulate the growth and differentiation of cultured human endometrial stromal cells. Endocrinology 1991;129(5):2385–2392.

68. Iwabe T, Harada T, Tsudo T et al. Pathogenetic significance of increased levels of interleukin-8 in the peritoneal fluid of patients with endometriosis. Fertil Steril 1998;69(5):924–930.

69. Gaetje R, Kotzian S, Herrmann G et al. Invasiveness of endometriotic cells in vitro. Lancet 1995;346(8988):1463–1464.

70. Gaetje R, Kotzian S, Herrmann G et al. Nonmalignant epithelial cells, potentially invasive in human endometriosis, lack the tumor suppressor molecule E-cadherin. Am J Pathol 1997;150(2):461–467.

71. Zeitvogel A, Baumann R, Starzinski-Powitz A. Identification of an invasive, N-cadherin-expressing epithelial cell type in endometriosis using a new cell culture model. Am J Pathol 2001;159(5):1839–1852.

72. Starzinski-Powitz A, Gaetje R, Zeitvogel A et al. Tracing cellular and molecular mechanisms involved in endometriosis. Hum Reprod Update 1998;4(5):724–729.

73. Rodgers RJ, Irving-Rodgers HF, Russell DL. Extracellular matrix of the developing ovarian follicle. Reproduction 2003;126(4):415–424.

74. Kyama CM, Debrock S, Mwenda JM et al. Potential involvement of the immune system in the development of endometriosis. Reprod Biol Endocrinol 2003;1(1):123.

75. Braun DP, Gebel H, Rana N et al. Cytolysis of eutopic and ectopic endometrial cells by peripheral blood monocytes and peritoneal macrophages in women with endometriosis. Fertil Steril 1998;69(6):1103–1108.

76. Chuang PC, Lin YJ, Wu MH et al. Inhibition of CD36-dependent phagocytosis by prostaglandin E2 contributes to the development of endometriosis. Am J Pathol 2010;176(2):850–860.

77. Badawy SZ, Marshall L, Gabal AA et al. The concentration of 13,14-dihydro-15-keto prostaglandin F2 alpha and prostaglandin E2 in peritoneal fluid of infertile patients with and without endometriosis. Fertil Steril 1982;38(2):166–170.

78. Dawood MY, Khan-Dawood FS, Wilson L Jr. Peritoneal fluid prostaglandins and prostanoids in women with endometriosis, chronic pelvic inflammatory disease, and pelvic pain. Am J Obstet Gynecol 1984;148(4):391–395.

79. Banu SK, Lee J, Starzinski-Powitz A et al. Gene expression profiles and functional characterization of human immortalized endometriotic epithelial and stromal cells. Fertil Steril 2008;90(4):972–987.

80. Jones RK, Bulmer JN, Searle RF. Phenotypic and functional studies of leukocytes in human endometrium and endometriosis. Hum Reprod Update 1998;4(5):702–709.

81. Tariverdian N, Siedentopf F, Rucke M et al. Intraperitoneal immune cell status in infertile women with and without endometriosis. J Reprod Immunol 2009;80(1–2):80–90.

82. Harada T, Iwabe T, Terakawa N. Role of cytokines in endometriosis. Fertil Steril 2001;76(1):1–10.

83. Lebovic DI, Mueller MD, Taylor RN. Immunobiology of endometriosis. Fertil Steril 2001;75(1):1–10.

84. Gazvani R, Templeton A. Peritoneal environment, cytokines and angiogenesis in the pathophysiology of endometriosis. Reproduction 2002;123(2):217–226.

85. Oral E, Olive DL, Arici A. The peritoneal environment in endometriosis. Hum Reprod Update 1996;2(5):385–398.

86. Kyama CM, Mihalyi A, Simsa P et al. Role of cytokines in the endometrial-peritoneal cross-talk and development of endometriosis. Front Biosci (Elite Ed) 2009;1:444–454.

87. Barczyk M, Carracedo S, Gullberg D. Integrins. Cell Tissue Res 2010;339(1):269–280.

88. Smith CW. 3. Adhesion molecules and receptors. J Allergy Clin Immunol 2008;121(2, Supplement 2):S375-S379.

89. Thiery JP. Cell adhesion in development: a complex signaling network. Curr Opin Genet Dev 2003;13(4):365–371.

90. Takeichi M. Morphogenetic roles of classic cadherins. Curr Opin Cell Biol 1995;7(5):619–627.

91. Bryant DM, Mostov KE. From cells to organs: building polarized tissue. Nat Rev Mol Cell Biol 2008;9(11):887–901.

92. Danen EH, Sonnenberg A. Integrins in regulation of tissue development and function. J Pathol 2003;200(4):471–480.

93. Zhang Y, Yeh J, Richardson PM et al. Cell adhesion molecules of the immunoglobulin superfamily in axonal regeneration and neural repair. Restor Neurol Neurosci 2008;26(2–3):81–96.

94. Makrilia N, Kollias A, Manolopoulos L et al. Cell adhesion molecules: role and clinical significance in cancer. Cancer Invest 2009;27(10):1023–1037.

95. Yilmaz M, Christofori G. EMT, the cytoskeleton, and cancer cell invasion. Cancer Metastasis Rev 2009;28(1–2):15–33.

96. Playford MP, Schaller MD. The interplay between Src and integrins in normal and tumor biology. Oncogene 2004;23(48):7928–7946.

97. Lyons AJ, Jones J. Cell adhesion molecules, the extracellular matrix and oral squamous carcinoma. Int J Oral Maxillofac Surg 2007;36(8):671–679.

98. Nair KS, Naidoo R, Chetty R. Expression of cell adhesion molecules in oesophageal carcinoma and its prognostic value. J Clin Pathol 2005;58(4):343–351.

99. Stemmler MP. Cadherins in development and cancer. Mol Biosyst 2008;4(8):835–850.

100. Van Roy F, Berx G. The cell-cell adhesion molecule E-cadherin. Cell Mol Life Sci 2008;65(23):3756–3788.

101. Velasco I, Acien P, Campos A et al. Interleukin-6 and other soluble factors in peritoneal fluid and endometriomas and their relation to pain and aromatase expression. J Reprod Immunol 2010;84(2):199–205.

102. Kalu E, Sumar N, Giannopoulos T et al. Cytokine profiles in serum and peritoneal fluid from infertile women with and without endometriosis. J Obstet Gynaecol Res 2007;33(4):490–495.

103. Khan KN, Masuzaki H, Fujishita A et al. Association of interleukin-6 and estradiol with hepatocyte growth factor in peritoneal fluid of women with endometriosis. Acta Obstet Gynecol Scand 2002;81(8):764–771.

104. Pizzo A, Salmeri FM, Ardita FV et al. Behaviour of cytokine levels in serum and peritoneal fluid of women with endometriosis. Gynecol Obstet Invest 2002;54(2):82–87.

105. Rodriguez DA, Tapia JC, Fernandez JG et al. Caveolin-1-mediated suppression of cyclooxygenase-2 via a beta-catenin-Tcf/Lef-dependent transcriptional mechanism reduced prostaglandin E2 production and survivin expression. Mol Biol Cell 2009;20(8):2297–2310.

106. Park JY, Pillinger MH, Abramson SB. Prostaglandin E2 synthesis and secretion: the role of PGE2 synthases. Clin Immunol 2006;119(3):229–240.

107. Ueda M, Yamashita Y, Takehara M et al. Survivin gene expression in endometriosis. J Clin Endocrinol Metab 2002;87(7):3452–3459.

108. Fujino K, Ueda M, Takehara M et al. Transcriptional expression of survivin and its splice variants in endometriosis. Mol Hum Reprod 2006;12(6):383–388.

109. Dohadwala M, Yang SC, Luo J et al. Cyclooxygenase-2-dependent regulation of E-cadherin: prostaglandin E(2) induces transcriptional repressors ZEB1 and snail in non-small cell lung cancer. Cancer Res 2006;66(10):5338–5345.

110. Hynes RO. Integrins: versatility, modulation, and signaling in cell adhesion. Cell 1992;69(1):11–25.

111. Burridge K, Chrzanowska-Wodnicka M. Focal adhesions, contractility, and signaling. Annu Rev Cell Dev Biol 1996;12:463–518.

112. Mainiero F, Pepe A, Yeon M et al. The intracellular functions of alpha6beta4 integrin are regulated by EGF. J Cell Biol 1996;134(1):241–253.

113. Stamenkovic I. Extracellular matrix remodelling: the role of matrix metalloproteinases. J Pathol 2003;200(4):448–464.

114. Kreis T, Vale R. Guidebook to the Extracellular Matrix, Anchor, and Adhesion Proteins, 2nd edn. Oxford: Sambrook & Tooze, 1999.

115. Iozzo RV. Matrix proteoglycans: from molecular design to cellular function. Annu Rev Biochem 1998;67:609–652.

116. Myllyharju J, Kivirikko KI. Collagens and collagen-related diseases. Ann Med 2001;33(1):7–21.

117. Stovall DW, Anners JA, Halme J. Immunohistochemical detection of type I, III, and IV collagen in endometriosis implants. Fertil Steril 1992;57(5):984–989.

118. Aplin JD, Charlton AK, Ayad S. An immunohistochemical study of human endometrial extracellular matrix during the menstrual cycle and first trimester of pregnancy. Cell Tissue Res 1988;253(1):231–240.

119. Iwahashi M, Muragaki Y, Ooshima A et al. Alterations in distribution and composition of the extracellular matrix during decidualization of the human endometrium. J Reprod Fertil 1996;108(1):147–155.

120. Stenback F. Collagen type III formation and distribution in the uterus: effects of hormones and neoplasm development. Oncology 1989;46(5):326–334.

121. Giannelli G, Sgarra C, di Naro E et al. Endometriosis is characterized by an impaired localization of laminin-5 and alpha3beta1 integrin receptor. Int J Gynecol Cancer 2007;17(1):242–247.

122. Beliard A, Donnez J, Nisolle M et al. Localization of laminin, fibronectin, E-cadherin, and integrins in endometrium and endometriosis. Fertil Steril 1997;67(2):266–272.

123. Harrington DJ, Lessey BA, Rai V et al. Tenascin is differentially expressed in endometrium and endometriosis. J Pathol 1999;187(2):242–248.

124. Faber M, Wewer U, Berthelsen J et al. Laminin production by human endometrial stromal cells relates to the cyclic and patholigic state of the endometrium. Am J Pathol 1986;124:384–398.

125. Tan O, Ornek T, Seval Y et al. Tenascin is highly expressed in endometriosis and its expression is upregulated by estrogen. Fertil Steril 2008;89(5):1082–1089.

126. Lessey BA, Damjanovich L, Coutifaris C et al. Integrin adhesion molecules in the human endometrium. Correlation with the normal and abnormal menstrual cycle. J Clin Invest 1992;90(1):188–195.

127. Van der Linden PJ, de Goeij AF, Dunselman GA et al. Expression of cadherins and integrins in human endometrium throughout the menstrual cycle. Fertil Steril 1995;63(6):1210–1216.

128. Lessey BA, Castelbaum AJ, Buck CA et al. Further characterization of endometrial integrins during the menstrual cycle and in pregnancy. Fertil Steril 1994;62(3):497–506.

129. Bridges JE, Prentice A, Roche W et al. Expression of integrin adhesion molecules in endometrium and endometriosis. Br J Obstet Gynaecol 1994;101(8):696–700.

130. Schwarzbauer J. Basement membranes: putting up the barriers. Curr Biol 1999;9(7):R242–244.

131. Hynes R. Fibronectins. In: Rich A (ed) Springer Series in Molecular Biology. New York: Springer, 1990.

132. Colognato H, Yurchenco PD. Form and function: the laminin family of heterotrimers. Dev Dyn 2000;218(2):213–234.

133. Preissner KT. Structure and biological role of vitronectin. Annu Rev Cell Biol 1991;7:275–310.

134. Fernandez-Shaw S, Marshall JM, Hicks B et al. Plasminogen activators in ectopic and uterine endometrium. Fertil Steril 1995;63(1):45–51.

135. Wenzl RJ, Heinzl H. Localization of matrix metalloproteinase-2 in uterine endometrium and ectopic implants. Gynecol Obstet Invest 1998;45(4):253–257.

136. Sillem M, Prifti S, Monga B et al. Soluble urokinase-type plasminogen activator receptor is over-expressed in uterine endometrium from women with endometriosis. Mol Hum Reprod 1997;3(12):1101–1105.

137. Chiquet-Ehrismann R, Kalla P, Pearson CA et al. Tenascin interferes with fibronectin action. Cell 1988;53(3):383–390.

138. Sage EH, Bornstein P. Extracellular proteins that modulate cell-matrix interactions. SPARC, tenascin, and thrombospondin. J Biol Chem 1991;266(23):14831–14834.

139. Orend G, Chiquet-Ehrismann R. Adhesion modulation by antiadhesive molecules of the extracellular matrix. Exp Cell Res 2000;261(1):104–110.

140. Taguchi M, Kubota T, Aso T. Immunohistochemical localization of tenascin and ki-67 nuclear antigen in human endometrium throughout the normal menstrual cycle. J Med Dent Sci 1999;46(1):7–12.

141. Chiquet-Ehrismann R, Mackie EJ, Pearson CA et al. Tenascin: an extracellular matrix protein involved in tissue interactions during fetal development and oncogenesis. Cell 1986;47(1):131–139.

142. Huang W, Chiquet-Ehrismann R, Moyano JV et al. Interference of tenascin-C with syndecan-4 binding to fibronectin blocks cell adhesion and stimulates tumor cell proliferation. Cancer Res 2001;61(23):8586–8594.

143. Sasano H, Nagura H, Watanabe K et al. Tenascin expression in normal and abnormal human endometrium. Mod Pathol 1993; 6(3):323–326.

144. Matsumoto E, Yoshida T, Kawarada Y et al. Expression of fibronectin isoforms in human breast tissue: production of extra domain A+/ extra domain B+ by cancer cells and extra domain A+ by stromal cells. Jpn J Cancer Res 1999;90(3):320–325.

145. Koukoulis GK, Howeedy AA, Korhonen M et al. Distribution of tenascin, cellular fibronectins and integrins in the normal, hyperplastic and neoplastic breast. J Submicrosc Cytol Pathol 1993;25(2):285–295.

146. Maatta M, Salo S, Tasanen K et al. Distribution of basement membrane anchoring molecules in normal and transformed endometrium: altered expression of laminin gamma2 chain and collagen type XVII in endometrial adenocarcinomas. J Mol Histol 2004;35(8–9):715–722.

147. Katayama M, Sekiguchi K. Laminin-5 in epithelial tumour invasion. J Mol Histol 2004;35(3):277–286.

148. Katayama M, Sanzen N, Funakoshi A et al. Laminin {gamma}2-chain fragment in the circulation: a prognostic indicator of epithelial tumor invasion. Cancer Res 2003;63(1):222–229.

149. Giannelli G, Falk-Marzillier J, Schiraldi O et al. Induction of cell migration by matrix metalloprotease-2 cleavage of laminin-5. Science 1997;277(5323):225–228.

150. Giannelli G, Bergamini C, Fransvea E et al. Laminin-5 with transforming growth factor-beta1 induces epithelial to mesenchymal transition in hepatocellular carcinoma. Gastroenterology 2005;129(5):1375–1383.

151. Mathias RA, Chen YS, Wang B et al. Extracellular remodelling during oncogenic Ras-induced epithelial-mesenchymal transition facilitates MDCK cell migration. J Proteome Res 2010;9(2):1007–1019.

152. Koks CA, Groothuis PG, Dunselman GA et al. Adhesion of shed menstrual tissue in an in-vitro model using amnion and peritoneum: a light and electron microscopic study. Hum Reprod 1999; 14(3):816–822.

153. Spuijbroek MD, Dunselman GA, Menheere PP et al. Early endometriosis invades the extracellular matrix. Fertil Steril 1992; 58(5):929–933.

154. Witz CA, Montoya-Rodriguez IA, Cho S et al. Composition of the extracellular matrix of the peritoneum. J Soc Gynecol Invest 2001;8(5):299–304.

155. Witz C, Doucet R, Honore G. Preferential endometrial stromal cell adhesion to collagen IV and collagen I is inhibited by echistatin. [Abstract no. O-026]. Fertil Steril 1997;Suppl:S14.

156. Sillem M, Prifti S, Monga B et al. Integrin-mediated adhesion of uterine endometrial cells from endometriosis patients to extracellular matrix proteins is enhanced by tumor necrosis factor alpha (TNF alpha) and interleukin-1 (IL-1). Eur J Obstet Gynecol Reprod Biol 1999;87(2):123–127.

157. Klemmt PA, Carver JG, Koninckx P et al. Endometrial cells from women with endometriosis have increased adhesion and proliferative capacity in response to extracellular matrix components: towards a mechanistic model for endometriosis progression. Hum Reprod 2007;22(12):3139–3147.

158. Vernet-Tomas Mdel M, Perez-Ares CT, Verdu N et al. The depolarized expression of the alpha-6 integrin subunit in the endometria of women with endometriosis. J Soc Gynecol Invest 2006;13(4):292–296.

159. Rai V, Hopkisson J, Kennedy S et al. Integrins alpha 3 and alpha 6 are differentially expressed in endometrium and endometriosis. J Pathol 1996;180(2):181–187.

160. Cano A, Perez-Moreno MA, Rodrigo I et al. The transcription factor snail controls epithelial-mesenchymal transitions by repressing E-cadherin expression. Nat Cell Biol 2000;2(2):76–83.

161. Takkunen M, Grenman R, Hukkanen M et al. Snail-dependent and -independent epithelial-mesenchymal transition in oral squamous carcinoma cells. J Histochem Cytochem 2006;54(11):1263–1275.

162. Batlle E, Sancho E, Franci C et al. The transcription factor snail is a repressor of E-cadherin gene expression in epithelial tumour cells. Nat Cell Biol 2000;2(2):84–89.

163. Haraguchi M, Okubo T, Miyashita Y et al. Snail regulates cell-matrix adhesion by regulation of the expression of integrins and basement membrane proteins. J Biol Chem 2008;283(35):23514–23523.

164. Sillem M, Prifti S, Neher M et al. Extracellular matrix remodelling in the endometrium and its possible relevance to the pathogenesis of endometriosis. Hum Reprod Update 1998;4(5):730–735.

165. Cox KE, Piva M, Sharpe-Timms KL. Differential regulation of matrix metalloproteinase-3 gene expression in endometriotic lesions compared with endometrium. Biol Reprod 2001;65(4):1297–1303.

166. Bokor A, Debrock S, Drijkoningen M et al. Quantity and quality of retrograde menstruation: a case control study. Reprod Biol Endocrinol 2009;7:123.

167. Witz CA, Allsup KT, Montoya-Rodriguez IA et al. Culture of menstrual endometrium with peritoneal explants and mesothelial monolayers confirms attachment to intact mesothelial cells. Hum Reprod 2002;17(11):2832–2838.

168. Witz CA, Cho S, Centonze VE et al. Time series analysis of transmesothelial invasion by endometrial stromal and epithelial cells using three-dimensional confocal microscopy. Fertil Steril 2003;79 Suppl 1:770–778.

169. Taylor RN, Yu J, Torres PB et al. Mechanistic and therapeutic implications of angiogenesis in endometriosis. Reprod Sci 2009; 16(2):140–146.

170. Harada T, Enatsu A, Mitsunari M et al. Role of cytokines in progression of endometriosis. Gynecol Obstet Invest 1999;47 Suppl 1:34–39; discussion 9–40.

171. Guo SW. Epigenetics of endometriosis. Mol Hum Reprod 2009;15(10):587–607.

172. Casslen B. Uterine fluid volume. Cyclic variations and possible extrauterine contributions. J Reprod Med 1986;31(6):506–510.

173. Acloque H, Adams MS, Fishwick K et al. Epithelial-mesenchymal transitions: the importance of changing cell state in development and disease. J Clin Invest 2009;119(6):1438–1449.

174. Thiery JP, Sleeman JP. Complex networks orchestrate epithelial-mesenchymal transitions. Nat Rev Mol Cell Biol 2006; 7(2):131–142.

12 Stem Cells in Endometriosis

Caroline E. Gargett[1,2], Hirotaka Masuda[2] and Gareth C. Weston[1]

[1]Department of Obstetrics and Gynaecology, Monash University, Melbourne, Australia
[2]The Ritchie Centre, Monash Institute of Medical Research, Melbourne, Australia

Properties of adult stem cells

Adult stem cells are undifferentiated cells present in most adult tissues. Increasingly adult stem cells are being identified in a wide variety of tissues and organs by demonstration of their defining functional properties of high proliferative potential, self-renewal, and differentiation into one or more lineages [1]. Other functional properties of adult stem cells include clonogenicity or colony-forming unit (CFU) activity, vital (Hoechst 33342) dye exclusion to identify the side population (SP) cells, tissue reconstitution *in vivo*, and DNA synthesis label (BrdU) retention for identifying label-retaining cells (LRC) [2]. These experimental approaches enable the identification of adult stem cell activity in the absence of known specific markers. Ongoing research, however, continues to focus on identifying markers of adult stem cells, although few are specific or defining. Adult stem cells maintain tissue homeostasis through provision of replacement cells in routine cellular turnover and repairing injured tissues [3]. The stem cell niche, comprising the adult stem cell, surrounding niche cell(s) and extracellular matrix, regulates adult stem cell fate decisions, balancing stem cell replacement and provision of differentiated mature cells necessary for organ function [3]. Thus the stem cell niche provides a protective environment for the resident stem cell to maintain genetic fidelity over the lifespan, at the same time maintaining capacity to rapidly respond to tissue needs for cellular replacement.

Endometrial stem/progenitor cells

Endometrial regeneration and the stem cell hypothesis
The mucosal lining of the human endometrium is structurally and functionally divided into two major regions. The upper two-thirds, comprising the functionalis containing glands lined with a pseudostratified columnar epithelium extending from the surface epithelium surrounded by a loose vascularized stroma, is shed at menses. The lower basalis containing the basal region of the glands, dense stroma and large vessels is not shed during menstruation and serves as a germinal compartment for generating the new functionalis each month [4]. The human endometrium is a dynamic remodeling tissue undergoing more than 400 cycles of regeneration, differentiation and shedding during a woman's reproductive years [2,5]. Each month 4–10 mm of mucosal tissue grows within 4–10 days during the proliferative stage of the menstrual cycle under the influence of increasing circulating estrogen levels. Endometrial regeneration also follows parturition and resection of the endometrium, and occurs in postmenopausal women taking estrogen replacement therapy [2,6]. In non-menstruating species such as rodents, the endometrial lining also undergoes cycles of growth and apoptosis as part of the estrus cycle, rather than physical shedding [2]. This level of new tissue growth is similar to the cellular turnover in other highly regenerative organs, including hemopoietic tissue, epidermis and intestinal epithelium. Adult stem cells are responsible for cellular production in these continuously regenerating tissues. Similarly, it has been hypothesized that human endometrial stem/progenitor cells are responsible for regenerating the functionalis each month, that they reside in the basalis, and are present in the atrophic endometrium of postmenopausal women (reviewed in Gargett [2]).

Endometrial epithelial stem/progenitor cells
Cell cloning
Cell cloning studies on human endometrium provided the first evidence for the existence of endometrial epithelial progenitor cells [7]. In these studies, 0.2% of single cell suspensions of epithelial cell adhesion molecule (EpCAM+) cells freshly isolated from hysterectomy tissues had CFU activity, with 0.09% forming large CFU and 0.14% forming small CFU. Clonogenic endometrial epithelial cells can be cultured in serum-free medium containing

either epidermal growth factor (EGF) or transforming growth factor-α (TGF-α), suggesting that they express EGF receptors [6–8]. Mouse fibroblast feeder layers were required for serum-free clonal culture, indicating the importance of the stem cell niche for endometrial epithelial progenitor cell activity.

Self-renewal and differentiation of epithelial colony-forming units

Subsequent studies on epithelial CFU indicated that individual large CFU had substantial self-renewal activity *in vitro*, undergoing serial subcloning 2.9 times at very low seeding densities (10 cells/cm^2), while small CFU subcloned 0.5 times [9]. The large epithelial CFU had high proliferative potential, undergoing 34 population doublings when cultured at bulk culture densities (2000 cells/cm^2), generating 6×10^{11} cells from the original cell, while small CFU produced six orders of magnitude fewer cells. Large epithelial CFU also differentiated into large cytokeratin-expressing gland-like structures when cultured in Matrigel [9]. The ability of large epithelial CFU to self-renew and differentiate suggests that they are initiated by epithelial progenitor cells which, we postulate, reside in the bases of the glands in the basalis (Fig. 12.1), while small CFU may be initiated by more mature transit amplifying cells, likely resident in the functionalis and responsible for the extensive proliferation observed in the first half of the menstrual cycle.

Monoclonality of endometrial glands

Evidence from several approaches suggests that endometrial glands are monoclonal in origin and therefore arise from a common ancestor or stem/progenitor cell. Monoclonality of individually dissected glands was demonstrated using a polymerase chain reaction (PCR)-based assay for the X-linked androgen receptor gene, which undergoes random X-linked inactivation [10]. Adjacent glands also shared clonality for areas up to 1 mm apart, indicating that well-circumscribed regions of the endometrium were derived from the same precursor, suggesting that single epithelial progenitor cells generated several glands, raising questions on the precise locality of these progenitor cells.

Monoclonal endometrial glands were also identified in the endometrium of female chimeric mice [11]. In mice carrying the GFP gene on the X chromosome, individual glands were either GFP positive or GFP negative and the surface epithelium showed clear demarcation of GFP-positive and -negative regions [10]. Further evidence comes from phosphatase and tensin homolog deleted on chromosome 10 (PTEN) immunostaining of normal human endometrium, which reveals that rare glands fail to express this tumor suppressor gene due to a mutation and/or deletion [12]. The PTEN-null gland clones persist in the basalis region between menstrual cycles and generate more PTEN-null glands in the functionalis in subsequent cycles. PTEN is an estrogen-responsive gene and the proportion of PTEN-null glands increases in the endometrium of women taking unopposed estrogen and in endometrial hyperplasia [13].

Together, these observations of endometrial glandular monoclonality suggest the existence of epithelial stem/progenitor

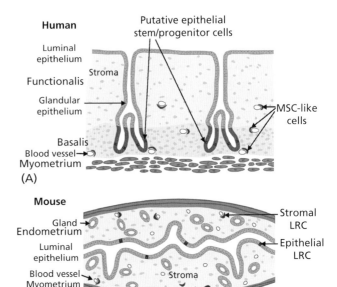

Figure 12.1 Possible location of endometrial stem/progenitor cells in human and mouse endometrium. (A) Human endometrium. It is hypothesized that epithelial progenitor cells will be located in the base of the glands in the basalis. MSC-like cells are located near blood vessels in both the basalis and the functionalis. (B) Mouse endometrium. LRC candidate epithelial and stromal stem/progenitor cells which rapidly proliferate during estrogen-stimulated endometrial growth are located in the luminal epithelium and mainly near blood vessels at the endometrial–myometrial junction, respectively. Reproduced from Gargett *et al* Mol Cell Endocrinol 2008;288:22–29 with permission from Elsevier.

cells at the base of individual glands (see Fig. 12.1A) that are responsible for generating single glandular units or a region comprising several glands.

Endometrial gland methylation patterns

Methylation patterns of genes in individual glands of human endometrium have been investigated to trace the history of epithelial stem cell kinetics [14]. Epigenetic markers arising during adult stem cell division are inherited by all the daughter cells and therefore persist, while those arising in the transit amplifying or more mature cells are lost when the functionalis layer is shed during menstruation. Thus the total number of stem cell divisions may be inferred from the numbers of somatic errors accumulated within individual glands [15]. This study showed that the extent of methylation of genes in endometrial glands increased with age until menopause, after which it remained relatively constant, indicating that the number of epigenetic errors was a reflection of the mitotic activity of endometrial stem cells [14]. Mathematical modeling of the data indicated that individual glands contain stem cell niches occupied by several long-lived stem cells. It would appear that symmetrical and asymmetrical cell divisions occurred in a stochastic manner to maintain a constant number of stem cells in the endometrial gland niche [14], arguing against the monoclonality concept.

Label-retaining cells in mouse endometrial epithelium

Label-retaining cells (LRC) have been identified as candidate adult stem cells *in vivo* in mouse endometrium [16–18]. The LRC approach is used to identify adult stem cells when specific markers are unknown, and relies on the relatively infrequent cell turnover of most adult stem cells in comparison to rapidly proliferating transit amplifying cells [2,16,19]. LRC are detected by pulse-labeling the majority of tissue cells with a DNA synthesis label (bromodeoxyuridine (BrdU)) when adult stem cells are proliferating, and subsequently chasing out the label over long periods of time. With each cell division, the incorporated BrdU is diluted 50% until it reaches undetectable levels after 3–4 cell divisions. Immuno histochemistry localizes BrdU-positive LRC, revealing their location and the stem cell niche. BrdU labeling during the postnatal period (days 3–5) showed that 3% of mouse endometrial epithelial cells were LRC located in the luminal rather than the glandular epithelium as well-separated estrogen receptor-alpha (ERα)-negative cells, suggesting that luminal epithelial stem/progenitor cells are responsible for the growth of glands during development and in cycling mice (see Fig. 12.1B) [16,20].

In ovariectomized prepubertal mice, the first cells to proliferate in estrogen-stimulated endometrial growth are the epithelial LRC, suggesting that they function as stem/progenitor cells to initiate epithelial regeneration [16]. However, in ovariectomized cycling mice, both epithelial LRC and non-LRC rapidly proliferated in response to estrogen to regenerate luminal and glandular epithelium [20]. Application of the LRC technique to a mouse model of menstrual breakdown and repair [21] showed that in adult female mice labeled with BrdU, ERα-negative glandular epithelial LRC may contribute to repair of the luminal epithelium when it is sloughed off in response to progesterone withdrawal. In this model, endometrial repair occurs in the absence of estrogen [22].

These various models of endometrial epithelial growth and repair suggest that LRC may reside in luminal or glandular epithelium at different stages of murine endometrial development, and that luminal LRC may have an important role in generating luminal epithelium during development, while glandular LRC have a key role in replenishing shed or lost luminal epithelium, as is expected in human endometrium.

Endometrial mesenchymal stromal/stem cells

In addition to epithelial progenitor cells, a rare population of mesenchymal stem/stromal cells (MSC) has also been identified in human and mouse endometrium. These MSC-like cells have properties and phenotype similar to bone marrow or adipose tissue MSC.

Cell cloning

Initial studies identified a small population of clonogenic stromal cells (1.25%) isolated from the EpCAM-negative fraction of freshly isolated single cell suspensions of endometrial cells obtained from hysterectomy tissues from cycling women [7]. Clonogenic stromal cells were also observed in freshly isolated inactive endometrium of peri/postmenopausal women and in women on oral contraceptives, suggesting that these stromal CFU may be responsible for regenerating the endometrium when women commence estrogen replacement therapy or cease oral contraceptive treatment, respectively [6,8]. Similar to the clonogenic epithelial progenitor, two types of stromal CFU were generated: large (0.02%) and small (1.23%). Endometrial stromal CFU are clonogenic in serum-free medium supplemented with either fibroblast growth factor-2 (FGF-2), EGF, TGF-α or platelet-derived growth factor-BB (PDGF-BB), suggesting that they express FGF receptors, EGFR and PDGF receptor-β (PDGF-Rβ) [7,8]. Clonogenic stromal cells have also been identified in bulk cultured and passaged endometrial stromal cells at a higher frequency than in freshly isolated cell populations [23], indicating that prior culture selects for clonogenic cells.

Self-renewal and multilineage differentiation of stromal colony-forming units

Subsequent studies of the large stromal CFU derived from freshly isolated hysterectomy endometrium demonstrated substantial self-renewal ability *in vitro*, as they underwent serial subcloning 3.3 times when seeded at very low seeding densities (10 cells/cm²), while small CFU serially cloned once [9]. Individual large stromal CFU had high proliferative potential, undergoing 30 population doublings when cultured at bulk culture density (2000 cells/cm²), generating 6.4×10^{11} cells from the original colony-initiating stromal cells, seven orders of magnitude more than produced by small CFU.

Single large stromal CFU derived from freshly isolated endometrial tissue underwent multilineage differentiation into four mesodermal lineages when cultured under appropriate conditions, including smooth muscle, fat, cartilage, and bone [9]. Passaged endometrial stromal cells also contain a population of cells that differentiate *in vitro* into adipocytes [23] or chondrocytes [24], and this chondrogenic differentiation does not occur in myometrium, fibroid, fallopian tube or uterosacral ligament. CFU obtained from freshly isolated or cultured endometrial stromal cells expressed typical MSC markers used to phenotype bone marrow and adipose tissue MSC; CD29, CD44, CD73, CD90, CD105, CD146 [25], but not STRO-1, CD31 (endothelial), CD34 (hemopoietic stem cell and endothelial), CD45 (leukocyte) or HLA-DR [9,23]. These studies indicate that multipotent MSC-like cells with properties and phenotype similar to bone marrow and adipose tissue MSC are present in the highly regenerative endometrial stroma, but not in neighboring reproductive tract tissues, suggesting that they may be responsible for regenerating the endometrial stroma each menstrual cycle.

Label-retaining cells in endometrial stroma

Candidate stromal stem/progenitor cells have been identified in mouse endometrium as stromal LRC [16–18]. Between 6% and 9% of the stromal cells were identified as LRC. A large proportion of these were located near blood vessels close to the endometrial–myometrial junction (see Fig. 12.1B) [16,17], correlating with their postulated basalis location in human endometrium. The endometrial–myometrial junction is a site of cyclic tissue remodeling in both human [26] and in a mouse model of menstruation and repair [22]. Stromal LRC did not express CD45 [16], suggesting thaat they were not leukocytes or of bone marrow origin. Some (0.6%) expressed Oct-4, a pluripotency marker, and c-kit, a hemopoietic stem cell marker [17]. In other studies, stromal LRC did not express the stem cell markers Sca-1 [16] or c-kit [18]. The majority of stromal LRC did not express ERα (84%) [16] and one-third of stromal LRC expressed α-smooth muscle actin (α-SMA) but not CD31, suggesting that they are pericytes or vascular smooth muscle cells and that they occupy a perivascular niche.

Human endometrial side population cells

Hemopoietic stem cells can be purified on the basis of differential staining of the fluorescent DNA binding vital dye, Hoechst 33342, using dual-emission wavelength fluorescence activated cell sorting (FACS) [27]. This small side population separates from the majority of the cells as a low Hoechst population due to their ability to efflux the dye through highly expressed ABCG2/Bcrp1 transporter proteins in the plasma membrane of adult stem cells [28]. ABCG2 was not essential for conferring stemness, but the SP phenotype is considered a universal marker of adult stem cell activity [29]. SP cells (0–5%) have been identified in freshly isolated [30,31,33] and short-term cultures [32] of human endometrial cells. Similar to CFU activity in human endometrium, the percentage of SP cells was highly variable between subjects, although higher in the menstrual [32] and proliferative [30,33] stages of the menstrual cycle. Freshly sorted human endometrial SP cells showed little growth in culture, likely because they were largely in G0 (85%) phase of the cell cycle, indicating their relative quiescence. In contrast, SP cells sorted from primary endometrial cultures were primarily in G1 and G1/M/S phases [30]. Endometrial SP cells, FACS sorted from short-term cultures, did not express endometrial epithelial (CD9) or stromal (CD13) cell differentiation markers, but re-expressed them in long-term Matrigel cultures, indicating capacity to differentiate into CD9-positive, E-cadherin-positive gland-like organoids and CD13-positive stromal clusters [32]. Both SP and non-SP cells differentiated into prolactin-secreting decidual cells [30]. Clonogenic endometrial cells were also enriched in the SP compared to the non-SP fraction [30], although toxic levels of Hoechst dye may affect CFU activity in non-SP cells.

Further analysis indicates that human endometrial SP cells are a mixed population, comprising endothelial, epithelial and stromal cells [30,33]. Immunostaining of full-thickness endometrial tissue for the SP marker ABCG2 revealed that ABCG2-positive cells lined blood vessels distributed throughout the functionalis and basalis layers [30,33], and co-localized with CD31-positive endothelial cells [33]. ABCG2-positive cells are located adjacent to endometrial MSC-like cells expressing PDGFRβ and CD146 [34], indicating the importance of the vascular niche for endometrial stem/progenitor cells [2]. Only freshly isolated human endometrial SP cells, but not non-SP cells, reconstituted

various endometrial tissue components or even the entire endometrium when transplanted under the kidney capsule of immunocompromised NOD/SCID/γ$_c$ null (NOG) mice [33].

Together, these data indicate that endometrial SP cells produce endometrial epithelial and stromal cells *in vitro* and *in vivo*, and because they are located in both basalis and functionalis, they may be shed during menstruation and could be candidate endometriosis-initiating cells. However, the hierarchical relationship between endometrial SP cells, clonogenic, CD146- positive PDGFRβ-positive and tissue reconstituting cells (see below) still remains to be clarified.

Endometrial tissue reconstituting cells

Demonstrating the regenerative capacity of putative endometrial adult stem cell populations by examining their ability to reconstitute endometrial tissue *in vivo* is an important goal and provides functional proof of adult stem cell activity. Transplantation of fully dissociated unfractionated human endometrial epithelial and stromal cell suspensions (5×10^5 cells) directly beneath the kidney capsule of ovariectomized and estrogen-supplemented NOG mice recapitulated well-organized endometrial and myometrial layers of functional endometrium comprising cytokeratin-positive CD9-positive glandular structures, CD10-positive CD13-positive stroma and α-SMA-positive myometrial layers [35]. This robust endometrial tissue reconstitution assay generated dozens of homogeneous xenografted mice from one sample. The endometrial xenografts responded to cyclical sex steroid hormones, forming tortuous glands and decidualized stroma when estrogen and progesterone were administered, as well as large blood-filled cysts similar to red spot lesions of active endometriosis after hormonal withdrawal (Plate 12.1) [35]. This animal model suggests that human endometrial cells have the capacity to grow endometriosis-like tissue when transplanted into an ectopic site.

Markers of endometrial stem/progenitor cells

Specific markers of endometrial stem/progenitor cells would greatly facilitate investigation into their possible role in initiating endometriosis lesions. It would also enable the identification of their location in shedding endometrium and endometriotic lesions. Currently no markers are known for endometrial epithelial stem/progenitor cells which cannot be distinguished from their mature progeny in the glands and luminal epithelium.

Mesenchymal/stromal stem cells

Mesenchymal stem cell-like cells were recently isolated from human endometrium by their co-expression of two perivascular cell markers, CD146 and PDGF-Rβ [34]. The FACS-sorted CD146-positive PDGF-Rβ-positive subpopulation of endometrial stromal cells was enriched eight-fold for CFU compared to unsorted stromal cells. The CD146-positive PDGF-Rβ-positive cells expressed typical MSC surface markers, CD29, CD44, CD73, CD90 and CD105 and were negative for hemopoietic and endothelial markers (CD31, CD34 and CD45) [34]. However,

STRO-1, a marker used to prospectively isolate bone marrow MSC [36], was not expressed by CD146-positive PDGF-Rβ-positive cells, nor by clonogenic stromal CFU [37]. The CD146-positive PDGF-Rβ-positive cells underwent multilineage differentiation into adipogenic, myogenic, chondrogenic and osteoblastic lineages when cultured in appropriate induction media [34]. CD146-positive PDGF-Rβ-positive cells were located perivascularly in both functionalis and basalis layers of human endometrium [34]. The CD146-positive PDGF-Rβ-positive subpopulation of endometrial stromal cells appear to be similar to bone marrow and fat MSC in differentiation potential and perivascular location. This finding also indicates that endometrial MSC-like cells are likely shed during menstruation.

Stem cell marker expression in endometrium

Stem cell marker expression in human and mouse endometrium has been examined in several studies by immunotechniques. Oct-4 (POU5F1), a marker of pluripotent human embryonic stem cells and some adult stem cells, was demonstrated in some human endometrial samples but the cell types and location was not determined [38].

The orphan receptor and Wnt target gene, leucine-rich repeat-containing G protein-coupled receptor-5 (Lgr-5), has recently been identified as a marker of mouse small intestine and colon epithelial stem cells located in the intestinal crypts [39]. Using genetic lineage tracing, Lgr-5-expressing cells were shown to generate all epithelial lineages in the intestine and hair follicles. Lgr-5 is dynamically regulated in endometrial epithelium, expressed only in immature and ovariectomized mice, and downregulated by estrogen [40]. Lgr-5 is also expressed in human endometrial epithelium [41]. The utility of Lgr-5 as a marker of human endometrial epithelial progenitor cells requires the development of quality antibodies to a surface epitope to purify the cells for subsequent assessment of adult stem cell function.

Musashi-1, an RNA binding protein in neural stem cells and an epithelial progenitor cell marker that regulates stem cell self-renewal signaling pathways, was recently immunolocalized to single epithelial and small clusters of stromal cells in human endometrium [42]. Musashi-1-positive cells were mainly found in the basalis in the proliferative stage of the menstrual cycle, suggesting their possible stem/progenitor cell function. Stromal Musashi-1-positive cells were not found in a perivascular location, although some were in a periglandular region, similar to some stromal LRC in mouse endometrium [16]. A large proportion of endometriotic glands expressed Musashi-1. Whether Musashi-1-positive endometriotic cells represent basalis-derived epithelium or stem/progenitor cells with CFU activity remains to be determined. It is also important to determine whether Musashi-1 is expressed in CD146-positive PDGF-Rβ-positive stromal cells and SP cells.

Cells with a hematopoietic stem cell phenotype (CD34-positive CD45-positive) co-expressing CD7 and CD56 have been identified in human endometrial cell suspensions and may be lymphoid progenitors [43]. Whether these cells function as hemopoietic

stem cells and generate endometrial leukocytes in the endometrium or contribute to the SP population is unknown. Neither is it known whether the cells expressing these markers function as endometrial stem/progenitor cells [2].

Source of endometrial stem/progenitor cells

Endometrial stem/progenitor cells may be derived from residual fetal stem cells [2], although emerging evidence suggests that bone marrow cells may also populate the endometrium and contribute to the pool of resident adult stem cells. Bone marrow stem cells, including hemopoietic stem cells, MSC and endothelial progenitor cells, circulate in very low numbers. Clinical and scientific evidence indicates that bone marrow stem cells and myeloid cells home to sites of tissue damage and incorporate into various organs, transdifferentiating into the cells of the new tissue in which they reside [44]. This concept of bone marrow stem cell plasticity is controversial and generally a rare event that may result from cell fusion or the paracrine action of growth factors released from MSC.

The first report on bone marrow cell contribution to endometrial regeneration demonstrated significant chimerism ranging from 0.2% to 52% in the endometrial glands and stroma of four women who received single-antigen HLA-mismatched bone marrow transplants [45]. Most glands consisted entirely of host or entirely donor-derived cells, indicating their monoclonality. However, some individual glands contained a mixture of donor and recipient cells [45], suggesting that a single gland may be composed of multiple clones. A similar study of the endometrium from three women who had received gender-mismatched bone marrow transplants also demonstrated chimeric endometrial glands containing a Y chromosome in 0.6–8.4% of the epithelial cells [46]. These XY-positive epithelial cells expressed ERα. Approximately 9% of stromal cells were XY positive, although it was technically difficult to distinguish CD45-positive bone marrow cells. These XY-positive endometrial cells appeared as individual cells and clonal expansion was not apparent, despite treatment with hormone replacement therapy for several cycles. It is not known if the source of donor bone marrow cells contributing to chimeric endometrial tissue is hemopoietic stem cells, MSC or even myeloid cells. Of interest is that estrogen plus progesterone induced bone marrow-derived MSC to differentiate down the endometrial fibroblast lineage *in vitro* [47]. These cells showed characteristic decidual cell morphology and expressed typical decidual markers, suggesting that bone marrow MSC have the capacity to differentiate into endometrial stromal cells under certain conditions.

Studies in mice provide further evidence for the contribution of bone marrow-derived cells to endometrial repair. In a gender-mismatched bone marrow transplant model, endometrial epithelial cells of recipient mice comprised <0.01% XY-positive cytokeratin positive cells and <0.1% XY-positive stromal cells [48]. Bone marrow cell contribution to endometrial repair is very modest and engraftment of the endometrium seems more likely during repair after injury. In a novel double reporter *CD45/*

Cre-Z/EG transgenic mouse model used to track the fate of CD45-positive green fluorescent protein (GFP) cells, circulating CD45-positive bone marrow cells contributed small numbers of GFP-positive endometrial luminal epithelial cells, ranging from 0% in 6-week-old to 6% in 20-week-old mice [49]. Although small numbers of animals were examined, these data suggest increasing incorporation rather than clonal expansion of bone marrow-derived cells into the endometrial epithelium over time. The lack of CD45 expression observed in epithelial and stromal LRC may be due to transdifferentiation into endometrial cells [16].

It is too early to draw conclusions on whether endometrial cells are derived from bone marrow cells or resident stem cells, or if both sources contribute. The apparent vascular location of endometrial SP cells and the fact that MSC are perivascular cells suggest that the endometrial stem cell niche is associated with blood vessels, a convenient portal of entry for bone-marrow derived cells. It is also unclear if an ultimate endometrial stem cell exists that has capacity to replace all endometrial cells, including epithelial, stromal, vascular cells, or whether there are separate epithelial and MSC. To date, the data suggest that there are two distinct endometrial stem/progenitor cells: an epithelial progenitor cell and a MSC-like cell.

Endometrial stem/progenitor cells in endometriosis

Currently the pathogenesis of endometriosis is poorly understood. The most widely accepted mechanism is Sampson's retrograde menstruation theory where viable endometrial fragments refluxed into the pelvic cavity attach to and invade the peritoneal mesothelium to establish ectopic growth of endometrial tissue [50]. It is not known why only 6–10% of women develop endometriosis when retrograde menstruation occurs in most women. An attractive hypothesis is that endometrial stem/progenitor cells are abnormally shed during menses, gaining access to the peritoneal cavity where they establish ectopic implants in those women who develop endometriosis (Fig. 12.2) [2,51–53]. Although long-term endometriotic lesions may develop from endometrial stem/progenitor cells, those that resolve may have established from mature transit amplifying cells. Alternatively, endometrial stem/progenitor cells with yet to be identified intrinsic abnormalities may have increased propensity to implant and establish an ectopic colony, or normal stem/progenitor cells implant more readily on an abnormal peritoneal mesothelium. No direct evidence for the role of endometrial stem/progenitor cells in the pathogenesis of endometriosis has been reported to date. However, there are numerous experiments showing that unfractionated human endometrial cells establish ectopic endometrial growth in the many models used for the study of endometriosis [52]. In baboons which menstruate, shed menstrual debris induces endometriosis spontaneously or under experimental conditions [54], suggesting the presence of stem/progenitor cells in the debris.

Monoclonality of ectopic endometriosis lesions

The demonstration that epithelial cells in some endometriosis lesions are monoclonal [55] provides a strong argument for single cell origin and the likelihood that the cell initiating endometriosis is an endometrial stem/progenitor cell. However, polyclonal lesions have also been reported, which has been attributed to contamination with polyclonal stromal cells, repeated seeding of the lesion with cells from other sources, including the bone marrow, or establishment from fragments of shed endometrium containing several stem/progenitor cells [56]. More careful analysis using microdissected ectopic endometrium has shown that multiple foci of monoclonal regions are present in the lesions [57]. Cellular lineages in a menstrual fragment of human endometrium has been reconstructed from methylation patterns, providing a cellular genealogy [58]. The cells in close proximity showed greater relatedness than those at greater distances and the data indicated that the number of endometrial stem/progenitor cells in the endometrium is likely to be very small.

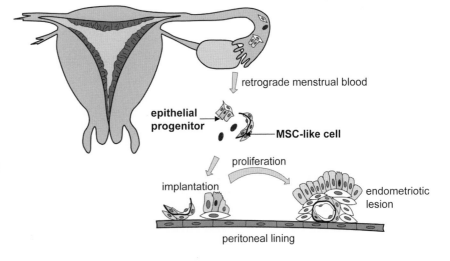

Figure 12.2 Possible role of endometrial stem/progenitor cells in the pathogenesis of endometriosis. It is postulated that endometrial epithelial progenitor cells and MSC-like cells together with their niche cells are shed into the peritoneal cavity via retrograde menstruation where they establish ectopic endometriotic lesions in women who endometriosis [68]. Adapted from Gargett and Guo [56] with permission from Jaypee Brothers Medical Publishers..

Stem/progenitor cells in menstrual blood

Given that endometrial MSC-like cells have been identified in both functionalis and basalis [34], it is not surprising that emerging evidence suggests that endometrial stem/progenitor cells are shed in menstrual blood [59–62]. Stromal cells have been cultured from menstrual blood in a manner similar to bone marrow-derived MSC but interestingly, epithelial cells have been overlooked, overgrown by stromal cells [63] or not been retrieved, indicating that epithelial progenitors are most likely resident in the basalis layer and are not normally shed during menstruation. Cells cultured from menstrual blood have broad differentiation capacity, producing all the mesodermal lineages including skeletal and cardiac muscle cells [59,60], but also neural lineages [62]. Our own unpublished studies have also demonstrated that menstrual blood contains clonogenic, multipotent cells with MSC activity [64]. It is not known if there are differences in the numbers of clonogenic MSC-like cells shed in menstrual blood between women with and without endometriosis, or whether women susceptible to endometriosis may have a higher propensity to shed endometrial stem/progenitor cells. Neither is it known whether endometrial stem/progenitor cells are shed in a retrograde manner in women with endometriosis.

A recent study assessing the peritoneal fluid of women with and without endometriosis at different stages of the cycle could not find an increase in endometrial cells in the peritoneal fluid either with menstruation or with endometriosis [65]. A difficulty experienced by this and previous studies examining peritoneal fluid for refluxed endometrial cells is that multiple markers are required to distinguish endometrial epithelial and stromal cells, mesothelial cells and leukocyte populations, which is technically very difficult using immunohistochemical approaches. However, if rare stem/progenitor cells are present in retrogradely shed endometrium, their concentrations will be even less compared to normal endometrial cells, but they would still be capable of forming endometriotic lesions due to their increased proliferative potential compared with more mature differentiated cells. These studies are technically difficult and highlight the importance of finding specific endometrial stem/progenitor cell markers. If endometrial stem/progenitor cells are shed in retrograde menstrual debris, it is likely they will only establish ectopic lesions when transported with their niche cells [2].

Role of the endometrial basalis

There is increasing evidence that women with endometriosis have a greater amount of basalis-type endometrium in their menstrual debris than women without endometriosis [51]. One group has postulated that this may be due to increased peristaltic contractions of the uterine muscle in women with endometriosis [66]. The excessive uterine muscular activity could result in both increased microtrauma to the basalis layer and increased transport of the fragments of basal endometrium retrogradely through the fallopian tubes into the peritoneal cavity. The basalis, but not the functionalis, retains ER and P450 aromatase expression in the secretory phase of the cycle. It has been demonstrated that in women with endometriosis, a much larger proportion of the endometrial fragments shed at menstruation are from the basalis than in healthy controls (75% versus 10% were ER positive). The authors also demonstrated that the endometrial tissue in endometriotic lesions displayed the same characteristics as basalis endometrium, providing further evidence that the retrogradely shed endometrial fragments may originate from basalis endometrium. The importance of basalis-type endometrium in endometriotic lesion formation may be related to the greater numbers of stem/progenitor cells.

Endometriosis-initiating cells

Just as tumor-initiating cells are considered to be cancer stem cells that initiate malignant tumors *in vivo*, it is postulated that human endometriosis-initiating cells reconstituting ectopic endometriotic lesions *in vivo* are likely to be endometrial stem/progenitor cells. Numerous animal models exist for investigating endometriosis lesion development, and as new, more severely immuno-compromised mouse strains have been developed, the longer the xenografted tissue fragments survive. In a recent model, singly dispersed human endometrial cells transplanted beneath the kidney capsule of NOG mice (lacking NK, T- and B-cells) fully reconstructed endometrial histoarchitecture and function, mimicking hormone-dependent processes such as cellular proliferation, differentiation (decidualization) and tissue breakdown [35]. In this model, progesterone withdrawal produced a large blood-filled cyst like a red spot lesion of endometriosis on the kidney surface (see Plate 12.1).

It is postulated that the endometrial stem/progenitor cells in the initial xenograft are also the endometriosis-initiating cells producing these endometriosis-like grafts. Furthermore, the mouse kidney parenchyma was invaded by human blood vessels which formed chimeric vessels with the host murine endothelium, providing a murine blood flow to the transplant [35]. This angiogenic potential of the endometrial endothelial cells is likely crucial for establishment and development of endometriosis, not only because the functional vascularization is required for maintenance of endometriotic lesion but because the endometrial MSC niche is perivascular [34]. This unique animal model is also suitable for the study of the pathogenesis of endometriosis through non-invasive, real-time, and quantitative assessment of ectopically reconstituted endometrium-like tissues and could potentially be applicable for drug testing and gene target validation in endometriosis [35].

Transdifferentiation, metaplasia of stem/progenitor cells

An area of controversy in the stem cell field is the concept of adult stem cell plasticity, mediated by nuclear reprogramming and alteration of transcriptional activity in key developmental genes. This process is a form of metaplasia which results from changes in the extracellular environment, and appears to occur in the setting of tissue damage [67]. Metaplasia of the peritoneal lining has been suggested as one possible cause of endometriosis. However, another source of the metaplastic cells with transdifferentiation capacity are bone marrow stem cells transported via the circulation into the pelvic cavity. In a mouse transplant model where genetically marked bone marrow-derived cells can be tracked, it was demonstrated that a small number incorporated into established endometriosis lesions and transdifferentiated into epithelial (<0.04%) and stromal (0.1%) cells [48]. However, bone marrow-derived cells did not appear to initiate endometriosis lesion development, but rather contributed to endometriosis progression.

Changing cell phenotype may involve epithelial-mesenchymal transition (EMT) or mesenchymal-epithelial transition (MET), processes known to occur during embryogenesis and recapitulated again in carcinogenesis. Changing cell phenotypes within endometriotic lesions may be responsible for the invasiveness of endometriotic cells. For example, endometriotic lesions contain a well-differentiated cytokeratin (CK)-positive E-cadherin-positive population, a CK-negative E-cadherin-negative stromal population and a more invasive CK-positive E-cadherin-negative N-cadherin-positive epithelial population, the latter with properties similar to early carcinoma micrometastasis [53]. In keeping with the similarity to early carcinoma, endometriotic lesions regress during estrogen depletion therapy but recur on cessation of therapy, suggesting that putative stem/progenitor cells in the lesion remain quiescent or dormant and then reactivate on subsequent estrogen replacement. Endometrial stem/progenitor cells within the lesions may also reseed subsequent lesions. Interestingly, clonogenic endometrial epithelial cells are weakly or negative for cytokeratin [7] and some SP cells do not express the epithelial maturation marker CD9 [32], also suggesting an epithelial–mesenchymal transition in these putative epithelial stem/progenitor cells.

Conclusion

A reasonable body of evidence indicates that rare populations of epithelial stem/progenitor cells and MSC-like cells are present in human and mouse endometrium. While there is some evidence for the monoclonality of individual endometrial glands, it is still not clear whether epithelial stem/progenitor cells exist as single or multiple cells in the bases of individual glands. There is much interest in the hypothesis that foci of endometriosis which are monoclonal in origin are initiated by retrogradely shed endometrial stem/progenitor cells and their niche cells in women who develop endometriosis. Genealogy studies on menstruated fragments, the recent evidence for the presence of MSC-like cells in menstrual blood, and the identification of markers that enable the prospective isolation and identification of endometrial MSC-like cells provide impetus for investigating the role of endometrial stem/progenitor cells in the pathogenesis of endometriosis. *In vivo* models are now available to investigate the role of endometriosis-initiating cells, characterize their stem/progenitor cell properties and examine the effects of new treatments that target self-renewal processes in shed endometrial stem/progenitor cells as novel therapeutic options for the treatment of endometriosis.

Acknowledgments

This work was supported by a grant from the National Health and Medical Research Council (NHMRC) of Australia (ID 545992) to CEG and GW. CEG is also supported by an NHMRC RD Wright Career Development Award (465121).

References

1. Eckfeldt CE, Mendenhall EM, Verfaillie CM. The molecular repertoire of the 'almighty' stem cell. Nature Rev Molec Cell Biol 2005; 6:726–737.

2. Gargett CE. Uterine stem cells: what is the evidence? Hum Reprod Update 2007;13:87–101.

3. Li L, Xie T. Stem cell niche: structure and function. Annu Rev Cell Dev Biol 2005;21:605–631.

4. Spencer TE, Hayashi K, Hu J, Carpenter KD. Comparative developmental biology of the mammalian uterus. Curr Top Dev Biol 2005; 68:85–122.

5. Jabbour HN, Kelly RW, Fraser HM, Critchley HOD. Endocrine regulation of menstruation. Endocrine Rev 2006;27:17–46.

6. Gargett CE. Identification and characterisation of human endometrial stem/progenitor cells. Aust NZ J Obstet Gynaecol 2006;46:250–253.

7. Chan RWS, Schwab KE, Gargett CE. Clonogenicity of human endometrial epithelial and stromal cells. Biol Reprod 2004;70:1738–1750.

8. Schwab KE, Chan RW, Gargett CE. Putative stem cell activity of human endometrial epithelial and stromal cells during the menstrual cycle. Fertil Steril 2005;84 (Suppl 2):1124–1130.

9. Gargett CE, Schwab KE, Zillwood RM, Nguyen HPT, Wu D. Isolation and culture of epithelial progenitors and mesenchymal stem cells from human endometrium. Biol Reprod 2009;80:1136–1145.

10. Tanaka M, Kyo S, Kanaya T et al. Evidence of the monoclonal composition of human endometrial epithelial glands and mosaic pattern of clonal distribution in luminal epithelium. Am J Pathol 2003;163:295–301.

11. Lipschutz JH, Fukami H, Yamamoto M et al. Clonality of urogenital organs as determined by analysis of chimeric mice. Cells Tiss Organs 1999;165:57–66.

12. Mutter GL, Lin MC, Fitzgerald JT, Kum JB, Eng C. Changes in endometrial PTEN expression throughout the human menstrual cycle. J Clin Endocrinol Metab 2000;85:2334–2338.

13. Mutter GL, Ince TA, Baak JPA, Kust GA, Zhou XP, Eng C. Molecular identification of latent precancers in histologically normal endometrium. Cancer Res 2001;61:4311–4314.

14. Kim JY, Tavare S, Shibata D. Counting human somatic cell replications: methylation mirrors endometrial stem cell divisions. Proc Natl Acad Sci USA 2005;102(49):17739–17744.

15. Ro S, Rannala B. Methylation patterns and mathematical models reveal dynamics of stem cell turnover in the human colon. Proc Natl Acad Sci USA 2001;98:10519–10521.

16. Chan RW, Gargett CE. Identification of label-retaining cells in mouse endometrium. Stem Cells 2006;24:1529–1538.

17. Cervello I, Martinez-Conejero JA, Horcajadas JA, Pellicer A, Simon C. Identification, characterization and co-localization of label-retaining

cell population in mouse endometrium with typical undifferentiated markers. Hum Reprod 2007;22:45–51.

18. Szotek PP, Chang HL, Zhang L et al. Adult mouse myometrial label-retaining cells divide in response to gonadotropin stimulation. Stem Cells 2007;25:1317–1325.

19. Gargett CE, Chan RW, Schwab KE. Endometrial stem cells. Curr Opin Obstet Gynecol 2007;19:377–383.

20. Chan RWS, Kaitu'u-Lino TJ, Gargett CE. Role of label-retaining cells in estrogen-induced endometrial regeneration. Reprod Sci 2011; DOI:10.1177/1933719111414207 .

21. Kaitu'u-Lino TJ, Ye L, Gargett CE. A model for investigating the contribution of mouse endometrial stem/progenitor cells to endometrial rengeneration following menstruation. Seventh International Meeting of the Society of Stem Cell Research, Barcelona, Spain, 2009, July 8–11.

22. Kaitu'u-Lino TJ, Morison NB, Salamonsen LA. Estrogen is not essential for full endometrial restoration after breakdown: lessons from a mouse model. Endocrinology 2007;148:5105–5111.

23. Dimitrov R, Timeva T, Kyurkchiev D et al. Characterisation of clonogenic stromal cells isolated from human endometrium. Reproduction 2008;135:551–558.

24. Wolff EF, Wolff AB, Du H, Taylor HS. Demonstration of multipotent stem cells in the adult human endometrium by in vitro chondrogenesis. Reprod Sci 2007;14:524–533.

25. Dominici M, Le BK, Mueller I et al. Minimal criteria for defining multipotent mesenchymal stromal cells. The International Society for Cellular Therapy position statement. Cytotherapy 2006;8:315–317.

26. Fujii S, Konishi I, Mori T. Smooth muscle differentiation at the endometrio-myometrial junction. Virchows Arch A Pathol Anat 1989;414:105–112.

27. Goodell MA, Brose K, Paradis G, Conner AS, Mulligan RC. Isolation and functional properties of murine hematopoietic stem cells that are replicating in vivo. J Exp Med 1997;183:1797–1806.

28. Zhou S, Schuetz JD, Bunting KD et al. The ABC transporter Bcrp1/ABCG2 is expressed in a wide variety of stem cells and is a molecular determinant of the side-population phenotype. Nature Med 2001;7:1028–1034.

29. Challen GA, Little MH. A side order of stem cells: the SP phenotype. Stem Cells 2006;24:3–12.

30. Tsuji S, Yoshimoto M, Takahashi K, Noda Y, Nakahata T, Heike T. Side population cells contribute to the genesis of human endometrium. Fertil Steril 2008;90:1528–1537.

31. Cervello I, Simon C. Somatic stem cells in the endometrium. Reprod Sci 2009;16:200–205.

32. Kato K, Yoshimoto M, Kato K et al. Characterization of side-population cells in human normal endometrium. Hum Reprod 2007;22:1214–1223.

33. Masuda H, Matsuzaki Y, Hiratsu E, Ono M, Nagashima T, Kajitani T, Arase T, Oda H, Uchida H, Asada H, Ito M, Yoshimura Y, Maruyama T, Okano H. Stem cell-like properties of the endometrial side population: implication in endometrial regeneration. PLoS One. 2010 Apr 28;5(4):e10387.

34. Schwab KE, Gargett CE. Co-expression of two perivascular cell markers isolates mesenchymal stem-like cells from human endometrium. Hum Reprod 2007;22:2903–2911.

35. Masuda H, Maruyama T, Hiratsu E et al. Noninvasive and real-time assessment of reconstructed functional human endometrium in NOD/SCID/γ_c^{null} immunodeficient mice. Proc Natl Acad Sci USA 2007;104:1925–1930.

36. Gronthos S, Simmons PJ. The growth factor requirements of STRO-1-positive human bone marrow stromal precursors under serum-deprived conditions in vitro. Blood 1995;85:929–940.

37. Schwab KE, Hutchinson P, Gargett CE. Identification of surface markers for prospective isolation of human endometrial stromal colony-forming cells. Hum Reprod 2008;23:934–943.

38. Matthai C, Horvat R, Noe M et al. Oct-4 expression in human endometrium. Mol Hum Reprod 2006;12:7–10.

39. Barker N, van Es JH, Kuipers J et al. Identification of stem cells in small intestine and colon by marker gene Lgr5. Nature 2007;449:1003–1007.

40. Sun X, Jackson L, Dey SK, Daikoku T. In pursuit of leucine-rich repeat-containing G protein-coupled receptor-5 regulation and function in the uterus. Endocrinology 2009;150:5065–5073.

41. Krusche CA, Kroll T, Beier HM, Classen-Linke I. Expression of leucine-rich repeat-containing G-protein-coupled receptors in the human cyclic endometrium. Fertil Steril 2007;87:1428–1437.

42. Götte M, Wolf M, Staebler A et al. Increased experssion of the adult stem cell marker Musashi-1 in endometriosis and endometrial carcinoma. J Pathol 2008;215:317–329.

43. Lynch L, Golden-Mason L, Eogan M, O'Herlihy C, O'Farrelly C. Cells with haematopoietic stem cell phenotype in adult human endometrium: relevance to infertility? Hum Reprod 2007;22:919–926.

44. Korbling M, Estrov Z. Adult stem cells for tissue repair – a new therapeutic concept? N Engl J Med 2003;349:570–582.

45. Taylor HS. Endometrial cells derived from donor stem cells in bone marrow transplant recipients. JAMA 2004;292:81–85.

46. Ikoma T, Kyo S, Maida Y et al. Bone marrow-derived cells from male donors can compose endometrial glands in female transplant recipients. Am J Obstet Gynecol 2009;201:608.

47. Aghajanova L, Horcajadas JA, Esteban FJ, Giudice LC. The bone marrow-derived human mesenchymal stem cell: potential progenitor of the endometrial stromal fibroblast. Biol Reprod 2010;82(6):1076–1087.

48. Du H, Taylor HS. Contribution of bone marrow-derived stem cells to endometrium and endometriosis. Stem Cells 2007;25:2082–2086.

49. Bratincsak A, Brownstein MJ, Cassiani-Ingoni R et al. CD45-positive blood cells give rise to uterine epithelial cells in mice. Stem Cells 2007;25:2820–2826.

50. Giudice LC, Kao LC. Endometriosis. Lancet 2004;364:1789–1799.

51. Leyendecker G, Herbertz M, Kunz G, Mall G. Endometriosis results from the dislocation of basal endometrium. Hum Reprod 2002; 17:2725–2736.

52. Sasson IE, Taylor HS. Stem cells and the pathogenesis of endometriosis. Ann NY Acad Sci 2008;1127:106–115.

53. Starzinski-Powitz A, Zeitvogel A, Schreiner A, Baumann R. In search of pathogenic mechanims in endometriosis: the challenge for molecular cell biology. Curr Molec Med 2001;1:655–664.

54. Fazleabas AT, Brudney A, Gurates B, Chai D, Bulun S. A modified baboon model for endometriosis. Ann NY Acad Sci 2002; 955:308–317.

55. Jimbo H, Hitomi Y, Yoshikawa H et al. Evidence for monoclonal expansion of epithelial cells in ovarian endometrial cysts. Am J Pathol 1997;150:1173–1178.

56. Gargett CE, Guo SW. Stem cells and clonality in endometriosis. In: Garcia-Velasco J, Rizk B (eds) Endometriosis: Current Management and Future Trends. New Delhi: Jaypee Brothers Medical Publishers, 2010, pp. 307–316.

57. Wu Y, Basir Z, Kajdacsy-Balla A et al. Resolution of clonal origins for endometriotic lesions using laser capture microdissection and the human androgen receptor (HUMARA) assay. Fertil Steril 2003;79:710–717.

58. Wu Y, Guo SW. Reconstructing cellular lineages in endometrial cells. Fertil Steril 2008;89:481–484.

59. Cui CH, Uyama T, Miyado K et al. Menstrual Blood-derived cells confer human dystrophin expression in the murine model of Duchenne muscular dystrophy via cell fusion and myogenic transdifferentiation. Mol Biol Cell 2007;18:1586–1594.

60. Hida N, Nishiyama N, Miyoshi S et al. Novel Cardiac precursor-like cells from human menstrual blood-derived mesenchymal cells. Stem Cells 2008;26:1695–1704.

61. Meng X, Ichim TE, Zhong J et al. Endometrial regenerative cells: a novel stem cell population. J Transl Med 2007;5:57.

62. Patel AN, Park E, Kuzman M, Benetti F, Silva FJ, Allickson JG. Multipotent menstrual blood stromal stem cells: isolation, characterization, and differentiation. Cell Transplant 2008;17:303–311.

63. Musina RA, Belyavski AV, Tarusova OV, Solovyova EV, Sukhikh GT. Endometrial mesenchymal stem cells isolated from the menstrual blood. Bull Exp Biol Med 2008;145:539–543.

64. Masuda H, Anwar S, Buhring HJ, Rao J, Gargett CE. A novel marker of human endometrial mesenchymal stem-like cells. Cell Transplantation 2011 (in press).

65. Bokor A, Debrock S, Drijkoningen M, Goossens W, Fulop V, 'Hooghe T. Quantity and quality of retrograde menstruation: a case control study. Reprod Biol Endocrinol 2009;7:123.

66. Leyendecker G, Kunz G, Herbertz M et al. Uterine peristaltic activity and the development of endometriosis. Ann NY Acad Sci 2004; 1034:338–355.

67. Tosh D, Slack JMW. How cells change their phenotype. Nature Rev Molec Cell Biol 2002;3:187–194

68. Gargett CE, Masuda H. Adult stem cells in the endometrium. Molec Hum Reprod 2010;16:818–834.

13 Role of Steroid Hormones: Estrogen and Endometriosis

Elke Winterhager

Institute of Molecular Biology, University Hospital Essen, Essen, Germany

Introduction

Endometrial functions are predominantly governed by both steroid hormones, estrogen and progesterone, in most mammalian species. Estrogens are classic hormones for the development and function of the female reproductive tract but estrogens are also ubiquitous acting hormones with effects on non-reproductive tissues such as bone, liver, colon, skin, and heart [1]. For the female reproductive tract, estrogen and progesterone seem to act in either partly synergistic or opposite ways to accomplish reproductive functions. The role of estrogen receptors (ER) and progesterone receptors (PR) and their ligands for female reproduction has been impressively demonstrated by generating mice deficient in the different receptors for estrogen, ERα and ERβ [2,3], or progesterone, PRA and PRB [4,5].

In humans and in non-human primates, both hormones play the key role in regulating the menstrual cycle and the dominance of progesterone is responsible for decidualization and maintenance of pregnancy [6]. An imbalance in both ligands or changes in their receptor expression levels and ratio are the main reasons for several gynecological disorders such as impaired fertility, leiomyomata, endometrial cancers and not least endometriosis. Though this chapter focuses on the action of estrogen, it should be borne in mind that estrogen action is closely linked to changes in the progesterone receptor function and levels, as reviewed by Bulun *et al* [7].

Endometriosis has long been considered as a predominantly estrogen-dependent disease because of several observations. Symptoms do not appear before menarche and lesions typically regress spontaneously after menopause [8], suggesting an important role for estrogen in the establishment and maintenance of endometriosis by supporting growth of ectopic endometrial implants. Regression of endometriotic lesions is combined with menopause, ovariectomy or chemical castration using gonadotropin-releasing hormone (GnRH) analogs which suppress ovarian steroidogenesis. Moreover, aromatase inhibitors that block estrogen formation as well as progestins are beneficial in this disease [9] (see Chapters 34 and 35). These observations have been corroborated by ample studies giving evidence for a crucial role of estrogen in this complex pathomechanism of endometriosis [10–12].

However, the defined pathomechanism of estrogen action for the development and maintenance of endometriosis and the effectiveness of the use of compounds with pure antiestrogenic effects for a therapeutic approach are still under debate.

What do we know about the impact of estrogen in the pathophysiology of endometriosis?

Changes in estrogen receptors

It is well established that estrogen acts via both ERα and ERβ receptors, members of the nuclear receptor superfamily, and both are expressed in human endometrial stromal and epithelial cells in a similar pattern. However, ERα represents the more prominent receptor type in the cycling endometrium [13,14] whereas ERβ is always expressed at lower levels [15]. ERβ is found predominantly in the predecidualized stromal cells in the late secretory phase, which suggests some specific role of this receptor during decidualization. Because it has been well recognized that there are no differences in estrogen serum levels in patients with endometriosis, it has always been considered that the endometrial response to estrogen may be impaired by changes in the amount of the two estrogen receptors or their function. However, the higher response to estrogen must not be mandatorily related to reduced estrogen receptor levels but to progesterone resistance which in turn leads to an imbalance of the steroid hormone interplay with a dominance in estrogen action [7].

Endometriosis: Science and Practice, First Edition. Edited by Linda C. Giudice, Johannes L.H. Evers and David L. Healy.
© 2012 Blackwell Publishing Ltd. Published 2012 by Blackwell Publishing Ltd.

Changes in estrogen receptor expression in eutopic endometria of patients with endometriosis and in endometrial lesions are still not universally agreed upon. While Hudelist *et al* [16] could not find any significant differences in endometrial ERα and ERβ immunostaining in endometriotic tissues, most studies documented that in endometriotic tissues the ratio between ERα and ERβ changes in favor of ERβ expression [17–20]. The imbalance in receptor expression could help to explain the pathophysiology of this disease because both receptors do not represent a redundant system but regulate different cellular processes.

Reasons for a shift in the expression levels of both ERs could be due to genetic or epigenetic alterations. There are several studies on the correlation with polymorphisms in the risk of endometriosis in different populations, but the results were not consistent [21,22]. Recently Luisi *et al* [23] showed the presence of gene polymorphisms of the estrogen receptor ERα (PvuII and XbaI) and a correlation between PvuII ERα gene polymorphism in recurrence of endometriosis but there is no common acceptance that genetic alterations play a major role in the development of this disease. There is more evidence for epigenetic modifications of the ERβ gene. Xue *et al* [19] identified CpG islands in the promoter of the ESR2 gene which are hypomethylated in endometriotic stromal cells compared to normal ones. They give further evidence that demethylation of the CpG islands confers higher ERβ expression.

However, the estrogen responsiveness gets more complex since splice variants of the estrogen-related protein ERRβ have been recently shown to modulated ERα activity in human endometrium [24]. ERRβ long variant overexpression induced c-myc and enhanced proliferation in Ishikawa cells whereas the short splice variant acts as a counterpart. Further studies are needed to confirm if these modulators are involved in impaired responsiveness of endometriotic endometrium.

Sources of local estrogen

Despite the variations in estrogen receptor function and expression levels, there has been a focus on the ligand and the possible local enhancement of estrogen within the endometrial tissue independent of the general estrogen sources. The local production of estrogen is thought to derive from impaired converting enzyme cascades including aromatase, 17β-hydroxysteroid dehydrogenase (HSD) type 1 and HSD type 2 enzymes [25]. Estrogens from C19 steroids are catalyzed by aromatase cytochrome P450 encoded by the Cyp19 gene. In human endometrium, it has been well established that androgens cannot be converted into estrogen because of the lack of aromatase [26]. In contrast, in eutopic as well as ectopic endometrium of patients suffering from endometriosis, numerous studies have described aberrantly high aromatase expression [27–30] and it appears that endometriotic implants use both the adipose-type promoter I.4 and gonadal-type promoter II for aromatase expression.

Since this disease is not correlated with elevated serum levels of estrogen, expression of aromatase in eutopic endometrial tissues from patients with endometriosis and endometriotic lesion suggests the possibility of local estrogen production in the diseased endometrium and implants. This mechanism could promote growth and maintenance of the ectopic lesions and could be responsible for infertility by changing the programming of the eutopic endometrium. However, these findings are not always consistent in the literature. Colette *et al* [31] reported the absence of aromatase in the endometrium of patients with endometriosis. We found a highly variant expression of aromatase mRNA in eutopic endometria completely independent of the disease [12, and unpublished results]. Our findings are supported by results from Dheenadayalu [32] who detected aromatase expression in endometriotic lesions; however, they also found high numbers of false-negative results in disease-free endometrium. Nevertheless, the clinical relevance of these findings of high aromatase was exemplified by the successful treatment of an unusual postmenopausal endometriosis patient using an aromatase inhibitor [33].

Another abnormality in endometriosis is the downregulation of 17β-HSD2 expression which impairs the inactivation of estradiol to estrone. The potent estrogen estradiol is promoted by 17β-HSD-1 and inactivated by 17β-HSD2 [34]. These enzyme aberrations favor an accumulation of increasing quantities of estradiol in endometriosis by the dominance of 17β-HSD-1 enzyme activity. Taken together, locally enhanced estrogen synthesis may be due to enhanced expression of the estrogen synthesizing enzyme aromatase [35] combined with reduced 17β-HSD-2 expression in the endometriotic endometrium [33].

Estrogen-dependent physiological and molecular changes in endometriosis

Changes in the endometrial estrogen ligand and receptor profile in endometriosis should result in a dysregulated gene profile of the endometrium and ectopic implants, thus explaining the physiological consequences.

Proliferation

It is well established that normal endometrial growth is estrogen dependent and that progesterone can inhibit the estrogen-mediated cell proliferation [36]. There is also evidence that steroid hormone concentrations influence the proliferation and differentiation of endometriotic tissue [37,38]. Klein *et al* [39] showed that endometriotic tissue displayed a lower proliferative activity than eutopic endometrium, but others have reported conflicting findings and revealed that ectopic endometrium proliferates more than eutopic endometrium [40,41]. The effect of estrogens in the development of endometriosis in murine models has also shown conflicting results. Some authors reported a clear estrogen effect on proliferation [42–45] while others found no effect at all [46,47]. Though the findings about estrogen action on proliferation in endometriosis are not convincing, there is increasing evidence that genes regulating the cell cycle are altered in ectopic endometrium. Recently it has been shown that c-fos, that has been reported to be related to estradiol-dependent cell proliferation, showed a more abundant distribution in the stroma of endometriotic tissue [48]. Furthermore, the expression levels of cyclin B1 and Plk1 in ectopic endometria were significantly higher than in eutopic endometria and expression levels of both were positively correlated with serum estrogen levels of patients [49]. Considering the role of estrogen in proliferation, it has to be taken into account that the majority of peritoneal endometriotic implants stay mostly limited in size and invasion. This suggests that estrogen is predominantly responsible for maintenance of these lesions but not for enhanced proliferation.

Aberrant endometrial gene expression upon estrogen

The genomic era has provided an excellent chance to identify candidate genes and gene patterns associated with endometriosis [12,50–52]. Among the genes found, there were several upregulated genes which are known to be estrogen regulated, such as 40S ribosomal protein S23, the early growth response gene EGR-1 [12,53], c-fos and jun-B [12]. Absenger et al [12] distinguished gene expression patterns between the proliferative and secretory phases and found a general shift of endometrial genes such as CYR61 characteristic for the proliferative phase now expressed in the secretory phase of endometriotic endometrium. However, like EGR-1, CYR61 is regulated not only by estrogen but by interleukins, tumor necrosis factor (TNF)-α and prostaglandin (PG) E_2 [54]. Endometriotic tissue clearly overexpresses prostaglandins and cytokines [55–57] and it has been shown that PGE_2 strikingly induces aromatase enzyme activity and formation of local estrogen in this tissue. Upregulation of estrogen in turn upregulates PGE_2 formation and thereby establishes a positive feedback cycle [58]. These findings confirm the close connection between estrogen and inflammatory molecules in regulating aberrant gene expression.

Therapeutic approaches based on estrogen action

Downregulation of estrogenic activity in the endometriotic endometrium, such as functional antiestrogen activity of progestins as well as of antiprogestins, has been in the focus of therapeutic approaches. Moreover, interference with estrogen synthesis pathways predominantly by suppressing aromatase is considered as a therapeutic target, as discussed in other chapters of this book. Another approach to downregulating local estrogen action is the development of 17β-HSD-1 inhibitors for endometriosis. Using the nude mouse model with engrafted human endometrium, we showed that downregulation of 17β-HSD-1 is correlated with reduced proliferation of the implants [59]. Many groups are now working on inhibitors specific for several of these 15 different 17β-HSD enzymes involved in steroid-dependent diseases, which are discussed in Day et al [60]. But at present none of the inhibitors has yet reached clinical trials for endometriosis.

The therapeutic potential of different selective ERβ agonists or antagonists represents another very promising approach [61]. Recently Minutolo et al [62] published a comprehensive review on ERβ ligands for clinical applications. They point out that there exist a group of newly selective steroidal and non-steroidal ERβ agonists but the remaining ligand-binding properties of ERα make it difficult to develop drugs with high selectivity.

Besides numerous synthetic selective ligands developed by different companies, phytoestrogens bind to both ERα and ERβ [63,64] but with a lower affinity [65], and act partly as selective estrogen receptor mediators or exhibit antiestrogenic properties. Phytoestrogens have received increasing attention due to the health benefits associated with their consumption [66]. There are no direct studies correlating the intake of phytoestrogens, e.g. soya, with a predisposition for endometriosis but in contrast, some studies have hinted at a benefit of phytoestrogens using experimental models [67,68]. Phytoestrogens like genestein and coumestrol, as well as liquiritigenin from *Glycyrrhizae uralensis* roots, are more selective for ERβ and reduce lesions in the nude mouse model [69]. However, ERβ selective agonists are active in the ovary [70] and thus side-effects for prolonged treatment in endometriosis have to be considered.

In general, these newly developed drugs modulating estrogen action do not cure endometriosis and thus do not prevent recurrence after withdrawal. Long-term treatment is prone to side-effects, predominantly on the ovary, which is detrimental for women who want to have children.

Conclusion

Despite conflicting studies, it seems that endometriosis is associated with an imbalance in estrogen action, such as higher local estrogen production, and changes in the balance between ERα and ERβ resulting in an aberrant gene expression pattern of endometriotic endometrium and implants. These aberrations, however, seem to be only a predisposition or stimulus in concert with all other factors such as progesterone resistance, immune factors, environmental risk, and genetic predisposition, and the complex cross-talk in the pathomechanisms of this disease will continue to challenge our research.

References

1. Murphy E, Korach KS. Actions of estrogen and estrogen receptors in non-classical target tissues. Ernst Schering Found Symp Proc 2006;13–24.

2. Hewitt MJ, Mutch P, Pratten MK. Potential teratogenic effects of benomyl in rat embryos cultured in vitro. Reprod Toxicol 2005;20:271–280.

3. Zhao C, Dahlman-Wright K, Gustafsson JA. Estrogen receptor beta: an overview and update. Nucl Recept Signal 2008;6:e003.

4. Mulac-Jericevic B, Mullinax RA, DeMayo FJ et al. Subgroup of reproductive functions of progesterone mediated by progesterone receptor-B isoform. Science 2000;289:1751–1754.

5. Mulac-Jericevic B, Lydon JP, DeMayo FJ et al. Defective mammary gland morphogenesis in mice lacking the progesterone receptor B isoform. Proc Natl Acad Sci USA 2003;100:9744–9749.

6. Ramathal CY, Bagchi IC, Taylor RN et al. Endometrial decidualization: of mice and men. Semin Reprod Med 2010;28:17–26.

7. Bulun SE, Cheng YH, Pavone ME et al. Estrogen receptor-beta, estrogen receptor-alpha, and progesterone resistance in endometriosis. Semin Reprod Med 2010;28:36–43.

8. Thomas JA. Falling sperm counts. Lancet 1995;346:635.

9. Bulun SE. Endometriosis. N Engl J Med 2009;360:268–279.

10. Kitawaki J, Kado N, Ishihara H et al. Endometriosis: the pathophysiology as an estrogen-dependent disease. J Steroid Biochem Mol Biol 2002;83:149–155.

11. Giudice LC, Kao LC. Endometriosis. Lancet 2004;364:1789–1799.

12. Absenger Y, Hess-Stumpp H, Kreft B et al. Cyr61, a deregulated gene in endometriosis. Mol Hum Reprod 2004;10:399–407.

13. Rey JM, Pujol P, Dechaud H et al. Expression of oestrogen receptor-alpha splicing variants and oestrogen receptor-beta in endometrium of infertile patients. Mol Hum Reprod 1998;4:641–647.

14. Matsuzaki S, Fukaya T, Suzuki T et al. Oestrogen receptor alpha and beta mRNA expression in human endometrium throughout the menstrual cycle. Mol Hum Reprod 1999;5:559–564.

15. Lecce G, Meduri G, Ancelin M et al. Presence of estrogen receptor beta in the human endometrium through the cycle: expression in glandular, stromal, and vascular cells. J Clin Endocrinol Metab 2001;86:1379–1386.

16. Hudelist G, Huber A, Knoefler M et al. beta-HCG/LH receptor (beta-HCG/LH-R) expression in eutopic endometrium and endometriotic implants: evidence for beta-HCG sensitivity of endometriosis. Reprod Sci 2008;15:543–551.

17. Brandenberger AW, Lebovic DI, Tee MK et al. Oestrogen receptor (ER)-alpha and ER-beta isoforms in normal endometrial and endo-metriosis-derived stromal cells. Mol Hum Reprod 1999;5:651–655.

18. Fujimoto J, Hirose R, Sakaguchi H et al. Expression of oestrogen receptor-alpha and -beta in ovarian endometriomata. Mol Hum Reprod 1999;5:742–747.

19. Xue Q, Lin Z, Cheng YH et al. Promoter methylation regulates estrogen receptor 2 in human endometrium and endometriosis. Biol Reprod 2007;77:681–687.

20. Smuc T, Pucelj MR, Sinkovec J et al. Expression analysis of the genes involved in estradiol and progesterone action in human ovarian endometriosis. Gynecol Endocrinol 2007;23:105–111.

21. Lee GH, Kim SH, Choi YM et al. Estrogen receptor beta gene +1730 G/A polymorphism in women with endometriosis. Fertil Steril 2007;88:785–788.

22. Wang Z, Yoshida S, Negoro K et al. Polymorphisms in the estrogen receptor beta gene but not estrogen receptor alpha gene affect the risk of developing endometriosis in a Japanese population. Fertil Steril 2004;81:1650–1656.

23. Luisi S, Galleri L, Marini F et al. Estrogen receptor gene polymorphisms are associated with recurrence of endometriosis. Fertil Steril 2006;85:764–766.

24. Bombail V, Collins F, Brown P et al. Modulation of ER alpha transcriptional activity by the orphan nuclear receptor ERR beta and evidence for differential effects of long- and short-form splice variants. Mol Cell Endocrinol 2010;314(1):53–61.

25. Zeitoun KM, Bulun SE. Aromatase: a key molecule in the pathophysiology of endometriosis and a therapeutic target. Fertil Steril 1999;72:961–969.

26. Bulun SE, Mahendroo MS, Simpson ER. Polymerase chain reaction amplification fails to detect aromatase cytochrome P450 transcripts in normal human endometrium or decidua. J Clin Endocrinol Metab 1993;76:1458–1463.

27. Noble LS, Simpson ER, Johns A et al. Aromatase expression in endometriosis. J Clin Endocrinol Metab 1996;81:174–179.

28. Hudelist G, Czerwenka K, Keckstein J et al. Expression of aromatase and estrogen sulfotransferase in eutopic and ectopic endometrium: evidence for unbalanced estradiol production in endometriosis. Reprod Sci 2007;14:798–805.

29. Bulun SE, Fang Z, Imir G et al. Aromatase and endometriosis. Semin Reprod Med 2004;22:45–50.

30. Maia H Jr, Casoy J, Valente Filho J. Is aromatase expression in the endometrium the cause of endometriosis and related infertility? Gynecol Endocrinol 2009;25:253–257.

31. Colette S, Lousse JC, Defrere S et al. Absence of aromatase protein and mRNA expression in endometriosis. Hum Reprod 2009;24:2133–2141.

32. Dheenadayalu K, Mak I, Gordts S et al. Aromatase P450 messenger RNA expression in eutopic endometrium is not a specific marker for pelvic endometriosis. Fertil Steril 2002;78:825–829.

33. Bulun SE, Zeitoun K, Sasano H et al. Aromatase in aging women. Semin Reprod Endocrinol 1999;17:349–358.

34. Gurates B, Bulun SE. Endometriosis: the ultimate hormonal disease. Semin Reprod Med 2003;21:125–134.

35. Zeitoun K, Takayama K, Sasano H et al. Deficient 17beta-hydroxysteroid dehydrogenase type 2 expression in endometriosis: failure to metabolize 17beta-estradiol. J Clin Endocrinol Metab 1998;83:4474–4480.

36. Ferenczy A, Bertrand G, Gelfand MM. Proliferation kinetics of human endometrium during the normal menstrual cycle. Am J Obstet Gynecol 1979;133:859–867.

37. Vierikko P, Kauppila A, Ronnberg L et al. Steroidal regulation of endometriosis tissue: lack of induction of 17 beta-hydroxysteroid dehydrogenase activity by progesterone, medroxyprogesterone acetate, or danazol. Fertil Steril 1985;43:218–224.

38. Gerbie AB, Merrill JA. Pathology of endometriosis. Clin Obstet Gynecol 1988;31:779–786.

39. Klein B, Lurie H, Stein M et al. Hereditary ovarian cancer: a dilemma in prognosis. Isr J Med Sci 1992;28:16–19.

40. Li SF, Nakayama K, Masuzawa H et al. The number of proliferating cell nuclear antigen positive cells in endometriotic lesions differs from that in the endometrium. Analysis of PCNA positive cells during the menstrual cycle and in post-menopause. Virch Arch A Pathol Anat Histopathol 1993;423:257–263.

41. Park JS, Lee JH, Kim M et al. Endometrium from women with endometriosis shows increased proliferation activity. Fertil Steril 2009;92:1246–1249.

42. Zamah NM, Dodson MG, Stephens LC et al. Transplantation of normal and ectopic human endometrial tissue into athymic nude mice. Am J Obstet Gynecol 1984;149:591–597.

43. Bergqvist A, Jeppsson S, Kullander S et al. Human endometrium transplanted into nude mice. Histologic effects of various steroid hormones. Am J Pathol 1985;119:336–344.

44. Fortin M, Lepine M, Merlen Y et al. Quantitative assessment of human endometriotic tissue maintenance and regression in a noninvasive mouse model of endometriosis. Mol Ther 2004;9:540–547.

45. Grummer R, Schwarzer F, Bainczyk K et al. Peritoneal endometriosis: validation of an in-vivo model. Hum Reprod 2001;16:1736–1743.

46. Zaino RJ, Satyaswaroop PG, Mortel R. Histologic response of normal human endometrium to steroid hormones in athymic mice. Hum Pathol 1985;16:867–872.

47. Bruner KL, Matrisian LM, Rodgers WH et al. Suppression of matrix metalloproteinases inhibits establishment of ectopic lesions by human endometrium in nude mice. J Clin Invest 1997;99:2851–2857.

48. Morsch DM, Carneiro MM, Lecke SB et al. C-fos gene and protein expression in pelvic endometriosis: a local marker of estrogen action. J Mol Histol 2009;40(1):53–58.

49. Tang L, Wang TT, Wu YT et al. High expression levels of cyclin B1 and Polo-like kinase 1 in ectopic endometrial cells associated with abnormal cell cycle regulation of endometriosis. Fertil Steril 2009;91:979–987.

50. Eyster KM, Lindahl R. Molecular medicine: a primer for clinicians. Part XII: DNA microarrays and their application to clinical medicine. S D J Med 2001;54:57–61.

51. Taylor RN, Lundeen SG, Giudice LC. Emerging role of genomics in endometriosis research. Fertil Steril 2002;78:694–698.

52. Kao LC, Germeyer A, Tulac S et al. Expression profiling of endometrium from women with endometriosis reveals candidate genes for disease-based implantation failure and infertility. Endocrinology 2003;144:2870–2881.

53. Lundeen GA, Vajda EG, Bloebaum RD. Age-related cancellous bone loss in the proximal femur of caucasian females. Osteoporos Int 2000;11:505–511.

54. Gashaw I. Proceedings of the International Symposium, Kobe, Japan 2007. In: Mara T, Mardon H, Stewart C (eds) Translational Research in Uterine Biology. Tokyo: Elsevier, 2008, pp. 31–40.

55. Tseng JF, Ryan IP, Milam TD et al. Interleukin-6 secretion in vitro is up-regulated in ectopic and eutopic endometrial stromal cells from women with endometriosis. J Clin Endocrinol Metab 1996;81:1118–1122.

56. Hornung D, Ryan IP, Chao VA et al. Immunolocalization and regulation of the chemokine RANTES in human endometrial and endometriosis tissues and cells. J Clin Endocrinol Metab 1997;82:1621–1628.

57. Noble LS, Takayama K, Zeitoun KM et al. Prostaglandin E2 stimulates aromatase expression in endometriosis-derived stromal cells. J Clin Endocrinol Metab 1997;82:600–606.

58. Bulun SE, Yang S, Fang Z et al. Estrogen production and metabolism in endometriosis. Ann N Y Acad Sci 2002;955:75–85; discussion 86–78, 396–406.

59. Fechner S, Husen B, Thole H et al. Expression and regulation of estrogen-converting enzymes in ectopic human endometrial tissue. Fertil Steril 2007;88:1029–1038.

60. Day JM, Tutill HJ, Purohit A et al. Design and validation of specific inhibitors of 17beta-hydroxysteroid dehydrogenases for therapeutic application in breast and prostate cancer, and in endometriosis. Endocr Relat Cancer 2008;15:665–692.

61. Harris HA. Preclinical characterization of selective estrogen receptor beta agonists: new insights into their therapeutic potential. Ernst Schering Found Symp Proc 2006;149–161.

62. Minutolo F, Bertini S, Granchi C et al. Structural evolutions of salicylaldoximes as selective agonists for estrogen receptor beta. J Med Chem 2009;52:858–867.

63. Mäkälä S, Savolainen H, Aavik E et al. Differentiation between vasculoprotective and uterotrophic effects of ligands with different binding affinities to estrogen receptors alpha and beta. Proc Natl Acad Sci USA 1999;96(12):7077–7082.

64. Ruh MF, Zacharewski T, Connor K et al. Naringenin: a weakly estrogenic bioflavonoid that exhibits antiestrogenic activity. Biochem Pharmacol 1995;50:1485–1493.

65. Kuiper GG, Gustafsson JA. The novel estrogen receptor-beta subtype: potential role in the cell- and promoter-specific actions of estrogens and anti-estrogens. FEBS Lett 1997;410:87–90.

66. Cederroth CR, Nef S. Soy, phytoestrogens and metabolism: a review. Mol Cell Endocrinol 2009;304:30–42.

67. Edmunds KM, Holloway AC, Crankshaw DJ et al. The effects of dietary phytoestrogens on aromatase activity in human endometrial stromal cells. Reprod Nutr Dev 2005;45:709–720.

68. Yavuz E, Oktem M, Esinler I et al. Genistein causes regression of endometriotic implants in the rat model. Fertil Steril 2007;88:1129–1134.

69. Harris HA, Bruner-Tran KL, Zhang X et al. A selective estrogen receptor-beta agonist causes lesion regression in an experimentally induced model of endometriosis. Hum Reprod 2005;20:936–941.

70. Hegele-Hartung C, Siebel P, Peters O et al. Impact of isotype-selective estrogen receptor agonists on ovarian function. Proc Natl Acad Sci USA 2000;101:5129–5134.

14 Role of Steroid Hormones: Progesterone Signaling

Shirin Khanjani, Marwa K. Al-Sabbagh, Luca Fusi and Jan J. Brosens

Institute of Reproductive and Developmental Biology, Imperial College London, London, UK

Introduction

It is commonly stated that endometriosis is foremost an estrogen-dependent disorder [1]. This is strictly correct but only in so far as all uterine tissues, ectopic or not, involute in the absence of estrogens. Whether aberrant estrogen signaling is causal to endometriosis is doubtful. After all, unopposed estrogens induce endometrial hyperplasia and cancer but not necessarily endometriosis. Although endometriosis is defined by the presence of visible endometrial implants, it is also a disorder characterized by abnormal cycle-dependent responses in all hormone-sensitive compartments of the female reproductive tract, including the ovary, fallopian tube, endometrium, and inner myometrium (also termed the uterine junctional zone) [2,3].

The rise and fall in ovarian progesterone production represent the master signal for ovulation, embryo implantation, decidualization, and menstrual shedding. However, the remodeling of target tissues that underpin these reproductive events is dependent on influx of distinct immune cells and controlled local inflammation. In other words, the physiological responses to progesterone are strictly intertwined with activation of inflammatory pathways. A salient feature of endometriosis is chronic pelvic inflammation and oxidative stress, which in turn represent powerful cues capable of modulating progesterone responses in target tissues. Remarkably, this "reprogramming" of progesterone responses in patients with endometriosis, often referred to as progesterone resistance, is not just transient but engraved in the memory of target cells [4,5].

This chapter summarizes our current understanding of progesterone actions in the female reproductive tract, focusing on endometrial cells. In addition, we will explore the possible mechanisms that underpin the programming events that govern the cellular responses to progesterone and define how perturbations in these systems contribute to the pathogenesis of endometriosis as a chronic disease.

Progesterone actions in the female reproductive tract

Progesterone elicits myriad responses in the female reproductive tract as well as in extrareproductive tissues, such as bone, cardiovascular and respiratory systems, kidney, adipose tissue, and the brain [6]. The ovary is not only the major source of progesterone production during the cycle but progesterone signaling is implicated in follicular growth, ovulation, and luteinization. Progesterone also has profound effects on the contraction waves of the junctional zone, on tubal transport function, and on cervical secretion, although its actions are perhaps most dramatic, and definitely most studied, in the endometrium.

The postovulatory rise in circulating progesterone levels normally triggers a highly co-ordinated endometrial response, characterized by inhibition of estrogen-dependent proliferation of epithelial cells, secretory transformation of the glands, followed by influx of various bone marrow-derived immune cells, including macrophages and uterine natural killer cells, and transformation of endometrial stromal cells into specialized epithelioid decidual cells [7]. During the mid-secretory phase, progesterone transiently induces a receptive phenotype in luminal endometrial epithelial cells, essential for embryo implantation, although this response is mediated by signals derived from the underlying stromal cells [8,9]. Spontaneous decidualization of the stromal compartment in the absence of pregnancy is a rare biological phenomenon, which, like spontaneous endometriosis, is confined to humans and the few other menstruating species [10,11]. Once the endometrium undergoes a decidual response, the integrity of the tissue becomes inextricably dependent upon continuous

Endometriosis: Science and Practice, First Edition. Edited by Linda C. Giudice, Johannes L.H. Evers and David L. Healy.
© 2012 Blackwell Publishing Ltd. Published 2012 by Blackwell Publishing Ltd.

progesterone signaling. In the absence of pregnancy, declining progesterone levels trigger a switch in the secretory repertoire of decidual stromal cells, now characterized by expression of proinflammatory cytokines, chemokines and matrix metalloproteinases, which activates a sequence of events leading to tissue breakdown of the superficial endometrial layer, focal bleeding and menstrual shedding [12,13].

The decidual phenotype is rather intriguing as on the one hand, these cells are programmed to undergo apoptosis upon progesterone withdrawal, yet on the other, they also acquire the ability to resist oxidative stress signals and to regulate local immune responses, and they display invasive potential [7,14,15], all of which are attributes that may promote the formation of ectopic implants upon retrograde menstruation.

Progesterone resistance in endometriosis

The term "progesterone resistance" was prompted by the observation that expression of a subset of progesterone-dependent genes is perturbed in eutopic secretory endometrium from patients with endometriosis [5,16–18]. Progesterone resistance is also a feature of ectopic implants and is likely to play a role in ovarian and tubal dysfunction associated with the disease [1,19,20]. Microarray studies have been particularly informative in delineating the nature and magnitude of impaired endometrial gene expression in patients with endometriosis. For example, Kao and colleagues identified in excess of 200 dysregulated genes in mid-secretory biopsies from women with minimal or mild endometriosis compared to disease-free controls [17]. A subsequent study showed that impaired gene expression in eutopic endometrium of patients with endometriosis encompasses the entire cycle, including the proliferative phase, although the most extensive perturbations were found in early-secretory endometrium. Many of the dysregulated genes identified during this phase of the cycle were not only *bona fide* progesterone targets but the overall signature suggested a persistent proliferative phenotype of the endometrium [16]. Importantly, while there is some, albeit controversial, evidence that the postovulatory surge in progesterone production is affected by endometriosis [21], the term "progesterone resistance" refers mostly to perturbations in signal transduction and expression of downstream progesterone target genes.

Genomic and non-genomic progesterone signaling

Many but not all progesterone actions are mediated through binding and activation of the progesterone receptors, PRA and PRB, members of the superfamily of ligand-activated transcription factors. Progesterone also elicits a variety of rapid signaling events, independently of transcriptional regulation or even the presence of its nuclear receptors [6]. Ultimately, it is the convergence and intertwining of these rapid non-genomic events and the slower transcriptional actions that determine the

---

> **Box 14.1 Validated and putative progesterone receptors**
>
> **Nuclear progesterone receptors**
> - PRA
> - PRB
> - Truncated PRs : PRC, PRM, PRS, PRT
> - Pregnane X receptor
>
> **Alternative progesterone receptors**
> - GABA type A
> - Oxytocin receptor
> - Progesterone receptor membrane component 1
> - Progestin and adipoO receptors
> - Sigma$_1$
> - Microtubule-associated protein 2

Source: Gellersen *et al* [6].

functional response to progesterone in a cell type- and environment-specific manner. While the genomic actions are increasingly defined, characterization of the mechanisms that relay rapid progesterone signaling has been fraught with difficulties and controversy. In fact, several putative progesterone-sensitive receptors (Box 14.1) have been identified in a variety of tissue, yet their roles in normal female reproductive physiology, or disorders such as endometriosis, remain largely elusive [6].

Progesterone receptor action: the classic model

As is the case for all other nuclear receptors, PR has a modular structure made up of distinct functional domains, which can be exchanged between related receptors without loss of function [22]. Both PR isoforms arise from different promoter usage in a single gene but PRB differs from PRA in that it contains an additional 164 amino acids at the amino terminus. A number of alternatively transcribed, translated or spliced isoforms have been described, including PRC, PRM or PRS, although it is doubtful that these truncated PR variants are actually expressed at physiologically relevant levels *in vivo* [23]. While PRA and -B display indistinguishable hormone- and DNA-binding affinities, their actions are remarkably divergent. Early functional studies, using reporter assays driven by simple or complex progesterone response elements (PREs), indicated that the liganded PRA has very limited intrinsic transcriptional activity and suggested that it functions primarily as a dominant inhibitor of PRB and various other steroid receptors, including the estrogen receptor [22,24]. However, this view is no longer sustainable. For example, PRA and -B were subsequently shown to govern distinct endogenous gene networks in progesterone-responsive cells [25]. More importantly, selective gene ablation studies in mice revealed that only PRA is indispensable for ovarian and uterine functions whereas PRB but not -A is critical for mammary gland development [22,26,27].

Like other steroid receptors, PR contains defined sequences, termed nuclear import and export signals, which enable the receptor to shuttle actively between the nuclear and cytoplasmic compartments. The unliganded receptor is assembled in a large multisubunit complex that contains various heat shock proteins (e.g. hsp90, hsp40, hsp70 and p23) and immunophilins (e.g. FKBP51 and FKBP52) [28–30]. These chaperone proteins maintain the receptor in conformation state that allows hormone binding and play a critical role in the dynamic shuttling of the receptor. Progesterone, which is lipophilic, freely crosses the cell membrane and triggers a conformational change in PR, which in turn leads to dissociation of the chaperone proteins, dimerization and binding of the receptor to specific DNA recognition sequences in the promoters of target genes, and finally activation or repression of transcription [22].

Progesterone receptor action: a changing paradigm

The classic model outlined above predicts that progesterone treatment of PR-expressing cells will modulate, in concert, the expression of numerous genes with accessible DNA response elements in their promoter region and that the level of the response correlates with the abundance of the receptor. Both predictions are, however, incorrect. For example, there are few, if any, genes regulated promptly by progesterone in purified primary endometrial cells or myocytes, despite the abundant expression of receptors in these cells. A case in point is decidualization, which denotes the differentiation of endometrial stromal cells (ESCs) into specialized decidual cells indispensable for pregnancy. While decidualization is unequivocally a progesterone-dependent process, ESCs become sensitive to progesterone signaling only if the protein kinase A pathway is first activated in response to rising intracellular cAMP levels [7,31]. *In vivo*, cAMP stimulation in ESCs is thought to be the result of a variety of factors upregulated in the secretory phase of the cycle, including prostaglandin E$_2$, corticotropin-releasing factor, and relaxin. In other words, additional levels of input are required to ensure that progesterone triggers a response that is appropriate and tailored to a particular cell in a specific environment.

Progesterone receptor co-regulators

Binding of an activated PR to DNA is in itself insufficient to alter gene expression. The reason for this is that nuclear receptors do not possess the necessary enzymatic activity to modify the chromatin in a way that it becomes either accessible or inaccessible for recruitment of the basal transcriptional machinery [32–34]. To modulate gene expression, PR and other transcription factors must therefore first bind to a protein complex with intrinsic histone- and DNA-modifying activities. Amazingly, it is less than 15 years since the discovery of the first such co-regulator, termed steroid receptor co-activator-1 (SRC-1) [35]. The number of co-regulators identified has since grown spectacularly and totals now over 300 different proteins. Co-regulators are broadly divided into co-activators and co-repressors, which promote or repress transcription respectively, although for some family members this distinction is rather blurred [32–34].

Based on their mechanisms of action, nuclear receptor co-activators can be categorized into three major function complexes: (i) the SWI/SNF complex, which remodels the local chromatin structure through adenosine triphosphate-dependent histone acetylation; (ii) the SRC complex, which contains acetyltransferases (e.g. CBP, p300, and the p300/CBP-associated factor) and methyltransferases (e.g. CARM1 and PRMT1); and (iii) the mediator complex, involved in the activation of RNA polymerase II and initiation of transcription. In addition to chromatin modification and remodeling, co-activators have been implicated in a variety of other processes, including initiation of transcription, elongation of RNA chains, mRNA splicing, and even proteolytic termination of the transcriptional response.

The prototypic nuclear receptor co-repressors are NCoR (nuclear receptor co-repressor) and SMRT (silencing mediator for retinoid and thyroid hormone), which exist in large protein complexes that include histone deacetylases [36]. Another putative co-repressor, RIP140, promotes the assembly of DNA- and histone-methyltransferases upon interaction with DNA-bound nuclear receptors, which further indicates that transcriptional repression is mediated primarily through epigenetic mechanisms, including nucleosomal condensation and DNA methylation [37]. However, to date NCoR and SMRT have only been shown to interact with antagonist-bound PR. Whether they are also involved in progesterone-dependent repression of target genes requires further clarification.

Cross-talk between the progesterone receptor and other transcription factors

Like other nuclear receptors, PR can modulate gene expression without interacting directly with DNA. This mechanism is referred to as transcription-factor "cross-talk" and is dependent on protein–protein interactions between steroid receptors and other sequence-specific transcription factors. A well-studied example of such cross-talk is the interaction of steroid receptors and AP1 transcription factors, which modulates the activity of gene promoters devoid of steroid receptor binding sites [38]. Another "classic" example involves binding of PR to the NF-κB family of proinflammatory transcription factors [39], which leads to mutual repression and contributes to the anti-inflammatory actions of progesterone.

Transcriptional cross-talk is critical for cycle-dependent endometrial differentiation. Initiation of the decidual response by cAMP involves activation of several transcription factors, including p53, FOXO1, HOXA10, HOXA11, STAT5, and C/EBPβ, capable of interacting directly or indirectly with PR [7,31]. This has led to the hypothesis that PRA in endometrial cells may serve as a platform for the formation of multimeric transcriptional complexes that regulate the expression of decidua-specific genes. In other words, by hijacking other transcription factors, the hormone-bound PR acquires the ability to regulate the expression of a multitude of genes that do not have consensus PR-binding elements in their promoter region. Importantly, many of these transcription factors are capable of interacting with PR even in the absence of ligand, although the resultant transcriptional complexes may be less productive.

Modification of the progesterone receptor

The activity of PR, as well as that of its transcriptional partners and co-regulators, is exquisitely determined by a number of post-translational modifications, including phosphorylation, sumoylation, ubiquitination, and acetylation. These modifications provide a rapid and dynamic mechanism to alter the behavior and activity of PR complex in response to changes in hormonal, growth factor, cytokine, and environmental stress signals [15,32,40]. For example, PR has numerous phosphorylation sites, 14 of which have been mapped. Some sites are modified in response to hormone binding and others by kinases, including mitogen-activated protein kinase (MAPK), casein kinase II, and cyclin-dependent protein kinase-2, upon growth factor signaling. The phosphorylation state of PR influences its subcellular localization, transcriptional activity, rate of turnover, protein complex formation, and target gene specificity [40]. An important feature of the activated PR in both endometrial and breast cells is that it regulates the expression of several genes that encode for intermediates of various signal transduction pathways [41,42], including the WNT/β-catenin, TGF-β/SMAD and STAT pathways. Thus, progesterone is capable of reprogramming the activity of growth factor and cytokine signal transduction, which in turn can alter its post-translational modification code and that of its co-regulators.

Sumoylation has emerged as another critical modification system that determines the activity of PR in the reproductive tract. Like ubiquitination, sumoylation denotes a process in which target proteins, mostly transcription factors, are modified by covalent attachment of a small peptide, SUMO (small ubiquitin modifier), in an enzymatic reaction [31]. While ubiquitination earmarks proteins for proteasomal degradation, binding of SUMO generally bestows transcription factors with repressive properties. In agreement, mutation of the single SUMO binding site in PRA converts this receptor isoform from a weak to a potent transcriptional activator. Interestingly, cAMP signaling in endometrial stromal cells alters the expression of many conjugating and deconjugating SUMO enzymes, resulting in a gradual loss of PRA sumoylation and increased receptor activity. A particular feature of the SUMO pathway is that it is very sensitive to a variety of environmental stress signals, including oxidative stress. In endometrial cells, relative low levels of free radicals are sufficient to induce global as well as PR-specific sumoylation, leading to loss of receptor activity. Strikingly, this coupling of oxidative stress signals to PR via enhanced sumoylation is disabled upon differentiation of ESCs into decidual cells [15].

Dynamic interactions with the chromatin landscape

Gene regulation by steroid hormones like progesterone is by and large a slow process that takes several hours and sometimes days to materialize. At first glance, the slow kinetics of the response fits well with the concept that the activated PR must first bind to the promoter of target genes, recruit co-regulators, assemble them in a multimeric complex that has the right enzymatic activity to modify the local chromatin structure, which in turn will lead to changes in the transcriptional machinery, efficacy of RNA synthesis, translation and, ultimately, protein levels.

This static model is being profoundly challenged by novel techniques that allow genome-wide mapping of binding of nuclear receptors to DNA and real-time monitoring of transcription [28,43]. First, the interaction of nuclear receptors and other transcription factors with the chromatin turned out to be a highly dynamic process, characterized by rapid cycles (measured in seconds [44]) of transient association and dissociation with the chromatin, which in turn leads to oscillating transcriptional events. Receptor turnover by ubiquitination and chaperone proteins is indispensable for this cyclic recruitment of PR to the chromatin template. Moreover, the nature of the ligand determines the kinetics of interaction with chromatin, characterized by rapid exchanges with agonist-bound PR but much slower interactions upon treatment with antagonists like RU486 [45].

Second, genome-wide mapping has revealed that the majority of nuclear receptors bind response elements located at a considerable distances from target promoters. Moreover, rather than the activated receptor inducing local chromatin remodeling to allow transcription, many of these sites are already "pre-existing" or constitutively accessible [43]. These observations indicate not only that long-range interactions between distant regulatory elements and promoters are fundamental to regulating gene expression but also that global epigenetic changes, which invariably occur upon commitment of stem/progenitor cells to a specific lineage, ultimately determine the subsequent cellular responses to steroid hormones.

Mechanisms of progesterone resistance in endometriosis

Induction of pelvic endometriosis in animal models, such as the baboon, is sufficient to disrupt the progesterone responses in the eutopic endometrium in a manner akin to the human situation [11]. From a molecular perspective, it is not too challenging to envisage mechanisms that would disrupt progesterone actions in target cells in the presence of chronic pelvic inflammation. For example, inflammatory signals could induce progesterone resistance by altering the expression of PR isoforms, chaperone proteins like FKBP52, or co-regulators such as HIC-5/ARA55. Activation of proinflammatory transcription factors could compete with PR for a limited pool of co-regulators or disrupt the interaction between the receptor and key transcriptional partners, such as FOXO1. Moreover, inflammation is invariably associated

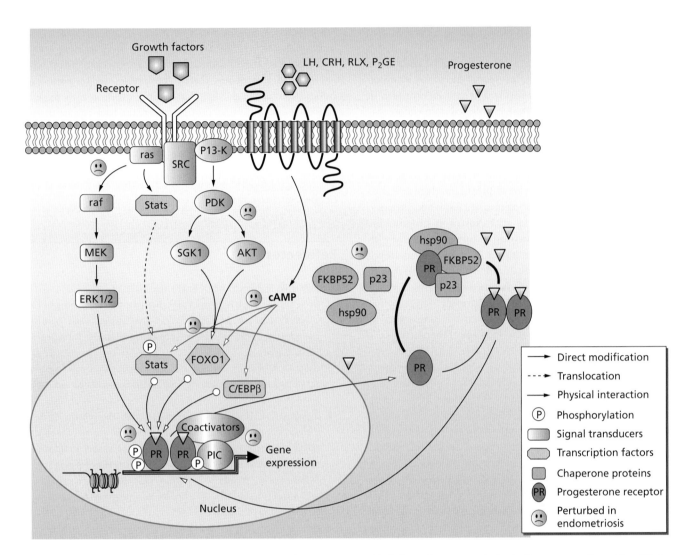

Figure 14.1 Regulation of progesterone responses in endometrium and endometriosis. For detailed explanation, see text. The sad faces indicate perturbations in progesterone signal transduction at different levels of control, including expression of PR isoforms, chaperone proteins involved in receptor recycling and ligand binding, co-regulators, transcriptional partners, and a variety of upstream signal transduction pathways capable of modifying PR and its co-regulators.

Table 14.1 Progesterone signal intermediates perturbed in endometriosis.

Mechanism of action	Protein	Reference
Receptor	PRB	[20,53]
Chaperone protein	FKBP52	[11,61]
Transcriptional partner	HOXA10	[18,50,54]
	HOXA11	[18,50,54]
	FOXO1	[55–57]
	NF-κB	[59]
	C/EBPβ	[62]
Receptor co-activator	SRC-1	[59]
	P300/CBP	[59]
	HIC-5/ARA55	[60]
Receptor co-repressor	RIP140	[58]
	NCoR	[59]
	SMRT	[59]

with free radical production and oxidative stress signals, which in turn will alter the post-translational code of PR. In fact, there is evidence to implicate most, if not all, of these mechanisms in progesterone resistance in endometriosis patients, as illustrated in Figure 14.1 and summarized in Table 14.1. This is not entirely surprising as progesterone signal transduction is tightly controlled at different levels, albeit by interconnected mechanisms.

Despite the overwhelming evidence in support of the paradigm outlined above, it does not entirely explain progesterone resistance in endometriosis for two reasons. First, the model suggests that suppression of endometriotic lesions and associated inflammation, for example upon prolonged treatment with GnRH analogs or after surgical ablation of the lesions, would suffice to restore normal steroid hormone responses and cure the disease, which is ostensibly not the case. Second, several studies have now shown that the decidual response in ESCs remains perturbed in patients with endometriosis even when these cells are purified and differentiated in extended cultures [4,46,47].

Importantly, aberrant gene expression in purified ESCs is not confined to differentiating cells. In a recent microarray study, no fewer than 245 genes were reportedly differentially expressed in unstimulated primary ESC cultures established from endometriosis patients and controls [4]. The results should be interpreted with some caution, not only because relatively few biological samples have been analyzed in this way to date but also because differences in gene expression may reflect not only the presence of endometriosis but the net sum of all prior reproductive events, including the number of preceding menstruations and pregnancies [10,48]. In addition to basal gene expression, progesterone and/or cAMP responses, endometriosis is further associated with perturbed gene expression upon human chorionic gonadotropin stimulation, both in eutopic human endometrial explants *in vitro* as well as in the baboon model of endometriosis *in vivo* [8,49].

The observations outlined above strongly suggest that progesterone resistance is likely to be as much a consequence of changes in the epigenetic chromatin landscape of endometrial cells as the result of intrinsic defects in PR or other signal transduction pathways. Inflammatory signals are established epigenetic modifiers, which raises the possibility that cyclic menstruation is important for "programming" hormonal responses in the uterus, especially prior to pregnancy [10]. Moreover, animal experiments demonstrated that induction of pelvic disease has long-lasting consequences for the chromatin landscape of eutopic endometrial cells by altering DNA methylation and histone tail modifications in proximal promoter regions of progesterone-dependent genes [48,50,51]. For example, Kim and co-workers demonstrated that induction of endometriosis in the baboon resulted in a gradual decrease in endometrial HOXA10 expression, a homeobox transcription factor involved in endometrial development and differentiation. Importantly, this downregulation was only significant 6–12 months after the induction of endometriosis and corresponded to increased methylation of the proximal promoter of HOXA10 [50]. In order to have a lasting effect on uterine function, inflammatory cues associated with menstruation or endometriosis must impact on basal endometrial cells, which contain the progenitor cells for the superficial endometrium as well as the junctional zone myometrium. It is indeed striking that the junctional zone myometrium is significantly thicker on T2-weighted magnetic resonance imaging (MRI) in patients with endometriosis when compared to age-matched controls [52].

Conclusion

As our understanding of nuclear receptor actions in general, and PR in specific, has expanded phenomenally in recent years, so have our insights into the pathological mechanisms that underpin endometriosis. It is increasingly apparent that steroid hormone responses in the endometrium are much more dynamic than previously appreciated and modified by the cumulative effects of reproductive events, such as menstruation and pregnancy. The cause of endometriosis may well reside in programming events that accentuate the inflammatory responses associated with cyclic endometrial remodeling, thereby promoting the formation of ectopic lesions and pelvic inflammation, which in turn renders endometriosis a chronic disorder by feeding back on the uterus and other reproductive organs.

Acknowledgment

We apologize to all those authors whose important work could not be referenced due to space constraints.

References

1. Bulun SE. Endometriosis. N Engl J Med 2009;360:268–279.
2. Brosens I, Derwig I, Brosens J, Fusi L, Benagiano G, Pijnenborg R. The enigmatic uterine junctional zone: the missing link between reproductive disorders and major obstetrical disorders? Hum Reprod 2010;25:569–574.
3. Gupta S, Goldberg JM, Aziz N, Goldberg E, Krajcir N, Agarwal A. Pathogenic mechanisms in endometriosis-associated infertility. Fertil Steril 2008;90:247–257.
4. Aghajanova L, Horcajadas JA, Weeks JL et al. The protein kinase a pathway-regulated transcriptome of endometrial stromal fibroblasts reveals compromised differentiation and persistent proliferative potential in endometriosis. Endocrinology 2010;151:1341–1355.
5. Aghajanova L, Velarde MC, Giudice LC. Altered gene expression profiling in endometrium: evidence for progesterone resistance. Semin Reprod Med 2010;28:51–58.
6. Gellersen B, Fernandes MS, Brosens JJ. Non-genomic progesterone actions in female reproduction. Hum Reprod Update 2009;15:119–138.
7. Gellersen B, Brosens IA, Brosens JJ. Decidualization of the human endometrium: mechanisms, functions, and clinical perspectives. Semin Reprod Med 2007;25:445–453.
8. Brosens JJ, Hodgetts A, Feroze-Zaidi F et al. Proteomic analysis of endometrium from fertile and infertile patients suggests a role for apolipoprotein A-I in embryo implantation failure and endometriosis. Mol Hum Reprod 2010;16(4):273–285.
9. Simon L, Spiewak KA, Ekman GC et al. Stromal progesterone receptors mediate induction of Indian Hedgehog (IHH) in uterine epithelium and its downstream targets in uterine stroma. Endocrinology 2009;150:3871–3876.
10. Brosens JJ, Parker MG, McIndoe A, Pijnenborg R, Brosens IA. A role for menstruation in preconditioning the uterus for successful pregnancy. Am J Obstet Gynecol 2009;200:615.
11. Fazleabas AT. Progesterone resistance in a baboon model of endometriosis. Semin Reprod Med 2010;28:75–80.
12. Brosens JJ, Gellersen B. Death or survival–progesterone-dependent cell fate decisions in the human endometrial stroma. J Mol Endocrinol 2006;36:389–398.
13. Jabbour HN, Kelly RW, Fraser HM, Critchley HO. Endocrine regulation of menstruation. Endocrine Rev 2006;27:17–46.

14. Gellersen B, Reimann K, Samalecos A, Aupers S, Bamberger AM. Invasiveness of human endometrial stromal cells is promoted by decidualization and by trophoblast-derived signals. Hum Reprod 2010;25(4):862–873.

15. Leitao B, Jones MC, Fusi L et al. Silencing of the JNK pathway maintains progesterone receptor activity in decidualizing human endometrial stromal cells exposed to oxidative stress signals. FASEB J 2010;24(5):1541–1551.

16. Burney RO, Talbi S, Hamilton AE et al. Gene expression analysis of endometrium reveals progesterone resistance and candidate susceptibility genes in women with endometriosis. Endocrinology 2007;148:3814–3826.

17. Kao LC, Germeyer A, Tulac S et al. Expression profiling of endometrium from women with endometriosis reveals candidate genes for disease-based implantation failure and infertility. Endocrinology 2003;144:2870–2881.

18. Taylor HS, Bagot C, Kardana A, Olive D, Arici A. HOX gene expression is altered in the endometrium of women with endometriosis. Hum Reprod 1999;14:1328–1331.

19. Wu Y, Kajdacsy-Balla A, Strawn E et al. Transcriptional characterizations of differences between eutopic and ectopic endometrium. Endocrinology 2006;147:232–246.

20. Wu Y, Strawn E, Basir Z, Halverson G, Guo SW. Promoter hypermethylation of progesterone receptor isoform B (PR-B) in endometriosis. Epigenetics 2006;1:106–111.

21. Koninckx PR, Brosens IA. Clinical significance of the luteinized unruptured follicle syndrome as a cause of infertility. Eur J Obstet Gynecol Reprod Biol 1982;13:355–368.

22. Brosens JJ, Tullet J, Varshochi R, Lam EW. Steroid receptor action. Best Pract Res 2004;18:265–283.

23. Samalecos A, Gellersen B. Systematic expression analysis and antibody screening do not support the existence of naturally occurring progesterone receptor (PR)-C, PR-M, or other truncated PR isoforms. Endocrinology 2008;149:5872–5887.

24. Vegeto E, Shahbaz MM, Wen DX, Goldman ME, O'Malley BW, McDonnell DP. Human progesterone receptor A form is a cell- and promoter-specific repressor of human progesterone receptor B function. Mol Endocrinol 1993;7:1244–1255.

25. Richer JK, Jacobsen BM, Manning NG, Abel MG, Wolf DM, Horwitz KB. Differential gene regulation by the two progesterone receptor isoforms in human breast cancer cells. J Biol Chem 2002;277:5209–5218.

26. Conneely OM, Mulac-Jericevic B, DeMayo F, Lydon JP, O'Malley BW. Reproductive functions of progesterone receptors. Recent Prog Hormone Res 2002;57:339–355.

27. Mulac-Jericevic B, Lydon JP, DeMayo FJ, Conneely OM. Defective mammary gland morphogenesis in mice lacking the progesterone receptor B isoform. Proc Natl Acad Sci USA 2003;100:9744–9749.

28. George AA, Schiltz RL, Hager GL. Dynamic access of the glucocorticoid receptor to response elements in chromatin. Int J Biochem Cell Biol 2009;41:214–224.

29. Kosano H, Stensgard B, Charlesworth MC, McMahon N, Toft D. The assembly of progesterone receptor-hsp90 complexes using purified proteins. J Biol Chem 1998;273:32973–32979.

30. Tranguch S, Wang H, Daikoku T, Xie H, Smith DF, Dey SK. FKBP52 deficiency-conferred uterine progesterone resistance is genetic background and pregnancy stage specific. J Clin Invest 2007;117:1824–1834.

31. Jones MC, Fusi L, Higham JH et al. Regulation of the SUMO pathway sensitizes differentiating human endometrial stromal cells to progesterone. Proc Natl Acad Sci USA 2006;103:16272–16277.

32. Han SJ, Lonard DM, O'Malley BW. Multi-modulation of nuclear receptor coactivators through posttranslational modifications. Trends Endocrinol Metab 2009;20:8–15.

33. Lonard DM, O'Malley BW. The expanding cosmos of nuclear receptor coactivators. Cell 2006;125:411–414.

34. Thakur MK, Paramanik V. Role of steroid hormone coregulators in health and disease. Hormone Res 2009;71:194–200.

35. Onate SA, Tsai SY, Tsai MJ, O'Malley BW. Sequence and characterization of a coactivator for the steroid hormone receptor superfamily. Science 1995;270:1354–1357.

36. Li J, Wang J, Wang J et al. Both corepressor proteins SMRT and N-CoR exist in large protein complexes containing HDAC3. EMBO J 2000;19:4342–4350.

37. Kiskinis E, Hallberg M, Christian M et al. RIP140 directs histone and DNA methylation to silence Ucp1 expression in white adipocytes. EMBO J 2007;26:4831–4840.

38. Bamberger AM, Bamberger CM, Gellersen B, Schulte HM. Modulation of AP-1 activity by the human progesterone receptor in endometrial adenocarcinoma cells. Proc Natl Acad Sci USA 1996;93:6169–6174.

39. McKay LI, Cidlowski JA. Cross-talk between nuclear factor-kappa B and the steroid hormone receptors: mechanisms of mutual antagonism. Mol Endocrinol 1998;12:45–56.

40. Dressing GE, Hagan CR, Knutson TP, Daniel AR, Lange CA. Progesterone receptors act as sensors for mitogenic protein kinases in breast cancer models. Endocr Relat Cancer 2009;16:351–361.

41. Cloke B, Huhtinen K, Fusi L et al. The androgen and progesterone receptors regulate distinct gene networks and cellular functions in decidualizing endometrium. Endocrinology 2008;149:4462–4474.

42. Li X, O'Malley BW. Unfolding the action of progesterone receptors. J Biol Chem 2003;278:39261–39264.

43. Biddie SC, John S, Hager GL. Genome-wide mechanisms of nuclear receptor action. Trends Endocrinol Metab 2009;21:3–9.

44. McNally JG, Muller WG, Walker D, Wolford R, Hager GL. The glucocorticoid receptor: rapid exchange with regulatory sites in living cells. Science 2000;287:1262–1265.

45. Rayasam GV, Elbi C, Walker DA et al. Ligand-specific dynamics of the progesterone receptor in living cells and during chromatin remodeling in vitro. Mol Cell Biol 2005;25:2406–2418.

46. Klemmt PA, Carver JG, Kennedy SH, Koninckx PR, Mardon HJ. Stromal cells from endometriotic lesions and endometrium from women with endometriosis have reduced decidualization capacity. Fertil Steril 2006;85:564–572.

47. Minici F, Tiberi F, Tropea A et al. Endometriosis and human infertility: a new investigation into the role of eutopic endometrium. Hum Reprod 2008;23:530–537.

48. Guo SW. Epigenetics of endometriosis. Mol Hum Reprod 2009;15:587–607.

49. Sherwin JR, Sharkey AM, Cameo P et al. Identification of novel genes regulated by chorionic gonadotropin in baboon endometrium during the window of implantation. Endocrinology 2007;148:618–626.

50. Kim JJ, Taylor HS, Lu Z et al. Altered expression of HOXA10 in endometriosis: potential role in decidualization. Mol Hum Reprod 2007;13:323–332.

51. Lee B, Du H, Taylor HS. Experimental murine endometriosis induces DNA methylation and altered gene expression in eutopic endometrium. Biol Reprod 2009;80:79–85.

52. Kunz G, Herbertz M, Beil D, Huppert P, Leyendecker G. Adenomyosis as a disorder of the early and late human reproductive period. Reprod Biomed Online 2007;15:681–685.

53. Attia GR, Zeitoun K, Edwards D, Johns A, Carr BR, Bulun SE. Progesterone receptor isoform A but not B is expressed in endometriosis. J Clin Endocrinol Metab 2000;85:2897–2902.

54. Wu Y, Halverson G, Basir Z, Strawn E, Yan P, Guo SW. Aberrant methylation at HOXA10 may be responsible for its aberrant expression in the endometrium of patients with endometriosis. Am J Obstet Gynecol 2005;193:371–380.

55. Labied S, Kajihara T, Madureira PA et al. Progestins regulate the expression and activity of the forkhead transcription factor FOXO1 in differentiating human endometrium. Mol Endocrinol 2006;20:35–44.

56. Kim JJ, Fazleabas AT. Uterine receptivity and implantation:the regulation and action of insulin-like growth factor binding protein-1 (IGFBP-1), HOXA10 and forkhead transcription factor-1 (FOXO-1) in the baboon endometrium. Reprod Biol Endocrinol 2004;2:34.

57. Shazand K, Baban S, Prive C et al. FOXO1 and c-jun transcription factors mRNA are modulated in endometriosis. Mol Hum Reprod 2004;10:871–877.

58. Caballero V, Ruiz R, Sainz JA et al. Preliminary molecular genetic analysis of the Receptor Interacting Protein 140 (RIP140) in women affected by endometriosis. J Exp Clin Assist Reprod 2005;2:11.

59. Suzuki A, Horiuchi A, Oka K, Miyamoto T, Kashima H, Shiozawa T. Immunohistochemical detection of steroid receptor cofactors in ovarian endometriosis: involvement of down-regulated SRC-1 expression in the limited growth activity of the endometriotic epithelium. Virchows Arch 2010;456(4):433–441.

60. Aghajanova L, Velarde MC, Giudice LC. The progesterone receptor coactivator Hic-5 is involved in the pathophysiology of endometriosis. Endocrinology 2009;150:3863–3870.

61. Hirota Y, Tranguch S, Daikoku T et al. Deficiency of immunophilin FKBP52 promotes endometriosis. Am J Pathol 2008;173:1747–1757.

62. Yang S, Fang Z, Suzuki T et al. Regulation of aromatase P450 expression in endometriotic and endometrial stromal cells by CCAAT/enhancer binding proteins (C/EBPs): decreased C/EBPbeta in endometriosis is associated with overexpression of aromatase. J Clin Endocrinol Metab 2002;87:2336–2345.

15 Early Origins of Endometriosis: Role of Endocrine Disrupting Chemicals

Germaine M. Buck Louis

Division of Epidemiology, Statistics & Prevention Research, Eunice Kennedy Shriver National Institute of Child Health and Human Development, National Institutes of Health, Bethesda, MD, USA

Introduction

The conceptual paradigm for assessing potential reproductive and/or developmental toxicants has undergone fundamental rethinking during the past few decades, which provides a framework for assessing the early origins of disease, including gynecological disorders. The first key conceptual change is recognition that human development is more than the unfolding of the rigid genome resulting in an invariant sequence of developmental stages, but rather one of developmental plasticity, which is conceptualized as continual multi-causal development [1]. As such, research has moved beyond studying exposures during critical windows in relation to structural changes such as birth defects to the study of exposures during sensitive windows and functional changes, including those that arise later during the life course [2]. Another important paradigm shift is the conceptualization of disease away from a simplistic to a complex set of processes. Complex diseases arise from the interplay of genes, proteins and environmental influences during sensitive windows of development, and have implications across the lifespan.

Within the complex disease conceptualization, two additional changes have occurred in our thinking: (1) greater recognition of the importance of time-varying parental and not just maternal exposures during sensitive windows and later onset adult diseases, and (2) the importance of low-dose additivity consistent with the manner in which most humans are exposed to a mixture of environmental contaminants [3–6]. Thus, the long-standing toxicological premise that the dose makes the poison in the simple disease paradigm is now being reconsidered.

In response to these and other conceptual changes, some authors have articulated the need for life course epidemiological methods that permit the study of biological, behavioral, and psychosocial exposures during gestation, childhood, adolescence, young adulthood, and later adulthood and disease across the life course [1].

That human health is shaped by environmental (non-genetic) influences is beyond dispute. In fact, the environment is believed to be the culprit responsible for the purported worldwide decline in human fecundity [7,8] partially fueled by the long-standing recognition of the effects of maternal (under)nutrition and pregnancy outcomes. Some authors argue that the reduction in fertility cannot sustain populations [9]. Still, opponents argue that declining worldwide fertility rates are driven by social phenomena and not biological or environmental factors.

Environmental effects on male fecundity recently have been synthesized as the testicular dysgenesis syndrome (TDS). This hypothesis posits that exposures during critical and sensitive windows that disrupt normal testicular and genital development may manifest in a spectrum of adverse outcomes such as hypospadias, cryptorchidism, testicular cancer, and decreased sperm counts [8]. The central aspect of TDS hypothesis is purported to be Leydig cell dysfunction with androgen insufficiency being either a cause or consequence of the disruption of testicular development. The increasing prevalence of these outcomes over time and place suggests an environmental etiology, particularly given the absence of identifiable genetic causes (e.g. Y chromosome deletions). Also, TDS can be produced experimentally in animals following exposure to endocrine disrupting chemicals such as phthalates during sensitive windows [10].

The TDS hypothesis is not a new concept *per se*, and builds upon the Barker [11] or thrifty phenotype hypotheses [12] that have purported associations between early development and later-onset disease. Developmental plasticity is consistent with epigenetic research in that epigenetic-induced changes may allow the embryo or fetus to adapt by altering organogenesis for anticipated needs later in life. As such, the developing organism may change structure and function in response to environmental cues during critical windows

Endometriosis: Science and Practice, First Edition. Edited by Linda C. Giudice, Johannes L.H. Evers and David L. Healy.
© 2012 Blackwell Publishing Ltd. Published 2012 by Blackwell Publishing Ltd.

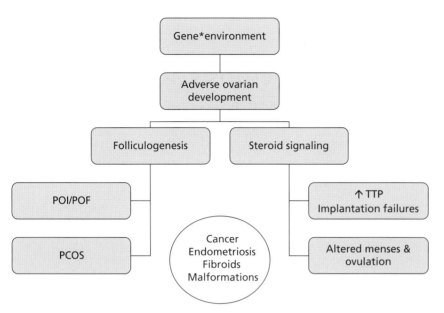

Figure 15.1 Ovarian dysgenesis syndrome – paradigm. *, interaction; PCOS, polycystic ovarian syndrome; POF, premature ovarian failure; POI, premature ovarian insufficiency; TTP, time to pregnancy.

[13]. If nutritional resources are limited during pregnancy, the fetus may be reprogrammed to expect fewer resources across the lifespan. In the context of adequate or excessive nutrition, the infant or adult becomes overweight from this early reprogramming or the so-called "mismatch" between fetal exposures and adult health, resulting in an inappropriate physiology for postnatal life [14,15]. For example, a compromised *in utero* nutritional environment may program the organism for a similar postnatal environment. In the context of adequate postnatal nutrition, the thrifty prenatal programming may result in child or adult obesity. While a number of names have evolved for fetal programming (e.g. fetal origins of disease, early origins of disease, developmental basis of health and disease), a common underlying assumption is that exposures during the periconception, *in utero* or other developmentally susceptible windows may affect later-onset disease manifesting in a spectrum of diseases across the lifespan such as coronary heart disease, type 2 diabetes, metabolic syndrome, mood disorders, and osteoporosis [16–18].

The TDS hypothesis prompted investigators to consider whether female fecundity or biological capacity for reproduction irrespective of pregnancy intentions and later adult health may be affected by time-sensitive exposure during early development, or the so-called ovarian dysgenesis syndrome (ODS) [2]. The ODS hypothesis posits that alterations in ovarian function arising from exposures during early development may compromise female fecundity and, thereby, predispose women to later-onset adult diseases as illustrated in Figure 15.1. Adverse ovarian development may affect folliculogenesis and/or steroid signaling manifesting as polycystic ovarian syndrome (PCOS), premature ovarian insufficiency (POI) or failure (POF), alterations in menstruation, ovulation or time to pregnancy (TTP), and pregnancy loss. As we move forward with the early origins of disease hypothesis, it is imperative to consider both males and females as possible susceptible populations in capturing time-varying exposures during critical and sensitive windows of development as noted below.

Critical and sensitive windows

Critical windows are time-limited intervals of development characterized by high rates of cell proliferation and changing metabolic capabilities [19]. Exposures during critical windows can exert an adverse or protective effect on development and subsequent disease, while exposures outside critical windows will have little effect. Embryonic development is a classic example of timed and inter-related critical windows for structural development, with birth defects being a classic example of adverse effects. Xenoestrogen exposures during critical windows produce changes in structure and reprogram gene expression in tissue to respond abnormally later in life, underscoring that phenotype is governed by parental genes and intrauterine environment. It is plausible that many health outcomes have more than one critical window, and closure of one critical window may result in the opening of others for other disease states.

Ben-Shlomo and Kuh have eloquently articulated the need to distinguish critical and sensitive windows, given that exposures during the latter may still adversely affect development, including later-onset adult diseases, though possibly with reduced magnitude [1]. For example, an exposure during critical embryonic windows may produce structural birth defects, whereas those occurring outside the critical window may produce non-structural or functional deficits, including those that manifest later in adult life. This recognition challenges investigators to look beyond structural defects and to consider a spectrum of endpoints in relation to exposures within critical or sensitive windows.

When considering critical or sensitive windows, it is important to keep susceptibility in mind in that not all exposed organisms or

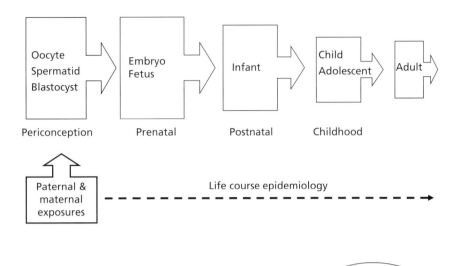

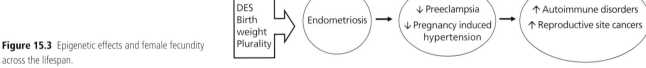

Figure 15.2 Sensitive windows for gynecological health.

Figure 15.3 Epigenetic effects and female fecundity across the lifespan.

individuals will be adversely affected. Also, severity of a particular outcome may vary across affected individuals. For example, there is considerable speculation that males are at greater risk to exposures during critical and sensitive windows resulting in their selective reduction from conception through birth as measured by sex ratios or the ratio of the number of male-to-female conceptions or births [20].

Figure 15.2 illustrates a paradigm for considering critical and sensitive windows for gynecological diseases inclusive of endometriosis that is consistent with epigenetics being involved in disease onset across the lifespan. Three assumptions underlie this paradigm. Firstly, parental exposures need to be considered, especially in the earliest stages of human development consistent with the couple-dependent nature of human reproduction and development. The male is now thought to contribute more to the conceptus than just the paternal genome. For example, sperm morphology is associated with blastomere cleavage rate [21] while centrosome defects are associated with fertilization and early developmental disorders [22], suggesting a paternal role in embryonic quality and, hence, survival. Also, the preimplantation embryo is sensitive to environmental exposures and epigenetic regulation [23] consistent with the probability that DNA exposure is high as well.

The second assumption underlying Figure 15.2 is that time-varying exposures can be captured with regard to the type, timing, and dose of an exposure(s). Fetal life is the most dynamic phase of ovarian development with initiation of oogenesis that is not completed until long after fertilization [24]. Prospective pregnancy cohort studies with preconception enrollment of women/couples have been shown to have utility and feasibility for capturing periconceptional and *in utero* exposures that may affect human reproduction and development, including gynecological health [25]. Periconception and *in utero* exposures coincide with

biological susceptibility of the developing organism as evident by its limited ability for DNA repair, an immature immune system, primitive liver metabolism, lack of a blood–brain barrier, and an increased metabolic rate. Time-varying exposures are a critical aspect of epigenetics, since chemical modifications of DNA and chromatin may affect genomic functions such as alterations in transcription, replication and recombination.

Finally, the third assumption underlying Figure 15.2 is the selective loss of embryos/fetuses/infants across sensitive windows as illustrated by the declining size of the windows. The selective survival advantage of females relative to men from conception through birth and the perimenopausal period provides evidence for such thinking [20]. To this end, if exposures are not properly captured relative to the sensitive windows, an exposure may result in embryonic demise while appearing protective for later outcomes or the so-called competing risk concept well known to epidemiologists and biostatisticians.

The literature for two environmental estrogenic exposures – bisphenol A (BPA) and diethylstilbestrol (DES) – has been globally synthesized relative to Figure 15.2 and are illustrated in Figure 15.3. Specifically, exposure of males and females during the periconception and *in utero* windows leads to epigenetic changes that result in alterations in gene expression or protein regulation via DNA methylation or chromatin remodeling, resulting in functional changes in specific organs or tissues that lead to adult susceptibilities, possibly across generations [26–29]. Estrogen-like exposures stimulate estrogen-sensitive gene expression, especially during estrogen low periods or when estrogen is not active. DES is the prototype for *in utero* estrogen exposure, given that it is a potent synthetic estrogen and is associated with a spectrum of adverse reproductive outcomes in females (also males) such as cervicovaginal carcinomas, genitourinary malformations, fecundity impairments, early menopause, breast cancer [30,31] and, possibly, transgenerational effects [32]. Many of these adverse relations have been corroborated in experimental animals [33] though exact mechanisms remain largely unknown.

Developmental origin of endometriosis

Endometriosis is hypothesized to arise from retrograde menstruation [34,35] despite long-standing recognition that the majority of menstruating women do not have endometriosis. Despite a plethora of hypotheses, the etiology of endometriosis remains speculative at best, but recently has shifted to consideration of a possible *in utero* origin. This conceptual change recognizes a substantial body of evidence suggestive of an *in utero* origin for other gynecological disorders such as *in utero* androgen exposure and polycystic ovarian syndrome [36] or DES exposure and fibroids [37]. There has been rather long-standing recognition that girls born small for gestational age have poorer ovarian development, smaller ovaries, diminished follicle-stimulating hormone responsiveness, and more anovulatory cycles than adequately sized girls, supporting the theory of *in utero* programming and later-onset fecundity impairments [38–41].

An *in utero* origin for endometriosis is consistent with developmental biology in that the müllerian ducts develop into the fallopian tubes, uterus, cervix, and upper vagina in the absence of anti-müllerian hormone at about 6–7 weeks' gestation, following co-ordinated gene expression and hormone exposure [42]. Estrogen is needed for such development, with its receptor being expressed in the mesenchyme of developing uterus early during the second trimester. Research is just beginning to identify the genes and hormonal exposures at critical or sensitive windows relevant for endometriosis or gynecological health, more generally.

Table 15.1 summarizes some of the available research focusing on fecundity outcomes, gravid health status and later-onset adult disease. While speculative and based largely on observational studies, there is evidence in support of an early origin for female fecundity, including endometriosis. The first suggested *in utero* exposure for endometriosis was reported by Missmer and colleagues [43]. Specifically, DES exposure was associated with an 80% increased risk of having an endometriosis diagnosis among women participating in the long-standing Nurses Health Study II. Using the same study cohort, a 30% increased risk of endometriosis was observed for women born weighing ≤5.5 pounds, and a 70% increase in risk if born as a part of a multiple birth in comparison to referent groups [43].

Hediger and colleagues reported an association between women with a leaner body habitus from adolescence through laparoscopy and diagnosis of endometriosis, suggesting an early origin of disease [44]. This finding was corroborated by Vitonis and colleagues who reported an inverse relation between childhood and early adulthood body size and incidence of laparo-

Table 15.1 Reproductive outcomes and later-onset adult diseases.

Reproductive outcome	Gravid disease	Adult disease
Early menarche		↑ Risk breast cancer
Earlier menopause		↑ Osteoporosis, cardiovascular disease and overall mortality
Late menopause		↑ Risk breast and endometrial cancer
Subfecundity	↑ Preeclampsia	
Parity	↑ Preeclampsia & preterm delivery	↓ Leiomyomas ↑ Risk cardiovascular death ↓ Cancer death
Low birthweight		↑ Leiomyomas
Small-for-gestational age		
Small-for-gestational age		↓ Responsiveness of follicle-stimulating hormone, poor ovarian development
Polycystic ovarian syndrome	↑ Preeclampsia	↑ Metabolic syndrome, coronary disease, type 2 diabetes
Endometriosis	↑ Gestational diabetes ↓ Preeclampsia ↓ Pregnancy-induced hypertension	↑ Autoimmune disorders ↑ Reproductive site cancers

Note: Based upon observational human studies.
↑ denotes increased risk; ↓ denotes decreased risk.

scopically confirmed endometriosis among women participating in the Nurses Health Study II [45]. *In utero* exposure to maternal cigarette smoking exerted a significant reduction in risk for an endometriosis diagnosis at laparoscopy (80–95% reduction), particularly among current smokers [46]. The authors suggested that smoking exposure may induce a hypoestrogenic state.

Endocrine disrupting chemicals and endometriosis

Overview

There is considerable public health concern about the impact of environmental chemicals on wildlife and human populations. The available evidence remains suggestive of adverse relations between some chemicals and human reproduction and development, necessitating clinicians to be informed so that they may properly communicate risk and uncertainty to the women who seek their services. Human exposure to environmental chemicals increased dramatically during the latter part of the 20th century, partly because of the tremendous increase in the number of synthetic compounds manufactured. To date, there are approximately 90,000 chemicals of which only 1000–2000 are reported to have good data (www.epa.gov/comptox/toxcast).

While most human exposure remains at background levels, certain subgroups of the population remain at higher risk based upon residence (e.g. proximity to hazardous waste sites), occupation or lifestyle (e.g. anglers). Background exposure does not denote safe concentrations *per se*, given the ability of chemicals such as endocrine disrupting chemicals (EDCs) to bio-accumulate and biomagnify within ecosystems such as our food chain [47]. Another consideration is that EDC exposure is ubiquitous, with many compounds being found in everyday products (e.g. plastic bottles, flame retardants, toys, and cosmetics) or food (e.g. animal fat, dairy products, and fish).

Endocrine disrupting chemicals are organochlorine substances that contain chemically combined carbon and chlorine, resulting in a strong binding that resists degradation by normal biochemical and physical processes, and long half-lives. Given their ability to cross the placenta and enter the embryonic circulation [48] and to change the epigenome by altering phenotypic expression [49], EDCs pose health risks for some of the most susceptible populations. While there are some naturally occurring organochlorine compounds produced by living organisms at low concentrations [104], much of the human exposure is through diet [50]. Humans have no mechanisms or biochemical pathways for detoxification and excretion; hence, many EDCs are stored and accumulate in lipids and fatty tissue [47].

Endocrine disrupting chemicals are exogenous agents that have a multitude of effects and, thereby, have a multitude of targets and pathways, in part reflecting their diverse chemical structure. EDCs modulate hormonal function by binding to receptors and mimicking or blocking the action of hormones or reacting (in) directly with hormone structure, thereby altering the function of hormone synthesis or modulation of hormone receptors [51]. In addition, they can act as agonists or antagonists for a given endocrine system [51]. EDCs mechanisms are diverse, as recently reviewed, and include:

- aromatase inhibition
- estrogen receptor agonism/antagonism
- androgen receptor agonism/antagonism
- arylhydrocarbon receptor agonism
- interactions with binding proteins
- involvement in hormone metabolism [52].

The main targets of EDCs are sex steroids and thyroid homeostasis, underscoring the potential for reproductive and developmental impairments. Chemicals with endocrine disrupting activity include (broadly defined) pesticides; food antioxidants; mycoestrogens; steroids; phytoestrogens; industrial chemicals and pollutants; and pharmaceuticals [53]. However, the spectrum of effects is dependent upon the characteristics of the exposure(s) such as route, timing, dose, and host susceptibility coupled with other stressors such as nutrition and lifestyle. The reproductive and/or developmental toxicity of EDCs have been reviewed, including with regard to endometriosis [54–58]. The EDCs of particular concern include naturally occurring estrogenic-like compounds such as the phytoestrogen genistein; synthetic estrogenic-like compounds such as BPA; dioxins such as polychlorinated

dibenzo-dioxins (PCDDs) and polychlorinated-dibenzo-furans (PCDFs); organochlorine pesticides such as dichlorodiphenyl-trichloroethane (DDT) or its metabolite dichlorodiphenyldichloroethylene (DDE); phthalates; and polychlorinated biphenyls (PCBs). To date, the literature on EDCs and endometriosis has largely focused on dioxin, PCB and phthalate exposures as summarized below.

Endocrine disrupting chemicals and endometriosis

There is considerable evidence supporting a relation between organochlorine exposure at critical windows and subsequent endometriosis in laboratory animals, particularly for compounds such as PCDDs, PCDFs, and PCBs [59]. Initial evidence stemmed from the work of Rier and colleagues [60] who reported a dose-dependent relationship between 2,3,7,8-tetrachlorodibenzo-*p*-dioxin (TCDD) and peritoneal endometriosis in rhesus monkeys, and later an association with dioxin-like PCBs [61]. PCB congeners 77, 105, 153, and 180 have been associated with an increased expression of type 1 collagen in normal human peritoneal and adhesion fibroblasts indicative of a possible role in the pathogenesis of tissue fibrosis [62]. TCDD has been shown to affect endometrial endothelial cell profileration, suggesting a role in endometrial angiogenesis [63].

While the mechanisms through which EDCs may initiate or promote development of endometriosis remain unknown, hypothesized mechanisms include altered progesterone action [64] or immune function [65] consistent with a hormonal and immunological basis for progression of endometriosis. Quaranta and colleagues reported that PCBs and p,p'-DDE downregulated natural killer (NK) cell cytotoxic activity and interleukin (IL)-1β and IL-12 production, which suggests that these exposures may change specific immune markers [66]. Also, EDCs may influence the developmental plasticity of uterine tissue toward enzymatic and signaling cascades that promote development of endometriosis in adulthood following estrogen exposure [67].

The weight of evidence for human research is equivocal, as summarized in Table 15.2. The table indicates that there are approximately 20 human studies published to date, not all of which meet the rigid criteria of epidemiological methods. Authors are often quick to point out that the equivocal literature may reflect differences in study samples or in the diagnosis of endometriosis. Other critical methodologica; aspects have received less attention and include: (1) choice of the study population which afects the percentage of the study sample with endometriosis as it relates to statistical power, which is particularly relevant for negative findings; (2) consideration of the mixtures to which women are exposed irrespective of how authors model such exposures; and (3) laboratory methodologies such as automatic substitution of values below the limits of detection (LOD) or automatic lipid adjustment of chemical concentrations that may bias findings toward the null [68–70]. As noted in Table 15.2, negative studies often have a low percentage of women with endometriosis relative to the size of the overall study sample, and do not utilize endometriosis diagnoses based on laparoscopic or

Table 15.2 Environmental contaminants and endometriosis – weight of human evidence.

Authors	Exposures	Observed association	No observed association	Comment
Metals				
Heilier et al 2004 [84]	Cadmium		✓	n = 59 women (42%); sampling framework and endometriosis definition not stated. Creatinine-adjusted concentrations
Jackson et al 2008 [85]	Lead, cadmium and mercury	✓		n = 2818 (2% endometriosis) women comprising representative sample US women aged 20–49. Cross-sectional design and analysis. Self-reported endometriosis and gynecological history
Dioxin (with or without other compounds)				
Mayani et al 1997 [86]	TCDD	✓		n = 79 (56% endometriosis) infertile women undergoing laparoscopy. Did not lipid-adjust concentrations
Eskenazi et al 2002 [87]	TCDD		✓	n = 601 (3% endometriosis) residential women. Elevated risk, not significant.
Pauwels et al 2001 [88]	Dioxins and co-planar PCBs		✓	Medical record/ultrasonography confirmation of endometriosis. Lipid-adjusted concentrations n = 69 (61% endometriosis) infertile women. Elevated risk, not significant. Sample restricted to infertile women; comparison group matched on operative indication. Lipid-adjusted concentrations
Fierens et al 2003 [89]	PCDD, PCDF and co-planar PCBs		✓	n = 142 (7% endometriosis) geographic residents. Self-reported endometriosis
DeFelip et al 2004 [90]	PCDD, PCDF and co-planar PCBs		✓	n = 40 (58% endometriosis) nulliparous women seeking clinical care. Pooled biospecimens; substitutes values <LOD and lipid-adjusted concentrations
Heilier et al 2005 [91]	PCDD, PCDF and PCBs	✓		n = 71 women (35% peritoneal endometriosis). Control women represent convenient sample and did not undergo laparoscopy. Lipid-adjusted concentrations
Tsukino et al 2005 [92]	PCDDs, PCDFs, PCBs		✓	139 infertile women with endometriosis categorized as "cases" (stages 2–4) or "controls" (stages 0–1). No unaffected comparison group. Lipid-adjusted concentrations
Phthalates				
Corbellis et al 2003 [93]	PE	✓		n = 59 (59% endometriosis) women undergoing laparoscopy. Histological confirmation of endometriosis. Did not lipid-adjust concentrations
Reddy et al 2006 [94,95]	PE	✓		n = 108 (45% endometriosis) women undergoing laparoscopy; two laparoscopic comparison groups of women
PCBs (with or without compounds)				

Study	Compounds			Comments
Gerhard & Runnebaum 1992 [96]	PCBs	✓		Not clear if endometriosis was laparoscopically or histologically confirmed
Lebel et al 1998 [97]	PCBs and chlorinated pesticides		✓	n = 156 (55%) women undergoing laparoscopy. Control women matched on surgical indication, possibly overadjusting and removing effect. Lipid-adjusted concentrations
Buck Louis et al 2005 [98]	PCBs	✓		n = 84 (38% endometriosis) women undergoing laparoscopy; two laparoscopic comparison groups of women. Did not automatically substitute values <LOD or lipid-adjust concentrations
Quanta et al 2006 [66]	PCBs and p,p'-DDE	✓		
Porpora et al 2006 [99]	PCBs	✓		n = 80 (50% endometriosis) women undergoing laparoscopy. Lipid-adjusted concentrations
Porpora et al 2009 [100]	PCBs	✓		n = 158 (51% endometriosis) women undergoing laparoscopy. Lipid-adjusted concentrations
Hoffman et al 2007 [101]	PBBs, PCBs		✓	n = 943 (8% endometriosis) women from Michigan Female Health Study. Self-reported endometriosis; 60% medical records verification. Substituted values <LOD; did not lipid-adjust concentrations. Suggestive association for PCBs and endometriosis
Niskar et al 2008 [102]	PCBs, DDE		✓	n = 90 (67% endometriosis) women undergoing laparoscopy, 34 additional controls not undergoing laparoscopy.
Trabert et al 2010 [103]	PCBs, DDE		✓	Lipid-adjusted and unadjusted concentrations n = 789 (32% endometriosis) women covered by one health plan. Controls did not undergo laparoscopy; randomly selected from health plan. Substituted values <LOD

Note: Not all studies meet the methodological rigor of epidemiological studies; rather, all involved human females.
DDE, dichlorodiphenyldichlorothylene; LOD, limits of detection; PBB, polybrominated biphenyl; PCB, polychlorinated biphenyl; PCDD, polychlorinated dibenzo-dioxin; PCDF, polychlorinated-dibenzo-furan; PE, phthalate esters; TCDD, 2,3,7,8-tetrachlorodibenzo-p-dioxin.

histological confirmation. Laboratory practices for these studies often automatically substitute values for concentrations <LOD and/or lipid-adjusted concentrations. This latter practice makes strong causal assumptions about the role of serum lipids, viz., it is an independent risk factor for disease and also associated with chemical exposures.

Although beyond the scope of this chapter, a definitive answer about the relation between EDCs and endometriosis in humans requires population-based matched exposure cohort designs that permit quantification of EDCs in operative cohorts (exposure cohort) who are matched to referent populations (unexposed cohort), allowing for the comparison of women with endometriosis to those without disease in both the operative and population cohorts. Such designs also provide an opportunity to quantify EDCs in lipophilic tissue for comparison with more commonly used proxy media such as serum or plasma.

Life course perspective for endometriosis

The literature supporting a possible *in utero* origin for endometriosis is still evolving as investigators increasingly appreciate the early origin of disease hypothesis and design etiological research responsive to this avenue of study. Figure 15.3 illustrates the available literature from *in utero* exposures associated with a lifetime diagnosis of endometriosis and its relation with gravid health status and later-onset diseases. As noted above, female fetuses with evidence of growth restriction as measured by a birth weight ≤5.5 pounds or born as a part of a multiple pregnancy may be at higher risk of developing endometriosis than unaffected fetuses [43]. While women with endometriosis are often assumed to have lower fecundity than women without the disease, affected women are reported to be at lower risk for developing preeclampsia or pregnancy-induced hypertension than unaffected women [71]. These findings contrast with the clinical perspective that women with subfecundity are typically at greater risk for pregnancy complications than fecund women. In this paradigm, endometriosis is no longer viewed as just a gynecological disorder with a finite period of time in which it manifests. For example, endometriosis is associated with high rates of autoimmune and endocrine disorders such as hypothyroidism, fibromyalgia, chronic fatigue syndrome, allergies, asthma [72] and, increasingly, cancer.

Despite long-standing recognition of the close morphological relationship between endometriosis and ovarian cancer as described by Sampson in 1925 [105], recent reports about the malignant transformation of endometriosis are gaining attention [73,74]. At the population level, Swedish women with a diagnosis of endometriosis were at greater risk of breast, ovarian and non-Hodgkin lymphoma than unaffected women [75]. When this cohort was expanded and followed for a longer period of time, elevated cancer risks were found for ovarian cancer, endocrine tumors, non-Hodgkin lymphoma, and brain tumors. Risk of ovarian cancer was increased for women with an earlier endometriosis diagnosis, and reduced if women had a hysterectomy before or at the time of diagnosis [76]. As summarized based upon the Swedish population, women with endometriosis have a high frequency (8%) of malignancies, especially ovarian cancer. Estrogenicity may be the mechanism underlying both reproductive and developmental toxicity and carcinogenesis.

The ODS hypothesis provides a framework for conceptualizing an early origin for endometriosis with health implications across the lifespan. ODS suggests that epigenetic mechanisms may lead to the permanent programming of functional changes, resulting in the occurrence of incident disease across the lifespan. To this end, gynecological disorders may be an early signal, including during pregnancy, of later-onset disease. Future challenges will be to identify and measure exposures during critical and sensitive windows while placing them in the broader context of lifestyle and behavior across human development. Modeling chemical mixtures in the context of lifestyle is challenging and underscores the importance of assessing non-linear (e.g. U-shaped or reversed U-shaped) relations such as those seen for hormones [77,78] when assessing EDCs and health outcomes. Suffice it to say, the degree of methodological rigor is high and will require specification of causal models that avoid overadjusting intermediates or factors in the causal pathway [79] or the so-called reversal paradox [80]. Life course epidemiological methods coupled with newer statistical (joint) models that can assess multiple outcomes [81] consistent with a possible spectrum of epigenetic effects offer promise for designing research sensitive to critical data gaps.

More recently, some authors have suggested that human health is at a critical tipping point [82], and that the increasing rate of testicular cancer is a whistleblower for male subfertility [83]. These questions point to another – is there a whistleblower for female fecundity and later-onset diseases?

References

1. Ben-Shlomo Y, Kuh D. A life course approach to chronic disease epidemiology: conceptual models, empirical challenges and interdisciplinary perspectives. Int J Epidemiol 2002;31:285–293.
2. Buck Louis GM, Cooney MA. Effects of environmental contaminants on ovarian function and fertility. In: González-Bulnes A (ed) Novel Concepts in Ovarian Endocrinology. Kerala, India: Transworld Research Newtwork, 2007, pp.249–268.
3. Rajapakse N, Silva E, Kortenkamp A. Combining xenoestrogens at levels below individual no-observed-effect concentrations dramatically enhances steroid hormone action. Environ Health Perspect 2002;110:917–921.
4. Rasmussen TH, Nielsen F, Andersen HR, Nielsen JB, Weihe P, Grandjean P. Assessment of xenoestrogenic exposure by a biomarker approach: application of the E-screen bioassay to determine estrogenic response of serum extracts. Environ Health 2003;2:12.
5. Koppe JG, Bartonova A, Bolte G et al. Exposure to multiple environmental agents and their effect. Acta Paediatr 2006;95(Suppl):106–113.

6. Patisaul HB, Adewale HB. Long-term effects of environmental endocrine disruptors on reproductive physiology and behavior. Front Behav Neurosci 2009;3:1–18.

7. Daguet F. Un Siecle de Fecondité Francaise: 1901–1999. Paris: INSEE, 2002.

8. Skakkebaek NE, Rajpert-DeMeyts E, Main KM. Testicular dysgenesis syndrome: an increasingly commond developmental disorder with environmental aspects. Hum Reprod 2001;16:972–978.

9. Lutz W, O'Neill BC, Scherbov S. Demographics. Europe's population at a turning point. Science 2003;299:1991–1992.

10. Gray LE Jr, Ostby J, Furr J, Price M, Veeramachaneni DN, Parks L. Perinatal exposure to the phthalates DEHP, BBP, and DINP, but not DEP, DMP, or DOTP, alters sexual differentiation of the male rat. Toxicol Sci 2000;58:350–365.

11. Barker DPJ. Mothers, Babies and Disease in Later Life. London: BMJ Publishing Group, 1984.

12. Hales CN, Barker DJP. Type 2 (non-insulin-dependent) diabetes mellitus: the thrify phenotype hypothesis. Diabetologia 1992; 35:595–601.

13. Gluckman PD, Hanson MA. Living with the past: evolution, development, and patterns of disease. Science 2004;305:1733–1736.

14. Bateson P. Developmental plasticity and evolutional biology. J Nutr 2007;137:1060–1062.

15. Tang WY, Ho SM. Epigenetic reprogramming and imprinting in origins of disease. Rev Endocr Metab Disord 2007;8:173–182.

16. Thompson C, Syddall H, Rodin I, Osmond C, Barker DJ. Birth weight and the risk of depressive disorder in late life. Br J Psychiatry 2001;179:450–455.

17. Dennison EM, Arden NK, Keen RW et al. Birthweight, vitamin D receptor genotype and the programming of osteoporosis. Paediatr Perinat Epidemiol 2001;15:211–219.

18. Gluckman PD, Hanson MA. Developmental plasticity and human disease: research directions. J Intern Med 2007;261:461–471.

19. Calabrese EJ. Sex differences in susceptibility to toxic industrial chemicals. Br J Ind Med 1986;43:577–579.

20. Pyeritz RE. Sex: what we make of it. JAMA 1998;279:269.

21. Salumets A, Suikkari AM, Möls T, Söderström-Anttila V, Tuuri T. Influence of oocytes and spermatozoa on early embryonic development. Fertil Steril 2002;78:1082–1087.

22. Asch R, Simerly C, Ord T, Ord VA, Schatten G. The stages at which human fertilization arrests: microtubule and chromosome configurations in inseminated oocytes which failed to complete fertilization and development in humans. Hum Reprod 1995;10:1897–1906.

23. Kafri T, Ariel M, Brandeis M et al. Developmental pattern of gene-specific DNA methylation in the mouse embryo and germ line. Genes Dev 1992;6:705–714.

24. Macklon NS, Fauser BC. Aspects of ovarian follicle development throughout life. Horm Res 1999;52:161–170.

25. Buck GM, Lynch CD, Stanford JB et al. Prospective pregnancy study designs for assessing reproductive developmental toxicants. Environ Health Perspect 2004;112:79–86.

26. Li S, Hansman R, Newbold R, Davis B, McLachlan J. Neonatal diethyl-stilbesterol exposure induces persistent elevation of *c-fos* expression and hypomethylation of its exon-4 in mouse uterus. Mol Carcinog 2003;38:78–84.

27. Ho SM, Tang WY, de Frausto JB, Prins GS. Developmental exposure to estradiol and bisphenol A increases susceptibility to prostate carcinogenesis and epigenetically regulates phosphodiesterase type 4 variant 4. Cancer Res 2006;66:5624–5632.

28. Heindel JJ. Role of exposure to environmental chemicals in the developmental basis of reproductive disease and dysfunction. Semin Reprod Med 2006;24:168–177.

29. Heindell JJ. Animal models for probing the developmental basis of disease and dysfunction paradigm. Basic Clin Pharmacol Toxicol 2008;102:76–78.

30. Herbst AL, Ulfelder H, Poskanzer DC. Adenocarcinoma of the vagina. Association of maternal stilbestrol therapy with tumor appearance in young women. N Engl J Med 1971;184:878–881.

31. Palmer JR, Hatch EE, Rosenberg CL et al. Risk of breast cancer in women exposed to diethylstilbesterol in utero: preliminary results (United States). Cancer Causes Control 2002;13:753–758.

32. Newbold RR, Padilla-Banks E, Jefferson WN. Adverse effects of the model environment estrogen diethylstilbesterol are transmitted to subsequent generations. Endocrinology 2006;147(6 Suppl):S11–17.

33. Newbold RR, Hanson RB, Jefferson WN, Bullock BC, Haseman J, McLachlan JA. Increased tumors but uncompromised fertility in the female descendents of mice exposed developmentally to diethyl-stilbesterol. Carcinogenesis 1998;19:1655–1663.

34. Halme J, Hammond MG, Hulka JF, Raj SG, Talbert LM. Retrograde menstruation in healthy women and in patients with endometriosis. Obstet Gynecol 1984;64:151–154.

35. Sampson JA. Peritoneal endometriosis due to menstrual dissemination of endometrial tissue into the peritoneal cavity. Am J Obstet Gynecol 1927;14:422–469.

36. Abbott DH, Dumesic DA, Franks S. Developmental origin of polycystic ovarian syndrome – a hypothesis. J Endocrinol 2002;174:1–5.

37. Baird DD, Newbold R. Prenatal diethystilbestrol (DES) exposure is associated with uterine leiomyoma development. Reprod Toxicol 2005;20:81–84.

38. De Bruin JP, Dorland M, Bruinse HW, Spliet W, Nikkels PGJ, te Velde ER. Fetal growth retardation as a cause of impaired ovarian development. Early Hum Dev 2000;51:39–46.

39. Ibáñez L, Potau N, de Zegher F. Ovarian hyporesponsiveness to follicle stimulating hormone in adolescent girls born small for gestational age. J Clin Endocrinol Metab 2000;85:2624–2626.

40. Ibáñez L, Potau N, Enríquez G, de Zegher F. Reduced uterine and ovarian size in adolescent girls born small for gestational age. Pediatr Res 2000;47:575–577.

41. Ibáñez L, Potau N, Ferrer A, Rodriguez-Hierro F, Marcos MV, de Zegher F. Reduced ovulation rate in adolescent girls born small for gestational age. J Clin Endocrinol Metab 2002;87:3391–3393.

42. Acién P. Embryological observations on the female genital tract. Hum Reprod 1992;7:437–444.

43. Missmer SA, Hankinson SE, Spiegelman D, Barbieri RL, Michels KB, Hunter DJ. In utero exposures and the incidence of endometriosis. Fertil Steril 2004;82:1501–1508.

44. Hediger ML, Hartnett HJ, Louis GM. Association of endometriosis with body size and figure. Fertil Steril 2005;84:1366–1374.

45. Vitonis AF, Baer HJ, Hankinson SE, Laufer MR, Missmer SA. A prospective study of body size during childhood and the incidence of endometriosis. Hum Reprod 2010;25:1325–1334.

46. Buck Louis GM, Hediger ML, Pena JB. Intrauterine exposures and risk of endometriosis. Hum Reprod 2007;22:3232–3236.

47. Fisher BE. Most unwanted persistent organic pollutants. Environ Health Perspect 1999;107:A18–A23.

48. Kanja LW, Skaare JU, Ojwang SBO et al. A comparison of organochlorine pesticide residues in maternal adipose tissue, maternal blood, cord blood, and human milk from mother/infant pairs. Arch Environ Contam Toxicol 1992;22:21–24.

49. Anway MD, Cupp AS, Uzumcu M, Skinner MK. Epigenetic transgenerational actions of endocrine disruptors and male fertility. Science 2005;308:1466–1469.

50. Hall RH. A new threat to public health: organochlorines and food. Nutr Health 1992;8:33–43.

51. Sonnenschein C, Soto AM. An updated review of environmental estrogen and androgen mimics and antagonists. J Steroid Biochem Mol Biol 1998;65:143–150.

52. Yang M, Park MS, Lee HS. Endocrine disrupting chemicals: human exposure and health risks. J Environ Sci Heath 2006;24:183–224.

53. Damgaard IN, Main KM, Toppari J, Skakkebaek NE. Impact of exposure to endocrine disrupters in utero and in childhood on adult reproduction. Best Pract Res Clin Endocrinol Metab 2002;16:289–309.

54. Miller KP, Borgeest C, Greenfeld C, Tomic D, Flaws JA. In utero effects of chemicals on reproductive tissues in females. Toxicol Appl Pharm 2004;198:111–131.

55. Torf G, Hagmar L, Giweercman A, Bonde JP. Epidemiological evidence on reproductive effects of persistent organochlorines in humans. Reprod Toxicol 2004;19:5–26.

56. McLachlan J, Simpson E, Martin M. Endocrine disrupters and female reproductive health. Best Pract Res Clin Endocrinol Metab 2006;20:63–75.

57. Buck Louis GM, Lynch CD, Cooney MA. Environmental influences on female fecundity and fertility. Sem Reprod Med 2006;24:147–155.

58. Mendola P, Messer LC, Rappazzo K. Science linking environmental contaminant exposures with fertility and reproductive health impacts in the adult female. Fertil Steril 2008;89(Suppl):e81–e94.

59. Birnbaum LS, Cummings AM. Dioxins and endometriosis: a plausible hypothesis. Environ Health Perspect 2002;110:15–21.

60. Rier SE, Martin DC, Bowman RE, Dmowski WP, Becker JL. Endometriosis in rhesus monkeys (*Macaca mulatta*) following chronic exposure to 2,3,7,8-tetrachlorodibenzo-*p*-dioxin. Fund Appl Toxicol 1993;21:433–441.

61. Rier SE, Turner WE, Martin DC, Morris R, Lucier GW, Clark GC. Serum levels of TCDD and dioxin-like chemicals in Rhesus monkeys chronically exposed to dioxin: correlation of increased serum PCB levels with endometriosis. Toxicol Sci 2001;59:147–159.

62. Diamond MP, Wirth JJ, Saed GM. PCBs enhance collagen I expression from human peritoneal fibroblasts. Fertil Steril 2008;90:1372–1375.

63. Bredhult C, Bäcklin B-M, Olovsson M. Effects of some endocrine disruptors on the proliferation and viability of human endometrial endothelial cells *in vitro*. Reprod Toxicol 2007;23:550–559.

64. Nayyar T, Bruner-Tran KL, Piestrzeniewicz-Ulanska D, Osteen KG. Developmental exposure of mice to TCDD elicits a similar uterine phenotype in adult animals as observed in women with endometriosis. Reprod Toxicol 2007;23:326–336.

65. Mueller MD, Vigne JL, Streich M et al. 2,3,7,8-Tetrachlorodibenzo-*p*-dioxin increases glycodelin gene and protein expression in human endometrium. J Clin Endocrinol Metab 2005;90:4809–4815.

66. Quaranta MG, Porpora MG, Mattioli B et al. Impaired NK-cell-mediated cytotoxic activity and cytokine production in patients with endometriosis: a possible role for PCBs and DDE. Life Sci 2006;79:491–498.

67. Crain DA, Janssen SJ, Edwards TM et al. Female reproductive disorders: the roles of endocrine-disrupting compounds and developmental timing. Fertil Steril 2008;90:911–940.

68. Richardson DB, Ciampi A. Effects of exposure measurement error when an exposure variable is constrained by a lower limit. Am J Epidemiol 2003;157:355–363.

69. Schisterman EF, Whitcomb BW, Louis GM, Louis TA. Lipid adjustment in the analysis of environmental contaminants and human health risks. Environ Health Perspect 2005;113:853–857.

70. Schisterman EF, Vexler A, Whitcomb BW, Liu A. The limitations due to exposure detection limits for regression models. Am J Epidemiol 2006;163:374–383.

71. Brosens IA, de Sutter P, Hamerlynck T et al. Endometriosis is associated with a decreased risk of pre-eclampsia. Hum Reprod 2007;22:1725–1729.

72. Sinaii N, Cleary SD, Ballweg ML, Nieman LK, Stratton P. High rates of autoimmune and endocrine disorders, fibromyalgia, chronic fatigue syndrome and atopic diseases among women with endometriosis: a survey analysis. Hum Reprod 2002;17:2715–2724.

73. Ogawa S, Kaku T, Amada S et al. Ovarian endometriosis associated with ovarian carcinoma: a clinicopathological and immunohistochemical study. Gynecol Oncol 2000;77:298–304.

74. Yoshikawa H, Jimbo H, Okada S et al. Prevalence of endometriosis in ovarian cancer. Gynecol Obstet 2000;50(Suppl 1):11–17.

75. Brinton LA, Gridley G, Persson I, Baron J, Bergqvist A. Cancer risk afer a hospital discharge diagnosis of endometriosis. Am J Obstet Gynecol 1997;176:572–579.

76. Melin A, Sparén P, Persson I, Bergqvist A. Endometriosis and the risk of cancer with special emphasis on ovarian cancer. Hum Reprod 2006;21:1237–1242.

77. Sheehan DM. No-threshold dose-response curves for nongenotoxic chemicals: findings and applications for risk assessment. Environ Res 2006;100:93–99.

78. Vandenberg LN, Wadia PR, Schaeberle CM, Rubin BS, Sonnenschein C, Soto AM. The mammary gland response to estradiol: monotonic at the cellular level, non-monotonic at the tissue-level of organization? J Steroid Biochem Mol Biol 2006;101:263–274.

79. Tu YK, West R, Ellison GTH, Gilthorpe MS. Why evidence for the fetal origins of adult disease might be a statistical artifact: the "reversal

paradox" for the relation between birth weight and blood pressure in later life. Am J Epidemiol 2005;161:27–32.

80. Stigler SM. Statistics on the Table. Cambridge, MA: Harvard University Press, 1999.

81. DeStavola BL, Nitsch D, dos Santos Silva I et al. Statistical issues in life course epidemiology. Am J Epidemiol 2005;163:84–96.

82. Andersson AM, Jorgensen N, Main KM et al. Adverse trends in male reproductive health: we may have reached a crucial 'tipping point'. Int J Andrology 2008;31(2):74-80.

83. Skakkebaek NE, Rajpert-De Meyts E, Jorgensen N et al. Testicular cancer trends as 'whistle blowers' of testicular developmental problems in populations. Int J Androl 2007;30:198–204.

84. Heilier JF, Verougstraete V, Nackers F, Tonglet R, Donnez J, Lison D. Assessment of cadmium impregnation in women suffering from endometriosis: a preliminary study. Toxicol Lett 2004;154:89–93.

85. Jackson LW, Zullo MD, Goldberg JM. The association between heavy metals, endometriosis and uterine myomas among premenopausal women: National Health and Nutrition Examination Survey 1999–2002. Hum Reprod 2008;23:679–687.

86. Mayani A, Barel S, Soback S, Almagor M. Dioxin concentrations in women with endometriosis. Hum Reprod 1997;12:373–375.

87. Eskenazi B, Mocarelli P, Warner M et al. Serum dioxin concentrations and endometriosis: a cohort study in Seveso, Italy. Environ Health Perspect 2002;110:629–634.

88. Pauwels A, Schepens PJ, D'Hooghe T et al. The risk of endometriosis and exposure to dioxins and polychlorinated biphenyls: a case-control study of infertile women. Hum Reprod 2001;16:2050–2055.

89. Fierens S, Mairesse H, Heilier JF et al. Dioxin/polychlorinated biphenyl body burden, diabetes and endometriosis: findings in a population-based study in Belgium. Biomarkers 2003;8:529–534.

90. De Felip E, Porpora MG, di Domenico A et al. Dioxin-like compounds and endometriosis: a study on Italian and Beligan women of reproductive age. Toxicol Lett 2004;150:203–209.

91. Heilier J-F, Nackers F, Verougstraete V, Tonglet R, Lison D, Donnez J. Increased dioxin-like compounds in the serum of women with peritoneal endometriosis and deep endometriotic (adenomyotic) nodules. Fertil Steril 2005;84:305–312.

92. Tsukino H, Hanaoka T, Sasaki H et al. Associations between serum levels of selected organochlorine compounds and endometriosis in infertile Japanese women. Environ Res 2005;99:118–125.

93. Cobellis L, Latini G, de Felice C et al. High plasma concentrations of di-(2-ethylhexyl)-phthalate in women with endometriosis. Hum Reprod 2003;18:1512–1515.

94. Reddy BS, Rozati R, Reddy BV, Raman NV. Association of phthalate esters with endometriosis in Indian women. Br J Obstet Gynaecol 2006;113:515–520.

95. Reddy BS, Rozati R, Reddy S, Kodampur S, Reddy P, Reddy R. High plasma concentrations of polychlorinated biphenyls and phathalate esters in women with endometriosis: a prospective case control study. Fertil Steril 2006;85:775–779.

96. Gerhard I, Runnebaum B. The limits of hormone substitution in pollutant exposure and fertility disorders. Zentralbl Gynakol 1992;114:593–602.

97. Lebel G, Dodin S, Ayotte P, Marcoux S, Ferron LA, Dewailly E. Organochlorine exposure and the risk of endometriosis. Fertil Steril 1998;69:221–228.

98. Buck Louis GM, Weiner JM, Whitcomb BW et al. Environmental PCB exposure and risk of endometriosis. Hum Reprod 2005;20:279–285.

99. Porpora MG, Ingelido AM, di Domenico A et al. Increased levels of polychlorinated biphenyls in Italian women with endometriosis. Chemosphere 2006;63:1361–1367.

100. Porpora MG, Medda E, Abballe A et al. Endometriosis and organochlorine environmental pollutants: a case control study on Italian women of reproductive age. Environ Health Perspect 2009;1117:1070–1075.

101. Hoffman CS, Small CM, Blanck HM, Tolbert P, Rubin C, Marcus M. Endometriosis among women exposed to polybrominated biphenyls. Ann Epidemiol 2007;17:503–510.

102. Niskar AS, Needham LL, Rubin C et al. Serum dioxins, polychlorinated biphenyls, and endometriosis: a case-control study in Atlanta. Chemosphere 2009;74:944–949.

103. Trabert B, de Roos AJ, Schwartz SM et al. Non-dioxin-like polychlorinated biphenyls and risk of endometriosis. Environ Health Perspect 2010;118:1280–1285.

104. Gribble GW. The natural production of chlorinated compounds. Environ Sci Technol 1994;28:A310-A318.

105. Sampson J. Endometrial carcinoma of the ovary. Arising in endometrial tissue in that organ. Arch Surg 1925;10:1–72.

16 Signaling Pathways in Endometriosis (Eutopic/Ectopic)

J. Julie Kim and Xunqin Yin

Department of Obstetrics and Gynecology, Division of Reproductive Biology Research, Robert H. Lurie Comprehensive Cancer Center, Northwestern University, Chicago, IL, USA

Introduction

A cell's response to external stimuli involves a tightly regulated orchestration of receptors, signaling cascades, and transcription factors which ultimately manifests as cellular processes such as proliferation, differentiation, and apoptosis. There has been much research focusing on each of these components of cellular activity which has provided an in-depth knowledge of how a cell responds to a growth factor, for example, and which signaling pathways are involved for a specific physiological response. In instances where a cell does not appropriately respond to stimuli and signals are not transferred correctly, as is the case for cells from a disease state, there are usually defects that can occur at any level from receptors all the way down to DNA that contribute to the induction or inhibition of signaling pathways. In cases where pathways are hyperactivated, inhibitors to specific kinases have been used to study the function of these kinases as well as clinically to treat malignant conditions.

In the field of endometriosis research, elucidation of signaling cascades has been relatively understudied. While it is not surprising that certain signaling pathways are perturbed in ectopic endometrial tissues/cells given that the environment is vastly different from that of the uterine cavity, it is intriguing that cells from the eutopic endometrium from women with endometriosis also exhibit aberrant signaling activities. In this chapter, we review studies that have been done on signaling pathways in endometriosis in both ectopic and eutopic tissues.

Endometriosis

The unique ability of endometrial tissue to proliferate, survive, and invade sites outside the uterine cavity contributes to its persistence and growth. Ectopic tissues occur mainly in the pelvic peritoneum, ovaries, and rectovaginal septum and although rare, endometrial tissue can be found in distant sites such as the heart, lung, and brain [1,2]/ Endometriosis is an estrogen-dependent disorder affecting up to 10% of the female population and 30–50% of infertile women, with no cure and few therapies [1,2]. It is often associated with pelvic pain and infertility, and there is increasing evidence of an elevated risk of developing ovarian cancer [3]. To date, medical therapies are limited to surgery and hormonal or non-steroidal anti-inflammatory agents. Contraceptive steroids, progestins, and gonadotropin releasing hormone (GnRH) agonists which are used to minimize or eliminate menstrual flow and/or lower circulating estradiol concentrations are used for a limited time due to their unacceptable side-effects, including osteoporosis [2]. There remains little consensus as to the most efficacious medical or surgical approach to treating endometriosis, and thus the development of better therapies is urgently needed.

Given that endometriosis is a hormone-dependent disorder, associated with inflammation and survival of ectopic tissues, numerous studies have examined the signaling pathways in endometriotic cells and have found, in general, an increased activation of the mitogen-activated protein kinase (MAPK) and v-akt murine thymoma viral oncogene (AKT) pathways with a blunted protein kinase A (PKA) response. While this area of investigation has not been as extensively studied in endometriosis as it has in the cancer field, the rationale for intervening at this level using kinase inhibitors to treat endometriosis is strong.

Signaling pathways

Manning *et al* first catalogued the protein kinase network as the "kinome" which is the complement of the human genome [4]. They identified 518 putative protein kinase genes as well as 106 protein kinase pseudogenes, underlining the elaborate and complex nature of signaling mechanisms. The signal transduction

Endometriosis: Science and Practice, First Edition. Edited by Linda C. Giudice, Johannes L.H. Evers and David L. Healy.
© 2012 Blackwell Publishing Ltd. Published 2012 by Blackwell Publishing Ltd.

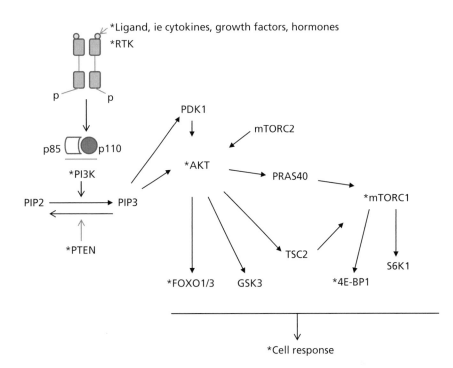

Figure 16.1 The PI3K/AKT pathway. See text for explanation. RTK, receptor tyrosine kinase.
*denotes demonstrated dysregulation in endometriosis.

pathways that have been characterized in detail include the MAPK, AKT, cyclic adenosine monophosphate (cAMP)-PKA, protein kinase C (PKC), inositol trisphosphate-diacylglycerol (IP3-DAG), phospholipase C (PLC), calcium, and cGMP-dependent protein kinase (PKG) pathways. Each pathway, its second messengers and protein kinases have been characterized extensively. The multiple cross-conversations and common receptors among the different pathways have contributed to the challenge of deciphering the roles of the kinases and the pathways in processes associated with normal and disease conditions [5–8]. However, genetic manipulation of the signaling proteins using animal and cell models has allowed for the identification of oncogenes, such as RAt Sarcoma (Ras), or tumor suppressors, such as phosphatase and tensin homolog (PTEN). Inhibitors of protein kinases have also been useful to elucidate their roles in cellular processes.

Here, a concise overview of three major signaling pathways, MAPK, AKT and PKA, is provided, given that these are the pathways that have been studied in endometriosis thus far. Each section is introduced by a brief overview of the major players involved and the sequential cascade of events that occur in the pathway under discussion.

PI3K/AKT

Background

The phosphoinositide-3-kinase (PI3K)/AKT pathway has been the focus of much research, given its role in promoting cell survival and proliferation, and is considered a likely driver of tumor progression in most carcinomas [9–11]. In many human solid tumors, including breast, endometrial, ovarian, prostate and colon, the AKT pathway is overactivated. This upregulation of AKT activity can occur due to amplification or mutations of AKT

itself, or in other members of this pathway, from receptor tyrosine kinases, PI3K, RAS, to PTEN.

The PI3K/AKT signaling pathway is initiated by growth factors, hormones, and cytokines through their corresponding receptors [12] (Fig. 16.1). PI3K consists of a regulatory subunit (p85) and a catalytic subunit (p110). When tyrosine kinase receptors bind to the SRC homology (SH) domain in the p85 subunit, they activate the kinase and then the p110 subunit phosphorylates the lipid substrate phosphatidylinositol (4,5) bisphosphate (PIP2) to produce phosphatidylinositol (3,4,5) trisphosphate (PIP3). PIP3 then binds to the pleckstrin homology domains of 3-phosphoinositide dependent protein kinase-1 (PDK1) and AKT and causes translocation of each kinase to the plasma membrane, where both are activated. AKT is partially activated through PDK1 but full activation requires a second phosphorylation event in the hydrophobic motif, which can be mediated by several kinases, including mammalian target of rapamycin complex 2 (mTORC2). mTORC2 is made up of mTOR, Rictor, and SIN1 as well as other proteins and is resistant to rapamycin. This is different from mTORC1 which consists of mTOR, Raptor and other proteins which make it sensitive to rapamycin and which acts downstream of AKT [13]. PTEN is a phosphatase that dephosphorylates PI3K phosphorylation products, PIP2 and PIP3, which in turn leaves Akt dephosphorylated and inactivated [14] (see Fig. 16.1). When PTEN is mutated, AKT becomes constitutively active, inhibiting several downstream targets through phosphorylation, such as forkhead box O1 (FOXO1), forkhead box O3 (FOXO3) and glycogen synthase kinase 3 beta (GSK3B.) It has been postulated that AKT phosphorylates over 9000 proteins [15,16] and thus is considered a critical regulator of cellular processes. Once activated, AKT plays a central role in modulating cell survival, proliferation, migration, differentiation, and apoptosis [12,15,16]. Its importance in promoting cell survival and inhibition of apoptosis has provided the rationale for studying this pathway in cancer.

PI3K/AKT in endometriosis

Global analysis of genes associated with the PI3K/AKT pathway has revealed some significant differences in expression patterns in endometriosis tissues. In a study using endometriosis tissues from four premenopausal and four postmenopausal women, Yagyu *et al* observed an increase in phospho-mTOR levels in endometriosis tissues from postmenopausal women but not in premenopausal women, for reasons which remain unclear [17]. Using micro fluidic gene array, Laudanski *et al* compared the expression of 15 tumor suppressor and oncogenes (neurofibromin 1 [NF1], Ras homolog enriched in brain [RHEB], mTOR, PTEN, tuberous sclerosis 1 [TSC1], tuberous sclerosis 2 [TSC2], v-Ki-ras2 Kirsten rat sarcoma viral oncogene homolog [KRAS], ribosomal protein S6 kinase [S6K1], tumor protein p53 [TP53], eukaryotic translation initiation factor 4E [EIF4E], serine/threonine kinase 11 [LKB1], phosphoinositide-3-kinase, catalytic, alpha polypeptide [PIK3CA], beclin 1, autophagy related [BECN1], eukaryotic translation initiation factor 4E binding protein 1 [4EBP1] and AKT1) in eutopic endometrium of 40 women with endometriosis, among whom 14 women had matched ovarian lesions, and 41 controls without endometriosis [18]. Significantly higher levels of AKT1 and the tumor suppressor gene 4EBP1 mRNAs were found in the eutopic endometrium of women with endometriosis compared with control patients, and immunohistochemistry confirmed upregulation at the protein level.

These data suggest that upregulation of AKT1 and 4EBP1 in eutopic endometrium contributes to increasing the AKT signaling pathway in endometriosis. Honda *et al* used the serial analysis of gene expression (SAGE) technique to identify genes specific to epithelial cells from ovarian endometrioma [19]. IGF2, ACTN4, AXL, and SHC1 were among the most upregulated genes. Furthermore, immunohistochemistry analysis revealed an increase in staining of ectopic endometriotic tissues for PI3KCA, pAKT, pmTOR, and pERK, strongly implicating the AKT and MAPK pathways in the pathogenesis of endometriosis. Others have also observed that phospho-AKT levels are higher in eutopic and ectopic endometrium of endometriosis compared with normal endometrium, *in vivo* [20]. In addition, *in vitro* studies demonstrated higher AKT phosphorylation in stromal cells from eutopic and ectopic endometrium from endometriosis, compared with normal cells [20] suggestive of significant inherent differences in this pathway in cells from endometriosis.

PTEN, which negatively regulates the AKT pathway (see Fig.16.1), has often been found to be mutated in cancers. In endometrial cancer, PTEN mutations are rampant and occur in up to 80% of endometrial adenocarcinoma [14,21,22]. Very little is known regarding the PTEN status in endometriosis. Treloar *et al* [23] genotyped single nucleotide polymorphisms (SNPs) to evaluate association between endometriosis and variations in PTEN and

EMX2, two genes that are found on chromosome 10, a region which has been linked to genetic susceptibility of endometriosis [24]. After analysis of a large cohort of women with and without endometriosis, they found no significant association between any SNPs or haplotypes and endometriosis for either of these genes [23].

Recently, Zhang *et al* demonstrated that PTEN was downregulated in both the eutopic and ectopic endometrial epithelial cells from endometriosis due to transcriptional and post-transcriptional regulation of the gene, rather than mutations [25]. They also found that pERK, pAKT and NFκB levels were higher in eutopic and ectopic epithelial cells compared to the normal counterpart and that estradiol enhanced this effect. Their proposed model described that in the eutopic and ectopic endometriotic epithelial cells, estradiol activates the PI3K/AKT, MAPK/ERK, and NFκB pathways, which then enhances NFκB binding to suppress PTEN transcription and expression, which thereby facilities the activity of PI3K/AKT. This then creates a positive feedback loop, in which the activated PI3K/AKT pathway can further promote suppression of PTEN through NFκB. The importance of PTEN as a tumor suppressor gene is further demonstrated in transgenic mice where heterozygous PTEN mice develop complex proliferative endometrial lesions [26] and PTEN conditional knockout mice develop endometrial cancer [27]. The first genetic model for endometriosis was shown by Dinulescu [28] where either Cre(causes recombination)-mediated inactivation of PTEN or activation of K-ras was sufficient for formation of "benign" endometriotic ovarian lesions. These studies strongly implicate the role of PI3K/AKT and/or MAPK (see below) pathways in the pathogenesis of endometriosis.

It has been well documented that the effect of hormones in the endometrium involves paracrine interactions between the epithelial and stromal cells [29–40]. For example, progesterone binds to the progesterone receptor (PR) on stromal cells to induce secretion of paracrine factor(s) that in turn stimulate neighboring epithelial cells to express the estradiol metabolizing enzyme 17β-hydroxysteroid dehydrogenase type 2 (HSD17β2) [29,41]. In endometriotic tissues, progesterone is incapable of inducing epithelial HSD17β2 expression mostly likely due to low PR levels in the stroma. Recently, Zhang *et al* demonstrated in endometriotic cells that stromal factors were able to inhibit phosphorylation of AKT and expression of survivin in epithelial cells and this was further enhanced by progesterone [42]. They observed this in both normal endometrial cells and eutopic endometrial cells from endometriosis. However, progesterone had little effect in the presence of stromal factors from ectopic endometriotic stromal cells to mediate the response in endometriotic epithelial cells and the authors concluded that this aberrant response may facilitate epithelial cell proliferation in endometriosis and promote the survival of endometriotic lesions.

Mitogen-activated protein kinase
Background

Mitogen-activated protein kinases (MAPKs) are serine-threonine kinases which form a signaling network that controls cellular processes in response to external stimuli. There are three members

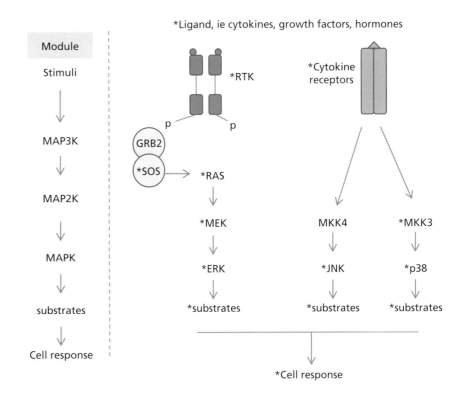

Figure 16.2 The MAPK pathway. See text for explanation. *denotes demonstrated dysregulation in endometriosis.

of the MAPK family: the extracellular signal-regulated kinase (ERK), p38, and c-Jun NH2-terminal kinase (JNK). Generally, the MAPK pathway involves a three-tiered module of sequentially acting kinases: a MAPK, MAPKK, and MAPKKK (Fig. 16.2) (reviewed in [43–45]). The kinases in each of these tiers occur in several similar isoforms, creating complexity and broadening the range of activity of the MAPK pathway. An example of sequential activation of kinases leading to phosphorylation of various substrate proteins can be shown using the ERK cascade (see Fig.16.2). Specifically, upon ligand binding of receptor tyrosine kinases (RTK), this leads to binding of adapter molecules such as Grb2 and Shc, which contain the SH2 domain. The adapters, through its N-terminal SH3 domain, then link the receptors to a proline-rich region of the guanine nucleotide exchange protein Son of sevenless (Sos) which enhances guanosine diphosphate (GDP) release and guanosine-5'-triphosphate (GTP) binding to Ras. Ras is a critical switch that controls the ERK cascade in that the GTP-bound form of Ras binds to Raf, bringing it to the plasma membrane where its protein kinase activity is increased and the kinase cascade is activated. Once activated, Raf phosphorylates and activates the dual-specificity protein kinases Mitogen-activated protein kinase kinase 1 (MEK1) and MEK2, which then activate ERK1 and ERK2. The activation of p38 and JNK follows a similar module and they are activated by MKK3 and MKK4 respectively. The MAPK pathway regulates a vast array of cellular processes, such as proliferation, differentiation, development, stress response, and apoptosis.

Mitogen-activated protein kinase and endometriosis

In endometriosis, the MAPK pathway, similar to the AKT pathway, remains relatively understudied but has been receiving more attention in the recent years. Microarray analysis performed by Matsuzaki *et al* [46,47] in eutopic endometrium from endometriosis patients identified genes involved in MAPK and PI3K signaling pathways to be significantly regulated. These genes included RON, SOS, 14-3-3 protein η, and uPAR in epithelial cells and KSR and PI3K p85 regulatory subunit α in stromal cells. Using laser capture microdissection and a cDNA microarray with 9600 genes/expressed sequence tags (ESTs), Wu *et al* [48] conducted a comprehensive profiling of gene expression differences between the ectopic and eutopic endometrium taken from women with endometriosis adjusted for menstrual phase and the location of the lesions. Specific genes clustered together that differentiated ovarian versus peritoneal endometriosis. Numerous pathways were identified by KEGG (Kyoto Encyclopedia of Genes and Genomes) and the MAPK signaling pathway was one of them. Thirteen genes were categorized under the MAPK pathway: DUSP5, AKT1, HSPB2, PDGFB, PDGFRA, PLA2G5, MAPK6, MAPK7, RAC1, RAF1, RPS6KA3, TGFB3, MKNK1. Significant differences in expression of these genes which converge on the MAPK pathway in endometriosis may explain the hyperactivation of this pathway in endometriotic cells.

Global analysis of genes performed by Burney *et al* [49] of eutopic endometrium of women with endometriosis identified genes associated with inactivation of MAPK signaling cascades to be decreased in endometriosis. Specifically, ERBB receptor feedback inhibitor 1 (ERRFI1, also known as MIG-6) and regulators of G protein signaling 1 (RGS1), which is an activator of GTPases that rapidly turns off G-protein-coupled receptor signaling pathways, were decreased. This led to the investigation of the MAPK pathway by Velarde et al [50], who found that phospho-ERK1/2 levels were elevated in eutopic endometrial stromal cells of women with disease compared to those without disease. Moreover, increased ERK1/2 activity interfered with 8-Br-cAMP-mediated downregulation of cyclin D1 in stromal cells from endometriosis and the inhibitor of MEK1/2, U0126, restored the response by 8-Br-cAMP. Furthermore, intense immunostaining of phospho-ERK1/2 was observed in early-secretory epithelial and stromal cells of the eutopic endometrium from those with disease whereas phospho-ERK1/2 levels were highest in the late-secretory epithelial and stromal cells in women without disease, demonstrating variation in cyclic regulation of phospho-ERK1/2 The authors suggest that this observation could explain the proliferative phenotype that is often associated with the eutopic endometrium of women with endometriosis during the secretory phase of the menstrual cycle.

Endometriosis is often accompanied by local inflammatory reactions in the peritoneal cavity and this has provided a strong rationale for studying signal transduction systems in endometriotic cells. Elevated levels of proinflammatory cytokines, such as interleukin (IL)-6, IL-8, and tumor necrosis factor (TNF), occur in the peritoneal fluid of women with endometriosis [51–54]. Yoshino et al [55] found that IL-1β, TNF-α and H2O2 stimulated the phosphorylation of ERK, p38, and JNK in endometriotic stromal cells. Others have shown that TNF-α significantly increased IL-6 protein in endometriotic stromal cells isolated from chocolate cysts [56] through activation of ERK1/2 and degradation of IκB.

Using a focused oligoarray, Taniguchi et al [57] identified TAK1 to be augmented in endometriotic stromal cells from ovarian endometriomas in response to TNF-α. TAK1 is a member of the MAPK kinase kinase (MAPKKK) family which can lead to activation of ERK1/2, p38, and IKK [58]. In endometriotic stromal cells, knocking down TAK1 using siRNA resulted in repression of TNF-α-induced phosphorylation of IκBα, JNK1/2, and p38MAPK, and a decrease in IL-6 and IL-8 expression, a decrease in the proportion of cells in S-phase and reduced proliferation. Another group demonstrated that the activation of protease-activated receptor 2 (PAR2) stimulated the phosphorylation of all three MAPK, ERK, p38, and JNK in endometriotic stromal cells [59]. Furthermore, activation of PAR2 stimulated secretion of IL-6 and IL-8 in a dose-dependent manner as well as stimulating the proliferation of endometriotic stromal cells.

Corresponding inhibitors to each of the MAPKs suppressed proliferation induced by PAR2 activation. Using an endometriotic epithelial cell line, Grund et al [60] demonstrated that MEK, p38, and IKK inhibitors blocked TNF-α-induced IL-8, IL-6, and granulocyte macrophage-colony stimulating factor (GM-CSF) secretion and cell invasion, while the PI3K inhibitors did not

demonstrate specificity of the pathways to a particular physiological response. Tagashira et al [61] demonstrated that addition of IL-10, an anti-inflammatory cytokine [62,63], to endometriotic stromal cells suppressed the expression of IL-6 induced by TNF-α. In turn, IL-10 attenuated TNF-α-induced phosphorylation of STAT3, ERK1/2, JNK1/2, and IκB.

The above studies clearly demonstrate that proinflammatory cytokines can activate the MAPK pathway resulting in additional cytokine release, and an increase in proliferation, invasion and potentially disease progression.

Protein kinase A
Background
The cAMP-PKA signaling system was the first mammalian second messenger system to be characterized and is highly conserved from yeast to mammals. This pathway is activated upon ligand binding to G-protein-coupled receptors which are bound to the G complex (Gβ or Gγ, and Gα subunits) (Fig. 16.3). After ligand binding, GTP binds to the Gα subunit in place of GDP, causing the Gα subunit to activate adenylate cyclase. This then catalyzes the conversion of adenosine triphosphate (ATP) to the second messenger cAMP which binds to the regulatory subunits of PKA, allowing for the release of the catalytic subunits. The active catalytic subunits are then able to phosphorylate target proteins such as cAMP response element binding protein (CREB) which can then bind to DNA and regulate genes. Ligand binding is transient and loss of binding to the receptor reverts it back to binding of Gα to GDP, resulting in an inactive state. There are hundreds, if not thousands of substrates identified for PKA which are involved in regulating cellular processes such as proliferation, glycogen metabolism and cortisol secretion, to name a few.

Protein kinase A signaling in endometriosis
There are only a few studies looking at the PKA pathway in endometriosis and this has been done primarily in the context of decidualization of the human endometrium. Decidualization, which is the transformation of the endometrial stromal cells to a secretory, epithelioid-like decidual cell, is initiated during the secretory phase of the menstrual cycle when progesterone levels are high [64]. Decidualization of the stromal cells has long been associated with the PKA pathway since endometrial stromal cells *in vitro* can be induced to decidualize by activation of PKA with cAMP agonists [64]. Prostaglandin (PG) E_2 can also increase intracellular cAMP and promote decidualization in normal endometrial stromal cells [65]. It was demonstrated by Carli et al [66] that macrophage migration inhibitory factor (MIF), a potent proinflammatory and growth-promoting factor found at elevated concentrations in the peritoneal fluid of women with endometriosis, stimulated the synthesis of cyclo-oxygenase-2 (COX-2), and the release of PGE_2. MIF was able to increase COX-2 synthesis through activation of ERK and p38 in endometriotic stromal cells, isolated from ectopic endometriotic tissues from stage I–III disease. Interestingly, this group demonstrated that while p38

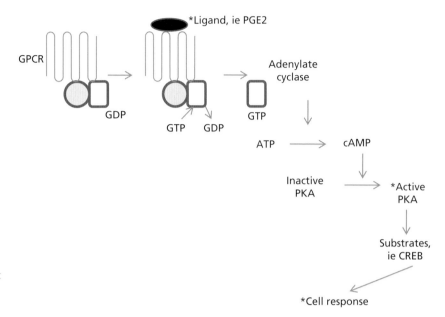

Figure 16.3 The cAMP-PKA signaling pathway. See text for explanation. *denotes demonstrated dysregulation in endometriosis.

inhibitors negatively affected the stimulated synthesis of COX-2 and PGE_2, ERK inhibitors decreased only the production of PGE_2. They proposed that p38 was involved in controlling activation of COX-2 for PGE_2 synthesis whereas ERK was involved in potentially activating the PGE synthase enzyme and thereby providing a complementary mechanism. Wu *et al* [67] reported evidence to demonstrate distinct regulation of COX-2 by IL-1β in normal versus endometriotic stromal cells. Ectopic endometriotic stromal cells were 100 times more sensitive to IL-1β, compared with its eutopic counterpart. Specifically, MAPK-dependent phosphorylation of CREB induced COX-2 promoter activity. Although these data suggest an increased sensitivity to decidualization, due to increased PGE_2 production through increased COX-2 synthesis in response to cytokines, we and others have observed the contrary in that decidualization is blunted in endometriotic stromal cells [68–70]. Given that cAMP agonists were used in these studies, it can be assumed that PKA is either not functioning as needed or that additional mechanisms regulating targets of PKA are dysfunctional.

Microarrays have been used to identify downstream targets of PKA in stromal cells from the eutopic endometrium of women with or without endometriosis [69]. This study revealed that in normal stromal cells, cyclin D1, cyclin-dependent kinase 6, and cell division cycle 2 were decreased while cyclin-dependent kinase inhibitor 1A increased. However, this was not the case for cells from eutopic endometrium with endometriosis, in that these cycle components were not responsive to PKA activation by 8-Br-cAMP treatment, resulting in persistence of a proliferative phenotype. The authors suggested that the increased proliferative potential of the eutopic endometrial stromal cells from endometriosis contributes to the establishment, survival, and proliferation of endometriosis lesions due to an inherent abnormality in the PKA pathway.

Protein kinase A has also been implicated in regulating the steroidogenic acute regulatory protein (StAR), which is involved in the first committed step in the biosynthesis of steroids. StAR, which has been shown to be aberrantly expressed in endometriotic implants [71,72], was shown to be regulated by PGE_2, through EP2 receptor-coupled activation of PKA. Sun *et al* also found that regulation of StAR was independent of ERK [73].

Despite the small number of studies looking at PKA in endometriosis, the observations are consistent in that PKA response during decidualization of stromal cells is blunted in endometriosis and PKA mediates the aberrant expression of StAR, a critical protein for the biosynthesis of steroids. Further investigation is needed to explore why PKA signaling is altered in endometriosis.

Conclusion

It is evident that activation of signaling cascades is different in endometriosis compared to normal endometrium. Overall, studies demonstrate that the MAPK and AKT pathways are overactive in endometriotic cells and tissues and the PKA response is blunted during decidualization, resulting in increased cell proliferation, survival, cytokine production, and decreased differentiation. *In vitro* studies have shown that inhibition of MAPK or AKT can reverse these physiological effects.

The reasons for the heightened activation of MAPK and AKT are multifactorial. Microarray studies have identified genes associated with the MAPK, AKT, and PKA pathways to be aberrantly expressed in endometriosis. Thus, the tight regulation that the cell has in place for controlling these pathways is lost. Furthermore, ligands to the receptors that activate MAPK, AKT, and PKA, i.e. cytokines and estradiol, may be present in overabundance in endometriosis given that this disease is accompanied by increased inflammation and endometriotic tissues can synthesis estradiol through increased aromatase activity [2]. Perhaps the number of receptors that activate the signaling pathways is increased due to heightened synthesis or decreased turnover, although this has yet to be shown.

What we know thus far is that the MAPK and AKT pathways are overactive in endometriosis. As is the case for other diseases that exhibit kinase dependency, there is potential to use kinase inhibitors to combat endometriosis. Inhibitors of kinases that target signaling pathways are currently being explored for the treatment of many malignant conditions [11,74,76]. This has led to the development of kinase inhibitors that are currently being tested in clinical trials or are used in the clinic [77–81]. The very first small-molecule kinase inhibitor on the market was imatinib mesylate, also known as Gleevec, which has been effective in treating chronic myeloid leukemia [77]. In such instances where there is constitutive activation of kinases, due to gene mutations, kinase inhibitors are effective.

While it is unclear whether mutations are involved in the increased activities of MAPK and AKT in endometriosis, epigenetic changes in genes associated with the pathways may play a role. Evidence has supported the view that endometriosis is an epigenetic disease [82]. Given that endometriosis is accompanied by increased levels of inflammatory cytokines and estradiol, it is not inconceivable to think that prolonged exposure to such stimuli over the many years that a woman has endometriosis can cause epigenetic changes that contribute to kinase dependency. Perhaps the use of inhibitors to MAPK and AKT pathways as a mode of treatment for endometriosis is not as far-fetched as one may think. The studies reviewed here provide a strong rationale for further research into testing the efficacy of such inhibitors in endometriosis.

References

1. Giudice LC, Kao LC. Endometriosis. Lancet 2004;364(9447): 1789–1799.
2. Bulun SE. Endometriosis. N Engl J Med 2009;360(3):268–279.
3. Swiersz LM. Role of endometriosis in cancer and tumor development. Ann N Y Acad Sci 2002;955:281–292; discussion 93–95, 396–406.
4. Manning G, Whyte DB, Martinez R, Hunter T, Sudarsanam S. The protein kinase complement of the human genome. Science 2002;298(5600):1912–1934.
5. Chiaradonna F, Balestrieri C, Gaglio D, Vanoni M. RAS and PKA pathways in cancer: new insight from transcriptional analysis. Front Biosci 2008;13:5257–5278.
6. Gerits N, Kostenko S, Shiryaev A, Johannessen M, Moens U. Relations between the mitogen-activated protein kinase and the cAMP-dependent protein kinase pathways: comradeship and hostility. Cell Signal 2008;20(9):1592–1607.
7. Moelling K, Schad K, Bosse M, Zimmermann S, Schweneker M. Regulation of Raf-Akt Cross-talk. J Biol Chem 2002;277(34): 31099–1106.
8. Karnoub AE, Weinberg RA. Ras oncogenes: split personalities. Nat Rev Mol Cell Biol 2008;9(7):517–531.
9. Altomare DA, Testa JR. Perturbations of the AKT signaling pathway in human cancer. Oncogene 2005;24(50):7455–7464.
10. Hennessy BT, Smith DL, Ram PT, Lu Y, Mills GB. Exploiting the PI3K/ AKT pathway for cancer drug discovery. Nat Rev Drug Discov 2005;4(12):988–1004.
11. Steelman LS, Stadelman KM, Chappell WH et al. Akt as a therapeutic target in cancer. Expert Opin Ther Targets 2008;12(9):1139–1165.
12. Datta SR, Brunet A, Greenberg ME. Cellular survival: a play in three Akts. Genes Dev 1999;13(22):2905–2927.
13. Bhaskar PT, Hay N. The two TORCs and Akt. Dev Cell 2007;12(4):487–502.
14. Brazil DP, Yang ZZ, Hemmings BA. Advances in protein kinase B signalling: AKTion on multiple fronts. Trends Biochem Sci 2004;29(5): 233–242.
15. Hay N. The Akt-mTOR tango and its relevance to cancer. Cancer Cell 2005;8(3):179–183.
16. Lawlor MA, Alessi DR. PKB/Akt: a key mediator of cell proliferation, survival and insulin responses? J Cell Sci 2001;114(Pt 16): 2903–2910.
17. Yagyu T, Tsuji Y, Haruta S et al. Activation of mammalian target of rapamycin in postmenopausal ovarian endometriosis. Int J Gynecol Cancer 2006;16(4):1545–1551.
18. Laudanski P, Szamatowicz J, Kowalczuk O, Kuzmicki M, Grabowicz M, Chyczewski L. Expression of selected tumor suppressor and oncogenes in endometrium of women with endometriosis. Hum Reprod 2009;24(8):1880–1890.
19. Honda H, Barrueto FF, Gogusev J, Im DD, Morin PJ. Serial analysis of gene expression reveals differential expression between endometriosis and normal endometrium. Possible roles for AXL and SHC1 in the pathogenesis of endometriosis. Reprod Biol Endocrinol 2008; 6:59.
20. Cinar O, Seval Y, Uz YH et al. Differential regulation of Akt phosphorylation in endometriosis. Reprod Biomed Online 2009;19(6): 864–871.
21. Risinger JI, Hayes AK, Berchuck A, Barrett JC. PTEN/MMAC1 mutations in endometrial cancers. Cancer Res 1997;57(21):4736–4738.
22. Hecht JL, Mutter GL. Molecular and pathologic aspects of endometrial carcinogenesis. J Clin Oncol 2006;24(29):4783–4791.
23. Treloar SA, Zhao ZZ, Le L et al. Variants in EMX2 and PTEN do not contribute to risk of endometriosis. Mol Hum Reprod 2007;13(8): 587–594.
24. Ali-Fehmi R, Khalifeh I, Bandyopadhyay S et al. Patterns of loss of heterozygosity at 10q23.3 and microsatellite instability in endometriosis, atypical endometriosis, and ovarian carcinoma arising in association with endometriosis. Int J Gynecol Pathol 2006;25(3): 223–229.
25. Zhang H, Zhao X, Liu S, Li J, Wen Z, Li M. 17betaE2 promotes cell proliferation in endometriosis by decreasing PTEN via NFkappaB-dependent pathway. Mol Cell Endocrinol 2010;317(1–2):31–43.
26. Podsypanina K, Ellenson LH, Nemes A et al. Mutation of Pten/ Mmac1 in mice causes neoplasia in multiple organ systems. Proc Natl Acad Sci USA 1999;96(4):1563–1568.

27. Daikoku T, Hirota Y, Tranguch S et al. Conditional loss of uterine Pten unfailingly and rapidly induces endometrial cancer in mice. Cancer Res 2008;68(14):5619–5627.

28. Dinulescu DM, Ince TA, Quade BJ, Shafer SA, Crowley D, Jacks T. Role of K-ras and Pten in the development of mouse models of endometriosis and endometrioid ovarian cancer. Nat Med 2005;11(1):63–70.

29. Cheng YH, Imir A, Fenkci V, Yilmaz MB, Bulun SE. Stromal cells of endometriosis fail to produce paracrine factors that induce epithelial 17beta-hydroxysteroid dehydrogenase type 2 gene and its transcriptional regulator Sp1: a mechanism for defective estradiol metabolism. Am J Obstet Gynecol 2007;196(4):391.

30. Cheng YH, Imir A, Suzuki T et al. SP1 and SP3 mediate progesterone-dependent induction of the 17beta hydroxysteroid dehydrogenase type 2 gene in human endometrium. Biol Reprod 2006;75(4):605–614.

31. Florio P, Rossi M, Sigurdardottir M et al. Paracrine regulation of endometrial function: interaction between progesterone and corticotropin-releasing factor (CRF) and activin A. Steroids 2003;68(10–13):801–807.

32. Yang S, Fang Z, Gurates B et al. Stromal PRs mediate induction of 17beta-hydroxysteroid dehydrogenase type 2 expression in human endometrial epithelium: a paracrine mechanism for inactivation of E2. Mol Endocrinol 2001;15(12):2093–2105.

33. Franco HL, Jeong JW, Tsai SY, Lydon JP, DeMayo FJ. In vivo analysis of progesterone receptor action in the uterus during embryo implantation. Semin Cell Dev Biol 2008;19(2):178–186.

34. Kurihara I, Lee DK, Petit FG et al. COUP-TFII mediates progesterone regulation of uterine implantation by controlling ER activity. PLoS Genet 2007;3(6):e102.

35. Rubel CA, Jeong JW, Tsai SY, Lydon JP, DeMayo FJ. Epithelial-stromal interaction and progesterone receptors in the mouse uterus. Semin Reprod Med 2010;28(1):27–35.

36. Simon L, Spiewak KA, Ekman GC et al. Stromal progesterone receptors mediate induction of Indian Hedgehog (IHH) in uterine epithelium and its downstream targets in uterine stroma. Endocrinology 2009;150(8):3871–3876.

37. Cunha GR, Cooke PS, Kurita T. Role of stromal-epithelial interactions in hormonal responses. Arch Histol Cytol 2004;67(5):417–434.

38. Kurita T, Cooke PS, Cunha GR. Epithelial-stromal tissue interaction in paramesonephric (Mullerian) epithelial differentiation. Dev Biol 2001;240(1):194–211.

39. Kurita T, Medina R, Schabel AB et al. The activation function-1 domain of estrogen receptor alpha in uterine stromal cells is required for mouse but not human uterine epithelial response to estrogen. Differentiation 2005;73(6):313–322.

40. Kurita T, Wang YZ, Donjacour AA et al. Paracrine regulation of apoptosis by steroid hormones in the male and female reproductive system. Cell Death Differ 2001;8(2):192–200.

41. Bulun SE, Cheng YH, Pavone ME et al. 17Beta-hydroxysteroid dehydrogenase-2 deficiency and progesterone resistance in endometriosis. Semin Reprod Med 2010;28(1):44–50.

42. Zhang H, Li M, Zheng X, Sun Y, Wen Z, Zhao X. Endometriotic stromal cells lose the ability to regulate cell-survival signaling in endometrial epithelial cells in vitro. Mol Hum Reprod 2009;15(10):653–663.

43. Rubinfeld H, Seger R. The ERK cascade: a prototype of MAPK signaling. Mol Biotechnol 2005;31(2):151–174.

44. Cobb MH. MAP kinase pathways. Prog Biophys Mol Biol 1999;71(3–4):479–500.

45. Bodart JF. Extracellular-regulated kinase-mitogen-activated protein kinase cascade: unsolved issues. J Cell Biochem 2010;109(5):850–857.

46. Matsuzaki S, Canis M, Vaurs-Barriere C, Boespflug-Tanguy O, Dastugue B, Mage G. DNA microarray analysis of gene expression in eutopic endometrium from patients with deep endometriosis using laser capture microdissection. Fertil Steril 2005;84(Suppl 2):1180–1190.

47. Matsuzaki S, Canis M, Pouly JL, Botchorishvili R, Dechelotte PJ, Mage G. Differential expression of genes in eutopic and ectopic endometrium from patients with ovarian endometriosis. Fertil Steril 2006;86(3):548–553.

48. Wu Y, Kajdacsy-Balla A, Strawn E et al. Transcriptional characterizations of differences between eutopic and ectopic endometrium. Endocrinology 2006;147(1):232–246.

49. Burney RO, Talbi S, Hamilton AE et al. Gene expression analysis of endometrium reveals progesterone resistance and candidate susceptibility genes in women with endometriosis. Endocrinology 2007;148(8):3814–3826.

50. Velarde MC, Aghajanova L, Nezhat CR, Giudice LC. Increased mitogen-activated protein kinase kinase/extracellularly regulated kinase activity in human endometrial stromal fibroblasts of women with endometriosis reduces 3′,5′-cyclic adenosine 5′-monophosphate inhibition of cyclin D1. Endocrinology 2009;150(10):4701–4712.

51. Gazvani MR, Christmas S, Quenby S, Kirwan J, Johnson PM, Kingsland CR. Peritoneal fluid concentrations of interleukin-8 in women with endometriosis: relationship to stage of disease. Hum Reprod 1998;13(7):1957–1961.

52. Harada T, Yoshioka H, Yoshida S et al. Increased interleukin-6 levels in peritoneal fluid of infertile patients with active endometriosis. Am J Obstet Gynecol 1997;176(3):593–597.

53. Pizzo A, Salmeri FM, Ardita FV, Sofo V, Tripepi M, Marsico S. Behaviour of cytokine levels in serum and peritoneal fluid of women with endometriosis. Gynecol Obstet Invest 2002;54(2):82–87.

54. Ryan IP, Tseng JF, Schriock ED, Khorram O, Landers DV, Taylor RN. Interleukin-8 concentrations are elevated in peritoneal fluid of women with endometriosis. Fertil Steril 1995;63(4):929–932.

55. Yoshino O, Osuga Y, Hirota Y et al. Possible pathophysiological roles of mitogen-activated protein kinases (MAPKs) in endometriosis. Am J Reprod Immunol 2004;52(5):306–311.

56. Yamauchi N, Harada T, Taniguchi F, Yoshida S, Iwabe T, Terakawa N. Tumor necrosis factor-alpha induced the release of interleukin-6 from endometriotic stromal cells by the nuclear factor-kappaB and mitogen-activated protein kinase pathways. Fertil Steril 2004;82(Suppl 3):1023–1028.

57. Taniguchi F, Harada T, Miyakoda H et al. TAK1 activation for cytokine synthesis and proliferation of endometriotic cells. Mol Cell Endocrinol 2009;307(1–2):196–204.

58. Srivastava AK, Qin X, Wedhas N et al. Tumor necrosis factor-alpha augments matrix metalloproteinase-9 production in skeletal muscle

cells through the activation of transforming growth factor-beta-activated kinase 1 (TAK1)-dependent signaling pathway. J Biol Chem 2007;282(48):35113–35124.

59. Hirota Y, Osuga Y, Hirata T et al. Activation of protease-activated receptor 2 stimulates proliferation and interleukin (IL)-6 and IL-8 secretion of endometriotic stromal cells. Hum Reprod 2005;20(12): 3547–3553.

60. Grund EM, Kagan D, Tran CA et al. Tumor necrosis factor-alpha regulates inflammatory and mesenchymal responses via mitogen-activated protein kinase kinase, p38, and nuclear factor kappaB in human endometriotic epithelial cells. Mol Pharmacol 2008;73(5): 1394–1404.

61. Tagashira Y, Taniguchi F, Harada T, Ikeda A, Watanabe A, Terakawa N. Interleukin-10 attenuates TNF-alpha-induced interleukin-6 production in endometriotic stromal cells. Fertil Steril 2009;91(5 Suppl):2185–2192.

62. Moore KW, de Waal Malefyt R, Coffman RL, O'Garra A. Interleukin-10 and the interleukin-10 receptor. Annu Rev Immunol 2001;19: 683–765.

63. Bogdan C, Vodovotz Y, Nathan C. Macrophage deactivation by interleukin 10. J Exp Med 1991;174(6):1549–1555.

64. Gellersen B, Brosens J. Cyclic AMP and progesterone receptor crosstalk in human endometrium: a decidualizing affair. J Endocrinol 2003;178(3):357–372.

65. Frank GR, Brar AK, Cedars MI, Handwerger S. Prostaglandin E2 enhances human endometrial stromal cell differentiation. Endocrinology 1994;134(1):258–263.

66. Carli C, Metz CN, Al-Abed Y, Naccache PH, Akoum A. Up-regulation of cyclooxygenase-2 expression and prostaglandin E2 production in human endometriotic cells by macrophage migration inhibitory factor: involvement of novel kinase signaling pathways. Endocrinology 2009;150(7):3128–3137.

67. Wu MH, Wang CA, Lin CC, Chen LC, Chang WC, Tsai SJ. Distinct regulation of cyclooxygenase-2 by interleukin-1beta in normal and endometriotic stromal cells. J Clin Endocrinol Metab 2005;90(1): 286–295.

68. Aghajanova L, Hamilton A, Kwintkiewicz J, Vo KC, Giudice LC. Steroidogenic enzyme and key decidualization marker dysregulation in endometrial stromal cells from women with versus without endometriosis. Biol Reprod 2009;80(1):105–114.

69. Aghajanova L, Horcajadas JA, Weeks JL et al. The protein kinase a pathway-regulated transcriptome of endometrial stromal fibroblasts reveals compromised differentiation and persistent proliferative potential in endometriosis. Endocrinology 2010;151(3):1341–1355.

70. Klemmt PA, Carver JG, Kennedy SH, Koninckx PR, Mardon HJ. Stromal cells from endometriotic lesions and endometrium from women with endometriosis have reduced decidualization capacity. Fertil Steril 2006;85(3):564–572.

71. Tian Y, Kong B, Zhu W, Su S, Kan Y. Expression of steroidogenic factor 1 (SF-1) and steroidogenic acute regulatory protein (StAR) in endometriosis is associated with endometriosis severity. J Int Med Res2009;37(5):1389–1395.

72. Attar E, Tokunaga H, Imir G et al. Prostaglandin E2 via steroidogenic factor-1 coordinately regulates transcription of steroidogenic genes necessary for estrogen synthesis in endometriosis. J Clin Endocrinol Metab 2009;94(2):623–631.

73. Sun HS, Hsiao KY, Hsu CC, Wu MH, Tsai SJ. Transactivation of steroidogenic acute regulatory protein in human endometriotic stromal-cells is mediated by the prostaglandin EP2 receptor. Endocrinology 2003;144(9):3934–3942.

74. Kim LC, Song L, Haura EB. Src kinases as therapeutic targets for cancer. Nat Rev Clin Oncol 2009;6(10):587–595.

75. McCubrey JA, Steelman LS, Abrams SL et al. Emerging Raf inhibitors. Expert Opin Emerg Drugs 2009;14(4):633–648.

76. McCubrey JA, Steelman LS, Franklin RA et al. Targeting the RAF/MEK/ERK, PI3K/AKT and p53 pathways in hematopoietic drug resistance. Adv Enzyme Regul 2007;47:64–103.

77. Druker BJ. STI571 (Gleevec) as a paradigm for cancer therapy. Trends Mol Med 2002;8(4 Suppl):S14–18.

78. Becker J. Signal transduction inhibitors – a work in progress. Nat Biotechnol 2004;22(1):15–18.

79. Carter CA, Kelly RJ, Giaccone G. Small-molecule inhibitors of the human epidermal receptor family. Expert Opin Invest Drugs 2009;18(12): 1829–1842.

80. Castaneda CA, Gomez HL. Pazopanib: an antiangiogenic drug in perspective. Future Oncol 2009;5(9):1335–1348.

81. Lane HA, Breuleux M. Optimal targeting of the mTORC1 kinase in human cancer. Curr Opin Cell Biol 2009;21(2):219–229.

82. Guo SW. Epigenetics of endometriosis. Mol Hum Reprod 2009;15(10): 587–607.

17 MicroRNAs in Endometriosis

M. Louise Hull[1] and Cristin G. Print[2]

[1]Research Centre for Reproductive Health, School of Paediatrics and Reproductive Health, University of Adelaide, Adelaide, Australia
[2]Department of Molecular Medicine and Pathology, and New Zealand Bioinformatics Institute, University of Auckland, Auckland, New Zealand

Introduction

A major barrier to the development of diagnostic and therapeutic tools for endometriosis is our poor understanding of the pathophysiology of this disease. Sampson's theory of retrograde menstruation is the most widely followed, proposing that endometriosis arises from endometrial fragments in menstrual fluid that pass retrogradely through the fallopian tubes into the pelvic cavity, where they attach and grow at an ectopic site [1]. Genetic factors and an estrogenic hormonal milieu augment the risk of developing endometriosis. There is increasing evidence that epigenetic mechanisms such as microRNAs (miRNAs) play important roles in the pathogenesis of this disease [2].

Microarray analyses of the messenger RNA (mRNA) profile of endometriosis have advanced our understanding of the endometriotic disease process. Comparisons of paired eutopic (that lines the endometrial cavity) and ectopic (endometriotic) endometrium reveal patterns of mRNA transcripts that provide an insight into the cellular processes unique to ectopic endometrium. Functional bio-informatic analyses of the ectopic transcriptome indicate that cell adhesion, inflammation, immune system regulation, cell migration, proliferation, extracellular matrix remodelling, and angiogenesis contribute to endometriotic disease [3–8].

Human endometrial samples only represent the moment in time when they were obtained so animal models are needed to ascertain longitudinal endometriotic lesion development. Data from microarray analyses of ectopic endometrial lesions from rodent models of endometriosis concord closely with mRNA profiles obtained from human endometriotic tissues [4,9]. These animal models have been used to formulate a new understanding of endometriotic lesion development. Displaced endometrial tissue in retrograde menstrual fluid is likely to progress through attachment, hypoxia, tissue degradation, acute inflammation, macrophage infiltration, tissue remodeling, neovascularization, neurogenesis and fibrosis, in order to become established at an ectopic site (Plate 17.1) [4,10].

Messenger RNA data only portray part of the complexity of endometriotic disease. In mRNA microarray studies, endometriosis-associated mRNA profiles display a high degree of individual variation. Furthermore, the power to detect endometriosis-associated mRNA expression patterns is low as only small numbers of individual women have been included in most published studies. Bio-informatic meta-analyses of multiple mRNA microarray studies comparing eutopic with ectopic endometrium reveal considerable variation between studies in the lists of mRNAs that were differentially expressed, but remarkable concordance between studies in the functional profiles of the proteins encoded by these mRNAs [11].

Although microarray studies have proved to be powerful and productive tools for investigating endometriosis, they are subject to numerous technical constraints. For example, in mRNA microarray studies involving small numbers of subjects, only large changes in mRNA abundance are readily detected. Small changes in mRNA abundance may not be detected but if they encode transcription or growth factors, may have a profound effect on cell function and cell fate. Additionally, Wren *et al* found a mismatch between mRNA abundance and protein activity in an *in silico* analysis of endometriosis [12], raising the possibility that epigenetic regulatory mechanisms and post-translational modifications may contribute to the disease process.

Epigenetic mechanisms alter mRNA abundance without altering the gene sequence and there is evidence that DNA methylation, histone modification and miRNAs may all contribute to the pathophysiology of endometriosis [13]. miRNAs are 19–22 nucleotide (nt) non-coding RNA sequences specifically binding to target mRNAs, repressing their translation into proteins. The first microRNAs were discovered in 1993, and since then there has been a rapid increase in our understanding of their role in physiological and pathological processes [2]. The number of microRNAs that have been identified has also risen dramatically and in the April 2010 release of the web-based microRNA registry, miRBase, 14,197 microRNAs had been registered in 115 species, 940 of which are present in *homo sapiens*. It has become clear that microRNAs are important, evolutionarily conserved, epigenetic regulators of gene expression.

The microRNA profile of ectopic tissues is different from that in the eutopic endometrium from women with endometriosis [14–16]. Furthermore, endometriosis-associated miRNAs have been identified in eutopic endometrial tissues [17]. This chapter will provide an overview of the current literature in the field of miRNAs in endometriosis. Postulations regarding the role of miRNAs in pathogeneic endometriosis and possible future diagnostic and therapeutic applications of endometriosis-associated miRNAs will also be discussed.

Studies exploring microRNA expression profiles in endometriosis

At the time of writing, there are four published original papers that have explored the expression profiles of miRNAs in endometriosis (Table 17.1) [14–17]. The first study that utilized deep sequencing techniques to explore miRNAs in endometrial tissues including endometriosis has also been published [18].

Eutopic versus ectopic analyses

Pan *et al* described a miRNA microarray comparison of four eutopic endometrial tissues from endometriosis-free volunteers, four paired eutopic and ectopic endometrial samples, and four additional unpaired ectopic endometrial tissue samples [14]. Although no direct comparisons were made of eutopic and ectopic endometrial tissues, a three-way ANOVA analysis revealed 48 miRNAs that were predominantly downregulated in endometriotic lesions in comparison to eutopic control tissue. Quantitative real-time-polymerase chain reaction (RT-PCR) was used to assess differential regulation of seven miRNAs because they targeted the endometriosis-associated genes for the transforming growth factor-β receptor 2 (TGF-βR2), estrogen receptor-α (ERα), estrogen receptor-β (ERβ) and the progesterone receptor (PR). In this study, only hsa-miR21, hsa-miR26a, and hsa-miR142–5p were confirmed as dysregulated in eutopic and ectopic endometrial tissues.

Our group was the first to perform a miRNA microarray analysis that directly compared paired eutopic and ectopic endometrium from seven women [15]. Fourteen miRNAs were upregulated, eight were downregulated in endometriosis with a cut-off fold change of ≥1.5 and $P \leq 0.05$, which was confirmed by quantitative RT-PCR for six transcripts (three up- and three downregulated) in eight women. Putative mRNA targets of these differentially abundant miRNAs were identified using the Pictar and TargetScan *in silico* target prediction tools. Functional information was obtained using a list of mRNAs (n = 673) that were both predicted targets of these miRNAs and shown to be

Table 17.1 MicroRNA microarray studies in endometriosis.

Study	Type of tissue studied (number in each group) *Phase of cycle*	Array type	Number of gene probes on array	Functional analysis	Upregulated in endometriosis	Downregulated in endometriosis	RT-PCR
Eutopic versus ectopic endometrium							
Pan *et al* 2007 [14]	Eutopic non-endometriosis (4) Eutopic endometriosis (4) Unpaired ectopic (4) *Early to mid secretory phase*	mirVana miRNA Bioarray Slides	287		0	48	2 validated in same 4 ectopic and 8 eutopic tissue samples
Ohlsson Teague *et al* 2008 [15]	Eutopic endometriosis (7) Paired ectopic (7) *All stages of menstrual cycle*	Custom-made mirVana miRNA microarrays	377	IPA GOSTAT	14	8	8 validated in 8 patients (paired samples)
Filigheddu *et al* 2010 [16]	Eutopic endometriosis (3) Paired ectopic (3) *Proliferative phase*	μParaflo microfluidic chip	475	IPA FatiGO Kegg pathway analysis	27	23	5 validated in 13 patients (paired samples)
Eutopic control versus eutopic endometriosis endometrium							
Burney *et al* 2009 [17]	Eutopic control (3) Eutopic endometriosis (4) *Early secretory phase*	miRCURY™ LNA Array	1488	IPA	0	6	3 validated (out of 4 tested) in same 7 tissue samples

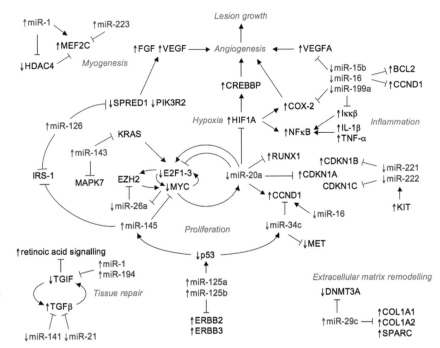

Figure 17.1 MicroRNA regulatory networks in endometriosis. Regulatory networks of differentially expressed miRNAs and their experimentally confirmed mRNA targets associated with endometriosis in the literature. Upregulated (″) and downregulated (#) miRNA and target mRNA/protein. The gene names in these networks are identified on the HUGO Gene Nomenclature Committee home page (www.genenames.org). Reproduced from Ohlsson-Teague et al [2] with permission from Oxford University Press.

differentially expressed in endometriosis in two independent mRNA microarray analyses [4,6]. These putative mRNA targets appeared to constitute 12 molecular networks driving cellular functions including cell death; connective tissue development, nervous and muscular system development and function; cellular movement; cell proliferation and the cell cycle; angiogenesis and reproductive/endocrine system disorders.

A similar miRNA microarray study directly compared proliferative stage eutopic and ectopic endometrium from three women [16]. Fifty miRNAs were dysregulated with a more than two-fold change ($P < 0.01$) in endometriosis (27 upregulated and 23 downregulated). The microarray findings were confirmed by RT-PCR for five miRNAs in 13 women. The TargetScan and PictarVERT methods predicted 3093 mRNA targets as being regulated by these miRNAs, which constituted 49 functional networks associated with endometriosis. Functional annotations included gene expression, cellular growth and proliferation, cellular development, cellular movement, cell death, cell cycle, cancer, and reproductive system disorders. The endometriosis subcategory of reproductive system disorders was over-represented in the data ($P = 6.1 \times 10^{-18}$) with 119 transcripts predicted to be regulated by miRNAs in this category.

There is considerable concordance between the three microarray studies in the identification of endometriosis-associated miRNAs (Fig. 17.1) [14–16]. Six miRNAs have been identified in all three studies (Box 17.1) and three of these (miR-145, miR-99a, and miR-126) have been validated by RT-PCR [15]. The 13 miRNAs that were present in both Ohsson Teague's and Filigheddu's miRNA lists were differentially expressed in the same direction (nine upregulated and four downregulated). However, in Pan's study, the direction of regulation (up or down) was discordant for all miRNAs except miR-17–5p, which was also downregulated in

Filigheddu's study. Sixty percent of the miRNAs identified in our analysis were concordant with Filigheddu's and 36% with Pan's analysis [15] (Fig. 17.2) (see Box 17.1).

Any differences seen between miRNA lists are likely to be due to the numbers of patients sampled, the menstrual cycle stage of sampling, the number and type of statistical methods used and the level of conservatism in determining fold change and P value cut-offs. However, the high correlation between the miRNA lists does indicate that these findings are likely to be

Box 17.1 Endometriosis-associated microRNAs that concur between studies

Present in Pan, Ohlsson Teague and Filigheddu	Present in Ohlsson Teague and Filigheddu only	
Upregulated*	*Upregulated*	*Downregulated*
miR-29c	miR-365	miR-200a[†]
miR-145[†]	miR-1	miR-200b[†]
miR-143[†]	miR-150	miR-20a
miR-99a[†]		miR-196b
miR-126[†]		
miR-100		

Present in Pan and Ohlsson Teague only	Present in Pan and Filigheddu only	
Upregulated*	*Upregulated**	*Downregulated*
miR-125a	miR199a	miR-17-5p[†]
miR-125b	miR-221	
	miR-30e-5p	

* Pan's study did not concur in the direction of regulation.
[†] Validated by RT-PCR.

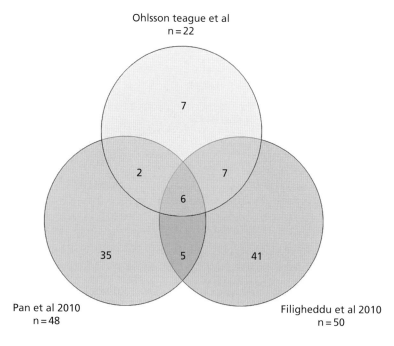

Ohlsson teague et al
n = 22

Pan et al 2010
n = 48

Filigheddu et al 2010
n = 50

Figure 17.2 A Venn diagram demonstrating the concurrence of miRNAs identified in the three microarray analyses of eutopic versus ectopic endometrium. Considerable overlap was demonstrated in the lists of endometriosis-associated miRNA from the Ohlsson Teague, Pan and Filigheddu papers. With one exception, all miRNAs from the Pan study did not concur in the direction of regulation with the other two analyses.

robust and suggests that a constant alteration of miRNA activity is associated with endometriosis.

Eutopic control versus eutopic endometriosis endometrium

Only one paper has compared eutopic endometrium from women with (n = 4) and without (n = 3) surgically diagnosed endometriosis [17]. Utilizing locked nucleic acid miRNA gene chips, six miRNAs were downregulated in the endometriosis-associated samples, which was confirmed by RT-PCR for three miRNAs (see Table 17.1). Two of these (miR-34b* and miR34c-5p) belong to the same broad category of miRNAs and regulate similar target genes. From this broad category, miR-34a was downregulated [16] and miR-34c upregulated [15] in eutopic endometrium compared to ectopic tissues from the same women.

In Burney's study [17], the TargetScan algorithm was used to predict target mRNAs of the dysregulated miRNAs and this list was cross-referenced to the list of dysregulated mRNAs in a large mRNA microarray study of eutopic endometrium from women with and without endometriosis. Both criteria were fulfilled by 156 mRNAs which were used to formulate *in silico* molecular networks postulated to participate in biological functions including cell death, cell cycle and cellular assembly and organization and the canonical pathways of molecular mechanisms of cancer, semaphorin signaling in neurons and cell cycle regulation.

Future studies using deep sequencing

There has been one paper that has used deep sequencing techniques to explore miRNAs in 13 different reproductive

tissues, including 10 endometriomas, 10 control eutopic and three eutopic endometriosis samples [18]. At this stage, Creighton's group has discovered seven confirmed and 51 confidently predicted novel miRNAs in the entire tissue database of 103 samples. It is likely that future comparisons will be made to identify differentially regulated miRNAs in endometriosis-associated tissue types and extensive new information regarding endometriosis-associated miRNAs may become available.

The role of microRNAs in endometriotic lesion development: a model

A comparison of eutopic and ectopic endometrium from the same women provides information regarding pathophysiological events unique to endometriosis. Molecular pathways revealed by web applications such as Gene Ontology and Ingenuity Pathway Analysis are likely to be both important in the endometriotic disease process and manipulable by iatrogenically introduced miRNAs (see Fig. 17.1). An *in silico* model of miRNA regulation in endometriosis was developed based only on endometriosis-associated miRNA/mRNA interactions previously validated by the luciferase assay (see Plate 17.1 and Fig. 17.1). As miRNA regulation of target transcripts has never been evaluated in endometrial cell lines, this model remains speculative and would be expected to oversimplify the complex inter-relationships between miRNAs, transcription factors and other epigenetic mechanisms that regulate gene expression and protein production in endometriosis. Nevertheless, this model is likely to be useful for providing specific hypotheses and determining the research directions in this complex field (see Plate 17.1).

Hypoxic injury

Hypoxia-induced factor-α (HIF-1α) activity appears to be upregulated in endometriotic lesions [19] and in a mouse model of endometriosis, ectopic endometrial lesions displayed markers of hypoxia early in development [20]. Hypoxia-induced responses appear to require finely tuned miRNA regulation in endometriosis, as several endometriosis-associated miRNAs control transcripts from HIF-1α pathways.

Hypoxia-induced factor-α is inhibited by miR-20a [21] which is downregulated in ectopic endometrial tissues, potentially contributing to HIF-1α's up-regulation. The CREB binding protein (CREBBP), a co-factor that enhances HIF-1α activity, is central to miRNA regulated molecular networks [15,16] and is found at high levels in endometriotic tissues [4]. Increased CREBBP mRNA levels may be the result of reduced miR-200b repression as this predicted regulator of CREBBP was found at low levels in endometriotic tissues [15,16].

Inflammation

The inflammatory modulators interleukin-1β (IL-1β) and tumor necrosis factor-α (TNF-α) activate nuclear factor κ B (NFκB), which in turn upregulates other factors including HIF-1α and cyclo-oxygenase (COX)-2 [22]. IL-1β, TNF-α [23], NFκB [24], HIF-1α [19] and COX-2 [25] are all found at high levels in endometriotic lesions, and inhibition of TNF-α [26] and COX-2 [27] has been shown to suppress endometriosis-like lesion development in primate and rodent models of endometriosis. A number of miRNAs that were differentially expressed in endometriosis were predicted to target members of this pathway. Furthermore, several miRNA-regulated molecular networks featured TNF-α, NFκB, its co-factor IκB and COX-2 [15,16]. miRNAs are therefore likely to 'fine tune' the critical effects of this proinflammatory pathway in endometriosis.

Cyclo-oxygenase 2 translation is suppressed by miR-199a* and miR-16 [28,29] and both of these miRNAs were downregulated in endometriosis [14]. miR-199a also negatively regulates IκB kinase-b (IκBKB), a co-factor required for NFκB activation [30]. Reduced expression of miR-199a and miR-16 in endometriosis is likely to enhance COX-2 protein production, resulting in enhanced prostaglandin production [31], neo-angiogenesis [32] and activation of the aromatase/COX-2 feedforward loop, leading to enhanced local estrogen levels [33].

Tissue repair and transforming growth factor-β-regulated pathways

Women with endometriosis have higher levels of TGF-β in their peritoneal fluid [34,35], serum [35] and ectopic endometrium in comparison to eutopic tissues [36]. TGF-β was a central component of several molecular networks identified in different endometriosis mRNA microarray studies [4,8]. Moreover, a deficiency of host-derived TGF-β1 led to a reduction in ectopic endometrial lesion size in a *tgfb-/-* null mutant mouse model of endometriosis [37] (unpublished data). It appears that TGF-β1 is critical to the normal development of endometriosis-like lesions and is likely to be highly controlled by miRNAs.

Several miRNAs that fine-tune TGF-β's bio-availability and signaling were altered in endometriosis. miR-200b, miR200c [15,16], miR-141 [15] and miR-21 [14] were downregulated in endometriotic tissues. Luciferase reporter assays have confirmed that miR-141 and miR-200c repress TGF-β2 and modulate TGF-β signaling pathways in cancer cell lines [38]. MiR-21 has also been experimentally confirmed to suppress TGF-β1.

Transforming growth factor-β signaling induces the transcription of TGF-β-induced factor (TGIF), which inhibits TGF-β transcription in a negative feedback loop [39]. miR-1 and miR-194 are both upregulated in endometriotic tissues [15] and predicted to suppress TGIF translation and therefore enhance TGF-β activity (see Plate 17.1). In microarray studies, TGIF mRNA transcripts were downregulated [4] and TGF-β signaling pathways augmented [15], suggesting a role for miR-1 and miR-194 in elevated TGF-β signaling in endometriosis.

In summary, downregulation of the TGF-β repressors, miR-141, miR-200b, miR-200c and miR-21 and upregulation of the miRNAs that suppress TGIF (miR-1 and miR-194) appear to enhance TGF-β activity in endometriosis.

Cell proliferation

Cellular proliferation appears to be important at least in the early stages of endometriotic lesion development as mouse models of endometriosis have revealed elevated numbers of mitotic cells [4] and high levels of the cellular proliferation marker ki-67 [40] in ectopic endometrial tissues. In contrast, Jones *et al* demonstrated a low proliferative index in endometriotic tissues, independent of menstrual cycle stage [41]. One reason for this discrepancy may be that there are tight regulatory control mechanisms that suppress uncontrolled cellular division as the lesion matures.

Many of the endometriosis-associated miRNAs that target mediators of cell proliferation are known to be differentially expressed in cancer [2]. However, the direction of their over- or underexpression in cancer is opposite to that seen in endometriosis. For example, v-erb-b2 erythroblastic leukemia viral oncogene homolog (ERBB) 2 and ERBB3 are oncogenes targeted by miR-125a and miR125b [42]. ERBB2 and ERBB3's oncogenic activity appears to be enhanced by low levels of miR-125a and miR-125b in ovarian endometrioid cancers [43], whereas in endometriosis, these two miRNAs are upregulated and are likely to repress ERBB2 and ERBB3 activity.

In endometriosis, miRNAs that control oncogenic proteins are abundant and likely to control cell growth. miRNA mir-143 is present at high levels in endometriosis and inhibits cell proliferation by suppression of mitogen-activated protein kinase 7 (MAPK7) [44] and v-Ki-ras2 Kirsten rat sarcoma viral oncogene homolog (KRAS) [45]. miR-126 and miR-145 [15,16] are also upregulated in endometriosis and repress insulin receptor substrate-1 (IRS1), a factor that promotes mitogenesis and cell proliferation [46].

Another mechanism of cell cycle control present in endometriosis appears to be the downregulation of miR-20a, miR-221 and miR-222 which target the cell cycle repressors cyclin-dependent kinase inhibitor 1A (CDKN1A/p21) [47], CDKN1B(p27) [48] and CDKN1C (p57) [49] respectively. These three miRNAs were identified at low levels [14–16] whereas their transcript targets were upregulated in endometriosis [4,50], enhancing their control of cellular proliferation.

Messenger RNA microarray studies of endometriosis have revealed an upregulation of tumor suppressor genes and a down-regulation of mRNAs associated with the cell cycle progression [3] and this is likely to be enhanced by microRNA activity in endometriotic lesions. We hypothesize that cellular proliferation is increased early in endometriotic lesion development, but is highly controlled by suppressors of the cell cycle. This mechanism would permit the cell division required to establish an endometriotic lesion but ensure that progression to malignancy was a rare event [51].

Extracellular matrix remodeling

In endometrial tissue, the extracellular matrix provides scaffolding and structure for proliferating glandular and stromal cells. Additionally, the extracellular matrix framework provides a surface for anchorage for migrating host-derived macrophages and myofibroblasts that infiltrate the lesion [52]. mRNA microarray studies have demonstated an overexpression of several extracellular matrix proteins including COL1A1 [4,6], COL1A2 [6], COL3A1, COL15A1 [5] and secreted protein, acidic, cysteine-rich, osteonectin (SPARC) [4].

Three miRNA-regulated ingenuity pathway analysis (IPA) analysis networks incorporated COL1A1, COL1A2, COL3A1, COL15A1 and SPARC in both the Ohlsson Teague [15] and Filigheddu [16] studies. These extracellular matrix molecules are all regulated by miR-29c [53] which was consistently upregulated in endometriosis, suggesting tight control of extracellular matrix production.

Angiogenesis

Gross and microscopic neovascularization is characteristic of endometriosis, and angiogenic growth factors, including vascular endothelial growth factor (VEGF)-A, are found at high levels in peritoneal fluid [54] and ectopic lesions from women with endometriosis [55]. Antiangiogenic agents have been shown to inhibit ectopic endometrial lesion development in animal models [20,56].

Downregulation of miR-15b and miR-16m occurs in hypoxic conditions, releasing their repressive effect on VEGF-A transcription [57]. In endometriosis, increased expression of VEGF-A may therefore result from low levels of miR-15b and miR-16 [58]. Elevated levels of miR-126 in endometriosis are also likely to enhance VEGF activity [59] by relieving the negative inhibitory effect of downstream suppressors of the VEGF-A pathway [2,60]. Vascular endothelial cell migration may also be promoted by the upregulation of MiR-143 and miR-145 which enhance the contraction of vascular smooth muscle cells *in vitro* [61].

Four miRNAs (miR-145, miR-126, miR-24, and miR-23a) are consistently associated with the vascular fragment of several tissue types [62] and all these miRNAs were upregulated in endometriosis compared to control tissues [14–16]. Three other miRNAs (miR-20a [63], miR-143 and miR-145 [61]) that have previously been associated with angiogeneic activity were also differentially expressed in endometriosis (see Box 17.1). The direction of regulation in all seven angiogenesis-associated miRNAs would promote vascular development and increase oxygen delivery, improving the ability of endometrial tissue to survive at an ectopic site.

MicroRNAs and risk factors for endometriosis

Genetic inheritance and an enhanced estrogenic environment are risk factors for endometriosis [64], but the mode of their effect is poorly understood. There is increasing evidence that the effect of genetic inheritance and elevated estrogen activity in endometriosis is mediated, at least in part, by miRNAs.

MicroRNAs and genetic inheritance in endometriosis

Epidemiological twin [65] and familial trait analysis [66] studies have demonstrated a polygenic inheritance pattern for endometriosis. Candidate gene studies have analyzed at least 76 genetic variants, but none has shown a consistent and replicable association with endometriosis [67]. An affected sibling pair analysis was undertaken recruiting sibling pairs with laparoscopically diagnosed endometriosis [68]. In this analysis, highly polymorphic microsatellite markers were genotyped in the DNA of more than 900 familial endometriosis cases and a similar number of controls, covering a linkage distance of more than 90% of the genome [67]. There is evidence to support an endometriosis-associated genetic linkage to chromosomes 7 [69]. and 10 [68] but the genes in these regions that contribute to the risk of endometriosis have not been identified.

Several researchers have demonstrated that single nucleotide polymorphisms (SNPs) in non-coding miRNA gene sequences or in the miRNA promoter sites of transcript targets can be associated with malignant disease [70,71]. Zhao *et al* [72] evaluated 102 SNPs in the predicted binding sites of 22 miRNAs that were differentially regulated in endometriosis by genotyping SNPs in 958 endometriosis cases and 959 controls from the endometriosis-affected sibling pair analysis database. Initial findings showed that SNPs in miR-99b and miR-125a-3p binding sites were associated with endometriosis-associated infertility and more severe stage of disease. These findings are the first to raise the possibility that some women may have a genetic susceptibility to endometriosis that is mediated via altered miRNA regulation of mRNA translation.

MicroRNAs and estrogen regulation in endometriosis

Epidemiological studies [73] and studies in primate models of endometriosis [74] provide evidence that an estrogenic milieu enhances the development of endometriosis. Bulun proposed that an aberrant feedforward loop upregulated local estrogen production in endometriotic disease, promoting disease progression [33]. In this loop, estrogen upregulates COX-2, enhancing prostaglandin production which further increases aromatase activity and estradiol levels in the ectopic endometrial tissues.

There is growing evidence that estrogen's complex cellular activity is highly regulated by miRNAs [75], and estrogen response elements (EREs) have been identified in miRNA promoter sites [76]. In animal models [77] and human cell lines [75], estrogen exposure does alter miRNA profiles, but the degree and direction of dysregulation appear to be tissue and cell line specific [78].

Estrogen also appears to mediate miRNA dysregulation in human endometrial tissues [79]. Using laser capture microdissection, Kuokkanen et al isolated luminal and glandular epithelial cells from four eutopic endometrial samples from the estrogenic late follicular phase and four biopsies from the progestogen exposed, mid-secretory phase from eight healthy volunteers with regular menstrual cycles [79]. Twelve miRNAs were upregulated and 12 downregulated in the late proliferative phase. Three of these miRNAs were present in a gene network controlled by ERα (miR-222, miR30B, miR-30D), suggesting that at least some of estrogen's influence on miRNA activity in endometriosis is mediated through the ERα receptor [80].

According to Bulun's theory of enhanced local estrogen production, a profound and consistent estrogenic effect would be expected in ectopic tissues [33]. However, steroid-mediated fluctuations in eutopic endometrial miRNA levels would alter the differential in miRNA levels in comparisons of eutopic and ectopic endometrial tissues. This effect can be assessed in a limited way as Filigheddu's eutopic-ectopic endometrial comparison was in the follicular stage of the cycle [16] and Pan et al [14] used early to midsecretory samples. In endometriotic tissues, miR-29c was upregulated in Filigheddu's proliferative phase study but downregulated in Pan's secretory phase analysis. The difference in miR-29c levels in ectopic tissues could have been confounded by steroid-modulated miRNA changes in the eutopic endometrium, because miR-29c was downregulated in the estrogenic, late proliferative phase endometrium [79]. Similarly, in Pan's paper 30b and 30d were upregulated in eutopic secretory tissues [14] but were downregulated in secretory ectopic tissues [79], which could solely reflect eutopic endometrial changes. However, the direction of regulation was opposite to that expected if eutopic endometrial steroid changes had a significant influence on miR-222 [14] and miR-200c, miR-503and miR-376a [16].

The effect of miRNA activity on the feedforward loop involving aromatase and COX-2 was specifically explored by measuring their respective regulators, miR-23a/miR-23b and MiR-542–3p in eutopic and ectopic tissues by quantitative polymerase chain reaction (PCR) [81]. All these miRNAs were downregulated, which is likely to have contributed to the enhancement of aromatase and COX-2 mRNA levels in ectopic tissues. Steroidogenic acute regulatory protein (StAR) is the rate-limiting enzyme in steroid production in endometrial cells and is upregulated in endometriosis. This enzyme appears to have complex regulatory controls as the miRNA predicted to target this enzyme, miR-17–5p, was up- rather than downregulated [81].

Diagnostic and therapeutic potential of microRNAs

Development of microRNA-based diagnostic tests

There is a significant lag time between the onset of endometriosis-associated symptoms and the diagnosis of endometriosis [82]. This may be because laparoscopic evaluation of endometriosis is currently the only reliable method of diagnosis. Laparoscopic surgery is costly, invasive and has a 2% risk of injury to pelvic organs and a small risk of mortality [83]. However, the specificity of diagnostic laparoscopy is low and only 70–75% of visually diagnosed lesions are confirmed histologically [84]. Additionally, the need for a non-invasive diagnostic test for endometriosis has been recognized internationally [85] and many researchers have attempted to identify new diagnostic modalities for this disease.

MicroRNAs hold great promise as diagnostic markers for endometriosis [86]. They are not subject to rapid degradation by RNAses and miRNA profiles reflect both physiological and pathological conditions more accurately than mRNA abundance profiles [86]. The high sensitivity and specificity displayed by miRNA biomarkers in cancer detection [87] are reflected by commercially available plasma miRNA-based diagnostic tests for cancers (www.rosettagenomics.com). Cellular processes such as cell survival, proliferation and cell motility are regulated by miRNAs in a cell lineage-dependent manner [88] and are characteristic of both cancer and endometriosis. It is therefore likely that endometriosis has a distinct miRNA profile.

A semi-invasive miRNA-based test for endometriosis could be developed by analyzing eutopic endometrial biopsies obtained at an outpatient clinic visit. Women with endometriosis have an altered eutopic endometrial environment compared to disease-free women [89] and baboon studies indicate that this is a response to endometriotic lesion establishment [90]. Although most endometriosis-associated endometrial proteins lack the sensitivity and specificity required for a diagnostic test, a notable exception has been positive PGP 9.5 nerve fiber immunostaining, which appears to accurately identify women with endometriotic disease in initial studies [91].

The Burney et al study identified four miRNAs that were differentially regulated in eutopic endometrium from women with endometriosis and these could prove useful in a diagnostic test [17]. Further investigation is needed as only one time point in the menstrual cycle was assessed, the numbers of participants were small and demographic factors such as age and fibroid status may have confounded the data. This early paper does, however, raise the possibility of a reliable diagnostic test for endometriosis based on eutopic endometrial miRNA profiles.

An alternative strategy is to examine plasma miRNA expression profiles from women with endometriosis as there is increasing evidence that plasma miRNA profiles can reflect disease activity

[92]. The expression levels of eight miRNAs found in ovarian cancer tissues correlated strongly with their plasma miRNA levels [88], implying that the plasma miRNAs were derived from ovarian cancer tissues. When human prostate cells were implanted into immunocompromised mice, two human-specific miRNAs (miR-629 and miR 660) were detected at high levels in the plasma of xenografted but not in control mice [93]. It appears that miRNAs can be secreted from tissues into the bloodstream as these human miRNAs could only be derived from the implanted human cells. Using multiplex RT-PCR, we have isolated and measured plasma miRNAs from eight healthy women at three stages of the menstrual cycle, revealing that plasma miRNAs were minimally affected by menstrual cycle changes (unpublished data). If endometriosis-specific miRNAs can be identified in the plasma, a non-invasive diagnostic blood test could be developed for endometriosis.

Therapeutic applications of microRNAs

Antagonism and augmentation of miRNA activity have emerged as strategies for miRNA manipulation in the field of miRNA-based therapeutics. Antagomirs are synthetic single-stranded RNA oligonucleotides that form stable heteroduplexes with complementary miRNAs, preventing their suppression of target mRNA translation. For example, miR-122 suppresses several genes in the liver that metabolize cholesterol, leading to high levels of plasma cholesterol. When an antagomir complementary to miR-122 was administered to mice [94] and non-human primates [95], it hybridized to miR-122, resulting in the upregulation of more than 11 genes involved in cholesterol biosynthesis and a long-lasting dose-dependent lowering of plasma cholesterol levels.

Synthetic miRNAs have also been generated that increase the translational repression of cancer promoting genes involved in prostate, liver and lung cancer [96]. MiR-16 is found at low levels in prostate cancer, and therefore provides minimal suppression of its target genes which include cyclin D1 (CCND1), wingless-type MMTV integration site family, member 3A (WNT3A), and B-cell CLL/lymphoma 2 (BCL2), all of which are implicated in prostate cancer progression. Systemic administration of a synthetic miR-16 conjugated to atenocollagen, in a xenograft mouse model of prostate cancer, resulted in delivery of miR-16 to the xenograft tumors, downregulation of the miR-16 regulated genes and suppression of cancer growth [96]. The successful regulation of specific target mRNAs by antagomirs and synthetic miRNAs in several *in vivo* models raises the possibility that miRNA manipulation could alter events critical to endometriotic lesion development that are under miRNA regulatory control.

Before miRNA-based technologies become a realistic treatment for endometriotic disease, a considerable amount of work is required. Firstly, endometriosis-associated miRNAs and their mRNA targets have to be localized to cell lineages in endometriotic lesions. Cell cultures then need to be developed and screened for expression of miRNAs of interest and their target mRNAs. The luciferase assay can then be used to confirm miRNA regulation of

transcripts *in vitro*. An antagomir or synthetic miRNA will need to be developed and delivered in an appropriate vector to lesions in rodent and non-human models of endometriosis. Finally, the possibility of unacceptable 'off target' effects or the insertional mutagenesis of a viral vector has to be excluded before miRNA-based therapies can be trialled in humans.

Conclusion

MicroRNA regulation fine tunes the activity of important mediators of many diseases. There is now good evidence of a role for miRNAs in endometriotic disease. We are just beginning to understand the full impact of miRNA technology, but as our knowledge of miRNA function develops and the methodologies to explore miRNAs become more sophisticated *in vitro* and *in vivo*, it is possible that these small non-coding RNAs may become an important branch of our medical armamentarium for diseases such as endometriosis.

Referennces

1. Sampson JA. Peritoneal endometriosis due to menstrual dissemination of endometrial tissue into the peritoneal cavity. Am J Obstet Gynecol 1927;14:442–469.
2. Ohlsson Teague EM, Print CG, Hull ML. The role of microRNAs in endometriosis and associated reproductive conditions. Hum Reprod Update 2010;16(2):142–165.
3. Borghese B, Mondon F, Noel JC et al. Gene expression profile for ectopic versus eutopic endometrium provides new insights into endometriosis oncogenic potential. Mol Endocrinol 2008;22(11):2557–2562.
4. Hull ML, Escareno CR, Godsland JM et al. Endometrial-peritoneal interactions during endometriotic lesion establishment. Am J Pathol 2008;173(3):700–715.
5. Eyster KM, Klinkova O, Kennedy V, Hansen KA. Whole genome deoxyribonucleic acid microarray analysis of gene expression in ectopic versus eutopic endometrium. Fertil Steril 2007;88(6):1505–1533.
6. Hever A, Roth RB, Hevezi P et al. Human endometriosis is associated with plasma cells and overexpression of B lymphocyte stimulator. Proc Natl Acad Sci USA 2007;104(30):12451–12456.
7. Matsuzaki S, Canis M, Pouly JL, Botchorishvili R, Dechelotte PJ, Mage G. Differential expression of genes in eutopic and ectopic endometrium from patients with ovarian endometriosis. Fertil Steril 2006;86(3):548–553.
8. Arimoto T, Katagiri T, Oda K et al. Genome-wide cDNA microarray analysis of gene-expression profiles involved in ovarian endometriosis. Int J Oncol 2003;22(3):551–560.
9. Pelch KE, Schroder AL, Kimball PA, Sharpe-Timms KL, Davis JW, Nagel SC. Aberrant gene expression profile in a mouse model of endometriosis mirrors that observed in women. Fertil Steril 2010;93(5):1615–1627.
10. Flores I, Rivera E, Ruiz LA, Santiago OI, Vernon MW, Appleyard CB. Molecular profiling of experimental endometriosis identified gene

expression patterns in common with human disease. Fertil Steril 2007;87(5):1180–1199.

11. Lam EYN, Print C. ReproMine: generating a web-based platform for meta-analysis of microarray studies on reproductive disorders. Queenstown Reproductive Biology Conference, Queenstown, New Zealand, 2009.

12. Wren JD, Wu Y, Guo SW. A system-wide analysis of differentially expressed genes in ectopic and eutopic endometrium. Hum Reprod 2007;22(8):2093–2102.

13. Guo SW. Epigenetics of endometriosis. Mol Hum Reprod 2009;15(10):587–607.

14. Pan Q, Luo X, Toloubeydokhti T, Chegini N. The expression profile of micro-RNA in endometrium and endometriosis and the influence of ovarian steroids on their expression. Mol Hum Reprod 2007;13(11):797–806.

15. Ohlsson Teague EM, van der Hoek KH, van der Hoek MB et al. MicroRNA-regulated pathways associated with endometriosis. Mol Endocrinol 2009;23(2):265–275.

16. Filigheddu N, Gregnanin I, Porporato PE et al. Differential expression of microRNAs between eutopic and ectopic endometrium in ovarian endometriosis. J Biomed Biotechnol 2010;2010:369549.

17. Burney RO, Hamilton AE, Aghajanova L et al. MicroRNA expression profiling of eutopic secretory endometrium in women with versus without endometriosis. Mol Hum Reprod 2009;15(10):625–631.

18. Creighton CJ, Benham AL, Zhu H et al. Discovery of novel microRNAs in female reproductive tract using next generation sequencing. PLoS One 2010;5(3):e9637.

19. Goteri G, Lucarini G, Zizzi A et al. Proangiogenetic molecules, hypoxia-inducible factor-1alpha and nitric oxide synthase isoforms in ovarian endometriotic cysts. Virchows Arch 2010;456(6):703–710.

20. Becker CM, Rohwer N, Funakoshi T et al. 2-methoxyestradiol inhibits hypoxia-inducible factor-1{alpha} and suppresses growth of lesions in a mouse model of endometriosis. Am J Pathol 2008;172(2):534–544.

21. Taguchi A, Yanagisawa K, Tanaka M et al. Identification of hypoxia-inducible factor-1 alpha as a novel target for miR-17–92 microRNA cluster. Cancer Res 2008;68(14):5540–5545.

22. Jung YJ, Isaacs JS, Lee S, Trepel J, Neckers L. IL-1beta-mediated up-regulation of HIF-1alpha via an NFkappaB/COX-2 pathway identifies HIF-1 as a critical link between inflammation and oncogenesis. FASEB J 2003;17(14):2115–2117.

23. Keenan JA, Chen TT, Chadwell NL, Torry DS, Caudle MR. IL-1 beta, TNF-alpha, and IL-2 in peritoneal fluid and macrophage-conditioned media of women with endometriosis. Am J Reprod Immunol 1995;34(6):381–385.

24. Ponce C, Torres M, Galleguillos C et al. Nuclear factor kappaB pathway and interleukin-6 are affected in eutopic endometrium of women with endometriosis. Reproduction 2009;137(4):727–737.

25. Tamura M, Sebastian S, Yang S et al. Up-regulation of cyclooxygenase-2 expression and prostaglandin synthesis in endometrial stromal cells by malignant endometrial epithelial cells. A paracrine effect mediated by prostaglandin E2 and nuclear factor-kappa B. J Biol Chem 2002;277(29):26208–26216.

26. Kyama CM, Overbergh L, Mihalyi A et al. Effect of recombinant human TNF-binding protein-1 and GnRH antagonist on mRNA expression of inflammatory cytokines and adhesion and growth factors in endometrium and endometriosis tissues in baboons. Fertil Steril 2008;89(5 Suppl):1306–1313.

27. Dogan E, Saygili U, Posaci C et al. Regression of endometrial explants in rats treated with the cyclooxygenase-2 inhibitor rofecoxib. Fertil Steril 2004;82(Suppl 3):1115–1120.

28. Chakrabarty A, Tranguch S, Daikoku T, Jensen K, Furneaux H, Dey SK. MicroRNA regulation of cyclooxygenase-2 during embryo implantation. Proc Natl Acad Sci USA 2007;104(38):15144–15149.

29. Shanmugam N, Reddy MA, Natarajan R. Distinct roles of heterogeneous nuclear ribonuclear protein K and microRNA-16 in cyclooxygenase-2 RNA stability induced by S100b, a ligand of the receptor for advanced glycation end products. J Biol Chem 2008;283(52):36221–36233.

30. Chen R, Alvero AB, Silasi DA et al. Regulation of IKKbeta by miR-199a affects NF-kappaB activity in ovarian cancer cells. Oncogene 2008;27(34):4712–4723.

31. Masferrer JL, Zweifel BS, Manning PT et al. Selective inhibition of inducible cyclooxygenase 2 in vivo is antiinflammatory and nonulcerogenic. Proc Natl Acad Sci USA 1994;91(8):3228–3232.

32. Masferrer JL, Leahy KM, Koki AT et al. Antiangiogenic and antitumor activities of cyclooxygenase-2 inhibitors. Cancer Res 2000;60(5):1306–1311.

33. Bulun SE, Yang S, Fang Z, Gurates B, Tamura M, Sebastian S. Estrogen production and metabolism in endometriosis. Ann N Y Acad Sci 2002;955:75–85; discussion 6–8, 396–406.

34. Oosterlynck DJ, Meuleman C, Waer M, Koninckx PR. Transforming growth factor-beta activity is increased in peritoneal fluid from women with endometriosis. Obstet Gynecol 1994;83(2):287–292.

35. Pizzo A, Salmeri FM, Ardita FV, Sofo V, Tripepi M, Marsico S. Behaviour of cytokine levels in serum and peritoneal fluid of women with endometriosis. Gynecol Obstet Invest 2002;54(2):82–87.

36. Tamura M, Fukaya T, Enomoto A, Murakami T, Uehara S, Yajima A. Transforming growth factor-beta isoforms and receptors in endometriotic cysts of the human ovary. Am J Reprod Immunol 1999;42(3):160–167.

37. Hull ML, Johan MZ, Robertson SA, Ingman WH. Host-derived TGFB1 deficiency suppresses endometriosis-like lesion formation in an in vivo model. 57th Annual Meeting of the Society for Gynaecological Investigation, Glasgow, Scotland, 2009.

38. Burk U, Schubert J, Wellner U et al. A reciprocal repression between ZEB1 and members of the miR-200 family promotes EMT and invasion in cancer cells. EMBO Rep 2008;9(6):582–589.

39. Chen F, Ogawa K, Nagarajan RP, Zhang M, Kuang C, Chen Y. Regulation of TG-interacting factor by transforming growth factor-beta. Biochem J 2003;371(Pt 2):257–263.

40. Grummer R, Schwarzer F, Bainczyk K et al. Peritoneal endometriosis: validation of an in-vivo model. Hum Reprod 2001;16(8):1736–1743.

41. Jones RK, Bulmer JN, Searle RF. Immunohistochemical characterization of proliferation, oestrogen receptor and progesterone receptor expression in endometriosis: comparison of eutopic and ectopic endometrium with normal cycling endometrium. Hum Reprod 1995;10(12):3272–3279.

42. Scott GK, Goga A, Bhaumik D, Berger CE, Sullivan CS, Benz CC. Coordinate suppression of ERBB2 and ERBB3 by enforced

expression of micro-RNA miR-125a or miR-125b. J Biol Chem 2007;282(2):1479–1486.

43. Yang H, Kong W, He L et al. MicroRNA expression profiling in human ovarian cancer: miR-214 induces cell survival and cisplatin resistance by targeting PTEN. Cancer Res 2008;68(2):425–433.

44. Akao Y, Nakagawa Y, Naoe T. MicroRNA-143 and -145 in colon cancer. DNA Cell Biol 2007;26(5):311–320.

45. Chen X, Guo X, Zhang H et al. Role of miR-143 targeting KRAS in colorectal tumorigenesis. Oncogene 2009;28(10):1385–1392.

46. Shi B, Sepp-Lorenzino L, Prisco M, Linsley P, deAngelis T, Baserga R. Micro RNA 145 targets the insulin receptor substrate-1 and inhibits the growth of colon cancer cells. J Biol Chem 2007;282(45):32582–325890.

47. Inomata M, Tagawa H, Guo YM, Kameoka Y, Takahashi N, Sawada K. MicroRNA-17–92 down-regulates expression of distinct targets in different B-cell lymphoma subtypes. Blood 2009;113(2):396–402.

48. Le Sage C, Nagel R, Egan DA et al. Regulation of the p27(Kip1) tumor suppressor by miR-221 and miR-222 promotes cancer cell proliferation. EMBO J 2007;26(15):3699–3708.

49. Fornari F, Gramantieri L, Ferracin M et al. MiR-221 controls CDKN1C/p57 and CDKN1B/p27 expression in human hepatocellular carcinoma. Oncogene 2008;27(43):5651–5661.

50. Matsuzaki S, Canis M, Murakami T, Dechelotte P, Bruhat MA, Okamura K. Expression of the cyclin-dependent kinase inhibitor p27Kip1 in eutopic endometrium and peritoneal endometriosis. Fertil Steril 2001;75(5):956–960.

51. Somigliana E, Vigano P, Parazzini F, Stoppelli S, Giambattista E, Vercellini P. Association between endometriosis and cancer: a comprehensive review and a critical analysis of clinical and epidemiological evidence. Gynecol Oncol 2006;101(2):331–341.

52. Schmidt S, Friedl P. Interstitial cell migration: integrin-dependent and alternative adhesion mechanisms. Cell Tissue Res 2010;339(1):83–92.

53. Sengupta S, den Boon JA, Chen IH et al. MicroRNA 29c is down-regulated in nasopharyngeal carcinomas, up-regulating mRNAs encoding extracellular matrix proteins. Proc Natl Acad Sci USA 2008;105(15):5874–5878.

54. McLaren J, Prentice A, Charnock-Jones DS, Smith SK. Vascular endothelial growth factor (VEGF) concentrations are elevated in peritoneal fluid of women with endometriosis. Hum Reprod 1996;11(1):220–223.

55. Fasciani A, d'Ambrogio G, Bocci G, Monti M, Genazzani AR, Artini PG. High concentrations of the vascular endothelial growth factor and interleukin-8 in ovarian endometriomata. Mol Hum Reprod 2000;6(1):50–54.

56. Hull ML, Charnock-Jones DS, Chan CL et al. Antiangiogenic agents are effective inhibitors of endometriosis. J Clin Endocrinol Metab 2003;88(6):2889–2899.

57. Hua Z, Lv Q, Ye W et al. MiRNA-directed regulation of VEGF and other angiogenic factors under hypoxia. PLoS One 2006;1:e116.

58. Gilabert-Estelles J, Ramon LA, Espana F et al. Expression of angiogenic factors in endometriosis: relationship to fibrinolytic and metalloproteinase systems. Hum Reprod 2007;22(8):2120–2127.

59. Nicoli S, Standley C, Walker P, Hurlstone A, Fogarty KE, Lawson ND. MicroRNA-mediated integration of haemodynamics and Vegf signalling during angiogenesis. Nature 2010;464(7292):1196–1200.

60. Kuhnert F, Mancuso MR, Hampton J et al. Attribution of vascular phenotypes of the murine Egfl7 locus to the microRNA miR-126. Development 2008;135(24):3989–3993.

61. Parmacek MS. MicroRNA-modulated targeting of vascular smooth muscle cells. J Clin Invest 2009;119(9):2526–2528.

62. Larsson E, Fredlund Fuchs P, Heldin J et al. Discovery of microvascular miRNAs using public gene expression data: miR-145 is expressed in pericytes and is a regulator of Fli1. Genome Med 2009;1(11):108.

63. Doebele C, Bonauer A, Fischer A et al. Members of the microRNA-17–92 cluster exhibit a cell intrinsic anti-angiogenic function in endothelial cells. Blood 2010;115(23):4944–4950.

64. Giudice LC, Kao LC. Endometriosis. Lancet 2004;364(9447):1789–1799.

65. Treloar SA, O'Connor DT, O'Connor VM, Martin NG. Genetic influences on endometriosis in an Australian twin sample. Fertil Steril 1999;71(4):701–710.

66. Simpson JL, Elias S, Malinak LR, Buttram VC Jr. Heritable aspects of endometriosis. I. Genetic studies. Am J Obstet Gynecol 1980;137(3):327–331.

67. Montgomery GW, Nyholt DR, Zhao ZZ et al. The search for genes contributing to endometriosis risk. Hum Reprod Update 2008;14(5):447–457.

68. Treloar SA, Wicks J, Nyholt DR et al. Genomewide linkage study in 1,176 affected sister pair families identifies a significant susceptibility locus for endometriosis on chromosome 10q26. Am J Hum Genet 2005;77(3):365–376.

69. Zondervan KT, Treloar SA, Lin J et al. Significant evidence of one or more susceptibility loci for endometriosis with near-Mendelian inheritance on chromosome 7p13–15. Hum Reprod 2007;22(3):717–728.

70. Ye Y, Wang KK, Gu J et al. Genetic variations in microRNA-related genes are novel susceptibility loci for esophageal cancer risk. Cancer Prev Res 2008;1(6):460–469.

71. Chin LJ, Ratner E, Leng S et al. A SNP in a let-7 microRNA complementary site in the KRAS 3' untranslated region increases non-small cell lung cancer risk. Cancer Res 2008;68(20):8535–8540.

72. Zhao ZZ, Nyholt DR, Treloar SA et al. Evaluation of polymorphisms in predicted target sites for micro-RNAs differentially expressed in endometriosis. Mol Hum Reprod 2011;17(2):92–103.

73. Cramer DW, Wilson E, Stillman RJ et al. The relation of endometriosis to menstrual characteristics, smoking, and exercise. JAMA 1986;255(14):1904–1908.

74. Dizerega GS, Barber DL, Hodgen GD. Endometriosis: role of ovarian steroids in initiation, maintenance, and suppression. Fertil Steril 1980;33(6):649–653.

75. Klinge CM. Estrogen regulation of MicroRNA expression. Curr Genomics 2009;10(3):169–183.

76. Song G, Wang L. A conserved gene structure and expression regulation of miR-433 and miR-127 in mammals. PLoS One 2009;4(11):e7829.

77. Cohen A, Shmoish M, Levi L, Cheruti U, Levavi-Sivan B, Lubzens E. Alterations in micro-ribonucleic acid expression profiles reveal a novel pathway for estrogen regulation. Endocrinology 2008;149(4):1687–1696.

78. Maillot G, Lacroix-Triki M, Pierredon S et al. Widespread estrogen-dependent repression of micrornas involved in breast tumor cell growth. Cancer Res 2009;69(21):8332–8340.

79. Kuokkanen S, Chen B, Ojalvo L, Benard L, Santoro N, Pollard JW. Genomic profiling of microRNAs and messenger RNAs reveals hormonal regulation in microRNA expression in human endometrium. Biol Reprod 2010;82(4):791–801.

80. Cicatiello L, Mutarelli M, Grober OM et al. Estrogen receptor alpha controls a gene network in luminal-like breast cancer cells comprising multiple transcription factors and microRNAs. Am J Pathol 2010;176(5):2113–2130.

81. Toloubeydokhti T, Pan Q, Luo X, Bukulmez O, Chegini N. The expression and ovarian steroid regulation of endometrial micro-RNAs. Reprod Sci 2008;15(10):993–1001.

82. Greene R, Stratton P, Cleary SD, Ballweg ML, Sinaii N. Diagnostic experience among 4,334 women reporting surgically diagnosed endometriosis. Fertil Steril 2009;91(1):32–39.

83. Chapron C, Cravello L, Chopin N, Kreiker G, Blanc B, Dubuisson JB. Complications during set-up procedures for laparoscopy in gynecology: open laparoscopy does not reduce the risk of major complications. Acta Obstet Gynecol Scand 2003;82(12):1125–1129.

84. Spaczynski RZ, Duleba AJ. Diagnosis of endometriosis. Semin Reprod Med 2003;21(2):193–208.

85. Rogers PA, D'Hooghe TM, Fazleabas A et al. Priorities for endometriosis research: recommendations from an international consensus workshop. Reprod Sci 2009;16(4):335–346.

86. Gilad S, Meiri E, Yogev Y et al. Serum microRNAs are promising novel biomarkers. PLoS One 2008;3(9):e3148.

87. Rosenfeld N, Aharonov R, Meiri E et al. MicroRNAs accurately identify cancer tissue origin. Nat Biotechnol 2008;26(4):462–469.

88. Resnick KE, Alder H, Hagan JP, Richardson DL, Croce CM, Cohn DE. The detection of differentially expressed microRNAs from the serum of ovarian cancer patients using a novel real-time PCR platform. Gynecol Oncol 2009;112(1):55–59.

89. Burney RO, Talbi S, Hamilton AE et al. Gene expression analysis of endometrium reveals progesterone resistance and candidate susceptibility genes in women with endometriosis. Endocrinology 2007;148(8):3814–3826.

90. Gashaw I, Hastings JM, Jackson KS, Winterhager E, Fazleabas AT. Induced endometriosis in the baboon (Papio anubis) increases the expression of the proangiogenic factor CYR61 (CCN1) in eutopic and ectopic endometria. Biol Reprod 2006;74(6):1060–1066.

91. Al-Jefout M, Dezarnaulds G, Cooper M et al. Diagnosis of endometriosis by detection of nerve fibres in an endometrial biopsy: a double blind study. Hum Reprod 2009;24(12):3019–3024.

92. Tsujiura M, Ichikawa D, Komatsu S et al. Circulating microRNAs in plasma of patients with gastric cancers. Br J Cancer 2010;102(7):1174–1179.

93. Mitchell PS, Parkin RK, Kroh EM et al. Circulating microRNAs as stable blood-based markers for cancer detection. Proc Natl Acad Sci USA 2008;105(30):10513–10518.

94. Krutzfeldt J, Rajewsky N, Braich R et al. Silencing of microRNAs in vivo with 'antagomirs'. Nature 2005;438(7068):685–689.

95. Elmen J, Lindow M, Silahtaroglu A et al. Antagonism of micro-RNA-122 in mice by systemically administered LNA-antimiR leads to up-regulation of a large set of predicted target mRNAs in the liver. Nucleic Acids Res 2008;36(4):1153–1162.

96. Takeshita F, Patrawala L, Osaki M et al. Systemic delivery of synthetic microRNA-16 inhibits the growth of metastatic prostate tumors via downregulation of multiple cell-cycle genes. Mol Ther 2010;18(1):181–187.

18 HOX Genes and Endometriosis

Jennifer L. Kulp, Hakan Cakmak and Hugh S. Taylor

Department of Obstetrics, Gynecology and Reproductive Sciences, Yale University School of Medicine, New Haven, CT, USA

Introduction

HOX genes impart segmental identity to the developing reproductive tract. HOX gene expression in adults is found in the endometrium with peak expression levels occuring in the mid- and late secretory phase of the menstrual cycle. HOXA10 is believed to be critical for uterine receptivity at the time of embryo implantation. Decreased expression of HOXA10 in eutopic endometrium is seen in animal models of endometriosis as well as in women with endometriosis, possibly secondary to epigenetic phenomena. This chapter will review HOX genes, their role in the endometrium and in the pathogenesis of endometriosis.

Introduction to HOX genes

Homeobox (HOX) genes were originally identified in *Drosophila melanogaster* where they function through a conserved homeodomain as transcriptional regulators to provide developmental identity to all the various body segments of the fly [1]. Drosophila has eight homeobox genes clustered in one region of its genome, referred to collectively as the homeotic complex [1]. The vertebrate genome also contains clustered homeobox genes, called Hox genes in non-primates and HOX genes in primates. In both primates and non-primates, 39 Hox genes have been identified that are homologs of the original *Drosophila* complex. They organized into four Hox loci, each localized on a different chromosome (HOXA at 7p15.3, HOXB at 17p21.3, HOXC at 12q13.3 and HOXD at 2q31) and containing from nine to 11 genes [2]. On the basis of sequence similarity and position on the locus, corresponding genes in the four clusters can be aligned with each other into 13 paralogous groups [3].

During mammalian development, Hox gene expression controls the identity of various regions along the body axis

according to the rules of temporal and spatial co-linearity, with 3′ Hox genes expressed early in development and controlling anterior regions, followed by progressively more 5′ genes expressed later and controlling more posterior regions [4]. Individual genes of the HOXA cluster assign distinct identity to each segment of the paramesonephric duct, resulting in the development of the fallopian tube (HOXA9), uterus (HOXA10), lower uterine segment and cervix (HOXA11), and upper vagina (HOXA13) [5].

When a homeobox gene is mutated, the body segment where it is normally expressed typically develops characteristics of the segment immediately anterior to it, an effect known as anterior transformation [6]. In *Drosophila*, mutation of a single homeotic gene results in a dramatic phenotypic transformation. However, in vertebrates, targeted mutation in a single Hox gene usually causes only a subtle transformation to resemble more anterior tissues [7]. This is because, compared with the eight genes of the *Drosophila* HOM-C complex, the 39 mammalian homeotic genes confer genetic duplication, and loss of function of a single mutated gene may be compensated for by a paralog [8]. For example, *in utero* exposure to diethylstilbestrol, a well-known teratogen, induces a posterior shift of murine Hox gene expression, resulting in the homeotic anterior transformations of the reproductive tract that mimic the abnormalities noted in humans [9].

HOX gene expression in the endometrium

HOX genes were originally considered to be expressed only during embryonic development. However, the persistent expression of HOX genes has been noted in the female reproductive tract [5,10].

HOXA10 and HOXA11 have evolved a unique temporal pattern of expression consistent with their role in functional differentiation of the endometrium [11,12]. HOXA10 and HOXA11 messenger RNA (mRNA) are both expressed in human endometrial

Endometriosis: Science and Practice, First Edition. Edited by Linda C. Giudice, Johannes L.H. Evers and David L. Healy.
© 2012 Blackwell Publishing Ltd. Published 2012 by Blackwell Publishing Ltd.

epithelial and stromal cells, and their expression is significantly higher in the mid- and late secretory phases, coinciding with the time of embryo implantation and high levels of estrogen and progesterone [11–13]. Moreover, in the case of successful implantation, the decidua of the early pregnancy continues to express high levels of HOXA10 and HOXA11 mRNA [11,12].

Menstrual cyclicity is regulated by timed expression of estrogen and progesterone receptors, which act both independently and in concert to upregulate HOXA10 and HOXA11 expression in endometrium. In endometrial stromal cells, 17β-estradiol significantly increased HOXA10 mRNA expression in a dose-dependent manner. A similar effect of 17β-estradiol on HOXA10 mRNA expression was also observed in Ishikawa cells, a well-differentiated endometrial adenocarcinoma cell line [11]. Likewise, HOXA10 mRNA levels were significantly increased in endometrial stromal cells treated with medroxyprogesterone acetate (MPA). This response to MPA was greater than to 17β-estradiol, and combination treatment of 17β-estradiol and MPA induced higher levels of HOXA10 mRNA expression compared to treatment with either hormone alone [11]. Progestational regulation of HOXA10 was blocked by RU486, a specific progesterone receptor antagonist, in primary endometrial cells [12,14]. A similar expression pattern of HOXA11 was also demonstrated in response to estrogen and progesterone in endometrial cells [12]. Furthermore, these effects of estrogen and progesterone are mediated through their cognate receptors binding to the regulatory regions of the HOXA10 or HOXA11 genes [12,14–16].

Roles of HOX genes in endometrium

During each reproductive cycle, endometrial epithelial and stromal cells display a well-defined pattern of functional differentiation that is necessary for successful pregnancy under the cyclic influence of estrogen and progesterone. Initial proliferation is followed by differentiation leading to a receptive state for embryo implantation. In the absence of implantation, however, apoptosis and degeneration of the endometrium are observed.

HOX genes are essential for endometrial growth, differentiation and receptivity by mediating some functions of the sex steroids during each reproductive cycle. As transcription factors, they regulate other downstream target genes, leading to proper development of the endometrium and receptivity to implantation.

A microarray analysis of progesterone-responsive genes in the endometrium of ovariectomized HOXA10 null versus wild-type mice shows that cell cycle inhibitory genes p15 and p57 are upregulated in the null mice, implicating a negative impact on cell proliferation in the absence of HOXA10 [17]. Similarly, it was reported that the downregulation of HOXA10 is correlated with the upregulation of p57 during the progression of differentiation of human endometrial stromal cells *in vitro*, suggesting that p57, acting as a downstream regulator of HOXA10, presumably controls the exit of cell cycle activity [18].

Both HOXA10 and HOXA11 are necessary for fertility in mice. Although HOXA10 or HOXA11 knockout mice produce a normal number of embryos and these embryos survive in a wild-type surrogate, wild-type embryos from the surrogate mice cannot implant in the HOXA10- and HOXA11-deficient mice, suggesting uterine factor infertility due to an implantation defect [10,19,20]. In female HOXA10 knockout mice, implantation site defects are common and frequently consist of hemorrhage within the site itself, as well as in the adjacent uterine lumen. Small implantation sites with disorganized embryos and empty decidua suggestive of early degeneration of a postimplantation embryo were also observed. Furthermore, the size of the decidual swellings is reduced compared with wild-type uteri [20]. Similar implantation defects with deficient endometrial stromal, glandular, and decidual cell development in early gestation are also seen in HOXA11 knockout mice [13]. In another study, to determine the necessity of HOXA10 expression in adult uterine function, uteri of wild-type mice were transfected in the peri-implantation period with constructs that altered HOXA10 expression levels [21]. *In vivo* uterine transfection with a HOXA10 antisense construct was used to decrease endometrial HOXA10 expression levels, whereas a full-length HOXA10 cDNA construct was used to increase HOXA10 expression. A significant reduction in litter size in antisense transfected mice (mean number of pups: 6.5) compared with controls (mean: 13.3) was observed. In contrast, mice transfected with HOXA10 cDNA consistently delivered large litters (11–14 pups) compared with controls (4–11) [21].

Impaired endometrial receptivity is considered to be a major limiting factor for the establishment of pregnancy. In an attempt to develop a clinically relevant and reproducible evaluation of endometrial function, a number of molecular and morphological markers specific to the implantation window have been identified. Some of these markers were shown to be regulated by HOX genes including pinopodes, β3 integrin and insulin-like growth factor binding protein-1 (IGFBP-1) [6].

Pinopodes are progesterone-dependent endometrial epithelial surface projections whose appearance coincides with the onset of the implantation window [22,23]. HOXA10 antisense treatment diminishes pinopod number, whereas an increase is observed when uterine HOXA10 expression is upregulated [24]. Pinopod development may therefore represent a morphological feature of HOXA10-induced endometrial functional differentiation.

Integrins are a family of cell adhesion molecules that function in both cell–cell and cell–substratum adhesion. The expression of αvβ3 integrin at the apical surface of luminal endometrial epithelium is critical; it is expressed during the secretory phase of the menstrual cycle after cycle day 20, around the time of embryo implantation, and has a role in the initial embryo–endometrial interaction [25,26]. HOXA10 has been shown to directly regulate the expression of β3 integrin through a consensus Abd-B type HOX binding site located 5′ of the β3 integrin gene within its regulatory region [27]. Human decidualized endometrial stromal cells express IGFBP-1 [28]. It has been hypothesized that a paracrine interaction at the maternal–fetal interface occurs between decidual IGFBP-1 and fetal trophoblast-expressed IGF-II that is necessary for embryo implantation [29]. In baboon and human endometrial stromal cells, HOXA10 interacts with the

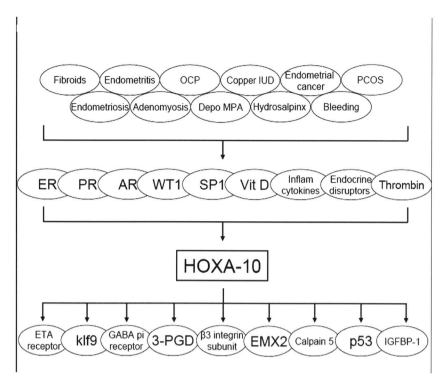

Figure 18.1 Modulators of HOXA10 gene expression and direct transcriptional target genes regulated by HOXA10. In multiple gynecological diseases and as a result of several birth control methods, HOXA10 gene expression is dysregulated, resulting in an inhospitable environment for blastocyst implantation. HOXA10 regulates other downstream target genes, leading to proper endometrial development and receptivity to implantation. AR, androgen receptor; ER, estrogen receptor; ETA, endothelin type A; GABA, γ-amino butyric acid; IGFBP, insulin-like growth factor binding protein; IUD, intrauterine device; MPA, medroxyprogesterone acetate; OCP, oral contraceptive; PCOS, polycystic ovarian syndrome; 3-PGD, 3-phosphoglycerate dehydrogenase; PR, progesterone receptor.

FOXO transcription factor FKHR, and together this heterodimer upregulates IGFBP-1 expression [30–32].

HOX gene expression in endometriosis

There are no documented human mutations in HOXA10 or HOXA11. However, the aberrant expression of HOX genes, as observed in endometriosis, is likely associated with endometrial functional deficiency manifest clinically as implantation defects [33].

Endometriosis is defined by the presence of viable endometrial tissue outside the uterine cavity. The prevalence of endometriosis is estimated to be 6–10% in the general reproductive age female population and 25–50% in women with infertility [34]. Moreover, among women with endometriosis, 30–50% are infertile [35]. There are multiple proposed mechanisms of subfertility in endometriosis including altered folliculogenesis, impaired fertilization, defective embryo implantation and poor oocyte quality [36–38].

The expression of both HOXA10 and HOXA11 rises dramatically in epithelial cells during the implantation window and remains elevated throughout the rest of the luteal phase [11,12]. However, the peak of HOXA10 and HOXA11 expression fails to occur in women with endometriosis [33]. Similarly, in mice and baboons with induced endometriosis, HOXA expression was downregulated in eutopic endometrium [32,39]. Furthermore, the expression of various other mediators of endometrial receptivity that are also mediated by HOX genes, such as pinopodes, αvβ3 integrin and IGFBP-1, is found to be decreased in endometriosis [39–46]. The expression of the Empty spiracles

homolog 2 (Emx2/EMX2) gene, that is associated with defective implantation, is repressed by elevated levels of HOXA in normal endometrium during the window of implantation [47]. However, the diminished HOXA10 expression in endometriosis results in elevated levels of endometrial EMX2 mRNA [48]. Consistent with the fact that high peri-implantation endometrial EMX2 levels are associated with a defective embryo implantation in patients with endometriosis, there is a significant 40% decrease in the litter size of mice transfected with EMX2 cDNA in the peri-implantation period [49]. A variety of disorders, medications, and endocrine disrupting chemicals affect HOXA10 expression, and dysregulation of HOXA10 results in altered expression of downstream targets (Fig. 18.1), which can affect uterine receptivity.

Mechanisms of altered HOX gene expression/ epigenetic regulation

Epigenetic modification is a common method by which gene expression is regulated. Epigenetic regulation occurs when there are inherited changes in gene expression which occur via methods other than changes in the underlying DNA sequence. The most common types of epigenetic regulation are DNA methylation and post-translational histone modifications. In humans, DNA methylation most commonly occurs at CpG dinucleotides, in which a cytosine is followed by a guanine. Methylation occurs at these sites when a methyl group is added to the cytosine ring by DNA methyltransferases. When promoter CpG islands are methylated, the end result is gene silencing due to decreased transcription of the gene. These patterns of methylation and resulting gene expression can be maintained through cell divisions. However, the methylation status of specific tissues or individual genes can also be modified by environmental or lifestyle factors or disease, which then may contribute to the development of abnormal phenotypes. In humans, multiple disease states have been associated with aberrant DNA methylation, such as cancers and imprinting disorders [50,51]. Recent evidence suggests that endometriosis may also be an epigenetic disease.

HOXA10 transcription is known to be decreased in endometriosis with associated poor uterine receptivity and embryo implantation rates. The downregulation of HOXA10 in endometriosis may be due to hypermethylation of the HOXA10 gene. In a mouse model of induced endometriosis, in which normal endometrium from donor mice was sutured into the peritoneum of recipient mice, decreased expression of HOXA10 was noted in the eutopic endometrium of the mice with induced endometriosis. There was a corresponding hypermethylation of HOXA10 in the endometrium of these mice, suggesting a possible mechanism for the observed downregulation of HOXA10 [39].

In a baboon model of induced endometriosis, significantly decreased HOXA10 mRNA in the eutopic endometrium was documented at 12 and 16 months. Hypermethylation of the F1 region of the HOXA10 promoter was found, again suggesting a possible mechanism for the decreased expression of HOXA10 seen in this disease state [32].

In humans, women with endometriosis are infertile due to multiple etiologies, including decreased embryo implantation rates. Numerous studies have demonstrated decreased implantation rates in women with endometriosis undergoing *in vitro* fertilization (IVF) embryo transfer cycles [52]. HOXA10 and HOXA11 are not upregulated in the midluteal phase in the endometrium of these women [33]. Data in humans with endometriosis have also demonstrated aberrant methylation of HOXA10 in eutopic endometrium compared to controls. Both the promoter region of the genes as wells as two CpG islands within intron 1 were found to have areas of hypermethylation [53]. This evidence suggests that aberrant methylation of HOXA10 may be responsible for the decreased HOXA10 expression seen in women with endometriosis. Further, a study examining expression levels of DNA methyltransferases, which catalyze DNA methylation, found that three genes that code for DNA methyltransferase (DNMT1, DNMT3A and DNMT3B) were overexpressed in ectopic endometriosis implants as compared to normal control or eutopic endometrium of women with endometriosis. In eutopic endometrium of women with endometriosis, there was an indication that one of the methyltransferases, DNMT3A, was upregulated. These findings support the hypothesis that endometriosis is an epigenetic disease [54].

Taken together, these studies show that across different models of endometriosis, either experimentally induced, as in the mouse or baboon, or spontaneous, as seen in human studies, eutopic endometrium has decreased receptivity and altered gene expression. There are changes in the markers of uterine receptivity, such as altered progesterone receptor ratios, as well as alterations

in HOXA10 expression. With experimentally induced models of endometriosis, it becomes clear that normal endometrium becomes defective in endometriosis and not that abnormal endometrium results in endometriosis. Perhaps the normal endometrium is rendered defective due to a signal from the ectopic endometrium. This theory has yet to be proven. However, evidence to date suggests that altered signal conduction pathways and epigenetic modification related to endometriosis result in changes in endometrial gene expression.

Correction of abnormal expression of HOXA10

If epigenetic phenomena contribute to poor uterine receptivity secondary to abnormal expression of HOXA10 in endometriosis patients, what therapies are available to reverse these changes? Traditional therapies for endometriosis include medical therapies such as oral contraceptive pills, progestin therapy and the use of gonadotropin-releasing hormone (GnRH) agonists. Yet with all of these therapies, the majority of patients will have recurrent symptoms such as pelvic pain upon discontinuation of the treatment. This suggests that while medical therapy may suppress endometriosis, it does not reverse the disease process. Medical therapies do not improve fertility.

Patients who have failed medical therapy may move on to surgical treatments such as ablation or resection of endometriotic lesions via laparoscopy. This may provide temporary relief from the pain symptoms, but after surgery endometriosis tends to return, again suggesting that the underlying disease process is not altered with surgical therapy [55,56].

Endometriosis is found in 20–50% of women with infertility. Without treatment, spontaneous monthly fecundity rates are between 2% and 3%. Surgery for endometriosis-associated infertility may result in a slightly increased monthly fecundity rate of 4.7% [57]. However, this is only a small improvement, and demonstrates that fertility remains poor even after surgical therapy in women with endometriosis. The limited success of both surgical and medical therapy in patients with endometriosis could be explained by the fact that epigenetic changes, such as methylation of the HOXA10 promoter, are unlikely to be fixed by these types of therapies.

Current research focuses on the role of stem cells in endometriosis. The human endometrium is renewed each menstrual cycle and this may be secondary to endometrial stem cells in the basalis layer which cyclically differentiate to form endometrium under hormonal direction [58–60]. Bone marrow-derived mesenchymal stem cells may also differentiate into endometrium and endometriosis [61]. These stem cells can be recruited to the endometrium where they differentiate into both endometrial stromal and epithelial cells. In women who have undergone bone marrow transplants, the endometrium contains a significant number of donor-derived endometrial cells. Also, bone marrow-derived stem cells may populate established endometriotic implants. In hysterectomized mice with endometriosis, endometriosis lesions contained bone marrow-derived endometrial cells [62]. This suggests that bone marrow-derived stem cells contribute to the persistence and progression of endometriosis. Stem cells are also known to play a role in the regeneration of damaged tissue. Possibly in the future, epigenetic modifications of the HOX gene could be treated with stem cells which could regenerate to replace the abnormally methylated uterine cells with healthy endometrium.

Conclusion

Expression of sufficient HOXA10 mRNA is known to be essential to endometrial receptivity and embryo implantation. Through animal model studies, we know that normal endometrium develops changes in gene expression patterns secondary to the presence of endometriosis. HOXA10 gene expression is downregulated in eutopic endometrium of patients with endometriosis. Aberrant methylation of promoter regions of HOXA10 is associated with downregulation of HOXA10 gene expression. Traditional treatments for endometriosis, such as medical and surgical therapies, likely do lead to correction of this aberrant methylation, which may explain why endometriosis persists and progresses at the cessation of treatment. Progressive understanding of the epigenetic mechanisms that regulate HOXA10 gene expression in endometriosis may lead to the development new therapeutic agents which can modify or correct disease-associated aberrant methylation, such as stem cell therapy.

References

1. Gehring WJ, Hiromi Y. Homeotic genes and the homeobox. Annu Rev Genet. 1986;20:147–173.

2. Apiou F, Flagiello D, Cillo C et al. Fine mapping of human HOX gene clusters. Cytogenet Cell Genet 1996;73:114–115.

3. Scott MP. Vertebrate homeobox gene nomenclature. Cell 1992;71: 551–553.

4. Dekker EE, Kitson RP. 2-Keto-4-hydroxyglutarate aldolase: purification and characterization of the homogeneous enzyme from bovine kidney. J Biol Chem 1992;267:10507–10514.

5. Taylor HS, Vanden Heuvel GB, Igarashi P. A conserved Hox axis in the mouse and human female reproductive system: late establishment and persistent adult expression of the Hoxa cluster genes. Biol Reprod 1997;57:1338–1345.

6. Daftary GS, Taylor HS. Endocrine regulation of HOX genes. Endocr Rev 2006;27:331–355.

7. Balling R, Mutter G, Gruss P et al. Craniofacial abnormalities induced by ectopic expression of the homeobox gene Hox-1.1 in transgenic mice. Cell 1989;58:337–347.

8. Hunt P, Gulisano M, Cook M et al. A distinct Hox code for the branchial region of the vertebrate head. Nature 1991;353:861–864.

9. Block K, Kardana A, Igarashi P et al. In utero diethylstilbestrol (DES) exposure alters Hox gene expression in the developing mullerian system. Faseb J 2000;14:1101–1108.

10. Benson GV, Lim H, Paria BC et al. Mechanisms of reduced fertility in Hoxa-10 mutant mice: uterine homeosis and loss of maternal Hoxa-10 expression. Development 1996;122:2687–2696.

11. Taylor HS, Arici A, Olive D et al. HOXA10 is expressed in response to sex steroids at the time of implantation in the human endometrium. J Clin Invest 1998;101:1379–1384.

12. Taylor HS, Igarashi P, Olive DL et al. Sex steroids mediate HOXA11 expression in the human peri-implantation endometrium. J Clin Endocrinol Metab 1999;84:1129–1135.

13. Gendron RL, Paradis H, Hsieh-Li HM et al. Abnormal uterine stromal and glandular function associated with maternal reproductive defects in Hoxa-11 null mice. Biol Reprod 1997;56:1097–1105.

14. Ma L, Benson GV, Lim H et al. Abdominal B (AbdB) Hoxa genes: regulation in adult uterus by estrogen and progesterone and repression in mullerian duct by the synthetic estrogen diethylstilbestrol (DES). Dev Biol 1998;197:141–154.

15. Akbas GE, Song J, Taylor HS. A HOXA10 estrogen response element (ERE) is differentially regulated by 17 beta-estradiol and diethylstilbestrol (DES). J Mol Biol 2004;340:1013–1023.

16. Martin R, Taylor MB, Krikun G et al. Differential cell-specific modulation of HOXA10 by estrogen and specificity protein 1 response elements. J Clin Endocrinol Metab 2007;92:1920–1926.

17. Yao MW, Lim H, Schust DJ et al. Gene expression profiling reveals progesterone-mediated cell cycle and immunoregulatory roles of Hoxa-10 in the preimplantation uterus. Mol Endocrinol. 2003;17:610–627.

18. Qian K, Chen H, Wei Y et al. Differentiation of endometrial stromal cells in vitro: down-regulation of suppression of the cell cycle inhibitor p57 by HOXA10? Mol Hum Reprod 2005;11:245–251.

19. Hsieh-Li HM, Witte DP, Weinstein M et al. Hoxa 11 structure, extensive antisense transcription, and function in male and female fertility. Development 1995;121:1373–1385.

20. Satokata I, Benson G, Maas R. Sexually dimorphic sterility phenotypes in Hoxa10-deficient mice. Nature 1995;374:460–463.

21. Bagot CN, Troy PJ, Taylor HS. Alteration of maternal Hoxa10 expression by in vivo gene transfection affects implantation. Gene Ther 2000;7:1378–1384.

22. Nikas G, Drakakis P, Loutradis D et al. Uterine pinopodes as markers of the 'nidation window' in cycling women receiving exogenous oestradiol and progesterone. Hum Reprod 1995;10: 1208–1213.

23. Singh MM, Chauhan SC, Trivedi RN et al. Correlation of pinopod development on uterine luminal epithelial surface with hormonal events and endometrial sensitivity in rat. Eur J Endocrinol 1996;135:107–117.

24. Bagot CN, Kliman HJ, Taylor HS. Maternal Hoxa10 is required for pinopod formation in the development of mouse uterine receptivity to embryo implantation. Dev Dyn 2001;222:538–544.

25. Lessey BA, Damjanovich L, Coutifaris C et al. Integrin adhesion molecules in the human endometrium. Correlation with the normal and abnormal menstrual cycle. J Clin Invest 1992;90:188–195.

26. Sueoka K, Shiokawa S, Miyazaki T et al. Integrins and reproductive physiology: expression and modulation in fertilization, embryogenesis, and implantation. Fertil Steril 1997;67:799–811.

27. Daftary GS, Troy PJ, Bagot CN et al. Direct regulation of beta3-integrin subunit gene expression by HOXA10 in endometrial cells. Mol Endocrinol 2002;16:571–579.

28. Hustin J, Philippe E, Teisner B et al. Immunohistochemical localization of two endometrial proteins in the early days of human pregnancy. Placenta 1994;15:701–708.

29. Irwin JC, Suen LF, Faessen GH et al. Insulin-like growth factor (IGF)-II inhibition of endometrial stromal cell tissue inhibitor of metalloproteinase-3 and IGF-binding protein-1 suggests paracrine interactions at the decidua:trophoblast interface during human implantation. J Clin Endocrinol Metab 2001;86:2060–2064.

30. Foucher I, Volovitch M, Frain M et al. Hoxa5 overexpression correlates with IGFBP1 upregulation and postnatal dwarfism: evidence for an interaction between Hoxa5 and Forkhead box transcription factors. Development 2002;129:4065–4074.

31. Kim JJ, Jaffe RC, Fazleabas AT. Insulin-like growth factor binding protein-1 expression in baboon endometrial stromal cells: regulation by filamentous actin and requirement for de novo protein synthesis. Endocrinology 1999;140:997–1004.

32. Kim JJ, Taylor HS, Lu Z et al. Altered expression of HOXA10 in endometriosis: potential role in decidualization. Mol Hum Reprod 2007;13:323–332.

33. Taylor HS, Bagot C, Kardana A et al. HOX gene expression is altered in the endometrium of women with endometriosis. Hum Reprod 1999;14:1328–1331.

34. Houston DE. Evidence for the risk of pelvic endometriosis by age, race and socioeconomic status. Epidemiol Rev 1984;6:167–191.

35. Strathy JH, Molgaard CA, Coulam CB et al. Endometriosis and infertility: a laparoscopic study of endometriosis among fertile and infertile women. Fertil Steril 1982;38:667–672.

36. Simon C, Gutierrez A, Vidal A et al. Outcome of patients with endometriosis in assisted reproduction: results from in-vitro fertilization and oocyte donation. Hum Reprod 1994;9:725–729.

37. Tummon IS, Maclin VM, Radwanska E et al. Occult ovulatory dysfunction in women with minimal endometriosis or unexplained infertility. Fertil Steril 1988;50:716–720.

38. Ulukus M, Cakmak H, Arici A. The role of endometrium in endometriosis. J Soc Gynecol Invest 2006;13:467–476.

39. Lee B, Du H, Taylor HS. Experimental murine endometriosis induces DNA methylation and altered gene expression in eutopic endometrium. Biol Reprod 2009;80:79–85.

40. Fazleabas AT, Brudney A, Chai D et al. Steroid receptor and aromatase expression in baboon endometriotic lesions. Fertil Steril 2003;80(Suppl 2):820–827.

41. Burney RO, Talbi S, Hamilton AE et al. Gene expression analysis of endometrium reveals progesterone resistance and candidate susceptibility genes in women with endometriosis. Endocrinology 2007;148:3814–3826.

42. Kamat AA, Younes PS, Sayeeduddin M et al. Protein expression profiling of endometriosis: validation of 2-mm tissue microarrays. Fertil Steril 2004;82:1681–1683.

43. Kao LC, Germeyer A, Tulac S et al. Expression profiling of endometrium from women with endometriosis reveals candidate genes for disease-based implantation failure and infertility. Endocrinology 2003;144:2870–2881.

44. Klemmt PA, Carver JG, Kennedy SH et al. Stromal cells from endometriotic lesions and endometrium from women with endometriosis have reduced decidualization capacity. Fertil Steril 2006;85:564–572.

45. Lessey BA, Castelbaum AJ, Sawin SW et al. Aberrant integrin expression in the endometrium of women with endometriosis. J Clin Endocrinol Metab 1994;79:643–649.

46. Vitiello D, Kodaman PH, Taylor HS. HOX genes in implantation. Semin Reprod Med 2007;25:431–436.

47. Troy PJ, Daftary GS, Bagot CN et al. Transcriptional repression of peri-implantation EMX2 expression in mammalian reproduction by HOXA10. Mol Cell Biol 2003;23:1–13.

48. Daftary GS, Taylor HS. EMX2 gene expression in the female reproductive tract and aberrant expression in the endometrium of patients with endometriosis. J Clin Endocrinol Metab 2004;89:2390–2396.

49. Taylor HS, Fei X. Emx2 regulates mammalian reproduction by altering endometrial cell proliferation. Mol Endocrinol 2005;19:2839–2846.

50. Reik W, Dean W, Walter J. Epigenetic reprogramming in mammalian development. Science 2001;293:1089–1093.

51. Robertson KD. DNA methylation and human disease. Nat Rev Genet 2005;6:597–610.

52. Barnhart K, Dunsmoor-Su R, Coutifaris C. Effect of endometriosis on in vitro fertilization. Fertil Steril 2002;77:1148–1155.

53. Wu Y, Halverson G, Basir Z et al. Aberrant methylation at HOXA10 may be responsible for its aberrant expression in the endometrium of patients with endometriosis. Am J Obstet Gynecol 2005;193:371–380.

54. Wu Y, Strawn E, Basir Z et al. Aberrant expression of deoxyribonucleic acid methyltransferases DNMT1, DNMT3A, and DNMT3B in women with endometriosis. Fertil Steril 2007;87:24–32.

55. Sutton CJ, Ewen SP, Whitelaw N et al. Prospective, randomized, double-blind, controlled trial of laser laparoscopy in the treatment of pelvic pain associated with minimal, mild, and moderate endometriosis. Fertil Steril 1994;62:696–700.

56. Sutton CJ, Pooley AS, Ewen SP et al. Follow-up report on a randomized controlled trial of laser laparoscopy in the treatment of pelvic pain associated with minimal to moderate endometriosis. Fertil Steril 1997;68:1070–1074.

57. Marcoux S, Maheux R, Berube S. Laparoscopic surgery in infertile women with minimal or mild endometriosis. Canadian Collaborative Group on Endometriosis. N Engl J Med 1997;337:217–222.

58. Chan RW, Gargett CE. Identification of label-retaining cells in mouse endometrium. Stem Cells 2006;24:1529–1538.

59. Chan RW, Schwab KE, Gargett CE. Clonogenicity of human endometrial epithelial and stromal cells. Biol Reprod 2004;70:1738–1750.

60. Dimitrov R, Timeva T, Kyurkchiev D et al. Characterization of clonogenic stromal cells isolated from human endometrium. Reproduction 2008;135:551–558.

61. Taylor HS. Endometrial cells derived from donor stem cells in bone marrow transplant recipients. JAMA 2004;292:81–85.

62. Du H, Taylor HS. Contribution of bone marrow-derived stem cells to endometrium and endometriosis. Stem Cells 2007;25:2082–2086.

19 Angiogenesis and Endometriosis

Patrick. G. Groothuis

Department of Women's Health, Merck Sharp and Dohme, Oss, The Netherlands

Introduction

Endometriosis was first described in 1860 [1], and Sampson was the first to suggest that endometriosis results from the implantation of disseminated menstrual tissue [2]. However, it took another 50 years until the first papers were published linking angiogenesis to the ectopic survival of endometrial tissue. It was the group of Stephen Smith which first recognized that endometrium and endometriotic tissues express angiogenic factors [3]. In that same year the group of Philippe Koninckx demonstrated in the chick chorio-allantoic membrane (CAM) model that peritoneal fluid from endometriosis patients was more angiogenic than peritoneal fluid from women without disease [4]. Key to the survival of ectopic endometrium tissue is an adequate blood supply. This chapter will summarize our current understanding of the development of the vasculature in endometrium and endometriotic lesions, and touch on novel emerging concepts in angiogenesis and vessel development.

Angiogenesis in the endometrium

Angiogenesis is a rare event in adult tissues, but plays a fundamental role in the ovary and uterine endometrium. Each menstrual cycle, the human endometrium undergoes periods of tissue repair, growth, differentiation, and breakbown. The initial stages of the postmenstrual repair process start while the shedding of the decidualized tissue is still ongoing, prior to any rise in follicular estrogen. The endometrium regenerates from the remaining deeper zones and re-epithelialization of the denuded surface occurs by outgrowth and spreading of the epithelium from the mouths of the residual glands [5–7].

Angiogenesis presumably plays prominent roles in all or most of the above-mentioned processes in the endometrial tissue. Yet there is surprisingly little evidence to support this. We know that the endometrium expresses a variety of receptors for vascular growth regulatory factors and that it is a major source of vascular growth regulatory factors itself [8,9]. This explains why transplanted human endometrial tissue is extremely angiogenic [10–14].

Angiogenesis in the endometrium can occur through different mechanisms: sprouting, intussusception (internal division of the vessel by endothelial cells resulting in the vessel splitting in two), elongation and widening (growth lengthwise without formation of new junctions), or incorporation of circulating endothelial (precursor) cells into endometrial vessels. Sprouting is the most frequently observed and studied angiogenic mechanism and this process is associated with increased proliferative activity in the sprouts. However, in contrast to the clear cycle-related changes in endothelial cell proliferation in the non-human primate endometrium [15], there is no clear evidence of cyclic peaks in endothelial proliferation in the human endometrium, and proliferating endothelial cells were always identified within vessels rather than associated with sprouts (reviewed in [9]). In contrast, Ferenczy et al [16] performed radio-autographic analysis of human endometrium after incubation with methyl-^{3}H thymidine in vitro and observed an increase in thymidine incorporation at cycle days 8–10, but only in the upper one-third of the functionalis. This probably explains why a correlation was not found when evaluating the endometrium as a whole. Evidence was provided that vessel elongation is a major angiogenic mechanism during the mid-proliferative phase of the menstrual cycle (Fig. 19.1). This changes during the progesterone-dominated early-to-midsecretory stage of the cycle, when the vascular density increases as a result of an increase in the vessel branch point density (reviewed in [9]).

Endometriosis: Science and Practice, First Edition. Edited by Linda C. Giudice, Johannes L.H. Evers and David L. Healy.
© 2012 Blackwell Publishing Ltd. Published 2012 by Blackwell Publishing Ltd.

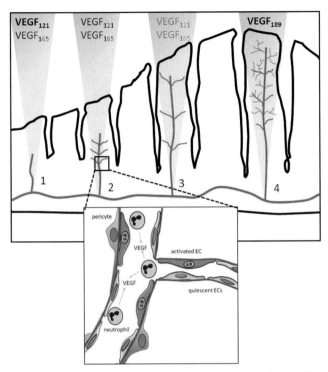

Figure 19.1 Vasculogenesis in the human endometrium. In the perimenstrual phase, VEGF121 and VEGF165 are the most abundantly expressed isoforms, and are most likely responsible for regulating initial vascular repair and the subsequent elongation process when the endometrium thickness increases later in the proliferative phase. Simultaneously, neutrophils are recruited to the endometrium and concentrate in vessels containing proliferating endothelial cells. In the secretory phase, VEGF189 is the predominant isoform, which is responsible for the extensive branching, leading to increased vascular density.

Vascular endothelial growth factor controls the angiogenic process in the endometrium

The only direct evidence of critical involvement of angiogenesis in endometrium regeneration, growth and function was provided in vascular endothelial growth factor (VEGF) intervention studies in rodents and non-human primate models. For example, immunoneutralization of VEGF prevented embryo implantation in adult rats [17]. In other studies, VEGF was inhibited using the VEGF Trap, also called aflibercept, a recombinant chimeric protein comprising portions of the extracellular domains of the human VEGF receptors 1 and 2 expressed in sequence with the Fc portion of human immunoglobulin G (IgG) [18]. In pseudopregnant mice and non-human primate models with induced menstrual cycles, VEGF Trap treatment at the time of or shortly after the induction of endometrial breakdown by progesterone withdrawal significantly impaired revascularization and re-epithelialization [7]. Pre-existing vessels in the basal zones or the myometrium were not affected, however, indicating that only the neo-angiogenic process was antagonized. These studies confirm that angiogenesis plays an important role in the early stages of postmenstrual repair and revascularization of the endometrium, and that VEGF is an important factor in this process.

Vascular endothelial growth factor is a member of the VEGF family of growth factors which comprises VEGF, VEGF-B, VEGF-C, VEGF-D, VEGF-E, placental growth factor (PlGF), and their receptors VEGFR-1, -2, and -3. Many of these proteins are abundantly expressed in the human and non-human primate endometrium. VEGF is considered the most relevant with regard to the regulation of endometrial angiogenesis. It binds to VEGFR-1 and VEGFR-2 and promotes endothelial cell proliferation, survival and recruitment of bone marrow-derived cells, vascular permeability and vasodilation.

The VEGF gene contains eight exons separated by seven introns, and by means of alternative splicing, at least three different splice variants are generated in mice: $VEGF_{120}$, $VEGF_{164}$, and $VEGF_{188}$. The isoforms differ in their ability to bind to heparin [19]. $VEGF_{188}$ binds to heparan sulfates with the highest affinity which leads to sequestration to the extracellular matrix (ECM). $VEGF_{120}$, however, is freely diffusible and thereby capable of acting over longer distances [19,20]. The most common variant, $VEGF_{164}$, has intermediate properties and is partly secreted, partly bound to the ECM. Both $VEGF_{164}$ and $VEGF_{188}$ can be released by proteolytic cleavage. The $VEGF_{121}$, $VEGF_{165}$, and $VEGF_{189}$ isoforms are also expressed in the human endometrium [8] and clearly have different spatiotemporal functions in the development of the endometrial vasculature (see Fig. 19.1). Studies in transgenic mice in which only $VEGF_{121}$ is expressed demonstrated that this diffusible isoform is responsible for vessel enlargement, at the expense of vessel branching [20,21]. During the menstrual, early and midproliferative phases of the menstrual cycle, $VEGF_{121}$ is the major isoform, which correlates well with the observed vessel growth through elongation of angiogenic vessels observed in this phase of the cycle. At the same time, $VEGF_{121}$ levels are elevated and the expression of the $VEGF_{165}$ isoform is increased as well [8].

Transgenic mice expressing only the $VEGF_{165}$ isoform develop normally, so this isoform can take over the roles of the other two. This indicates that this isoform may be expressed in the endometrium as a safety mechanism. Transgenic mice expressing only $VEGF_{189}$ showed no significant elongation of large vessels, but displayed supernumerary branching of smaller vessels [20,21]. This corresponds well with the fact that from the late proliferative phase on, expression of the $VEGF_{121}$ and $VEGF_{165}$ isoforms disappears, whereas expression of the $VEGF_{189}$ isoform increases [8], which corresponds with the observed increase in the number of vessel branching points in the secretory phase of the menstrual cycle [9] (see Fig. 19.1).

In contrast to what was observed in the non-human primate endometrium, there is no clear evidence of cyclical peaks in endothelial proliferation in the human endometrium [9] and no relation between the expression of VEGF in the endometrium and endothelial cell proliferation [22]. However, endometrial endothelial cell proliferation did correlate with the presence of foci of intense VEGF immunostaining during the proliferative phase. The foci were located mainly in the blood vessels in the subepithelial capillary plexus and were shown to be marginating and adherent neutrophils [23] (see Fig. 19.1). Even though the neutrophils mostly expressed $VEGF_{121}$ and $VEGF_{165}$ mRNA, the major isoform released during degranulation is $VEGF_{189}$ [24].

Why the neutrophils accumulate at these locations remains to be elucidated. E-selectin, intercellular adhesion molecule-1 (ICAM-1) and vascular cell adhesion molecule-1 (VCAM-1) are involved in the adhesion and extravasation of neutrophils. VEGF was shown to upregulate ICAM-1 and VCAM-1 expression on endothelial cells, whereas estrogen promotes neutrophil influx in mice and enhances leukocyte binding to tumor necrosis factor-α (TNF-α)-induced endothelial cells via increases in E-selectin, ICAM-1, and VCAM-1 [25–27].

Steroid hormones and hypoxia control vascular endothelial growth factor production

Although the changes in the endometrium are under the overall control of estrogen and progesterone, it remains to be demonstrated whether these steroids act directly or indirectly on endometrial endothelial cells, meaning that the changes are secondary to hormone-dependent tissue degradation and growth which possibly lead to hypoxia [7].

In tumors, tissue hypoxia, primarily mediated by hypoxia-inducible factor (HIF)-1, is a key regulator of VEGF expression [28,29]. The presence of hypoxia in the damaged, regenerating perimenstrual endometrium appears also to be related to the production of VEGF. HIF is a heterodimeric transcription factor that is ubiquitously expressed and activates gene expression in response to reduced cellular oxygen concentrations. The activity of HIF-1 is mostly regulated through the stabilization of the proteins. In non-hypoxic cells, HIF-1β protein is detected in both the nucleus and cytoplasm, but when the cells are exposed to 1% oxygen there is progressive nuclear translocation. The HIF-1α protein, however, is not detected in the absence of hypoxia but is considerably increased in the nucleus following 4–8 h of continuous hypoxia [8]. On return to 20% oxygen, the HIF-1β subunit reappears in the cytoplasm while the HIF-1α disappears completely. Increasing evidence implicates HIF-1α as the major regulator of the vascular network in mammals. Stabilization of HIF induces, directly or indirectly, a plethora of angiogenic mediators including, but not limited to, VEGF, PlGF, their receptors VEGFR-1 and VEGFR-2, platelet-derived growth factor (PDGF), angiopoietin-2 and matrix metalloproteinases [30]. Several studies support a role for hypoxia and HIF-1α in the regulation of VEGF production in the damaged, regenerating perimenstrual human endometrium [8,19,31–35].

Next to the fact that hypoxia is a strong inducer of VEGF production, there is also good evidence that the production of VEGF and its receptors is regulated directly by estrogen [36–42]. The finding that estradiol induces VEGF production is consistent with the fact that the promoter region of the VEGF gene contains eight half-palindromic estrogen response elements [40]. Koos and co-workers [40,41] demonstrated that estrogen rapidly induced the recruitment of HIF-1α and HIF-1β to the region of the VEGF promoter containing the HIF response elements to induce transcription, analogous to what happens during hypoxia.

This binding was transient, matching the pattern of estrogen-induced VEGF expression.

In the second part of the menstrual cycle, the secretory phase, the major VEGF isoform is $VEGF_{189}$ [8,24]. The production of this isoform is clearly regulated by progesterone and parallels the expression pattern of other decidualization markers such as insulin-like growth factor binding protein (IGFBP)-1 [42]. This VEGF isoform sequesters in the ECM and can be released by proteolysis. Licht *et al* [43], using a uterine microdialysis device, showed that intrauterine VEGF levels significantly increased in the premenstrual phase, at the same time as progesterone levels dropped, allowing massive activation of matrix metalloproteinases [44]. This is probably the reason why this isoform was prominently present in the menstrual endometrium [8].

Vessel maturation in the human endometrium

The angiopoietin (Ang)-1/Tie-2 system is in large part responsible for the last stage of blood vessel development, the stabilization and maturation of the newly formed vessels in the endometrium. The Tie-2 receptor is almost exclusively expressed by endothelial cells and hematopoietic stem cells, whereas its ligand Ang-1 is constitutively expressed in pericytes, smooth muscle cells and fibroblasts (reviewed in [45]). In normal tissues, Ang-1-induced activation of the Tie-2 receptor is required to maintain the quiescent resting state of the endothelium. Ang-2 is almost undetectable in the quiescent vasculature and is stored in Weibel-Palade bodies. However, Ang-2 is released when endothelial cells become activated through VEGF, fibroblast growth factor (FGF)-2 or TNF-α, or environmental cues such as hypoxia, high glucose levels, and superoxides. The release of Ang-2 results in rapid destabilization of the endothelium, allowing induction of angiogenesis by VEGF. When Ang-2 is released, it competes with Ang-1 for binding to Tie-2 and functions as a natural antagonist of Ang-1. The effect of Ang-2 on the endothelial cells is, however, context dependent. It facilitates angiogenesis only in the presence of VEGF; in the absence of VEGF, vessels regress.

The expression of Ang-2 is highest in the menstrual/early proliferative phase when VEGF levels are high as well, so vessels are destabilized and fragile. Ang-2 expression decreases during the menstrual cycle, and the expression of Ang-1 increases significantly in the secretory phase which results in vessel stabilization [46,47]. In women with menorrhagia, a decrease in Ang-1 levels causes imbalance in the Ang-1/Ang-2 expression ratio, and as a result the blood vessels become very fragile [48].

Maintenance of the resting endothelial cell phenotype requires tight association with periendothelial cells, the pericytes. The best characterized endothelial cell-derived pericyte-recruiting factor is platelet-derived growth factor (PDGF)-BB upon interacting with its receptor PDGFR-β [49,50], but until recently it was unclear how PDGF-BB co-ordinates the recruitment of pericytes. PDGF and PDGF-β receptor (PDGFR-β) are expressed in the human endometrium [51], and contribute to the revascularization of ectopic endometrium [52]. Recently, it became clear that PDGF-BB, through interaction with PDGFR-β, induces the expression of stromal-derived factor (SDF)-1α in endothelial cells, resulting in the formation of a SDF-1α chemotaxis gradient [53]. Blocking the SDF-1α/CXCR4 axis prevents PDGF-BB-induced pericyte recruitment *in vitro* and *in vivo*. SDF-1α/*Cxcl-12* and its receptor CXCR-4 are both expressed in the human endometrium [54,55]. These new findings warrant further investigation of the role of PDGF-BB in vessel stabilization in human endometrium in health and disease.

Angiogenesis in the endometriotic lesion

During laparoscopy active endometriotic lesions are readily identifiable by an abundance of vessels in the proximity of the lesions. In addition, red lesions, considered to be the earliest forms of endometriosis and the most active lesions, have a higher vascular density and higher mitotic index than the more advanced black and white lesions [56,57]. The vessel maturation index, however, as determined by the percentage of microvessels co-localizing with α-smooth muscle actin-positive cells (pericytes), is lower. These are strong indications of an ongoing neovascularization process in early lesions.

The endometrial tissue which is shed during the menstrual cycle is able to elicit angiogenic responses at the locations to which it translocates. This is clearly illustrated by the angiogenic responses induced by the menstrual endometrial tissue transplanted onto the growing CAM model. The number of vessels growing towards the transplanted tissue is significantly increased, and application of angiogenesis inhibitors prevents this process and inhibits lesion development as well [11,12]. Revascularization of lesions after transplantation of human endometrium into immunodeficient mice is completed in approximately 2 weeks [13,14]. The human resident vessels in the lesions disappeared and the grafts were repopulated with murine vessels [14]. Most of these vessels consist of endothelial cells only; a pericyte layer typical of vessel maturation was lacking. In these xenograft models, lesion development could also be effectively blocked by treatment with substances known to inhibit angiogenesis, including TNP-470, anginex, endostatin, angiostatin, and selective cyclo-oxygenase (COX)-2 inhibitors [58–62].

Non-human primate models are generally considered to be the most biologically relevant models for endometriosis, because most species have regular menstrual cycles and a normally functioning immune system and they spontaneously develop the disease [63]. In rhesus macaques in which endometriosis was induced by autotransplantation of endometrial tissue, the disease burden could be significantly reduced by treating the animals with a blocking antibody against the VEGF receptor-2 (Flk1) [64]. Taken together, these studies clearly demonstrate the importance of the angiogenic process during early lesion formation and development, and confirm a significant role for VEGF.

Revascularization of ectopic endometrium
The revascularization of ectopic endometrial tissue is the result of a multitude of processes that commence upon the arrival of menstrual blood into the abdominal cavity. Prior to menstruation,

a marked influx of bone marrow-derived cells in the human endometrium is observed [65]. These cells produce large amounts of growth factors and inflammatory cytokines. The shed endometrial tissue including these immune cells is transported by the blood to the abdominal cavity [66,67]. In addition, an inflammatory response is elicited in the abdominal cavity aimed at the clearance of the endometrial tissue [68]. This first-line defense against the ectopic endometrial cells is not foolproof, since microscopic endometriosis can be found intermittently in all women with patent fallopian tubes [69]. The peritoneal fluid is angiogenic, as was demonstrated in, for instance, the CAM model [70], which indicates that the vasoactive substances in the exudate could potentially affect vessels in the peritoneal lining.

Ang/Tie system and vessel destabilization
The matured capillaries in the peritoneum are protected by a sheath of pericytes, and under these circumstances vessel branching cannot be induced by VEGF. As discussed earlier, the angiopoietin (Ang)/Tie system is key in regulating vascular integrity and quiescence [45]. The most important vasoactive factor is undoubtedly VEGF, which is elevated in the peritoneal fluid and endometriotic lesions of endometriosis patients [71–73]. In a mouse tumor model, it was demonstrated that VEGF in the abdominal cavity affects the peritoneal lining by increasing the vascular permeability of blood vessels [74]. This suggests that VEGF is able to activate the vessels of the peritoneal lining prior to the attachment of the endometrial tissue to the peritoneal surface. The activated vessels release Ang-2 which disrupts the endothelial cell–pericyte interactions, upon which the endothelial cells become susceptible to the action of vasoactive factors (Fig. 19.2).

The role of hypoxia-inducible factor-1α
The revascularization of human endometrium fragments transplanted into the abdomen of immunodeficient mice is completed in approximately 1–2 weeks [13,14]. A recent study in the mouse showed that hypoxia is a very important trigger for the initial angiogenic responses in transplanted uterine tissue [75]. HIF-1α protein was rapidly and transiently upregulated, which corresponded closely with a transient increase in the expression of the HIF-1α target genes, glucose transporter-1 (Glut-1) and VEGF. Inhibition of HIF-1α expression resulted in a decrease in Glut-1 and VEGF expression and a dose-dependent inhibition of the growth of the endometriotic lesions. These studies clearly demonstrate that the early vascular events at the endometrium–peritoneum interface are orchestrated by HIF-1α originating from the endometrium tissue.

Hypoxia-inducible factor-1α is a ubiquitously expressed transcription factor in mammalian cells. Under normoxic conditions, HIF-1α is hydroxylated at prolyl and asparaginyl residues, binds to the von Hippel–Lindau (vHL) protein and undergoes proteosomal degradation. Under low oxygen levels, HIF-1α is not hydroxylated, avoiding binding to the vHL protein and thereby inhibiting ubiquitination and proteosomal degradation [28,29].

While HIFs are the executors of the response to hypoxia, oxygen-sensing enzymes are responsible for the sensing of oxygen

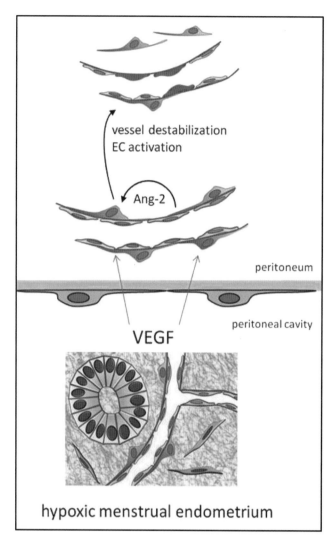

Figure 19.2 VEGF produced by the hypoxic menstrual endometrium and activated leukocytes in the peritoneal exudates activates endothelial cells in vessels in the peritoneal lining. This results in the release of Ang-2, which leads to the dissociation of pericytes in the immediate vicinity, and consequently the cells become susceptible to proangiogenic factors.

tension and in turn regulate HIF activity in an oxygen-dependent way, the oxygen-sensing prolyl hydroxylase domain proteins (PHD-1, -2, and -3), and the factor inhibiting HIF (FIH) [76,77]. Under well-oxygenated conditions, PHDs hydroxylate conserved proline residues in HIFs, upon which they bind to the vHL protein which is part of an E3 ubiquitin ligase complex. The HIF protein is then ubiquitinated and targeted for proteosomal degradation. The FIH hydroxylates a C-terminal asparaginyl residue in HIF-1α which impairs the interaction with the co-activator p300, thereby silencing transcription of hypoxia-inducible genes. When oxygen levels drop, the hydroxylation activity of the PHDs and FIH is reduced, which results in the accumulation and activation of HIF-1α.

Hypoxia-inducible factor-1α is mainly catalyzed by PHD-2, also referred to as egl nine homolog-1 (*C. elegans*) or EGLN-1. EGLN-1 mRNA and protein were shown to be constitutively expressed

in both proliferative and secretory phase endometrium [78], indicating that an oxygen-sensing mechanism which controls the degradation of HIF-1α is also present in the endometrium.

Branch formation

The development of new vessel branches (sprouting) has been studied in great detail in recent years. Specialized endothelial cells, called "tip" cells, are selected and lead the sprout at the forefront of the vessel branches [79]. These cells highly express VEGFR-2, are highly polarized and use filopodia to guide a sprouting vessel towards an angiogenic stimulus, usually VEGF. This cell is highly motile, tubeless, and proliferates minimally or not at all. The elongation of the new branch relies on proliferation of endothelial "stalk" cells, which trail behind the pioneering "tip" cell. In the stalk a lumen is created. The new branch then connects with another branch through "tip" cell fusion to form a lumen for initiation of blood flow. Following the "stalk" cells are the "phalanx" cells. These are non-proliferating endothelial cells that form a tube, which can sense and regulate the perfusion of the persistent sprout. The "phalanx" cells are also responsible for vessel stabilization and maturation by the recruitment of pericytes, deposition of ECM, tightening of cellular junctions and induction of quiescence. Once the branch is formed and perfused, the normalizing oxygen levels reduce VEGF concentrations, and the maintenance of low VEGF levels secures the survival of the quiescent "phalanx" cells and vascular homeostasis (Fig. 19.3).

The "tip" cells are designated through δ-like ligand-4 (Dll-4)/ Notch signaling [79] (see Fig. 19.3). This is a mechanism by which cells instruct neighboring cells to adopt a distinct fate. VEGF induces the expression of Dll-4, and since VEGF concentrations are highest at the vascular front, Dll-4 expression is highest in the "tip" cell. Notch signaling activity, however, is strongest in the "stalk" cells. In turn, the Dll-4 activates Notch in the neighboring cells, leading to downregulation of VEGFR-2 and VEGR-3, upregulation of VEGFR-1, and inhibition of the migratory response. In addition, elongation of the branch requires "stalk" cell proliferation, but Notch signaling is known to induce cell cycle arrest. To overcome this, Notch induces the expression of Notch-regulated ankyrin repeat protein (Nrarp) in the "stalk" cells. Nrarp acts downstream from Notch and induces degradation of the Notch intracellular domain, thus antagonizing the cell cycle inhibitory activity of Notch. Simultaneously, Nrarp also induces Wnt signaling which promotes proliferative activity as well as stalk stability by tightening intercellular junctions.

Vasculogenesis in the graft

The repopulation of the endometrial tissue with new blood vessels is a key process in the establishment of endometriotic lesions. Growing tumors and tumor metastases induce an angiogenic response once the critical tumor mass of ~1 mm³ is reached. The requirement for oxygen and nutrients for endometrial tissue may be more acute, however, since only fragments of menstrual endometrium large enough to preserve the original tissue architecture were shown to have invasive and angiogenic properties [80].

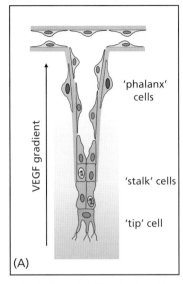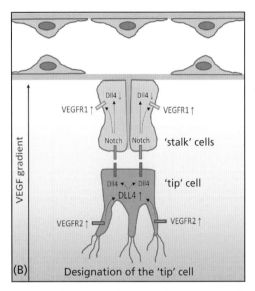

Figure 19.3 Branch formation. (A) The first endothelial cell activated becomes the "tip" cell. This cell is migratory but does not proliferate. It expresses high levels of VEGFR-2 and migrates towards a VEGF gradient. The cells trailing the "tip" cells are the "stalk" cells, which are less migratory but they do proliferate and contribute to the elongation of the branch. Once the branch is completed, a lumen is formed and blood flow is restored, oxygen levels are normalized. This leads to normalization of VEGF concentrations and endothelial cells return back to their quiescent state which allows them to recruit pericytes. (B) The "tip" cell is designated by the level of Dll4 expression. Dll4 expression is induced by VEGF, so the endothelial cell exposed to the highest VEGF concentrations will have the highest Dll4 expression. High expression of Dll4 signals activates the Notch expressed in the neighboring cells, which leads to a downregulation of VEGFR-2, upregulation of VEGFR-1, and inhibition of the migratory response.

Once the endothelial cells in the peritoneum are activated and the branching process is initiated, and the vessel branches reach the endometrial tissue, the endothelial cells most likely follow a gradient of proangiogenic and vasoactive factors that are produced by the endometrial tissue, i.e. VEGF, PlGF, FGF-2, CNN1/Cyr61, prostaglandins, and inflammatory cytokines. However, this process is not well understood.

The fastest way for the vessels to grow is to follow a path with the lowest resistance (Fig. 19.4). This means that the endometrial tissue is repopulated with endothelial cells from the host environment and this is orchestrated by the ECM deposited by the progressively regressing resident vessels in the graft [14,81]. Studies by Demarchez and co-workers [82] elegantly showed that in skin grafts in nude mice, the original endothelial cells of the transplanted tissue progressively disappeared, while murine endothelial cells invaded the graft, using the basement membrane of the pre-existing vessels as a scaffold. Murine collagen IV progressively appeared in the graft, and co-localized with the human collagen IV.

Xenograft transplantation studies in the mouse showed that upon transplantation of human endometrium tissue, the human resident vessels progressively regress and that the grafts are completely repopulated with endothelial cells from the host [14]. The high degree of organization [13] strongly suggests that the murine vessels are also employing the pre-existing network of ECM deposited by the human vessels. Whether the murine endothelial cells are also employing the basement membrane of the human vessels as a guidance cue has not yet been confirmed.

Recent studies indicate that stem or adult progenitor cells have the capacity to form or contribute to functional vascular networks

in vivo [83]. It was shown that the endothelium in the endometrium is partially reconstituted by stem cells [84], and that menstrual blood also contains endothelium regenerating cells. However, it is not likely that these cells play a significant role in the neovascularization of the early endometriotic lesions because the numbers of progenitor cells found in the blood vessels of the endometrium were very low, even after 2 years [85].

The final step in the revascularization process is vessel restabilization. As discussed before, the Ang-1/Tie-2 system is responsible for vessel stabilization. However, it also regulates the restoration of the expression of junctional proteins controlling endothelial barrier functions, i.e. VE-cadherin and N-cadherin, as well as junctional adhesion molecules in tight junctions [86,87].

After the vessel branch is formed and tissue oxygenation has been restored, local VEGF levels decrease spontaneously. The endothelium switches back to the quiescent state. This is illustrated by, for instance, the high expression of VE-cadherin in the "phalanx" cells [79]. As a result of the reducing VEGF levels, Ang-2 release ceases and the protein is stored again in the Weibel–Palade bodies. Subsequently, Ang-1/Tie-2 complexes are installed at the interendothelial cell junctions to transduce survival signals. The interactions between the endothelial cells and pericytes recruited through the PDGF-BB/SDF-1α/CXCR-4 mechanism are also restored through Ang-1/Tie-2 interactions [88].

There is not much information with regard to the expression of Ang-1, Ang-2 and Tie-2 in endometriotic lesions. Ang-2 mRNA and protein were found to be higher in eutopic and ectopic endometrium of patients compared to controls [89]. Drenkhahn and co-workers [90] showed that after transplantation of human

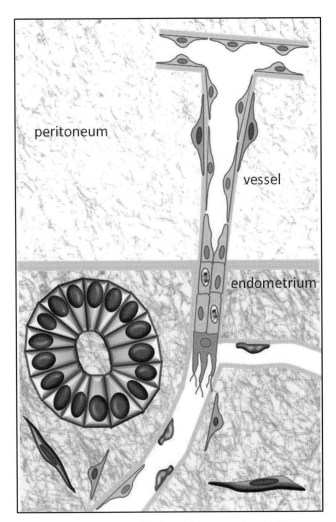

Figure 19.4 Revascularization of endometrial fragments adhered to the peritoneal lining. The quickest way to restore the vascular supply is for growing branches of the peritoneum to make use of the existing network of basement membrane-coated channels, that become available as the resident endothelial cells regress. Observations in mouse xenograft models after transplantation of endometrium tissue support this. An even quicker way is for the peritoneal vessels to anastomose with the vessels in the human endometrium but there is no evidence to support this.

endometrium on the CAM, the expression of Ang-1 and Ang-2 mRNA decreased. However, the Ang-2/Ang-1 expression ratio increased considerably, most likely due to the activation of endothelial cells under these hypoxic conditions.

Conclusion

Hypoxia and VEGF are key regulators in the revascularization process. Endothelial cells in vessels of the peritoneal lining are activated by the proangiogenic factors produced in response to hypoxia in the endometrium and inflammatory environment, and the angiogenic process is initiated. Even though the evidence

is circumstantial, it is likely that the ectopic endometrium is revascularized by repopulating the existing vascular channels with peritoneal endothelial cells, once the resident endothelial cells have regressed.

Our understanding of the revascularization process of the endometriotic lesions, however, is not nearly detailed enough. We must develop more ingenious models and experiments, and in addition, study peri- and post-transplantation events in peritoneal lining and endometrium grafts at the cellular level. This can be done, for instance, by including transgenic animals in the study designs, which will allow the study of single-gene effects in this complex process.

References

1. Von Rokitansky C. Ueber Uterusdrüsen-Neubildung in Uterus und Ovarial-Sarcomen. Zeitschr KK Gesellschaft der Aerzte zu Wien 1860;37:577–581.
2. Sampson JA Peritoneal endometriosis due to the menstrual dissemination of endometrial tissue into the peritoneal cavity. Am J Obstet Gynecol 1927;14:422–469.
3. Ferriani RA, Charnock-Jones DS, Prentice A et al. Immunohistochemical localization of acidic and basic fibroblast growth factors in normal human endometrium and endometriosis and the detection of their mRNA by polymerase chain reaction. Hum Reprod 1993;8:11–16.
4. Oosterlynck DJ, Cornillie FJ, Waer M, Koninckx PR. Immunohistochemical characterization of leucocyte subpopulations in endometriotic lesions. Arch Gynecol Obstet 1993;253:197–206.
5. Ferenczy A. Studies on the cytodynamics of human endometrial regeneration. II. Transmission electron microscopy and histochemistry. Am J Obstet Gynecol 1976;124:582–595.
6. Ludwig H, Spornitz UM. Microarchitecture of the human endometrium by scanning electron microscopy, menstrual desquamation and remodeling. Ann N Y Acad Sci 1991;622:28–46.
7. Fan X, Krieg S, Kuo CJ et al. VEGF blockade inhibits angiogenesis and reepithelialization of endometrium. FASEB J 2008;22:3571–3580.
8. Punyadeera C, Thijssen VL, Tchaikovski S et al. Expression and regulation of vascular endothelial growth factor ligands and receptors during menstruation and post-menstrual repair of human endometrium. Mol Hum Reprod 2006;12:367–375.
9. Girling JE, Rogers PA. Recent advances in endometrial angiogenesis research. Angiogenesis 2005;8(2):89–99.
10. Print C, Valtola R, Evans A et al. Soluble factors from human endometrium promote angiogenesis and regulate the endothelial cell transcriptome. Hum Reprod 2004;19:2356–2366.
11. Maas JW, Groothuis PG, Dunselman GAJ et al. Endometrial angiogenesis throughout the human menstrual cycle. Hum Reprod 2001;16:1557–1561.
12. Nap AW, Dunselman GA, Griffioen AW et al. Angiostatic agents prevent the development of endometriosis-like lesions in the chicken chorioallantoic membrane. Fertil Steril 2005;83:793–795.

13. Grümmer R, Schwarzer F, Bainczyk K et al. Peritoneal endometriosis, validation of an in-vivo model. Hum Reprod 2001;16:1736–1743.

14. Eggermont J, Donnez J, Casanas-Roux F et al. Time course of pelvic endometriotic lesion revascularization in a nude mouse model. Fertil Steril 2005;84:492–499.

15. Nayak NR, Brenner RM. Vascular proliferation and the vascular endothelial growth factor expression in the rhesus macaque endometrium. J Clin Endocrinol Metab 2002;87:1845–1855.

16. Ferenczy A, Bertrand G, Gelfand MM. Proliferation kinetics of human endometrium during the normal menstrual cycle. Am J Obstet Gynecol 1979;133:859–867.

17. Rabbani ML, Rogers PA. Role of vascular endothelial growth factor in endometrial vascular events before implantation in rats. Reproduction 2001;122:85–90.

18. Holash J, Davis S, Papadopoulos N et al. VEGF-Trap, a VEGF blocker with potent antitumor effects. Proc Natl Acad Sci USA 2002;99:11393–11398.

19. Carmeliet P. VEGF as a key mediator of angiogenesis in cancer. Oncology 2005;69(Suppl 3):4–10.

20. Loges S, Roncal C, Carmeliet P. Development of targeted angiogenic medicine. J Thromb Haemost 2009;7:21–33.

21. Carmeliet P, Tessier-Lavigne M. Common mechanisms of nerve and blood vessel wiring. Nature 2005;436:193–200.

22. Gargett CE, Lederman F, Lau TM et al. Lack of correlation between vascular endothelial growth factor production and endothelial cell proliferation in the human endometrium. Hum Reprod 1999;14:2080–2088.

23. Gargett CE, Lederman F, Heryanto B et al. Focal vascular endothelial growth factor correlates with angiogenesis in human endometrium. Role of intravascular neutrophils. Hum Reprod 2001;16:1065–1075.

24. Ancelin M, Chollet-Martin S, Hervé MA et al. Vascular endothelial growth factor VEGF189 induces human neutrophil chemotaxis in extravascular tissue via an autocrine amplification mechanism. Lab Invest 2004;84:502–512.

25. Zhang H, Issekutz AC. Growth factor regulation of neutrophil-endothelial cell interactions. J Leukoc Biol 1994;70:225–232.

26. Choi EY, Santoso S, Chavakis T. Mechanisms of neutrophil transendothelial migration. Front Biosci 2009;14:1596–1605.

27. Cid MC, Kleinman HK, Grant DS et al. Estradiol enhances leukocyte binding to tumor necrosis factor (TNF)-stimulated endothelial cells via an increase in TNF-induced adhesion molecules E-selectin, intercellular adhesion molecule type 1, and vascular cell adhesion molecule type 1. J Clin Invest 1994;93:17–25.

28. Semenza GL. HIF-1, mediator of physiological and pathophysiological responses to hypoxia. J Appl Physiol 2000;88:1474–1480.

29. Semenza GL. Targeting HIF-1 for cancer therapy. Nat Rev Cancer 2003;3:721–732.

30. Kelly BD, Hackett SF, Hirota K et al. Cell type-specific regulation of angiogenic growth factor gene expression and induction of angiogenesis in nonischemic tissue by a constitutively active form of hypoxia-inducible factor 1. Circ Res 2003;93:1074–1081.

31. Graubert MD, Ortega MA, Kessel B et al. Vascular repair after menstruation involves regulation of vascular endothelial growth factor-receptor phosphorylation by sFLT-1. Am J Pathol 2001;158: 1399–1410.

32. Charnock-Jones DS, Sharkey AM, Rajput-Williams J et al. Identification and localization of alternately spliced mRNAs for vascular endothelial growth factor in human uterus and estrogen regulation in endometrial carcinoma cell lines. Biol Reprod 1993;48:1120–1128.

33. Nayak NR, Critchley HO, Slayden OD et al. Progesterone withdrawal up-regulates vascular endothelial growth factor receptor type 2 in the superficial zone stroma of the human and macaque endometrium, potential relevance to menstruation. J Clin Endocrinol Metab 2000;85:3442–3452.

34. Sharkey AM, Day K, McPherson A et al. Vascular endothelial growth factor expression in human endometrium is regulated by hypoxia. J Clin Endocrinol Metab 2000;85:402–409.

35. Popovici RM, Irwin JC, Giaccia AJ, Giudice LC. Hypoxia and cAMP stimulate vascular endothelial growth factor (VEGF) in human endometrial stromal cells, potential relevance to menstruation and endometrial regeneration. J Clin Endocrinol Metab 1999;84:2245–2248.

36. Fraser HM, Wilson H, Silvestri A et al. The role of vascular endothelial growth factor and estradiol in the regulation of endometrial angiogenesis and cell proliferation in the marmoset. Endocrinology 2008;149:4413–4420.

37. Albrecht ED, Babischkin JS, Lidor Y et al. Effect of estrogen on angiogenesis in co-cultures of human endometrial cells and microvascular endothelial cells. Hum Reprod 2003;18:2039–2047.

38. Rees MC, Bicknell R. Angiogenesis in the endometrium. Angiogenesis 1998;2:29–35.

39. Hervé MA, Meduri G, Petit FG et al. Regulation of the vascular endothelial growth factor (VEGF) receptor Flk-1/KDR by estradiol through VEGF in uterus. J Endocrinol 2006;188:91–99.

40. Koos RD, Kazi AA, Roberson MS, Jones JM. New insight into the transcriptional regulation of vascular endothelial growth factor expression in the endometrium by estrogen and relaxin. Ann N Y Acad Sci 2005;1041:233–247.

41. Kazi AA, Molitoris KH, Koos RD. Estrogen rapidly activates the PI3K/AKT pathway and hypoxia-inducible factor 1 and induces vascular endothelial growth factor A expression in luminal epithelial cells of the rat uterus. Biol Reprod 2009;81:378–387.

42. Ancelin M, Buteau-Lozano H, Meduri G et al. A dynamic shift of VEGF isoforms with a transient and selective progesterone-induced expression of VEGF189 regulates angiogenesis and vascular permeability in human uterus. Proc Natl Acad Sci USA 2002; 99:6023–6028.

43. Licht P, Russu V, Lehmeyer S et al. Cycle dependency of intrauterine vascular endothelial growth factor levels is correlated with decidualization and corpus luteum function. Fertil Steril 2003; 80:1228–1233.

44. Salamonsen LA, Butt AR, Hammond FR et al. Production of endometrial matrix metalloproteinases, but not their tissue inhibitors, is modulated by progesterone withdrawal in an in vitro model for menstruation. J Clin Endocrinol Metab 1997;82:1409–1415.

45. Fiedler U, Augustin HG. Angiopoietins, a link between angiogenesis and inflammation. Trends Immunol 2006;27:552–558.

46. Papetti M, Herman IM. Mechanisms of normal and tumor-derived angiogenesis. Am J Physiol Cell Physiol 2002;282:C947–970.

47. Hirchenhain J, Huse I, Hess A et al. Differential expression of angiopoietins 1 and 2 and their receptor Tie-2 in human endometrium. Mol Hum Reprod 2003;9:663–669.

48. Hewett P, Nijjar S, Shams M et al. Down-regulation of angiopoietin-1 expression in menorrhagia. Am J Pathol 2002;160:773–780.

49. Lindahl P, Betsholtz C. Not all myofibroblasts are alike, revisiting the role of PDGF-A and PDGF-B using PDGF-targeted mice. Curr Opin Nephrol Hypertens 1998;7:21–26.

50. Kaminski WE, Lindahl P, Lin NL et al. Basis of hematopoietic defects in platelet-derived growth factor (PDGF)-B and PDGF beta-receptor null mice. Blood 2001;97:1990–1998.

51. Chegini N, Rossi MJ, Masterson BJ. Platelet-derived growth factor (PDGF), epidermal growth factor (EGF), and EGF and PDGF beta-receptors in human endometrial tissue, localization and in vitro action. Endocrinology 1992;130:2373–2385.

52. Laschke MW, Elitzsch A, Vollmar B et al. Combined inhibition of vascular endothelial growth factor (VEGF), fibroblast growth factor and platelet-derived growth factor, but not inhibition of VEGF alone, effectively suppresses angiogenesis and vessel maturation in endometriotic lesions. Hum Reprod 2006;21:262–268.

53. Song N, Huang Y, Shi H et al. Overexpression of platelet-derived growth factor-BB increases tumor pericyte content via stromal-derived factor-1alpha/CXCR4 axis. Cancer Res 2009;69:6057–6064.

54. Gelmini S, Mangoni M, Castiglione F et al. The CXCR4/CXCL12 axis in endometrial cancer. Clin Exp Metastasis 2009;26:261–268.

55. Glace L, Grygielko ET, Boyle R et al. Estrogen-induced stromal cell-derived factor-1 (SDF-1/Cxcl12) expression is repressed by progesterone and by Selective Estrogen Receptor Modulators via estrogen receptor alpha in rat uterine cells and tissues. Steroids 2009;74:1015–1024.

56. Nisolle M, Casanas-Roux F, Anaf V et al. Morphometric study of the stromal vascularization in peritoneal endometriosis. Fertil Steril 1993;59:681–684.

57. Matsuzaki S, Canis M, Murakami T et al. Immunohistochemical analysis of the role of angiogenic status in the vasculature of peritoneal endometriosis. Fertil Steril 2001;76:712–716.

58. Hull ML, Charnock-Jones DS, Chan CL et al. Antiangiogenic agents are effective inhibitors of endometriosis. J Clin Endocrinol Metab 2003;88:2889–2899.

59. Nap AW, Griffioen AW, Dunselman GA et al. Antiangiogenesis therapy for endometriosis. J Clin Endocrinol Metab 2004;89:1089–1095.

60. Dabrosin C, Gyorffy S, Margetts P et al. Therapeutic effect of angiostatin gene transfer in a murine model of endometriosis. Am J Pathol 2002;161:909–918.

61. Dogan E, Saygili U, Posaci C et al. Regression of endometrial explants in rats treated with the cyclooxygenase-2 inhibitor rofecoxib. Fertil Steril 2004;82(Suppl 3):1115–1120.

62. Becker CM, Sampson DA, Rupnick MA et al. Endostatin inhibits the growth of endometriotic lesions but does not affect fertility. Fertil Steril 2005;84(Suppl 2):1144–1155.

63. D'Hooghe TM, Kyama CM, Chai D et al. Nonhuman primate models for translational research in endometriosis. Reprod Sci 2009;16:152–161.

64. Park A, Chang P, Ferin M et al. Inhibition of endometriosis development in Rhesus monkeys by blocking VEGF receptor, a novel treatment for endometriosis. Fertil Steril 2004;82:S71.

65. Salamonsen LA, Lathbury LJ. Endometrial leukocytes and menstruation. Hum Reprod Update 2000;6:16–27.

66. Halme J, Hammond MG, Hulka JF et al. Retrograde menstruation in healthy women and in patients with endometriosis. Obstet Gynecol 1984;64:151–154.

67. Liu DT, Hitchcock A. Endometriosis, its association with retrograde menstruation, dysmenorrhoea and tubal pathology. Br J Obstet Gynaecol 1986;93:859–862.

68. D'Hooghe TM, Bambra CS, Xiao L et al. Effect of menstruation and intrapelvic injection of endometrium on inflammatory parameters of peritoneal fluid in the baboon (Papio anubis and Papio cynocephalus). Am J Obstet Gynecol 2001;184:917–925.

69. Koninckx PR. Is mild endometriosis a condition occurring intermittently in all women? Hum Reprod 1994;9:2202–2205.

70. Maas JW, Calhaz-Jorge C, ter Riet G et al. Tumor necrosis factor-alpha but not interleukin-1 beta or interleukin-8 concentrations correlate with angiogenic activity of peritoneal fluid from patients with minimal to mild endometriosis. Fertil Steril 2001;75:180–185.

71. McLaren J, Prentice A, Charnock-Jones DS, Smith SK. Vascular endothelial growth factor (VEGF) concentrations are elevated in peritoneal fluid of women with endometriosis. Hum Reprod 1996;11:220–223.

72. Di Carlo C, Bonifacio M, Tommaselli GA et al. Metalloproteinases, vascular endothelial growth factor, and angiopoietin 1 and 2 in eutopic and ectopic endometrium. Fertil Steril 2009;91:2315–2323.

73. Kim HO, Yang KM, Kang IS et al. Expression of CD44s, vascular endothelial growth factor, matrix metalloproteinase-2 and Ki-67 in peritoneal, rectovaginal and ovarian endometriosis. J Reprod Med 2007;52:207–213.

74. Nagy JA, Masse EM, Herzberg KT et al. Pathogenesis of ascites tumor growth, vascular permeability factor, vascular hyperpermeability, and ascites fluid accumulation. Cancer Res 1995;55:360–368.

75. Becker CM, Rohwer N, Funakoshi T et al. 2-methoxyestradiol inhibits hypoxia-inducible factor-1{alpha} and suppresses growth of lesions in a mouse model of endometriosis. Am J Pathol 2008;172:534–544.

76. Kaelin WG Jr, Ratcliffe PJ. Oxygen sensing by metazoans, the central role of the HIF hydroxylase pathway. Mol Cell 2008;30:393–402.

77. Appelhoff RJ, Tian YM, Raval RR et al. Differential function of the prolyl hydroxylases PHD1, PHD2, and PHD3 in the regulation of hypoxia-inducible factor. J Biol Chem 2004;279:38458–38465.

78. Kato H, Inoue T, Asanoma K et al. Induction of human endometrial cancer cell senescence through modulation of HIF-1alpha activity by EGLN1. Int J Cancer 2006;118:1144–1153.

79. Carmeliet P, de Smet F, Loges S, Mazzone M. Branching morphogenesis and antiangiogenesis candidates, tip cells lead the way. Nat Rev Clin Oncol 2009;6:315–326.

80. Nap AW, Groothuis PG, Demir AY et al. Tissue integrity is essential for ectopic implantation of human endometrium in the chicken chorioallantoic membrane. Hum Reprod 2003;18:30–34.

81. Anderson CR, Ponce AM, Price RJ. Immunohistochemical identification of an extracellular matrix scaffold that microguides capillary sprouting in vivo. J Histochem Cytochem 2004;52:1063–1072.

82. Demarchez M, Hartmann DJ, Prunieras M. An immunohistological study of the revascularization process in human skin transplanted onto the nude mouse. Transplantation 1987;43:896–903.

83. Melero-Martin JM, Khan ZA, Picard A et al. In vivo vasculogenic potential of human blood-derived endothelial progenitor cells. Blood 2007;109:4761–4768.

84. Mints M, Jansson M, Sadeghi B et al. Endometrial endothelial cells are derived from donor stem cells in a bone marrow transplant recipient. Hum Reprod 2008;23:139–143.

85. Meng X, Ichim TE, Zhong J et al. Endometrial regenerative cells, a novel stem cell population. J Transl Med 2007;5:57.

86. Lampugnani MG, Dejana E. Interendothelial junctions, structure, signalling and functional roles. Curr Opin Cell Biol 1997; 9:674–682.

87. Luo Y, Radice GL. N-cadherin acts upstream of VE-cadherin in controlling vascular morphogenesis. J Cell Biol 2005;169:29–34.

88. Augustin HG, Koh GY, Thurston G, Alitalo K. Control of vascular morphogenesis and homeostasis through the angiopoietin-Tie system. Nat Rev Mol Cell Biol 2009;10:165–177.

89. Jingting C, Yangde Z, Yi Z et al. Expression of heparanase and angiopoietin-2 in patients with endometriosis. Eur J Obstet Gynecol Reprod Biol 2008;136:199–209.

90. Drenkhahn M, Gescher DM, Wolber EM et al. Expression of angiopoietin 1 and 2 in ectopic endometrium on the chicken chorioallantoic membrane. Fertil Steril 2004;81(Suppl 1):869–875.

Uterine Peristalsis and the Development of Endometriosis and Adenomyosis

Gerhard Leyendecker[1] and Ludwig Wildt[2]

[1]Kinderwunschzentrum (Fertility Center) Darmstadt, Darmstadt, Germany
[2]University Clinic of Gynecological Endocrinology and Reproductive Medicine, Department of Obstetrics and Gynecology, Medical University Innsbruck, Innsbruck, Austria

Introduction

In our understanding of the pathophysiology of endometriosis and adenomyosis, a reanalysis of both structure and function of the non-pregnant uterus turned out to be of the utmost importance [1–4]. With uterine peristalsis and directed (sperm) transport, a novel uterine function has been discovered [5–12]. It became evident that the non-pregnant uterus is constantly active throughout the reproductive period of life and thereby, like other mechanically active organs of the body such as the skeletal and cardiovascular systems, inevitably subjected to mechanical strain. Research performed in recent years has demonstrated a crucial role of mechanical strain in normal and pathological function of various tissues. Moreover, it became apparent that the molecular mechanisms associated with mechanical strain, injury and repair display a pattern that is quite similar in different tissues and involves the expression of P450 aromatase and the local production of estrogen [13]. The sequels of tissue injury and repair, however, may be very specific, depending on the structure and functions of the tissues and organs involved, such as tendons and cartilage in the skeleton and the intima in the cardiovascular system. This is of particular importance when, as is the case with the uterus, the tissue is physiologically highly estrogen sensitive and when injury is chronic in character [14]. Chronic mechanical strain sustains an inflammatory process. Meyer has hinted at the inflammatory character of ectopic endometrial lesions [15].

The concept of the archimetra and its structure and function

The uterus is composed of two different organs: the inner archimetra and the outer neometra [1,4] (Plate 20.1). Phylogenetically and ontogenetically, the archimetra or endometrial-subendometrial unit constitutes the oldest part of the uterus (hence its denomination) and is composed of the epithelial and stromal endometrium and the underlying stratum subvasculare of the myometrium (archimyometrium [2]) with a predominantly circular arrangement of muscular fibers. While both the endometrium and the subendometrial myometrium display a marked cyclical pattern of steroid hormone receptor expression, the two other layers of the myometrium, the outer stratum supravasculare with a predominantly longitudinal arrangement of muscular fibers and the stratum vasculare consisting of a three-dimensional mesh of short muscular bundles [2,3], show a more or less continuously high receptor expression throughout the cycle [4,16]. Only the archimetra is of paramesonephric origin, while the outer layers, the neometra, are of non-müllerian origin [2].

The archimyometrium

The archimyometrium extends from the lower part of the cervix through the uterine corpus into the cornua, where it continues as the muscular layer of the fallopian tubes [3]. In high-resolution sonography and magnetic resonance imaging (MRI), the archimyometrium can be visualized as a hypodense "halo" and a hypointense "junctional zone" with 4–8 mm of width encircling the endocervix as well as the endometrium (see Plate 20.1D,E). The anlage of the archimyometrium can be identified during the first trimester of gestation (hence its denomination) [2,4]. Circular mesenchymal layers surround the fused paramesonephric ducts and develop into muscular fibers during midgestation. Short longitudinal fibers branch off the circular ones [2], presumably providing coherence of the circular fibers in the longitudinal direction and thereby adding physical strength to the archimyometrium. In the adult, co-ordinated contractions of the circular and short longitudinal fibers result in thickening of the archimyometrium that moves from the cervix to the fundal part of the uterus and that can be visualized in cine MRI as a wave of focal and symmetrical enlargements of the junctional zone.

Endometriosis: Science and Practice, First Edition. Edited by Linda C. Giudice, Johannes L.H. Evers and David L. Healy.
© 2012 Blackwell Publishing Ltd. Published 2012 by Blackwell Publishing Ltd.

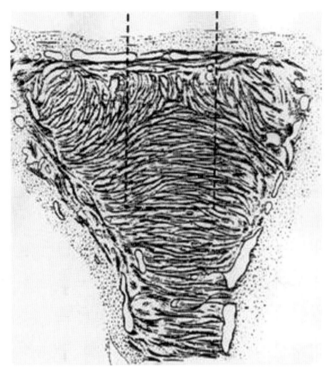

Figure 20.1 Modified original drawing from Werth and Grusdew showing the architecture of the subendometrial myometrium (archimyometrium) in a human fetal uterus. The specific orientation of the circular fibers of the archimyometrium results from the fusion of the two paramesonephric ducts forming a fundocornual raphe in the midline (*dashed rectangle*). The peristaltic pump of the uterus, which is continuously active during the menstrual cycle, is driven by co-ordinated contractions of these muscular fibers. Directed sperm transport into the dominant tube is made possible by differential activation of these fibers. The region of the fundocornual raphe is considered the predominant site of mechanical strain. Modified from Werth and Grusdew [2] with permission from Springer-Verlag.

The ontogenetically early formation of the archimyometrium is pertinent to its function and is in particular exemplified by the fundocornual raphe that results from the fusion of the two paramesonephric ducts and their mesenchymal elements to form the primordial uterus [2,17]. The bipartition of the circular subendometrial myometrium in the upper part of the uterine corpus and its separate continuation through the cornua into the respective tubes are the morphological basis of directed sperm transport into the tube ipsilateral to the dominant follicle (Fig. 20.1).

The production of smooth muscle cells by stromal metaplasia occurring during the first trimester of gestation [2] is a property of the basal endometrial stroma that is also retained in the adult. Cyclical metaplasia of the basal endometrial stromal cells into myofibroblasts and back into stromal cells is constantly taking place at the endometrial–myometrial junction [18,19]. This metaplastic potential of the basal endometrial mesenchyme is of particular importance with respect to the metaplastic production of smooth muscle cells in endometriotic lesions and their possible further development in deeply infiltrating foci (see Plate 20.1B). There is indirect evidence derived from immunohistochemical

studies that the archimyometrium and the muscular fibers of ectopic endometrial lesions constitute homologous tissues [16].

Functional versus basal endometrium

Improved immunostaining could extend previous data about the cylical pattern of estradiol receptor (ER) and progesterone receptor (PR) expression in the endometrium during the menstrual cycle [16] (Fig. 20.2). In both the functional and basal layers, there is a cyclical pattern of ER-α and PR expression. While within the functionalis, the receptor expression of both steroids steadily declines during the secretory phase, with immunoreactive scores (IRS) tending virtually towards zero immediately prior to menstruation, in the basal endometrium, after an intermediate fall, there is a steady increase of the IRS of ER-α and PR during the secretory phase that extends into the next proliferative phase (Fig. 20.3). This is of importance in characterizing the tissue fragments that are shed during menstruation and potentially seeded within the peritoneal cavity by retrograde transport. Judging by cytomorphological criteria, tissue fragments devoid of receptor expression (functional endometrium) are destined for cellular death while those with positive staining (basal endometrium) appear to be highly vital [16].

The archimetra and the outer layers of the uterus have different functions during the process of reproduction. While the stratum supravasculare and the stratum vasculare, sequentially acquired during evolution in meeting the requirements for the appropriate forces during parturition [4], only subserve the expulsion of the conceptus, the archimetra has extra fundamental functions in the very early processes of reproduction. These functions may be summarized as proliferation and differentiation of the endometrium for implantation, uterine peristalsis for directed rapid and sustained sperm transport and inflammatory defense [1]. In order to meet these functions, the components of the archimetra, the epithelial and stromal endometrium as well as the subendometrial myometrium constantly undergo fundamental structural and biochemical changes throughout the cycle [4,19].

Uterine peristalsis

Peristaltic activity of the non-pregnant uterus is a fundamental function in the early process of reproduction [8,9,20]. Uterine peristalsis only involves the stratum subvasculare of the myometrium and exhibits cyclical changes in direction, frequency, and intensity [5,6,8] (Fig. 20.4). During menstruation the contraction waves with lowest frequency and intensity are directed towards the cervix, while during the other phases of the cycle cervicofundal peristalsis prevails, with highest frequency and intensity during the periovulatory phase [6]. Rapid as well as sustained sperm transport [8,20] constitutes the predominant reproductive function of uterine peristalsis. Also high fundal implantation of the embryo is considered a function of uterine peristalsis during the luteal phase [5]. Vaginal discharge of the menstrual debris may be effected by fundocervical peristalsis and additional contractile activity of the stratum vasculare that increases the tone of the uterus during this phase of the cycle. Retrograde menstruation is probably scant and may only constitute a "side effect" of the low cervicofundal contractile activity during

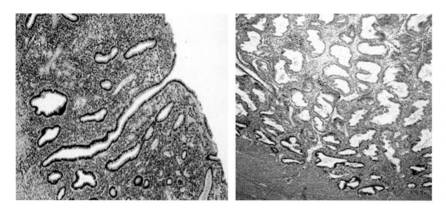

Figure 20.2 Representative sections of the endometrium of healthy women in the late proliferative and late secretory phases of the cycle, immunostained for ERs. During the proliferative phase of the cycle, the ERs of the endometrial epithelium and the stroma are evenly distributed over all endometrial zones, whereas during the late secretory phase, positive staining for epithelial and stromal estrogen receptors is confined to the small basal endometrial fringe. Reproduced from Leyendecker *et al* [16] with permission from Oxford University Press.

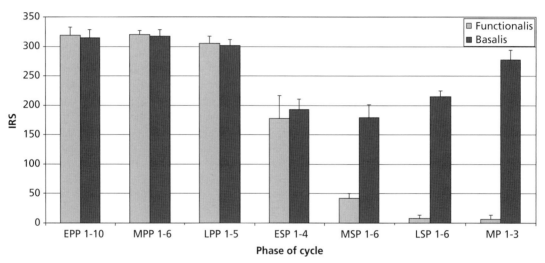

Figure 20.3 Immunoreactive scores (IRS) of ERα expression in the functionalis and basalis, during the menstrual cycle. Modified from Leyendecker *et al* [16] with permission from Oxford University Press.

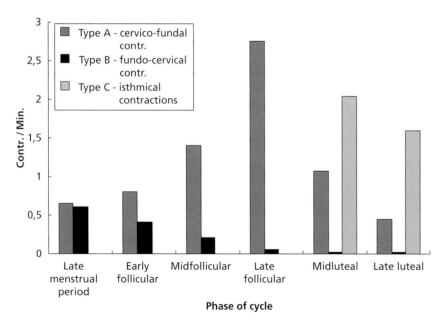

Figure 20.4 Histogram demonstrating the frequency of uterine peristaltic waves during menstruation, the early, mid- and late follicular and mid- and late luteal phases of the cycle, as obtained from video sonography of uterine peristalsis in healthy women. The relative distribution of cervicofundal (type A) versus fundocervical (type B) and isthmical (type C) contractions is also shown. The graph clearly demonstrates the increase in frequency of type A contractions with the progression of the follicular phase reaching a maximum during the late follicular phase and the decrease during the luteal phase of the cycle. With progression of the menstrual cycle, type B contraction waves almost disappear. Type C contractions prevail during the luteal phase. These contractions do not extend beyond the isthmical or lower corporal part of the uterus, rendering the fundocornual part of the uterus a zone of relative peristaltic quiescence during the period of embryo implantation. Modified from Kunz *et al* [28] with permission from Monduzzi Editore.

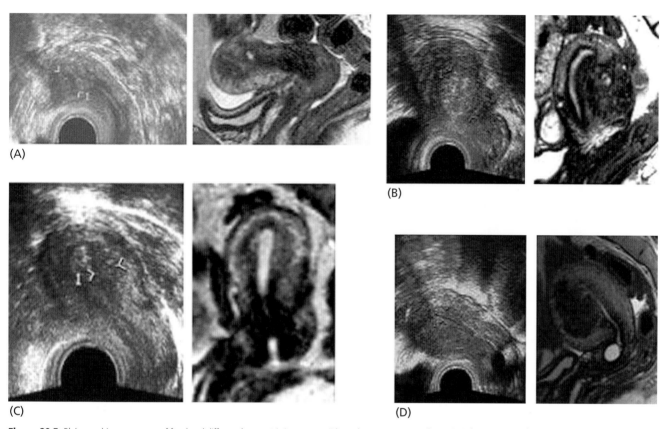

Figure 20.5 Pleiomorphic appearance of focal and diffuse adenomyosis in women with moderate to severe endometriosis (27–31 years of age; A-C). In patient (D) (37 years of age), because of low sperm count of the husband, no laparoscopy was performed. She had curettage at the age of 22. The transvaginal sonography (TVS) was apparently normal. Meticulous analysis, however, showed asymmetry of the uterine walls and no "halo" could be demonstrated. MRI revealed focal to diffuse adenomyosis of the anterior wall and incipient adenomyosis of the posterior wall of the uterus. Sagittal scans of the uterine midline are shown.

this phase of the cycle. Retrograde shedding of blood might, however, be significant under the pathological conditions of cervicofundal uterine hyperperistalsis, such as in endometriosis, and juvenile dysfunctional bleeding, helping to preserve the iron content of the body in the latter situation [21].

During the follicular phase, cervicofundal peristalsis is controlled by the rising tide of follicular estradiol [22], which induces within the archimetra a cascade of transcriptional events such as the expression of endometrial oxytocin (OT) and oxytocin receptor (OTR) mRNA [23,24]. OT has been shown to increase uterine peristaltic activity [22]. As soon as a dominant ovarian structure can be visualized by ultrasound sperm transport is directed preferentially into the tube ipsilateral to the dominant follicle [8]. Directed sperm transport by uterine peristalsis is made possible by the specific structure of the stratum subvasculare in the fundal and cornual region [2,17,21,25] as well as by the specific endocrine stimuli that reach the upper part of the uterus by means of the utero-ovarian counter-current system [26] and are superimposed on those reaching the uterus via the systemic circulation [22,27]. This enables the uterus, though having become an unpaired organ during evolution and embryogenesis, to function asymmetrically as a paired one. During the luteal phase, the contractile activity of the archimyometrium decreases and changes

in character. This results in a zone of relative quiescence in the fundal region of the uterine cavity. The cyclical functions of the archimetra can be completely mimicked by the sequential administration of estradiol and estradiol plus progesterone that yields physiological blood levels of these hormones, thus underlining the ovarian role in the control of archimetral function [28].

The role of the uterus in the disease process

There are several lines of evidence for the notion that dysfunctions of the uterus play a crucial role in the pathophysiology of endometriosis.

- Fragments of basal endometrium were found in the menstrual effluent with a higher prevalence in women with endometriosis than in controls. On the basis of these and other findings, it was suggested that pelvic endometriosis results from the transtubal dislocation of fragments of basal endometrium [16].
- There is a significant association of pelvic endometriosis with uterine adenomyosis in women and in the baboon with life-long infertility. In women, the reported prevalence, however, differs according to the study population chosen and the criteria applied to the interpretation of MRI findings [1,29–34] (Fig. 20.5).

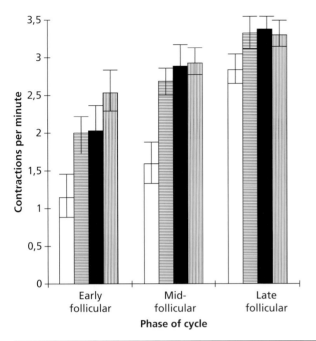

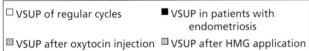

Figure 20.6 The frequency of uterine peristaltic contractions during the follicular phase of the menstrual cycle in healthy women, in those with endometriosis, in those treated with HMG (human menopausal gonadotropin), resulting in unphysiologically high levels of estradiol in serum, and normal women treated with an intravenous bolus of oxytocin. The data show that high estradiol levels and bolus injections of oxytocin, respectively, simulate the significantly increased uterine peristalsis in patients with endometriosis in comparison to healthy women. Values are mean ± SEM (standard error of the mean). VSUP, vaginal sonography of uterine peristalsis. Reproduced from Leyendecker *et al* [1] with permission from Oxford University Press.

- The uterine function of rapid and directed sperm transport into the "dominant tube" is dysfunctional in women with endometriosis and is characterized by hyper- and dysperistalsis [20,35–39] (Plate 20.2, Fig. 20.6).

It has been suggested that this uterine dysfunction in women with endometriosis and adenomyosis is a result of archimetral hyperestrogenism [1,20,21,25]. There are several lines of evidence that support this notion.

- In comparison to normal controls and in contrast to peripheral blood, estradiol levels are elevated in menstrual blood of women with endometriosis and adenomyosis [40].
- The expression of P450 aromatase is increased in adenomyotic tissue and in ectopic and eutopic endometrium of women with endometriosis [41–47].
- A highly estrogen-dependent gene, Cyr61, is upregulated in eutopic endometrium in women with endometriosis and also in ectopic lesions as well as in experimental endometriosis [48,49].
- The peristaltic activity of the subendometrial myometrium can be dramatically increased by elevated peripheral levels of estradiol

as they are observed during controlled ovarian hyperstimulation. The intensity of uterine peristaltic activity in women with endometriosis resembles that of women during controlled ovarian hyperstimulation although the peripheral estradiol levels are within the normal range [1,20,22] (Fig. 20.6).

Tissue injury and repair – archimetral hyperestrogenism

The local production of estrogen at the level of both eutopic endometrium in women with endometriosis and ectopic lesions is central to understanding the pathophysiology of the disease. The etiology of this increased estrogen-producing "glandular" potential of these tissues, however, is still enigmatic.

Recent studies have increasingly shown that estradiol is of the utmost importance in the process of wound healing [50–52]. This action of estrogens appears to be mainly mediated by ERβ. Animal experiments with chemotoxic or mechanic stress to astroglia [13,53,54], urinary bladder tissue as well as studies with isolated connective tissue such as fibroblasts and cartilage [55–57] have revealed that tissue injury and inflammation with subsequent healing are associated with a specific physiological process that involves the local production of estrogen from its precursors. Interleukin (IL)-1-induced activation of the cyclo-oxygenase-2 (COX-2) enzyme results in the production of prostaglandin E_2 (PGE_2), which in turn activates steroidogenic acute regulatory protein (StAR) and P450 aromatase. Thus, with the increased transport of cholesterol to the inner mitochondrial membrane, testosterone can be formed and aromatized into estradiol that exerts its proliferative and healing effects via ERβ. In studies with fibroblasts, it was shown that the first steps of this cascade could be activated by seemingly minor biophysical strain [55]. Following termination of unphysiological strain and healing, this process is downregulated and the local production of estrogen or upregulation of estrogen-dependent genes ceases [55–58]. This cascade can even be activated in tissue that normally does not express P450 aromatase, indicating the basic physiological significance of the local production of estrogen in tissue injury and repair (TIAR) [59]. The similarity of the molecular biology of TIAR in various tissues to that described in endometriosis [45–47,60–63] strongly suggests that this represents the common underlying mechanism of both processes (Fig. 20.7).

Mechanism of disease: uterine autotraumatization

It is understandable that myometrial fibers and fibroblasts at the endometrial–myometrial interface near the fundocornual raphe are subjected to increased mechanical strain during midcycle, because not only is the ovarian estradiol secretion at its peak at

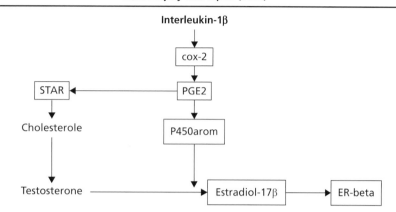

Figure 20.7 The basic aspects of the molecular biology of the physiological mechanism of TIAR as demonstrated in mesenchymal tissue such as astrocytes, tendons, and cartilage. Reproduced from Leyendecker *et al* [14] with permission from Springer-Verlag.

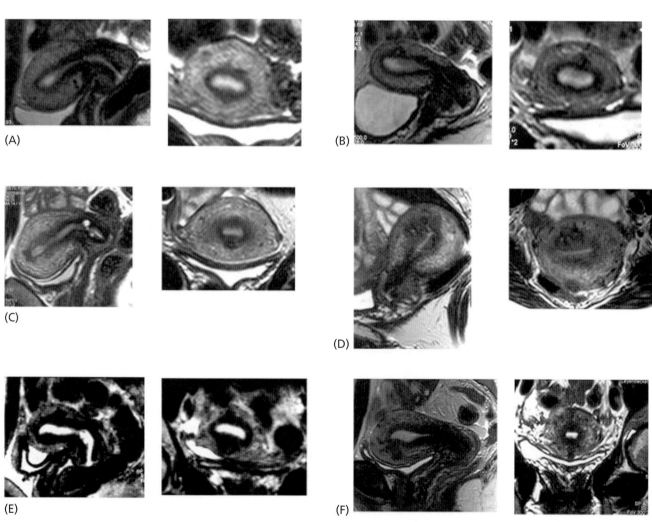

(A)

(B)

(C)

(D)

(E)

(F)

Figure 20.8 Examples of uterine adenomyosis in six patients as presented by MRI. Representative sagittal and coronary scans are shown. In the infertile, non-parous women (A–E) (30–32 years of age), pelvic endometriosis of grade I–IV was demonstrated by laparoscopy. In the parous woman (F) (40 years of age), no laparoscopy was performed. In all scans preponderance of the adenomyotic lesions (expanded junctional zone) in the midline close to the fundocornual raphe of the archimyometrium can be demonstrated. In the first three scans (A–C), the diagnosis of adenomyosis would not meet the established radiological criteria for MRI. In a scientific context, however, the irregularities of the junctional zone are characteristic of incipient adenomyosis. Reproduced from Leyendecker *et al* [14] with permission from Springer-Verlag.

that time, but also additional mechanical strain is imposed on these cells due to estradiol that reaches the uterus via the utero-ovarian counter-current system and controls the direction of the upward transport [27]. Directed sperm transport begins during the midfollicular phase of the cycle when the dominant follicle becomes visible [8]. The fundocornual raphe as a site of predilection of mechanical strain is documented by the observation that early adenomyosis usually evolves in the sagittal midline of the midcorporal and fundal part of the uterus (Fig. 20.8; see Fig. 20.1). Even in more advanced cases of adenomyosis, the expansion of the junctional zone in MRI often shows preponderance at these locations [21].

"First-step" injury: microtraumatization

Experiments with cultivated fibroblasts have shown that mechanical strain within certain limits is physiological to such cells. However, even minor increments in mechanical strain resulted in the activation of COX-2 and the production of PGE_2, the basic biochemical mechanisms underlying tissue injury [55], and also in the production of IL-8 [64]. Thus, with respect to the subendometrial myometrium, deviations from the normal cyclical endocrine pattern with increases or prolongations of estradiol stimulation of uterine peristalsis could impose supraphysiological mechanical strain on the cells near the fundocornual raphe. It has been attempted to relate irregularities of the menstrual cycle to the development of endometriosis, without clear-cut evidence [65]. The irregularities under discussion, however, are not easily determined and might escape self-observation and recording of patient history.

It is tempting to speculate that events such as prolonged follicular phases, anovulatory cycles or periods of follicular persistency and also the presence of large antral follicles in both ovaries before definite selection of the dominant follicle would impose, by increased or prolonged estrogenic stimulation, stronger mechanical strain to the muscular fibers and fibroblasts. That a prolonged period of estrogenic stimulation might promote the development of endometriosis is documented in a study aiming at examining the hereditary component of endometriosis in colonized rhesus monkeys. Only a history of application of estrogen patches (in addition to a history of trauma by hysterotomy) showed a significant association with endometriosis [66]. The cyclical irregularities discussed above, that might also have a hereditary background, occur frequently during the early period of reproductive life. This concurs with an early onset of endometriosis in most cases [67]. But other factors should also be taken into consideration that might increase the susceptibility to mechanical strain and tissue injury.

In any event, repeated and sustained overstretching and injury of the myocytes and fibroblasts at the endometrial–myometrial interface close to the fundocornual raphe would activate the TIAR system focally with increased local production of estradiol. This process starts on a microscopic level and complete healing might be possible, particularly if the mechanical strain with subsequent tissue injury happened to be only a singular

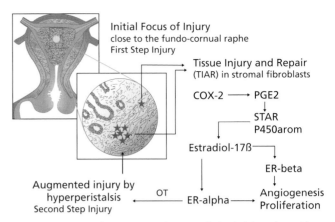

Figure 20.9 Model of tissue injury and repair on the level of the endometrial–myometrial interface at the fundocornual raphe. The mechanisms of first- and second-step injury are depicted. Persistent uterine peristaltic activity and hyperperistalsis are responsible for perpetuation of injury with permanently increased paracrine estrogen action. Reproduced from Leyendecker *et al* [14] with permission from Springer-Verlag.

event or followed by a longer phase of uterine quiescence such as during pregnancy and breastfeeding.

During such a singular phase of "first-step" injury transtubal dislocation of fragments of basal endometrium might occur. In addition to the very low probability of transtubal seeding of fragments of basal endometrium in normal women, such single events could contribute to the development of asymptomatic pelvic endometriosis [16,21,68]. In case of accidental implantation at an unfavorable site, such as the ovaries, severe intraperitoneal endometriosis could develop without further involvement of the uterus in the disease process, as indicated by a completely normal junctional zone in MRI.

With continuing hyperperistaltic activity and sustained injury, however, healing at the fundocornual raphe will not ensue and an increasing number of foci are involved in this process of chronic injury, proliferation, and inflammation. The expansion or accumulation of such sites with an activated TIAR system provokes local areas of the basal endometrium to function as an endocrine gland that produces estradiol (Figs 20.9, 20.10).

"Second-step" injury: autotraumatization by hyperperistalsis

Focal estrogen production might reach a tissue level that, in a paracrine fashion, acts upon the archimyometrium and increases uterine peristaltic activity presumably mediated by endometrial oxytocin and its receptor [22,23,24]. Hyperperistalsis constitutes a mechanical trauma resulting in increased desquamation of fragments of basal endometrium [16] and, in combination with an increased retrograde uterine transport capacity [20], in enhanced transtubal dissemination of these vital fragments [16]. The development of peritoneal endometriotic lesions from fragments of basal endometrium is in fact a process of transplantation and represents to a certain extent Sampson's aspect of the disease development [69].

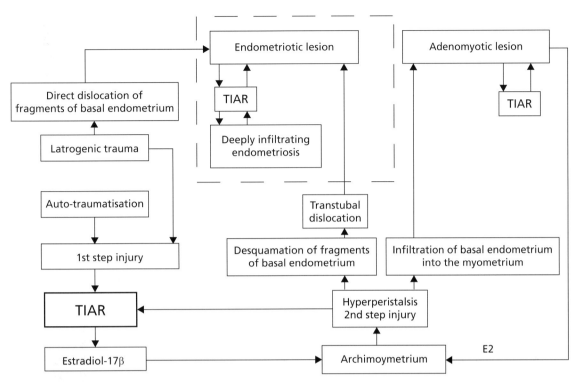

Figure 20.10 Model of the pathophysiology of endometriosis and adenomyosis. Tissue injury in the depth of the endometrium and the activation of the TIAR system constitute the prime movers in disease development. This pertains to spontaneously developing endometriosis/adenomyosis as well as to that induced by iatrogenic trauma. The dashed rectangle depicts the extrauterine sites of the disease process. Reproduced from Leyendecker *et al* [14] with permission from Springer-Verlag.

The development of uterine adenomyosis is a continuation of the process that is initiated by the "first-step" injury. With the extension or accumulation of the sites of injury and the ensuing hyperperistalsis following paracrine estrogen effects, this inflammatory process of tissue injury and repair is reinforced and perpetuated, resulting in the proliferation of connective tissue with the inherent potential of smooth muscle metaplasia. That is why adenomyotic lesions, in contrast to superficial endometriotic lesions, display a more fibromuscular character. While even short periods of transtubal seeding might result in peritoneal lesions, such as in experimental endometriosis with inoculation of endometrial material in the peritoneal cavity, the development of adenomyosis is a more prolonged process. In any event, the initiation of the TIAR mechanism in the depth of the endometrial stroma and its possible perpetuation constitute the initial events in the development of both endometriosis and adenomyosis.

Premenarcheal endometriosis

Pelvic endometriosis has been described in adolescent girls prior to menarche and coelomic metaplasia had been suggested as the underlying mechanism [70]. However, it should be borne in mind that with the progression of puberty, there is an increasing nocturnal hypothalamo-pituitary activity with secretory bursts of luteinizing hormone (LH) and follicle-stimulating hormone

(FSH) [71]. As in low-grade hypothalamic amenorrhea, large antral follicles are observed in the ovaries of premenarcheal girls which, following nocturnal gonadotropic stimulation, intermittently secrete estradiol during the morning hours that presumably in turn stimulates uterine peristalsis [72–74]. Thus, detachment and upward transport of fragments of basal endometrium from the more or less unstimulated endometrium in these girls have to be considered as well.

In this respect, the significance of menstruation in the disease process [69] should be more precisely defined. It is not menstruation *per se* but rather the fact that, following detachment of the functionalis, the basal endometrium is maximally exposed. In the presence of hyperperistalsis, this facilitates both detachment of fragments of basal endometrium and their upward transport [16,20,25].

Iatrogenic injury

Iatrogenic traumata to the uterus are considered to increase the risk for development of endometriosis and adenomyosis [75]. A history of hysterotomy in colonized rhesus monkeys showed a significant association with the later development of endometriosis in these animals [66]. The underlying mechanism of induction of endometriosis by iatrogenic trauma such as curettage and other ablative techniques appears to be very similar to those described above. Such surgical interventions might result in extended lesions with an enhanced TIAR reaction. The rapidly increasing local estrogen levels during the process of healing interfere with the ovarian control over uterine peristaltic activity, leading rapidly to "second-step" injury with ensuing autotraumatization and perpetuation of the disease process.

Thus, within the context of our model, iatrogenic lesions that result in the development of endometriosis and adenomyosis can be viewed as strong one-time "first-step" injuries. In the baboon model, experimental endometriosis was induced by inoculation of endometrial fragments that were obtained by endometrial biopsies during the menstrual phase of the animals. In the endometriotic lesions Cyr61, a highly estrogen-dependent gene, was soon upregulated [49]. Surprisingly, Cyr61 started to be upregulated also in the eutopic endometrium of these primarily healthy animals. Most probably, the activation of Cyr61 in the eutopic endometrium resulted from activation of the TIAR system with local production of estrogen following tissue injury that was caused by the biopsy rather than from "cross-talk" between the endometriotic lesions and the eutopic endometrium, as suggested by the authors.

Ectopic lesions

In both endometriotic lesions and eutopic endometrium of women with endometriosis, the cellular and molecular components of the regulatory systems that enable the tissue to produce estradiol have been shown to be expressed. While this has been convincingly shown for peritoneal lesions, data concerning the eutopic endometrium of women with endometriosis are unequivocal in this respect. Fragments of basal endometrium constitute injured tissue. The expression of acute and inflammatory cytokines such as IL-1β, IL-6 and IL-8 [65,76] facilitates implantation. As autotransplants, however, the fragments should implant without inflammatory sequels. Due to the cyclical strain imposed upon the peritoneal endometriotic lesions, the TIAR system is repeatedly and chronically activated. Immunhistochemistry has also demonstrated a dramatic upregulation of ERα [16]. In superficial lesions this chronic inflammatory process might calm down and healing might be possible [77]. The recent finding of nerve fibers in ectopic lesions and eutopic endometrium of affected women and their regression following gestagen administration is in harmony with the view that chronic strain sustains an inflammatory process [78–82].

Superficial lesions usually display the glandular character of the parent tissue and are surrounded by muscular fibers [16,83] that result from the inherent potential of the basal mesenchyme to form muscular tissue [16]. Superficial endometriotic lesions have, therefore, been described as "microuteri" or "microarchimetras" [16] (see Fig. 20.1B, C). However, in most cases the unfavorable environment does not allow for even a truncated simulation of the cyclical events seen in the parent tissue, such as proliferation and secretory transformation. Therefore, the glandular epithelium and stroma of the lesions display the immunohistochemical character of the basalis layer of the eutopic endometrium [16].

Deeply infiltrating lesions develop at sites that are also subjected to chronic mechanical irritation, such as the rectosigmoid fixed to the pelvic wall or uterus, the sacrouterine ligaments, the urinary bladder, ovaries fixed to the pelvic wall, the rectovaginal septum as well as the abdominal wall. It appears that chronic trauma to the ectopic lesions maintains the inflammatory process and results in the same tissue response as seen in uterine adenomyosis [21]. These are in fact the extrauterine sites of adenomyoma described by Cullen [84]. As outlined above, the peristromal fibromuscular tissue of endometriotic lesions is homologous to the respective tissue within the archimetra and probably in the same way susceptible to mechanical strain. Chronic mechanical strain results in proliferation and preponderance of fibromuscular tissue, both characteristic of deeply infiltrating endometriosis and uterine adenomyosis [85]. Deeply infiltrating lesions tend to persist, while superficial lesions might heal. That is why long-lasting endometriosis usually presents with deeply infiltrating lesions [77] and also uterine adenomyosis [21–30].

As delineated above, the disease process starts focally in the depth of the basal endometrium. Thus, endometrial biopsies might miss the focus with an activated TIAR system. With the progression of the disease, the area of alteration might be expanded. This is in keeping with the observation that the molecular markers associated with endometriosis could be more consistently demonstrated in more advanced stages of the disease [46].

With respect to the molecular biology of the eutopic endometrium in endometriosis, it has to be taken into consideration that the endometrium, as has been pointed out before, is composed morphologically and functionally of at least two distinct layers: the basalis and the functionalis [16,86–88]. This is not sufficiently taken into account when studies on molecular biology are performed with material taken from more or less random endometrial biopsies [45–47,89]. The basal endometrium in women with endometriosis is twice as thick as in healthy women [16,25]. Moreover, while in healthy women the endometrial/ myometrial lining is smooth and regular, it is irregular and sometimes polypoid in affected women [21,90]. Thus, biopsies taken from women with endometriosis might to a variable and unknown extent be "contaminated" with basal endometrium and may even contain basal endometrial stroma that is altered by the TIAR process. This might at least in part explain the finding of "progesterone resistance" [46,91,92] and an impaired estradiol metabolism in the endometrium of women with endometriosis [47,89].

Using immunohistochemistry of ERα and PR, no progesterone resistance could be observed in the late secretory phase of the functional endometrium of affected women. As in healthy women, with the progression of the secretory phase, ER and PR expression declined in the functionalis and steadily rose in the basalis as well as in the endometriotic lesions [16]. The latter findings suggest physiological progesterone resistance in the basal endometrium and also in the endometriotic lesions as they are derived from implanted fragments of basal endometrium.

Moreover, clinical studies with oocyte donation do not support a generally impeded implantation in women with endometriosis [93]. With respect to the expression of 17β-hydroxysteroid dehydrogenase type 2, no data are available that distinguish between functionalis and basalis [94].

Conclusion

Pelvic endometriosis, deeply infiltrating endometriosis and uterine adenomyosis share a common pathophysiology and may now be integrated into the pyhsiological mechanism and new nosological concept of "tissue injury and repair" (TIAR) and may, in this context, represent the extreme of a basically physiological, estrogen-related mechanism, that is pathologically exaggerated in an extremely estrogen-sensitive reproductive organ.

Accumulating evidence suggests that endometriosis and adenomyosis are caused by trauma. In the spontaneously developing disease, chronic uterine peristaltic activity or phases of hyperperistalsis induce, at the endometrial–myometrial interface near the fundocornual raphe, microtraumatizations with the activation of the TIAR mechanism. This results in the local production of estrogen. With ongoing peristaltic activity, such sites might accumulate and the estrogens increasingly produced interfere in a paracrine fashion with ovarian control over uterine peristaltic activity, resulting in permanent hyperperistalsis and self-perpetuation of the disease process. Overt autotraumatization of the uterus with dislocation of fragments of basal endometrium into the peritoneal cavity and infiltration of basal endometrium into the depth of the myometrial wall ensues. In most cases of endometriosis/adenomyosis, a causal event early in the reproductive period of life must be postulated, leading rapidly to uterine hyperperistalsis. In late premenopausal adenomyosis, such an event might not have occurred. However, as indicated by the high prevalence of the disease, it appears to be unavoidable that, with time, chronic normoperistalsis throughout the reproductive period of life accumulates to the same extent of microtraumatization. With the activation of the TIAR mechanism followed by chronic inflammation and infiltrative growth, endometriosis/adenomyosis of the younger woman and premenopausal adenomyosis share in principle the same pathophysiology.

References

1. Leyendecker G, Kunz G, Noe M et al. Endometriosis: a dysfunction and disease of the archimetra. Hum Reprod Update 1998;4:752–762.
2. Werth R, Grusdew W. Untersuchungen über die Entwicklung und Morphologie der menschlichen Uterusmuskulatur. Arch Gynäkol 1898;55:325–409.
3. Wetzstein R. Der Uterusmuskel: Morphologie. Arch Gynecol 1965;202:1–13.
4. Noe M, Kunz G, Herbertz M et al. The cyclic pattern of the immuno-cytochemical expression of oestrogen and progesterone receptors in human myometrial and endometrial layers: characterisation of the endometrial-subendometrial unit. Hum Reprod 1999;14:101–110.
5. De Vries K, Lyons EA, Ballard G et al. Contractions of the inner third of the myometrium. Am J Obstet Gynecol 1990;162:679–682.
6. Lyons EA, Taylor PJ, Zheng XH et al. Characterisation of subendometrial myometrial contractions throughout the menstrual cycle in normal fertile women. Fertil Steril 1991;55:771–775.
7. Williams M, Hill CJ, Scudamore I et al. Sperm numbers and distribution within the human fallopian tube around ovulation. Hum Reprod 1993;8:2019–2026.
8. Kunz G, Beil D, Deininger H et al. The dynamics of rapid sperm transport through the female genital tract. Evidence from vaginal sonography of uterine peristalsis (VSUP) and hysterosalpingoscintigraphy (HSSG). Hum Reprod 1996;11:627–632.
9. Wildt L, Kissler S, Licht P et al. Sperm transport in the human female genital tract and its modulation by oxytocin as assessed by hysterosalpingography, hysterotonography, electrohysterography and Doppler sonography. Hum Reprod Update 1998;4:655–666.
10. Schmiedehausen K, Kat S, Albert N et al. Determination of velocity of tubar transport with dynamic hysterosalpingoscintigraphy. Nucl Med Commun 2003;24:865–870.
11. Zervomanolakis I, Ott HW, Hadziomerovic D et al. Physiology of upward transport in the human female genital tract. Ann N Y Acad Sci 2007;1101:1–20.
12. Zervomanolakis I, Ott HW, Müller J et al. Uterine mechanisms of ipsilateral directed spermatozoa transport: evidence for a contribution of the utero-ovarian countercurrent system. Eur J Obstet Gynecol Reprod Biol 2009;144(Suppl 1):45–49.
13. Garcia-Segura LM. Aromatase in the brain: not just for reproduction anymore. J Neuroendocrinol 2008;20:705–712.
14. Leyendecker G, Wildt L, Mall G. The pathophysiology of endometriosis and adenomyosis. Tissue injury and repair. Arch Gynecol Obstet 2009;280:529–538.
15. Meyer R. Über den Stand der Frage der Adenomyositis und Adenome im allgemeinen und insbesondere über Adenomyositis seroepithelialis und Adenomyometritis sarcomatosa. Zbl Gynäkol 1919;43:745–750.
16. Leyendecker G, Herbertz M, Kunz G et al. Endometriosis results from the dislocation of basal endometrium. Hum Reprod 2002;17:2725–2736.
17. Leyendecker G. Endometriosis is an entity with extreme pleiomorphism. Hum Reprod 2000;15:4–7.
18. Bird CC, Willis RA. The production of smooth muscle by the endometrial stroma of the adult human uterus. J Path Bact 1965;90:75–81.
19. Fujii S, Konishi I, Mori T. Smooth muscle differentiation at endometrio-myometrial junction. An ultrastructural study. Virchows Archiv Anat Pathal Anat 1989;414:105–112.
20. Leyendecker G, Kunz G, Wildt L et al. Uterine hyperperistalsis and dysperistalsis as dysfunctions of the mechanism of rapid sperm transport in patients with endometriosis and infertility. Hum Reprod 1996;11:1542–1551.
21. Leyendecker G, Kunz G, Kissler S et al. Adenomyosis and reproduction. Best Pract Res Clin Obstet Gynaecol 2006;20:523–546.

22. Kunz G, Noe M, Herbertz M et al. Uterine peristalsis during the follicular phase of the menstrual cycle. Effects of oestrogen, antioestrogen and oxytocin. Hum Reprod Update 1998;4:647–654.

23. Zingg HH, Rosen F, Chu K et al. Oxytocin and oxytocin receptor gene expression in the uterus. Recent Progr Hormone Res 1995;50:255–273.

24. Mitzumoto Y, Furuya K, Makimura N et al. Gene expression of oxytocin receptor in human eutopic endometrial tissues. Adv Exp Med Biol 1995;395:491–493.

25. Leyendecker G, Kunz G, Herbertz M et al. Uterine peristaltic activity and the development of endometriosis. Ann NY Acad Sci 2004;1034:338–355.

26. Einer-Jensen N. Countercurrent transfer in the ovarian pedicle and its physiological implications. Oxford Rev Reprod Biol 1988; 10:348–381.

27. Kunz G, Herbertz M, Noe M et al. Sonographic evidence of a direct impact of the ovarian dominant structure on uterine function during the menstrual cycle. Hum Reprod Update 1998;4:667–672.

28. Kunz G, Kissler S, Wildt L et al. Uterine peristalsis: directed sperm transport and fundal implantation of the blastocyst. In: Filicori M (ed) Endocrine Basis of Reproductive Function. Bologna: Monduzzi Editore, 2000.

29. Kunz G, Beil D, Huppert P et al. Structural abnormalities of the uterine wall in women with endometriosis and infertility visualized by vaginal sonography and magnetic resonance imaging. Hum Reprod 2000;15:76–82.

30. Kunz G, Beil D, Huppert P et al. Adenomyosis in endometriosis – prevalence and impact on fertility. Evidence from magnetic resonance imaging. Hum Reprod 2005;20:2309–2316.

31. Kunz G, Herbertz M, Beil D et al. Adenomyosis as a disorder of the early and late human reproductive period. Reprod Biomed Online 2007;15:681–685.

32. Dueholm M, Lundorf E, Hansen ES et al. Magnetic resonance imaging and transvaginal ultrasonography for the diagnosis of adenomyosis. Fertil Steril 2001;76:588–594.

33. Dueholm M, Lundorf E. Transvaginal ultrasound or MRI for diagnosis of adenomyosis. Curr Opin Obstet Gynecol 2007;19:505–512.

34. Barrier BF, Malinowski MJ, Dick EJ Jr et al. Adenomyosis in the baboon is associated with primary infertility. Fertil Steril 2004;82(Suppl 3):1091–1094.

35. Mäkäräinen L. Uterine contractions in endometriosis: effects of operative and danazol treatment. Obstet Gynecol 1988;9:134–138.

36. Salamanca A, Beltran E. Subendometrial contractility in menstrual phase visualised by transvaginal sonography in patients with endometriosis. Fertil Steril 1995;64:193–195.

37. Bulletti C, de Ziegler D, Polli V et al. Characteristics of uterine contractility during menses in women with mild to moderate endometriosis. Fertil Steril 2002;77:156–161.

38. Kissler S, Hamscho N, Zangos S et al. Uterotubal transport disorder in adenomyosis and endometriosis – a cause for infertility. Br J Obstet Gynaecol 2006;113:902–908.

39. Kissler S, Zangos S, Wiegratz I et al. Utero-tubal sperm transport and its impairment in endometriosis and adenomyosis. Ann N Y Acad Sci 2007;1101:38–48.

40. Takahashi K, Nagata H, Kitao M. Clinical usefulness of determination of estradiol levels in the menstrual blood for patients with endometriosis. Acta Obstet Gynecol Jpn 1989;41:1849–1850.

41. Yamamoto T, Noguchi T, Tamura T et al. Evidence for oestrogen synthesis in adenomyotic tissues. Am J Obstet Gynecol 1993;169: 734–738.

42. Noble LS, Simpson ER, Johns A et al. Aromatase expression in endometriosis. J Clin Endocrinol Metab 1996;81:174–179.

43. Noble LS, Takayama K, Zeitoun KM et al. Prostaglandin E2 stimulates aromatase expression in endometriosis-derived stromal cells. J Clin Endocrinol Metab 1997;82:600–606.

44. Kitawaki J, Noguchi T, Amatsu T et al. Expression of aromatase cytochrome P450 protein and messenger ribonucleic acid in human endometriotic and adenomyotic tissues but not in normal endometrium. Biol Reprod 1997;57:514–519.

45. Hudelist G, Czerwenka K, Keckstein J et al. Expression of aromatase and estrogen sulfotransferase in eutopic and ectopic endometrium: evidence for unbalanced estradiol production in endometriosis. Reprod Sci 2007;14:798–805.

46. Aghajanova L, Hamilton A, Kwintkiewicz J et al. Steroidogenic enzyme and key decidualization marker dysregulation in endometrial stromal cells from women with versus without endometriosis. Biol Reprod 2009;80:105–114.

47. Bulun SE. Endometriosis. N Engl J Med 2009;360:268–279.

48. Absenger Y, Hess-Stumpp H, Kreft B et al. Cyr61, a deregulated gene in endometriosis. Mol Hum Reprod 2004;10:399–407.

49. Gashaw I, Hastings JM, Jackson KS et al. Induced endometriosis in the baboon (Papio anubis) increases the expression of the proangiogenic factor CYR61 (CCN1) in eutopic and ectopic endometria. Biol Reprod 2006;74:1060–1066.

50. Ashcroft GS, Ashworth JJ. Potential role of estrogens in wound healing. Am J Clin Dermatol 2003;4:737–743.

51. Gilliver SC, Ashworth JJ, Ashcroft GS. The hormonal regulation of cutaneous wound healing. Clin Dermatol 2007;25:56–62.

52. Mowa CN, Hoch R, Montavon CL et al. Estrogen enhances wound healing in the penis of rats. Biomed Res 2008;29:267–270.

53. Sierra A, Lavaque E, Perez-Martin M et al. Steroidogenic acute regulatory protein in the rat brain: cellular distribution, developmental regulation and overexpression after injury. Eur J Neurosci 2003;18:1458–1467.

54. Lavaque E, Sierra A, Azcoitia I et al. Steroidogenic acute regulatory protein in the brain. Neuroscience 2006;138:741–747.

55. Yang G, Im HJ, Wang JH. Repetitive mechanical stretching modulates IL-1beta induced COX-2, MMP-1 expression, and PGE2 production in human patellar tendon fibroblasts. Gene 2005;363: 166–172.

56. Jeffrey JE, Aspden RM. Cyclooxygenase inhibition lowers prostaglandin E2 release from articular cartilage and reduces apoptosis but not proteoglycan degradation following an impact load in vitro. Arthritis Res Ther 2007;9:R129.

57. Shioyama R, Aoki Y, Ito H et al. Long-lasting breaches in the bladder epithelium lead to storage dysfunction with increase in bladder PGE2 levels in the rat. Am J Physiol Regul Integr Comp Physiol 2008;295:R714–718.

58. Hadjiargyrou M, Ahrens W, Rubin CT. Temporal expression of the chondrogenic and angiogenic growth factor CYR61 during fracture repair. J Bone Miner Res 2000;15:1014–1023.

59. Garcia-Segura LM, Wozniak A, Azcoitia I et al. Aromatase expression by astrocytes after brain injury: implications for local estrogen formation in brain repair. Neuroscience 1999;89:567–578.

60. Gurates B, Bulun SE. Endometriosis: the ultimate hormonal disease. Semin Reprod Med 2003;21:125–134.

61. Kissler S, Schmidt M, Keller N et al. Real-time PCR analysis for estrogen receptor beta and progesterone receptor in menstrual blood samples – a new approach to a non-invasive diagnosis for endometriosis. Hum Reprod 2005;20(Suppl 1):i179 (P-496).

62. Attar E, Bulun SE. Aromatase and other steroidogenic genes in endometriosis: translational aspects. Hum Reprod Update 2006;12:49–56.

63. Attar E, Tokunaga H, Imir G et al. Prostaglandin E2 via steroidogenic factor-1 coordinately regulates transcription of steroidogenic genes necessary for estrogen synthesis in endometriosis. J Clin Endocrinol Metab 2009;94:623–631.

64. Harada M, Osuga Y, Hirota Y et al. Mechanical stretch stimulates interleukin-8 production in endometrial stromal cells: possible implications in endometrium-related events. J Clin Endocrinol Metab 2005;90:1144–1148.

65. Mahmood TA, Templeton A. Pathophysiology of mild endometriosis: review of literature. Hum Reprod 1990;5:765–784.

66. Hadfield RM, Yudkin PL, Coe CL et al. Risk factors for endometriosis in the rhesus monkey (Macaca mulatta): a case-control study. Hum Reprod Update 1997;3:109–115.

67. Greene R, Stratton P, Cleary SD et al. Diagnostic experience among 4,334 women reporting surgically diagnosed endometriosis. Fertil Steril 2009;91:32–39.

68. Moen MH, Muus KM. Endometriosis in pregnant and non-pregnant women at tubal sterilisation. Hum Reprod 1991;6:699–702.

69. Sampson JA. Peritoneal endometriosis due to the menstrual dissemination of endometrial tissue into the peritoneal cavity. Am J Obstet Gynecol 1927;14:422–429.

70. Marsh EE, Laufer MR. Endometriosis in premenarcheal girls who do not have an obstructive anomaly. Fertil Steril 2005;83:758–760.

71. Goji K. Twenty-four-hour concentration profiles of gonadotropin and estradiol (E2) in prepubertal and early pubertal girls: the diurnal rise of E2 is opposite the nocturnal rise of gonadotropin. J Clin Endocrinol Metab 1993;77:1629–1635.

72. Leyendecker G, Wildt L, Hansmann M. Pregnancies following chronic intermittent (pulsatile) administration of GnRH by means of a portable pump (Zyklomat) – a new approach to the treatment of infertility in hypothalamic amenorrhea. J Clin Endocrinol Metab 1980;51:1214–1216.

73. Leyendecker G, Wildt L. Induction of ovulation with chronic-intermittent (pulsatile) administration of GnRH in hypothalamic amenorrhea. J Reprod Fertil 1983;69:397–409.

74. Peters H. The human ovary in childhood and early maturity. Eur J Obstet Gynecol Reprod Biol 1977;9:137–144.

75. Counseller VS. Endometriosis. A clinical and surgical review. Am J Obstet Gynecol 1938;36:877–886.

76. Tseng JF, Ryan IP, Milam TD et al. Interleukin-6 secretion in vitro is up-regulated in ectopic and eutopic endometrial stromal cells from women with endometriosis. J Clin Endocrinol Metab 1996;81:1118–1122.

77. Vercellini P, Aimi G, Panazza S et al. Deep endometriosis conundrum: evidence in favor of a peritoneal origin. Fertil Steril 2000;73:1043–1046.

78. Tokushige N, Markham R, Russell P et al. High density of small nerve fibres in the functional layer of the endometrium in women with endometriosis. Hum Reprod 2006;21:782–787.

79. Tokushige N, Markham R, Russell P et al. Nerve fibres in peritoneal endometriosis. Hum Reprod 2006;21:3001–3007.

80. Tokushige N, Markham R, Russell P et al. Effect of progestogens and combined oral contraceptives on nerve fibers in peritoneal endometriosis. Fertil Steril 2009;92:1234–1239.

81. Salo PT, Beye JA, Seerattan RA et al. Plasticity of peptidergic innervation in healing rabbit medial collateral ligament. Can J Surg 2008;51:167–172.

82. Ackermann PW, Salo PT, Hart DA. Neuronal pathways in tendon healing. Front Biosci 2009;14:5165–5187.

83. Anaf V, Simon P, Fayt I et al. Smooth muscles are frequent components of endometriotic lesions. Hum Reprod 2000;15:767–771.

84. Cullen TS. The distribution of adenomyoma containing uterine mucosa. Arch Surg 1920;1:215–283.

85. Brosens IA, Brosens JJ. Redefining endometriosis: is deep endometriosis a progressive disease? Hum Reprod 2000;15:1–3.

86. Kaiserman-Abramof IR, Padykula HA. Ultrastructural epithelial zonation of the primate endometrium (rhesus monkey). Am J Anat 1989;184:13–30.

87. Padykula HA, Coles LG, Okulicz WC et al. The basalis of the primate endometrium: a bifunctional germinal compartment. Biol Reprod 1989;40:681–690.

88. Okulicz WC, Balsamo M, Tast J. Progesterone regulation of endometrial estrogen receptor and cell proliferation during the late proliferative and secretory phase in artificial menstrual cycles in the rhesus monkey. Biol Reprod 1993;49:24–32.

89. Delvoux B, Groothuis P, D'Hooghe T et al. Increased production of 17beta-estradiol in endometriosis lesions is the result of impaired metabolism J Clin Endocrinol Metab 2009;94:876–883.

90. McBean JH, Gibson M, Brumsted JR. The association of intrauterine filling defects on hysterosalpingogram with endometriosis. Fertil Steril 1996;66:522–526.

91. Bulun SE, Cheng YH, Yin P et al. Progesterone resistance in endometriosis: link to failure to metabolize estradiol. Mol Cell Endocrinol 2006;248:94–103.

92. Burney RO, Talbi S, Hamilton AE et al. Gene expression analysis of endometrium reveals progesterone resistance and candidate susceptibility genes in women with endometriosis. Endocrinology 2007;148:3814–3826.

93. Simon C, Gutierrez A, Vidal A et al. Outcome of patients with endometriosis in assisted reproduction: results from in-vitro fertilization and oocyte donation. Hum Reprod 1994;9:725–729.

94. Zeitoun K, Takayama K, Sasano H et al. Deficient 17ß-hydroxysteroid dehydrogenase type 2 expression in endometriosis: failure to metabolize 17ß-estradiol. J Clin Endocrinol Metab 1998;83:4474–4480.

21 Pelvic Mechanisms Involved in the Pathophysiology of Pain in Endometriosis

Ian S. Fraser, Natsuko Tokushige, Alison J. Hey-Cunningham, Marina Berbic and Cecilia H.M. Ng

Department of Obstetrics, Gynaecology and Neonatology, Queen Elizabeth II Research Institute for Mothers and Infants, University of Sydney, Sydney, Australia

Introduction

Pelvic pain is universally recognized as the classic symptom associated with endometriosis [1–4]. This is the primary reason why most endometriosis patients present for medical assistance. Although many patients with endometriosis will first present with infertility, on specific questioning most of them will also have some symptoms of pelvic pain. Most doctors have been taught to think solely in terms of the classic endometriosis pain triad of dysmenorrhea, dyspareunia and pain with a bowel motion, but in reality the range and combination of pain types are much more complex [4].

Endometriosis is an extraordinarily variable condition. Variable in the age and manner of presentation, in the severity, site, cyclicity and nature of the pains, in the occurrence of other types of symptoms, in the response to different treatments, in the likelihood and rate of recurrence, and in the natural history of symptoms over time. This variability is probably reflective of the complex genetic and environmental factors which influence the process in individual women, and it does make the study of pain and its origins challenging.

Surprisingly, relatively little is known about the mechanisms which trigger the sensations of pelvic pain in endometriosis [2,3]. For some time it has been recognized that endometriosis has features of an "inflammatory" process with alterations in the presence and function of certain leukocytes [5–7]. Attention has generally been focused on the ectopic lesions themselves, and especially on the obvious changes in those ubiquitous leukocytes, macrophages, in peritoneal fluid and in the tissue of the ectopic lesions. In reality, there are highly significant changes in a wide range of different immune cells in and around the lesions. The fact that these immune cell changes ("inflammatory changes") may have direct effects on pain is supported by the fact that the lesions themselves may sometimes be exquisitely tender to touch, reflected in the occurrence of deep dyspareunia and tenderness on digital examination. Many immune cells have been shown to have the capacity to secrete molecules which can stimulate pain sensations. Although the lesions have usually been the main focus of study, it is being increasingly recognized that the eutopic endometrium in endometriosis functions quite differently from that of women without endometriosis, and that endometriosis may actually be an "endometrial disease."

One assumes that pain stimuli are always mediated through the presence of nociceptors and sensory nerve fibers in relevant tissues, and the recent characterization of large numbers of sensory and autonomic nerve fibers in the ectopic lesions and eutopic endometrium and myometrium of endometriosis sufferers provides a plausible route for painful stimuli. On the other hand, it is somewhat surprising that nerve fibers are rarely found in the endometrium of women with no endometriosis (even if other benign gynecological diseases like adenomyosis, uterine fibroids, endometrial polyps or chronic endometritis are present). It is recognized that a number of molecules which are capable of stimulating pain sensations through nociceptors are strongly expressed in endometrium and in ectopic lesions of women with endometriosis, but little is known about the actual mechanisms of pain generation.

Symptoms and signs

Pelvic pain is the primary complaint of women with endometriosis, but the nature of the pain is highly variable and the severity ranges from the most severe that a woman can imagine down to no pain at all [4,8]. It is commonly stated that some women with endometriosis will not have any pain, but on direct questioning very few women will actually have none. Many of these women do have pain but have accepted it as "normal" and have not complained. Others will have complained of a wide range of different types of pains

Endometriosis: Science and Practice, First Edition. Edited by Linda C. Giudice, Johannes L.H. Evers and David L. Healy.

Box 21.1 Different types of pain associated with endometriosis

1. **Types of menstrual cycle pain**
   - Premenstrual – general pelvic, back
   - Perimenstrual – uterine and general, back
   - Midcycle – uterine and ovarian
   - Back, leg and loin pain – referred
   - Bowel pain – from closely located lesions, painful abdominal bloating
   - Peri- and postmicturition pain – from closely located peritoneal lesions or from bladder

2. **Perimenstrual pain (dysmenorrhea)**
   - Dominant pain described as intense, unbearable, miserable, cramping, gnawing (89%)
   - Dominant sites of pain:
     – central/low abdomen (92%), deep pelvic area (41%), low back (50%)
     – thighs, loins, rectal area, umbilicus
   - Much more severe than in women with no specific gynecological disease

3. **Nerve entrapment**
   - Pain due to anatomical nerve distortion by scarred, but often active, endometriotic lesions with referred pain along the path of the trapped nerve
   - Distortion of small nerve trunks in dense enteric and endometriotic nerve plexuses within highly fibrotic deep pelvic endometriosis lesions may have similar effects

4. **Neuropathic pains**
   - Arises from damage to nerves (peripheral or central); may occur in endometriosis and be exacerbated by repeated surgery; therapies are often only partially successful

5. **Other pains**
   - Hyperalgesia; allodynia, myofascial dysfunction (trigger points)
   - Lowered pain pressure threshold
   - These are evidence of CNS sensitization

Source: Adapted from Fraser [4].

---

above and beyond the classic triad of dysmenorrhea, dyspareunia and pain with a bowel motion. The pains of endometriosis are part of a unique, diverse symptom complex (Box 21.1). Pains related to the gastrointestinal tract, bladder, referral to distant sites, nerve entrapment, neuropathic pain, hyperalgesia and allodynia all merit a greater degree of attention and understanding than hitherto given.

Anatomical pathways of pain

The nervous system is broadly divided into the central nervous system (CNS) and peripheral nervous system (PNS). The CNS comprises the brain and the spinal cord, where information transmitted from the periphery by nerve fibers is processed, interpreted and perceived at a conscious level. All other parts of the nervous system belong to the PNS. The lower abdomen and pelvis, with associated viscera, muscles, bone, and skin, are innervated by the somatic and visceral (autonomic) nervous systems, containing both motor and sensory elements. The efferent (motor) and afferent (sensory) nuclei and their pathways in the brain and spinal cord are in the CNS, whereas efferent and afferent nerve fibers and autonomic and sensory ganglia extending to the target organs are part of the PNS. The autonomic nervous system, further divided into the sympathetic and parasympathetic nervous systems, innervates the pelvic viscera, blood vessels and glands. In the pelvis, the sympathetic nervous system constricts blood vessels and raises blood pressure while the parasympathetic nervous system stimulates smooth muscle and gland activity, and relaxes sphincters.

Intermediary connections between different neurological structures in the body are provided by ganglia. Ganglia contain cell bodies of neurons in the PNS, and often interconnect with other ganglia to form complex systems, known as neural plexuses. The two major groups of ganglia are the dorsal root (or spinal) ganglia (DRG) and the autonomic ganglia. The DRG are positioned alongside the spinal cord and contain the cell bodies of sensory (afferent) nerves (including pain afferents), both somatic and visceral. Sensory ganglion cells in the dorsal root give off both centrally and peripherally directed processes, and do not have synapses on their cell bodies. Peripheral processes of visceral afferent neurons are distributed through autonomic ganglia and plexuses.

Female pelvic organ innervation

The pelvic organs receive afferent innervation from the autonomic nervous system (Fig. 21.1). This innervation is derived in a complex manner from the superior hypogastric plexus, sympathetic chain, parasympathetic fibers (S2–4) and the sacral plexus (sacral splanchnic nerves, S1–5).

The superior hypogastric plexus or presacral nerve is formed by intermesenteric nerves and fibers from the inferior mesenteric (primarily from the aortic plexus, but also receives input from the second and splanchnic lumbar nerves) and lumbar sympathetic ganglia (made up of the first, second and sometimes third lumbar ventral spinal rami and have fibers which travel to the lumbar spinal nerves). It is embedded in loose areolar tissue beneath the visceral peritoneum at the bifurcation of the aorta, overlying the middle sacral vessels and the bodies of the fourth and fifth lumbar vertebrae. The superior hypogastric plexus is usually broad, flattened and made up of two or three partially fused trunks. In 20–24% of individuals, however, it consists of a single nerve trunk. Fine nerve fibers from the lumbar sympathetic ganglia travel beneath the common iliac vessels to join the presacral nerve. The right ureter is also in close proximity [9,10].

In some individuals, a middle hypogastric plexus is also present overlying and just below the sacral promontory. Following the superior and middle hypogastric plexuses, the fibers divide into the inferior hypogastric plexuses or hypogastric nerves – two long, narrow strands. The inferior hypogastric plexus also receives

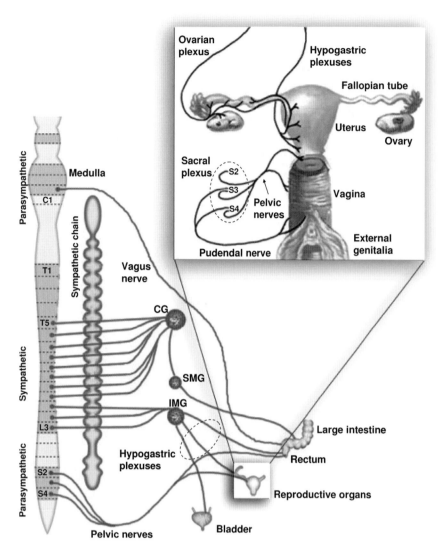

Figure 21.1 Afferent (sensory) innervation of the female pelvic organs. CG, celiac ganglion; IMG, inferior mesenteric ganglion; SMG, superior mesenteric ganglion. Compiled with data from Netter 1965 [9], Williams *et al* 1995 [18], Hollabaugh Jr *et al* 2001 [14], and Aguado 2002 [17]. The authors acknowledge Ned Berbic for creating this figure.

sacral splanchnic nerves from the sympathetic trunk. The hypogastric nerves travel along the internal iliac vessels, downward and outward near the sacral attachments of the uterosacral ligaments and then forward over the lateral aspect of the rectal ampulla and upper vagina as the pelvic plexuses [9,11–13].

These pelvic plexuses receive fibers from the sacral ganglia of the sympathetic trunk and parasympathetic input from the second to fourth sacral spinal nerves (also known as nervi erigentes or pelvic nerves). Each plexus covers around 2–3 cm² and contains interlacing nerve fibers and a number of minute ganglia. The pelvic plexuses are divided into rectal, uterovaginal and vesical plexuses [9,14–16]. The uterosacral ligament conveys elements of the inferior hypogastric plexus to the uterus and vagina [13]. The middle and upper rectum also receives afferent nerves of the superior rectal plexus which travel with the superior rectal artery and vein from the inferior mesenteric plexus [10].

The lower vagina, perineum and anus are innervated by the somatic branches of the pudendal nerve, derived from the second to fourth sacral root ganglia [9,14]. The dorsal rami derived from

these segments innervate the lower back, which is a common region of referred gynecological pain.

Fibers from the aortic and renal plexuses accompany the ovarian vessels in the suspensory ligament of the ovary (or infundibulopelvic ligament) and form the meshwork of the ovarian plexuses. These innervate the ovaries, fimbrial aspect of the fallopian tubes and broad ligaments [9,17]. Nerves traveling with the uterine arteries also supply the uterine body and tube, connecting with the tubal nerves from the inferior hypogastric plexus and with the ovarian plexus [18].

These complex neural structures make up the first of various relays which transmit pain sensations from pelvic organs to the brain. It should be recognized that neural interconnections can also occur in these neural plexuses, and also that nerve fibers supplying pelvic organs may link with the complex enteric nerve plexus which supplies the gastrointestinal tract. The cell bodies of sympathetic nerve trunks are located in a thoracolumbar distribution, and those of parasympathetic fibers are in the sacral DRG [19].

Peritoneal innervation

Parietal peritoneum, attached to the abdominal wall, derives its nerve supply from the somatic afferent nerves from T10 to L2 supplying the muscles and skin of the abdominal wall [18,20,21]. Pain originating from the parietal peritoneum can be caused by various types of mechanical, chemical or thermal stimulation [18]. Visceral peritoneum is an integral part of the organ it covers, and is supplied by autonomic (visceral) afferent fibers. The visceral peritoneum and the viscera themselves are not sensitive to the same stimuli as parietal peritoneum, but tension, muscle spasms, ischemia and presumably certain unknown factors can evoke pain [18].

Pelvic pain neuropathways

There are a minimum of six distinct neuropathways which transmit sensory afferent signals from noxious stimuli out of the pelvis to the CNS, leading to the potential perception of pain. These pathways are detailed below.
- From the pelvic plexuses or subsequent inferior hypogastric plexuses along the hypogastric nerves to the superior hypogastric plexus.
- From the nervi erigentes (which often pass through the inferior hypogastric plexus) along to the dorsal roots of S2–4.
- From the sacral (sympathetic) splanchnic nerves, through the inferior hypogastric plexus to the sacral extension of the paravertebral sympathetic ganglia.
- From the superior rectal plexus traveling with the superior rectal artery and vein to the inferior mesenteric plexus.
- From the ovarian plexus of nerves in the suspensory ligament of the ovary traveling from the ovary to the origin of the ovarian arteries at the aorta and then to the spinal levels of T11–12.
- From the somatic afferent nerves supplying the parietal peritoneum to the anterior primary rami of T10–12 and the ventral rami of L1–2.

While both the sympathetic and parasympathetic systems are involved in visceral sensation and reflexes, the major pathways for pelvic organ pain are in the sympathetic nerve trunk. Signals from noxious stimuli originating in the pelvis travel up the sensory (afferent) fibers along the pathways detailed above, to the DRG and into the spinal cord to the brain where the perception of pain occurs [10,18,22].

Pregnancy and uterine innervation

The spontaneous denervation of the myometrium during pregnancy has been well documented, with an almost complete absence of nerve fibers observed in the term uterus [23–28] and the uterus during labor [29,30]. It has been hypothesized that this denervation is a prerequisite for the low contractile activity of the myometrium until late pregnancy, but the denervation may also promote a hypersensitivity to catecholamines in connection with labor. After delivery, recovery of innervation occurs [31] but it appears that this takes a considerable period of time and may not be complete [27].

Pelvic innervations and pelvic surgery

The complex anatomical relationships of female pelvic innervation are of particular importance in terms of surgical management of endometriosis. Surgical treatment of endometriosis can involve excision of endometriotic lesions from the parietal and visceral peritoneum and from deep pelvic areas, division of adhesions or hysterectomy. Damage to pelvic nerves during some types of pelvic surgery can be associated with bladder dysfunction, sexual dysfunction and colorectal motility disorders. The importance of minimizing nerve damage during pelvic surgery in order to decrease undesirable side-effects is becoming increasingly apparent [32]. Preservation of sexual function and urinary and fecal continence is increasingly a priority for hysterectomy procedures [15,16,33,34]. Various surgical approaches have been investigated to minimize nerve damage in pelvic surgery and have prompted further study of neural anatomical relationships in the pelvis [11,12,14,16,33,35,36]. Nerve-sparing hysterectomy has shown promising results in terms of preservation of function [34,35,37,38], but further studies are required to confirm its effectiveness compared to conventional techniques and a significant decrease in long-term complications [39].

Peritoneal adhesions are common following pelvic surgery for endometriosis and can occasionally lead to complications such as intestinal obstruction, infertility, and chronic pain. Adhesions themselves have been shown to be frequently innervated [40,41] and to contain sensory nerve fibers [42], suggesting that they are capable of transmitting pain signals.

A further implication of a precise understanding of the anatomical pathways of pelvic pain is deliberate, planned pelvic denervation surgery for pain relief. The late 1980s and early 1990s saw a rapid growth in the performance of uterosacral nerve ablation and presacral neurectomy for alleviation of pelvic pain, especially in patients with endometriosis [10]. More recently, however, it has been recognized that quality evidence is lacking to support the use of surgical denervation for pain relief in the female pelvis [43]. Only a certain portion of uterine innervation is via the uterosacral ligament and the majority of visceral afferents from the uterus and vagina travel initially with the uterine vessels.

There is also increasing concern that repeated pelvic surgery for persistent or recurrent endometriosis may result in nerve damage of the type which may set up repetitive neuronal discharges capable of establishing neuropathic pain [4].

Pathophysiological mechanisms relevant to pain within the eutopic endometrium and myometrium

The fact that endometriosis may be an "endometrial disease" is becoming increasingly clearly established. Many molecular pathways show increased, decreased or disturbed expression in women with endometriosis and may play major roles in the pathophysiological and etiological mechanisms related to endometriosis pain. When viable endometrial cells are deposited in the peritoneal cavity via menstrual reflux, these endometrial cells carry with them the characteristics of "dysfunctional" mechanisms which allow establishment of nerve, vascular and lymphatic supply, as well as the ability to escape immune surveillance and with reduced apoptosis, which allow continued proliferation outside the uterus.

The following sections briefly highlight the multifactorial functional mechanisms within the eutopic endometrium and myometrium that may lead to the development of endometriosis and thus some of the pelvic pain mechanisms of this debilitating disease. Some of the key changes in structure and function addressed in the following sections are summarized in Table 21.1. These disturbances in molecular function are probably all important in establishment of the "inflammatory milieu" which may be a prerequisite for the development of sensory nerve fibers and pain stimuli.

Cell structure

Differential upregulation of cell structural and cytoskeletal molecules leads to a fundamental change in the cell wall and cytoplasmic structure, potentially allowing viable refluxed endometrial cells to induce attachment and adhesion to the peritoneum at ectopic sites and develop and grow into endometriotic lesions.

Cellular adhesion, invasion and proliferation

Attachment of viable endometrial cells to the peritoneal surface is the first step in the development of endometriosis at ectopic sites. Following initial attachment and adherence, the endometrial cells in women with endometriosis exhibit inherent dysregulated properties, which allow invasion of the surface peritoneal mesothelium to instigate cellular propagation and proliferation. These processes involve a number of molecules, such as integrins, cellular adhesion molecules (CAMs) and proteases (e.g. matrix metalloproteinases (MMPs) and their tissue inhibitors (TIMPs)), facilitate cell adhesion, migration and invasion into the peritoneal extracellular matrix (ECM) [44–46] (see Table 21.1).

Apoptosis

Apoptosis is a precisely regulated process of programmed cell death which does not elicit an inflammatory response and is decreased in the eutopic endometrium of women with endometriosis [47–51].

Immune factors and inflammatory mediators

Normal endometrium contains numerous leukocyte populations, which undergo significant changes during the menstrual cycle. These leukocytes provide immune protection for the uterine mucosal surface and play major roles during the processes of menstruation, embryonic implantation and the maintenance of early pregnancy [52]. Early studies of general immune cell populations reported no significant differences in the eutopic endometrium in endometriosis [6,53–55]. However, more recent studies have shown a range of subtle but significant differences

in specific leukocyte subsets throughout the menstrual cycle [52,56–60]. Some of these differences are outlined in Table 21.1.

While macrophage numbers are increased in eutopic endometrium in women with endometriosis, their phagocytic function against shed endometrial fragments is likely to be compromised [61]. Dysregulated dendritic cell (DC) expression in endometriosis further suggests that components of antigen capture and DC maturation may be defective in endometriosis [59]. In addition to this, Foxp3+ regulatory T-cells (Tregs), which play crucial roles in regulating a wide variety of immunological responses, have been shown to be significantly upregulated during the secretory phase in women with endometriosis. These immune cell types may be exerting immunosuppressive effects on newly recruited endometrial leukocytes, thus affecting their ability to effectively target shed endometrial fragments [60]. Dysregulated immune cell function in the eutopic endometrium of women with endometriosis is likely to contribute to increased synthesis and secretion of immunological and inflammatory mediators in endometriosis [57,62,63]. These mediators are likely to create a suitable microenvironment for attachment and invasion of viable endometrial cells and tissue fragments. These immune cells almost certainly play important roles in the generation of pain stimuli (see Table 21.1).

Angiogenesis

The process of new blood vessel formation, which is crucial to survival and growth of endometriotic lesions, is probably due primarily to the overexpression of various angiogenic factors in the eutopic endometrium. These ensure that neo-angiogenesis enables rapid vascularization of developing lesions, and probably also contribute to growth of nerve fibers. Angiogenic factors leading to the increase in vascularity around endometriotic lesions include vascular endothelial growth factor (VEGF), endoglin, tumor necrosis factor-α (TNF-α), epidermal growth factor (EGF), fibroblast growth factor (FGF), platelet endothelial cell adhesion molecule (PECAM) and integrin $\alpha v\beta 3$ [64–68] (see Table 21.1).

Oxidative stress

Oxidative stress reflects a fault in the antioxidant scavenger ability of a tissue, leading to excess production of reactive oxygen species (oxygen free radicals). This process is enhanced by disturbance of relevant enzyme systems in eutopic endometrium [69–74], and leads to stimulation of various immune cells and inflammatory mediators, potentiating a vicious circle of persistent oxidative stress (see Table 21.1).

Steroidogenesis

Endometriosis is recognized to be a hormone-dependent disease, in which estrogens are mitogens for endometriotic lesion development and progesterone antagonizes the mitogenic effects of estrogen. Aromatase and 17β-hydroxysteroid dehydrogenase (17β-HSD) enzymes are crucial to the biosynthesis of these steroid hormones. Aromatase converts androstenedione and testosterone to estrone (E_1) and estradiol (E_2) and 17β-HSD type 2 converts E_2 to the

Table 21.1 Pathophysiological dysregulation in the eutopic endometrium of women with endometriosis.

Molecular system	Dysregulations in the eutopic endometrium in women with endometriosis
Cell structure	Increased expression of molecules such as vimentin, cyclophilin, forkhead associated domain, actin, β-actin, microtubule-associated protein 6, tropomyosin, prefoldin and ARPC2 [168,170].
Cellular adhesion, invasion and proliferation	CAMs promote cell attachment to proteins on the ECM, facilitating cell migration and invasion [173,174].
	Increase in intracellular CAM-1 expression [56,174–176] may promote adhesion in immunological and inflammatory reactions.
	Increase in L1CAM in endometriosis may contribute to nerve growth and pain symptoms [177]
	Downregulation of integrins – $\alpha_v\beta_3$ [178,179], CD166 [170], annexin A2 [169], IL-11, leukemia inhibiting factor (LIF) [180], may play roles in endometriosis-associated infertility
	Increases in MMP-2 (which degrades type 4 collagen) and MMP-9 (which has been reported to be involved in vascular growth and may play a role in tumor metastasis) [44–46]
	Decrease in MMP-2 and MMP-9 inhibitors (TIMP-1 and TIMP-2) [44–46]
	Increased proliferation through stimulation of Wnt pathway [181,182]
Apoptosis	Reduced apoptotic potential, but studies are conflicting
	Increased expression of B-cell lymphoma-2 may account for increased endometrial resistance to apoptosis in endometriosis; may serve as a permissive factor contributing to survival of endometrial fragments [47, 48]
Immune factors	The following immune cell populations are significantly increased in eutopic endometrium in women with endometriosis:
	CD4+ T helper cells [183]; γδ T cells [56]; monocytes [56]
	Macrophages during proliferative [58,184] and secretory [184] phases of the menstrual cycle
	Immature CD1a+ DC during the proliferative phase [59]
	Foxp3+ Tregs during the secretory phase [60]
	The following immune cell populations are significantly decreased:
	CD83+ DC during all phases of the cycle [59]
Inflammatory mediators	Upregulation of IL-6 (stimulates lymphocyte proliferation) [185], IL-8 (promotes proliferation and adhesion of endometrial cells) [63], monocyte chemotactic protein-1 [186], TNF-α (inflammatory response) [63], macrophage migration inhibiting factor and altered and enhanced PG metabolism [57]
	Downregulation of IL-1 agonist receptor (increases IL-1 activity) [187], IL-18 (promotes T helper response and NK cytotoxicity) [188], IL-11 and LIF (altering uterine receptivity during implantation) [180]
Angiogenesis	Increased expression of VEGF, endoglin promoting neovascularization.
	VEGF, a potent angiogenic factor that promotes nerve fiber growth and neovascularization through vascular endothelial cells, is increased [64,65, 67,68]
	Endoglin, a transmembrane homodimer glycoprotein component of the transforming growth factor-β1 receptor-1 complex, plays an important role in angiogenesis [66]
Oxidative stress	Increased production of reactive oxygen species and their enzymes – endothelial nitric oxide synthase, cooper, zinc superoxide dismutase (SOD), manganese SOD, catalase, xanthine oxidase and nitric oxide [69–74] – may mediate increased sensitivity to pain stimuli
Steroidogenesis	Increased local estrogen synthesis by aromatase, 17β-HSD type 1 and PGs [75, 76]
	P resistance through absence of 17β-HSD type 2 (normally lowers E_2 action) and levels and lack of PRB expression [54,77]
Neurogenesis	Greatly increased production and expression of neurotropins: NGF, BDNF, NT3, NT4 and their receptors, Trk-A and NGFRp75
	Large numbers of sensory and autonomic nerve fibers in the functional and basal layers of eutopic endometrium, expressing PGP9.5, VIP, NPY, SP, CGRP and other neurotransmitters and neuromodulators
	Lack of expression of NF and myelinated nerve fibers

ARPC2, actin-related protein 2/3 complex subunit 2; BDNF, brain-derived neurotropic factor; CAM, cell adhesion molecule; CGRP, calcitonin gene-related peptide; ECM, extracellular matrix; DC, dendritic cell; HSD, hydroxysteroid dehydrogenase; IL, interleukin; MMP, matrix metalloproteinase; NF, neurofilament; NGF, nerve growth factor; NK, natural killer; NPY, neuropeptide Y; NT, neurotropin; P, progesterone; PG, prostaglandin; PGP, protein gene product; PRB, progesterone receptor B; SP, substance P; TIMP, tissue inhibitor of metalloproteinase; TNF, tumor necrosis factor; Treg, regulatory T-cell; VEGF, vascular endothelial growth factor; VIP, vasoactive intestinal polypeptide.

biologically less active E_1, and is impaired in eutopic endometrium. Under normal conditions, aromatase expression is not detected in the eutopic endometrium; however, it is aberrantly highly expressed in the eutopic endometrium and higher still in endometriotic implants [75,76]. Thus, endometriotic lesions are able to produce their own local estrogen supply, and with reduced metabolism, further potentiating lesion growth.

Prostaglandin E_2 (PGE_2) is a known potent inducer of aromatase activity in stromal endometriotic cells. This positive feedback loop of estrogen and local PG stimulation and production promotes further proliferation and an inflammatory reaction within the pelvis, thus creating an inflamed environment for further release of growth factors, inflammatory mediators, cytokines and MMPs.

Progesterone (P) is the main stimulator of 17β-HSD type 2 in the eutopic endometrium and normally plays a protective role to balance the actions of E_2. However, the eutopic endometrium of women with endometriosis is partially resistant to the action of P [77]. The failure of P action in endometriosis leads to impaired secretory transformation, decreased apoptosis and increase in proliferation of endometrial cells in the peritoneal cavity [77]. An explanation for P resistance may be partly due to the lack of expression of the P receptor, PRB, in the eutopic endometrium and lesions compared to the expression of PRA [54,77].

Neurogenesis

In normal women, nerve fibers can be detected in the myometrium, the endometrial–myometrial interface and occasionally in the deeper portion of the basal layer of endometrium, but nerve fibers are completely absent from the superficial two-thirds of the endometrium in the normal human uterus [78,79]. We have demonstrated small unmyelinated nerve fibers in the functional layer of endometrium in virtually all women with endometriosis (Plate 21.1), with a mean density ± SD 10 ± 7/mm^2 [79]. However, these nerve fibers were never seen in the functional layer in women without endometriosis. The density of nerve fibers in the basal layer of endometrium and myometrium in women with endometriosis was also highly significantly greater (4–20-fold greater) than in women without endometriosis (0.2/mm^2 and 0.9 ± 0.8/mm^2, respectively) [79].

Nerve fibers in the functional layer of endometrium in women with endometriosis expressed cholinergic (vasointestinal peptide (VIP)), adrenergic (neuropeptide Y (NPY)) and sensory (substance P (SP) and calcitonin gene-related peptide (CGRP)) markers, but not the myelination marker, neurofilament (NF). The nerve fiber density of autonomic markers VIP and NPY was much higher than that of SP and CGRP. In women with endometriosis, nerve fibers in the basal layer of endometrium expressed all markers including NF, but women without endometriosis had very small numbers of C nerve fibers and no NF in the basal layer. Nerve fibers expressing all markers were present in myometrium, but the density of all these nerve fibers was much higher (5–8-fold) in endometriosis [80].

The function of these nerve fibers in endometrium and myometrium in women with endometriosis is not known. SP induces contraction in the human myometrium [81] but CGRP is a potent vasodilator [82] and inhibitor of spontaneous contractile activity in the human uterus [81]. NPY is considered to regulate vascular tone and exert inhibitory effects on myometrial contractility [83], and VIP is a potent vasodilator of the uterine artery and is involved in smooth muscle relaxation, blood flow, and secretion [82]. Hence, many of these endometrial nerve fibers in endometriosis may be involved in vascular function, although there is no physiological evidence to point to alteration of these functions in the eutopic endometrium in endometriosis. It seems highly probable that those nerve fibers expressing SP and CGRP (and some with NF) are involved in mechanisms of pain generation and signaling within the uterus and elsewhere.

Expression of neurotropins and receptors in eutopic endometrium

In women with endometriosis, the neurotropin nerve growth factor (NGF) is dramatically expressed in endometrial glands, stromal cells, blood vessels and nerve fibers in both functional and basal layers of endometrium. NGF is also strongly expressed in smooth muscle cells, blood vessels and nerve fibers in the myometrium in women with endometriosis. In women without endometriosis, NGF is not expressed in the functional layer of endometrium. However, NGF is weakly expressed in endometrial glands, stroma, blood vessels and nerve fibers in the basal layer of normal endometrium. In normal myometrium, NGF is moderately expressed in blood vessels and nerve fibers [84]. One study has reported that NGF was more highly expressed in the glands and stroma in the proliferative phase than in the secretory phase in women with endometriosis ($P < 0.001$) [85], so neurotropins such as NGF may be influenced by local concentrations of estrogens and P.

When NGF binds to two different receptors, a high-affinity receptor, tyrosine kinase-A (Trk-A) and a low-affinity receptor, p75, which are expressed on peripheral nerve fibers, the neurotropic action of NGF is induced. NGF and other neurotropins are produced by a number of immune cells such as macrophages, mast cells, B-cells and T-cells [86].

There was dramatically stronger staining with NGFRp75 and Trk-A in endometrium and myometrium in women with endometriosis. Nerve fibers, blood vessels and endometrial stromal cells in the functional and basal layers of endometrium and myometrium in women with endometriosis were strongly stained with NGFRp75 [84]. There was no NGFRp75 immunoreactivity in nerve fibers or blood vessels in the functional layer of endometrium in women without endometriosis, and little expression in the basal layer or myometrium [84].

Our results have shown that there are more nerve fibers expressing the sympathetic nerve fiber marker NPY than the sensory C markers SP or CGRP in the functional layer of endometrium from women with endometriosis presenting pain symptoms [80]. It is well recognized that activation of sympathetic postganglionic fibers and intracutaneous injection of norepinephrine can induce pain, while activation of α-adrenoceptors or administration of guanethidine can alleviate pain [87]. These results suggest that norepinephrine released from sympathetic postganglionic fibers may activate or sensitize nociceptors. Also, when peptidergic nociceptors in endometrium and myometrium are activated by noxious stimuli, neuropeptides including SP and CGRP can be released from the peripheral terminals [88]. These neuropeptides, in turn, may induce neurogenic inflammation, pain and intense smooth muscle contraction in women with endometriosis.

The observation that NGF and its receptors p75 and Trk-A (and other neurotropins) are so highly overexpressed in endometrium and myometrium in women with endometriosis compared with women without endometriosis suggests that neutropins play a primary role in neurogenesis and nociceptor stimulation. NGF has been recognized as a potent sensitizer of nociceptors and can increase the production of SP and CGRP in nociceptors [89,90]. There is evidence that other neurotropins such as brain-derived neurotropic factor (BDNF) and neurotropins 3 and 4 (NT-3, NT-4) can also sensitize nociceptors and induce intense pain [90–92].

Pathophysiological mechanisms in ectopic lesions

Viable endometrial fragments which reach the peritoneal cavity via retrograde flow are likely to have intrinsic properties which facilitate attachment, invasion and the establishment of a new functional blood supply. Components of the immune environment almost certainly facilitate such establishment and progression. Early studies demonstrated that immune cell expression is quite different between the eutopic and ectopic endometrium of women with endometriosis and between eutopic endometrium and the endometrium of women without endometriosis [6,7,93]. Recent studies have shown that ectopic peritoneal lesions are infiltrated by a number of immune cell subsets. Large numbers of CD68+ macrophages [94] and CD1a+ immature DCs [59] are present at the site of the ectopic endometriotic growths, and it is believed that these antigen-presenting cells are recruited to the lesion site in an attempt to initiate clearance of invading ectopic fragments [59]. Certain immune cell populations, such as Tregs, have been identified in some but not all peritoneal lesions, and their expression may be related to specific characteristics of certain endometriotic lesions, such as the stage of lesion development and the rate of progression [60].

Numerous factors may promote adhesion and progression of ectopic growth, including cell-surface MMPs [95], increased expression of fibronectin receptors ($\alpha4\beta1$, $\alpha5\beta2$) [96,97], increased adhesion molecules and insulin-like growth factor (IGF)-1 expression [98], while ECM components like fibronectin, collagen types I and IV, endometrial glycoprotein and laminin may contribute to endometrial cell implantation [99].

Ectopic endometriotic lesions secrete and respond to a range of immunological mediators and growth factors, such as interleukin (IL)-1β, IL-6, TNF-α and hepatocyte growth factor (HGF) [5,100,101] which interfere with and affect normal immunological processes [5], including a degree of resistance to macrophage-mediated destruction [102] and inhibition of natural killer (NK) cell-mediated cytolysis [103]. Intrinsic properties of ectopic lesions, including vascular and neuronal networks, may influence local immunological responses [104], facilitate survival of ectopic implants and facilitate pain mechanisms. The nerve fibers which innervate endometriotic lesions are almost certainly initiating and modulating pain. The immune cell populations are capable of stimulating nerve fiber and vascular growth.

Angiogenic factors, such as VEGF-A, which promote vascularization and establishment of new blood supply are essential for survival and growth of ectopic endometrial tissue [105,106]. VEGF further functions to promote growth of nerve fibers, and increased expression of VEGF has been noted in both the eutopic [64,107–109] and ectopic [64,108–110] endometrium in women with endometriosis. VEGF may regulate Tregs expression [111] and inhibit DC development [112], both of these being immune cell types which are noted in the eutopic endometrium of women with endometriosis [59,60]. Other immunological mediators like IL-1β and IL-6 may mediate VEGF expression and are likely to facilitate neovascularization of endometriotic lesions [67]. IL-8, another potent angiogenic factor which is upregulated in the peritoneal cavity in women with endometriosis, can assist endometrial cell adhesion to peritoneal and other ectopic surfaces [113]. Thus, angiogenic factors play important roles not only in promoting neovascularization and neurogenesis and ensuring viability of ectopic lesions; they also interfere with efficient immune cell adhesion [114] and are likely to contribute to defective immune response in endometriosis.

Increased aromatase activity in endometriosis enhances local estrogen biosynthesis at the lesion site, and plays a role in supporting the proliferation and growth of these endometriotic fragments [115,116]. Macrophages particularly express aromatase [117] and in doing so encourage disease progression [5]. While ectopic endometriotic tissue is histologically similar to eutopic endometrium, the immune cell expression and function within these two tissue types are quite different [6]. Factors in the local environment, particularly peritoneal fluid, may substantially interfere with and dysregulate immune cell expression and function within lesions. On the other hand, certain similarities between the eutopic and ectopic endometrium in endometriosis, such as the presence of sensory nerve fibers, suggest that inflammatory factors may influence growth of nerve fibers and facilitate propagation of pain.

Nerve fibers in ectopic endometriotic lesions

We have demonstrated numerous nerve fibers in peritoneal lesions (Plate 21.2) (mean density $\pm$ SD: 16.3 $\pm$ 10.0/mm^2) compared with normal peritoneum from women without endometriosis (2.5 $\pm$ 1.3/mm^2; n = 36) or peritoneal endosalpingiosis (3.8 $\pm$ 0.9/mm^2; n = 9). Nerve fibers in peritoneal lesions expressed cholinergic, adrenergic, and sensory markers. Peritoneal nerve fibers were present in increased density, even at a long distance from lesions, and in microscopically normal peritoneum in women with confirmed endometriosis [118].

We have reported substantially more nerve fibers in deep infiltrating endometriosis (uterosacral ligaments, cul-de-sac, and peritoneal side wall) than in peritoneal lesions [119]. The nerve plexuses were particularly dense in deep lesions infiltrating bowel (rectum, sigmoid colon and appendix), where nerve densities were around a mean of 170 fibers/mm^2. These nerve fibers also expressed cholinergic, adrenergic and sensory markers [120].

One study has reported that myelinated nerve fibers could not be detected in ovarian endometriomas or in the endometrioma-containing ovaries, whereas nerve fibers stained with NF were detected in dermoid cysts [121]. However, other studies have reported that the expression of NGF and neural cell adhesion molecule (NCAM) was greater in ovarian endometriomas than in peritoneal endometriotic lesions [122]. By contrast, we have demonstrated the presence of large numbers of nerve fibers in ovarian endometriomas (55.6 ± 11.8/mm²; n = 29) and this was much greater than in normal ovarian cortex from both women with ovarian endometriomas (6.7 ± 1.0/mm²; n = 10) and women without endometriosis (1.5 ± 0.3/mm²; n = 10, $P < 0.001$). Nerve fibers in ovarian endometriomas expressed cholinergic, adrenergic, sensory and myelination markers. It is likely that both sensory afferent fibers and sympathetic afferent fibers may be involved in pain generation in endometriomas [123].

In endometriotic cysts in a rat model, the density of sympathetic nerve fibers (but not sensory fibers) and levels of NGF and VEGF were increased in proestrus, a time when severity of hyperalgesia (an excessive response to painful stimuli) was greatest, suggesting that sympathetic afferent fibers play important roles in such pain generation [124,125].

Expression of neurotropins and receptors in ectopic lesions

Nerve growth factor is essential for growth, differentiation, survival and regeneration of sensory and sympathetic fibers in the PNS and for cholinergic neurons in the CNS [126,127]. Although BDNF is mainly synthesized in the CNS, it is located at low levels in the PNS and can induce axonal outgrowth and regeneration of sensory fibers [128] but acts negatively on sympathetic neuronal survival [129] in the PNS. NT-3 can support the growth and survival of sympathetic and sensory neurons in the PNS [130], and also potentiates neurotransmitter release [131]. Little is known about NT-4, but it is considered to be required for the survival of sensory and sympathetic fibers [132]. There was an intense immunoreactivity for NGF and its receptors near endometriotic glands and stroma in peritoneal and deep endometriotic lesions [118]. The expression of NGF and Trk-A correlated with the density of nerve fibers. There were large numbers of NGFRp75-positive nerve fibers in the stroma and near the endometriotic glands [123]. Other neurotropins stained weakly in endometriotic stroma and glandular epithelium as well as in superficial ovarian cortex. In our limited experience, it seems unlikely that these molecules are playing as significant a role in pain generation as NGF and its receptors [123].

Local mechanisms related to mediation of pain in endometrium and endometriotic lesions

Nociceptors and sensory nerve fibers

Nociceptors are "silent" receptors found on sensory neurons in skin, muscle, joints, and viscera. They only respond to noxious stimuli, which have the potential to harm the organism. Nociceptors develop on sensory neurons arising from neural crest stem cells and their cell bodies are located outside the spinal column in the DRG [133]. Cell bodies with the largest diameters give rise to myelinated Aβ-δ fibers, and medium and small diameter cell bodies give rise to myelinated Aδ and non-myelinated C-fibers, respectively [134]. Most myelinated Aβ-δ fibers detect innocuous mechanical stimuli (light touch and pressure) and do not contribute to pain. These are not found in pelvic viscera. In contrast to myelinated Aβ-δ fibers, myelinated Aδ fibers transmit sharp, pricking pain and non-myelinated C-fibers usually transmit burning and throbbing pain. Nociceptors can be divided into four categories, namely mechanical, chemical, thermal and polymodal [135]. Polymodal nociceptors respond to a range of high-intensity stimuli including mechanical, thermal and chemical substances.

Myelinated Aδ fibers are about 2–5 μm in diameter, covered with thin myelin sheaths and have a fast conduction velocity (5–40 m/s). Non-myelinated C-fibers are 0.4–1.2 μm in diameter and have a slow conduction velocity (0.5 -2.0 m/sec). Myelinated Aδ fibers can be divided into two groups (type I and II); type I responds to both mechanical and chemical stimuli but has high heat thresholds (>50°C). Type II has much lower heat thresholds but a very high mechanical threshold [88]. Most C-fibers have polymodal nociceptors and detect a range of high-intensity mechanical, thermal and chemical stimuli, but some are only responsive to noxious heat. It is not known what nociceptors in the reproductive tract respond to.

Non-myelinated C-fibers include both peptidergic and non-peptidergic fibers [88]. When peptidergic fibers are activated by noxious stimuli, peripheral nociceptors release neuropeptides such as SP and CGRP from vesicles in the peripheral terminals. The release of neuropeptides can proliferate keratinocytes, stimulate immune cells, degranulate mast cells, and initiate vasodilation, plasma extravasation, and smooth muscle contraction [88]. Tissue injury can induce the release of numerous endogenous regulatory molecules, which can activate or sensitize the terminals of nociceptors (Table 21.2). For example, damaged cells and tissues in the vicinity of the injury can release NGF, bradykinin, serotonin, histamine, PGs, TNF-α and oxygen free radicals which can alter the sensitivity of nociceptor terminals.

Role of immune cells

Nerve fibers which innervate the ectopic endometriotic lesions [118,136,137], and perhaps more importantly the eutopic endometrium [79,138,139], are likely to contribute to mediation of pain, and may also be modifying local immune cell function and response. The nociceptors of these nerve fibers can potentially be stimulated by a number of inflammatory substances, including histamine, serotonin, bradykinin, PGs, leukotrienes, ILs, acetylcholine (ACh), VEGF, TNF-α, EGFs, platelet-derived growth factor and NGF, many of which can be secreted by a range of immune cell populations. In turn, the neurotropic factors themselves are capable of enhancing proliferation and function of immune cells and may play a role in modulating the inflammatory response and cytokine production in endometriosis [140].

Table 21.2 Activation effects of various mediators released by specific cells or organelles with effects on sensory neurons.

Substance	Main sources	Effects on sensory neurons and nociceptors
NGF	Schwann cells, fibroblasts	Sensitization
PGs	Mast cells, endothelial cells	Sensitization
Histamine	Mast cells, neutrophils	Activation
Serotonin	Platelets, mast cells	Activation
Bradykinin	Plasma kininogen	Activation
Adenosine triphosphate	Mitochondria	Activation
Acetylcholine	Parasympathetic and some sympathetic fibers	Sensitization
Nitric oxide	Endothelial cells and immune cells	Sensitization

NGF, nerve growth factor; PG, prostglandin.

Various immune cell populations, including T-cells, B-cells, macrophages, NK cells, mast cells and DCs, are capable of secreting a range of neurotropic factors [127,141–144] and consequently may play a role in facilitating development and function of nerve fibers in lesions and in eutopic endometrium in endometriosis. Macrophages particularly play important roles in facilitating development, growth and repair of nerve fibers [145]. The growth of nerve fibers is regulated by many substances, including NGF, BDNF, NT-3, NT-4 and their receptors, as well as VEGF. Synthesis of these substances is also affected by immune cell activities. NGF, which is released from endometriotic lesions [85] as well as many other cell types including macrophages, is well documented as a substance that is important in the development of the PNS and CNS. The synthesis of NGF can be upregulated by IL-1 [146,147] and basic FGF [148], both of which can substantially increase the content of NGF mRNA in astrocytes [149]. BDNF, another neurotropin which plays a crucial role in growth and differentiation of the PNS [150,151], is also secreted by activated macrophages. Recent studies have demonstrated that VEGF, produced by macrophages, can also act as a potent neurotropic factor in addition to its effects on small vessel growth [107,152].

Thus the evidence which suggests that the immune cell populations, particularly macrophages, are likely to play crucial roles in growth and survival of nerve fibers in endometriosis is compelling, and indicates that certain inflammatory mechanisms may substantially contribute to generation of pain in endometriosis.

Neurotropins and pain

There is substantial evidence that NGF can produce pain and hyperalgesia by increasing the sensitivity of nociceptors. NGF also increases the production of neuropeptides (e.g. SP, CGRP and neurokinins) in sensory nerve fibers [153]. Exogenous administration of NGF produces hyperalgesia to noxious stimuli in the adult rat [89] and anti-NGF treatment reduces hypersensitivity during inflammation [154]. BDNF induces spinal hyperalgesia and intrathecal BDNF antisense treatment attenuates hyperalgesia in a mouse model [155]. NT-4 evokes hyperalgesia and acute nerve fiber sensitization when injected locally into the skin [156,157]. It seems probable that NGF and other neurotropic factors play important roles in the generation of pain stimuli through nociceptors in the uterus and in endometriotic pelvic lesions.

Neuropathic pain

Neuropathic pain develops when nerves themselves are damaged by injury or disease and may be caused by tissue damage, nerve inflammation or injury to the PNS or CNS [158]. This damage causes the nerve fibers to misfire and send abnormal signals. The symptoms include allodynia (pain resulting from a stimulus that is normally non-painful), hyperalgesia and spontaneous pain. Little is known about the mechanisms underlying neuropathic pain, but increased excitability of sensory fibers and sensitization of nerve fibers in the dorsal horn of the spinal cord are considered to be associated with neuropathic pain [159].

Accumulating evidence suggests that inflammatory and immune cells are involved in neuropathic pain following peripheral nerve injury [158]. At the site of injury in injured nerves, mast cells are degranulated and release inflammatory mediators such as histamine and TNF-α and other substances which can sensitize nociceptors. Some inflammatory mediators can recruit neutrophils and macrophages and release other inflammatory mediators such as PGE$_2$, resulting in further sensitization of nociceptors. Nerve injury also induces the release of NGF, TNF-α and PGE$_2$ from the Schwann cells associated with myelinated axons, and recruitment of T-cells, which can secrete several cytokines to further sensitize nociceptors and induce pain hypersensitivity.

Injury to a peripheral nerve can also initiate the release of neuropeptides such as SP and CGRP from the nerve terminal [88]. These neuropeptides activate microglia and astrocytes in the dorsal horn of the spinal cord and release various inflammatory mediators. These inflammatory mediators can further activate microglia and astrocytes to produce more inflammatory mediators, which can sensitize nerve fibers in the dorsal horn and induce central pain sensations.

In our studies, we hypothesized that unmyelinated sensory and adrenergic fibers in endometrium and myometrium of women with endometriosis may be involved in pain generation. Since there were many more nerve fibers expressing NPY than SP or CGRP, a large amount of norepinephrine released from adrenergic fibers may alter the sensitivity of nociceptors. When SP and CGRP are released from the nociceptive terminals, these neuropeptides can promote non-neuronal cells and vascular tissues to release inflammatory mediators, which may further activate or sensitize nociceptors.

The activation and sensitization of nociceptors by neurotropins and other neurotropic factors may be pivotal in terms of pain generation, since NGF and its receptors are highly expressed in endometrium and myometrium in women with endometriosis. It is unclear whether nerve fibers in endometrium may be permanently damaged by repeated trauma during partial shedding at the time of menstruation.

Pain perception is very variable in women with endometriosis. Some women have severe pelvic pain, while others do not present with any pain symptoms. This may be due to the presence of different types of nerve fibers, different expression of neurotropins in endometrium, myometrium and endometriotic lesions or differences in central processing of signals. Further research is required to define the roles of nerve fibers and neurotropins in different tissues in women with endometriosis.

Linkage of peripheral pain signaling with central mechanisms

The primary processing of impulses arising with sensory nerve fibers generally occurs within the DRG where the relevant cell bodies of these axons lie. Some complex processing of signals may also occur within the various plexuses which lie within the pelvis, although these influences are not well understood. Synaptic transmission of impulses within the DRG allows for processing of the signal before it is passed into the spinothalamic tracts of the spinal cord for projection to higher centers within the brain.

Peptidergic fibers can also release neuropeptides from their afferent terminals when activated. Neuropeptides stimulate interneurons to carry the pain signals up the spinal cord via the spinothalamic and spinomesencephalic tracts to the reticular formation, the thalamus, and the somatosensory cortex. The reticular formation is involved in alertness associated with the noxious stimuli. The pain signals are then sent to the thalamus, in which pain perception occurs. The somatosensory cortex is considered to be involved with sensory and discriminative aspects of pain perception including pain localization [160] and when the pain signals reach the somatosensory cortex from the thalamus, individuals are fully aware of the pain. The limbic system includes the hypothalamus, hippocampus, and amygdala. When the thalamus and the reticular formation are interconnected to the limbic system, behavioral and emotional responses to pain are elicited and unpleasant pain perception can be induced.

Implications for clinical management of pelvic pain

Currently, management of endometriosis pain focuses around four broad approaches.
- Surgical excision of lesions
- Suppression of ovarian E_2 secretion
- Suppression of "inflammatory" and other disturbed molecular activity in ectopic lesions by action of high doses of progestogens
- Attempts to treat pain directly by the administration of analgesic drugs.

All of these approaches are reasonably effective in many women, highly effective in a minority and ineffective in a substantial minority. In most cases we really do not understand clearly why a particular approach works well – or does not work – in a particular woman. Indeed, we often do not understand where the pain is coming from or how it is arising. Visceral pain arising from any organ is complex, and its management can often be difficult, especially with endometriosis [2]. It seems crucial that we try to understand the specific attributes and origins of visceral pain involving the reproductive organs and peritoneum – and local nerve fiber function – before the specific and focused treatments can be developed.

It seems highly likely that enhanced expression of neurotropins, such as NGF, is a primary determinant of nociceptor activity, enhanced by disturbances of PG release and other molecular combinations not well characterized. It may well be that future approaches to medical management require combinations of therapies targeted at different mechanisms.

There is increasing current concern that repeated and incomplete surgical excision (especially with cautery) of endometriotic lesions may repeatedly damage nerve fibers and set up conditions favorable to the development of neuropathic pain. There is little specific evidence to support this concern but it remains an important field for investigation, especially in women with persistent and atypical pain.

Future directions in research into pelvic pain mechanisms

Current understanding regarding the debilitating and chronic pain symptoms experienced by women suffering from endometriosis is still poor. The relationships of pain to the severity of pelvic organ involvement, to the presence of nerve fibers in the eutopic endometrium and lesions of women with endometriosis and to understanding the origin and role the nerve fibers play in endometriosis lesion development and perception of pain are all unclear and need to be further explored, defined, and investigated. The need for novel directions in pain research in endometriosis has been highlighted by a prestigious international group of endometriosis researchers [161].

Several recent studies have shown that the genome of women with endometriosis is aberrantly regulated compared to women without endometriosis [63,162–167] and attempts to identify candidate genes to elucidate the pathogenesis of endometriosis have been extensive. However, these attempts have been largely unsuccessful. Simultaneously, the endometriosis proteome has also been thoroughly investigated [168–171]. Protein expression is the end-product of gene translation and needs to be linked specifically with gene expression and regulation, with specific focus on those molecular systems which control pain stimuli. This may require highly sensitive, high-throughput molecular technologies which can target low abundance markers.

Identifying genes of neuronal interest will enable animal models of gene knockout to be developed. There is a real need to also pursue the links between different types of immune cells and their potential to influence nerve fiber growth and function. Genotyping of the neurotransmitter and neurotropin systems may help to explain the major interindividual variability in pain symptoms of endometriosis seen in the clinic. Better recognition of specific neurogenic and neurostimulatory factors could identify potential therapeutic targets in the management of endometriosis in women with chronic persistent pelvic pain. Epigenetic aspects of hormone (estrogen and/or P) regulation of neurotropic gene activation or silencing are being increasingly recognized as having importance in endometriosis [172] and merit further active research.

The conscious perception of pain occurs in the thalamus and limbic system in the brain, with intermediate processing in the DRG and spinal cord. Effective, targeted interruption or modulation of these signals could be a valuable adjunct to chronic pelvic pain management, and merits a much greater research effort. The need for this has been highlighted by recent observations that women with endometriosis may experience hyperalgesia, allodynia and related sensory perception changes pointing to altered central processing of pain signals [4].

Conclusion

Pelvic pain is universally recognized as the key symptom in endometriosis but is highly variable in expression from one woman to another. Mechanisms of the generation of pelvic pain signals, their processing and perception are very poorly understood, and urgently require a major research investment before improved evidence-based medical therapies are likely to be designed. A hypothetical sequence of mechanisms which may be involved in the generation of pelvic pain in women with endometriosis is presented in Box 21.2. The observation that large numbers of new sensory and autonomic nerve fibers are present in the endometrium, myometrium and ectopic lesions in endometriosis sufferers, but not in sufferers from other reproductive conditions which can cause pain (such as fibroids, adenomyosis and endometritis), suggests that the pelvic pain suffered by women with endometriosis has different origins and characteristics compared with other types of pelvic pain. In spite of the fact that endometriosis has been recognized as a specific pathological condition

---

Box 21.2 Hypothetical sequence of mechanisms involved in the generation of pelvic pain in women with endometriosis

- Activation of the endometrial genes responsible for synthesis of NGF, other neurotropins and their receptors.

- Ingrowth and extensive branching (neurites) of sensory and autonomic nerve fibers from pre-existing uterine nerves throughout eutopic endometrium and myometrium.

- NGF stimulates BDNF and both of these factors sensitize existing nerve fibers (and nociceptors) to pain stimuli.

- Release of PGs within the endometrium and myometrium in the pre- and perimenstrual phases further sensitizes and may trigger pain stimuli through uterine nociceptors.

- Ectopic peritoneal and other endometriotic lesions develop over time (through the effects of other disturbed molecular mechanisms in the endometrium).

- These ectopic lesions synthesize neurotropins, which encourage the ingrowth and branching of nerve fibers. Local release of neurotropins and PGs and other pain-mediating substances in the perimenstrual phase now triggers pain stimuli within the lesions. Ingrowth and activation of certain immune cells increase the capability of the ectopic tissue to sensitize and stimulate nociceptors.

- Processing of nociceptor stimuli occurs in the DRG and the sacral and lumbar regions of the spinal cord. After initial processing, certain impulses are allowed to enter the anterior spinothalamic tracts of the spinal cord for final processing and "perception" of pain in higher centers.

- Repeated nerve damage around ectopic lesions may lead to persistent or repetitive nociceptor activation with the setting up of abnormal spinal cord pain circuits and the development of neuropathic pain.

---

for well over 100 years, we are still only at the very beginning of understanding its most prominent and distressing symptom.

References

1. Giudice LC, Kao LC. Endometriosis. Lancet 2004;364(9447): 1789–1799.

2. Fraser IS, Tokushige N, Al-Jefout M et al. Endometriosis and visceral pain. In: Bjorling DE (ed) Visceral Pain. Kerala, India: Research Signpost; 2009.

3. Howard FM. Endometriosis and mechanisms of pelvic pain. J Minim Invasive Gynecol 2009;16(5):540–550.

4. Fraser IS. Mysteries of endometriosis pain: Chien-Tien Hsu Memorial Lecture 2009. J Obstet Gynaecol Res 2010;36(1):1–10.

5. Braun DP, Dmowski WP. Endometriosis: abnormal endometrium and dysfunctional immune response. Curr Opin Obstet Gynecol 1998;10(5):365–369.

6. Jones RK, Bulmer JN, Searle RF. Phenotypic and functional studies of leukocytes in human endometrium and endometriosis. Hum Reprod Update 1998;4(5):702–709.

7. Dmowski WP, Braun DP. Immunology of endometriosis. Best Pract Res Clin Obstet Gynaecol 2004;18(2):245–263.

8. Kennedy S, Bergqvist A, Chapron C et al. ESHRE guideline for the diagnosis and treatment of endometriosis. Hum Reprod 2005;20(10):2698–2704.

9. Netter FH. A Compilation of Paintings on the Normal and Pathologic Anatomy of the Reproductive System, 2nd edn. New York: Ciba Pharmaceutical Company, 1965.

10. Rogers RM Jr. Pelvic denervation surgery: what the evidence and anatomy teach us. Clin Obstet Gynecol 2003;46(4):767–772.

11. Butler-Manuel SA, Buttery LD, A'Hern RP et al. Pelvic nerve plexus trauma at radical hysterectomy and simple hysterectomy: the nerve content of the uterine supporting ligaments. Cancer 2000;89(4):834–841.

12. Butler-Manuel SA, Buttery LD, A'Hern RP et al. Pelvic nerve plexus trauma at radical and simple hysterectomy: a quantitative study of nerve types in the uterine supporting ligaments. J Soc Gynecol Invest 2002;9(1):47–56.

13. McBride AW, Li J, Gutman R. Anatomy of the pelvis. J Pelvic Med Surg 2003;9(3):103–123.

14. Hollabaugh RS Jr, Steiner MS, Dmochowski RR. Neuroanatomy of the female continence complex: clinical implications. Urology 2001;57(2):382–388.

15. Mauroy B, Bizet B, Bonnal JL et al. Systematization of the vesical and uterovaginal efferences of the female inferior hypogastric plexus (pelvic): applications to pelvic surgery on women patients. Surg Radiol Anat 2007;29(3):209–217.

16. Mauroy B, Demondion X, Bizet B et al. The female inferior hypogastric (= pelvic) plexus: anatomical and radiological description of the plexus and its afferences – applications to pelvic surgery. Surg Radiol Anat 2007;29(1):55–66.

17. Aguado LI. Role of the central and peripheral nervous system in the ovarian function. Microsc Res Tech 2002;59(6):462–473.

18. Williams PL, Bannister LH, Berry MM et al (eds). Gray's Anatomy: The Anatomical Basis of Medicine and Surgery, 38th edn. New York: Churchill Livingstone; 1995.

19. Rapkin AJ. Neuroanatomy, neurophysiology, and neuropharmacology of pelvic pain. Clin Obstet Gynecol 1990;33(1):119–129.

20. Roberts M. Clinical neuroanatomy of the abdomen and pelvis: implications for surgical treatment of prolapse. Clin Obstet Gynecol 2005;48(3):627–638.

21. Ahluwalia HS, Burger JP, Quinn TH. Anatomy of the anterior abdominal wall. Oper Tech Gen Surg 2004;6(3 SPEC.ISS.):147–155.

22. Rogers RM Jr. Basic neuroanatomy for understanding pelvic pain. J Am Assoc Gynecol Laparosc 1999;6(1):15–29.

23. Owman C, Sjoberg NO. Effect of pregnancy and sex hormones on the transmitter level in uterine short adrenergic neurons. Biochem Pharmacol 1974;23(Suppl 2):657–663.

24. Thorbert G, Alm P, Björklund AB et al. Adrenergic innervation of the human uterus. Disappearance of the transmitter and transmitter-forming enzymes during pregnancy. Am J Obstet Gynecol 1979;135(2):223–226.

25. Wikland M, Lindblom B, Dahlström A et al. Structural and functional evidence for the denervation of human myometrium during pregnancy. Obstet Gynecol 1984;64(4):503–509.

26. Bryman I, Norström A, Dahlström A et al. Immunohistochemical evidence for preserved innervation of the human cervix during pregnancy. Gynecol Obstet Invest 1987;24(2):73–79.

27. Morizaki N, Morizaki J, Hayashi RH et al. A functional and structural study of the innervation of the human uterus. Am J Obstet Gynecol 1989;160(1):218–228.

28. Marzioni D, Tamagnone L, Capparuccia L et al. Restricted innervation of uterus and placenta during pregnancy: evidence for a role of the repelling signal semaphorin 3A. Dev Dyn 2004;231(4):839–848.

29. Tingaker BK, Ekman-Ordeberg G, Forsgren S. Presence of sensory nerve corpuscles in the human corpus and cervix uteri during pregnancy and labor as revealed by immunohistochemistry. Reprod Biol Endocrinol 2006;4:45.

30. Tingaker BK, Johansson O, Cluff AH et al. Unaltered innervation of the human cervix uteri in contrast to the corpus during pregnancy and labor as revealed by PGP 9.5 immunohistochemistry. Eur J Obstet Gynecol Reprod Biol 2006;125(1):66–71.

31. Quinn MJ, Kirk N. Differences in uterine innervation at hysterectomy. Am J Obstet Gynecol 2002;187(6):1515–1519; discussion 1519–1520.

32. Zakashansky K, Bradley WH, Chuang L et al. Recent advances in the surgical management of cervical cancer. Mt Sinai J Med 2009;76(6):567–576.

33. Maas CP, Kenter GG, Trimbos JB et al. Anatomical basis for nerve-sparing radical hysterectomy: immunohistochemical study of the pelvic autonomic nerves. Acta Obstet Gynecol Scand 2005;84(9):868–874.

34. Ito E, Kudo R, Saito T et al. A new technique for radical hysterectomy with emphasis on preservation of bladder function. J Gynecol Surg 2000;16(4):133–140.

35. Fujii S, Takakura K, Matsumura N et al. Anatomic identification and functional outcomes of the nerve sparing Okabayashi radical hysterectomy. Gynecol Oncol 2007;107(1):4–13.

36. Ercoli A, Delmas V, Gadonneix P et al. Classical and nerve-sparing radical hysterectomy: an evaluation of the risk of injury to the autonomous pelvic nerves. Surg Radiol Anat 2003;25(3–4):200–206.

37. Skret-Magierlo J, Naróg M, Kruczek A et al. Radical hysterectomy during the transition period from traditional to nerve-sparing technique. Gynecol Oncol 2010;116(3):502–505.

38. Cibula D, Velechovska P, Sláma J et al. Late morbidity following nerve-sparing radical hysterectomy. Gynecol Oncol 2010;116(3):506–511.

39. Dursun P, Ayhan A, Kuscu E. Nerve-sparing radical hysterectomy for cervical carcinoma. Crit Rev Oncol Hematol 2009;70(3):195–205.

40. Tulandi T, Chen MF, Al-Took S et al. A study of nerve fibers and histopathology of postsurgical, postinfectious, and endometriosis-related adhesions. Obstet Gynecol 1998;92(5):766–768.

41. Herrick SE, Mutsaers SE, Ozua P et al. Human peritoneal adhesions are highly cellular, innervated, and vascularized. J Pathol 2000;192(1):67–72.

42. Sulaiman H, Gabella G, Davis MC et al. Presence and distribution of sensory nerve fibers in human peritoneal adhesions. Ann Surg 2001;234(2):256–261.

43. Proctor ML, Latthe PM, Farquhar CM et al. Surgical interruption of pelvic nerve pathways for primary and secondary dysmenorrhoea. Cochrane Database Syst Rev 2005;19(4):CD001896.

44. Salamonsen LA, Zhang J, Hampton A et al. Regulation of matrix metalloproteinases in human endometrium. Hum Reprod 2000;15(Suppl 3):112–119.

45. Chung HW, Lee JY, Moon HS et al. Matrix metalloproteinase-2, membranous type 1 matrix metalloproteinase, and tissue inhibitor of metalloproteinase-2 expression in ectopic and eutopic endometrium. Fertil Steril 2002;78(4):787–795.

46. Collette T, Bellehumeur C, Kats R et al. Evidence for an increased release of proteolytic activity by the eutopic endometrial tissue in women with endometriosis and for involvement of matrix metalloproteinase-9. Hum Reprod 2004;19(6):1257–1264.

47. Dufournet C, Uzan C, Fauvet R et al. Expression of apoptosis-related proteins in peritoneal, ovarian and colorectal endometriosis. J Reprod Immunol 2006;70(1–2):151–162.

48. Harada T, Kaponis A, Iwabe T et al. Apoptosis in human endometrium and endometriosis. Hum Reprod Update 2004;10(1):29–38.

49. Gebel HM, Braun DP, Tambur A et al. Spontaneous apoptosis of endometrial tissue is impaired in women with endometriosis. Fertil Steril 1998;69(6):1042–1047.

50. Dmowski WP, Gebel H, Braun DP. Decreased apoptosis and sensitivity to macrophage mediated cytolysis of endometrial cells in endometriosis. Hum Reprod Update 1998;4(5):696–701.

51. Meresman GF, Vighi S, Buquet RA et al. Apoptosis and expression of Bcl-2 and Bax in eutopic endometrium from women with endometriosis. Fertil Steril 2000;74(4):760–766.

52. Bulmer JN, Jones RK, Searle RF. Intraepithelial leukocytes in endometriosis and adenomyosis: comparison of eutopic and ectopic endometrium with normal endometrium. Hum Reprod 1998;13(10):2910–2915.

53. Fernández-Shaw S, Clarke MT, Hicks B et al. Bone marrow-derived cell populations in uterine and ectopic endometrium. Hum Reprod 1995;10(9):2285–2289.

54. Jones RK, Bulmer JN, Searle RF. Immunohistochemical characterization of proliferation, oestrogen receptor and progesterone receptor expression in endometriosis: comparison of eutopic and ectopic endometrium with normal cycling endometrium. Hum Reprod 1995;10(12):3272–3279.

55. Klentzeris LD, Bulmer JN, Liu DT, Morrison L. Endometrial leukocyte subpopulations in women with endometriosis. Eur J Obstet Gynecol Reprod Biol 1995;63(1):41–47.

56. Ota H, Igarashi S, Tanaka T. Expression of gamma delta cells and adhesion molecules in endometriotic tissue in patients with endometriosis and adenomyosis. Am J Reprod Immunol 1996;35(5):477–482.

57. Akoum A, Metz CN, Al-Akoum M, Kats R. Macrophage migration inhibitory factor expression in the intrauterine endometrium of women with endometriosis varies with disease stage, infertility status, and pelvic pain. Fertil Steril 2006;85(5):1379–1385.

58. Berbic M, Schulke L, Markham R et al. Macrophage expression in endometrium of women with and without endometriosis. Hum Reprod 2009;24(2):325–332.

59. Schulke L, Berbic M, Manconi F et al. Dendritic cell populations in the eutopic and ectopic endometrium of women with endometriosis. Hum Reprod 2009;24(7):1695–1703.

60. Berbic M, Hey-Cunningham AJ, Ng C et al. The role of Foxp3+ regulatory T-cells in endometriosis, a potential controlling mechanism for a complex, chronic immunological condition. Hum Reprod 2010;25(4):900–907.

61. Chuang PC, Wu MH, Shoji Y, Tsai SJ. Downregulation of CD36 results in reduced phagocytic ability of peritoneal macrophages of women with endometriosis. J Pathol 2009;219(2):232–241.

62. Harada T, Iwabe T, Terakawa N. Role of cytokines in endometriosis. Fertil Steril 2001;76(1):1–10.

63. Kyama CM, Overbergh L, Debrock S et al. Increased peritoneal and endometrial gene expression of biologically relevant cytokines and growth factors during the menstrual phase in women with endometriosis. Fertil Steril 2006;85(6):1667–1675.

64. Donnez J, Smoes P, Gillerot S et al. Vascular endothelial growth factor (VEGF) in endometriosis. Hum Reprod 1998;13(6):1686–1690.

65. Print C, Valtola R, Evans A et al. Soluble factors from human endometrium promote angiogenesis and regulate the endothelial cell transcriptome. Hum Reprod 2004;19(10):2356–2366.

66. Kim SH, Choi YM, Chae HD et al. Increased expression of endoglin in the eutopic endometrium of women with endometriosis. Fertil Steril 2001;76(5):918–922.

67. Ulukus M, Cakmak H, Arici A. The role of endometrium in endometriosis. J Soc Gynecol Invest 2006;13(7):467–476.

68. Bourlev V, Volkov N, Pavlovitch S et al. The relationship between microvessel density, proliferative activity and expression of vascular endothelial growth factor-A and its receptors in eutopic endometrium and endometriotic lesions. Reproduction 2006;132(3):501–509.

69. Ota H, Igarashi S, Hatazawa J, Tanaka T. Endothelial nitric oxide synthase in the endometrium during the menstrual cycle in patients with endometriosis and adenomyosis. Fertil Steril 1998;69(2):303–308.

70. Ota H, Igarashi S, Hatazawa J, Tanaka T. Endometriosis and free radicals. Gynecol Obstet Invest 1999;48(Suppl 1):29–35.

71. Ota H, Igarashi S, Hatazawa J, Tanaka T. Immunohistochemical assessment of superoxide dismutase expression in the endometrium in endometriosis and adenomyosis. Fertil Steril 1999;72(1):129–134.

72. Ota H, Igarashi S, Tanaka T. Xanthine oxidase in eutopic and ectopic endometrium in endometriosis and adenomyosis. Fertil Steril 2001;75(4):785–790.

73. Ota H, Igarashi S, Sato N et al. Involvement of catalase in the endometrium of patients with endometriosis and adenomyosis. Fertil Steril 2002;78(4):804–809.

74. Wu MY, Chao KH, Yang JH. Nitric oxide synthesis is increased in the endometrial tissue of women with endometriosis. Hum Reprod 2003;18(12):2668–2671.

75. Bulun SE, Zeitoun K, Takayama K et al. Estrogen production in endometriosis and use of aromatase inhibitors to treat endometriosis. Endocr Relat Cancer 1999;6(2):293–301.

76. Bulun SE, Fang Z, Imir G et al. Aromatase and endometriosis. Semin Reprod Med 2004;22(1):45–50.

77. Bulun SE, Cheng YH, Yin P et al. Progesterone resistance in endometriosis: link to failure to metabolize estradiol. Mol Cell Endocrinol 2006;248(1–2):94–103.

78. Coupland RE. The distribution of cholinergic and other nerve fibres in the human uterus. Postgrad Med J 1969;45(519):78–79.

79. Tokushige N, Markham R, Russell P, Fraser IS. High density of small nerve fibres in the functional layer of the endometrium in women with endometriosis. Hum Reprod 2006;21(3):782–787.

80. Tokushige N, Markham R, Russell P, Fraser IS. Different types of small nerve fibers in eutopic endometrium and myometrium in women with endometriosis. Fertil Steril 2007;88(4):795–803.

81. Samuelson UE, Dalsgaard CJ, Lundberg JM, Hökfelt T. Calcitonin gene-related peptide inhibits spontaneous contractions in human uterus and fallopian tube. Neurosci Lett 1985;62(2):225–230.

82. Sato S, Hayashi RH, Garfield RE. Mechanical responses of the rat uterus, cervix, and bladder to stimulation of hypogastric and pelvic nerves in vivo. Biol Reprod 1989;40(2):209–219.

83. Rodriguez R, Pozuelo JM, Martin R et al. Stereological quantification of nerve fibers immunoreactive to PGP 9.5, NPY, and VIP in rat prostate during postnatal development. J Androl 2005;26(2):197–204.

84. Tokushige N, Markham R, Russell P, Fraser IS. Effects of hormonal treatment on nerve fibers in endometrium and myometrium in women with endometriosis. Fertil Steril 2008;90(5):1589–1598.

85. Anaf V, Simon P, El Nakadi I et al. Hyperalgesia, nerve infiltration and nerve growth factor expression in deep adenomyotic nodules, peritoneal and ovarian endometriosis. Hum Reprod 2002;17(7):1895–1900.

86. Braun A, Lommatzsch M, Renz H. The role of neurotrophins in allergic bronchial asthma. Clin Exp Allergy 2000;30(2):178–186.

87. Jänig W, Baron R. Complex regional pain syndrome is a disease of the central nervous system. Clin Auton Res 2002;12(3):150–164.

88. Julius D, Basbaum AI. Molecular mechanisms of nociception. Nature 2001;413(6852):203–210.

89. Malcangio M. Nerve growth factor treatment increases stimulus-evoked release of sensory neuropeptides in the rat spinal cord. Eur J Neurosci 1997;9(5):1101–1104.

90. Pezet S, McMahon SB. Neurotrophins: mediators and modulators of pain. Annu Rev Neurosci 2006;29:507–538.

91. Carroll P, Lewin GR, Koltzenburg M et al. A role for BDNF in mechanosensation. Nat Neurosci 1998;1(1):42–46.

92. Schmelz M. Itch and pain. Dermatol Ther 2005;18(4):304–307.

93. Chiang CM, Hill JA. Localization of T cells, interferon-gamma and HLA-DR in eutopic and ectopic human endometrium. Gynecol Obstet Invest 1997;43(4):245–250.

94. Tran LVP, Tokushige N, Berbic M et al. Macrophages and nerve fibres in peritoneal endometriosis. Hum Reprod 2009;24(4):835–841.

95. Mulayim N, Savlu A, Guzeloglu-Kayisli O et al. Regulation of endometrial stromal cell matrix metalloproteinase activity and invasiveness by interleukin-8. Fertil Steril 2004;81(Suppl 1):904–911.

96. Béliard A, Donnez J, Nisolle M, Foidart JM. Localization of laminin, fibronectin, E-cadherin, and integrins in endometrium and endometriosis. Fertil Steril 1997;67(2):266–272.

97. Kauma S, Clark MR, White C, Halme J. Production of fibronectin by peritoneal macrophages and concentration of fibronectin in peritoneal fluid from patients with or without endometriosis. Obstet Gynecol 1988;72(1):13–18.

98. Sbracia M, Zupi E, Alo P et al. Differential expression of IGF-I and IGF-II in eutopic and ectopic endometria of women with endometriosis and in women without endometriosis. Am J Reprod Immunol 1997;37(4):326–329.

99. Olive DL, Schwartz LB. Medical progress: endometriosis. N Engl J Med 1993;328(24):1759–1769.

100. Akoum A, Lemay A, Paradis I et al. Secretion of interleukin-6 by human endometriotic cells and regulation by proinflammatory cytokines and sex steroids. Hum Reprod 1996;11(10):2269–2275.

101. Sugawara J, Fukaya T, Murakami T et al. Increased secretion of hepatocyte growth factor by eutopic endometrial stromal cells in women with endometriosis. Fertil Steril 1997;68(3):468–472.

102. Braun DP, Gebel H, Rana N, Dmowski WP. Cytolysis of eutopic and ectopic endometrial cells by peripheral blood monocytes and peritoneal macrophages in women with endometriosis. Fertil Steril 1998;69(6):1103–1108.

103. Somigliana E, Viganò P, Gaffuri B et al. Modulation of NK cell lytic function by endometrial secretory factors: potential role in endometriosis. Am J Reprod Immunol 1996;36(5):295–300.

104. Bedaiwy MA, Falcone T. Laboratory testing for endometriosis. Clin Chim Acta 2004;340(1–2):41–56.

105. Vinatier D, Orazi G, Cosson M, Dufour P. Theories of endometriosis. Eur J Obstet Gynecol Reprod Biol 2001;96(1):21–34.

106. Hull ML, Charnock-Jones DS, Chan CL et al. Antiangiogenic agents are effective inhibitors of endometriosis. J Clin Endocrinol Metab 2003;88(6):2889–2899.

107. Gilabert-Estellés J, Ramón LA, España F et al. Expression of angiogenic factors in endometriosis: relationship to fibrinolytic and metalloproteinase systems. Hum Reprod 2007;22(8):2120–2127.

108. Takehara M, Ueda M, Yamashita Y et al. Vascular endothelial growth factor A and C gene expression in endometriosis. Hum Pathol 2004;35(11):1369–1375.

109. Tan XJ, Lang JH, Liu DY et al. Expression of vascular endothelial growth factor and thrombospondin-1 mRNA in patients with endometriosis. Fertil Steril 2002;78(1):148–153.

110. Shifren JL, Tseng JF, Zaloudek CJ et al. Ovarian steroid regulation of vascular endothelial growth factor in the human endometrium: implications for angiogenesis during the menstrual cycle and in the pathogenesis of endometriosis. J Clin Endocrinol Metab 1996;81(8):3112–3118.

111. Li B, Lalani AS, Harding TC et al. Vascular endothelial growth factor blockade reduces intratumoral regulatory T cells and enhances the efficacy of a GM-CSF-secreting cancer immunotherapy. Clin Cancer Res 2006;12(22):6808–6816.

112. Gabrilovich D, Ishida T, Oyama T et al. Vascular endothelial growth factor inhibits the development of dendritic cells and dramatically affects the differentiation of multiple hematopoietic lineages in vivo. Blood 1998;92(11):4150–4166.

113. Gazvani MR, Christmas S, Quenby S et al. Peritoneal fluid concentrations of interleukin-8 in women with endometriosis: relationship to stage of disease. Hum Reprod 1998;13(7):1957–1961.

114. Giatromanolaki A, Bates GJ, Koukourakis MI et al. The presence of tumor-infiltrating FOXP3+ lymphocytes correlates with intratumoral angiogenesis in endometrial cancer. Gynecol Oncol 2008;110(2):216–221.

115. Zeitoun K, Takayama K, Sasano H et al. Deficient 17beta-hydroxysteroid dehydrogenase type 2 expression in endometriosis: failure to metabolize 17beta-estradiol. J Clin Endocrinol Metab 1998;83(12):4474–4480.

116. Bulun SE, Yang S, Fang Z et al. Role of aromatase in endometrial disease. J Steroid Biochem Mol Biol 2001;79(1–5):19–25.

117. Brosens I, Puttemans P, Campo R, Gordts S. Endometriosis: a uterine disease with extrauterine lesions? Rev Gynaecol Pract 2003;3(3): 115–119.

118. Tokushige N, Markham R, Russell P, Fraser IS. Nerve fibres in peritoneal endometriosis. Hum Reprod 2006;21(11):3001–3007.

119. Wang G, Tokushige N, Markham R, Fraser IS. Rich innervation of deep infiltrating endometriosis. Hum Reprod 2009;24(4): 827–834.

120. Wang G, Tokushige N, Russell P et al. Hyperinnervation in intestinal deep infiltrating endometriosis. J Minim Invas Gynecol 2009;16(6): 713–719.

121. Al-Fozan H, Bakare S, Chen MF et al. Nerve fibers in ovarian dermoid cysts and endometriomas. Fertil Steril 2004;82(1):230–231.

122. Odagiri K, Konno R, Fujiwara H et al. Smooth muscle metaplasia and innervation in interstitium of endometriotic lesions related to pain. Fertil Steril 2009;92(5):1525–1531.

123. Tokushige N, Russell P, Black K et al. Nerve fibers in ovarian endometriomas. Fertil Steril 2010;94(5):1944–1947.

124. Zhang G, Dmitrieva N, Liu Y et al. Endometriosis as a neurovascular condition: estrous variations in innervation, vascularization, and growth factor content of ectopic endometrial cysts in the rat. Am J Physiol Regul Integr Comp Physiol 2008;294(1):R162–171.

125. Berkley KJ, Zalcman SS, Simon VR. Sex and gender differences in pain and inflammation: a rapidly maturing field. Am J Physiol Regul Integr Comp Physiol 2006;291(2):R241–244.

126. Brodie C, Gelfand EW. Functional nerve growth factor receptors on human B lymphocytes: interaction with IL-2. J Immunol 1992; 148(11):3492–3497.

127. Mitsuma N, Yamamoto M, Iijima M et al. Wide range of lineages of cells expressing nerve growth factor mRNA in the nerve lesions of patients with vasculitic neuropathy: an implication of endoneurial macrophage for nerve regeneration. Neuroscience 2004;129(1): 109–117.

128. Song X-Y, Li F, Zhang F-H et al. Peripherally-derived BDNF promotes regeneration of ascending sensory neurons after spinal cord injury. PLoS One 2008;3(3):e1707.

129. Krizsan-Agbas D, Pedchenko T, Hasan W, Smith PG. Oestrogen regulates sympathetic neurite outgrowth by modulating brain derived neurotrophic factor synthesis and release by the rodent uterus. Eur J Neurosci 2003;18(10):2760–2768.

130. Okragly AJ, Niles AL, Saban R et al. Elevated tryptase, nerve growth factor, neurotrophin-3 and glial cell line-derived neurotrophic factor levels in the urine of interstitial cystitis and bladder cancer patients. J Urol 1999;161(2):438–442.

131. He XP, Yang F, Xie ZP, Lu B. Intracellular Ca2+ and Ca2+/calmodulin-dependent kinase II mediate acute potentiation of neurotransmitter release by neurotrophin-3. J Cell Biol 2000;149(4):783–791.

132. Roosen A, Schober A, Strelau J et al. Lack of neurotrophin-4 causes selective structural and chemical deficits in sympathetic ganglia and their preganglionic innervation. J Neurosci 2001;21(9): 3073–3084.

133. Mantyh PW, Clohisy DR, Koltzenburg M, Hunt SP. Molecular mechanisms of cancer pain. Nat Rev Cancer 2002;2(3):201–209.

134. Paik SK, Park KP, Lee SK et al. Light and electron microscopic analysis of the somata and parent axons innervating the rat upper molar and lower incisor pulp. Neuroscience 2009;162(4):1279–1286.

135. Basbaum AI, Bautista DM, Scherrer G, Julius D. Cellular and molecular mechanisms of pain. Cell 2009;139(2):267–284.

136. Tulandi T, Felemban A, Chen MF. Nerve fibers and histopathology of endometriosis-harboring peritoneum. J Am Assoc Gynecol Laparosc 2001;8(1):95–98.

137. Tamburro S, Canis M, Albuisson E et al. Expression of transforming growth factor beta1 in nerve fibers is related to dysmenorrhea and laparoscopic appearance of endometriotic implants. Fertil Steril 2003;80(5):1131–1136.

138. Al-Jefout M, Andreadis N, Tokushige N et al. A pilot study to evaluate the relative efficacy of endometrial biopsy and full curettage in making a diagnosis of endometriosis by the detection of endometrial nerve fibers. Am J Obstet Gynecol 2007;197(6):578.

139. Bokor A, Kyama CM, Vercruysse L et al. Density of small diameter sensory nerve fibres in endometrium: a semi-invasive diagnostic test for minimal to mild endometriosis. Hum Reprod 2009;24(12): 3025–3032.

140. Gulati AK. Immune response and neurotrophic factor interactions in peripheral nerve transplants. Acta Haematol 1998;99(3):171–174.

141. Leon A, Buriani A, Dal Toso R et al. Mast cells synthesize, store, and release nerve growth factor. Proc Natl Acad Sci USA 1994;91(9): 3739–3743.

142. Torcia M, Bracci-Laudiero L, Lucibello M et al. Nerve growth factor is an autocrine survival factor for memory B lymphocytes. Cell 1996;85(3):345–356.

143. Kerschensteiner M, Gallmeier E, Behrens L et al. Activated human T cells, B cells, and monocytes produce brain-derived neurotrophic factor in vitro and in inflammatory brain lesions: a neuroprotective role of inflammation? J Exp Med 1999;189(5):865–870.

144. Noga O, Peiser M, Altenähr M et al. Differential activation of dendritic cells by nerve growth factor and brain-derived neurotrophic factor. Clin Exp Allergy 2007;37(11):1701–1708.

145. Fawcett JW, Keynes RJ. Peripheral nerve regeneration. Ann Rev Neurosci 1990;13:43–60.

146. Lindholm D, Heumann R, Hengerer B, Thoenen H. Interleukin 1 increases stability and transcription of mRNA encoding nerve growth factor in cultured rat fibroblasts. J Biol Chem 1988; 263(31):16348–16351.

147. Bandtlow CE, Meyer M, Lindholm D et al. Regional and cellular codistribution of interleukin 1 beta and nerve growth factor mRNA in the adult rat brain: possible relationship to the regulation of nerve growth factor synthesis. J Cell Biol 1990;111(4):1701–1711.

148. Vigé X, Costa E, Wise BC. Mechanism of nerve growth factor mRNA regulation by interleukin-1 and basic fibroblast growth factor in primary cultures of rat astrocytes. Mol Pharmacol 1991;40(2): 186–192.

149. Spranger M, Lindholm D, Bandtlow C et al. Regulation of nerve growth factor (NGF) synthesis in the rat central nervous system: comparison between the effects of interleukin-1 and various growth factors in astrocyte cultures and in vivo. Eur J Neurosci 1990; 2(1):69–76.

150. Conover JC, Yancopoulos GD. Neurotrophin regulation of the developing nervous system: analyses of knockout mice. Rev Neurosci 1997;8(1):13–27.

151. Lu B, Figurov A. Role of neurotrophins in synapse development and plasticity. Rev Neurosci 1997;8(1):1–12.

152. Pupo-Nogueira A, de Oliveira RM, Petta CA et al. Vascular endothelial growth factor concentrations in the serum and peritoneal fluid of women with endometriosis. Int J Gynaecol Obstet 2007;99(1):33–37.

153. Lewin GR, Rueff A, Mendell LM. Peripheral and central mechanisms of NGF-induced hyperalgesia. Eur J Neurosci 1994;6(12): 1903–1912.

154. Andreev NY, Dimitrieva N, Koltzenburg M, McMahon SB. Peripheral administration of nerve growth factor in the adult rat produces a thermal hyperalgesia that requires the presence of sympathetic post-ganglionic neurones. Pain 1995;63(1):109–115.

155. Nicholas RS, Winter J, Wren P et al. Peripheral inflammation increases the capsaicin sensitivity of dorsal root ganglion neurons in a nerve growth factor-dependent manner. Neuroscience 1999;91(4): 1425–1433.

156. Groth R, Aanonsen L. Spinal brain-derived neurotrophic factor (BDNF) produces hyperalgesia in normal mice while antisense directed against either BDNF or trkB, prevent inflammation-induced hyperalgesia. Pain 2002;100(1–2):171–181.

157. Shu XQ, Mendell LM. Neurotrophins and hyperalgesia. Proc Natl Acad Sci USA 1999;96(14):7693–7696.

158. Moalem G, Tracey DJ. Immune and inflammatory mechanisms in neuropathic pain. Brain Res Rev 2006;51(2):240–264.

159. Woolf CJ. Dissecting out mechanisms responsible for peripheral neuropathic pain: implications for diagnosis and therapy. Life Sci 2004;74(21):2605–2610.

160. Bushnell MC, Duncan GH, Hofbauer RK et al. Pain perception: is there a role for primary somatosensory cortex? Proc Natl Acad Sci USA 1999;96(14):7705–7709.

161. Rogers PAW, D'Hooghe TM, Fazleabas A et al. Priorities for endometriosis research: recommendations from an international consensus workshop. Reprod Sci 2009;16(4):335–346.

162. Giudice LC. Genomics' role in understanding the pathogenesis of endometriosis. Semin Reprod Med 2003;21(2):119–124.

163. Eyster KM, Boles AL, Brannian JD et al. DNA microarray analysis of gene expression markers of endometriosis. Fertil Steril 2002; 77(1):38–42.

164. Eyster KM, Klinkova O, Kennedy V, Hansen KA. Whole genome deoxyribonucleic acid microarray analysis of gene expression in ectopic versus eutopic endometrium. Fertil Steril 2007;88(6): 1505–1533.

165. Kao LC, Germeyer A, Tulac S et al. Expression profiling of endometrium from women with endometriosis reveals candidate genes for disease-based implantation failure and infertility. Endocrinology 2003;144(7):2870–2881.

166. Borghese B, Mondon F, Noël JC et al. Gene expression profile for ectopic versus eutopic endometrium provides new insights into endometriosis oncogenic potential. Mol Endocrinol 2008;22(11):2557–2562.

167. Burney RO, Talbi S, Hamilton AE et al. Gene expression analysis of endometrium reveals progesterone resistance and candidate susceptibility genes in women with endometriosis. Endocrinology 2007; 148(8):3814–3826.

168. Ten Have S, Fraser I, Markham R et al. Proteomic analysis of protein expression in the eutopic endometrium of women with endometriosis. Proteomics Clin Appl 2007;1(10):1243–1251.

169. Fowler PA, Tattum J, Bhattacharya S et al. An investigation of the effects of endometriosis on the proteome of human eutopic endometrium: a heterogeneous tissue with a complex disease. Proteomics 2007;7(1):130–142.

170. Zhang H, Niu Y, Feng J et al. Use of proteomic analysis of endometriosis to identify different protein expression in patients with endometriosis versus normal controls. Fertil Steril 2006;86(2):274–282.

171. Li CY, Lang JH, Liu HY, Zhou HM. Expression of annexin-1 in patients with endometriosis. Chin Med J (Engl) 2008;121(10):927–931.

172. Guo SW. Epigenetics of endometriosis. Mol Hum Reprod 2009;15(10):587–607.

173. Sharpe-Timms KL. Endometrial anomalies in women with endometriosis. Ann N Y Acad Sci 2001;943:131–147.

174. Witz CA. Cell adhesion molecules and endometriosis. Semin Reprod Med 2003;21(2):173–182.

175. Viganò P, Gaffuri B, Somigliana E et al. Expression of intercellular adhesion molecule (ICAM)-1 mRNA and protein is enhanced in endometriosis versus endometrial stromal cells in culture. Mol Hum Reprod 1998;4(12):1150–1156.

176. Wang F, He YL, Peng DX, Liu MB. Expressions of nuclear factor-kappaB and intercellular adhesion molecule-1 in endometriosis. Acad J First Medical College PLA 2005;25(6):703–705.

177. Finas D, Huszar M, Agic A et al. L1 cell adhesion molecule (L1CAM) as a pathogenetic factor in endometriosis. Hum Reprod 2008;23(5):1053–1062.

178. Healy DL, Rogers PA, Hii L, Wingfield M. Angiogenesis: a new theory for endometriosis. Hum Reprod Update 1998;4(5):736–740.

179. Sharkey AM, Smith SK. The endometrium as a cause of implantation failure. Best Pract Res Clin Obstet Gynaecol 2003; 17(2):289–307.

180. Dimitriadis E, Stoikos C, Stafford-Bell M et al. Interleukin-11, IL-11 receptoralpha and leukemia inhibitory factor are dysregulated in endometrium of infertile women with endometriosis during the implantation window. J Reprod Immunol 2006; 69(1):53–64.

181. Gaetje R, Holtrich U, Karn T et al. Characterization of WNT7A expression in human endometrium and endometriotic lesions. Fertil Steril 2007;88(6):1534–1540.

182. Eyster KM. New paradigms in signal transduction. Biochem Pharmacol 2007;73(10):1511–1519.

183. Antsiferova YS, Sotnikova NY, Posiseeva LV, Shor AL. Changes in the T-helper cytokine profile and in lymphocyte activation at the systemic and local levels in women with endometriosis. Fertil Steril 2005;84(6):1705–1711.

184. Khan KN, Masuzaki H, Fujishita A et al. Differential macrophage infiltration in early and advanced endometriosis and adjacent peritoneum. Fertil Steril 2004;81(3):652–661.

185. Buyalos RP, Funari VA, Azziz R et al. Elevated interleukin-6 levels in peritoneal fluid of patients with pelvic pathology. Fertil Steril 1992;58(2):302–306.

186. Jolicoeur C, Boutouil M, Drouin R et al. Increased expression of monocyte chemotactic protein-1 in the endometrium of women with endometriosis. Am J Pathol 1998;152(1):125–133.

187. Akoum A, Lawson C, Herrmann-Lavoie C, Maheux R. Imbalance in the expression of the activating type I and the inhibitory type II interleukin 1 receptors in endometriosis. Hum Reprod 2007;22(5):1464–1473.

188. Luo Q, Ning W, Wu Y et al. Altered expression of interleukin-18 in the ectopic and eutopic endometrium of women with endometriosis. J Reprod Immunol 2006;72(1–2):108–117.

22 Neuroendocrine Aspects of Endometriosis-Associated Pain

Pamela Stratton[1] and Karen J. Berkley[2]

[1]Program in Reproductive and Adult Endocrinology, Intramural Program, Eunice Kennedy Shriver National Institute of Child Health and Human Development, National Institutes of Health, Bethesda, MD, USA

[2]Program in Neuroscience, Florida State University, Tallahassee, FL, USA

Introduction

Most women experiencing endometriosis-associated pain have chronic pelvic pain. Pain symptoms ascribed to endometriosis and their severity correlate poorly with lesion characteristics and occur in women without endometriosis. Both endometriosis lesions and endometriosis-ascribed pain symptoms are modulated by estrogens and progestogens. Because the nervous system determines the experience of pain and an endometriosis lesion can develop its own nerve supply, the interplay between the nervous and endocrine systems is an important modulator of endometriosis-ascribed pain. Lesions and the nervous system have a direct and two-way interaction that provides a mechanism by which the dynamic and hormonally responsive central and peripheral nervous systems can produce a variety of individual variations in pain that can become independent of endometriosis itself in some women. Improving understanding and alleviating endometriosis-associated pain will likely occur if the emphasis changes from the lesions to pain and studies the interactions between the nervous and endocrine systems in this condition.

The spectrum of endometriosis-associated pain

The association between endometriosis and chronic pelvic pain is demonstrated by finding endometriosis lesions in one-third of women who undergo laparoscopy for chronic pelvic pain (CPP), but only 5% of those having surgery with neither CPP nor infertility [1,2]. Endometriosis lesions of any type, superficial peritoneal lesions, endometriomas and deeply infiltrating lesions are all associated with chronic pelvic pain [3]. In carefully documented studies, however, lesion extent and location bear minimal relation to pain location or severity [3-6].

Pain symptoms attributed to endometriosis vary between individuals but usually include dysmenorrhea. Other pain symptoms include dyspareunia and non-menstrual chronic pelvic-abdominal muscle pain that may persist over the month or occur only during specific times, such as at ovulation. Dysuria, dyschezia, other chronic musculoskeletal conditions like fibromyalgia, temporomandibular joint disorder or chronic fatigue syndrome, other chronic pelvic visceral pain syndromes like painful bladder syndrome/interstitial cystitis or irritable bowel syndrome may or may not be associated with endometriosis. These pain symptoms and their chronicity, their patterns in relation to the menstrual cycle, and their association with other types of visceral pain reflect changing actions and hormonal modulation of the nervous system [7].

Endocrine influences on endometriosis-associated pain

As endometriosis is regarded as an estrogen-dependent disease, most treatments suppress ovarian function [8], but do not resolve lesions. The finding that nearly all women taking gonadotropin-releasing hormone (GnRH) agonists and progestagens have lesions, despite having relief of symptoms, is well known [9]. This situation reinforces the perplexing lack of correspondence between lesions and pain location or severity.

The observation that endometriosis-associated chronic pelvic pain can be reduced or heightened by various hormonal therapies suggests a relationship between hormones and neural or other aspects of endometriosis, rather than simply the lesions themselves. For example, in randomized double-blind, placebo-controlled clinical trials, leuprolide acetate relieved pain in women with endometriosis, but was also effective in those who did not have endometriosis [10,11].

Another example of hormonal effects on pain is that the selective estrogen receptor modulator raloxifene, when taken after endometriosis excision, significantly shortens time to return of pain, as shown in a randomized, double-blind, placebo-controlled study [12]. Most women in both the treatment and placebo groups had endometriosis when they underwent surgery because the pain had returned or after 2 years of being pain-free. Because raloxifene use was associated with return of pain, but recurrence of endometriosis lesions was not, and an increase in estrogen level occurs at this dosage [13], estrogens or factors other than lesions likely were associated with their returned pelvic pain. An additional explanation may be that most agents suppress ovulation and alter endometrium, frequently causing amenorrhea. When medical therapies are stopped, ovulation and menstruation are restored and symptoms often return. This situation suggests that the contribution of these reproductive functions to symptoms is independent of lesions, perhaps by altering the neuroinflammatory-peritoneal environment.

Hormonal treatments that reduce estradiol or change progesterone levels can lessen pain in women with endometriosis. This hormonal responsiveness supports the idea that estradiol contributes to pain symptoms and that progestogens may contribute to decreased symptoms [14-16]. However, how ovarian hormones actually effect endometriosis-ascribed pain is poorly understood. "Progesterone resistance" is one possible contributor [17,18].

Surgical influences on endometriosis-associated pain

The relationship between endometriosis and the central nervous system is also illustrated by surgery. Randomized studies on the efficacy of surgery for symptomatic endometriosis show that 20% of patients do not have relief after surgery [19]. While surgical treatment of lesions permanently alleviates pain in some patients, indicating that lesions contribute to pain in those patients, surgical treatment does not alleviate pain long term in ~50% of carefully selected patients [20]. In patients whose pain was relieved by surgically treating lesions, pain sometimes returns without evidence of new lesions [20,21]. Patients with minimal or mild endometriosis are more likely to re-experience pain soon after surgery [22]. Thus, those with few endometriosis lesions who experience pain symptoms or who have a return of symptoms without evidence of endometriosis may have a remodeling of the central nervous system (CNS) that is not affected by removing lesions.

Nervous system mechanisms of endometriosis-associated pain

The endocrine and surgical influences on endometriosis-associated pain are affected by neural mechanisms. Innervation of ectopic endometrial growths by sensory and sympathetic fibers was shown in endometriosis growths from a rat model [23] and lesions from women [24]. Endometriosis lesions must be vascularized to attach

and survive [25]. Blood vessels are innervated by sensory and sympathetic fibers [26]. Factors that act on sprouting blood vessels also act on nerve fibers (vascular endothelial growth factor (VEGF), nerve growth factor (NGF), semaphorins, netrins, slits, and membrane-bound ephrins [27-29]). Thus, when angiogenesis occurs to vascularize developing lesions, neural spouting may also occur, thereby enabling nerves to invade lesions.

A new conceptualization of mechanisms underlying pain in endometriosis has evolved from the finding that lesions can be *directly* innervated by attracting nerve fibers innervating nearby structures to sprout branches into the lesions. The conceptualization is that the variable association between endometriosis lesions and pain arises from attributes of the ectopic lesions' newly formed nerve supply and the resulting two-way communication between the lesions and CNS [7,24]. Neural sprouting, especially sprouting associated with NGF, can sensitize sensory fibers [30], meaning that they are more easily activated by noxious stimulation or their spontaneous activity is greater.

It is therefore likely that hormonal and neural influences comprise important, interacting factors that affect pain symptomatology in endometriosis patients.

Rethinking endometriosis-associated chronic pelvic pain: neuroendocrine mechanisms of endometriosis-associated pain

Neuroendocrine aspects of endometriosis-associated pain are illustrated by evidence from the endometriosis (ENDO) rat model concerning how the ectopic growths' nerve supply could contribute to pain in endometriosis via peripheral and central factors (Plate 22.1) [7]. In this model, pieces of uterine horn are autotransplanted onto abdominal arteries that develop into cyst-like lesions that become vascularized, stabilize by 2 months, and remain viable for ~10 months [31]. The control model (shamENDO) involves autotransplanting fat to these vessels; no lesions develop. Similar to the pain symptoms that occur in women with endometriosis, the ENDO rat model develops symptoms that do not correlate with the amount of ectopic growth [32]. One such symptom is vaginal hyperalgesia that may correspond to dyspareunia symptoms [33] and is associated with increased abdominal muscle (external oblique) activity [32]. Table 22.1 compares the rat ENDO model with endometriosis in women.

Severity of ENDO-induced vaginal hyperalgesia in rats varies with their ovarian cycle and is accompanied by changes in lesions [34]. As severity decreases, the lesions' sympathetic innervation, VEGF, and NGF significantly decrease. These changes do not occur in the rat's eutopic uterus. Both sympathetic and sensory fibers in lesions are labeled by antibodies to the NGF receptor (Trk-A), indicating that NGF can act on both fiber types [35]. The hormonal effects on innervation of these lesions suggest that a two-way communication exists between the lesions and the CNS such that the lesions are directly transmitting hormonally modifiable information to the CNS while simultaneously

Table 22.1 Rodent model of endometriosis: comparison with endometriosis in women.

Lesions/symptoms/innervation of lesions	Rat model of endometriosis	Women with endometriosis	References rat	References human
Lesions				
Etiology of lesions	Surgically induced	Endogenous origin (several hypotheses)	[31]	[133,134]
Location of lesions	Restricted to abdomen	Varied, but predominantly pelvic cavity	[31]	[133,135]
Appearance/composition of lesions	Cystic; includes full uterine horn (i.e. endometrium, myometrium and stroma)	Varied appearance (see text): mainly endometrium and stroma	[31]	[3,135]
Symptoms				
Dysmenorrhea	Rats do not menstruate	Yes		[3]
Dyspareunia/vaginal hyperalgesia	Yes (vaginal hyperalgesia)	Yes (dyspareunia)	[33]	[136]
Ovarian cyclicity of dyspareunia	Correlates with estradiol levels and uterine contractions	Unknown	[33,137]	
Referred muscle hyperalgesia	Yes	Yes	[32]	[138]
Location of referred muscle pain	Abdomen	Pelvic regions/abdomen	[32]	[138]
Ovarian cyclicity of referred hyperalgesia	Yes: correlates with estradiol levels and uterine contractions	Unknown	[32,137]	
Urological symptoms	Hyper-reflexia	Increased frequency/urgency	[72]	[139,140]
Pain associated with kidney stones	Increased	Likely increased; becomes more cyclic	[73]	[37]
Innervation of lesions				
Sensory innervation of cysts/lesions	Yes	Yes	[23]	[24,141]
Sympathetic innervation of cysts/lesions	Yes	Yes	[23]	[24,141]
Hormonal influences on cyst/lesion innervation	Correlates with estradiol levels, dyspareunia symptoms, and uterine contractions	Innervation is reduced by Rx with progestagens or combined oral contraceptives	[34,137]	[142]

Reproduced from Stratton and Berkley [7] with permission from Oxford University Press.

receiving hormonally modifiable information from the CNS (see Plate 22.1, Part 1).

Other animal and human neuropathic and chronic pain conditions have similar functional interlinking between sympathetic and sensory innervation [36]. Like headache, endometriosis is a neurovascular endocrine condition [34], a concept also suggested clinically [37-40]. The ENDO model data suggest that at least four features contribute to severity of endometriosis pain: (a) systemic and local hormonal environment; (b) lesions' sensory and sympathetic innervation; (c) vascularity; and (d) local growth factor environment.

Sympathetic nerve involvement in endometriosis lesions and its modulation by estradiol are being studied in women. In recto-vaginal DIE lesions, nerve fibers, vascularity, estrogen receptor α (ERα), and progesterone receptors (PR) are significantly correlated [41]. Nearly all (92%) women in this study had chronic pelvic pain, but immunohistochemical findings did not correlate with symptoms, disease score, or hormonal contraceptive use. The association between raloxifene use and accelerated return of pain after surgery [12] also suggests a potential role of peripheral and/or central estradiol modulation because raloxifene use may increase circulating estradiol levels [13]. Possover [42] found a strong association between sympathetic fibers and blood vessels

in endometriosis lesions infiltrating uterosacral ligaments, but correlation with patients' symptoms or hormone levels was not assessed.

Central factors, general and hormonal

The ENDO rat model findings illustrate the interplay not only between hormones and the peripheral innervation of the lesions, but also between hormones and the CNS consequences of this innervation, likely triggered by sensitized innervation of the growths (see Plate 22.1, Part 2). First, vaginal hyperalgesia and abdominal muscle activity are increased more significantly when estradiol is high than when it is low in the ENDO model. Rather than resulting from estradiol's direct effects on the lesions or peritoneal environment [32,33], these effects may signify estradiol modulation of neuronal processing within the CNS [43-47]. Second, the ENDO model influences nociception associated with pelvic/abdominal regions (bladder, vagina, abdominal muscle, mid-ureter; see Table 22.1). The neural entry from the surgically induced lesions in this model is to the thoracic spinal cord, which is distant from the neural entry from the bladder and vagina to the lumbar cord, suggesting that intersegmental processing is the relevant mechanism (see Plate 22.1, Part 3). Third, the CNS contribution to vaginal hyperalgesia is illustrated by the observation that bladder distension increases activation of spinal neurons located in the L6–S1 spinal segments in ENDO rats, but not shamENDO rats [48]. Fourth, ENDO-induced vaginal hyperalgesia is mitigated by completely removing the lesions. However, vaginal hyperalgesia returns when rats experience reproductive senescence [49], when their estradiol levels, unlike those in women and mice, increase significantly [50,51]. Thus, the CNS preserves a "memory" of central neuronal changes induced by the lesions' neural input, and that "memory" can be "summoned up" by the actions of estradiol on CNS neuron activity. Fifth, when lesions are not completely removed, ENDO-induced vaginal hyperalgesia increases, which is associated with increases in the lesions' innervation [49]. Furthermore, the increased vaginal hyperalgesia persists even when estradiol levels are low, suggesting that CNS neurons can be released from estradiol modulation in ENDO rats.

Peripheral factors, peripheral sensitization

Sensory fibers innervating the ENDO model ectopic growths immunostain with antibodies to calcitonin gene-related peptide (CGRP) [23,24]. CGRP-positive fibers include C-fiber nociceptors [52]. Nociceptors are peripheral sensory nerves that respond to a noxious stimulus, denoting a stimulus that can potentially or actually injure [53,54]. C-fiber nociceptors are frequently "silent" [55,56]. When activated by noxious events such as inflammation, in addition to conveying information to the CNS through an afferent function, C-fibers can also discharge substance P, somatostatin, CGRP, nitric oxide, tachykinins and other factors into the local environment through an efferent function. Once activated, C-fibers can become sensitized, meaning that after inflammation abates, they are no longer silent [57] (see Plate 22.1, Part 1). Efferent actions of C-fiber nociceptors also include increasing local vascular permeability and inflammation, a process called "neurogenic inflammation" [58,59]. Pre-existing nerve fibers that innervate adjacent regions branch to innervate ENDO rats' ectopic growths [34]. This sprouting of CGRP-positive sensory fibers strongly suggests that the nerve fibers have become sensitized [36] and therefore have ongoing electrical activity [60].

Central factors, central sensitization

These ENDO model findings suggest that central sensitization, a process considered to underlie pain hypersensitivity, is an important mechanism contributing to the association between endometriosis and chronic pelvic pain [44,61-69] (see Plate 22.1, Parts 2–5, asterisks). Central sensitization means the central nervous system has changed such that a normal stimulus now evokes an exaggerated response [66]. Clinical research suggests that this concept applies to endometriosis-associated pain in women [70].

Central sensitization, initiated by peripheral sensitization (see Plate 22.1), can be maintained by continued input to the central nervous system from sensitized sensory afferent fibers [71]. The activity of peripherally sensitized fibers can be altered by estradiol and sympathetic modulation in the ENDO model which, in turn, can modulate activity of centrally sensitized

neurons affecting pain severity [71]. Removal of the ectopic growths could eliminate or reduce the sensitized input, thereby relieving pain. In other poorly understood circumstances, however, central neural processing can be modified by the initial peripheral sensitization so that what was initially peripherally maintained central sensitization becomes independent of peripheral input [71]. Under these circumstances, therapies directed at the periphery, such as removing endometriosis lesions or medical therapy to alter the lesion characteristics, fail to relieve pain, and pain becomes difficult to treat.

Viscero-visceral central nervous system connections or cross-organ effects

At times, women with endometriosis-associated pain have other pelvic pain syndromes such as irritable bowel syndrome or painful bladder syndrome, which suggests that neural mechanisms underlying cross-talk between viscera contribute to pain, a finding observed in the ENDO model [72,73]. ENDO but not shamENDO surgery (i) induces bladder inflammation and bladder hyperactivity [72], (ii) induces vaginal hyperalgesia [74], (iii) increases pain behaviors produced by ureteral calculosis [73], and (iv) induces hyperactivity in abdominal muscles [32]. These findings strongly support engagement of the central nervous system (see Plate 22.1).

Summary: neuroendocrine aspects of endometriosis: peripheral sensitization, central sensitization, central neural circuitry, and estradiol

Peripheral sensitization in endometriosis can significantly influence information processing via highly interconnected CNS circuitry (see Plate 22.1). Thus, sensitized inputs from endometriosis lesions can affect neuronal activity throughout the CNS by unmasking latent processes or by altering existing inhibitory or excitatory processes. Some central effects are sustained by persistent input from the endometriosis lesions' sensory fibers which themselves are modulated by activity in sympathetic fibers and estradiol. Local peritoneal factors produced by lesions themselves or during ovulation or menstruation may also contribute to maintaining continued input to the CNS. Furthermore, as a result of long-term modification of CNS functioning, central actions can become autonomous of any peripheral input from endometriosis lesions. All central effects can be modulated by estradiol.

Most central sensitization happens in the same spinal region as the sensitized peripheral afferent fibers (see Plate 22.1, Part 2). Thus, in women, pain occurs mostly in the pelvis because most endometriosis lesions are located there [4,75]. However, pain can be experienced not only in association with innervated lesions in pelvic reproductive organs but also by referral to bladder, colon and abdominopelvic muscles. Importantly, because of the vast CNS interconnectivity and long-ranging peripheral sensory fibers, remote central sensitization can also take place from widely disparate parts of the body (see Plate 22.1, Parts 3–5). For women, remote central sensitization could explain the co-morbidity of pelvic pain with other pain syndromes such as migraine, fibromyalgia or temporomandibular joint disorder [76,77].

Further, estradiol dependence of endometriosis's pain symptoms can be partly explained by estradiol's effects on central neural functioning, reviewed in the next section.

Neuroimmune and neuroendocrine factors

Estradiol's influence on nervous system function

Nervous system activity in pain states appears to be modulated by estradiol [78,79]. Pain modulation by estrogens is complex such that in different settings, estrogens may either worsen or alleviate pain [80]. In most experimental pain settings, menstrual variation in pain in healthy women appears to be related to hormone levels [81-83], but this relationship is reported as minimal in some studies [84]. This inconsistency may arise from varying methods of determining menstrual cycle phase, whether hormones are measured, and where or how pain is measured. Also possible is that short-term experimental pain paradigms have less modulation by estrogens compared to chronic pain states. Thus, the estrogen modulation of pain may depend on the type and chronicity of pain, as well as estrogen type, level and stability [80]. Whether pain modulation by estrogens is dose-dependent is not yet clear, nor is it clear how different estrogens might affect pain differently. An added level of complexity is the tissue-specific actions of estrogens that undoubtedly influence pain modulation by estrogen in the setting of different types of pain.

In rodent models, the genital sensory field increases with estradiol treatment and the estrus cycle, suggesting that estradiol modifies the sensitivity of peripheral sensory neurons [85-88]. The ERα agonist propyl pyrazole triol elicited neurite growth from dorsal root ganglia (DRG) neurons and estradiol induced neural sprouting from unmyelinated neurons harvested from newborn rats [89]. Further, alterations in circulating estradiol produce complex alterations in how neurons in the thalamus process information concerning the reproductive organs, colon, and skin [90].

While estrogens and estrogen receptors are likely involved in pain modulation in endometriosis, this area has been poorly studied. However, ERα gene polymorphisms have been associated with various pain conditions including a higher risk of osteo-arthritis in women and higher pain levels in women with temporomandibular joint osteo-arthritis [80]. ERα expression was reported to be increased in vulvar tissue in those with vulvodynia compared to controls in one study [91], but not in others [92]. While systemic and tissue ERα polymorphisms are associated with development and maintenance of endometriosis [17,93,94] and are suppressed in endometriosis lesions by some treatments [95], it is unknown whether or how ERα polymorphisms might be associated with pain from endometriosis. In other chronic pain states, there appears to be a relationship between estrogen level and pain symptoms. As with endometriosis, menstrual migraine can be significantly improved by use of leuprolide acetate, implying that ovarian hormones may be responsible for development of both types of pain [96]. The estrogen effects may be strongly influenced by specific serum

estradiol levels. In the late luteal phase, a decline in estrogen levels below 45–50 pg/mL triggers menstrual migraine [97]. Also, high serum estrogen levels observed during pregnancy or with use of high-potency estrogens (e.g. oral contraceptive pills) may exacerbate migraine in some patients [97].

The timing of headache symptoms in relation to hormone levels may also be important. In the previously cited study using leuprolide [96], headache was more frequent in the first 2 days of using a transdermal estradiol patch compared to the fifth and sixth days, although estradiol level varied little with a level of 50 pg/mL at 2 days and 42 pg/mL at 5 days. Thus, either women with pain are unusually sensitive to small changes in serum estradiol concentration, or tolerance or adaptation to estradiol level occurs over time.

A similar relationship between estradiol and pain is seen in women with temporomandibular joint disorder. For example, pain in women is highest at times of lowest estradiol levels just before menses, but rapid estradiol change observed with the midcycle rise may also be associated with increased pain [98].

Progesterone also likely modulates pain. For example, progesterone has been shown to attenuate inflammation-induced thermal hyperalgesia [99]. The intricate relationship between estrogen and progesterone, in which progesterone receptors are influenced by estradiol levels and receptors, makes any discussion of the effects of progesterone on pain inextricably linked to various estrogens. The combined effects of estradiol and progestagens likely differ from the effects of estradiol alone. In some cases, progesterone reverses the effects of estradiol, as seen in formalin-induced nociception [100], and in other instances, estradiol reverses the effects of progesterone, as seen in apoptotic injury in experimental allergic encephalitis [101]. Because many women with endometriosis frequently take estrogen-progestin combinations, these ovarian hormones likely interact to affect pain ascribed to endometriosis.

Proinflammatory cytokines, sickness response and sensitivity to pain

Sickness responses include physiological and behavioral changes of fever, increased white blood cell count, decreased food and water intake, increased sleep, and endocrine changes, including activation of the hypothalamo-pituitary adrenal axis and sympathetic nervous system [102-104]. These responses are adaptive because they result in increasing energy production while decreasing energy use that aids in developing fever. Fever, in turn, enhances the immune system while decreasing the replication of pathogens. Pain (body aches), evidenced as a sickness-induced increased sensitivity to noxious stimuli or hyperalgesia, is also an integral component of the sickness syndrome.

Proinflammatory cytokines (tumor necrosis factor (TNF), interleukin (IL)-1 and IL-6) are key mediators for the induction of hyperalgesia and, in fact, all other sickness responses[105]. Elevated proinflammatory cytokines are an important facet of chronic pain states. Animal models of chronic pain each have increased proinflammatory cytokines in systemic circulation

[105-108]. Infusing proinflammatory cytokines TNF-α, IL-1 and IL-6 in rodents induces both the sickness response and hyperalgesia [105,109,110]. Lipopolysaccharide (LPS) induces proinflammatory cytokine expression and marked hyperalgesia in rodents, an effect that is mitigated by peripheral dosing with an IL-1 receptor antagonist [111-113] or TNF-α antagonist [110,114]. However, TNF-α antagonist treatment has not been effective for endometriosis-associated pain [115,116].

Prostaglandins are released from the endometrium into the systemic circulation when progesterone falls at the end of the luteal phase of the menstrual cycle. These same proinflammatory cytokines are elevated in peritoneal fluid [117,118] in women with painful endometriosis and likely elevated in their menses. This "prostaglandin release" appears to play a role in the pathophysiology of other pain states like menstrual migraine [119]. First, injections of prostaglandin E in non-migraineurs can trigger migraine-like headaches [120]. Second, serum obtained from women during menstruation that is later infused back to them can induce dysmenorrhea and headache [121]. Third, medications that are prostaglandin inhibitors can prevent menstrual migraine [122]. Thus, increased levels of proinflammatory cytokines are an important facet of central sensitization [105].

Hypothalamic-pituitary-adrenal axis and pain

Pain is a stressful experience such that the hypothalamic-pituitary-adrenal (HPA) axis is activated in animal models experiencing either phasic or tonic pain [111]. Nociceptive transmission is suppressed in the brainstem by monoaminergic neurons. In the setting of HPA activation, the increase in glucocorticoid secretion produces loss of monoaminergic tone because of monoamine depletion [123], and thus can result in increased pain.

Similarly, chronic stress is associated with heightened pain symptoms [124]. Chronic stress resulting in the continuous, prolonged activation of the HPA axis disrupts the negative feedback loop, leading to either enhanced hormone production and release or resistance to circulating glucocorticoids [123]. Additionally, chronic stress is associated with loss of glucocorticoid receptor expression that, in turn, can result in loss of the glucocorticoid inhibition of proinflammatory cytokines and ultimately in increased cytokine levels [125]. The resulting chain of events can contribute to peripheral sensitization and, eventually, central sensitization.

Dysfunctional HPA responsivity has been observed in clinical studies on chronic pain states such as rheumatoid arthritis, fibromyalgia, and several autoimmune inflammatory diseases [126-131]. Alterations in the HPA axis may also occur in endometriosis and chronic pain [132].

Conclusion

The nervous system determines the experience of pain, and an endometriosis lesion can develop its own sensory and sympathetic nerve supply. Persistent input to the CNS from the lesions' sensory fibers is modulated by activity in sympathetic fibers and estradiol, and likely sustains some central effects. Thus, the endocrine and nervous systems, and their inter-relationships, are important modulators of endometriosis-ascribed pain. Peripheral and central nervous system sensitization can both significantly influence pain ascribed to endometriosis (see Plate 22.1). Local peritoneal cytokines and other factors produced during menstruation or ovulation, or by implants themselves, may also contribute to sensitization. Further, central actions can become independent of peripheral input from endometriosis lesions, indicating long-term modification of CNS functioning. Thus, the hormonally responsive communication between the lesions and the CNS that is created by the lesions' innervation creates a substrate that permits the development of individual variations in pain that can, in some cases, become independent of endometriosis itself. Improvements in understanding and alleviating endometriosis-associated pain will likely occur from a change in emphasis from the lesions to pain and the dynamic interplay between the nervous and endocrine systems.

References

1. Howard FM. The role of laparoscopy in chronic pelvic pain: promise and pitfalls. Obstet Gynecol Surv 1993;48(6):357–387.
2. Howard FM. Endometriosis and mechanisms of pelvic pain. J Min Invas Gynecol 2009;16(5):540–550.
3. Fauconnier A, Chapron C. Endometriosis and pelvic pain: epidemiological evidence of the relationship and implications. Hum Reprod Update 2005;11(6):595–606.
4. Vercellini P, Fedele L, Aimi G, Pietropaolo G, Consonni D, Crosignani PG. Association between endometriosis stage, lesion type, patient characteristics and severity of pelvic pain symptoms: a multivariate analysis of over 1000 patients. Hum Reprod 2007; 22(1):266–271.
5. Vercellini P, Trespidi L, de Giorgi O, Cortesi I, Parazzini F, Crosignani PG. Endometriosis and pelvic pain: relation to disease stage and localization. Fertil Steril 1996;65(2):299–304.
6. Chapron C, Fauconnier A, Dubuisson JB, Barakat H, Vieira M, Breart G. Deep infiltrating endometriosis: relation between severity of dysmenorrhoea and extent of disease. Hum Reprod 2003;18(4): 760–766.
7. Stratton P, Berkley KJ. Chronic pelvic pain and endometriosis: translational evidence of the relationship and implications. Hum Reprod Update 2011;17(3):327–346.
8. Kennedy S, Bergqvist A, Chapron C et al. ESHRE guideline for the diagnosis and treatment of endometriosis. Hum Reprod 2005;20(10):2698–2704.
9. Nisolle-Pochet M, Casanas-Roux F, Donnez J. Histologic study of ovarian endometriosis after hormonal therapy. Fertil Steril 1988;49(3):423–426.
10. Ling FW. Randomized controlled trial of depot leuprolide in patients with chronic pelvic pain and clinically suspected endometriosis. Pelvic Pain Study Group. Obstet Gynecol 1999;93(1):51–58.

11. Jenkins TR, Liu CY, White J. Does response to hormonal therapy predict presence or absence of endometriosis? J Min Invas Gynecol 2008;15(1):82–86.

12. Stratton P, Sinaii N, Segars J et al. Return of chronic pelvic pain from endometriosis after raloxifene treatment: a randomized controlled trial. Obstet Gynecol 2008;111(1):88–96.

13. Baker VL, Draper M, Paul S et al. Reproductive endocrine and endometrial effects of raloxifene hydrochloride, a selective estrogen receptor modulator, in women with regular menstrual cycles. J Clin Endocrinol Metab 1998;83(1):6–13.

14. Aghajanova L, Hamilton A, Kwintkiewicz J, Vo KC, Giudice LC. Steroidogenic enzyme and key decidualization marker dysregulation in endometrial stromal cells from women with versus without endometriosis. Biol Reprod 2009;80(1):105–114.

15. Fedele L, Somigliana E, Frontino G, Benaglia L, Vigano P. New drugs in development for the treatment of endometriosis. Expert Opin Invest Drugs 2008;17(8):1187–1202.

16. Huang HY. Medical treatment of endometriosis. Chang Gung Med J 2008;31(5):431–440.

17. Bulun SE, Cheng YH, Pavone ME et al. Estrogen receptor-beta, estrogen receptor-alpha, and progesterone resistance in endometriosis. Semin Reprod Med 2010;28(1):36–43.

18. Osteen KG, Bruner-Tran KL, Eisenberg E. Reduced progesterone action during endometrial maturation: a potential risk factor for the development of endometriosis. Fertil Steril 2005;83(3):529–537.

19. Abbott J, Hawe J, Hunter D, Holmes M, Finn P, Garry R. Laparoscopic excision of endometriosis: a randomized, placebo-controlled trial. Fertil Steril 2004;82(4):878–884.

20. Vercellini P, Crosignani PG, Abbiati A, Somigliana E, Vigano P, Fedele L. The effect of surgery for symptomatic endometriosis: the other side of the story. Hum Reprod Update 2009;15(2):177–188.

21. Abbott JA, Hawe J, Clayton RD, Garry R. The effects and effectiveness of laparoscopic excision of endometriosis: a prospective study with 2–5 year follow-up. Hum Reprod 2003;18(9):1922–1927.

22. Sutton CJ, Ewen SP, Whitelaw N, Haines P. Prospective, randomized, double-blind, controlled trial of laser laparoscopy in the treatment of pelvic pain associated with minimal, mild, and moderate endometriosis. Fertil Steril 1994;62(4):696–700.

23. Berkley KJ, Dmitrieva N, Curtis KS, Papka RE. Innervation of ectopic endometrium in a rat model of endometriosis. Proc Natl Acad Sci USA 2004;101(30):11094–11098.

24. Berkley KJ, Rapkin AJ, Papka RE. The pains of endometriosis. Science 2005;308(5728):1587–1589.

25. May K, Becker CM. Endometriosis and angiogenesis. Minerva Ginecol 2008;60(3):245–254.

26. Burnstock G. Autonomic neurotransmission: 60 years since sir Henry Dale. Ann Rev Pharmacol Toxicol 2009;49:1–30.

27. Carmeliet P, Tessier-Lavigne M. Common mechanisms of nerve and blood vessel wiring. Nature 2005;436(7048):193–200.

28. Raab S, Plate KH. Different networks, common growth factors: shared growth factors and receptors of the vascular and the nervous system. Acta Neuropathol 2007;113(6):607–626.

29. Jones CA, Li DY. Common cues regulate neural and vascular patterning. Curr Opin Genet Dev 2007;17(4):332–336.

30. Mendell LM, Albers KM, Davis BM. Neurotrophins, nociceptors, and pain. Microsc Res Techn 1999;45(4–5):252–261.

31. Vernon MW, Wilson EA. Studies on the surgical induction of endometriosis in the rat. Fertil Steril 1985;44(5):684–694.

32. Nagabukuro H, Berkley KJ. Influence of endometriosis on visceromotor and cardiovascular responses induced by vaginal distention in the rat. Pain 2007;132(Suppl 1):S96–103.

33. Cason AM, Samuelsen CL, Berkley KJ. Estrous changes in vaginal nociception in a rat model of endometriosis. Hormones Behav 2003;44(2):123–131.

34. Zhang G, Dmitrieva N, Liu Y, McGinty KA, Berkley KJ. Endometriosis as a neurovascular condition: estrous variations in innervation, vascularization, and growth factor content of ectopic endometrial cysts in the rat. Am J Physiol 2008;294(1):R162–171.

35. Sofroniew MV, Howe CL, Mobley WC. Nerve growth factor signaling, neuroprotection, and neural repair. Ann Rev Neurosci 2001;24:1217–1281.

36. Janig W, Levine JD, Michaelis M. Interactions of sympathetic and primary afferent neurons following nerve injury and tissue trauma. Progr Brain Res 1996;113:161–184.

37. Giamberardino MA, de Laurentis S, Affaitati G, Lerza R, Lapenna D, Vecchiet L. Modulation of pain and hyperalgesia from the urinary tract by algogenic conditions of the reproductive organs in women. Neurosci Lett 2001;304(1–2):61–64.

38. Bendtsen L. Central and peripheral sensitization in tension-type headache. Curr Pain Headache Rep 2003;7(6):460–465.

39. Calandre EP, Hidalgo J, Garcia-Leiva JM, Rico-Villademoros F. Trigger point evaluation in migraine patients: an indication of peripheral sensitization linked to migraine predisposition? Eur J Neurol 2006;13(3):244–2449.

40. Evans S, Moalem-Taylor G, Tracey DJ. Pain and endometriosis. Pain 2007;132(Suppl 1):S22–25.

41. Signorile PG, Campioni M, Vincenzi B, d'Avino A, Baldi A. Rectovaginal septum endometriosis: an immunohistochemical analysis of 62 cases. In Vivo 2009;23(3):459–464.

42. Possover M, Tersiev P, Angelov DN. Comparative study of the neuropeptide-Y sympathetic nerves in endometriotic involved and noninvolved sacrouterine ligaments in women with pelvic endometriosis. J Min Invas Gynecol 2009;16(3):340–343.

43. Tang B, Ji Y, Traub RJ. Estrogen alters spinal NMDA receptor activity via a PKA signaling pathway in a visceral pain model in the rat. Pain 2008;137(3):540–549.

44. Ji Y, Murphy AZ, Traub RJ. Estrogen modulates the visceromotor reflex and responses of spinal dorsal horn neurons to colorectal stimulation in the rat. J Neurosci 2003;23(9):3908–3915.

45. Ji Y, Tang B, Traub RJ. Modulatory effects of estrogen and progesterone on colorectal hyperalgesia in the rat. Pain 2005;117(3):433–442.

46. Evrard HC, Balthazart J. Rapid regulation of pain by estrogens synthesized in spinal dorsal horn neurons. J Neurosci 2004;24(33):7225–7229.

47. Evrard HC, Balthazart J. Aromatase (estrogen synthase) activity in the dorsal horn of the spinal cord: functional implications. Ann NY Acad Sci 2003;1007:263–271.

48. McGinty KA, Zhang G, McAllister SL et al. Endometriosis (ENDO) and co-morbidity with bladder dysfunction in the rat: influence of ENDO and shamENDO on spinal c-Fos expression induced by distention of the uninflamed and inflamed bladder. Society for Neuroscience. Washington, D.C. 2009.

49. McAllister SL, McGinty KA, Resuehr D, Berkley KJ. Endometriosis-induced vaginal hyperalgesia in the rat: role of the ectopic growths and their innervation. Pain 2009;147:255–264.

50. Berkley KJ, McAllister SL, Accius BE, Winnard KP. Endometriosis-induced vaginal hyperalgesia in the rat: effect of estropause, ovariectomy, and estradiol replacement. Pain 2007;132 (Suppl 1):S150–159.

51. Lu KH, Hopper BR, Vargo TM, Yen SS. Chronological changes in sex steroid, gonadotropin and prolactin secretions in aging female rats displaying different reproductive states. Biol Reprod 1979;21(1):193–203.

52. Snider WD, McMahon SB. Tackling pain at the source: new ideas about nociceptors. Neuron 1998;20(4):629–632.

53. Sherrington CS. The Integrative Action of the Nervous System. New York: Scribner, 1906.

54. Merskey H, Bogduk N. Classification of Chronic Pain. Descriptions of Chronic Pain Syndromes and Definitions of Pain Terms, 2nd edn. Seattle, WA: IASP Press, 1994.

55. Cervero F, Janig W. Visceral nociceptors: a new world order? Trends Neurosci 1992;15(10):374–378.

56. Michaelis M, Habler HJ, Jaenig W. Silent afferents: a separate class of primary afferents? Clin Exper Pharmacol Physiol 1996;23(2):99–105.

57. Gebhart GF. Peripheral contributions to visceral hyperalgesia. Can J Gastroenterol 1999;13(Suppl A):37A–41A.

58. Szolcsanyi J. Forty years in capsaicin research for sensory pharmacology and physiology. Neuropeptides 2004;38(6):377–384.

59. Holzer P. Neurogenic vasodilatation and plasma leakage in the skin. Gen Pharmacol 1998;30(1):5–11.

60. Dmitrieva N, Nikonov A, Berkley KJ. Endometriosis (ENDO) in the rat: sensitization of afferent fibers that innervate the ectopic growths. *Society for Neuroscience*. Washington, D.C. 2009.

61. Woolf CJ, Ma Q. Nociceptors – noxious stimulus detectors. Neuron 2007;55(3):353–364.

62. Melzack R, Coderre TJ, Katz J, Vaccarino AL. Central neuroplasticity and pathological pain. Ann NY Acad Sci 2001;933:157–174.

63. DeLeo JA. Basic science of pain. J Bone Joint Surg 2006;88 (Suppl 2):58–62.

64. Ren K, Dubner R. Central nervous system plasticity and persistent pain. J Orofacial Pain 1999;13(3):155–163; discussion 64–71.

65. Ren K, Dubner R. Neuron-glia crosstalk gets serious: role in pain hypersensitivity. Curr Opin Anaesthesiol 2008;21(5):570–579.

66. Woolf CJ. Evidence for a central component of post-injury pain hypersensitivity. Nature 1983;306(5944):686–688.

67. Giamberardino MA, Valente R, Affaitati G, Vecchiet L. Central neuronal changes in recurrent visceral pain. Int J Clin Pharmacol Res 1997;17(2–3):63–66.

68. Coderre TJ, Katz J, Vaccarino AL, Melzack R. Contribution of central neuroplasticity to pathological pain: review of clinical and experimental evidence. Pain 1993;52(3):259–285.

69. McMahon SB. Mechanisms of sympathetic pain. Br Med Bull 1991;47(3):584–600.

70. Bajaj P, Madsen H, Arendt-Nielsen L. Endometriosis is associated with central sensitization: a psychophysical controlled study. J Pain 2003;4(7):372–380.

71. Woolf CJ, Salter MW. Neuronal plasticity: increasing the gain in pain. Science 2000;288(5472):1765–1769.

72. Morrison TC, Dmitrieva N, Winnard KP, Berkley KJ. Opposing viscerovisceral effects of surgically induced endometriosis and a control abdominal surgery on the rat bladder. Fertil Steril 2006;86 (4 Suppl):1067–1073.

73. Giamberardino MA, Berkley KJ, Affaitati G et al. Influence of endometriosis on pain behaviors and muscle hyperalgesia induced by a ureteral calculosis in female rats. Pain 2002;95(3):247–257.

74. Bradshaw HB, Temple JL, Wood E, Berkley KJ. Estrous variations in behavioral responses to vaginal and uterine distention in the rat. Pain 1999;82(2):187–197.

75. Bricou A, Batt RE, Chapron C. Peritoneal fluid flow influences anatomical distribution of endometriotic lesions: why Sampson seems to be right. Eur J Obstet Gynecol Reprod Biol 2008;138(2):127–134.

76. DeSantana JM, Sluka KA. Central mechanisms in the maintenance of chronic widespread noninflammatory muscle pain. Curr Pain Headache Rep 2008;12(5):338–343.

77. Sinaii N, Cleary SD, Ballweg ML, Nieman LK, Stratton P. High rates of autoimmune and endocrine disorders, fibromyalgia, chronic fatigue syndrome and atopic diseases among women with endometriosis: a survey analysis. Hum Reprod 2002;17(10):2715–2724.

78. Craft RM, Mogil JS, Aloisi AM. Sex differences in pain and analgesia: the role of gonadal hormones. Eur J Pain 2004;8(5):397–411.

79. Greenspan JD, Craft RM, LeResche L et al. Studying sex and gender differences in pain and analgesia: a consensus report. Pain 2007;132(Suppl 1):S26–45.

80. Craft RM. Modulation of pain by estrogens. Pain 2007;132 (Suppl 1):S3–12.

81. Riley JL 3rd, Robinson ME, Wise EA, Price DD. A meta-analytic review of pain perception across the menstrual cycle. Pain 1999;81(3):225–235.

82. Giamberardino MA, Berkley KJ, Iezzi S, de Bigontina P, Vecchiet L. Pain threshold variations in somatic wall tissues as a function of menstrual cycle, segmental site and tissue depth in non-dysmenorrheic women, dysmenorrheic women and men. Pain 1997;71(2):187–197.

83. Fillingim RB, Maixner W, Girdler SS et al. Ischemic but not thermal pain sensitivity varies across the menstrual cycle. Psychosom Med 1997;59(5):512–520.

84. Kowalczyk WJ, Sullivan MA, Evans SM, Bisaga AM, Vosburg SK, Comer SD. Sex differences and hormonal influences on response to mechanical pressure pain in humans. J Pain 2010;11(4):330–342.

85. Adler NT, Davis PG, Komisaruk BR. Variation in the size and sensitivity of a genital sensory field in relation to the estrous cycle in rats. Hormones Behav 1977;9(3):334–344.

86. Komisaruk BR, Adler NT, Hutchison J. Genital sensory field: enlargement by estrogen treatment in female rats. Science 1972;178(67):1295–1298.

87. Kow LM, Pfaff DW. Effects of estrogen treatment on the size of receptive field and response threshold of pudendal nerve in the female rat. Neuroendocrinology 1973;13(4):299–313.

88. Kaur G, Janik J, Isaacson LG, Callahan P. Estrogen regulation of neurotrophin expression in sympathetic neurons and vascular targets. Brain Res 2007;1139:6–14.

89. Chakrabarty A, Blacklock A, Svojanovsky S, Smith PG. Estrogen elicits dorsal root ganglion axon sprouting via a renin-angiotensin system. Endocrinology 2008;149(7):3452–3460.

90. Reed WR, Chadha HK, Hubscher CH. Effects of 17-{beta} estradiol on responses of viscerosomatic convergent thalamic neurons in the ovariectomized female rat. J Neurophysiol 2009;102(2):1062–1074.

91. Johannesson U, Sahlin L, Masironi B et al. Steroid receptor expression and morphology in provoked vestibulodynia. Am J Obstet Gynecol 2008;198(3):311.

92. Goetsch MF, Morgan TK, Korcheva VB, Li H, Peters D, Leclair CM. Histologic and receptor analysis of primary and secondary vestibulodynia and controls: a prospective study. Am J Obstet Gynecol 2010;202(6):614.

93. Attia GR, Zeitoun K, Edwards D, Johns A, Carr BR, Bulun SE. Progesterone receptor isoform A but not B is expressed in endometriosis. J Clin Endocrinol Metab 2000;85(8):2897–2902.

94. Govindan S, Shaik NA, Vedicherla B, Kodati V, Rao KP, Hasan Q. Estrogen receptor-alpha gene (T/C) Pvu II polymorphism in endometriosis and uterine fibroids. Dis Markers 2009;26(4):149–154.

95. Gomes MK, Rosa-e-Silva JC, Garcia SB et al. Effects of the levonorgestrel-releasing intrauterine system on cell proliferation, Fas expression and steroid receptors in endometriosis lesions and normal endometrium. Hum Reprod 2009;24(11):2736–2745.

96. Martin V, Wernke S, Mandell K et al. Medical oophorectomy with and without estrogen add-back therapy in the prevention of migraine headache. Headache 2003;43(4):309–321.

97. Martin VT, Behbehani M. Ovarian hormones and migraine headache: understanding mechanisms and pathogenesis – part 2. Headache 2006;46(3):365–386.

98. LeResche L, Mancl L, Sherman JJ, Gandara B, Dworkin SF. Changes in temporomandibular pain and other symptoms across the menstrual cycle. Pain 2003;106(3):253–261.

99. Ren K, Wei F, Dubner R, Murphy A, Hoffman GE. Progesterone attenuates persistent inflammatory hyperalgesia in female rats: involvement of spinal NMDA receptor mechanisms. Brain Res 2000;865(2):272–277.

100. Kuba T, Wu HB, Nazarian A et al. Estradiol and progesterone differentially regulate formalin-induced nociception in ovariectomized female rats. Hormones Behav 2006;49(4):441–419.

101. Hoffman GE, Le WW, Murphy AZ, Koski CL. Divergent effects of ovarian steroids on neuronal survival during experimental allergic encephalitis in Lewis rats. Exp Neurol 2001;171(2):272–284.

102. Hart BL. Biological basis of the behavior of sick animals. Neurosci Biobehav Rev 1988;12(2):123–137.

103. Maier SF, Watkins LR. Cytokines for psychologists: implications of bidirectional immune-to-brain communication for understanding behavior, mood, and cognition. Psychol Rev 1998;105(1):83–107.

104. Kent S, Bluthe RM, Kelley KW, Dantzer R. Sickness behavior as a new target for drug development. Trends Pharmacol Sci 1992;13(1):24–28.

105. Wieseler-Frank J, Maier SF, Watkins LR. Central proinflammatory cytokines and pain enhancement. Neuro-Signals 2005;14(4):166–174.

106. Walters ET. Injury-related behavior and neuronal plasticity: an evolutionary perspective on sensitization, hyperalgesia, and analgesia. Int Rev Neurobiol 1994;36:325–427.

107. Watkins LR, Maier SF, Goehler LE. Immune activation: the role of pro-inflammatory cytokines in inflammation, illness responses and pathological pain states. Pain 1995;63(3):289–302.

108. Watkins LR, Maier SF, Goehler LE, Walters ET. Injury-related behaviour and neuronal plasticity: an evolutionary perspective on sensitization, hyperalgesia and analgesia. Int Rev Neurobiol 1995;36:325–327.

109. Berczi I, Chow DA, Sabbadini ER. Neuroimmunoregulation and natural immunity. Domest Anim Endocrinol 1998;15(5):273–281.

110. Coelho A, Fioramonti J, Bueno L. Brain interleukin-1beta and tumor necrosis factor-alpha are involved in lipopolysaccharide-induced delayed rectal allodynia in awake rats. Brain Res Bull 2000;52(3):223–228.

111. Taylor BK, Akana SF, Peterson MA, Dallman MF, Basbaum AI. Pituitary-adrenocortical responses to persistent noxious stimuli in the awake rat: endogenous corticosterone does not reduce nociception in the formalin test. Endocrinology 1998;139(5):2407–2413.

112. Maier SF, Watkins LR. Immune-to-central nervous system communication and its role in modulating pain and cognition: implications for cancer and cancer treatment. Brain Behav Immunol 2003;17 (Suppl 1):S125–131.

113. Maier SF, Wiertelak EP, Martin D, Watkins LR. Interleukin-1 mediates the behavioral hyperalgesia produced by lithium chloride and endotoxin. Brain Res 1993;623(2):321–324.

114. Safieh-Garabedian B, Dardenne M, Kanaan SA, Atweh SF, Jabbur SJ, Saade NE. The role of cytokines and prostaglandin-E(2) in thymulin induced hyperalgesia. Neuropharmacology 2000;39(9):1653–1661.

115. Barrier BF, Bates GW, Leland MM, Leach DA, Robinson RD, Propst AM. Efficacy of anti-tumor necrosis factor therapy in the treatment of spontaneous endometriosis in baboons. Fertil Steril 2004;81 (Suppl 1):775–779.

116. Koninckx PR, Craessaerts M, Timmerman D, Cornillie F, Kennedy S. Anti-TNF-alpha treatment for deep endometriosis-associated pain: a randomized placebo-controlled trial. Hum Reprod 2008;23(9): 2017–2023.

117. Minici F, Tiberi F, Tropea A et al. Paracrine regulation of endometriotic tissue. Gynecol Endocrinol 2007;23(10):574–580.

118. Koninckx PR, Kennedy SH, Barlow DH. Endometriotic disease: the role of peritoneal fluid. Hum Reprod Update 1998;4(5):741–751.

119. Silberstein SD, Merriam GR. Estrogens, progestins, and headache. Neurology 1991;41(6):786–793.

120. Carlson LA, Ekelund LG, Oro L. Clinical and metabolic effects of different doses of prostaglandin E1 in man. Prostaglandin and related factors. Acta Med Scand 1968;183(5):423–430.

121. Irwin J, Morse E, Riddick D. Dysmenorrhea induced by autologous transfusion. Obstet Gynecol 1981;58(3):286–290.

122. Sances G, Martignoni E, Fioroni L, Blandini F, Facchinetti F, Nappi G. Naproxen sodium in menstrual migraine prophylaxis: a double-blind placebo controlled study. Headache 1990;30(11): 705–709.

123. Blackburn-Munro G, Blackburn-Munro R. Pain in the brain: are hormones to blame? Trends Endocrinol Metab 2003;14(1):20–27.

124. Romero LM, Sapolsky RM. Patterns of ACTH secretagog secretion in response to psychological stimuli. J Neuroendocrinol 1996;8(4): 243–258.

125. Sapolsky RM, Romero LM, Munck AU. How do glucocorticoids influence stress responses? Integrating permissive, suppressive, stimulatory, and preparative actions. Endocrine Rev 2000;21(1):55–89.

126. Bellometti S, Galzigna L. Function of the hypothalamic adrenal axis in patients with fibromyalgia syndrome undergoing mud-pack treatment. Int J Clin Pharmacol Res 1999;19(1):27–33.

127. Griep EN, Boersma JW, Lentjes EG, Prins AP, van der Korst JK, de Kloet ER. Function of the hypothalamic-pituitary-adrenal axis in patients with fibromyalgia and low back pain. J Rheumatol 1998;25(7):1374–1381.

128. Torpy DJ, Papanicolaou DA, Lotsikas AJ, Wilder RL, Chrousos GP, Pillemer SR. Responses of the sympathetic nervous system and the hypothalamic-pituitary-adrenal axis to interleukin-6: a pilot study in fibromyalgia. Arthritis Rheum 2000;43(4):872–880.

129. Lentjes EG, Griep EN, Boersma JW, Romijn FP, de Kloet ER. Glucocorticoid receptors, fibromyalgia and low back pain. Psychoneuroendocrinology 1997;22(8):603–614.

130. Crofford LJ. The hypothalamic-pituitary-adrenal axis in the pathogenesis of rheumatic diseases. Endocrinol Metab Clin North Am 2002;31(1):1–13.

131. Buyalos RP, Funari VA, Azziz R, Watson JM, Martinez-Maza O. Elevated interleukin-6 levels in peritoneal fluid of patients with pelvic pathology. Fertil Steril 1992;58(2):302–306.

132. Stegmann BJ, Gemmill J, Japp E, Chrousos G, Ballweg ML, Stratton P. Changes in the HPA axis associated with chronic pelvic pain. World Congress on Endometriosis, Melbourne, Australia, 2008.

133. Giudice LC, Kao LC. Endometriosis. Lancet 2004;364(9447):1789–1799.

134. Bulun SE. Endometriosis. N Engl J Med 2009;360(3):268–279.

135. Stegmann BJ, Funk MJ, Sinaii N et al. A logistic model for the prediction of endometriosis. Fertil Steril 2009;91(1):51–55.

136. Anaf V, Simon P, El Nakadi I et al. Hyperalgesia, nerve infiltration and nerve growth factor expression in deep adenomyotic nodules, peritoneal and ovarian endometriosis. Hum Reprod 2002;17(7):1895–1900.

137. Wray S, Noble K. Sex hormones and excitation-contraction coupling in the uterus: the effects of oestrous and hormones. J Neuroendocrinol 2008;20(4):451–461.

138. Jarrell J. Myofascial dysfunction in the pelvis. Curr Pain Headache Rep 2004;8(6):452–456.

139. Heitkemper M, Jarrett M. Overlapping conditions in women with irritable bowel syndrome. Urol Nurs 2005;25(1):25–30; quiz 1.

140. Vercellini P, Somigliana E, Vigano P, Abbiati A, Barbara G, Fedele L. Chronic pelvic pain in women: etiology, pathogenesis and diagnostic approach. Gynecol Endocrinol 2009;25(3):149–158.

141. Tokushige N, Markham R, Russell P, Fraser IS. Nerve fibres in peritoneal endometriosis. Hum Reprod 2006;21(11):3001–3007.

142. Tokushige N, Markham R, Russell P, Fraser IS. Effect of progestogens and combined oral contraceptives on nerve fibers in peritoneal endometriosis. Fertil Steril 2009;92(4):1234–1239.

23 Pathophysiology of Infertility in Endometriosis

Bruce A. Lessey[1] and Steven L. Young[2]

[1]Division of Reproductive Endocrinology and Infertility, Department of Obstetrics and Gynecology, University Medical Group, University of South Carolina, Greenville, SC, USA
[2]Division of Reproductive Endocrinology and Infertility, Department of Obstetrics and Gynecology, University of North Carolina at Chapel Hill, Chapel Hill, NC, USA

Introduction

Infertility is a common problem encountered by one in five couples and is defined as the inability to conceive after 1 year of unprotected intercourse. Up to 7.3 million couples in the United States experience infertility [1]. The yearly estimated cost for diagnosis and treatment of endometriosis-associated infertility and pain and loss productivity is approximately $22 billion in the US alone [2]. The underlying causes of infertility are multifactorial, involving both the male and female partner. Human reproduction is relatively inefficient compared to other species [3]. Five major categories account for the bulk of infertility cases seen clinically:
- male factor problems usually associated with sperm number, motility or morphology
- structural or biochemical problems involving the cervix or cervical mucus
- damaged or obstructed fallopian tubes or acquired or congenital uterine defects
- ovulatory dysfunction
- peritoneal factors including pelvic adhesions and endometriosis.

It is estimated that up to 50% of women with endometriosis are infertile [4]. Despite a seemingly clear association between endometriosis and infertility, the biological mechanisms linking them remain uncertain and controversial. The objective of this chapter is to review the literature regarding endometriosis in the context of human infertility and discuss what is known about the pathophysiology of this disorder that contributes to infertility and pregnancy loss. Recent and exciting research has focused on the apparent alterations in the eutopic endometrium of women with this disorder, suggesting endometrial progesterone resistance. Describing how those changes alter the potential for embryo implantation and favor the establishment, maintenance and recurrence of the ectopic lesions is a secondary goal of this chapter.

Implantation and endometrial receptivity

Embryo implantation is a tightly controlled process that is regulated by estrogen and progesterone in most mammalian species [5–13]. The timing of initial embryo attachment in the human corresponds to a narrow window of implantation that occurs on days 20–24, based on multiple perspectives [5,14–17]. One of the earliest studies on the timing of implantation in the human was performed in hysterectomy samples from women trying to conceive prior to surgery [18]. In that study, all identified embryos had attached after day 21 of the menstrual cycle while those from hysterectomy samples before day 19 were still free-floating in the fallopian tubes or uterine cavity. Using donor embryos placed in prepared recipients, Navot and colleagues demonstrated that the timing of transfer was also critical for success [15]. Furthermore, a delay in implantation appears to be a risk factor for implantation failure [17], consistent with earlier reports in animal models showing the importance of synchrony between embryo and endometrium [19].

Successful implantation requires a balance between estrogen and progesterone action, mediated by specific cognate receptors, whose levels fluctuate in response to changing serum levels of estradiol and progesterone [20]. Progesterone, in particular, is essential for the initiation and maintenance of pregnancy [21]; secretory phase estrogen appears to be non-essential [22,23]. In fact, in all species studied, a concerted loss of endometrial estrogen receptors (and therefore the ability to respond to estrogen) appears to be a sentinel event associated with the timing of the window of implantation [24].

The endometrium undergoes well-demarcated changes in its histological development [25]. A delay in endometrial progression, known as luteal phase defect (LPD), was first suggested as a cause of infertility in 1949 [26] and only later associated with

Endometriosis: Science and Practice, First Edition. Edited by Linda C. Giudice, Johannes L.H. Evers and David L. Healy.
© 2012 Blackwell Publishing Ltd. Published 2012 by Blackwell Publishing Ltd.

endometriosis [27]. Early loss of corpus luteal support or an endogenous resistance to progesterone could delay the window of implantation or prematurely shorten its duration, leading to infertility and/or early pregnancy loss.

Endometriosis overview

Endometriosis is defined as the presence of endometrial epithelial and/or stromal cells outside the uterine cavity. Endometriosis is found in 2–8% of the general population [28] but is more common in infertile women [29–31]. Endometriosis is present in 25–40% of women with infertility [29,32–34]. It also appears that 30–50% of women with endometriosis are infertile [35]. Logically, severe endometriosis might adversely affect fertility by virtue of adhesions and distortion of pelvic anatomy. Mild endometriosis is frequently identified (20–60%) in female partners of couples with infertility [32,33,36–38]. Others have demonstrated similar amounts of endometriosis in women unable to conceive due to profound male factor as in those infertile women with normal partners [39]. There remains collective skepticism regarding the association between mild cases of endometriosis and infertility.

A second obstacle to gaining a consensus on endometriosis and infertility has been the heterogeneity of endometriosis and variations in the phenotype of women who have it. Up to 50% of women with mild endometriosis will conceive with expectant management alone, while the rest are infertile. According to Olive, expectant management alone allows half of patients with mild disease to conceive, but only 25% with moderate endometriosis and just a few with severe disease [40]. Failure to account for this substantial effect of even mild disease has limited many studies on endometriosis and fertility, including the studies that examine the effect of medical therapy [41].

The most accepted theory of endometriosis pathogenesis remains that of retrograde menstruation [42,43]. Since most women shed endometrial cells into the peritoneal cavity during normal menstruation, it is likely that clinical endometriosis is due to an intrinsic or acquired abnormality of the eutopic endometrium, peritoneum, or clearance mechanisms of menstrual debris [44]. The intraperitoneal lesions of endometriosis or secondary inflammation might alter the phenotype of eutopic endometrium [45–50]. Eutopic endometrial abnormalities include dysregulation of biomarkers of endometrial receptivity [24,51–54], increased cell proliferation [55] and decreased apoptosis [45,56]. These changes reflected in the shed endometrium likely play a major role in the pathogenesis of endometriosis and its contribution to infertility [46,53,57–60].

The risk factors for the development of endometriosis are numerous. Women at risk for development of endometriosis include those with no prior pregnancy [30,31], women with a suboptimum immune response [61], women with excessive vaginal bleeding [62], including short cycle interval or prolonged bleeding episodes [63–65], and women with obstruction of their cervix [66–68]. Additionally, women with existing endometriosis appear to be at risk for recurrence or exacerbation of their disease. Places where lesions have already formed might be a site where newly deposited menstrual debris is able to attach and invade. Genetics appears to play a role in the occurrence of endometriosis [69–71]. Reduced physical activity and higher Body Mass Index (BMI) are associated with endometriosis [72,73], as well as socio-economic status, psychological traits, race and age [74]. This disorder has also been linked to environmental exposures, including dioxins [75–77].

Diagnosis of endometriosis

There are many signs and symptoms of endometriosis aside from infertility that can hasten the diagnosis of this disorder, including dysmenorrhea, dyspareunia or dyschezia. Studies suggest that a majority of cases of interstitial cystitis and irritable bowel syndrome are actually endometriosis [78–81]. Signs and symptoms, however, may be misleading or unreliable for an accurate diagnosis [82]. Furthermore, women without signs or symptoms of endometriosis can still harbor the disease [28,83–85].

Laparoscopy is the only recognized method for diagnosing endometriosis. Even with a surgical diagnosis, the prevalence of endometriosis can vary according to the clinical presentation, experience of the operator, year of the surgery, type of equipment used, and even time of the menstrual cycle. The likelihood of finding endometriosis is dependent on the clinical reasons for laparoscopy. In general, endometriosis is more frequently diagnosed in the setting of pelvic pain and infertility [86]. Teenagers with pelvic pain or severe dysmenorrhea already have endometriosis over 60% of the time [87,88]. Sadly, the diagnosis of endometriosis is often delayed, especially in the United States, compared to other countries [89,90].

Subtle forms of endometriosis may be the most active biologically and therefore more likely to reduce fertility [91]. Recognition of subtle endometriosis depends on the quality of the laparoscope used but also can be influenced by the operator's experience and training. Subtle or even invisible endometriosis has been described and is part of the continuum between a normal pelvis and stage IV endometriosis [92–99]. Methods have been described to increase the probability of finding endometriosis, including assessment of demographic and lifestyle data [100] or the use of special filters [101,102]. A response to GnRH agonist therapy has been suggested as a non-surgical indicator that endometriosis is present [103]. Various biomarkers have also been investigated for the diagnosis of endometriosis, including CA-125, autoendometrial antibodies, and members of the integrin family of proteins [52–54,104–114]. Finally proteomics and genomics are now establishing the basis for future biomarker development related to endometriosis [46,59,115–118].

Infertility and endometriosis

Infertility is defined as the inability of a couple to conceive despite 1 year of unprotected intercourse. In normal couples the probability of achieving a pregnancy in any single month is

15–20%, while in untreated women with endometriosis, this number falls to 2–10% [119–122]. There have been many efforts to develop staging systems that standardize the degree of endometriosis [123–125], but each method has been faulted for not predicting outcomes related to cycle fecundability. Recently, factors that contribute to the endometriosis-associated effects on fertility have been formulated into a new paradigm for assessing the risk of infertility – the Endometriosis Fertility Index (EFI). The EFI predicts pregnancy rates in patients with surgically documented endometriosis based on the revised American Society for Reproductive Medicine (rASRM) staging, a least function score of tubal and ovarian function at the end of surgery, and historical patient data, including age, duration of infertility and pregnancy history [126]. All staging systems are affected by the inherent heterogeneity of the disease and the variations in how endometriosis is treated by surgical or medical interventions.

There are several lines of evidence that support an association between infertility and endometriosis even in its mildest forms [127,128]. First, normal fertile women appear to have a lower incidence of endometriosis than women with infertility [32,33]. Women undergoing tubal ligation are an ideal fertile control group to study. A consensus of many studies on fertile women undergoing tubal ligation found that the prevalence of endometriosis ranged from 4% to 8% compared to recent estimates of endometriosis in infertile populations at 33% [28].

Animal models have replicated an association between endometriotic implants and subfertility [57,129–135]. Hahn demonstrated that intraperitoneal injection of peritoneal fluid from affected animals reproduced the decrease in implantation rates in normal animals, suggesting that a transferrable substance associated with endometriosis is present [57]. We reproduced this effect in the mouse model using human peritoneal fluid injected into otherwise fertile mice [136]. D'Hooghe demonstrated that cycle fecundibility was lower in baboons with mild, moderate and severe endometriosis compared to animals that did not harbor the disease [134] but similar to controls for minimal disease [135]. In a prospective study, Fazleabas showed a rapid change in eutopic endometrium of baboons after endometriosis was initiated, suggesting a possible communication between the extra- and intrauterine environment [50,58,137–139].

A third line of evidence comes from the collective experience with donor sperm insemination in couples with male factor infertility. Normal annualized pregnancy rate using donor sperm was reported to vary by age, but ranged from 54% to 75% with an average monthly fecundity rate (MFR) of 0.05–0.13 (5–13% per month) [119] using donor insemination. Uncontrolled trials have reported a normal MFR of 0.20 and clinical pregnancy rate (CPR) of 80% in women with untreated endometriosis [140,141] but in prospective trials, the evidence is more convincing. Jansen reported a MFR of 0.12 in normal women compared to a 0.036 in women with mild endometriosis [142]. Hammond performed a

similar larger study showing similar results, with a cycle fecundity of 0.102 in unaffected women but only 0.04 in women with endometriosis. Toma [121] showed similar results but noted that treatment did not alter the outcome in subsequent intrauterine insemination (IUI) cycles. Using frozen donor sperm in a prospective randomized study design, Byrd and colleagues showed that both intracervical and intrauterine insemination were more successful in women without endometriosis compared to those with this disease [143].

The fourth line of evidence comes from assisted reproductive technologies (ART) including hyperstimulation and *in vitro* fertilization. In an early meta-analysis, Hughes showed that endometriosis was associated with a worse prognosis than male factor infertility using gonadotropin hyperstimulation and IUI treatment [144] Surgical treatment versus expectant management provides a favorable outcome for women with endometriosis receiving gonadotropins and IUI [145]. In a prospective controlled trial, Deaton reported nearly a three-fold increase in pregnancy rates in laparoscopically treated women with endometriosis undergoing clomiphene citrate/IUI compared to similar treatments in the non-surgical group [146] In the setting of *in vitro* fertilization (IVF), the reports have been mixed, with some centers observing a detrimental effect of endometriosis [147–149] while others found no effect of endometriosis on IVF success rates [150–152]. Endometriosis reduced success rates in gamete intrafallopian tube transfer (GIFT) [153]. Meta-analyses suggest that endometriosis has a dose effect, reducing IVF success rates in a direct relationship to stage of disease [154]. Confounding these studies is the effect of downregulation prior to IVF that might influence the effect of endometriosis on cycle outcome. Prolonged luteal suppression with gonadotropin-releasing hormone agonists (GnRHa) appears to be an effective treatment and improves outcomes compared to cycles in which shorter courses of luteal suppression were used [41].

Mechanisms of infertility in endometriosis

Despite the supporting literature, a cause-and-effect relationship between endometriosis and infertility has yet to be firmly established. It is difficult to reconcile the findings of minimal or subtle peritoneal lesions with long-standing infertility. Furthermore, diagnostic accuracy can vary widely between observers. Finally, many women with mild forms of endometriosis might have been misdiagnosed or remain undiagnosed. Unfortunately, the presence or absence of disease cannot routinely be judged by histological confirmation, since pathological diagnosis can be unreliable and frequently lacks correlation with the laparoscopic findings [28,155]. When these problems are coupled with the fact that up to 50% of women with mild endometriosis conceive with expectant management alone, it is difficult to gain universal agreement on how endometriosis contributes to infertility.

Table 23.1 Proposed mechanisms of loss of fertility by endometriosis.

Presentation	Proposed mechanism	References
Folliculogenesis or ovulation	Abnormal follicular growth or oocyte function	[156–159]
Corpus luteum function	Altered CL function, enzymatic capacity or CL lifespan, elevated progesterone during proliferative phase	[160–162]
Ovulation	Luteinized unruptured follicle syndrome (LUFS)	[132,133,269,270]
Mechanical causes/egg pick-up	Adhesions, anatomical distortion, ovarian cysts	[132,163,164]
Altered immune function/inflammation	T-regulatory cells, embryonic tolerance or rejection, NK cells	[88,271–273]
Endometrial receptivity/changes in the eutopic endometrium	Progesterone resistance or estrogen dominance, aromatase expression	[47,48,50,59,118,137,139,158,274]
Altered sperm quality or function	Decreased motility, fertilization capacity, acrosome reaction, macrophage sequestration of sperm	[158,165–169]
Embryo quality	Endometriosis-mediated changes in the embryo	[159,170,171]
Peritoneal factors	Inappropriate signaling, growth factor or cytokine signaling, inflammatory changes, alterations in fallopian tube, gametes, endometrium	[169,173–179,180–185,189–196]

CL, corpus luteum; NK, natural killer.

Mechanisms that account for a negative impact of endometriosis on fertility (Table 23.1) include altered folliculogenesis or ovulation [156–159], defects in luteal phase function [160–162], mechanical distortion of pelvic anatomy, impaired oocyte release or pick-up [163,164], altered sperm quality or function [158,165–169], decreased embryo quality [159,170,171] and disturbances in uterine contractility [172]. Peritoneal factors are dramatically altered in the presence of endometriosis [173–179], and inflammatory effects associated with activated macrophages or alterations of immune function or cytokine production have also been reported [180–185]. A variety of bio-active factors has been shown to affect ovulation, fertilization, embryo quality and implantation [57,136,166,168–170,186–198].

Most recently, an altered endocrine/cytokine milieu and a new focus on progesterone resistance have been suggested [47,59,139,158], providing an explanation for both the fertility problems associated with endometriosis and its etiology and recurrence. Given the essential role of progesterone as a brake for estrogen action and for the success of pregnancy [21], progesterone resistance could account for suspected implantation failure in women with infertility and endometriosis [24]. Structural and biochemical alterations in the endometrium of women with endometriosis have been well described [199–201]. An increased proliferative phenotype of the eutopic endometrium has been reported as well [55,59], along with a faulty downregulation of estrogen receptors in the secretory phase [48]. These changes appear to arise by paracrine regulatory mechanisms involved in epithelial-mesenchymal cross-talk [202].

If a common theme is present, it is likely to be based on inflammatory changes arising in response to the endometriotic implant itself. Superficial lesions are more active than powder burn or scarred lesions [91,203–206]. Despite the widespread disagreement about mild forms of endometriosis and its relationship to infertility, studies exist that suggest that superficial endometriosis affects fertility, at least in a subset of women. Littman and colleagues reported finding endometriosis frequently in women with unexplained infertility and IVF failure. A high percentage of women (75%) conceived after surgical treatment [207]. The HOXA10 gene is a known regulator of a biomarker for uterine receptivity, $\alpha v \beta 3$ [208]. Both HOXA10 and $\alpha v \beta 3$ are significantly reduced in the eutopic endometrium of women with mild, but not moderate or severe endometriosis [52,205], perhaps accounting for the altered fertility in this group of patients. Together, there is increasing evidence that mild forms of endometriosis do cause infertility and that increased inflammatory changes within the peritoneal fluid and alterations in the eutopic endometrium may lead to implantation failure [209].

Endometriosis and progesterone resistance

The remainder of this chapter will focus on progesterone resistance. Embryo implantation is a tightly controlled process that is regulated by estrogen and progesterone in most mammalian species [5–13]. A delay in implantation appears to be a risk factor for implantation failure [17], consistent with earlier reports in animal models showing the importance of synchrony between embryo and endometrium [19].

Successful implantation requires a balance between estrogen and progesterone action. The actions of these sex steroids are mediated by specific cognate receptors, whose levels fluctuate in response to changing serum levels of estradiol and progesterone [20]. Progesterone, in particular, is essential for the initiation and maintenance of pregnancy [21]; secretory phase estrogen appears non-essential [210,211]. In fact, in all species studied, a concerted loss of endometrial epithelial estrogen receptors (and therefore the ability to respond to estrogen) appears to be a sentinel event associated with the timing of the window of implantation [24].

Table 23.2 Endometrial factors involved in P action and embryo receptivity.

Paracrine or autocrine	Transcription	Nuclear receptor co-activators & chaperones
Bone morphogenic protein 2 (BMP2)	Estrogen receptor α (ERα)	FK506 binding protein 5 (FKBP51)
Indian hedgehog (IHH)	Progesterone receptor (PR)	FK506 binding protein 4 (FKBP52)
Wingless (Wnt) family: Wnt4, Wnt5a, Wnt7a	Homeobox A10 and A11 (HOXA10 and HOXA11)	Steroid receptor co-activator 2 (SRC−2)
Transforming growth factor β (TGF-β)	CCAAT enhancer binding protein- β (C/EBPβ)	Hydrogen peroxide-inducible clone 5 protein (Hic5, TGFB1I1)
Epidermal growth factor (EGF) ligand family	Krüppel-like family 9 (KLF9)	Melanoma antigen gene protein−11 (MAGE−11)
Vascular endothelial growth factor (VEGF)	Chicken ovalbumin upstream promoter-transcription factor II (COUP-TFII)	
Interleukin-1, 6, and 11	Forkhead box O1 (FOXO1)	
Insulin-like growth factor (IGF)		
Leukemia inhibitor factor (LIF)		
Hepatocyte growth factor (HGF)		
Heparin binding EGF-like growth factor (HB-EGF)		

See [24,253,275,276].

There is little evidence that serum progesterone is reduced in women with endometriosis, so the endometrial dysfunction noted in endometriosis is likely due to a diminished endometrial response to progesterone. Perhaps one of the earliest observations that endometriosis is associated with progesterone resistance came from Ann Wentz, who reported premenstrual spotting in women with endometriosis [212]. Premature expression of endometrial bleeding associated factor (EBAF) (a progesterone suppressed protein), also associated with endometriosis and unexplained infertility [213–216], might contribute to such bleeding.

Other changes in gene expression patterns have been seen in eutopic endometrium of women with endometriosis, reflecting defective progesterone action and an exaggerated influence of estrogen [46–48,59,118,217–219]. A diminishing negative effect of progesterone on estrogen action leads to hyperproliferative and antiapoptotic changes observed in eutopic endometrium. When menses does occur, any shed menstrual tissue that undergoes retrograde efflux might be more likely to attach and grow; thus the changes in the eutopic endometrium promote the establishment, maintenance, and recurrence of ectopic endometrial lesions, leading to worsening or persistence of disease.

Altered actions of sex steroid hormones could be reflected in the steroid receptor concentrations that in turn change the orchestration of gene expression seen during the normal menstrual cycle [220]. Progesterone resistance would impede the expression of progesterone-induced proteins critical for implantation and endometrial receptivity (Table 23.2) that also might contribute to endometriosis-related infertility [53,219,221]. Progesterone acts via its cognate progesterone receptor (PR), which was the first factor implicated in progesterone resistance [222]. PR exists primarily in two forms, PRA and PRB [223], each resulting from mRNA transcripts produced from different transcriptional start sites on the same gene [224]. PRA and PRB exert different effects on gene expression and PRA, but not PRB, is required for murine embryo implantation.

Interestingly, specific suppression of PRB, but not PRA, due to promoter hypermethylation has been reported in women with endometriosis, suggesting a possible mechanism for P resistance [225–227]. In endometriosis, there is a failure of midsecretory downregulation of epithelial PR [20,228], which would alter PR action.

A second potential mechanism for P resistance is an alteration of expression or function of PR chaperones and co-chaperones that are bound to PR prior to activation [229]. After ligand binding, PR is released from chaperones, allowing it to mediate mRNA transcription. Evidence exists for a role of co-activators in endometrial receptivity [230,231], overexpression of co-chaperone FKBP51 [232] or lack of co-chaperone FKBP52 [137,233–236] causing P resistance in experimental models. High FKBP51 expression appears to be responsible for the relative P resistance seen in normal squirrel monkeys [232] but it also leads to glucocorticoid and androgen resistance, which has not been described in women with endometriosis. FKBP52 gene knockout in mice leads to P resistance and embryo implantation failure, which is mild enough to be overcome with supplemental P, mirroring the degree of resistance likely seen in some women with endometriosis [235]. Furthermore, endometriotic lesions from endometrium of mice carrying this deletion are reported to have increased growth and angiogenesis [236] and endometrium from women as well as baboon models of endometriosis show deficient FKBP52 expression [137].

Progesterone receptor modulates gene expression via interaction with co-activators and co-repressors and transcription factors, providing another potential mechanism for P resistance. A steroid receptor co-activator, Hic-5, has recently been shown to be deficient in the stroma of proliferative and late-secretory endometrium of women with endometriosis [237] and null mutations in the PR co-activator, steroid receptor co-activator 2 (SRC-2), cause mice to have severe defects in endometrial receptivity. Another possible mediator of P resistance is KLF9, which directly interacts with PR at specific gene promoters. Murine null mutations in KLF9 result in partial P resistance, subfertility, and reduced HOXA10 expression [238–240]. Furthermore, eutopic endometrium from a mouse model of endometriosis shows reduced expression of KLF9 [241]. However, no specific information is available describing altered endometrial expression of either SRC-2 or KLF9 in women.

Recent data also point to the role of microRNAs (miRNAs) in P action with cyclic regulation of key miRNAs in human endometrial epithelium correlating with decreased abundance of estrogen-induced miRNA targets [118,242–244]. MicroRNA expression appears to be P-regulated in a cell type-specific manner in normal endometrium [242] and differences between women with and without endometriosis have now been reported [118,245,246]. Notably, a single miRNA species can effect translation and stability of multiple mRNA species, suggesting both an important role in endometrial function and expansion of potential therapeutic approaches.

A novel and largely unexplored cause of P resistance is excessive estrogen (E) action, as evidenced by increased secretory phase endometrial estrogen receptor (ER)α expression [48] and proliferation [55]. The primary cause of increased E may be aromatase, a critical enzyme for synthesis of E [247,248], that is overexpressed in human endometrial stroma due to a stable, epigenetic change [44]. Local and inappropriate production of E by the endometrium could counteract P in several different ways, including alterations in the PRA/B ratio [227], increased (premature) expression of the transforming growth factor (TFG)-β antagonist LEFTY [213,215,249], reduced interleukin (IL)-6 expression by stroma [250], alterations in ERβ or other accessory estrogen-induced proteins such as erythroblastic leukemia viral oncogene homolog (ERBB) receptor feedback inhibitor-1 (Errfi1) [251], reduction in co-activator proteins (MAGE-11) [252] or PR chaperones (FKBP52) [137,233–235]. The cytokine IL-6 is interesting to consider in this regard, since it is normally low during the proliferative phase, high during the window of implantation but reduced in the midsecretory phase of women with recurrent pregnancy loss [253]. TGF-β is a known mediator of progesterone action in the secretory phase [254] and modulates expression of critical endometrial proteins, including leukemia inhibitor factor (LIF) [255], suggesting a mechanism by which an anti-TGF-β molecule like EBAF could reduce fertility.

Progesterone receptor may also act indirectly, by inducing expression of intracrine, autocrine, juxtacrine or paracrine factors including MIG-6 [59,256]. This antiproliferative, P-induced protein, whose absence results in hyperplasia [257], shows reduced expression in the endometrium of women with endometriosis [59]. Whether reduced MIG-6 expression is a primary cause or downstream effect of the disease, increased endometrial proliferation may contribute to endometriotic proliferation, once MIG-6 is reduced.

The use of biomarkers has furthered our understanding of the pathogenesis of endometriosis [24,258], but none has been shown to have sufficient specificity and sensitivity for clinical use.

A recent consensus statement described biomarkers as the highest priority in endometriosis research because the lack of non-surgical diagnostic markers is contributing to the delay in diagnosis and opportunity for timely intervention [259].

Improving studies on endometriosis on infertility

Studies on endometriosis must be viewed carefully because of pitfalls that arise regarding observer bias, study design and selection of control groups. Problems fall into four major categories: temporal relationship of treatment to measured outcomes, heterogeneity of the disease, lack of adequate control groups, and differences in observer bias or expertise.

Selection of the study subjects is critical to obtaining reliable results. Often patients previously diagnosed with endometriosis are included. It appears that once endometriosis is diagnosed, the outcome of prospective studies changes. Daya reviewed how the observed relationship between pregnancy loss and endometriosis exists only before the subjects are diagnosed by laparoscopy [260]. Once the diagnosis of endometriosis is made and the disease partially or completely treated, this association can no longer be demonstrated. Diagnosed patients with endometriosis may become unavailable because they were successful at achieving pregnancy or some may receive more aggressive therapy such as IVF. If diagnosis and treatment occur at the time of surgery, the patient no longer resembles the population from which she arose.

The second related problem is patient heterogeneity. Up to 50% of women with endometriosis will conceive without treatment [261]. While the percentage will depend on the severity of disease, this positive outcome has been used as an argument that endometriosis does not cause infertility. Such heterogeneity might also enlighten us about the unanswered questions related to endometriosis and infertility. What determines the difference between the fertile woman with endometriosis and the one that is infertile? The opportunity to better understand the underlying defect associated with endometriosis that leads to infertility lies within this heterogeneity. More importantly, inclusion of women with endometriosis who conceive in studies on infertility will alter the outcome and conclusions of the studies. Comparing two prospective surgical studies on outcome demonstrates this point. Nowroozi required a patient to have 8 months of expectant management before enrollment [262] while the Canadian EndoCan study enrolled everyone at laparoscopy [263]. The former found a greater success rate with surgery than the latter, with far fewer patients.

In terms of evidence-based medicine, this heterogeneity becomes a problem. For example, medical treatment for infertility associated with endometriosis has never been convincingly demonstrated [41]. Despite evidence that suppression with GnRH agonist increases fertility in the setting of IVF and endometriosis [264,265], menstrual suppression of endometriosis patients for 6 months does not improve fertility in natural cycles. Heterogeneity may explain this phenomenon. If 50% of women conceive without treatment (0.30 cycle fecundity), then 6 months of GnRH agonist therapy will decrease their cycle fecundity by half (0.15). In the infertile group with endometriosis, cycle fecundity is near 0.0. If GnRH agonist therapy were helpful in this group, cycle fecundity might be increased after 6 months of treatment (0.15). The net outcome of any study involving this heterogeneous group would never show benefit, since the average cycle fecundity of the treatment and placebo groups remains at 0.15 no matter how many patients are enrolled.

A third problem with many studies involving endometriosis is the lack of a comparable control group. Women with a history of fertility are often considered as a suitable control group for those with endometriosis. A study by Moen [84] showed that the time from last pregnancy to sterilization appeared to be directly associated with the likelihood of finding endometriosis. Thus, women with a pregnancy are not necessarily protected from endometriosis if the interval between delivery and the time of the study is sufficiently long. The thoroughness of the inspection at tubal ligation is not the same as that done for pelvic pain or infertility, making the tubal ligation control less reliable than one assumes. In women who have been treated for endometriosis, the amount of disease can change over time. Recurrence rates of 20–80% have been described [266,267]. Investigations relying on previous assessment of the pelvis, the choice of fertile controls, or studies involving the effect of prior laparoscopy must consider the variable of time in design of the study.

The fourth problem with many studies is heterogeneity of the observers. It is difficult to control for operator experience or expertise. Learned attitudes about what constitutes "active" endometriosis may bias the reporting of disease or influence how aggressively endometriosis is excised or cauterized. Methods for removing or just cauterizing endometriosis can vary between operator based on training and experience. Centers with greater proficiency at complete resection of implants including both deep nodular endometriosis as well as active red or non-pigmented lesions will likely report different outcomes compared to centers where only surface lesions are cauterized or ablated with a laser. When comparing the effectiveness of surgery, data are not generally presented on the methodology or thoroughness of the surgery. If a small amount of endometriosis causes infertility, as some studies suggest [207], then leaving a small amount of endometriosis behind might be equivalent to not performing the surgery at all. Perhaps this is why recent studies in which all endometriosis was completely resected at the time of surgery [207] appear to show better results than other RCTs with more patients [263,268].

Conclusion

The effect of mild endometriosis on fertility is inconsistent between individuals with the disease. Fertility is severely compromised in some women with even very mild or subtle forms of endometriosis, while in others the effect appears to be minimal.

Controversy and resistance to accepting a putative "cause and effect" on fertility have produced a scientific literature that is confusing and often self-contradictory. Variability in how endometriosis is diagnosed and treated has further contributed to the controversy. The study of women with a prior treatment of endometriosis may be quite different from studies on women prior to diagnosis. Studies are slowly reaching a consensus that the eutopic endometrium of women with endometriosis acquires defects in gene expression consistent with resistance to the actions of progesterone. This loss of balance between the effects of estrogen and progesterone likely contributes to a loss of synchrony required for normal implantation. Future studies using well-controlled inclusion and exclusion criteria and biomarkers will likely advance our understanding of this enigmatic disease and provide the long awaited answers to important questions that remain unanswered about endometriosis and infertility.

References

1. Chandra A, Martinez GM, Mosher WD et al. Fertility, family planning and reproductive health of U.S. women: data from the 2002 National Survey of Family Growth. Vital Health Stat 2005;23(25):1–160.

2. Simoens S, Hummelshoj L, D'Hooghe T. Endometriosis: cost estimates and methodological perspective. Hum Reprod Update 2007;13(4):395–404.

3. Strauss JF, III, Lessey BA. The structure, function, and evaluation of the female reproductive tract. In: Strauss JF, III, Barbieri RL (eds) Reproductive Endocrinology: Physiology, Pathophysiology, and Clinical Management. Philadelphia, PA: Saunders Elsevier, 2009, pp. 191–233.

4. Practice Committee of the American Society for Reproductive Medicine. Endometriosis and infertility. Fertil Steril 2006; 86(4):S156–S160.

5. Carson DD, Bagchi I, Dey SK et al. Embryo implantation. Dev Biol 2000;223(2):217–237.

6. Psychoyos A. Hormonal control of ovoimplantation. Vitam Horm 1973;31:201–256.

7. Anderson TL, Hodgen GD. Uterine receptivity in the primate. Prog Clin Biol Res 1989;294:389–399.

8. Rogers PAW, Murphy CR, Yoshinaga K. Uterine receptivity for implantation: human studies. In: Yoshinaga K (ed) Blastocyst Implantation: Serono Symposia. Boston: Adams Publishing Group, 1989, pp. 231–238.

9. Finn CA, Martin L. The control of implantation. J Reprod Fertil 1974;39:195–206.

10. Beier HM. Oviducal and uterine fluids. J Reprod Fertil 1974; 37:221–237.

11. Hodgen GD. Surrogate embryo transfer combined with estrogen-progesterone therapy in monkeys: implantation, gestation, and delivery without ovaries. JAMA 1983;250:2167–2171.

12. Shapiro SS, Johnson MH Jr. Progesterone altered amino acid accumulation by human endometrium in vitro. Biol Reprod 1989;40:555–565.

13. Navot D, Anderson TL, Droesch K et al. Hormonal manipulation of endometrial maturation. J Clin Endocrinol Metab 1989; 68:801–807.

14. Navot D, Bergh P. Preparation of the human endometrium for implantation. Ann N Y Acad Sci 1991;622:212–219.

15. Navot D, Bergh PA, Williams M et al. An insight into early reproductive processes through the in vivo model of ovum donation. J Clin Endocrinol Metab 1991;72:408–414.

16. Navot D, Mausher SJ, Oehninger S et al. The value of in vitro fertilization for the treatment of unexplained infertility. Fertil Steril 1988;49:854–857.

17. Wilcox AJ, Baird DD, Wenberg CR. Time of implantation of the conceptus and loss of pregnancy. N Engl J Med 1999;340:1796–1799.

18. Hertig AT, Rock J, Adams EC. A description of 34 human ova within the first 17 days of development. Am J Anat 1956;98:435–493.

19. Pope WF. Uterine asynchrony: a cause of embryonic loss. Biol Reprod 1988;39:999–1003.

20. Lessey BA, Killam AP, Metzger DA et al. Immunohistochemical analysis of human uterine estrogen and progesterone receptors throughout the menstrual cycle. J Clin Endocrinol Metab 1988;67:334–340.

21. Baulieu EE. Contragestion and other clinical applications of RU-486, an antiprogesterone at the receptor. Science 1989;245:1351–1357.

22. De Ziegler D, Cornel C, Bergeron C et al. Controlled preparation of the endometrium with exogenous estradiol and progesterone in women having functioning ovaries. Fertil Steril 1991;56:851–855.

23. De Ziegler D, Bergeron C, Cornel C et al. Effects of luteal estrogen on the secretory transformation of human endometrium and plasma gonadotropins. J Clin Endocrinol Metab 1992 74:322–331.

24. Donaghay M, Lessey BA. Uterine receptivity: alterations associated with benign gynecological disease. Semin Reprod Med 2007; 25(6):461–475.

25. Noyes RW, Hertig AI, Rock J. Dating the endometrial biopsy. Fertil Steril 1950;1:3–25.

26. Jones GS. Some newer aspects of management of infertility. JAMA 1949;141:1123–1129.

27. Pittaway DE, Maxson W, Daniell J et al. Luteal phase defects in infertility patients with endometriosis. Fertil Steril 1983;39:712–713.

28. D'Hooghe TM, Debrock S, Hill JA, Meuleman C. Endometriosis and subfertility: is the relationship resolved? Semin Reprod Med 2003; 21(2):243–254.

29. Kirshon B, Poindexter AN III, Fast J. Endometriosis in multiparous women. J Reprod Med 1989;34:215–217.

30. Berube S, Marcoux S, Maheux R, Canadian Collaborative Group on Endometriosis. Characteristics related to the prevalence of minimal or mild endometriosis in infertile women. Epidemiology 1998; 9(5):504–510.

31. Matalliotakis I, Cakmak H, Dermitzaki D et al. Increased rate of endometriosis and spontaneous abortion in an in vitro fertilization program: no correlation with epidemiological factors. Gynecol Endocrinol 2008;24(4):194–198.

32. Strathy JH, Molgaard CA, Coulam CB, Melton LJ. Endometriosis and infertility: a laparoscopic study of endometriosis among fertile and infertile women. Fertil Steril 1982; 38:667–672.

33. Verkauf BS. Incidence, symptoms, and signs of endometriosis in fertile and infertile women. J Fla Med Assoc 1987;74:671–675.

34. Houston DE, Noller KL, Melton LJ III et al. Incidence of pelvic endometriosis in Rochester, Minnesota, 1970-1979. Am J Epidemiol 1987;125(6):959–969.

35. Counsellor V. Endometriosis a clinical and surgical review. Am J Obstet Gynecol 1938;36:877–885.

36. Hasson HM. Incidence of endometriosis in diagnostic laparoscopy. J Reprod Med 1976;16:135–138.

37. Drake TS, Grunert GM. The unsuspected pelvic factor in the infertility investigation. Fertil Steril 1980;34(1):27–31.

38. Tsuji I, Ami K, Miyazaki A et al. Benefit of diagnostic laparoscopy for patients with unexplained infertility and normal hysterosalpingography findings. Tohoku J Exp Med 2009;219(1):39–42.

39. Matorras R, Rodriguez F, Pijoan JI et al. Women who are not exposed to spermatozoa and infertile women have similar rates of stage I endometriosis. Fertil Steril 2001;76(5):923–928.

40. Olive DL, Stohs GF, Metzger DA, Franklin RR. Expectant management and hydrotubations in the treatment of endometriosis-associated infertility. Fertil Steril 1985;44(1):35–41.

41. Lessey BA. Medical management of endometriosis and infertility. Fertil Steril 2000;73:1089–1096.

42. Sampson JA. Benign and malignant endometrial implants in the peritoneal cavity and their relation to certain ovarian tumors. Surg Gynecol Obstet 1924;38:287–311.

43. Sampson JA. Metastatic or embolic endometriosis, due to menstrual dissemination of endometrial tissue into venous circulation. Am J Pathol 1927;3:93–110.

44. Bulun SE. Endometriosis. N Engl J Med 2009;360(3):268–279.

45. Meresman GF, Vighi S, Buquet RA et al. Apoptosis and expression of Bcl-2 and Bax in eutopic endometrium from women with endometriosis. Fertil Steril 2000;74(4):760–766.

46. Kao LC, Germeyer A, Tulac S et al. Expression profiling of endometrium from women with endometriosis reveals candidate genes for disease-based implantation failure and infertility. Endocrinology 2003;144:2870–2881.

47. Bulun SE, Cheng YH, Yin P et al. Progesterone resistance in endometriosis: link to failure to metabolize estradiol. Mol Cell Endocrinol 2006;248(1-2):94–103.

48. Lessey BA, Palomino WA, Apparao KB et al. Estrogen receptor-alpha (ER-alpha) and defects in uterine receptivity in women. Reprod Biol Endocrinol 2006;4(Suppl 1):S9.

49. Bromer JG, Aldad TS, Taylor HS. Defining the proliferative phase endometrial defect. Fertil Steril 2009;91(3):698–704.

50. Wang C, Mavrogianis PA, Fazleabas AT. Endometriosis is associated with progesterone resistance in the baboon (Papio anubis) oviduct: evidence based on the localization of oviductal glycoprotein 1 (OVGP1). Biol Reprod 2009;80(2):272–278.

51. Ilesanmi AO, Hawkins DA, Lessey BA. Immunohistochemical markers of uterine receptivity in the human endometrium. Microsc Res Tech 1993;25(3):208–222.

52. Lessey BA, Castelbaum AJ, Sawin SW et al. Aberrant integrin expression in the endometrium of women with endometriosis. J Clin Endocrinol Metab 1994;79(2):643–649.

53. Wei Q, St Clair JB, Fu T et al. Reduced expression of biomarkers associated with the implantation window in women with endometriosis. Fertil Steril 2009;91(5):1686–1691.

54. Pan XY, Li X, Weng ZP, Wang B. Altered expression of claudin-3 and claudin-4 in ectopic endometrium of women with endometriosis. Fertil Steril 2009;91(5):1692–1699.

55. Park JS, Lee JH, Kim M et al. Endometrium from women with endometriosis shows increased proliferation activity. Fertil Steril 2009;92(4):1246–1249.

56. Gebel HM, Braun DP, Tambur A et al. Spontaneous apoptosis of endometrial tissue is impaired in women with endometriosis. Fertil Steril 1998;69:1042–1047.

57. Hahn DW, Carraher RP, Foldesy RG, McGuire JL. Experimental evidence for failure to implant as a mechanism of infertility associated with endometriosis. Am J Obstet Gynecol 1986;155:1109–1113.

58. Gashaw I, Hastings JM, Jackson KS et al. Induced endometriosis in the baboon (Papio anubis) increases the expression of the proangiogenic factor CYR61 (CCN1) in eutopic and ectopic endometria. Biol Reprod 2006;74(6):1060–1066.

59. Burney RO, Talbi S, Hamilton AE et al. Gene expression analysis of endometrium reveals progesterone resistance and candidate susceptibility genes in women with endometriosis. Endocrinology 2007;148(8):3814–3826.

60. Meola J, Rosa ES, Dentillo DB et al. Differentially expressed genes in eutopic and ectopic endometrium of women with endometriosis. Fertil Steril 2010;93(6):1750–1773.

61. Giudice LC, Kao LC. Endometriosis. Lancet 2004;364(9447):1789–1799.

62. Halme J, Becker S, Wing R. Accentuated cyclic activation of peritoneal macrophages in patients with endometriosis. Am J Obstet Gynecol 1984;148:85–90.

63. Arumugam K, Lim JMH. Menstrual characteristics associated with endometriosis. Br J Obstet Gynaecol 1997;104:948–950.

64. Cramer DW, Wilson E, Stillman RJ et al. The relation of endometriosis to menstrual characteristics, smoking, and exercise. JAMA 1986;255:1904–1908.

65. Vercellini P, De Giorgi O, Aimi G et al. Menstrual characteristics in women with and without endometriosis. Obstet Gynecol 1997;90:264–268.

66. Barbieri RL, Callery M, Perez SE. Directionality of menstrual flow: cervical os diameter as a determinant of retrograde menstruation. Fertil Steril 1992;57(4):727–730.

67. Olive DL, Henderson DY. Endometriosis and mullerian anomalies. Obstet Gynecol 1987;69:412–415.

68. Fedele L, Bianchi S, Di Nola G et al. Endometriosis and nonobstructive mullerian anomalies. Obstet Gynecol 1992;79:515–517.

69. Kennedy S. The genetics of endometriosis. J Reprod Med 1998;43 Suppl:263–268.

70. Lattuada D, Somigliana E, Vigano P et al. Genetics of endometriosis: a role for the progesterone receptor gene polymorphism PROGINS? Clin Endocrinol (Oxf) 2004;61(2):190–194.

71. Matalliotakis IM, Cakmak H, Krasonikolakis GD et al. Endometriosis related to family history of malignancies in the Yale series. Surg Oncol 2009;19:33–37.

72. Vitonis AF, Hankinson SE, Hornstein MD, Missmer SA. Adult physical activity and endometriosis risk. Epidemiology 2010;21(1):16–23.

73. Yi KW, Shin JH, Park MS et al. Association of body mass index with severity of endometriosis in Korean women. Int J Gynaecol Obstet 2009;105(1):39–42.

74. O'Connor DT. Epidemiology. In: Endometriosis. Edinburgh: Churchill Livingstone, 1987, pp. 7–23.

75. Rier S, Foster WG. Environmental dioxins and endometriosis. Toxicol Sci 2002;70(2):161–170.

76. Rier SE, Martin DC, Bowman RE, Becker JL. Immunoresponsiveness in endometriosis: implications of estrogenic toxicants. Environ Health Perspect 1995;103(Suppl 7):151–156.

77. Rier SE, Martin DC, Bowman RE et al. Endometriosis in rhesus monkeys (Macaca mulatta) following chronic exposure to 2,3,7,8-tetrachlorodibenzo-p-dioxin. Fundam Appl Toxicol. 1993;21:433–441.

78. Ferrero S, Camerini G, Ragni N, Remorgida V. Endometriosis and irritable bowel syndrome: co-morbidity or misdiagnosis? Br J Obstet Gynaecol 2009;116(1):129; author reply 130.

79. Maroun P, Cooper MJ, Reid GD, Keirse MJ. Relevance of gastrointestinal symptoms in endometriosis. Aust N Z J Obstet Gynaecol 2009;49(4):411–414.

80. Seaman HE, Ballard KD, Wright JT, de Vries CS. Endometriosis and its coexistence with irritable bowel syndrome and pelvic inflammatory disease: findings from a national case-control study – Part 2. Br J Obstet Gynecol 2008;115(11):1392–1396.

81. Chung MK, Chung RP, Gordon D. Interstitial cystitis and endometriosis in patients with chronic pelvic pain: The "Evil Twins" syndrome. JSLS 2005;9(1):25–29.

82. Muse K. Clinical manifestations and classification of endometriosis. Clin Obstet Gynecol 1988;31(4):813–822.

83. Dmowski WP. Pitfalls in clinical, laparoscopic and histologic diagnosis of endometriosis. Acta Obstet Gynecol Scand 1984;123(Suppl):61–66.

84. Moen MH. Endometriosis in women at interval sterilization. Acta Obstet Gynecol Scand 1987;66(5):451–454.

85. Lessey BA, Miller PB, Forstein DA. Laparoscopic surgery improves outcome and diagnostic accuracy in unexplained infertility. Fertil Steril 2010;94(4):3.

86. Pittaway DE. Diagnosis of endometriosis. In: Diamond MP (ed) Infertility and Reproductive Medicine Clinics of North America. Philadelphia: W.B. Saunders, 1992, pp. 619–631.

87. Templeman C. Adolescent endometriosis. Obstet Gynecol Clin North Am 2009;36(1):177–185.

88. Solnik MJ. Chronic pelvic pain and endometriosis in adolescents. Curr Opin Obstet Gynecol 2006;18(5):511–518.

89. Hadfield R, Mardon H, Barlow D, Kennedy S. Delay in the diagnosis of endometriosis: a survey of women from the USA and the UK. Hum Reprod 1996;11:878.

90. Greene R, Stratton P, Cleary SD et al. Diagnostic experience among 4,334 women reporting surgically diagnosed endometriosis. Fertil Steril 2009;91(1):32–39.

91. Khan KN, Masuzaki H, Fujishita A et al. Higher activity by opaque endometriotic lesions than nonopaque lesions. Acta Obstet Gynecol Scand 2004;83(4):375–382.

92. Redwine DB. Is "microscopic" peritoneal endometriosis invisible? Fertil Steril 1988;50(4):665–666.

93. Redwine DB, Yocom LB. A serial section study of visually normal pelvic peritoneum in patients with endometriosis. Fertil Steril 1990;54:648–651.

94. Nakamura M, Katabuchi H, Tohya T et al. Scanning electron microscopic and immunohistochemical studies of pelvic endometriosis. Hum Reprod 1993;8:2218–2226.

95. Murphy AA, Green WR, Bobbie D et al. Unsuspected endometriosis documented by scanning electron microscopy in visually normal peritoneum. Fertil Steril 1986;46:522–524.

96. Evers JLH, Land JA, Dunselman GAJ et al. "The Flemish Giant", reflections on the defense against endometriosis, inspired by Professor Emeritus Ivo A. Brosens. Eur J Obstet Gynecol Reprod Biol 1998;81:253–258.

97. D'Hooghe TM. Invisible microscopic endometriosis: how wrong is the sampson hypothesis of retrograde menstruation to explain the pathogenesis of endometriosis? Gynecol Obstet Invest 2003; 55(2):61–62.

98. Redwine DB. 'Invisible' microscopic endometriosis: a review. Gynecol Obstet Invest 2003;55(2):63–67.

99. Donnez J, Van Langendonckt A. Typical and subtle atypical presentations of endometriosis. Curr Opin Obstet Gynecol 2004; 16(5):431–437.

100. Missmer SA, Hankinson SE, Spiegelman D et al. Incidence of laparoscopically confirmed endometriosis by demographic, anthropometric, and lifestyle factors. Am J Epidemiol 2004; 160(8):784–796.

101. Buchweitz O, Wulfing P, Staebler A, Kiesel L. Detection of nonpigmented endometriotic lesions with 5-aminolevulinic acid-induced fluorescence. J Am Assoc Gynecol Laparosc 2004; 11(4):505–510.

102. Demco L. Laparoscopic spectral analysis of endometriosis. J Am Assoc Gynecol Laparosc 2004;11(2):219–222.

103. Barbieri RL. Primary gonadotropin-releasing hormone agonist therapy for suspected endometriosis: a nonsurgical approach to the diagnosis and treatment of chronic pelvic pain. Am J Manag Care 1997;3(2):285–290.

104. Cho S, Ahn YS, Choi YS et al. Endometrial osteopontin mRNA expression and plasma osteopontin levels are increased in patients with endometriosis. Am J Reprod Immunol 2009;61(4):286–293.

105. Sha G, Zhang Y, Zhang C et al. Elevated levels of gremlin-1 in eutopic endometrium and peripheral serum in patients with endometriosis. Fertil Steril 2009;91(2):350–358.

106. Barbieri RL, Bast RC, Niloff JM et al. Evaluation of a serological test for the diagnosis of endometriosis using a monoclonal antibody OC-125. SGI Annual Meeting, 1985.

107. Eskenazi B, Warner M, Bonsignore L, Olive D, Samuels S, Vercellini P. Validation study of nonsurgical diagnosis of endometriosis. Fertil Steril 2001;76:929–935.

108. Gagne D, Rivard M, Page M et al. Development of a nonsurgical diagnostic tool for endometriosis based on the detection of endometrial leukocyte subsets and serum CA-125 levels. Fertil Steril 2003;80(4):876–885.

109. Gupta S, Agarwal A, Sekhon L et al. Serum and peritoneal abnormalities in endometriosis: potential use as diagnostic markers. Minerva Ginecol 2006;58(6):527–551.

110. Othman Eel D, Hornung D, Salem HT et al. Serum cytokines as biomarkers for nonsurgical prediction of endometriosis. Eur J Obstet Gynecol Reprod Biol 2008;137(2):240–246.

111. Pittaway DE, Fayez JA. The use of CA-125 in the diagnosis and management of endometriosis. Fertil Steril 1986;46:790–795.

112. Pittaway DE. The use of serial CA 125 concentrations to monitor endometriosis in infertile women. Am J Obstet Gynecol 1990;163:1032–1035.

113. Pittaway DE, Rondinone D, Miller KA, Barnes K. Clinical evaluation of CA-125 concentrations as a prognostic factor for pregnancy in infertile women with surgically treated endometriosis. Fertil Steril 1995;64:321–324.

114. Bohler HC, Gercel-Taylor C, Lessey BA, Taylor DD. Endometriosis markers: immunologic alterations as diagnostic indicators for endometriosis. Reprod Sci 2007;14(6):595–604.

115. Taylor RN, Lundeen SG, Giudice LC. Emerging role of genomics in endometriosis research. Fertil Steril 2002;78(4):694–698.

116. Eyster KM, Boles AL, Brannian JD, Hansen KA. DNA microarray analysis of gene expression markers of endometriosis. Fertil Steril 2002;77:38–42.

117. Matsuzaki S, Canis M, Vaurs-Barriere C et al. DNA microarray analysis of gene expression in eutopic endometrium from patients with deep endometriosis using laser capture microdissection. Fertil Steril 2005;84(Suppl 2):1180–1190.

118. Burney RO, Hamilton AE, Aghajanova L et al. MicroRNA expression profiling of eutopic secretory endometrium in women with versus without endometriosis. Mol Hum Reprod 2009; 15(10):625–631.

119. Schwartz D, Mayaux MJ. Female fecundity as a function of age: results of artificial insemination in 2193 nulliparous women with azoospermic husbands. Federation CECOS. N Engl J Med 1982;306(7):404–406.

120. Hughes EG, Fedorkow DM, Collins JA. A quantitative overview of controlled trials in endometriosis-associated infertility. Fertil Steril 1993;59:963–970.

121. Toma SK, Stovall DW, Hammond MG. The effect of laparoscopic ablation or danocrine on pregnancy rates in patients with stage I or II endometriosis undergoing donor insemination. Obstet Gynecol 1992;80:253–256.

122. Olive DW, Stohs GF, Metzger DA, Franklin RR. Expectant management and hydrotubations in the treatment of endometriosis-associated infertility. Fertil Steril 1985;44:35–41.

123. Acosta AA, Buttram VC, Cesch PK. A proposed classification of pelvic endometriosis. Obstet Gynecol 1973;42:14–25.

124. American Fertility Society. Classification of endometriosis. Fertil Steril 1979;32(6):633–636.

125. American Fertility Society. Revised American Fertility Society classification of endomtriosis: 1985. Fertil Steril 1985;43:351–355.

126. Adamson GD, Pasta DJ. Endometriosis fertility index: the new, validated endometriosis staging system. Fertil Steril 2010; 94(5):1609–1615.

127. Bancroft K, Vaughan Williams CA, Elstein M. Minimal/mild endometriosis and infertility. A review. Br J Obstet Gynaecol 1989;96:454–460.

128. Endometriosis and infertility. Fertil Steril 2006;86(4):S156–S160.

129. Vernon MW. Experimental endometriosis in laboratory animals as a research model. Prog Clin Biol Res 1990;323:49–60.

130. Vernon MW, Wilson EA. Studies on the surgical induction of endometriosis in the rat. Fertil Steril 1985;44:684–694.

131. Schenken RS, Williams RF, Hodgen GD. Effect of pregnancy on surgically induced endometriosis in cynomolgus monkeys. Am J Obstet Gynecol 1987;157:1392.

132. Schenken RS, Asch RH, Williams RF, Hodgen GD. Etiology of infertility in monkeys with endometriosis: luteinized unruptured follicles, luteal phase defects, pelvic adhesions, and spontaneous abortions. Fertil Steril 1984;41:122–130.

133. Barragan JC, Brotons J, Ruiz JA, Acien P. Experimentally induced endometriosis in rats: effect on fertility and the effects of pregnancy and lactation on the ectopic endometrial tissue. Fertil Steril 1992;58:1215.

134. D'Hooghe TM, Bambra CS, Koninckx PR. Cycle fecundity in baboons of proven fertility with minimal endometriosis. Gynecol Obstet Invest 1994;37:63.

135. D'Hooghe TM, Bambra CS, Raeymaekers BM et al. The cycle pregnancy rate is normal in baboons with stage I endometriosis but decreased in primates with stage II and stage III-IV disease. Fertil Steril 1996;66(5):809–813.

136. Illera MJ, Juan L, Stewart CL et al. Effect of peritoneal fluid from women with endometriosis on implantation in the mouse model. Fertil Steril 2000;74(1):41–48.

137. Jackson KS, Brudney A, Hastings JM et al. The altered distribution of the steroid hormone receptors and the chaperone immunophilin FKBP52 in a baboon model of endometriosis is associated with progesterone resistance during the window of uterine receptivity. Reprod Sci 2007;14(2):137–150.

138. Kim JJ, Taylor HS, Lu Z et al. Altered expression of HOXA10 in endometriosis: potential role in decidualization. Mol Hum Reprod 2007;13(5):323–332.

139. Wang C, Mavrogianis PA, Fazleabas AT. Endometriosis is associated with progesterone resistance in the baboon (Papio anubis) oviduct: evidence based on the localization of oviductal glycoprotein 1 (OVGP1). Biol Reprod 2009;80(2):272–278.

140. Portuondo JA, Echanojauregui AD, Herran C, Alijarte I. Early conception in patients with untreated mild endometriosis. Fertil Steril 1983;39:22.

141. Rodriguez-Escudero FJ, Neyro JL, Corcostegui B, Benito JA. Does minimal endometriosis reduce fecundity? Fertil Steril 1988; 50(3):522–524.

142. Jansen RP. Minimal endometriosis and reduced fecundability: prospective evidence from an artificial insemination by donor program. Fertil Steril 1986;46:141–143.

143. Byrd W, Bradshaw K, Carr B et al. A prospective randomized study of pregnancy rates following intrauterine and intracervical insemination using frozen donor sperm. Fertil Steril 1990;53(3): 521–527.

144. Hughes EG. The effectiveness of ovulation induction and intrauterine insemination in the treatment of persistent infertility: a meta-analysis. Hum Reprod 1997;12:1865–1872.

145. Karabacak O, Kambic R, Gursoy R, Ozeren S. Does ovulation induction affect the pregnancy rate after laparoscopic treatment of endometriosis? Int J Fertil Womens Med 1999;44(1):38–42.

146. Deaton JL, Gibson M, Blackmer KM et al. A randomized, controlled trial of clomiphene citrate and intrauterine insemination in couples with unexplained infertility or surgically corrected endometriosis. Fertil Steril 1990;54:1083–1088.

147. Yovich JL, Matson PL. The influence of infertility etiology on the outcome of IVF-ET and GIFT treatments. Int J Fertil 1990;35:26–33.

148. Arici A, Oral E, Bukulmez O et al. The effect of endometriosis on implantation: results from the Yale University in vitro fertilization and embryo transfer program. Fertil Steril 1996;65:603–607.

149. Matson PL, Yovich JL. The treatment of infertility associated with endometriosis by in vitro fertilization. Fertil Steril 1986;46:432.

150. Chillik CF, Acosta AA, Garcia JE et al. The role of in vitro fertilization in infertile patients with endometriosis. Fertil Steril 1985;44:56.

151. Olivennes F, Feldberg D, Liu HC et al. Endometriosis: A stage by stage analysis – the role of in vitro fertilization. Fertil Steril 1995;64:392–398.

152. Alsalili M, Yuzpe A, Tummon I et al. Cumulative pregnancy rates and pregnancy outcome after in-vitro fertilization: > 5000 cycles at one centre. Hum Reprod 1995;10(2):470–474.

153. Guzick DS, Yao YAS, Berga SL et al. Endometriosis impairs the efficacy of gamete intrafallopian transfer: results of a case-control study. Fertil Steril 1994;62:1186–1191.

154. Barnhart KT, Dunsmoor R, Coutifaris C. The effect of endometriosis on in vitro fertilization. Fertil Steril 2002;77:1148–1155.

155. Balasch J, Creus M, Fábregues F et al. Visible and non-visible endometriosis at laparoscopy in fertile and infertile women and in patients with chronic pelvic pain: a prospective study. Hum Reprod 1996;11:387–391.

156. Doody MC, Gibbons WE, Buttram VC Jr. Linear regression analysis of ultrasound follicular growth series: evidence for an abnormality of follicular growth in endometriosis patients. Fertil Steril 1988;49:47–51.

157. Wardle PG, Mitchell JD, McLaughlin EA et al. Endometriosis and ovulatory disorder: reduced fertilisation in vitro compared with tubal and unexplained infertility. Lancet 1985;2(8449):236–239.

158. Soules MR, Makinak LR, Bury R, Poindexter A. Endometriosis and anovulation: a coexisting problem in the infertile female. Am J Obstet Gynecol 1976;125:412–417.

159. Pellicer A, Oliveira N, Ruiz A et al. Exploring the mechanism(s) of endometriosis-related infertility: an analysis of embryo development and implantation in assisted reproduction. Hum Reprod 1995;10(Suppl 2):91–97.

160. Cheesman KL, Cheesman SD, Chatterton RT Jr, Cohen MR. Alterations in progesterone metabolism and luteal function in infertile women with endometriosis. Fertil Steril 1983; 40:590–595.

161. Ayers JW, Birenbaum DL, Menon KM. Luteal phase dysfunction in endometriosis: elevated progesterone levels in peripheral and ovarian veins during the follicular phase. Fertil Steril 1987; 47:925–929.

162. Cheesman KL, Ben-Nun I, Chatterton RT Jr, Cohen MR. Relationship of luteinizing homrone, pregnanediol-3-glucoronide and estriol-16-glucuronide in urine of infertile women with endometriosis. Fertil Steril 1982;38:542–548.

163. Suginami H, Yano K, Nakahashi N, Takeda Y. Fallopian tube and fimbrial function in endometriosis: with a special reference to an ovum capture inhibitor. Prog Clin Biol Res 1990;323:81–97.

164. Drake TS, O'Brien WF, Ramwell PW, Metz SA. Peritoneal fluid thromboxane B2 and 6-Keto-prostaglandin F2 alpha in endometriosis. Am J Obstet Gynecol 1981;140:401–404.

165. Muscato JJ, Haney AF, Weinberg JB. Sperm phagocytosis by human peritoneal macrophages: a possible cause of infertility in endometriosis. Am J Obstet Gynecol 1982;144:503–510.

166. Soldati G, Piffaretti-Yanez A, Campana A et al. Effect of peritoneal fluid on sperm motility and velocity distribution using objective measurements. Fertil Steril 1989;52:113–119.

167. Chacho KJ, Chacho MS, Andresen PJ, Scommegna A. Peritoneal fluid in patients with and without endometriosis: prostanoids and macrophages and their effect on the spermatozoa penetration assay. Am J Obstet Gynecol 1986;154:1290.

168. Sueldo CE, Lambert H, Steinleitner A et al. The effect of peritoneal fluid from patients with endometriosis on murine sperm-oocyte interaction. Fertil Steril 1987;48:697–699.

169. Coddington CC, Oehninger S, Cunningham DS et al. Peritoneal fluid from patients with endometriosis decreases sperm binding to the zona-pellucida in the hemizona assay: a preliminary report. Fertil Steril 1992;57:783–786.

170. Morcos RN, Gibbons WE, Findley WE. Effect of peritoneal fluid on in vitro cleavage of 2-cell mouse embryos: possible role in infertility associated with endometriosis. Fertil Steril 1986;44:678–683.

171. Damewood MD, Hesla JS, Schlaff WD et al. Effect of serum from patients with minimal to mild endometriosis on mouse embryo development in vitro. Fertil Steril 1990;54:917–920.

172. Bulletti C, de Ziegler D. Uterine contractility and embryo implantation. Curr Opin Obstet Gynecol 2006;18(4):473–484.

173. Drake TS, Metz SA, Grunert GM, O'Brien WF. Peritoneal fluid volume in endometriosis. Fertil Steril 1980;34:280–281.

174. Badawy SZA, Cuenca V, Marshall L et al. Cellular components in peritoneal fluid in infertile patients with and without endometriosis. Fertil Steril 1984;42:704–708.

175. Koninckx PR, Riittinen L, Seppala M, Cornillie FJ. CA-125 and placental protein-14 concentrations in plasma and peritoneal fluid of women with deeply infiltrating pelvic endometriosis. Fertil Steril 1992;57:523–530.

176. Oosterlynck DJ, Meuleman C, Waer M et al. The natural killer activity of peritoneal fluid lymphocytes is decreased in women with endometriosis. Fertil Steril 1992;58:290–295.

177. Fairbanks F, Abrao MS, Podgaec S et al. Interleukin-12 but not interleukin-18 is associated with severe endometriosis. Fertil Steril 2009;91(2):320–324.

178. Ferrero S, Gillott DJ, Remorgida V et al. Proteomic analysis of peritoneal fluid in fertile and infertile women with endometriosis. J Reprod Med 2009;54(1):32–40.

179. Tariverdian N, Siedentopf F, Rucke M et al. Intraperitoneal immune cell status in infertile women with and without endometriosis. J Reprod Immunol 2009;80(1–2):80–90.

180. Halme J, Mathur S. Local autoimmunity in mild endometriosis. Int J Fertil 1987;32:309–311.

181. Haney AF, Muscata JJ, Weinberg JB. Peritoneal fluid cell populations in infertility patients. Fertil Steril 1981;35:696–698.

182. Haney AF, Weinberg JB. Reduction of the intraperitoneal inflammation associated with endometriosis by treatment with medroxyprogesterone acetate. Am J Obstet Gynecol 1988;159:450–454.

183. Halme J. Role of peritoneal inflammation in endometriosis-associated infertility. Ann N Y Acad Sci 1991;622:266–272.

184. Haney AF, Jenkins S, Weinberg JB. The stimulus responsible for the peritoneal fluid inflammation observed in infertile women with endometriosis. Fertil Steril 1991;56:408–413.

185. Scholl B, Bersinger NA, Kuhn A, Mueller MD. Correlation between symptoms of pain and peritoneal fluid inflammatory cytokine concentrations in endometriosis. Gynecol Endocrinol 2009; 25(11):701–706.

186. Morcos RN, Gibbons WE, Findley WE. Effect of peritoneal fluid on in vitro cleavage of 2-cell mouse embryos: possible role in infertility associated with endometriosis. Fertil Steril 1985;44:678–683.

187. Oak MK, Chantler EN, Williams CA, Elstein M. Sperm survival studies in peritoneal fluid from infertile women with endometriosis and unexplained infertility. Clin Reprod Fertil 1985; 3:297–303.

188. Suginami H, Yano K, Watanabe K, Matsuura S. A factor inhibiting ovum capture by the oviductal fimbriae present in endometriosis peritoneal fluid. Fertil Steril 1986;46:1140–1146.

189. Prough SG, Aksel S, Gilmore SM, Yeoman RR. Peritoneal fluid fractions from patients with endometriosis do not promote two-cell mouse embryo growth. Fertil Steril 1990;54:927–930.

190. Steinleitner A, Lambert H, Kazensky C, Danks P. Peritoneal fluid from endometriosis patients affects reproductive outcome in an in vivo model. Fertil Steril 1990;53:926–929.

191. Surrey ES, Halme J. Effect of peritoneal fluid from endometriosis patients on endometrial stromal cell proliferation in vitro. Obstet Gynecol 1990;76:792–797.

192. Taketani Y, Kuo TM, Mizuno M. Comparison of cytokine levels and embryo toxicity in peritoneal fluid in infertile women with untreated or treated endometriosis. Am J Obstet Gynecol 1992; 167:265–270.

193. Bielfeld P, Graf MA, Jeyendran RS et al. Effects of peritoneal fluids from patients with endometriosis on capacitated spermatozoa. Fertil Steril 1993;60:893–896.

194. Tasdemir M, Tasdemir I, Kodama H, Tanaka T. Effect of peritoneal fluid from infertile women with endometriosis on ionophore-stimulated acrosome loss. Hum Reprod 1995;10:2419–2422.

195. Aeby TC, Huang T, Nakayama RT. The effect of peritoneal fluid from patients with endometriosis on human sperm function in vitro. Am J Obstet Gynecol 1996;174:1779–1783.

196. Oral E, Arici A, Olive DL, Huszar G. Peritoneal fluid from women with moderate or severe endometriosis inhibits sperm motility: the role of seminal fluid components. Fertil Steril 1996;66: 787–792.

197. Seli E, Zeyneloglu HB, Senturk LM et al. Basic fibroblast growth factor: peritoneal and follicular fluid levels and its effect on early embryonic development. Fertil Steril 1998;69:1145–1148.

198. Selam B, Arici A. Implantation defect in endometriosis: endometrium or peritoneal fluid. J Reprod Fertil 2000; 55(Suppl):121–128.

199. Fedele L, Marchini M, Bianchi S et al. Structural and ultrastructural defects in preovulatory endometrium of normo-ovulating infertile women with minimal or mild endometriosis. Fertil Steril 1990; 53:989–993.

200. Weed JC, Arguembourg PC. Endometriosis: can it produce an auto-immune response resulting in infertility? Clin Obstet Gynecol 1980;23:885–893.

201. Sharpe-Timms KL. Endometrial anomalies in women with endometriosis. Ann N Y Acad Sci 2001;943:131–144.

202. Aghajanova L, Hamilton A, Kwintkiewicz J et al. Steroidogenic enzyme and key decidualization marker dysregulation in endometrial stromal cells from women with versus without endometriosis. Biol Reprod 2009;80(1):105–114.

203. Nisolle M, Donnez J. Peritoneal endometriosis, ovarian endometriosis, and adenomyotic nodules of the rectovaginal septum are three different entities. Fertil Steril 1997;68:585–596.

204. Fujishita A, Hasuo A, Khan KN et al. Immunohistochemical study of angiogenic factors in endometrium and endometriosis. Gynecol Obstet Invest 1999;48(Suppl 1):36–44.

205. Matsuzaki S, Canis M, Darcha C et al. HOXA-10 expression in the mid-secretory endometrium of infertile patients with either endometriosis, uterine fibromas or unexplained infertility. Hum Reprod 2009;24(12):3180–3187.

206. Donnez J, Nisolle M, Smoes P et al. Peritoneal endometriosis and "endometriotic" nodules of the rectovaginal septum are two different entities. Fertil Steril 1996;66:362–368.

207. Littman E, Giudice L, Lathi R et al. Role of laparoscopic treatment of endometriosis in patients with failed in vitro fertilization cycles. Fertil Steril 2005;84(6):1574–1578.

208. Daftary GS, Troy PJ, Bagot CN et al. Direct regulation of beta3-integrin subunit gene expression by HOXA10 in endometrial cells. Mol Endocrinol 2002;16(3):571–579.

209. Giudice LC, Telles TL, Lobo S, Kao L. The molecular basis for implantation failure in endometriosis: on the road to discovery. Ann N Y Acad Sci 2002;955:252–264; discussion 293–295, 396–406.

210. De Ziegler D. Endometrial receptivity for implantation. Hormonal control of endometrial receptivity. Hum Reprod 1995;10:4–7.

211. De Ziegler D, Bergeron C, Cornel C et al. Effects of luteal estradiol on the secretory transformation of human endometrium and plasma gonadotropins. J Clin Endocrinol Metab 1992;74:322–331.

212. Wentz AC. Premenstrual spotting: its association with endometriosis with no luteal phase inadequacy. Fertil Steril 1980;34:605–607.

213. Tabibzadeh S, Shea W, Lessey BA, Satyaswaroop PG. Aberrant expression of ebaf in endometria of patients with infertility. Mol Hum Reprod 1998;4:595.

214. Tabibzadeh S, Shea W, Lessey BA, Broome J. From endometrial receptivity to infertility. Semin Reprod Endocrinol 1999; 17(3):197–203.

215. Tabibzadeh S, Mason JM, Shea W et al. Dysregulated expression of ebaf, a novel molecular defect in the endometria of patients with infertility. J Clin Endocrinol Metab 2000;85(7):2526–2536.

216. Cornet PB, Picquet C, Lemoine P et al. Regulation and function of LEFTY-A/EBAF in the human endometrium. mRNA expression during the menstrual cycle, control by progesterone, and effect on matrix metalloprotineases. J Biol Chem 2002;277(45): 42496–42504.

217. Isaacson KB, Galman M, Coutifaris C, Lyttle CR. Endometrial synthesis and secretion of complement component-3 by patients with and without endometriosis. Fertil Steril 1990;53:836–841.

218. Bruner-Tran KL, Zhang Z, Eisenberg E et al. Down-regulation of endometrial matrix metalloproteinase-3 and -7 expression in vitro and therapeutic regression of experimental endometriosis in vivo by a novel nonsteroidal progesterone receptor agonist, tanaproget. J Clin Endocrinol Metab 2006;91(4):1554–1560.

219. Minici F, Tiberi F, Tropea A et al. Endometriosis and human infertility: a new investigation into the role of eutopic endometrium. Hum Reprod 2008;23(3):530–537.

220. Talbi S, Hamilton AE, Vo KC et al. Molecular phenotyping of human endometrium distinguishes menstrual cycle phases and underlying biological processes in normo-ovulatory women. Endocrinology 2006;147(3):1097–1121.

221. Lessey BA. Implantation defects in infertile women with endometriosis. Ann N Y Acad Sci 2002;955:265–280; discussion 293–295, 396–406.

222. Chrousos GP, MacLusky NJ, Brandon DD et al. Progesterone resistance. Adv Exp Med Biol 1986;196:317–328.

223. Lessey BA, Alexander S, Horwitz KB. The subunit structure of human breast cancer progesteorne receptor: characterization by chromatography and photoaffinity labeling. Endocrinology 1982; 112:1267.

224. Conneely OM, Jericevic BM. Progesterone regulation of reproductive function through functionaliy distinct progesterone receptor isoforms. Rev Endocr Metab Disord 2002;3:201–209.

225. Attia GR, Zeitoun K, Edwards D et al. Progesterone receptor isoform A but not B is expressed in endometriosis. J Clin Endocrinol Metab 2000;85(8):2897–2902.

226. Wu Y, Halverson G, Basir Z et al. Aberrant methylation at HOXA10 may be responsible for its aberrant expression in the endometrium of patients with endometriosis. Am J Obstet Gynecol 2005; 193(2):371–380.

227. Igarashi TM, Bruner-Tran KL, Yeaman GR et al. Reduced expression of progesterone receptor-B in the endometrium of women with endometriosis and in cocultures of endometrial cells exposed to 2,3,7,8-tetrachlorodibenzo-p-dioxin. Fertil Steril 2005;84(1):67–74.

228. Lessey BA, Yeh I, Castelbaum AJ et al. Endometrial progesterone receptors and markers of uterine receptivity in the window of implantation. Fertil Steril 1996;65(3):477–483.

229. Rowan BG, O'Malley BW. Progesterone receptor coactivators. Steroids 2000;65(10–11):545–549.

230. Gregory CW, Wilson EM, Apparao KB et al. Steroid receptor coactivator expression throughout the menstrual cycle in normal and abnormal endometrium. J Clin Endocrinol Metab 2002; 87(6):2960–2966.

231. Quezada S, Avellaira C, Johnson MC et al. Evaluation of steroid receptors, coregulators, and molecules associated with uterine receptivity in secretory endometria from untreated women with polycystic ovary syndrome. Fertil Steril 2006;85(4):1017–1026.

232. Hubler TR, Denny WB, Valentine DL et al. The FK506-binding immunophilin FKBP51 is transcriptionally regulated by progestin and attenuates progestin responsiveness. Endocrinology 2003;144(6):2380–2387.

233. Tranguch S, Cheung-Flynn J, Daikoku T et al. Cochaperone immunophilin FKBP52 is critical to uterine receptivity for embryo implantation. Proc Natl Acad Sci USA 2005;102(40):14326–14331.

234. Tranguch S, Smith DF, Dey SK. Progesterone receptor requires a cochaperone for signalling in uterine biology and implantation. Reprod Biomed Online 2006;13(5):651–660.

235. Tranguch S, Wang H, Daikoku T et al. FKBP52 deficiency-conferred uterine progesterone resistance is genetic background and pregnancy stage specific. J Clin Invest 2007;117(7):1824–1834.

236. Hirota Y, Tranguch S, Daikoku T et al. Deficiency of immunophilin FKBP52 promotes endometriosis. Am J Pathol 2008;173(6): 1747–1757.

237. Aghajanova L, Velarde MC, Giudice LC. The progesterone receptor coactivator Hic-5 is involved in the pathophysiology of endometriosis. Endocrinology 2009;150(8):3863–3870.

238. Zhang XL, Zhang D, Michel FJ et al. Selective interactions of Kruppel-like factor 9/basic transcription element-binding protein with progesterone receptor isoforms A and B determine transcriptional activity of progesterone-responsive genes in endometrial epithelial cells. J Biol Chem 2003;278(24):21474–21482.

239. Simmen RC, Simmen FA. Progesterone receptors and Sp/Kruppel-like family members in the uterine endometrium. Front Biosci 2002;7:1556–1565.

240. Simmen RC, Zhang XL, Michel FJ et al. Molecular markers of endometrial epithelial cell mitogenesis mediated by the Sp/Kruppel-like factor BTEB1. DNA Cell Biol 2002;21(2):115–128.

241. Lee B, Du H, Taylor HS. Experimental murine endometriosis induces DNA methylation and altered gene expression in eutopic endometrium. Biol Reprod 2009;80(1):79–85.

242. Kuokkanen S, Chen B, Ojalvo L et al. Genomic profiling of microRNAs and messenger RNAs reveals hormonal regulation in MicroRNA expression in human endometrium. Biol Reprod 2010;82(4):791–801.

243. Pan Q, Luo X, Toloubeydokhti T, Chegini N. The expression profile of micro-RNA in endometrium and endometriosis and the influence of ovarian steroids on their expression. Mol Hum Reprod 2007;13(11):797–806.

244. Pan Q, Chegini N. MicroRNA signature and regulatory functions in the endometrium during normal and disease states. Semin Reprod Med 2008;26(6):479–493.

245. Ohlsson Teague EM, Print CG, Hull ML. The role of microRNAs in endometriosis and associated reproductive conditions. Hum Reprod Update 2010;16(2):142–165.

246. Ohlsson Teague EM, van der Hoek KH, van der Hoek MB et al. MicroRNA-regulated pathways associated with endometriosis. Mol Endocrinol 2009;23(2):265–275.

247. Kitawaki J, Kusuki I, Koshiba H et al. Detection of aromatase cytochrome P-450 in endometrial biopsy specimens as a diagnostic test for endometriosis. Fertil Steril 1999;72:1100–1106.

248. Noble LS, Simpson ER, Johns A, Bulun SE. Aromatase expression in endometriosis. J Clin Endocrinol Metab 1996;81:174–179.

249. Tabibzadeh S, Lessey B, Satyaswaroop PG. Temporal and site-specific expression of transforming growth factor-beta4 in human endometrium. Mol Hum Reprod 1998;4(6):595–602.

250. Pottratz ST, Bellido T, Mocharla H et al. 17 beta-Estradiol inhibits expression of human interleukin-6 promoter-reporter constructs by a receptor-dependent mechanism. J Clin Invest 1994;93:944.

251. Kim TH, Lee DK, Franco HL et al. ERBB receptor feedback inhibitor 1 regulation of estrogen receptor activity is critical for uterine implantation in mice. Biol Reprod 2010;82(4):706–713.

252. Bai S, Grossman G, Yuan L et al. Hormone control and expression of androgen receptor coregulator MAGE-11 in human endometrium during the window of receptivity to embryo implantation. Mol Hum Reprod 2008;14(2):107–116.

253. Guzeloglu-Kayisli O, Kayisli UA, Taylor HS. The role of growth factors and cytokines during implantation: endocrine and paracrine interactions. Semin Reprod Med 2009;27(1):62–79.

254. Bruner KL, Rodgers WH, Gold LI et al. Transforming growth factor beta mediates the progesterone suppression of an epithelial metalloproteinase by adjacent stroma in the human endometrium. Proc Natl Acad Sci USA 1995;92(16):7362–7366.

255. Mazella J, Tang M, Tseng L. Disparate effects of relaxin and TGFbeta1: relaxin increases, but TGFbeta1 inhibits, the relaxin receptor and the production of IGFBP-1 in human endometrial stromal/decidual cells. Hum Reprod 2004;19(7):1513–1518.

256. Jeong J-W, Lee HS, Lee KY et al. Mig-6 modulates uterine steroid receptor responsiveness and exhibits altered expression in endometrial disease. Proc Natl Acad Sci USA 2009;106:8677–8682.

257. Jin N, Gilbert JL, Broaddus RR et al. Generation of a Mig-6 conditional null allele. Genesis 2007;45(11):716–721.

258. Aghajanova L, Hamilton AE, Giudice LC. Uterine receptivity to human embryonic implantation: histology, biomarkers, and transcriptomics. Semin Cell Dev Biol 2008;19(2):204–211.

259. Rogers PA, D'Hooghe TM, Fazleabas A et al. Priorities for endometriosis research: recommendations from an international consensus workshop. Reprod Sci 2009;16(4):335–346.

260. Daya S. Endometriosis and spontaneous abortion. Inf Reprod Med Clin North Am 1996;7:759–773.

261. Evers JL. The pregnancy rate of the no-treatment group in randomized clinical trials of endometriosis therapy. Fertil Steril 1989;52:906–907.

262. Nowroozi K, Chase JS, Check JH, Wu CH. The importance of laparoscopic coagulation of mild endometriosis in infertile women. Int J Fertil 1987;32(6):442–444.

263. Marcoux S, Maheux R, Berube S. Laparoscopic surgery in infertile women with minimal or mild endometriosis. Canadian Collaborative Group on Endometriosis. N Engl J Med 1997;337(4):217–222.

264. Surrey ES, Silverberg KM, Surrey MW, Schoolcraft WB. Effect of prolonged gonadotropin-releasing hormone agonist therapy on the outcome of in vitro fertilization-embryo transfer in patients with endometriosis. Fertil Steril 2002;78:699–704.

265. Kim CH, Cho YK, Mok JE. Simplified ultralong protocol of gonadotrophin-releasing hormone agonist for ovulation induction with intrauterine insemination in patients with endometriosis. Hum Reprod 1996;11:398–402.

266. Musich JR, Behrman SJ. Infertility laparoscopy in perspective: review of five hundred cases. Am J Obstet Gynecol 1982; 143(3):293–303.

267. Guo SW. Recurrence of endometriosis and its control. Hum Reprod Update 2009;15(4):441–461.

268. Parazzini F, Di Cintio E, Chatenoud L et al. Ablation of lesions or no treatment in minimal-mild endometriosis in infertile women: a randomized trial. Hum Reprod 1999;14:1332–1334.

269. Hulme VA, van der Merwe JP, Kruger TF. Gamete intrafallopian transfer as treatment for infertility associated with endometriosis. Fertil Steril 1990;53:1095.

270. Brosens IA, Koninckx PR, Corveleyn PA. A study of plasma progesterone, oestradiol-17·, prolactin and LH levels, and of the luteal phase appearance of the ovaries in patients with endometriosis and infertility. Br J Obstet Gynaecol 1978;85:246–250.

271. Bullock JL, Massey FM, Gambrell RD. Symptomatic endometriosis in teenagers. A reappraisal. Obstet Gynecol 1974;43:896–900.

272. Cunanan RG Jr, Courey NG, Lippes J. Laparoscopic findings in patients with pelvic pain. Am J Obstet Gynecol 1983; 146(5):589–591.

273. Kresch AJ, Seifer DB, Sachs LB et al. Laparoscopy in 100 women with chronic pelvic pain. Obstet Gynecol 1984;64:672.

274. Lessey BA, Castelbaum AJ, Sawin SJ et al. Aberrant integrin expression in the endometrium of women with endometriosis. J Clin Endocrinol Metab 1994;79:643–649.

275. Dey SK, Lim H, Das SK et al. Molecular cues to implantation. Endocr Rev 2004;25(3):341–373.

276. Ramanthal CY, Bagchi IC, Taylor RN et al. Endometrial decidualization: of mice and men. Semin Reprod Endocrinol 2010; 28(1):17–26.

24 Inflammation and Endometriosis

Daniela Hornung and Ursula von Wussow

Department of Obstetrics and Gynecology, University of Schleswig-Holstein, Lübeck, Germany

Implantation hypothesis

Although multiple theories exist regarding the etiology of endometriosis, the implantation hypothesis of Sampson is the most commonly accepted. Retrograde menstruation and peritoneal dispersion of viable endometrial epithelial cells occur frequently in women of reproductive age. Only 7–15% of these women develop clinical evidence of this syndrome.

Shed endometrial fragments are supposed to adhere to peritoneal surfaces, get into contact with the submesothelial matrix, proliferate and invade deeply into the subperitoneal space. Thus, sustaining factors must support the persistence of endometriotic lesions within the peritoneum of affected women. Furthermore, a malfunctioning immune surveillance may support the attachment and progression of ectopic endometrial tissue in these women. Several studies have indicated immune cell suppression or dysfunction in endometriosis.

C-reactive protein and serum amyloid A

C-reactive protein (CRP) and serum amyloid A (SAA) are serum protein markers arising during acute inflammatory phases. Increased CRP resulting from acute inflammatory processes seems to be directly proportional to the amount of tissue damage and is basically used as a marker in rheumatic diseases. The clinical application for SAA as a serum marker currently ranges from systemic amyloidosis to other inflammatory incidents. Although extensively studied in recent years, the role of the acute phase proteins CRP and SAA in endometriosis is sparsely documented. There are reports of increased serum levels of CRP and SAA in patients with stage III and IV endometriosis compared to those of healthy women [1]. An increase in both proteins with an elevation of interleukin (IL)-1, IL-6 and tumor necrosis factor (TNF)-α [2,3] and the correlation between increased CRP and vascular endothelial growth factor (VEGF) levels in endometriosis allow inference of the disease [4]. Although Lermann and colleagues found no correlation between CPR and disease stage in endometriosis, the protein has been shown to have marker potential to exclude endometriosis [5]. However, CRP and SAA are elevated in the majority of inflammatory processes and using them as a diagnostic tool for endometriosis necessitates exclusion of any other inflammatory cause [6].

Complement system and immunoglobulins

In 1980, Weed and Arquembourg first suggested the idea of endometriosis as an autoimmune response to local activation and consumption of complement factors by antigen-antibody complexes. This theory could not be definitely confirmed, since results of immunoglobulins and complement factors are very inhomogeneous. With regard to serum and peritoneal concentrations of immunoglobulin, some authors reported decreased [7], others increased [8,9] concentrations, even with correlation between the concentration and the clinical stage of the disease [10], and others reported no difference in concentrations at all [11–13]. Complement factor measurements also revealed inequalities. For women suffering from endometriosis, C3 and C4 levels have been increased in some reports [10,14], identical to those of healthy women in other studies [12,13,15] or even decreased [7,8].

Immunoglobulin (Ig) G precipitation in the conducted experiments was very unspecific and can be found in other pelvic inflammatory diseases [14,15]. In addition, factors regulating the activation of complement have been identified in endometrial cells [16]. Since it has become evident that endometrial cells are capable of producing complement factors by themselves [17–19], the presence of antibodies and activated complement factors cannot act as proof of a specific immune response.

Cellular immunity

Endometriosis is proposed to be associated with a dysfunction of immune cells, which mostly have been studied in the peritoneal

Endometriosis: Science and Practice, First Edition. Edited by Linda C. Giudice, Johannes L.H. Evers and David L. Healy.
© 2012 Blackwell Publishing Ltd. Published 2012 by Blackwell Publishing Ltd.

cavity [20,21]. Under normal conditions, peritoneal leukocytes delete ectopic endometrial cells, but in women suffering from endometriosis, the elimination ability of peritoneal leukocytes is significantly decreased. In a cascade of deteriorating events, the response of the immune cells promotes implantation, proliferation and development of endometrial cells into endometriosis and thereby assists in recruiting and activating peritoneal macrophages [20].

In several studies, the ratio of leukocyte populations in peritoneal fluid of healthy women and patients with endometriosis was compared to determine if the dysfunction of immune cells contributes to a change in their population number [21–24]. In additional studies, those changes were also measurable in the peripheral blood of patients with endometriosis [6,21,25,26].

One of the important changes in the peritoneal fluid of women suffering from endometriosis is the significant increase in activated macrophages [6,11,27–32]. Most of these macrophages derive from monocytes of the peripheral blood, migrated through the endothelial wall. Gagné *et al* showed a significant increase of monocytes co-expressing CD14+ and high levels of CD44 (HDLR) as well as subsets of CD14+ monocytes in the blood of patients with endometriosis compared with healthy women [26]. Considering that CD44 is a known adhesion molecule with pivotal functions in activation and homing of immune cells to inflammatory sites [6,33], it seems to be conclusive that increased levels of CD14+ CD44+ blood monocytes are activated and recruited to inflammatory sites in the peritoneal cavity. It has been postulated that activated blood monocytes from patients with endometriosis could also promote the adherence of endometrial cells in the peritoneal cavity and the development of endometriotic lesions [34,35]. Ho *et al* [21], Wu *et al* [23] and Gagné *et al* [26] reported slight but significant decreases in CD3+ T-lymphocytes and B-lymphocytes in the peritoneal fluid and peripheral blood of patients with endometriosis in contrast to healthy women, whereas others found increased serum levels of B-lymphocyte stimulator (BlyS) in patients with endometriosis [36].

The activity of natural killer (NK) cells is decreased in the peritoneal fluid of women with endometriosis [37], and significant correlations between the level of decrease and the disease stage have also been found [25]. Moreover, NK cell cytotoxicity in the peritoneal fluid of women with endometriosis stage III and IV was significantly reduced in relation to controls [38]. However, in the peripheral blood no changes in the number or activity of NK cells were detectable [26,39,40].

Cytokines and growth factors

Cytokines and growth factors are proteins or glycoproteins usually expressed by leukocytes and other cells and secreted into the extracellular environment, where they exert autocrine or paracrine effects. As some of these cytokines are able to circulate, they may also exert endocrine activities. Under certain circumstances, cytokines are present in cell membrane-associated forms, where they also affect adjacent cells in a juxtacrine way.

In general, intercellular communication within the immune system is mediated by cytokines. They act on a variety of target cells by proliferation, cell cycle arrest, chemoattraction or differentiation. Their biological activity normally ranges in high pM concentrations and is mostly coupled to intracellular signaling and second messenger pathways through specific high-affinity receptors on their target cells.

RANTES and CCR1

RANTES (Regulated on Activation, Normal T-Cell Expressed and Secreted) is a cytokine of the C-C chemokine family discovered in the early 1990s. It is a selective and very potent monocyte, macrophage, T-lymphocyte and eosinophil chemoattractant *in vivo* and *in vitro* [41]. First identified as secreted by hematopoietic cells, RANTES has been shown to be secreted by epithelial and mesenchymal cells and is a crucial mediator in acute and chronic inflammation. Regulation of the RANTES gene takes place through various potential binding sites for transcription factors. Specific early- and late-activating transcription factor complexes have been described [42–44].

In unaffected endometrium, RANTES protein is mainly found in the stromal compartment. *In vitro*, stromal cell cultures synthesize RANTES mRNA and secrete the protein after TNF-α and interferon (INF)-γ stimulation, whereas the epithelial cells synthesize neither transcripts nor protein. The inconsistency between basal RANTES expression *in vivo* and *in vitro*, and the requisition of cytokine stimulation in the cell cultures for expression of the chemokine suggest that cytokines from local immune cells stimulate these paracrine effects *in vivo*. To achieve significant increases in RANTES gene expression in the culture of purified cells, exogenous TNF-α has to be added [45].

In endometriotic lesions, RANTES protein distribution was similar to that found by immunolocalization in normal endometrium [45]. However, there are several differences between normal endometrial stromal cell cultures and those derived from endometriotic tissues. Even under the same culture conditions, stromal cells derived from endometriotic tissues secrete significantly higher levels of RANTES compared to stromal cells from endometrium [46]. Thus, peritoneal implants might contribute to the significant increase of RANTES measured in the peritoneal fluid of patients with endometriosis. In addition, the chemokine levels correlate to the severity of disease [27].

Furthermore, around 70% of the monocyte chemotactic activity in the peritoneal fluid from women with endometriosis is mediated by RANTES [29]. Lebovic and colleagues reported a feedforward regulatory loop in the pathogenesis of endometriosis: IL-1β produced by activated macrophages leads to further macrophage recruitment via RANTES production in endometrial stromal cells [47,48]. Fang *et al* [49] showed increased RANTES expression and higher monocyte chemotactic activity after IL-1β stimulation in endometrial stromal cells.

The cognate chemokine receptor (CCR) 1 is a 7 transmembrane domain G-protein-coupled receptor with high affinity for RANTES. CCR1 is expressed on the surface of neutrophil/mononuclear leukocytes [50,51]. Currently, there are no reported data about increased RANTES levels in the serum of women with endometriosis. Kalu *et al* reported slight but not significant differences in RANTES serum concentrations between healthy women and those with endometriosis [52], but Agic *et al* reported significantly higher levels of CCR mRNA in peripheral blood leukocytes of patients with endometriosis compared to controls [53]. Furthermore, Wieser *et al* found higher concentrations of CCR1 protein in peritoneal macrophages form patients with endometriosis compared to healthy controls [54]. These results led to the suggested use of CCR1 mRNA as a serum marker for the diagnosis or exclusion of endometriosis in combination with MCP1 and CA-125 protein [55].

Tumor necrosis factor-α

Tumor necrosis factors are pleiotropic cytokines that play a pivotal role in the inflammatory process. TNFs exert a wide range of beneficial and hazardous effects, depending on the amount and tissue localization of the cytokine, as well as the local activity of TNF-binding proteins. TNF-α is produced by neutrophils, activated lymphocytes, macrophages, NK cells and several other non-hematopoietic cells, whereas TNF-β is produced by lymphocytes. Initially identified for their ability to kill cell lines, their essential function is the initiation of the cytokine cascade and other factors associated with inflammatory responses.

In the human endometrium, TNF-α has been implicated in the physiological endometrial proliferation and shedding, with highest expression of mRNA and protein in the epithelial cells during the secretory phase [56]. Expression of TNF-α in stromal cells is present predominantly during the proliferative phase, suggesting differential local and hormonal regulation of the cytokine [57].

The secretion of TNF-α in cultured epithelial cells is modulated by IL-1, progesterone and PP14 (endometrial placental protein) [58]. TNF-α has been shown to increase prostaglandin production by cultured endometrial epithelial cells and to promote the adherence of cultured stromal cells to the mesothelium [59,60]. Generally, TNF-α is involved in the genesis of adherence since it leads to fibroblast proliferation and precipitation of collagen [14]. Iwabe *et al* demonstrated that TNF-α stimulates the proliferation of endometriotic stromal cells through the induction of IL-8 gene and protein expression and concluded that TNF-α may therefore be one of the essential factors for the pathogenesis of endometriosis [61]. Several investigators have shown elevated TNF-α levels in the peritoneal fluid of patients with endometriosis, and that this increase correlates to the stage of the disease [62,63]. In addition, numerous studies reported higher TNF-α serum levels in women suffering from endometriosis compared to healthy controls, especially in the early stages of the disease. These findings point to the involvement and importance of acute inflammatory processes in the onset of endometriosis [64,65].

Monocyte chemotactic protein-1

Monocyte chemotactic protein (MCP)-1 is a potent chemotactic and monocyte activation factor [28]. It is secreted by different cell types including endothelial cells, fibroblasts, and leukocytes. Fibroblasts secrete MCP-1 dependent on platelet-derived growth factor (PDGF) stimulation [66], whereas leukocyte MCP-1 secretion is induced by phytohemagglutinin (PHA), lipopolysaccharide (LPS) and IL-1 [67]. Under normal conditions, increased MCP-1 levels are seen in the peritoneal fluid obtained from women in the proliferative phase of their cycle in contrast to peritoneal fluid of women in the secretory phase. More severe increases were measurable in peritoneal fluid from patients with endometriosis, and a correlation with severity of disease was observable [68].

High levels of MCP-1 are likely to play a role in the maintenance and growth of ectopic endometrial lesions by stimulating macrophages to secrete cytokines and growth factors and by direct stimulation of the proliferation [68]. Several investigators have found significantly increased levels of MCP-1 in serum or peritoneal fluid of women with endometriosis compared to healthy controls [52,64,69–72]. Akoum *et al* [69] and Pizzo *et al* [64] reported large increases in peritoneal fluid at the early stages, decreasing with severity of disease. The early observed increases in MCP-1 and IL-8 could also be due to the involvement of circulating monocytes and massive amounts of cytokines [52,64,71]. Furthermore, the reported rise in protease-activated receptor proteins (PARs) could activate and induce the secretion of inflammatory cytokines from endometrial stromal cells and may enhance the proliferation of stromal cells in endometrial lesions. PAR1 is reported to stimulate the production of proinflammatory cytokines in stromal cells and PAR2 induces IL-8 production and thereby supports the further production of chemoattractant cytokines in the peritoneal fluid [71]. Gmyrek *et al* found an increase in MCP-1 levels in peripheral blood and monocytes of women with advanced endometriosis, suggesting that different immune cell activity in women with advanced endometriosis might be more a result of the disease than a cause [70,73].

Transforming growth factor-β

Transforming growth factor (TGF)-β is an extremely potent chemoattractant cytokine for macrophages, mononuclear leukocytes and fibroblasts [74]. It is known to regulate various cellular activities, including cell growth, differentiation, apoptosis, inflammatory and immune responses, extracellular matrix deposition, adhesion molecules, proteases, and protease inhibitor expression. In endometrium, TGF-ß regulates its own expression and that of extracellular matrix, adhesion molecules and proteases that are implicated in trophoblast invasion, angiogenesis and tumor metastasis during embryo implantation, endometriosis, irregular uterine bleeding, and endometrial cancer [75]. TGF-β stimulates the proliferation of stromal cells of the endometrium and an excess of the cytokine leads to defective scars and adherence [76]. As mentioned before, TGF-β stimulates tumoral angiogenesis. Endometriosis is only able to develop and proliferate in a vascularized environment. Oosterlynck *et al* showed stimulation of angiogenesis on chorio-allantoic membranes by peritoneal fluid of women with endometriosis, which could be explained by the concentrations of TGF-α and TGF-β in the peritoneal fluid of these patients [77]. Furthermore, TGF-β was reported to be strongly increased in the peritoneal fluid of patients with endometriosis compared to healthy controls. It has also been shown that TGF-β induces the expression of macrophage colony-stimulating factor gene and cell surface expression and enhances transmesothelial invasion into endometrial epithelial cells *in vitro* [78].

Interleukins

Currently, only IL-1, IL-6, and IL-8 have been investigated in the pathogenesis of endometriosis. Most of the studies analyzed the concentrations of interleukins in the peritoneal fluid, but some of the reports also provide information about changes in the peripheral blood [6,61,79–83].

Interleukin–1

Interleukin-1 plays a pivotal role in the regulation of inflammation and immune response. Primarily discovered as a secretion product of activated macrophages, IL-1 is known to have a great impact on T-lymphocyte activation and B-lymphocyte proliferation. Although the two receptor agonists, IL-α and IL-β, share only a small amount of amino acid homogeneity, they bind to the same receptors and exert similar biological activities [46,84]. High levels of IL-1 have been found in the peritoneal fluid of women with endometriosis [21,85,86], whereas Bedaiwy *et al* found no significant differences between serum IL-1 concentrations in patients with endometriosis and controls [65].

Interleukin-6

The pleiotrope cytokine IL-6 is an important regulator of inflammation and immunity by linking the endocrine and immune systems. Like IL-1, IL-6 affects the secretion of other cytokines, promotes the activation of T-lymphocytes and the proliferation of B-lymphocytes and inhibits the growth of several human cell lines. It is produced by miscellaneous cell types, including lymphocytes, monocytes, fibroblasts, endothelial cells, vascular smooth muscle cells, keratinocytes, mesangial cells and endometrial stromal and epithelial cells. Furthermore, it is produced by a number of endocrine glands, including the pancreas and pituitary [87–89]. Macrophages secrete IL-6 in response to several substances in the peritoneal fluid, including IL-1 [6,90], and IL-6 itself is an activator of macrophages [91] and promotes the cellular proliferation of endometrium [92].

Endometrial epithelial and stromal cells produce IL-6 depending on hormonal and immunological activators. IL-1α, IL-1β, INF-γ, TNF, and PDGF induce IL-6 protein expression in endometrial stromal cells [88,93]. Some investigators have reported the inhibition of the proliferation of endometrial stromal cells by IL-6 during the secretory phase [94,95], but these observation were only found in eutopic endometrium *in vitro* and not in endometriotic lesions. Increased levels of IL-6 have been found in the peritoneal fluid of women with endometriosis and in ectopic endometrial tissue cultures [52,80,96], whereas other investigators have found no significant elevations [97,98]. Furthermore, there are reports of increased IL-6 levels in the peripheral blood of patients with endometriosis, suggesting that this cytokine is a promising serum marker for the non-surgical prediction of endometriosis [99–101].

Interleukin–8

Interleukin-8 is a very potent angiogenic, proinflammatory and growth-promoting cytokine, which acts as a chemoattractant for neutrophils and induces the expression of a variety of cell adhesion molecules [82,99,102]. IL-8 can also activate neutrophils and therefore may contribute to the pathogenesis of inflammatory diseases like endometriosis [103,104]. There are many reports about increases in IL-8 concentrations in the peritoneal fluid and serum of women with endometriosis compared to healthy controls. Most of these increases were suggested to be derived from peritoneal macrophages [52,64,81,104]. Some investigators reported IL-8 increases in the peritoneal fluid correspondent with severity of disease [64], while others reported increases particularly in the early stages [81]. In contrast, serum levels of IL-8 decreased with severity of disease, but nevertheless were higher in patients with endometriosis compared to healthy controls [64]. In turn, others did not found any differences in IL-8 concentrations in the serum of patients with endometriosis compared to healthy women [52].

Vascular endothelial growth factor

Vascular endothelial growth factor (VEGF) is one of the most specific and potent angiogenic growth factors, whose biochemistry and molecular biology are well described [105]. Binding of VEGF to a family of tyrosine kinase receptors leads to dimerization and autophosphorylation of the receptor and thereby to the activation of mitogen-activated protein kinases [46]. It is a potent selective endothelial mitogen and survival factor, which delays or reverses the senescence of endothelial cells [105]. In normal endometrium, VEGF expression was found to be highest in the secretory phase of the cycle, with localization predominantly in the endometrial glands. The expression of VEGF in normal human endometrial cells is acutely upregulated by estradiol *in vitro* [106–108]. Other factors known to enhance VEGF expression include hypoxia, PDGF, prostaglandin E$_2$, estrogen, progesterone, IL-1β and IL-6 [93,108-111]. Angiogenesis induced by VEGF promotes the restoration of endometrium following menstruation and seems to increase microvascular permeability, thereby allowing the formation of a fibrin matrix for endothelial migration and proliferation. This results in local edema by increased fluid and protein extravasation, which supports endometrium preparation for possible embryo implantation [46,108,112].

Vascular endothelial growth factor is one of the most prominent and studied proangiogenic factors in endometriosis. It is generally accepted that this factor is the main stimulus for angiogenesis and increased vessel permeability in this disease [113]. It has been shown that VEGF is highly expressed by endometriotic lesions, macrophages, and neutrophils. There are significantly increased levels of VEGF in the peritoneal fluid and in endometriotic lesions, particularly in hemorrhagic red implants of women with endometriosis compared to healthy controls [108,114–116].

Platelet-derived growth factor and epidermal growth factor

Platelet-derived growth factor (PDGF) and epidermal growth factor (EGF) play important roles in the proliferation of endometrial stromal and epithelial cells. EGF is induced by estrogen, whereas PDGF promotes cell proliferation through autocrine interaction with its receptor PDGF-R during the proliferative phase, suggesting a role for estrogen [117].

Platelet derived growth factor was found to be upregulated in the peritoneal fluid of women with endometriosis, thereby activating the FasL expression of endometrial cells [52,118]. The proinflammatory nature of the peritoneal fluid of women with endometriosis induces FasL expression by regurgitated endometrial cells, and signals Fas-mediated cell death of activated immune cells. This could be a mechanism for endometrial cells to escape immune surveillance, adhere, implant, and grow.

Adhesion molecules

Intercellular adhesion molecule-1

The membrane-bound molecule intercellular adhesion molecule-1 (ICAM-1) belongs to the immunoglobulin supergene family that is involved in immunological functions [119,120]. ICAM-1 is a co-receptor for the cell surface integrin ligand expressed on several immune cells.

Shedding of membrane-bound ICAM-1 leads to the generation of soluble ICAM-1 (sICAM-1), which can interfere with the immunocyte-endometrial implant recognition by binding leukocyte-associated ligands, thus competing for the ability of these leukocytes to participate in cell–cell interactions [46]. Furthermore, ICAM-1-mediated cell–cell adhesion is indispensable for a variety of immunological functions, including NK cell cytotoxicity against endometrium.

In the peritoneal fluid of women with endometriosis, the levels of sICAM-1 were found to be increased, combined with reduced NK cell activity. These findings suggest an impairment of NK cell activity by high sICAM levels and progression of the disease [121,122].

Several investigators reported significant increases in sICAM-1 in the serum of patients with endometriosis, particularly in the advanced stages of disease [122-124]. In contrast, Barrier *et al* found decreases in sICAM-1 in the serum of patients with endometriosis stages III and IV [125]. De Placido *et al* reported significantly higher sICAM-1 serum levels in revised American Fertility Society (rAFS) stages I and II [126].

An increase in the early stages could be due to increased shedding of ICAM-1 molecules under the influence of proinflammatory cytokines in the peritoneal fluid. On the other hand, advanced stages may reflect a chronic inflammatory process with inhibited release of soluble ICAM-1 due to different cytokine profiles. The different findings may be caused by variable patient recruitment throughout several investigations.

References

1. Abrao MS, Podgaec S, Filho BM et al. The use of biochemical markers in the diagnosis of pelvic endometriosis Hum Reprod 1997;12:2523–2527.
2. Gleicher N, Pratt D, Dudkiewicz A. What do we really know about autoantibody abnormalities and reproductive failure: a critical review. Autoimmunity 1993;16:115–140.
3. Dmowski WP. Immunological aspects of endometriosis. Int J Gynaecol Obstet 1995;50(Suppl 1):S3-10.
4. Xavier P, Belo L, Beires J et al. Serum levels of VEGF and TNF-alpha and their association with C-reactive protein in patients with endometriosis. Arch Gynecol Obstet 2006;273:227–231.
5. Lermann J, Mueller A, Korber F et al. Evaluation of high-sensitivity C-reactive protein in comparison with C-reactive protein as biochemical serum markers in women with endometriosis. Fertil Steril 2010;93(7):2125–2129.
6. Agic A, Xu H, Finas D et al. Is endometriosis associated with systemic subclinical inflammation? Gynecol Obstet Invest 2006;62:139–147.
7. Meek SC, Hodge DD, Musich JR. Autoimmunity in infertile patients with endometriosis. Am J Obstet Gynecol 1988;158:1365–1373.
8. Gleicher N, El Roeiy A, Confino E et al. Is endometriosis an autoimmune disease? Obstet Gynecol 1987;70:115–122.
9. Badawy SZ, Cuenca V, Kaufman L et al. The regulation of immunoglobulin production by B cells in patients with endometriosis. Fertil Steril 1989;51:770–773.
10. Taylor PV, Maloney MD, Campbell JM et al. Autoreactivity in women with endometriosis. Br J Obstet Gynaecol 1991;98:680–684.
11. Badawy SZ, Cuenca V, Marshall L et al. Cellular components in peritoneal fluid in infertile patients with and without endometriosis. Fertil Steril 1984;42:704–708.
12. Gilmore SM, Aksel S, Hoff C et al. In vitro lymphocyte activity in women with endometriosis – an altered immune response? Fertil Steril 1992;58:1148–1152.
13. Nomiyama M, Hachisuga T, Sou H et al. Local immune response in infertile patients with minimal endometriosis. Gynecol Obstet Invest 1997;44:32–37.
14. Vinatier D, Dufour P, Oosterlynck D. Immunological aspects of endometriosis. Hum Reprod Update 1996;2:371–384.
15. Bartosik D, Damjanov I, Viscarello RR et al. Immunoproteins in the endometrium: clinical correlates of the presence of complement fractions C3 and C4. Am J Obstet Gynecol 1987;156:11–15.
16. D'Cruz OJ, Wild RA Evaluation of endometrial tissue specific complement activation in women with endometriosis. Fertil Steril 1992;57:787–795.
17. Isaacson KB, Galman M, Coutifaris C et al. Endometrial synthesis and secretion of complement component-3 by patients with and without endometriosis. Fertil Steril 1990;53:836–841.
18. Isaacson KB, Xu Q, Lyttle CR. The effect of estradiol on the production and secretion of complement component 3 by the rat uterus and surgically induced endometriotic tissue. Fertil Steril 1991;55:395–402.
19. Bischof P, Planas-Basset D, Meisser A et al. Investigations on the cell type responsible for the endometrial secretion of complement component 3 (C3). Hum Reprod 1994;9:1652–1659.

20. Braun DP, Gebel H, House R et al. Spontaneous and induced synthesis of cytokines by peripheral blood monocytes in patients with endometriosis. Fertil Steril 1996;65:1125–1129.

21. Ho HN, Wu MY, Yang YS. Peritoneal cellular immunity and endometriosis. Am J Reprod Immunol 1997;38:400–412.

22. Oosterlynck DJ, Meuleman C, Lacquet FA et al. Flow cytometry analysis of lymphocyte subpopulations in peritoneal fluid of women with endometriosis. Am J Reprod Immunol 1994;31:25–31.

23. Wu MY, Chao KH, Chen SU et al. The suppression of peritoneal cellular immunity in women with endometriosis could be restored after gonadotropin releasing hormone agonist treatment. Am J Reprod Immunol 1996;35:510–516.

24. Becker JL, Widen RH, Mahan CS et al. Human peritoneal macrophage and T lymphocyte populations in mild and severe endometriosis. Am J Reprod Immunol 1995;34:179–187.

25. Oosterlynck DJ, Meuleman C, Waer M et al. The natural killer activity of peritoneal fluid lymphocytes is decreased in women with endometriosis. Fertil Steril 1992;58:290.

26. Gagné D, Rivard M, Page M et al. Blood leukocyte subsets are modulated in patients with endometriosis. Fertil Steril 2003;80:43–53.

27. Khorram O, Taylor RN, Ryan IP et al. Peritoneal fluid concentrations of the cytokine RANTES correlate with the severity of endometriosis. Am J Obstet Gynecol 1993;169:1545–1549.

28. Oral E, Olive DL, Arici A The peritoneal environment in endometriosis. Hum Reprod Update 1996;2:385–398.

29. Hornung D, Bentzien F, Wallwiener D et al. Chemokine bioactivity of RANTES in endometriotic and normal endometrial stromal cells and peritoneal fluid. Mol Hum Reprod 2001;7:163–168.

30. Gazvani R, Templeton A. Peritoneal environment, cytokines and angiogenesis in the pathophysiology of endometriosis. Reproduction 2002;123:217–226.

31. Lousse JC, van Langendonckt A, Gonzalez-Ramos R et al. Increased activation of nuclear factor-kappa B (NF-kappaB) in isolated peritoneal macrophages of patients with endometriosis. Fertil Steril 2008;90:217–220.

32. Nowak NM, Fischer OM, Gust TC et al. Intraperitoneal inflammation decreases endometriosis in a mouse model. Hum Reprod 2008;23:2466–2474.

33. Nagano O, Saya H. Mechanism and biological significance of CD44 cleavage. Cancer Sci 2004;95:930–935.

34. Braun DP, Muriana A, Gebel H et al. Monocyte-mediated enhancement of endometrial cell proliferation in women with endometriosis. Fertil Steril 1994;61:78–84.

35. Griffith JS, Liu YG, Tekmal RR et al. Menstrual endometrial cells from women with endometriosis demonstrate increased adherence to peritoneal cells and increased expression of CD44 splice variants. Fertil Steril 2010;93(6):1745–1749.

36. Hever A, Roth RB, Hevezi P et al. Human endometriosis is associated with plasma cells and overexpression of B lymphocyte stimulator. Proc Natl Acad Sci USA 2007;104:12451–12456.

37. Ulukus M, Arici A. Immunology of endometriosis. Minerva Ginecol 2005;57:237–248.

38. Ho HN, Chao KH, Chen HF et al. Peritoneal natural killer cytotoxicity and CD25+ CD3+ lymphocyte subpopulation are decreased in women with stage III-IV endometriosis. Hum Reprod 1995;10:2671–2675.

39. Oosterlynck DJ, Cornillie FJ, Waer M et al. Women with endometriosis show a defect in natural killer activity resulting in a decreased cytotoxicity to autologous endometrium. Fertil Steril 1991;56:45–51.

40. Hassa H, Tanir HM, Tekin B et al. Cytokine and immune cell levels in peritoneal fluid and peripheral blood of women with early- and late-staged endometriosis. Arch Gynecol Obstet 2009;279:891–895.

41. Schall TJ, Bacon K, Toy KJ et al. Selective attraction of monocytes and T lymphocytes of the memory phenotype by cytokine RANTES. Nature 1990;347:669–671.

42. Ortiz BD, Krensky AM, Nelson PJ et al. Kinetics of transcription factors regulating the RANTES chemokine gene reveal a developmental switch in nuclear events during T-lymphocyte maturation. Mol Cell Biol 1996;16:202–210.

43. Nikolcheva T, Pyronnet S, Chou SY et al. A translational rheostat for RFLAT-1 regulates RANTES expression in T lymphocytes. J Clin Invest 2002;110:119–126.

44. Ahn YT, Huang B, McPherson L et al. Dynamic interplay of transcriptional machinery and chromatin regulates "late" expression of the chemokine RANTES in T lymphocytes. Mol Cell Biol 2007;27:253–266.

45. Hornung D, Ryan IP, Chao VA et al. Immunolocalization and regulation of the chemokine RANTES in human endometrial and endometriosis tissues and cells. J Clin Endocrinol Metab 1997;82:1621–1628.

46. Lebovic DI, Mueller MD, Taylor RN. Immunobiology of endometriosis. Fertil Steril 2001;75:1–10.

47. Lebovic DI, Chao VA, Martini JF et al. IL-1beta induction of RANTES (regulated upon activation, normal T cell expressed and secreted) chemokine gene expression in endometriotic stromal cells depends on a nuclear factor-kappaB site in the proximal promoter. J Clin Endocrinol Metab 2001;86:4759–4764.

48. Lebovic DI, Chao VA, Taylor RN. Peritoneal macrophages induce RANTES (regulated on activation, normal T cell expressed and secreted) chemokine gene transcription in endometrial stromal cells. J Clin Endocrinol Metab 2004;89:1397–1401.

49. Fang CL, Han SP, Fu SL et al. Ectopic, autologous eutopic and normal endometrial stromal cells have altered expression and chemotactic activity of RANTES. Eur J Obstet Gynecol Reprod Biol 2009;143:55–60.

50. Rossi D, Zlotnik A. The biology of chemokines and their receptors. Annu Rev Immunol 2000;18:217–242.

51. Nagase H, Miyamasu M, Yamaguchi M et al. Regulation of chemokine receptor expression in eosinophils. Int Arch Allergy Immunol 2001;125(Suppl 1):29–32.

52. Kalu E, Sumar N, Giannopoulos T et al. Cytokine profiles in serum and peritoneal fluid from infertile women with and without endometriosis. J Obstet Gynaecol Res 2007;33:490–495.

53. Agic A, Xu H, Rehbein M et al. Cognate chemokine receptor 1 messenger ribonucleic acid expression in peripheral blood as a diagnostic test for endometriosis. Fertil Steril 2007;87:982–984.

54. Wieser F, Dogan S, Klingel K et al. Expression and regulation of CCR1 in peritoneal macrophages from women with and without endometriosis. Fertil Steril 2005;83:1878–1881.

55. Agic A, Djalali S, Wolfler MM et al. Combination of CCR1 mRNA, MCP1, and CA125 measurements in peripheral blood as a diagnostic test for endometriosis. Reprod Sci 2008;15:906–911.

56. Philippeaux MM, Piguet PF. Expression of tumor necrosis factor-alpha and its mRNA in the endometrial mucosa during the menstrual cycle. Am J Pathol 1993;143:480–486.

57. Hunt JS, Chen HL, Hu XL et al. Tumor necrosis factor-alpha messenger ribonucleic acid and protein in human endometrium. Biol Reprod 1992;47:141–147.

58. Laird SM, Tuckerman EM, Saravelos H et al. The production of tumour necrosis factor alpha (TNF-alpha) by human endometrial cells in culture. Hum Reprod 1996;11:1318–1323.

59. Chen DB, Yang ZM, Hilsenrath R et al. Stimulation of prostaglandin (PG) F2 alpha and PGE2 release by tumour necrosis factor-alpha and interleukin-1 alpha in cultured human luteal phase endometrial cells. Hum Reprod 1995;10:2773–2780.

60. Zhang RJ, Wild RA, Ojago JM. Effect of tumor necrosis factor-alpha on adhesion of human endometrial stromal cells to peritoneal mesothelial cells: an in vitro system. Fertil Steril 1993;59:1196–1201.

61. Iwabe T, Harada T, Tsudo T et al. Tumor necrosis factor-alpha promotes proliferation of endometriotic stromal cells by inducing interleukin-8 gene and protein expression. J Clin Endocrinol Metab 2000;85:824–829.

62. Eisermann J, Gast MJ, Pineda J et al. Tumor necrosis factor in peritoneal fluid of women undergoing laparoscopic surgery. Fertil Steril 1988;50:573–579.

63. Calhaz-Jorge C, Costa AP, Barata M et al. Tumour necrosis factor alpha concentrations in the peritoneal fluid of infertile women with minimal or mild endometriosis are lower in patients with red lesions only than in patients without red lesions. Hum Reprod 2000;15:1256–1260.

64. Pizzo A, Salmeri FM, Ardita FV et al. Behaviour of cytokine levels in serum and peritoneal fluid of women with endometriosis. Gynecol Obstet Invest 2002;54:82–87.

65. Bedaiwy MA, Falcone T, Sharma RK et al. Prediction of endometriosis with serum and peritoneal fluid markers: a prospective controlled trial. Hum Reprod 2002;17:426–431.

66. Yoshimura T, Leonard E. Secretion by human fibroblasts of monocyte chemoattractant protein-1, the product of gene JE. J Immunol 1990;144:2377–2383.

67. Yoshimura T, Yuhki N, Moore SK et al. Human monocyte chemoattractant protein-1 (MCP-1). Full-length cDNA cloning, expression in mitogen-stimulated blood mononuclear leukocytes, and sequence similarity to mouse competence gene JE. FEBS Lett 1989;244:487–493.

68. Arici A, Oral E, Attar E et al. Monocyte chemotactic protein-1 concentration in peritoneal fluid of women with endometriosis and its modulation of expression in mesothelial cells. Fertil Steril 1997;67:1065–1072.

69. Akoum A, Lemay A, McColl SR et al. Increased monocyte chemotactic protein-1 level and activity in the peripheral blood of women with endometriosis. Le Groupe d'Investigation en Gynecologie. Am J Obstet Gynecol 1996;175:1620–1625.

70. Gmyrek GB, Sieradzka U, Goluda M et al. Flow cytometric evaluation of intracellular cytokine synthesis in peripheral mononuclear cells of women with endometriosis. Immunol Invest 2008;37:43–61.

71. Osuga Y, Hirota Y, Taketani Y. Basic and translational research on proteinase-activated receptors: proteinase-activated receptors in female reproductive tissues and endometriosis. J Pharmacol Sci 2008;108:422–425.

72. Ulukus M, Ulukus EC, Tavmergen Goker EN et al. Expression of interleukin-8 and monocyte chemotactic protein 1 in women with endometriosis. Fertil Steril 2009;91:687–693.

73. Gmyrek GB, Sozanski R, Jerzak M et al. Evaluation of monocyte chemotactic protein-1 levels in peripheral blood of infertile women with endometriosis. Eur J Obstet Gynecol Reprod Biol 2005;122:199–205.

74. Haddad GF, Jodicke C, Thomas MA et al. Case series of rosiglitazone used during the first trimester of pregnancy. Reprod Toxicol 2008;26:183–184.

75. Luo X, Xu J, Chegini N. The expression of Smads in human endometrium and regulation and induction in endometrial epithelial and stromal cells by transforming growth factor-beta. J Clin Endocrinol Metab 2003;88:4967–4976.

76. Hammond MG, Oh ST, Anners J et al. The effect of growth factors on the proliferation of human endometrial stromal cells in culture. Am J Obstet Gynecol 1993;168:1131–1136.

77. Oosterlynck DJ, Meuleman C, Sobis H et al. Angiogenic activity of peritoneal fluid from women with endometriosis. Fertil Steril 1993;59:778–782.

78. Liu YG, Tekmal RR, Binkley PA et al. Induction of endometrial epithelial cell invasion and c-fms expression by transforming growth factor beta. Mol Hum Reprod 2009;15:665–673.

79. Keenan JA, Chen TT, Chadwell NL et al. IL-1 beta, TNF-alpha, and IL-2 in peritoneal fluid and macrophage-conditioned media of women with endometriosis. Am J Reprod Immunol 1985;34:381–385.

80. Punnonen J, Teisala K, Ranta H et al. Increased levels of interleukin-6 and interleukin-10 in the peritoneal fluid of patients with endometriosis. Am J Obstet Gynecol 1986;174:1522–1526.

81. Gazvani MR, Christmas S, Quenby S et al. Peritoneal fluid concentrations of interleukin-8 in women with endometriosis: relationship to stage of disease. Hum Reprod 1998;13:1957–1961.

82. Garcia-Velasco JA, Arici A. Interleukin-8 expression in endometrial stromal cells is regulated by integrin-dependent cell adhesion. Mol Hum Reprod 1999;5:1135–1140.

83. Wu MY, Ho HN. The role of cytokines in endometriosis. Am J Reprod Immunol 2003;49:285–296.

84. Senturk LM, Arici A. Immunology of endometriosis. J Reprod Immunol 1999;43:67–83.

85. Sokolov DI, Solodovnikova NG, Pavlov OV et al. Study of cytokine profile and angiogenic potential of peritoneal fluid in patients with external genital endometriosis. Bull Exp Biol Med 2005;140:541–544.

86. Akoum A, Al Akoum M, Lemay A et al. Imbalance in the peritoneal levels of interleukin 1 and its decoy inhibitory receptor type II in endometriosis women with infertility and pelvic pain. Fertil Steril 2008;89:1618–1624.

87. Tabibzadeh SS, Santhanam U, Sehgal PB et al. Cytokine-induced production of IFN-beta 2/IL-6 by freshly explanted human endometrial stromal cells. Modulation by estradiol-17 beta. J Immunol 1989;142:3134–3139.

88. Laird SM, Li TC, Bolton AE. The production of placental protein 14 and interleukin 6 by human endometrial cells in culture. Hum Reprod 1993;8:793–798.

89. Ray P, Ghosh SK, Zhang DH et al. Repression of interleukin-6 gene expression by 17 beta-estradiol: inhibition of the DNA-binding activity of the transcription factors NF-IL6 and NF-kappa B by the estrogen receptor. FEBS Lett 1997;409:79–85.

90. Sironi M, Breviario F, Proserpio P et al. IL-1 stimulates IL-6 production in endothelial cells. J Immunol 1989;142:549–553.

91. Akira S, Taga T, Kishimoto T. Interleukin-6 in biology and medicine. Adv Immunol 1993;54:1–78.

92. Giudice LC Growth factors and growth modulators in human uterine endometrium: their potential relevance to reproductive medicine. Fertil Steril 1994;61:1–17.

93. Lebovic DI, Bentzien F, Chao VA et al. Induction of an angiogenic phenotype in endometriotic stromal cell cultures by interleukin-1beta. Mol Hum Reprod 2000;6:269–275.

94. Zarmakoupis PN, Rier SE, Maroulis GB et al. Inhibition of human endometrial stromal cell proliferation by interleukin 6. Hum Reprod 1995;10:2395–2399.

95. Yoshioka H, Harada T, Iwabe T et al. Menstrual cycle-specific inhibition of the proliferation of endometrial stromal cells by interleukin 6 and its soluble receptor. Am J Obstet Gynecol 1999;180:1088–1094.

96. Keenan JA, Chen TT, Chadwell NL et al. Interferon-gamma (IFN-gamma) and interleukin-6 (IL-6) in peritoneal fluid and macrophage-conditioned media of women with endometriosis. Am J Reprod Immunol 1994;32:180–183.

97. Buyalos RP, Funari VA, Azziz R et al. Elevated interleukin-6 levels in peritoneal fluid of patients with pelvic pathology. Fertil Steril 1992;58:302–306.

98. Rapkin A, Morgan M, Bonpane C et al. Peritoneal fluid interleukin-6 in women with chronic pelvic pain. Fertil Steril 2000; 74:325–328.

99. Koch AE, Polverini PJ, Kunkel SL et al. Interleukin-8 as a macrophage-derived mediator of angiogenesis. Science 1992;258:1798–1801.

100. Martinez S, Garrido N, Coperias JL et al. Serum interleukin-6 levels are elevated in women with minimal-mild endometriosis. Hum Reprod 2007;22:836–842.

101. Othman E, Hornung D, Salem HT et al. Serum cytokines as biomarkers for nonsurgical prediction of endometriosis. Eur J Obstet Gynecol Reprod Biol 2008;137:240–246.

102. Ryan IP, Tseng JF, Schriock ED et al. Interleukin-8 concentrations are elevated in peritoneal fluid of women with endometriosis. Fertil Steril 1995;63:929–932.

103. Leonard EJ, Yoshimura T. Human monocyte chemoattractant protein-1 (MCP-1). Immunol Today 1990;11:97–101.

104. Rana N, Braun DP, House R et al. Basal and stimulated secretion of cytokines by peritoneal macrophages in women with endometriosis. Fertil Steril 1996;65:925–930.

105. Becker CM, d'Amato RJ. Angiogenesis and antiangiogenic therapy in endometriosis. Microvasc Res 2007;74:121–130.

106. Li XF, Gregory J, Ahmed A. Immunolocalisation of vascular endothelial growth factor in human endometrium. Growth Factors 1994;11:277–282.

107. Torry DS, Holt VJ, Keenan JA et al. Vascular endothelial growth factor expression in cycling human endometrium. Fertil Steril 1996;66:72–80.

108. Shifren JL, Tseng JF, Zaloudek CJ et al. Ovarian steroid regulation of vascular endothelial growth factor in the human endometrium: impli-

cations for angiogenesis during the menstrual cycle and in the pathogenesis of endometriosis. J Clin Endocrinol Metab 1996;81:3112–3118.

109. Brogi E, Wu T, Namiki A et al. Indirect angiogenic cytokines upregulate VEGF and bFGF gene expression in vascular smooth muscle cells, whereas hypoxia upregulates VEGF expression only. Circulation 1994;90:649–652.

110. Ben-Av P, Crofford LJ, Wilder RL et al. Induction of vascular endothelial growth factor expression in synovial fibroblasts by prostaglandin E and interleukin-1: a potential mechanism for inflammatory angiogenesis. FEBS Lett 1995;372:83–87.

111. Lin YJ, Lai MD, Lei HY et al. Neutrophils and macrophages promote angiogenesis in the early stage of endometriosis in a mouse model. Endocrinology 2006;147:1278–1286.

112. Hornung D, Lebovic DI, Shifren JL et al. Vectorial secretion of vascular endothelial growth factor by polarized human endometrial epithelial cells. Fertil Steril 1998;69:909–915.

113. Taylor RN, Lebovic DI, Mueller MD. Angiogenic factors in endometriosis. Ann N Y Acad Sci 2002;955:89–100.

114. McLaren J, Prentice A, Charnock-Jones DS et al. Vascular endothelial growth factor (VEGF) concentrations are elevated in peritoneal fluid of women with endometriosis. Hum Reprod 1996;11:220–223.

115. McLaren J, Prentice A, Charnock-Jones DS et al. Vascular endothelial growth factor is produced by peritoneal fluid macrophages in endometriosis and is regulated by ovarian steroids. J Clin Invest 1996;98:482–489.

116. Donnez J, Smoes P, Gillerot S et al. Vascular endothelial growth factor (VEGF) in endometriosis. Hum Reprod 1998;13:1686–1690.

117. Gargett CE, Chan RW, Schwab KE. Hormone and growth factor signaling in endometrial renewal: role of stem/progenitor cells. Mol Cell Endocrinol 2008;288:22–29.

118. Garcia-Velasco JA, Arici A, Zreik T et al. Macrophage derived growth factors modulate Fas ligand expression in cultured endometrial stromal cells: a role in endometriosis. Mol Hum Reprod 1999;5:642–650.

119. Springer TA. Adhesion receptors of the immune system. Nature 1990;346:425–434.

120. Koninckx PR, Kennedy SH, Barlow DH. Endometriotic disease: the role of peritoneal fluid. Hum Reprod Update 1998;4:741–751.

121. Fukaya T, Sugawara J, Yoshida H et al. Intercellular adhesion molecule-1 and hepatocyte growth factor in human endometriosis: original investigation and a review of literature. Gynecol Obstet Invest 1999;47(Suppl 1):11–16.

122. Daniel Y, Geva E, Amit A et al. Do soluble cell adhesion molecules play a role in endometriosis? Am J Reprod Immunol 2000;43:160–166.

123. Wu MH, Yang BC, Hsu CC et al. The expression of soluble intercellular adhesion molecule-1 in endometriosis. Fertil Steril 1998;70:1139–1142.

124. Leng J, Lang J, Zhao D et al. Serum levels of soluble intercellular molecule 1 (sICAM-1) in endometriosis. Zhonghua Yi Xue Za Zhi 2002;82:189–190.

125. Barrier BF, Sharpe-Timms KL. Expression of soluble adhesion molecules in sera of women with stage III and IV endometriosis. J Soc Gynecol Invest 2002;9:98–101.

126. De Placido G, Alviggi C, di Palma G et al. Serum concentrations of soluble human leukocyte class I antigens and of the soluble intercellular adhesion molecule-1 in endometriosis: relationship with stage and non-pigmented peritoneal lesions. Hum Reprod 1998;13:3206–3210.

5   Models of Endometriosis

25 Models of Endometriosis: *In vitro* and *In vivo* Models

Ruth Grümmer

Institute of Molecular Biology, University Hospital Essen and University of Duisburg-Essen, Essen, Germany

Introduction

Alhough endometriosis is a prevalent gynecological disorder, little is known about the cell biological mechanisms leading to the development of this disease. Current therapies focus on treating the symptoms rather than curing the causes [1] and there is a substantial need for molecular and cellular research to unravel the pathogenic mechanisms of endometriosis as a basis for developing novel diagnostic and therapeutic concepts. Since the development of endometriosis is a very complex multifactorial process, the decoding of these mechanisms is challenging. Causal defects may originate in the eutopic endometrium as well as in factors of the extrauterine localizations [1,2]. Because in the majority of cases menstrual shedding is a requirement for the development of this disease, endometriosis occurs spontaneously only in humans and non-human primates. Thus, sophisticated experimental models have been established to evaluate fundamental mechanisms by which menstrual endometrium adheres, invades and establishes lesions in ectopic sites as well as to develop new therapeutical approaches. These range from simplistic *in vitro* models to complex animal models of induced endometriosis. This chapter will give a summarizing overview of these experimental systems.

In vitro models

In vitro systems offer the advantage of unraveling the molecular base of impaired signaling cascades in endometriotic cells by using primary cells or cell lines. Moreover, the interaction between endometrial cells and peritoneal mesothelium, which represents one major step in the establishment of this disease, can be studied in co-culture models.

Primary cells or cell lines

Endometrial epithelial and stromal cells have been isolated from endometrial biopsies as well as from endometriotic lesions and can be distinguished by specific markers [3–8]. In addition, immortalized human endometriotic epithelial and stromal cells have been established to study signaling cascades for non-estrogen-targeted therapies [9]. Comparing cells of eutopic endometrium of women with and without endometriosis, differences in their progesterone response [5] and their capacity to decidualize *in vitro* [6] were observed. In addition, a stimulatory effect of peritoneal fluid and macrophages from women with endometriosis and of inflammatory cytokines on proliferation of eutopic and ectopic endometrial cells was shown [10–12].

To investigate the interaction between endometrial cells and the peritoneum, primary mesothelial cells [13–15] or established cell lines have been used [15]. It has been demonstrated that adhesion of endometrial stromal cells to mesothelium is not dependent on the source of mesothelial cells but on the origin of endometrial cells [15], and stromal cells from ectopic and eutopic endometrium from diseased women are more adhesive to immobilized extracellular matrix (ECM) than eutopic endometrial cells from healthy women [16]. This endometrial–peritoneal adhesion can be increased by cytokines [13]. Transmesothelial invasion of endometrial cells has been investigated by culturing primary endometrial epithelial and stromal cells [7,8] or the endometrial cell line EM42 [7,8,17] on Matrigel [7] or on mesothelial LP9 cells grown on Matrigel-coated invasion chambers [8,17]. Invasion of primary endometrial cells was increased by the presence of peritoneal mesothelial cells [7] and activin A [8], whereas a peroxisome proliferator-activated receptor (PPAR)-γ agonist had no suppressive effect on invasion of EM42 cells through LP9 monolayer [17].

Endometriosis: Science and Practice, First Edition. Edited by Linda C. Giudice, Johannes L.H. Evers and David L. Healy.
© 2012 Blackwell Publishing Ltd. Published 2012 by Blackwell Publishing Ltd.

Organ culture

Since a three-dimensional tissue architecture containing epithelial and stromal cells seems to be important for endometrial physiology [14], several studies used three-dimensional organ cultures of endometrial tissue which was mechanically dissected from endometrial biopsies [8,14,18-22] or from menstrual effluent [23] and was co-cultured with amniotic membranes [18,19,24] or autologous peritoneum [20–22] as the mesothelial counterpart. While the mesothelium may act as a barrier to the attachment of endometrium [18,19,24], adhesion of both stromal and epithelial endometrial cells to peritoneal epithelium has been described independent of cycle phase or the presence and stage of endometriosis [22], while transmesothelial invasion was only observed for endometrial stromal cells [21]. When cultured on isolated ECM compounds, attachment of menstrual endometrium to collagen IV and I could be blocked by anti-integrin-β1 [23].

In summary, *in vitro* models offer valuable experimental systems for studying the molecular and cellular processes underlying endometrial–peritoneal interaction by comparing human endometrial and mesothelial cells of different locations from women with and without endometriosis. Epithelial and stromal cells can be easily manipulated, e.g. by transfection or by functional interference by small interfering RNA (siRNA) or blocking antibodies, respectively. However, it has to be considered that the cell physiology may have changed during *in vitro* culture, especially in transformed cell lines.

Chorio-allantoic membrane assay

In order to study cellular and molecular processes involved in adhesion, invasion and angiogenesis in a more complex setting, the chicken chorio-allantoic membrane (CAM) assay has been established as a model for endometriosis by culturing fragments of human endometrial tissue on the CAM of fertilized chicken eggs [24,25]. Heterologous tissue can be easily cultured on the CAM due to the host's immature immune system [26]. Endometrial fragments of all cycle stages invade the epithelium and develop endometriosis-like lesions, and vessels grow from the CAM into the xenotransplants [24,27]. During this process, expression of matrix metalloproteinases (MMPs) is upregulated in the endometrial fragments [28] and their invasion capacity can be reduced by inhibiting MMP activity [27].

The dense microvascular network of the CAM allows analysis of blood vessel development in ectopic endometrium and evaluation of antiangiogenic treatment strategies [29]. Formation of endometriotic lesions was significantly impaired after treatment with angiogenesis inhibitors [30] and a higher angiogenic potential of peritoneal fluid from women with endometriosis compared to peritoneal fluid of women without endometriosis could be proven [31]. In contrast, endometrial fragments of women with and without endometriosis showed no differences in angiogenic induction [32].

The CAM assay is well suited for the investigation of mechanisms involved in adhesion, invasion and angiogenesis during the establishment of endometriotic lesions. The ectopic lesions are easily accessible and can be simply monitored during the course of an experiment. However, this endometriosis model is not applicable for the investigation of immunological or inflammatory responses or systemic effects of drugs, and the time period for experiments is limited to approximately 10 days [29].

In vivo models

Because of the considerable limitations of *in vitro* models, animal models are indispensable to study mechanisms of endometriosis pathogenesis and the efficacy of treatment strategies before their introduction into clinical practice. Because endometriosis occurs spontaneously only in humans and some non-human primates, models of induced endometriosis have been developed in rodents and non-human primates by transplantation of endometrial tissue to ectopic sites. Since this book contains separate chapters on rodents and non-human primates as models for endometriosis, this review will just give a compressed overview of commonly used animal models.

Rodent models
Autologous rodent models

Since rodents do not menstruate and thus do not develop endometriosis spontaneously, autologous rodent models have been developed in rats and mice by intraperitoneal or subcutaneous transplantation of endometrial tissue of the same or of syngeneic animals. Biopsies of uterine tissue develop endometriosis-like lesions after transplantation at ectopic sites showing typical endometrial histomorphology. Implantation rate, localization, and graft size as well as histological and molecular changes within the ectopic lesions can be analyzed over time [29,33,34].

This model has been used to investigate various aspects of endometriosis pathogenesis. Angiogenesis, one of the predispositions for the establishment of this disease, as well as the efficacy of antiangiogenic agents on the establishment and growth of the ectopic lesions have been extensively studied in this experimental model [35,36]. In addition, it has been widely used to determine the responsiveness of ectopic lesions to steroid hormones, as well as to drugs interfering with steroid hormone action [34], and the effect of environmental toxicants on the establishment of ectopic uterine implants has been investigated [37].

Moreover, this model provides an intact immune system and thus is used to study the effect of immune-modulating drugs and anti-inflammatory agents on endometriotic lesions [34]. Furthermore, the influence of endometriotic lesions on pain nociception has been investigated [38] and a reduced fecundity was observed after artificial induction of endometriosis [39,40], which could be due to an increased number of luteinized unruptured ovarian follicles [40] or to a feedback effect of the ectopic lesions on gene expression in the eutopic endometrium [41].

One of the outstanding advantages of this rodent model is the possibility of using genetic modifications of specific target genes. Activation of the oncogene K-ras in ovarian surface epithelial cells resulted in the development of benign ovarian and peritoneal lesions with histomorphological features of human endometriosis [42] whereas mice homozygous for a CSF-1 mutation developed significantly fewer endometriotic lesions than syngeneic controls [43].

The autologous rodent model does not authentically reflect the situation in humans since rodents do not menstruate, and do not develop endometriosis spontaneously. In spite of this limitation, these models offer significant advantages. Apart from the limited costs and the opportunity to use large groups of genetically similar animals, long-term studies can be performed since there is no rejection of the autotransplanted ectopic tissue. Impact on inflammation, pain behavior, and fecundity can be investigated. Evaluation of therapeutic effects will be improved by advanced methods of *in vivo* imaging of ectopic lesions in these animal models [44,45]. Above all, with regard to new insights into the etiology of endometriosis obtained by genomic and proteomic approaches, transgenic mice models might gain importance in the examination of functions driven by single genes.

Humanized mouse models

To overcome the differences in endometrial physiology in autologous rodent models compared to humans an alternative experimental approach has been developed by transplanting human endometrial tissue into immunocomprised mice. Various immunodeficient mice strains have been used for these studies [34]. Eutopic endometrium from women with and without endometriosis as well as tissue from endometriotic lesions have been successfully transplanted and maintain endometrial characteristics at ectopic sites in terms of macroscopical and histological appearance and steroid hormone responsiveness, whereas the stage of the menstrual cycle of the human tissue seemed to have no impact on lesion development [29,34].

Revascularization of human xenografts occurs by invasion of host vessels in parallel with the disappearance of native graft vessels [46–48]. Interestingly, a large number of these ingrown vessels are immature, consisting of endothelial cells without an extensive pericytic layer [47], but recruitment of pericytes can be enhanced by progestins [49]. This model has been extensively used to study the effect of antiangiogenic compounds on preventing implantation and growth of ectopic endometrium [29].

Moreover, this heterologous mouse model offers the potential to analyze cell biological mechanisms in response to drug therapy in ectopic human endometrial tissue. Suppression of matrix metalloproteinases could be shown to inhibit the establishment of ectopic lesions in nude mice [50] and transcription of estrogen metabolizing enzymes is regulated by exogenously applied drugs interfering with estrogen metabolism [51].

With regard to the role of the immune system in the development of endometriosis, the simultaneous transplantation of human endometrial tissue and injection of immune cells of the same women revealed that immune cells from disease-free women limit the extent of intraperitoneal disease in this model [52].

Recently, it has been shown that human immortalized endometriotic epithelial and stromal cells establish peritoneal endometriosis-like lesions when xenografted into nude mice [53], providing, for example, the opportunity to analyze the effect of targeted genetic manipulation of these cells on lesion development.

In conclusion, in addition to low costs, the humanized mouse models offer the possibility to investigate human eutopic endometrium from women with and without endometriosis as well as endometriotic tissue. Regulatory mechanisms and effects of therapeutic drugs can be evaluated in the human ectopic tissue in an *in vivo* situation. To overcome the differences in reproductive endocrinology, the human menstrual cycle can be mimicked in ovariectomized animals. The use of this model is limited by the availability of human tissue, and by the restricted duration of culture due to the residual immunological response of the host.

Non-human primate models

Non-human primates have been extensively used as experimental models for endometriosis. Most studies have been performed in rhesus macaques and baboons [554,55]. Because spontaneous endometriosis develops with low frequency in monkeys, endometriosis usually is induced by intrapelvic injection of endometrium. Laparoscopic appearances, pelvic localization and microscopic aspects of spontaneous as well as induced endometriosis are similar to those in women [54,56]. In this model, the role of the immune response in the development and progression of endometriosis [2], as well as the effect of endometriosis on fecundity [57,58] and on endometrial gene expression [59,60], has been extensively investigated.

The various aspects of endometriosis pathophysiology which have been investigated in this model are reviewed in Chapter 27 of this book.

The non-human primate model of endometriosis unquestionably matches most closely the situation in women, revealing similar reproductive endocrinology and immunology. It yields a valuable tool for better understanding of the role of endometrium, peritoneum and peritoneal fluid in the onset and development of endometriosis.

However, ethical considerations as well as the very high costs of animal handling limit the use of non-human primates as an experimental model.

Conclusion

In vitro and *in vivo* models of endometriosis are of great value and are indispensable for the evaluation of pathophysiological mechanisms underlying the development of this prevalent gynecological disease. New advances will be provided by improved methods of *in vivo* imaging of ectopic lesions in animal models as well as by the use of genetically manipulated mice or cell lines. Since no single model absolutely replicates all aspects of the human disease, advantages and limitations should be thoroughly considered when deciding which particular model system is to be used for targeted evaluation of scientific questions. Bearing this in mind, these models will help to develop novel diagnostic tools and improved therapeutic strategies for a better treatment of endometriosis in women.

References

1. Giudice LC, Kao LC. Endometriosis. Lancet 2004;364:1789–1799.

2. Kyama CM, Mihalyi A, Simsa P et al. Role of cytokines in the endometrial-peritoneal cross-talk and development of endometriosis. Front Biosci (Elite Ed) 2009;1:444–454.

3. Osteen KG, Hill GA, Hargrove JT et al. Development of a method to isolate and culture highly purified populations of stromal and epithelial cells from human endometrial biopsy specimens. Fertil Steril 1989;52:965–972.

4. Ryan IP, Schriock ED, Taylor RN. Isolation, characterization, and comparison of human endometrial and endometriosis cells in vitro. J Clin Endocrinol Metab 1994;78:642–649.

5. Bruner-Tran KL, Zhang Z, Eisenberg E et al. Down-regulation of endometrial matrix metalloproteinase-3 and -7 expression in vitro and therapeutic regression of experimental endometriosis in vivo by a novel nonsteroidal progesterone receptor agonist, tanaproget. J Clin Endocrinol Metab 2006;91:1554–1560.

6. Klemmt PA, Carver JG, Kennedy SH et al. Stromal cells from endometriotic lesions and endometrium from women with endometriosis have reduced decidualization capacity. Fertil Steril 2006;85:564–572.

7. Nair AS, Nair HB, Lucidi RS et al. Modeling the early endometriotic lesion: mesothelium-endometrial cell co-culture increases endometrial invasion and alters mesothelial and endometrial gene transcription. Fertil Steril 2008;90:1487–1495.

8. Ferreira MC, Witz CA, Hammes LS et al. Activin A increases invasiveness of endometrial cells in an in vitro model of human peritoneum. Mol Hum Reprod 2008;14:301–307.

9. Banu SK, Lee J, Speights VO et al. Selective inhibition of prostaglandin E2 receptors EP2 and EP4 induces apoptosis of human endometriotic cells through suppression of ERK1/2, AKT, NFkappaB, and beta-catenin pathways and activation of intrinsic apoptotic mechanisms. Mol Endocrinol 2009;23:1291–1305.

10. Loh FH, Bongso A, Fong CY et al. Effects of peritoneal macrophages from women with endometriosis on endometrial cellular proliferation in an in vitro coculture model. Fertil Steril 1999;72:533–538.

11. Iwabe T, Harada T, Tsudo T et al. Tumor necrosis factor-alpha promotes proliferation of endometriotic stromal cells by inducing interleukin-8 gene and protein expression. J Clin Endocrinol Metab 2000;85:824–829.

12. Braun DP, Ding J, Dmowski WP. Peritoneal fluid-mediated enhancement of eutopic and ectopic endometrial cell proliferation is dependent on tumor necrosis factor-alpha in women with endometriosis. Fertil Steril 2002;78:727–732.

13. Zhang RJ, Wild RA, Ojago JM. Effect of tumor necrosis factor-alpha on adhesion of human endometrial stromal cells to peritoneal mesothelial cells: an in vitro system. Fertil Steril 1993;59:1196–1201.

14. Wild RA, Zhang R, Medders D et al. Endometrial fragments form characteristics of in vivo endometriosis in a mesothelial cell co-culture system: an in vitro model of the histogenesis of endometriosis. J Soc Gynecol Invent 1994;1:165–168.

15. Lucidi RS, Witz CA, Chrisco M et al. A novel in vitro model of the early endometriotic lesion demonstrates that attachment of endometrial cells to mesothelial cells is dependent on the source of endometrial cells. Fertil Steril 2005;84:16–21.

16. Klemmt PA, Carver JG, Koninckx P et al. Endometrial cells from women with endometriosis have increased adhesion and proliferative capacity in response to extracellular matrix components: towards a mechanistic model for endometriosis progression. Hum Reprod 2007;22:3139–3147.

17. Kavoussi SK, Witz CA, Binkley PA et al. Peroxisome-proliferator activator receptor-gamma activation decreases attachment of endometrial cells to peritoneal mesothelial cells in an in vitro model of the early endometriotic lesion. Mol Hum Reprod 2009;15:687–692.

18. Van der Linden PJ, de Goeij AF, Dunselman GA et al. Endometrial cell adhesion in an in vitro model using intact amniotic membranes. Fertil Steril 1996;65:76–80.

19. Groothuis PG, Koks CA, de Goeij AF et al. Adhesion of human endometrium to the epithelial lining and extracellular matrix of amnion in vitro: an electron microscopic study. Hum Reprod 1998;13:2275–2281.

20. Groothuis PG, Koks CA, de Goeij AF et al. Adhesion of human endometrial fragments to peritoneum in vitro. Fertil Steril 1999;71:1119–1124.

21. Witz CA, Dechaud H, Montoya-Rodriguez IA et al. An in vitro model to study the pathogenesis of the early endometriosis lesion. Ann N Y Acad Sci 2002;955:296–307.

22. Debrock S, Vander Perre S, Meuleman C et al. In-vitro adhesion of endometrium to autologous peritoneal membranes: effect of the cycle phase and the stage of endometriosis. Hum Reprod 2002;17:2523–2528.

23. Koks CA, Groothuis PG, Dunselman GA et al. Adhesion of menstrual endometrium to extracellular matrix: the possible role of integrin alpha(6)beta(1) and laminin interaction. Mol Hum Reprod 2000;6:170–177.

24. Koks CA, Groothuis PG, Dunselman GA et al. Adhesion of shed menstrual tissue in an in-vitro model using amnion and peritoneum: a light and electron microscopic study. Hum Reprod 1999;14:816–822.

24. Maas JW, Groothuis PG, Dunselman GA et al. Development of endometriosis-like lesions after transplantation of human endometrial fragments onto the chick embryo chorioallantoic membrane. Hum Reprod 2001;16:627–631.

25. Malik E, Meyhofer-Malik A, Berg C et al. Fluorescence diagnosis of endometriosis on the chorioallantoic membrane using 5-aminolaevulinic acid. Hum Reprod 2000;15:584–588.

26. Leene W, Duyzings MJ, van Steeg C. Lymphoid stem cell identification in the developing thymus and bursa of Fabricius of the chick. Z Zellforsch Mikrosk Anat 1973;136:521–533.

27. Nap AW, Dunselman GA, de Goeij AF et al. Inhibiting MMP activity prevents the development of endometriosis in the chicken chorioallantoic membrane model. Hum Reprod 2004;19:2180–2187.

28. Juhasz-Boss I, Hofele A, Lattrich C et al. Matrix metalloproteinase messenger RNA expression in human endometriosis grafts cultured on a chicken chorioallantoic membrane. Fertil Steril 2010;94(1):40–45.

29. Laschke MW, Menger MD. In vitro and in vivo approaches to study angiogenesis in the pathophysiology and therapy of endometriosis. Hum Reprod Update 2007;13:331–342.

30. Nap AW, Dunselman GA, Griffioen AW et al. Angiostatic agents prevent the development of endometriosis-like lesions in the chicken chorioallantoic membrane. Fertil Steril 2005;83:793–795.

31. Oosterlynck DJ, Meuleman C, Sobis H et al. Angiogenic activity of peritoneal fluid from women with endometriosis. Fertil Steril 1993;59:778–782.

32. Gescher DM, Siggelkow W, Meyhoefer-Malik A et al. A priori implantation potential does not differ in eutopic endometrium of patients with and without endometriosis. Arch Gynecol Obstet 2005;272:117–123.

33. Story L, Kennedy S. Animal studies in endometriosis: a review. Ilar J 2004;45:132–138.

34. Grümmer R. Animal models in endometriosis research. Hum Reprod Update 2006;12:641–649.

35. Van Langendonckt A, Donnez J, Defrere S et al. Antiangiogenic and vascular-disrupting agents in endometriosis: pitfalls and promises. Mol Hum Reprod 2008;14:259–268.

36. Becker CM, d'Amato RJ. Angiogenesis and antiangiogenic therapy in endometriosis. Microvasc Res 2007;74:121–130.

37. Anger DL, Foster WG. The link between environmental toxicant exposure and endometriosis. Front Biosci 2008;13:1578–1593.

38. Berkley KJ, Cason A, Jacobs H et al. Vaginal hyperalgesia in a rat model of endometriosis. Neurosci Lett 2001;306:185–188.

39. Vernon MW, Wilson EA. Studies on the surgical induction of endometriosis in the rat. Fertil Steril 1985;44:684–694.

40. Stilley JA, Woods-Marshall R, Sutovsky M et al. Reduced fecundity in female rats with surgically induced endometriosis and in their daughters: a potential role for tissue inhibitors of metalloproteinase 1. Biol Reprod 2009;80:649–656.

41. Lee B, Du H, Taylor HS. Experimental murine endometriosis induces DNA methylation and altered gene expression in eutopic endometrium. Biol Reprod 2009;80:79–85.

42. Dinulescu DM, Ince TA, Quade BJ et al. Role of K-ras and Pten in the development of mouse models of endometriosis and endometrioid ovarian cancer. Nat Med 2005;11:63–70.

43. Jensen JR, Witz CA, Schenken RS et al. A potential role for colony-stimulating factor 1 in the genesis of the early endometriotic lesion. Fertil Steril 2010;93:251–256.

44. Defrere S, Colette S, Lousse JC et al. Review: luminescence as a tool to assess pelvic endometriosis development in murine models. Reprod Sci 2009;16:1117–1124.

45. Laschke MW, Körbel C, Rudzitis-Auth J et al. High-resolution ultrasound imaging: a novel technique for the noninvasive in vivo analysis of endometriotic lesion and cyst formation in small animal models. Am J Pathol 2010;176:585–593.

46. Grümmer R, Schwarzer F, Bainczyk K et al. Peritoneal endometriosis: validation of an in-vivo model. Hum Reprod 2001;16:1736–1743.

47. Hull ML, Charnock-Jones DS, Chan CL et al. Antiangiogenic agents are effective inhibitors of endometriosis. J Clin Endocrinol Metab 2003;88:2889–2899.

48. Eggermont J, Donnez J, Casanas-Roux F et al. Time course of pelvic endometriotic lesion revascularization in a nude mouse model. Fertil Steril 2005;84:492–499.

49. Mönckedieck V, Sannecke C, Husen B et al. Progestins inhibit expression of MMPs and of angiogenic factors in human ectopic endometrial lesions in a mouse model. Mol Hum Reprod 2009;15:633–643.

50. Bruner KL, Matrisian LM, Rodgers WH et al. Suppression of matrix metalloproteinases inhibits establishment of ectopic lesions by human endometrium in nude mice. J Clin Invest 1997;99:2851–2857.

51. Fechner S, Husen B, Thole H et al. Expression and regulation of estrogen-converting enzymes in ectopic human endometrial tissue. Fertil Steril 2007;88:1029–1038.

52. Bruner-Tran KL, Carvalho-Macedo AC, Duleba AJ et al. Experimental endometriosis in immunocompromised mice after adoptive transfer of human leukocytes. Fertil Steril 2010;93(8):2519–2524.

53. Banu SK, Starzinski-Powitz A, Speights VO et al. Induction of peritoneal endometriosis in nude mice with use of human immortalized endometriosis epithelial and stromal cells: a potential experimental tool to study molecular pathogenesis of endometriosis in humans. Fertil Steril 2009;91(Suppl):2199–2209.

54. Fazleabas AT. A baboon model for inducing endometriosis. Methods Mol Med 2006;121:95–99.

55. D'Hooghe TM, Kyama CM, Chai D et al. Nonhuman primate models for translational research in endometriosis. Reprod Sci 2009;16:152–161.

56. D'Hooghe TM, Debrock S. Endometriosis, retrograde menstruation and peritoneal inflammation in women and in baboons. Hum Reprod Update 2002;8:84–88.

57. D'Hooghe TM, Bambra CS, Raeymaekers BM et al. The cycle pregnancy rate is normal in baboons with stage I endometriosis but decreased in primates with stage II and stage III-IV disease. Fertil Steril 1996;66:809–813.

58. Braundmeier AG, Fazleabas AT. The non-human primate model of endometriosis: research and implications for fecundity. Mol Hum Reprod 2009;15:577–586.

59. Gashaw I, Hastings JM, Jackson KS et al. Induced endometriosis in the baboon (Papio anubis) increases the expression of the proangiogenic factor CYR61 (CCN1) in eutopic and ectopic endometria. Biol Reprod 2006;74:1060–1066.

60. Winterhager E, Grummer R, Mavrogianis PA et al. Connexin expression pattern in the endometrium of baboons is influenced by hormonal changes and the presence of endometriotic lesions. Mol Hum Reprod 2009;15:645–652.

26 Models of Endometriosis: Animal Models I – Rodent-based Chimeric Models

Kaylon L. Bruner-Tran, Melinda E. McConaha and Kevin G. Osteen

Department of Obstetrics and Gynecology, Women's Reproductive Health Research Center, Vanderbilt University School of Medicine, Nashville, TN, USA

Introduction

The presence of endometrial glands and stroma outside the uterus was first described in the medical literature in the late 1800s [1,2], but another 40 years would pass before the disease would be given the name endometriosis by Dr John Sampson. In a landmark paper of 1927, Sampson recognized the link between menstruation and endometriosis, proposing that development of the disease was due to ectopic implantation of refluxed menstrual tissue [3]. Although numerous studies support his retrograde menstruation theory as a contributor to the development of endometriosis [4–6], simple mechanical transfer of menstrual tissue to the peritoneal cavity cannot account for all incidences of disease. Additionally, since retrograde menstruation is believed to occur in most reproductive-age women [7–9], why do only a fraction develop endometriosis? Alternative explanations of the etiology of endometriosis include the coelomic metaplasia theory [10–13] and development of disease following activation of embryonic cell rests [14,15], the latter of which may explain the rare occurrence of endometriosis in men [16,17]. Other factors which may affect an individual's risk for development of endometriosis include a genetic predisposition, immune dysregulation, and/or a previous environmental toxicant exposure [18]. Furthermore, we and others have proposed that toxicant exposure during early development may predispose one to the development of endometriosis via epigenetic modifications that persist into adulthood, resulting in alterations in reproductive tract gene expression [19–21]. Despite these recent perspectives, our current understanding of the basic biological mechanisms explaining the development of endometriosis in only a subset of women is limited; thus, exploring the pathophysiology of this disease remains an active area of research.

Although considered a benign condition, the spread of endometriosis within the peritoneal cavity and to distal sites exhibits many cancer-like elements, and the symptoms associated with this disease can be equally devastating. Endometriosis is often emotionally and physically debilitating, as patients may suffer from chronic pelvic pain, dyspareunia, dysmenorrhea and subfertility. An unequivocal diagnosis of endometriosis requires surgical observation via laparoscopy, followed by confirmation of endometrial cell identity by a pathologist. Early diagnosis of endometriosis is often difficult as symptoms generally do not present themselves until the disease is well established; furthermore, the delay between onset of symptoms and diagnosis averages 8–11 years for most women [22]. Approximately 10–15% of American women of reproductive age are estimated to have endometriosis, but as many as 40% of infertile women in the United States may have the condition [23]. Although controversial at this juncture, environmental factors have been suggested to contribute to an even higher percentage of disease among infertile women in certain populations [24–26].

Regardless of its etiology, treatment options for women with endometriosis are limited and frequently involve either hormonal manipulation and/or surgery. For many women, the side-effects of medical therapy can be as unpleasant as the symptoms of endometriosis and surgical treatment is generally non-curative, with a high recurrence rate [27–36]. Thus, the development of improved diagnostic and treatment strategies for women with endometriosis is also a high priority for research.

Autologous models of experimental endometriosis

Certainly, retrograde menstruation cannot explain all incidences of endometriosis; nevertheless, the disease only occurs in menstruating species, and only humans and other primates

Endometriosis: Science and Practice, First Edition. Edited by Linda C. Giudice, Johannes L.H. Evers and David L. Healy.
© 2012 Blackwell Publishing Ltd. Published 2012 by Blackwell Publishing Ltd.

spontaneously develop this condition. In the mid-1950s, Sampson's retrograde menstruation theory was examined in humans by Atlanta physicians John H. Ridley and I. Keith Edwards when they attempted to establish experimental endometriosis in women prior to undergoing scheduled surgeries for uterine fibroids [4]. Although not ethical by modern medical research standards, these investigators sought to initiate endometrioisis by intraperitoneal injection of autologous menstrual tissue from volunteers several months prior to their scheduled leiomyomectomies. At the time of fibroid surgery, the patients were examined for the presence of ectopic peritoneal lesions, and two of 13 women (15%) developed endometriotic disease. Although these findings provide support for Sampson's retrograde menstruation theory, this human experimental endometriosis model provided no insight into the cellular or tissue mechanisms involved in early disease establishment. Given the obvious limitations of human experimentation, current endometriosis researchers rely on animal models in order to investigate elements of disease pathophysiology that may lead to the development of better diagnostic or therapeutic strategies.

Humans and certain other primates share a similar menstrual cycle length as well as cyclical endometrial changes, including menstruation [37]. Importantly, primates in captivity have been observed to develop endometriosis spontaneously, and ectopic endometriotic lesions developing in non-human primates are histologically similar to those observed in women with the disease [38,39]. Similar to the Ridley and Edwards studies noted above, researchers have used baboons and other primates to surgically induce retrograde menstruation or inject menstrual tissues intraperitoneally in order to examine establishment and progression of endometriosis [40–43]. As observed in women, endometriosis in non-human primates is associated with decreased fertility [44], and recent research suggests that the loss of progesterone sensitivity that has been noted in the human endometrium [18,45] also occurs in the experimental baboon model [46].

Although there are clear advantages to using non-human primates to model endometriosis, these animals can be prohibitively expensive, severely limiting the scope of experimental questions. Equally importantly, although the disease occurs spontaneously in approximately 27% of primates in captivity [47], it must be induced in these animals for them to be practically useful. Most primates, such as macaques, do not reach reproductive maturity until 3 years of age, making transgenerational studies difficult. For these and other reasons, many researchers have turned to various rodent models of endometriosis, including the use of human tissue to establish disease in immunocompromised mice. The capacity to directly investigate human endometrial tissues growing *in vivo* makes chimeric models of experimental endometriosis particularly useful for preclinical testing, fostering the development of better therapeutic agents. Experimental endometriosis models using autologous uterine tissues have also been developed using rats, mice, rabbits, and hamsters [48–51], and are also valuable for examining multiple aspects of this disease. As will be discussed below, since these animals do not naturally develop ectopic sites of endometrial growth, each rodent model of experimental endometriosis has both benefits and limitations.

Of the various approaches adopted for examining endometriosis, perhaps the most commonly used *in vivo* model is the autologous rat model, first developed by Vernon and Wilson [48]. Although studies using this system require surgical induction of endometriosis, this model has provided significant insight into the mechanisms by which endometriosis may lead to infertility [52]. Of particular note, Sharpe-Timms and colleagues have recently used this model to demonstrate that establishment of experimental endometriosis not only affects the reproductive status of the experimental female herself, but can also adversely affect the fecundity of her adult female offspring [20]. Specifically, following surgical induction of endometriosis, female rats were mated and multiple fertility-related outcomes were examined; some pregnant mice were allowed to continue to term. Female offspring of rats with surgically induced endometriosis exhibited a similar decrease in fertility and disrupted ovarian phenotype as observed in dams with endometriosis. For example, the F1 daughters displayed impaired reproductive capability; two of three were infertile, and the single individual that became pregnant had a reduced litter size and increased number of spontaneous pregnancy losses compared to control animals.

These data suggest that *in utero* exposure to the presence of maternal endometriosis can result in an "endometriosis-like" uterine and ovarian phenotype in later generations, raising the possibility of epigenetic alterations associated with this experimental rodent model. Supporting this possibility, we have recently demonstrated a similar outcome in a murine model of early-life toxicant exposure to an environmental endocrine disruptor, 2,3,7,8-tetrachlorodibenzo-p-dioxin (TCDD). We found that *in utero* exposure to this toxicant is associated with the development of a uterine phenotype which is remarkably similar to that described in women with endometriosis [53]; this "endometriosis phenotype" was associated with decreased fertility for multiple generations [19].

Clearly, compared to human or primate studies, rodent models will continue to be extremely useful for transgenerational studies directed at understanding the potential impact of endometriosis on future fertility. Rodent models are equally valuable for developmental toxicology studies that are often not practical in primates and are unethical prospectively in humans. These and numerous other studies using non-chimeric rodent models of endometriosis highlight the important contributions these animal models continue to make to our understanding of the pathophysiology of this disease [54]. Nevertheless, a major limitation of autologous rodent models is that the rodent uterus naturally exhibits neither menstruation nor ectopic growth. Since rodents do not spontaneously develop endometriosis, establishment of endometriotic-like disease in these animals requires that fragments of uterine tissues be sutured to the recipient animal's peritoneal surface, near sites of existing vasculature (commonly, on the surface of the mesentery). Thus, very early events associated with

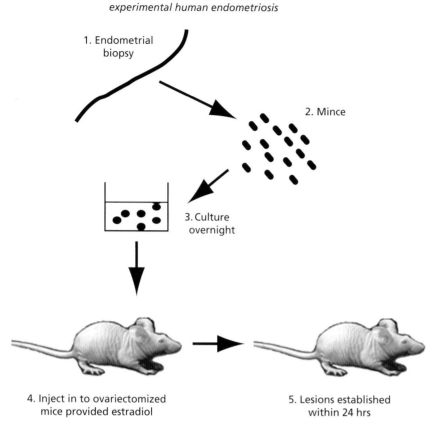

*Overview of the nude mouse model of
experimental human endometriosis*

1. Endometrial
biopsy

2. Mince

3. Culture
overnight

4. Inject in to ovariectomized
mice provided estradiol

5. Lesions established
within 24 hrs

Figure 26.1 Overview of the nude mouse model of experimental human endometriosis. Endometrial tissue, most commonly proliferative phase endometrium obtained by biopsy, is minced and cultured overnight in estradiol (1 nM) with or without additional compounds (i.e. a therapeutic test agent). After the incubation period, tissues are washed in PBS and injected into mice (subcutaneous or intraperitoneal). Lesions can be visualized as early as 4 h after injection and are well established by 24 h.

endometriosis, such as invasion and vascularization, cannot be examined in this model.

Experimental endometriosis in immunocompromised mice

In order to better understand the tissue characteristics and cellular mechanisms of ectopic implantation and survival, several laboratories, including ours, have developed chimeric mouse models of endometriosis using human endometrial tissue and immunocompromised mice [55–58]. Immunocompromised mice lack a fully competent immune system so they can accept human tissue xenografts, making them useful for examining many aspects of this disease. Immunocompromised mouse strains include athymic (nude) mice, severe combined immunodeficient (SCID) mice and recombinant activating gene 2/common cytokine receptor γ chain (γc) double null (rag2γ(c))mice (see Table 26.1 for overview).

As shown in Figure 26.1, in our model of experimental endometriosis using nude mice, human endometrial tissues are obtained by biopsy and prepared as organ cultures. Following overnight incubation in media containing estradiol, tissues are washed in

phosphate buffer saline (PBS) to remove occult blood and injected intraperitoneally or subcutaneously along the ventral midline. As shown in Plate 26.1, lesions which establish are markedly similar to spontaneous disease in women, exhibiting the classic characteristics of endometriosis both grossly and microscopically. Experimental endometriosis can also be established using tissues obtained via collection of menstrual effluent or from surgical specimens obtained from women with endometriosis [59–62], and these studies have revealed important differences between eutopic endometrial tissues obtained from women with endometriosis compared to similar tissue obtained from disease-free women.

In order to understand the pathophysiology of endometriosis, it is necessary to identify the specific elements of human endometrial tissue biology that promote the capacity for ectopic invasion and growth. In our studies, peritoneal attachment of human tissues in nude mice has been noted to occur as early as 4 h after injection of endometrial fragments, with initial host vascular development apparent by 24 h. Extensive vascularization and tissue remodeling of the ectopic lesion occur by about 5 days post injection (Plate 26.2) [63]. Since various experimental endometriosis models have been successfully established using human endometrial or endometriosis tissue in nude, SCID and rag2γ(c) mice, the capacity for successful ectopic invasion is likely

Table 26.1 Characteristics of selected immunocompromised mice.

	Athymic nude	Congenic SCID	Rag2γ(c)
Origin	Spontaneous mutation of Foxn1 (chromosome 11)	Spontaneous autosomal recessive mutation of Prkdc (DNA repair enzyme)(chromosome 16)	Targeted double mutation obtained by crossing γc knockout and Rag2 deficient mice (C57Bl/6 background)
First use/discovery	Discovered in 1962 in Virus Laboratory, Ruchill Hospital, Glasgow, Scotland	Developed in 1980 by Bosma and associates in BALB/c-Igh^bmice at Fox Chase Cancer Center	Mazurier *et al*, 1999 Université Victor Segalen, Bordeaux, France
Hairless	Yes	No	No
Lacking T-lymphocytes	Yes	Yes	Yes
Lacking B-lymphocytes	No	Yes	Yes
Lacking natural killer cells	No	No	Yes
Lacking macrophages	No	No	No
Lacking PMN	No	No	No
Develop extrathymic immunity	Yes	Yes	No
Short lifespan	No; 8.5 months to 1 year	Yes; develop lethal thymomas	No
Effects on reproduction	Homozygous – underdeveloped mammary glands	Can be limited by shorter lifespan	None known
Ability to perform long-term xenograft studies	No	No	Yes
Human endometrial xenograft survival	Up to 21 days, "take-rate" of 60%	Up to 28 days, "take-rate" of 100%	Up to 112 days, "take-rate" of 100%
Other uses in research	Cancer/tumors, angiogenesis, T-cell lymphocytes	HIV, vaccine development, cancer/tumors	HIV, cancer/tumor, infectious diseases

HIV, human immunodeficiency virus; PMN, polymorphonuclear neutrophils; SCID, severe combined immunodeficient.

an innate characteristic of human endometrium rather than a characteristic of the murine peritoneum. Thus, immunocompromised mice have allowed for the analysis of specific aspects of human endometrial cell and tissue function which act to either allow or perhaps actively promote the establishment of ectopic disease. Below, we will discuss these animal models in more detail as well as describe data obtained utilizing these mice to investigate multiple aspects of endometriosis.

Experimental endometriosis in nude mice

Athymic nude mice have been used in research since their discovery in the Virus Laboratory at Ruchill Hospital in Scotland in 1962. The nude mouse was a product of breeding a closed stock of outbred albino mice, which resulted in a spontaneous mutation in the forkhead box N1 (Foxn1) gene. In the late 1960s, this mutation was determined to be autosomal recessive and resulted in thymic dysgenesis [64–66]. As a result of an underdeveloped thymus and severely compromised number of T-cells, these animals are unable to mount most types of immune response (i.e. antibody formation, cell-mediated responses, delayed hypersensitivity, graft rejection). As shown in Table 26.1, homozygous nude mice have a normal complement of B-cells; however, the lack of T-cells prevents complete B-cell maturation. Nude mice are also slightly "leaky" and develop extrathymic immunity as they age, slowly expressing surface markers CD3, CD4, CD5, CD8, and Thy-1 around 3–4

months of age [67]. Later in life, nude mice also begin to express the proinflammatory cytokine interleukin (IL)-2 but still display an inability to sufficiently respond to mitogens [68]. As a result of developing extrathymic immunity, studies utilizing nude mice must be completed before the animals reach 3 months of age, severely limiting the duration of some experimental studies.

Prior to the discovery of nude mice, researchers interested in immunological components of the thymus had to thymectomize mice at birth [69]. Since the discovery of these unique animals, researchers have been able to utilize their immunocompromised state to study a variety of immunological diseases, making these mice a valuable contributor to many areas of study. As a result of their genetic mutation, hair follicle keratinization is disrupted in these mice, preventing normal eruption of hair from the follicle; thus athymic mice appear hairless which gives them their characteristic "nude" appearance. Heterozygous litter mates of nude mice are immune competent, have no defects in keratinization and have white fur. Importantly, care of nude mice, as with all immunodeficient animals, requires special precautions, including maintaining a sterile environment, in order to prevent opportunistic infections. To this end, mice are typically either housed in barrier facilities or maintained in specific pathogen-free (SPF) cages; food and water must be autoclaved or irradiated for sterility. Husbandry of nude mice also requires special consideration since female homozygous nude mice are unable to lactate;

therefore heterozygous females are typically mated to homozygous males to propagate a colony [70].

The first reported use of nude mice for establishment of experimental endometriosis was by Zamah and colleagues [59]. This group introduced eutopic and ectopic endometrium from women with and without endometriosis into the peritoneal space of nude mice; half of the mice were treated with estrogen. The authors described development of endometriotic-like disease in most mice, with the animals receiving both estrogen treatment and ectopic tissues from women with endometriosis exhibiting more extensive disease than mice receiving normal endometrium, regardless of steroid support. Following this study, Bergqvist *et al* [60] similarly introduced eutopic and ectopic endometrial tissue into nude mice treated with synthetic estrogen. Grafts were allowed to establish, then groups of mice were subjected to different steroid regimens (estrogen with or without medroxyprogesterone acetate or danazol) and growth was assessed histologically after 8 weeks. The authors concluded that histological changes in the grafts varied according to the treatment schedule, but were very similar in both types of tissue, suggesting that differences between endometrium and endometriotic tissue may be due to variations in the peritoneal environment. Both these early studies provided support for Sampson's theory of retrograde menstruation as a mechanical cause of endometriosis [3] as well as the utility of nude mice to examine aspects of this disease.

As noted above, a key element of early establishment of endometriosis is the ability of human endometrial tissue to rapidly attach and establish an invasive site on the peritoneal wall or surface of various organs within the peritoneum. Thus, our laboratory initially established our chimeric human/mouse model system of experimental endometriosis to investigate a possible role for matrix metalloproteinases (MMPs) in the invasive establishment of experimental endometriosis in nude mice [55,71]. The MMPs are highly regulated enzymes which are necessary for normal and pathological tissue remodeling such as that which occurs during tumor metastasis [72]. Additionally, these early studies using human tissues in nude mice provided one of the first demonstrations that this model could be utilized not only for the study of disease establishment but also for the development of therapeutic intervention strategies. We demonstrated that therapeutic intervention which blocked MMP expression or action prevented the establishment of human endometrial growth at ectopic sites within the peritoneum [55]. Our laboratory has continued to utilize this nude mouse model of experimental endometriosis to examine various therapeutic agents that hold promise for the treatment of this disease [62, 73].

Numerous other laboratories have also adopted or modified our basic experimental endometriosis model for therapeutic testing, and a number of significant advancements have resulted from a series of collaborations. For example, Fortin *et al* [74] labeled human endometrial tissues with green fluorescent protein prior to injection into nude mice. Since these mice are hairless, tissues could be non-invasively visualized through the skin of live mice via fluorescent imaging. Another adaptation of the nude mouse model has been the utilization of the kidney capsule for various studies rather than the random sites of growth observed following intraperitoneal injection of human tissues. The renal capsule is highly vascular, and human endometrial tissues or isolated and recombined endometrial cells can be readily inserted under the kidney capsule and recovered at later times [75]. Significantly, renal grafting permits various combinations of endometrial cells to be studied, potentially allowing a more precise examination of each endometrial cell type during growth in the nude mouse.

Together, the studies noted above and other similar studies using modifications of the nude mouse experimental model have greatly contributed to our understanding of endometriosis, particularly with regard to early lesion establishment. In all likelihood, this model will continue to provide a valuable tool in which to examine specific cellular pathways that may have potential as therapeutic targets. Finally, these docile mice are exceptionally easy to handle and, since they are hairless, surgical manipulations and various imaging paradigms are simplified. Perhaps for these reasons, despite immunological limitations, the nude mouse remains the most frequent choice for xenograft studies of experimental endometriosis.

Experimental endometriosis in severe combined immunodeficient mice

Severe combined immunodeficiency (SCID) occurs in many species, including humans [76]. This condition results from a severe genetic disorder characterized by the inability of the adaptive immune system to mount or sustain an appropriate immune response due to absent/dysfunctional T- and B-lymphocytes. In mice, the condition results from a rare, recessive mutation which gives rise to limited activity of a DNA repair enzyme, protein kinase, DNA activated, catalytic polypeptide (Prkdc), which ultimately leads to a failed maturation of either the humoral or cellular immune systems. In 1980, Bosma and associates at Fox Chase Cancer Center first described an autosomal recessive mutation in BALB/c-Ighb mice, resulting in the SCID phenotype [77]. As summarized in Table 26.1, SCID mice exhibit an impaired ability to make T- or B-lymphocytes and cannot efficiently fight infections or reject tumors. Additionally, they lack natural killer (NK) cells and all lymphocytes. For these reasons, SCID mice are also suitable animals for establishing experimental endometriosis using human tissues. Similar to nude mice, SCID mice often exhibit a degree of age-related compensatory immunity, limiting the duration of studies in these animals. Fertility is not affected in these mice, and propagation of a colony is rather simple, via mating of homozygous animals.

Only limited numbers of experimental endometriosis studies have been conducted in SCID mice, perhaps due to their increased susceptibility to opportunistic infections (both viral and bacterial) compared to nude mice. Nevertheless, Aoki *et al* [78] established experimental endometriosis using human tissues in both SCID and nude mice; these investigators suggested that experimental endometriosis in SCID mice was superior to the nude mouse model due to a significantly greater survival rate of human tissues. However, the SCID mouse model of human endometriosis was patented in 2002 [79], perhaps limiting its broad availability for general use in endometriosis-related studies.

Experimental endometriosis in recombinant activating gene 2/common cytokine receptor γ chain (γc) double null mice

Recombinant activating gene 2/common cytokine receptor γ chain (γc) double null mice (rag2γ(c)) are more completely immunosuppressed compared to nude or SCID mice, demonstrating an absence of B-cells, T-cells, NK cell activity and all lymphocytes (see Table 26.1). These mice were first described by Mazurier *et al* [80] who crossed the common γc knockout mouse [81] with the recombinase activating gene-2 (rag2) deficient mouse [82]. Although rag2γ(c) mice demonstrate more aggressive behavior compared to nude mice, they do not demonstrate the same age-related compensatory immunity as other immunocompromised mice. Thus, xenographic studies conducted in rag2γ(c) mice can be of much longer duration than those which can be conducted in nude or SCID mice.

Greenberg and Slayden [57] were the first to report the xenotransplantation of endometrial tissues into rag2γ(c) mice. In this study, human endometrium was transplanted into mice and subjected to up to four artificial menstrual cycles. Even after four 28-day cycles, the majority of mice exhibited endometriotic-like disease, supporting the use of this model system for long-term studies. Another advantage of these animals is that human immune cells can be adoptively transferred into the blood circulation as a component of an experimental endometriosis model, as we have recently reported [58]. Although the results of our study will be discussed in more detail later in this chapter, the addition of human immune cells to a human/murine chimeric model may provide a more natural experimental endometriosis model compared to the immunocompromised state of either the nude or SCID mouse.

Unfortunately, rag2γ(c) mice are available for research studies in limited supply and can currently only be obtained from Taconic Farms (Germantown, NY, USA) or through the maintenance of a colony. However, female mice do not exhibit the lactation defects noted in nude mice, so establishing and maintaining a rag2γ(c) colony is not prohibitively difficult for most researchers.

Preclinical therapeutic testing

A major need within the reproductive medical community is for more effective endometriosis therapies with fewer side-effects than those currently available to patients. As noted above, while each experimental model of endometriosis has utility as a research tool, the growth of human tissues in immunocompromised mice is particularly well suited for conducting preclinical testing of novel agents that may specifically target human endometrial cells. For example,

chimeric models of endometriosis allow scientists to examine the possibility that current medications being utilized for other human diseases might have potential use in endometriosis therapy.

Role of steroid modulation in experimental endometriosis

Since the publication of our first study utilizing the nude mouse model of experimental endometriosis in which we reported that progesterone treatments inhibited lesion development [55], a number of laboratories have utilized similar techniques to test various pharmacological and biological agents for therapeutic efficacy. It has long been known that progesterone exposure is a negative risk factor for the development of endometriosis [83,84]; thus, it is not surprising that we found that progesterone treatment of mice bearing normal tissue xenografts reduced the extent of experimental disease [55]. Progesterone is a potent differentiation agent and human endometrial tissue recovered from the peritoneal cavity of recipient mice undergoing treatment with the synthetic progestin levonorgestrol exhibits decidual changes reflective of the late secretory phase [85]. We have also observed similar decidual-like changes in human tissue lesions following short-term treatment of mice with the synthetic progestin medroxyprogesterone acetate (Plate 26.3A), while longer-term treatment with this steroid prevents normal endometrium from establishing disease [62].

These studies suggest that endometrial tissues, growing at an ectopic site in the peritoneum of nude mice, largely retain a similar level of responsiveness to progesterone that would be observed within the normal eutopic endometrium. In contrast, progesterone therapy fails to prevent the establishment and progression of experimental endometriosis when the ectopic sites of peritoneal growth are established with eutopic endometrial tissue obtained from women with endometriosis [62,86]. The failure of progesterone to limit the development of experimental disease by tissue acquired from patients appears to be related to the reduced degree of endometrial progesterone responsiveness noted in these women [62,86]. Thus, the decidual-like changes noted at ectopic sites of control human endometrial tissue growth in our experimental model are not observed in tissues acquired from endometriosis patients following treatment of mice with either natural progesterone or medroxyprogesterone acetate (Plate 26.3B). Given these findings, we examined whether a potent non-steroidal progesterone receptor agonist would have a better therapeutic profile compared to natural progesterone. In this study, tanaproget, a selective progesterone receptor modulator, was found to be more effective than either progesterone or medroxyprogesterone acetate in reducing experimental endometriosis in our model when ectopic disease was established by eutopic endometrial tissues acquired from women with endometriosis [62].

In addition to our studies examining natural progesterone or pharmaceutical progestins as a therapeutic strategy, we have also utilized ERB-041, a selective estrogen receptor-β (ERβ) agonist with anti-inflammatory activity, in our nude mouse model [87]. For this study, nude mice were injected with tissue fragments of control human endometrium and, following establishment of ectopic lesions for 11–14 days, the mice were treated with ERB-041 for up to 17 days. ERB-041 treatment was associated with complete lesion regression in the majority of mice; however, the effectiveness of ERB-041 therapy in this study was found to be dependent upon the site of human tissue growth. Specifically, intraperitoneal sites of ectopic lesions appeared to be more sensitive to ERB-041 therapy compared to subcutaneous sites of growth. Although the reasons for such a differential effect of lesion location were not fully explored in this study, one interpretation of the data is that ERB-041 may be more effective in inducing activity of immune surveillance within the peritoneum than at subcutaneous sites. For example, a group of investigators has explored the effects of ERB-041 on isolated macrophages from women with endometriosis, demonstrating that this agent inhibits activation of NFκB via prevention of nuclear translocation [88]. Additionally, this study described an increased expression of ERβ in macrophages derived from women with endometriosis compared to control patients. Taken together, these studies using an ERβ agonist suggest a role for macrophages in clearance of displaced human endometrium and support the use of ERB-041 and possibly other similar agents targeted toward immune cells in the treatment of endometriosis [87,88].

Antiangiogenesis therapy in experimental endometriosis

Ectopic survival of endometrial lesions requires a vascular supply; thus, it has been suggested that inhibitors of angiogenesis could be effective in preventing the early development of the disease. Blood vessels which are immature and have limited associations with pericyte cells can be most easily targeted by angiogenic inhibitors. Thus, a collaborative study with our laboratory [89] demonstrated that pericyte-free vessels supplied the human endometrial lesions in the nude mouse model of experimental endometriosis, as observed in the early native human disease. Moreover, this study also demonstrated that treatments with soluble flt-1, a vascular endothelial growth factor (VEGF) receptor antagonist, prevented the formation of ectopic human lesions in mice, suggesting that the use of angiogenesis inhibitors may be a useful therapeutic strategy following surgical removal of ectopic disease.

However, therapeutic *regression* of established lesions is perhaps of greater utility to most women with endometriosis, and would potentially decrease the need for surgical intervention. In this regard, established lesions were targeted by a more recent collaborative study with our group that examined the potential therapeutic efficacy of Icon, an immunoconjugate molecule, on experimental endometriosis in nude mice [90]. Icon binds with high affinity and specificity to tissue factor (TF) expressed inappropriately by endothelial cells. Icon has been found in other studies to induce a cytolytic immune response that eradicates tumor and choroidal blood vessels which also aberrantly express TF [91–95]. In this study, Krikun *et al* [90] demonstrated that endothelial cells in

experimental endometriotic lesions also exhibit anomalous expression of TF. Using the nude mouse model of human disease, lesions were allowed to establish for 10–12 days prior to the initiation of treatment with Icon. It was found that Icon treatment of established lesions eliminated disease in most mice, largely by disruption of the vascular supply via destruction of endothelial cells.

Several other studies using chimeric mouse models have also explored the efficacy of a variety of agents which modulate angiogenesis for the treatment of endometriosis. In a comprehensive study, Nap *et al* [96] tested anti-hVEGF, TNP-470, endostatin, and anginex treatment on existing endometriotic lesions in nude mice. Mice bearing both subcutaneous and intraperitoneal lesions were treated for 5 weeks with individual compounds. Although endostatin was most effective, all four treatments significantly reduced the number of lesions and microvessel density (MVD) of surviving lesions. Furthermore, lesions that remained after treatment displayed fewer pericyte-protected vessels, suggesting an impaired ability to undergo angiogenesis. A similar study was conducted by Jiang et al [97] using eutopic endometrium from women with endometriosis transplanted into SCID mice. For this study, ectopic lesions were allowed to establish for 2 weeks prior to mice receiving therapy with recombinant human endostatin (YH-16). Mice receiving endostatin treatment for 14 days exhibited fewer and smaller lesions; significantly lesions which were recovered in these mice were necrotic with reduced expression of VEGF and minimal MVD compared to controls.

Interestingly, epigallocatechin gallate (EGCG), a green tea extract with potent antiangiogenic properties, has also been tested as a therapeutic agent in a SCID mouse model of experimental endometriosis. In this study, Xu *et al* [88] treated mice implanted with endometrial tissues from women with endometriosis with EGCG at 5 or 50 mg/kg. The authors found that following treatment with the highest dose of EGCG, endometriotic-like lesions were smaller than control ($P < 0.05$) with underdeveloped vessels and reduced VEGF expression compared to lesions in control mice. To translate this therapeutically to humans, the higher dose would be equivalent to approximately 30 cups of green tea per day; however, supplemental extracts are readily available. An advantage of green tea catechins is their lengthy half-life, large volume of distribution, and ability to be easily tolerated even at high doses.

The studies described above using various pharmaceutical and natural agents that act as angiogenesis inhibitors indicate that such compounds can effectively interfere with both the maintenance and growth of endometriotic lesions in experimental endometriosis models and support investigating the use of angiostatic agents as potential therapies for women with endometriosis.

Anti-inflammatory agents in experimental endometriosis

Endometriosis, like many complex diseases, has a multifaceted etiology and pathophysiology which, while creating clinical challenges, suggests that various therapeutic approaches may have promise for the treatment of this disease. For example, the initial establishment and progression of this peritoneal disease requires that several related biological events, including peritoneal attachment, matrix degradation and neovascularization, occur in rapid fashion. Although targeting any one of these processes may be a useful therapeutic strategy for women with endometriosis, targeting multiple processes with one agent should be even more effective. Since inflammatory mediators can affect each of the processes known to be necessary for establishment of endometriosis, we and others have investigated the utility of anti-inflammatory agents as a therapuetic strategy.

Inflammatory cytokines and the inflammation pathway have been implicated in the development of endometriosis by a number of studies [98,99]. As noted in studies discussed above, steroid receptor modulators, including progestins and ERβ antagonists, can exert anti-inflammatory activity, effectively limiting the experimental disease in mice. These studies and others suggest that inflammation may represent a key component in the establishment of experimental endometriosis; however, a recent study by Donnez and colleagues has provided more direct evidence of the utility of targeting inflammation in experimental endometriosis. This group established experimental endometriosis in nude mice via intraperitoneal injection of menstrual endometrium; mice were either untreated or provided one of two NFκB inhibitors (BAY 11-7085 and SN-50) every other day for a total of three treatments [100]. Ectopic lesions were recovered and quantified on day 5. Analysis included the number and mass of endometriotic lesions, their fluorimetry and surface morphometry, as well as immunohistochemical analyses of NFκB activation, intercellular adhesion molecule (ICAM)-1 expression, apoptosis and cell proliferation. The authors reported a significant reduction in the number and size of lesions in both NFκB inhibitor-treated groups compared to control mice. Furthermore, NFκB activation and ICAM-1 expression of endometriotic lesions were significantly reduced in treated mice, while apoptosis was increased.

These results support a specific role for the NFκB pathway in the development of experimental endometriosis and implicate this pathway in the development of human disease. Clearly, anti-inflammatory agents which interfere with the NFκB pathway would likely also inhibit processes necessary for the establishment and progression of experimental endometriosis. Equally important, the success of therapuetic agents such as these provides important insights into how and why this disease occurs. The greater our understanding of the mechanisms by which endometriosis initially develops, the better able we are to design more effective therapeutic strategies. Thus, preclincal therapeutic studies and studies designed to examine disease mechanisms can be conducted in tandem, creating a positive, feedforward experimental system.

Experimental endometriosis models and examination of disease mechanism

As stated previously, immunocompromised mouse models of experimental endometriosis allow for the invasive growth of human endometrial tissue at ectopic peritoneal sites and provide an opportunity to explore multiple aspects of the disease which cannot be ethically examined in women. Due to their unique, chimeric nature, experimental human/mouse model systems have been invaluable in identifying cell-specific factors expressed during peritoneal invasion by the different cell types residing within the invading endometrial tissue (human origin), the invaded host site (mouse peritoneum) or cells that migrate to the invasion site (various immune cells and vascular cells). Each of these tissue-specific cell types plays an important role in determining the success or failure of experimental disease establishment. Below, we will briefly describe some key observations made using experimental models of endometriosis as we have explored the cellular processes that allow establishment and progression of disease. The goal of our studies is to provide insight into the mechanisms of disease which can then be translated into development of better therapeutic strategies.

Matrix metalloproteinases and experimental endometriosis

Endometriosis is an invasive disease requiring penetration of the mesothelial lining of the peritoneal cavity for establishment of ectopic lesions. Thus, the expression of enzymes capable of breaking down the extracellular matrix (ECM) at sites of endometrial attachment is likely an important prerequisite for development of endometriosis. However, numerous normal reproductive processes also require tissue remodeling, and researchers have demonstrated that multiple members of the MMP family are transiently expressed in both a cell-specific and site-specific manner within the female reproductive tract. Precisely controlled expression of these enzymes is required for important reproductive processes, including ovulation and menstruation [101]; however, these enzymes can also participate in disease processes, including cancer metastasis [72] and the benign but invasive establishment of endometriosis [45].

Our group has studied the MMP enzyme family in the female reproductive tract for more than 20 years, and we were among the first to describe the cyclical expression of several of these enzymes during the human menstrual cycle. Specifically, we demonstrated extensive expression of MMPs during menstrual tissue breakdown and a more modest expression during estrogen-mediated regrowth within the proliferative phase [102,103]. We further demonstrated that the messenger RNAs (mRNAs) for most of these MMPs were absent during the progesterone-dominated secretory phase of the menstrual cycle [102,103].

Following our initial *in vivo* analysis of the MMP system, *in vitro* studies further revealed that, within the normal endometrium, progesterone acts to suppress endometrial MMP expression via direct and indirect mechanisms requiring stromal-epithelial communication [104,105]. Not surprisingly, the highest levels of MMP enzyme expression within the human endometrium are found during the inflammatory process of menstruation (102,103,106). Taken together, the findings of a number of research groups interested in endometrial MMP expression strongly suggested that these enzymes play an important role in peritoneal invasion associated with the establishment of endometriosis. To more definitively assess the potential role of MMP expression and action in early peritoneal invasion and ectopic lesion survival, we established our nude mouse model of experimental endometriosis. In these studies, we found that proliferative phase endometrial tissues obtained from disease-free women and injected into the peritoneal cavity of nude mice readily established ectopic lesions in the presence of continuous estradiol exposure. However, a brief 16-h exposure of human endometrial fragments to progesterone prior to introduction into the peritoneal cavity of nude mice significantly decreased the ability of the human tissue to establish ectopic sites of peritoneal growth [55]. Importantly, we found that treatment of mice with recombinant tissue inhibitor of metalloproteinases (TIMP)-1, a natural inhibitor of MMP action, also reduced ectopic lesion formation even in the absence of progesterone exposure, strongly suggesting that the establishment of experimental endometriosis in our nude mouse model required the expression and action of these matrix-degrading enzymes.

Although our initial experiments using the nude mouse model were designed to determine the potential role of MMPs in the invasive establishment of ectopic lesions, our findings also suggested that the ability of progesterone to downregulate the endometrial MMP system may partially explain the protective role of this steroid in reducing the risk of developing endometriosis. Moreover, we found that eutopic endometrial tissues acquired from women with endometriosis exhibited a reduced sensitivity to progesterone *in vitro*; consequently, these tissues expressed higher levels of MMPs, and were able to establish ectopic lesions within the peritoneum of nude mice regardless of progesterone treatment [85].

Reduced endometrial progesterone response has emerged as an important component of the disease process in women with endometriosis [18,45] so understanding the pathophysiology of this defect is an important goal of future studies. In this regard, studies to date have revealed that reduced endometrial progesterone responsiveness noted in women with endometriosis is related to altered expression of progesterone receptor (PR) isoforms. Specifically, both eutopic and ectopic tissues from women with endometriosis have been shown to have reduced PRB expression, but abundant PRA expression [107,108]. This alteration in the PRA/PRB ratio is significant, since PRA can act as a dominant repressor of progesterone action, while PRB is generally associated with the differentiation effects of progesterone [109–111].

Although many endometrial proteins are expressed in response to progesterone, we have focused considerable attention on secondary mediators that are known to be involved in regulation of the endometrial MMP system. For example, members of the transforming growth factor (TGF)-β family are well-known regulators of the MMPs in numerous tissues [112,113]; thus, it is not surprising that the ability of differentiation agents, including progesterone or retinoic acid, to downregulate the endometrial MMP system depends on TGF-β signaling [105,114]. Not

unexpectedly, in our experimental model of endometriosis, we found that pretreatment of endometrial tissues acquired from women with endometriosis with a combination of progesterone, all-trans retinoic acid and TGF-β2 effectively suppressed the expression of MMP-3 and MMP-7 *in vitro* and subsequently blocked the establishment of ectopic lesions following injection into the peritoneal cavity of nude mice [86]. Certainly, such a combination of agents would not be therapeutically feasible in patients with endometriosis; however, this finding does provide insight into the important roles that progesterone-mediated endometrial growth factors and cytokines likely play in the regulation of the MMP system during reproductive processes.

As a more practical approach to the development of therapeutics for women with endometriosis, as mentioned earlier, we have demonstrated that the non-steroidal PR agonist tanaproget was more effective than medroxyprogesterone acetate in preventing experimental disease established by tissues from women with endometriosis. Perhaps this is not surprising given that tanaproget was highly effective *in vitro* in terms of suppressing MMPs secretion in endometrial tissues acquired from women with endometriosis [62]. As a better understanding of the biological origins of reduced progesterone responsiveness within the eutopic endometrium of women with endometriosis emerges, it is likely that new therapeutic targets will also be identified that can be tested in models of experimental disease.

Impact of the peritoneal microenvironment on experimental endometriosis

Peritoneal fluid, which bathes and lubricates the pelvic organs, is a rich source of growth factors, cytokines, steroids, and proteases [115–118]. Importantly, proteases within the peritoneal fluid of normal women are thought to prevent adhesion of refluxed menstrual tissue due to both degradation of endometrial tissue fragments into single cells and reduction in expression of cell adhesion molecules [119]. However, in women with endometriosis, the peritoneal fluid is essentially a proinflammatory matrix exhibiting increased concentrations of activated leukocytes and proinflammatory cytokines [120–123]. Thus, cross-talk between the peritoneal fluid and retrogradely shed endometrium may play a role in determining why only certain women develop endometriosis [124].

In contrast to biological agents that suppress the MMP system, peritoneal factors which promote expression or activity of endometrial MMPs following retrograde menstruation could also play an important role in the development of endometriosis. Indeed, among the first observations we made in our experimental model of endometriosis was that proinflammatory cytokines that induce endometrial MMP expression *in vitro* also promote the establishment of experimental endometriosis in nude mice [125]. Clearly, cytokines and growth factors present within the peritoneal cavity can have a profound influence on establishment of experimental disease in our model; similar mechanisms are likely at play in the human disease. For example, mice in our experimental model are routinely ovariectomized prior to establishment of ectopic sites of human tissue growth within the peritoneal cavity, allowing us to modulate the steroid environment via exogenous estradiol. The ovariectomy procedure results in a transient inflammatory peritoneal environment due to the surgical injury. Thus, we explored the impact of this injury-induced proinflammatory microenvironment on the development of experimental endometriosis [126]. For this study, proliferative-phase endometrial tissues from women with no history of endometriosis were established as organ cultures and treated overnight with estradiol. Tissues were injected intraperitoneally into mice at various times following surgery (i.e. less than 24 h or more than 5 days). We found that a recent surgical injury within the peritoneal cavity significantly enhanced the development of experimental endometriosis. Specifically, endometrial tissues injected within 16 h of surgery track to the wound site and established much larger lesions than those developing in sham-operated mice or mice which had undergone surgery more than 24 h previously (Plate 26.4). Although the inflammatory reactions associated with ovariectomy in our model may not reflect the degree of peritoneal injury normally occurring during surgery in women, our findings do suggest that peritoneal surgery near the time of menses may not be clinically wise in women of reproductive age, especially those who may be at risk for developing endometriosis.

Given the dramatic impact of wound-related inflammation on the development of experimental endometriosis, it was of interest to determine if an anti-inflammatory agent might have a protective effect against disease development. To explore this possibility, we examined the effect of simvastatin, a cholesterol-lowering drug with potent anti-inflammatory actions, on regulation of endometrial MMPs and prevention of the ectopic establishment of experimental endometriosis in our model [63]. We determined that simvastatin is effective in suppressing expression of MMP-3 *in vitro* in isolated human endometrial stromal cells, even in the presence of a potent proinflammatory cytokine, IL-1α. We also demonstrated that simvastatin significantly reduced the number and size of endometriotic-like lesions in our experimental model.

In women with endometriosis and a highly inflammatory peritoneal microenvironment, multiple immune system defects have been described [127]. Whether or not these alterations are a cause or consequence of the disease is not known; however, our data indicated that normal immune function is critical to preventing the development of experimental disease. Specifically, we recently established experimental human endometriosis in rag2γ(c) mice following the adoptive transfer of autologous human immune cells. As noted earlier, the severity and stability of the immune defects of the rag2γ(c) animals allow the introduction of elements of a human immune system [128,129], thereby enabling the examination of the effects of this system in experimental endometriosis [58]. Using these animals, our study clearly indicated that the presence of immune cells from women with no history of endometriosis impedes the growth of intraperitoneal experimental lesions, suggesting an important role of a robust immune system in preventing the development of this

disease. Thus, an important future direction will be to determine whether or not anti-inflammatory agents, such as simvastatin, can act to modulate the immune system of women with endometriosis and promote disease regression.

Influence of the environmental toxicants on the development of experimental endometriosis

The above data indicate that understanding the mechanisms associated with the development of endometriosis will require a better knowledge of the contributions of both the biology of the endometrial cells entering the peritoneal cavity and the influence of the peritoneal microenvironment itself. Certainly, as a discovery tool, the chimeric mouse model of experimental endometriosis has begun to reveal numerous potential targets that merit further examination for clinical utility. However, another area of research in which models of experimental endometriosis are not only useful but necessary is in the field of reproductive toxicology. We have utilized our chimeric models to explore the potential role of environmental toxicants on the development of endometriosis.

Although human exposure to environmental toxicants is common, experimentally connecting one's exposure to the risk for developing a specific disease is difficult and prospective human studies are not possible. For example, 2,3,7,8-tetrachlorodibenzo-p-dioxin (TCDD) a known endocrine disruptor, has been suspected to promote the development of endometriosis in women for more than a decade, yet no conclusive data have emerged [19]. Previously published data from our laboratory and others have demonstrated that many of the classic, genomic effects of TCDD on human cells are mediated via inflammatory cytokines and chemokines [107,130,131]. Through a series of *in vitro* studies with human endometrial cells and *in vivo* studies using a murine model of early-life TCDD exposure [53], we are beginning to uncover a plausible biological explanation that could link human exposure to toxicants with TCDD-like action and the development of endometriosis [19]. More specifically, we have shown that *in vitro* exposure of human endometrial cells to this toxicant both reduces levels of PRB expression relative to PRA and promotes increased levels of endometrial MMP-3 secretion, essentially inducing the endometrial phenotype observed in women with endometriosis [107]. Also, early-life exposure of mice to TCDD leads to the development of an endometriosis-like phenotype as these animals reach sexual maturity.

As noted above, we have shown that the phenotype of the eutopic human endometrial fragments can significantly influence the outcome in our nude mouse model of experimental endometriosis, largely by stimulating the host vascular response. For example, we have found that control endometrial tissues acquired from women with no history of endometriosis and maintained in the presence of estradiol prior to introduction in nude mice required several days to develop a robust vascular network (see Plate 26.2). As shown in Plate 26.2A and Plate 26.5A, control tissues readily attach to the murine peritoneum and, at 4 h after injection, have not acquired any significant vascularization. In contrast, endometrial tissues acquired from the endometrium of women with endometriosis more quickly establish an extensive vascular network which is apparent as early as 4 h post injection (Plate 26.5B).

Using the same approach in our experimental endometriosis model, we have shown that a 16-h *in vitro* exposure of control human endometrial fragments to TCDD causes these otherwise normal endometrial tissues to establish a highly aggressive experimental disease *in vivo*, similar to the activity of tissues acquired from endometriosis patients [73]. Results to date suggest that exposure of control human endometrial tissues to TCDD prior to injection into mice affects the murine vascular response by increasing the murine neutrophils to the invasion site. In experimental human lesions established in the peritoneum of mice in the absence of toxicant exposure, few neutrophils were present within the stromal compartment of the human tissue during invasion but rather were located in the lumen of glands, as is commonly seen in normal secretory-phase human endometrium. In contrast, numerous neutrophils of murine origin were observed within the stromal compartment of TCDD-exposed human tissues. The attraction of neutrophils by toxicant-treated human endometrial fragments may be particularly important since these cells can trigger inflammation at the invasive site and are also a major source of VEGF [89,127,132–135].

Significantly, in a collaborative study, we conducted an extensive immunohistochemical analysis of vessels in established experimental disease in our model which revealed the presence of both human and murine endothelial cells [89], suggesting that cytokines and growth factors released by the human tissue actively recruit the murine vasculature. Supporting these findings, the formation of chimeric vessels in human experimental endometriosis in SCID mice was similarly demonstrated by Alvarez Gonzalez *et al* [136].

Whether TCDD exposure affects the development of endometriosis in humans continues to be unclear; nevertheless, this toxicant remains a useful tool as we elucidate cellular mechanisms within the peritoneal cavity which may influence disease establishment and survival. Clearly, even in the absence of toxicant exposure, numerous studies have demonstrated that the host site response during ectopic invasion is a critical determinant in the establishment and survival of experimental endometriosis.

Conclusion

Despite being a recognized medical condition for more than a century, endometriosis remains enigmatic, with a poorly understood etiology. Nevertheless, advances in our understanding of disease processes necessary for its establishment and survival have been made. Due in large measure to use of immunocompromised, chimeric models of human endometriosis, we now have a much broader understanding of the role of the tissue phenotype and communication with the peritoneal microenvironment which prevent or promote disease establishment. These interactions affect matrix degradation, host angiogenic response and activa-

tion of the immune system which ultimately determine whether or not an individual develops endometriosis. These data, taken in concert with studies examining human tissues for genetic and epigenetic alterations which are associated with endometriosis, can further enhance our understanding of how and why this disease develops. Understanding the mechanisms which promote the development of endometriosis provides the best opportunity to develop therapeutic strategies which are more effective and with fewer side-effects. Ultimately, identifying factors which predispose an individual to the development of endometriosis would potentially open the door to preventing this enigmatic disease.

Acknowledgments

The human endometrial biopsies used in our experiments described above are most frequently obtained from volunteers. We are indebted to these women, as well as the physicians within the Vanderbilt Women's Center who perform these critical biopsies. We also express our grateful appreciation to Ms Dana Glore for expert assistance in preparing this chapter.

References

1. Diesterweg A. Ein fall von cystofibroma uteri verum. Z. Geburtshilfe 1883;9:191–195.

2. Benagiano G, Brosens I. The history of endometriosis: identifying the disease. Hum Reprod 1991;6:963–968.

3. Sampson JA. Peritoneal endometriosis due to menstrual dissemination of endometrial tissues into the peritoneal cavity. Am J Obstet Gynecol 1927;14:422–469.

4. Ridley JH, Edwards IK. Experimental endometriosis in the human. Am J Obstet Gynecol 1958;76:783–789; discussion 789–790.

5. TeLinde RW, Scott RB. Experimental endometriosis. Am J Obstet Gynecol 1950;60:1147–1173.

6. Sørensen SS, Andersen LF, Lose G. Endometriosis by implantation: a complication of endometrial ablation. Lancet 1994;343:1226.

7. Blumenkrantz MJ, Gallagher N, Bashore RA, Tenckhoff H. Retrograde menstruation in women undergoing chronic peritoneal dialysis. Obstet Gynecol 1981;57:667–670.

8. Halme J, Hammond MG, Hulka JF, Raj SG, Talbert LM. Retrograde menstruation in healthy women and in patients with endometriosis. Obstet Gynecol 1984;64:151–154.

9. Eskenazi B, Warner ML. Epidemiology of endometriosis. Obstet Gynecol Clin North Am 1997;24:235–258.

10. Meyer R. Ueber eine adenomatose. Wucherung der serosa in einer Banchuabe. Zeit Geburt Gynak 1903;49:32–38.

11. Meyer R. Ueber den stand der Frage der Adenomyositis und Adenomyome in algemeinen und insbesondere iiber Adenomyositis serosoepithelialis und Adenomyometritis sarcomatosa. Zentralbl Gyndkol 1919;43:745–750.

12. El–Mahgoub S, Yaseen S. A positive proof for the theory of coelomic metaplasia. Am J Obstet Gynecol 1980;137:137–140.

13. Nakamurma H, Nakamura M, Katabuchi H et al. Scanning electron microscopic and immunohistochemical studies of pelvic endometriosis. Hum Reprod 1993;8:2218–2226.

14. Batt RE, Smith RA. Embryologic theory of histogenesis of endometriosis in peritoneal pockets. Obstet Gynecol Clin North Am 1989;16:15–28.

15. Batt RE, Smith RA, Buck GM, Severino MF, Naples JD. Müllerianosis. Prog Clin Biol Res 1990;323:413–426.

16. Schrodt GR, Alcorn MO, Ibanez J. Endometriosis of the male urinary system: a case report. J Urol 1980;124:722–723.

17. Witz CA. Current concepts in the pathogenesis of endometriosis. Clin Obstet Gynecol 1999;42:566–585.

18. Bulun SE. Endometriosis. N Engl J Med 2009;360:268–277.

19. Bruner–Tran KL, Ding T, Osteen KG. Dioxin and endometrial progesterone resistance. Semin Reprod Med 2010;28:59–68.

20. Stilley JA, Woods–Marshall R, Sutovsky M, Sutovsky P, Sharpe-Timms KL. Reduced fecundity in female rats with surgically induced endometriosis and in their daughters: a potential role for tissue inhibitors of metalloproteinase 1. Biol Reprod 2009;80:649–656.

21. Guo SW. Epigenetics of endometriosis. Mol Hum Reprod 2009;15: 587–607.

22. Sinaii N, Cleary SD, Ballweg ML, Nieman LK, Stratton P. High rates of autoimmune and endocrine disorders, fibromyalgia, chronic fatigue syndrome and atopic diseases among women with endometriosis: a survey analysis. Hum Reprod 2002;17:2715–2724.

23. Cramer DW, Wilson E, Stillman RJ et al. The relation of endometriosis to menstrual characteristics, smoking, and exercise. JAMA 1986;255: 1904–1908.

24. Koninckx PR, Braet P, Kennedy SH, Barlow DH. Dioxin pollution and endometriosis in Belgium. Human Reprod 1994;9:1001–1002.

25. Heilier JF, Donnez J, Lison D. Organochlorines and endometriosis: a mini-review. Chemosphere 2008;71:203–210.

26. Yoshida K, Ikeda S, Nakanishi J. Assessment of human health risk of dioxins in Japan. Chemosphere 2000;40:177–185.

27. Kettel LM, Murphy AA. Combination medical and surgical therapy for infertile patients with endometriosis. Obstet Gynecol Clin North Am 1989;16:167–177.

28. Howard FM. The role of laparoscopy in chronic pelvic pain: promise and pitfalls. Obstet Gynecol Surv 1993;48:357–387.

29. Hughes EG, Fedorkow DM, Collins JA. A quantitative overview of controlled trials in endometriosis-associated infertility. Fertil Steril 1993;59:963–970.

30. Farquhar CM. Extracts from the "clinical evidence". Endometriosis. BMJ 2000;320:1449–1452.

31. Harrison RF, Barry-Kinsella C. Efficacy of medroxyprogesterone treatment in infertile women with endometriosis: a prospective, randomized, placebo controlled study. Fertil Steril 2000;74:24–30.

32. Chwalisz K, Garg R, Brenner RM, Schubert G, Elger W. Selective progesterone receptor modulators (SPRMs): a novel therapeutic concept in endometriosis. Ann N Y Acad Sci 2002;955:373–388; discussion 389–393, 396–406.

33. Abbott JA, Hawe J, Clayton RD, Garry R. The effects and effectiveness of laparoscopic excision of endometriosis: a prospective study with 2–5 year followup. Hum Reprod 2003;18:1922–1927.

34. D'Hooghe TM. Immunomodulators and aromatase inhibitors: are they the next generation of treatment for endometriosis? Curr Opin Obstet Gynecol 2003;15:243–249.

35. Donnez J, Pirard C, Smets M, Jadoul P, Squifflet J. Pre- and post-surgical management of endometriosis. Semin Reprod Med 2003; 21:235–242.

36. Garry R. The effectiveness of laparoscopic excision of endometriosis. Curr Opin Obstet Gynecol 2004;16:299–303.

37. Hendrickx A. Reproduction: methods. In: Hendrickx A (ed) Embryology of the Baboon. Chicago: University of Chicago Press, 1971, pp.1–44.

38. Merrill JA. Spontaneous endometriosis in the Kenya baboon (Papio doguera). Am J Obstet Gynecol 1968;101:569–570.

39. Folse DS, Stout LC. Endometriosis in a baboon (Papio doguera). Lab Anim Sci 1978;28:217–219.

40. TeLinde RW, Scott RB. Diagnosis and treatment of endometriosis. GP 1952;5:61–65.

41. D'Hooghe TM. Clinical relevance of the baboon as a model for the study of endometriosis. Fertil Steril 1997;68:613–625.

42. D'Hooghe TM, Bambra CS, Xiao L, Peixe K, Hill JA. Effect of menstruation and intrapelvic injection of endometrium on inflammatory parameters of peritoneal fluid in the baboon (Papio anubis and Papio cynocephalus). Am J Obstet Gynecol 2001;184:917–925.

43. Fazleabas AT, Brudney A, Gurates B, Chai D, Bulun S. A modified baboon model for endometriosis. Ann N Y Acad Sci 2002;955: 308–317; discussion 340–342, 396–406.

44. Hastings JM, Jackson KS, Mavrogianis PA, Fazleabas AT. The estrogen early response gene FOS is altered in a baboon model of endometriosis. Biol Reprod 2006;75:176–182.

45. Osteen KG, Bruner-Tran KL, Eisenberg E. Reduced progesterone action during endometrial maturation: a potential risk factor for the development of endometriosis. Fertil Steril 2005;83:529–537.

46. Fazleabas AT. Progesterone resistance in a baboon model of endometriosis. Semin Reprod Med 2010;28:75–80.

47. D'Hooghe TM, Bambra CS, de Jonge I, Lauweryns JM, Koninckx PR. The prevalence of spontaneous endometriosis in the baboon (Papio anubis, Papio cynocephalus) increases with the duration of captivity. Acta Obstet Gynecol Scand 1996;75:98–101.

48. Vernon MW, Wilson EA. Studies on the surgical induction of endometriosis in the rat. Fertil Steril 1985;44:684–694.

49. Cummings AM, Metcalf JL. Induction of endometriosis in mice: a new model sensitive to estrogen. Reprod Toxicol 1995;9:233–238.

50. Schenken RS, Asch RH. Surgical induction of endometriosis in the rabbit: effects on fertility and concentrations of peritoneal fluid prostaglandins. Fertil Steril 1980;34:581–587.

51. Steinleitner A, Lambert H, Suarez M, Serpa N, Robin B, Cantor B. Periovulatory calcium channel blockade enhances reproductive performance in an animal model for endometriosis-associated subfertility. Am J Obstet Gynecol 1991;164:949–952.

52. Sharpe KL, Vernon MW. Polypeptides synthesized and released by rat ectopic uterine implants differ from those of the uterus in culture. Biol Reprod 1993;48:1334–1340.

53. Nayyar T, Bruner-Tran KL, Piestrzeniewicz-Ulanska D, Osteen KG. Developmental exposure of mice to TCDD elicits a similar uterine

phenotype in adult animals as observed in women with endometriosis. Reprod Toxicol 2007;23:326–336.

54. Grümmer R. Animal models in endometriosis research. Hum Reprod Update 2006;12:641–649.

55. Bruner KL, Matrisian LM, Rodgers WH, Gorstein F, Osteen KG. Suppression of matrix metalloproteinases inhibits establishment of ectopic lesions by human endometrium in nude mice. J Clin Invest 1997;99:2851–2857.

56. Awwad JT, Sayegh RA, Tao XJ, Hassan T, Awwad ST, Isaacson K. The SCID mouse: an experimental model for endometriosis. Hum Reprod 1999;14:3107–3111.

57. Greenberg LH, Slayden OD. Human endometriotic xenografts in immunodeficient RAG–2/gamma(c)KO mice. Am J Obstet Gynecol 2004;190:1788–1795; discussion 1795–1796.

58. Bruner-Tran KL, Carvalho-Macedo AC, Duleba AJ, Crispens MA, Osteen KG. Experimental endometriosis in immunocompromised mice after adoptive transfer of human leukocytes. Fertil Steril 2010; 93(8):2519–2524.

59. Zamah NM, Dodson MG, Stephens LC, Buttram VC Jr, Besch PK, Kaufman RH. Transplantation of normal and ectopic human endometrial tissue into athymic nude mice. Am J Obstet Gynecol 1984;149:591–597.

60. Bergqvist A, Jeppsson S, Kullander S, Ljungberg O. Human uterine endometrium and endometriotic tissue transplanted into nude mice. Morphologic effects of various steroid hormones. Am J Pathol 1985; 121:337–341.

61. Nisolle M, Casanas-Roux F, Donnez J. Early-stage endometriosis: adhesion and growth of human menstrual endometrium in nude mice. Fertil Steril 2000;74:306–312.

62. Bruner-Tran KL, Zhang Z, Eisenberg E, Winneker RC, Osteen KG. Down-regulation of endometrial matrix metalloproteinase-3 and -7 expression in vitro and therapeutic regression of experimental endometriosis in vivo by a novel nonsteroidal progesterone receptor agonist, tanaproget. J Clin Endocrinol Metab 2006;91:1554–1560.

63. Bruner-Tran KL, Osteen KG, Duleba AJ. Simvastatin protects against the development of endometriosis in a nude mouse model. J Clin Endocrinol Metab 2009;94:2489–2494.

64. Flanagan SP. 'Nude', a new hairless gene with pleiotropic effects in the mouse. Genet Res 1966;8:295–309.

65. Pantelouris EM. Absence of thymus in a mouse mutant. Nature 1968;217:370–371.

66. Rygaard J. Thymus and Self. Immunobiology of the Mouse Mutant Nude. New York: John Wiley, 1973.

67. MacDonald HR, Blanc C, Lees RK, Sordat B. Abnormal distribution of T cell subsets in athymic mice. J Immunol 1986;136:4337–4339.

68. Kung JT, Thomas CA 3rd. Athymic nude CD4+8– T cells produce IL-2 but fail to proliferate in response to mitogenic stimuli. J Immunol 1988;141:3691–3696.

69. Metcalf D. Histologic and transplantation studies on preleukemic thymus of the AKR mouse. J Natl Cancer Inst 1966;37:425–442.

70. Hetherington CM, Hegan MA. Breeding nude (nu/nu) mice. Lab Anim 1975;9:19–20.

71. Bruner KL, Eisenberg E, Gorstein F, Osteen KG. Progesterone and transforming growth factor-beta coordinately regulate suppression of

endometrial matrix metalloproteinases in a model of experimental endometriosis. Steroids 1999;64:648–653.

72. VanSaun MN, Matrisian LM. Matrix metalloproteinases and cellular motility in development and disease. Birth Defects Res C Embryo Today 2006;78:69–79.

73. Bruner-Tran KL, Rier SE, Eisenberg E, Osteen KG. The potential role of environmental toxins in the pathophysiology of endometriosis. Gynecol Obstet Invest 1999;48(Suppl 1):45–56.

74. Fortin M, Lépine M, Pagé M et al. An improved mouse model for endometriosis allows noninvasive assessment of lesion implantation and development. Fertil Steril 2003;80(Suppl 2):832–838.

75. Kurita T, Medina R, Schabel AB et al. The activation function-1 domain of estrogen receptor alpha in uterine stromal cells is required for mouse but not human uterine epithelial response to estrogen. Differentiation 2005;73:313–322.

76. De Villartay JP. 9.V(D)J recombination deficiencies. Adv Exp Med Biol 2009;650:46–58.

77. Bosma GC, Owen J, Easton G, Marshall G, Dewitt C, Bosma MJ. Concentration of IgG1 and IgG2a allotypes in serum of nude and normal allotype-congenic mice. J Immunol 1980;124:879–884.

78. Aoki D, Katsuki Y, Shimizu A, Kakinuma C, Nozawa S. Successful heterotransplantation of human endometrium in SCID mice. Obstet Gynecol 1994;83:220–228.

79. Boyd J, Strauss J, van Deerlin P, Yamamoto K. Endometriosis mouse model. United States, 2002. Patent # 6429353. www.freepatentsonline.com/6429353.html.

80. Mazurier F, Fontanellas A, Salesse S et al. A novel immunodeficient mouse model – RAG2 × common cytokine receptor gamma chain double mutants – requiring exogenous cytokine administration for human hematopoietic stem cell engraftment. J Interferon Cytokine Res 1999;19:533–541.

81. Cao X, Kozak CA, Liu YJ, Noguchi M, O'Connell E, Leonard WJ. Characterization of cDNAs encoding the murine interleukin 2 receptor (IL-2R) gamma chain: chromosomal mapping and tissue specificity of IL-2R gamma chain expression. Proc Natl Acad Sci USA 1993;90:8464–8468.

82. Alt FW, Rathbun G, Oltz E, Taccioli G, Shinkai Y. Function and control of recombination-activating gene activity. Ann N Y Acad Sci 1992;651:277–294.

83. Olive DL. Role of progesterone antagonists and new selective progesterone receptor modulators in reproductive health. Obstet Gynecol Surv 2002;57(11 Suppl 4):S55–63.

84. Hemmings R, Rivard M, Olive DL et al. Evaluation of risk factors associated with endometriosis. Fertil Steril 2004;81:1513–1521.

85. Alvarez Gonzalez ML, Galant C, Frankenne F et al. Development of an animal experimental model to study the effects of levonorgestrel on the human endometrium. Hum Reprod 2009;24:697–704.

86. Bruner-Tran KL, Eisenberg E, Yeaman GR, Anderson TA, McBean J, Osteen KG. Steroid and cytokine regulation of matrix metalloproteinase expression in endometriosis and the establishment of experimental endometriosis in nude mice. J Clin Endocrinol Metab 2002;87:4782–4791.

87. Harris HA, Bruner-Tran KL, Zhang X, Osteen KG, Lyttle CR. A selective estrogen receptor-beta agonist causes lesion regression in an

experimentally induced model of endometriosis. Hum Reprod 2005;20:936–941.

88. Xu H, Lui WT, Chu CY, Ng PS, Wang CC, Rogers MS. Anti-angiogenic effects of green tea catechin on an experimental endometriosis mouse model. Hum Reprod 2009;24:608–618.

89. Hull ML, Charnock-Jones DS, Chan CL et al. Antiangiogenic agents are effective inhibitors of endometriosis. J Clin Endocrinol Metab 2003;88:2889–2899.

90. Krikun G, Hu Z, Osteen K et al. The immunoconjugate "icon" targets aberrantly expressed endothelial tissue factor causing regression of endometriosis. Am J Pathol 2010;176:1050–1056.

91. Hu Z, Sun Y, Garen A. Targeting tumor vasculature endothelial cells and tumor cells for immunotherapy of human melanoma in a mouse xenograft model. Proc Natl Acad Sci USA 1999;96:8161–8166.

92. Hu Z, Garen A. Intratumoral injection of adenoviral vectors encoding tumor-targeted immunoconjugates for cancer immunotherapy. Proc Natl Acad Sci USA 2000;97:9221–9225.

93. Hu Z, Garen A. Targeting tissue factor on tumor vascular endothelial cells and tumor cells for immunotherapy in mouse models of prostatic cancer. Proc Natl Acad Sci USA 2001;98:12180–12185.

94. Bora PS, Hu Z, Tezel TH et al. Immunotherapy for choroidal neovascularization in a laser-induced mouse model simulating exudative (wet) macular degeneration. Proc Natl Acad Sci USA 2003;100:2679–2684.

95. Tezel TH, Bodek E, Sonmez K et al. Targeting tissue factor for immunotherapy of choroidal neovascularization by intravitreal delivery of factor VII-Fc chimeric antibody. Ocul Immunol Inflamm 2007;15:3–10.

96. Nap AW, Griffioen AW, Dunselman GA et al. Antiangiogenesis therapy for endometriosis. J Clin Endocrinol Metab 2004;89:1089–1095.

97. Jiang HQ, Li YL, Zou J. Effect of recombinant human endostatin on endometriosis in mice. Chin Med J (Engl) 2007;120:1241–1246.

98. Guo SW. Nuclear factor-kappab (NF-kappaB): an unsuspected major culprit in the pathogenesis of endometriosis that is still at large? Gynecol Obstet Invest 2007;63:71–97.

99. González-Ramos R, van Langendonckt A, Defrère S et al. Involvement of the nuclear factor-kappaB pathway in the pathogenesis of endometriosis. Fertil Steril 2010;94(6):1985–1994.

100. González-Ramos R, van Langendonckt A, Defrère S et al. Agents blocking the nuclear factor-kappaB pathway are effective inhibitors of endometriosis in an in vivo experimental model. Gynecol Obstet Invest 2008;65:174–186.

101. Curry TE Jr, Osteen KG. The matrix metalloproteinase system: changes, regulation, and impact throughout the ovarian and uterine reproductive cycle. Endocr Rev 2003;24:428–465.

102. Rodgers WH, Osteen KG, Matrisian LM, Navre M, Giudice LC, Gorstein F. Expression and localization of matrilysin, a matrix metalloproteinase, in human endometrium during the reproductive cycle. Am J Obstet Gynecol 1993;168(1 Pt 1):253–260.

103. Rodgers WH, Matrisian LM, Giudice LC et al. Patterns of matrix metalloproteinase expression in cycling endometrium imply differential functions and regulation by steroid hormones. J Clin Invest 1994;94:946–953.

104. Osteen KG, Rodgers WH, Gaire M, Hargrove JT, Gorstein F, Matrisian LM. Stromal-epithelial interaction mediates steroidal regulation of metalloproteinase expression in human endometrium. Proc Natl Acad Sci USA 1994;91:10129–10133.

105. Bruner KL, Rodgers WH, Gold LI et al. Transforming growth factor beta mediates the progesterone suppression of an epithelial metalloproteinase by adjacent stroma in the human endometrium. Proc Natl Acad Sci USA 1995;92:7362–7366.

106. Salamonsen LA, Woolley DE. Menstruation: induction by matrix metalloproteinases and inflammatory cells. J Reprod Immunol 1999;44:1–27.

107. Attia GR, Zeitoun K, Edwards D, Johns A, Carr BR, Bulun SE. Progesterone receptor isoform A but not B is expressed in endometriosis. J Clin Endocrinol Metab 2000;85:2897–2902.

108. Igarashi TM, Bruner-Tran KL, Yeaman GR et al. Reduced expression of progesterone receptor-B in the endometrium of women with endometriosis and in cocultures of endometrial cells exposed to 2,3,7,8-tetrachlorodibenzo-p-dioxin. Fertil Steril 2005;84:67–74.

109. Tora L, Gronemeyer H, Turcotte B, Gaub MP, Chambon P. The N-terminal region of the chicken progesterone receptor specifies target gene activation. Nature 1988;333:185–188.

110. Tung L, Mohamed MK, Hoeffler JP, Takimoto GS, Horwitz KB. Antagonist-occupied human progesterone B-receptors activate transcription without binding to progesterone response elements and are dominantly inhibited by A-receptors. Mol Endocrinol 1993;7: 1256–1265.

111. Vegeto E, Shahbaz MM, Wen DX, Goldman ME, O'Malley BW, McDonnell DP. Human progesterone receptor A form is a cell- and promoter-specific repressor of human progesterone receptor B function. Mol Endocrinol 1993;7:1244–1255.

112. Yan C, Boyd DD. Regulation of matrix metalloproteinase gene expression. J Cell Physiol 2007;211:19–26.

113. Neth P, Ries C, Karow M, Egea V, Ilmer M, Jochum M. The Wnt signal transduction pathway in stem cells and cancer cells: influence on cellular invasion. Stem Cell Rev 2007;3:18–29.

114. Osteen KG, Keller NR, Feltus FA, Melner MH. Paracrine regulation of matrix metalloproteinase expression in the normal human endometrium. Gynecol Obstet Invest 1999;48(Suppl 1):2–13.

115. Punnonen J, Teisala K, Ranta H, Bennett B, Punnonen R. Increased levels of interleukin-6 and interleukin-10 in the peritoneal fluid of patients with endometriosis. Am J Obstet Gynecol 1996;174:1522–1526.

116. Harada T, Enatsu A, Mitsunari M et al. Role of cytokines in progression of endometriosis. Gynecol Obstet Invest 1999;47(Suppl 1):34–40.

117. Harada T, Iwabe T, Terakawa N. Role of cytokines in endometriosis. Fert Steril 2001;76:1–10.

118. Gazvani R, Templeton A. Peritoneal environment, cytokines and angiogenesis in the pathophysiology of endometriosis. Reproduction 2002;123:217–226.

119. Jeffrey JJ. Collagen synthesis and degradation in the uterine decidu-oma: regulation of collagenase activity by progesterone. Coll Relat Res 1981;1:257–268.

120. Halme J, Becker S, Hammond MG, Raj S. Pelvic macrophages in normal and infertile women: the role of patent tubes. Am J Obstet Gynecol 1982;142:890–895.

121. Oral E, Olive DL, Arici A. The peritoneal environment in endometriosis. Hum Reprod Update 1996;2:385–398.

122. Szamatowicz J, Laudański P, Tomaszewska I, Szamatowicz M. Chemokine growth-regulated-alpha: a possible role in the pathogenesis of endometriosis. Gynecol Endocrinol 2002;16:137–141.

123. Gilabert-Estellés J, Estellés A, Gilabert J et al. Expression of several components of the plasminogen activator and matrix metalloproteinase systems in endometriosis. Hum Reprod 2003;18:1516–1522.

124. Herington JN, Bruner-Tran KL, Osteen KG. Matrix metalloproteinases and endometriosis. In: Arici A, Matalliotakis I (eds) Endometriosis-Adenomyosis. Athens: PM Publications, 2010.

125. Bruner KL, Keller NK, Osteen KG. Interleukin-1α opposes suppression of human endometrial matrix metalloproteinases by progesterone in a model of experimental endometriosis. In: Lemay A, Maheux R (eds) Understanding and Managing Endometriosis: Advances in Research and Practice. New York: Parthenon Publishing, 1999.

126. Crispens MA, Herington JL, Carvalho-Macedo AC, Lebovic DI, Osteen KG. Postsurgical development of adhesions in a chimeric model of experimental endometriosis and inhibition by pioglitazone. J Clin Endocrin Metab 2011;95(4):1295–1301.

127. Dmowski PW, Braun DP. Immunology of endometriosis. Best Pract Res Clin Obstet Gynaecol 2004;18:245–263.

128. Van Rijn RS, Simonetti ER, Hagenbeek A et al. A new xenograft model for graft-versus-host disease by intravenous transfer of human peripheral blood mononuclear cells in RAG2-/- gammac-/- double-mutant mice. Blood 2003;102:2522–2531.

129. Goldman JP, Blundell MP, Lopes L, Kinnon C, DiSanto JP, Thrasher AJ. Enhanced human cell engraftment in mice deficient in RAG2 and the common cytokine receptor gamma chain. Br J Haematol 1998;103:335–342.

130. Vogel CF, Nishimura N, Sciullo E, Wong P, Li W, Matsumura F. Modulation of the chemokines KC and MCP-1 by 2,3,7,8-tetrachlorodibenzo-p-dioxin (TCDD) in mice. Arch Biochem Biophys 2007;461:169–175.

131. Kobayashi S, Okamoto H, Iwamoto T et al. A role for the aryl hydrocarbon receptor and the dioxin TCDD in rheumatoid arthritis. Rheumatology (Oxford) 2008;47:1317–1322.

132. Gargett CE, Rogers PA. Human endometrial angiogenesis. Reproduction 2001;121:181–186.

133. Mueller MD, Lebovic DI, Garrett E, Taylor RN. Neutrophils infiltrating the endometrium express vascular endothelial growth factor: potential role in endometrial angiogenesis. Fertil Steril 2000;74:107–112.

134. Nozawa H, Chiu C, Hanahan D. Infiltrating neutrophils mediate the initial angiogenic switch in a mouse model of multistage carcinogenesis. Proc Natl Acad Sci USA 2006;103:12493–12498.

135. Tee MK, Vigne JL, Taylor RN. All-trans retinoic acid inhibits vascular endothelial growth factor expression in a cell model of neutrophil activation. Endocrinology 2006;147:1264–1270.

136. Alvarez Gonzalez ML, Frankenne F, Galant C et al. Mixed origin of neovascularization of human endometrial grafts in immunodeficient mouse models. Hum Reprod 2009;24:2217–2224.

Models of Endometriosis: Animal Models II – Non-human Primates

Asgerally T. Fazleabas

Department of Obstetrics, Gynecology and Reproductive Biology, and Center for Women's Health Research, Michigan State University, Grand Rapids, MI, USA

Introduction

Endometriosis is a gynecological disease that affects one in ten reproductively aged women [1]. It is pathologically defined as the development of endometrial glands and stroma outside the uterine cavity [2]. Laparoscopic evaluation followed by histological confirmation is the gold standard for diagnosis of endometriosis.

Currently there are three theories that describe the etiology of endometriosis. The first is the embryonic rest theory which proposes that at puberty, there is activation of cells of müllerian duct origin at various sites in the pelvic cavity [3,4]. The second theory is that of coelomic metaplasia which states that substances in menstrual fluid can induce peritoneal tissues to form endometrial cells, suggesting that there is a factor found in menstrual fluid that is a precursor for the disease [5]. The third and most widely accepted theory is the Sampson hypothesis of retrograde menstruation [6] which states that endometrial fragments are displaced into the peritoneal cavity. Retrograde menstruation occurs in the majority (70–90%) [1,7] of women but only a small percentage (10%) of these women develop endometriosis, which suggests that the peritoneal environment or the endometrium of women with endometriosis may be altered compared to that of healthy women [6].

Endometriosis is associated with symptoms such as chronic pelvic pain, dysmenorrhea, dyspareunia and subfertility [8]. The mechanisms associated with the initiation of endometriosis are difficult to evaluate in women because of the extended period of time for diagnosis which is between 8–11 years [9]. Treatment for endometriosis involves both pharmacological and surgical intervention, either individually or combined [10]. Medical treatments available for endometriosis include oral contraceptives (OCPs), gonadotropin-releasing hormone (GnRH) analogs, progesterone analogs and aromatase inhibitors. Surgically, endometriosis has been treated by the excision or ablation of endometriotic lesions and the removal of adhesions in the peritoneal cavity. However, all these treatment modalities only offer a mechanism of suppression but not a cure. Currently there is no universally acceptable, standard treatment protocol for endometriosis so treatment is individualized for each patient, with mixed outcomes. Thus, the establishment of an animal model with experimentally inducible endometriosis would allow investigators to characterize factors involved in the early onset of disease and throughout disease progression, allowing for the evaluation of molecular changes that cause infertility and chronic pelvic pain. The experimentally induced model would also aid investigation of the efficacy of therapeutic intervention strategies.

Primate models of endometriosis

Although the use of rodents is cost-effective and it does allow for the generation of animals with specific gene deletions, the disadvantages are numerous. Ectopic lesions are very small and are not physiologically similar to those found in advanced stages of human disease. Also the use of immunocompromised rodents eliminates the investigation of any immunoregulatory component involved in the pathogenesis of disease. Additionally, these animals do not develop spontaneous disease since they are a nonmenstruating species. However, the rodent model is cost-effective for preliminary efficacy trials of medical therapies.

The presence of lesions resembling human endometriosis, both clinically and pathologically, has been documented in several species of non-human primates (NHP) [11]. The use of NHP is advantageous for the study of endometriosis because they are phylogenetically similar to the human. Additional studies in the NHP, particularly, the baboon have demonstrated that endometriosis is a dynamic process that undergoes cycles of development, regression and remodeling, and demonstrated a strong relationship between the immune system and the establishment and progression of

Endometriosis: Science and Practice, First Edition. Edited by Linda C. Giudice, Johannes L.H. Evers and David L. Healy.
© 2012 Blackwell Publishing Ltd. Published 2012 by Blackwell Publishing Ltd.

endometriosis [12]. Although spontaneous endometriosis in NHP is the most suitable model for studying the pathophysiology of endometriosis, this would be difficult to accomplish due to the limited incidence and slow progression of the disease, which is similar to that observed in women. Thus, this necessitates the development of an induced model of the disease. We have chosen the baboon (*Papio anubis*) as the preferred model because of its size and similar reproductive anatomy and physiology to the human female [13]. In addition, baboons also develop spontaneous endometriosis in which ectopic lesions resemble those of humans [14,15]. Endometriosis can also be induced in baboons by injecting autologous menstrual effluent into the pelvic cavity [16,17]. The intraperitoneal injection of menstrual tissue mimics the normal physiological process of retrograde menstruation and permits the study of disease progression from the initial onset of disease [18]. A further advantage of the baboon model is that it allows for multiple and complex surgical procedures and repeated collection of biological samples during the time course of the disease. Therefore, the baboon provides an excellent model for studying the pathogenesis of endometriosis, including the identification of molecules that may contribute to the establishment and development of lesions and provide an understanding of the mechanisms that alter the eutopic endometrial environment that could lead to infertility. This chapter will summarize the current findings and ongoing studies utilizing the experimentally induced baboon model of endometriosis.

Development and survival of ectopic lesions

The first steps in the pathogenesis of endometriosis require attachment and invasion of the peritoneal lining by endometrial fragments. The mechanism by which invasion of the peritoneum occurs is not fully understood. Some investigators propose that the peritoneal mesothelium acts as a barrier to refluxed endometrium, suggesting that endometrial attachment only occurs at sites of peritoneal damage. However, other investigators have shown rapid attachment and invasion through peritoneal surfaces by endometrial stromal and epithelial cells. Subsequently, mesothelial cells are thought to integrate into the endometriotic tissues within the peritoneal layer by a process referred to as re-epithelialization [19,20]. These processes mediating the initial establishment of disease are clearly invasive events that require breakdown of the peritoneal basement membrane and underlying extracellular matrix (ECM). Figure 27.1 summarizes the mechanisms that we propose lead to the establishment of lesion development.

Matrix metalloproteinases (MMPs) are essential for remodeling of the ECM in development, growth and repair of normal tissues and in inflammatory and degenerative diseases. Endometrial expression of the MMPs, and their tissue inhibitors (TIMPs), is normally tightly regulated throughout the menstrual cycle. The precise role of the MMPs in the pathophysiology of endometriosis is not fully understood. However, aberrant patterns of MMP and TIMP protein and mRNA expression in eutopic and ectopic endo-

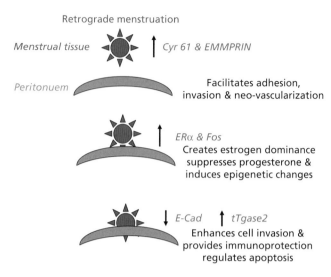

Figure 27.1 Postulated mechanism of lesion development. The increase in CYR61 and EMMPRIN in menstrual tissue of baboons with induced endometriosis enhances the ability of this tissue to attach and invade the peritoneum. During lesion development ERα is the dominant steroid hormone receptor that regulates the expression of other genes to facilitate further invasion and prevent apoptosis.

metriotic tissues are evident, specifically relating to MMP-7 in peritoneal endometriotic lesions. One mechanism by which MMPs could be activated during lesion formation would be by ECM metalloproteinase inducer (EMMPRIN) which is aberrantly expressed in both the eutopic and ectopic endometrium of baboons with endometriosis. Furthermore, EMMPRIN expression is markedly increased in the menstrual tissue of baboons with induced endometriosis, which could further facilitate the invasion process [21].

Angiogenesis is the formation of new blood vessels from existing vessels and the process is tightly regulated in the adult. However, the primate endometrium undergoes profound vascular remodeling during each menstrual cycle and it has been proposed that angiogenesis is important in the pathophysiology of endometriosis. Our studies have demonstrated that endometriotic lesions appear to be surrounded by peritoneal blood vessels and increased levels of numerous angiogenic factors are well documented in the peritoneal fluid of women with endometriosis [22,23]. The angiogenic factor CYR61, a member of the CCN family of growth factors involved in development, proliferation and tumorigenesis, has been shown to be upregulated in eutopic and ectopic endometria of women with endometriosis [24]. CYR61 is cyclically regulated in the baboon endometrium, with maximal mRNA levels observed in shed menstrual endometrium [25]. In the ectopic endometriotic lesions, the mean expression levels of CYR61 mRNA are significantly increased compared to the eutopic endometrium of both diseased and control animals. The highest levels of CYR61 mRNA were observed in the highly vascularized red lesions while white ectopic lesions, which are thought to represent the less active sites of disease, demonstrated the lowest levels of CYR61. The increased levels of CYR61 correlate with increased levels of vascular endothelial growth factor (VEGF) in both the ectopic and eutopic endometrium of baboons with experimental endometriosis and may contribute to lesion establishment.

The decrease in E-cadherin in the ectopic lesions of baboons [26] confirms previous studies which also reported a significant reduction in E-cadherin in the ectopic lesions obtained from women [27,28]. Furthermore, the differential expression of E-cadherin in eutopic and ectopic lesions observed in our studies has also been reported in women, which further validates the importance of our baboon model of endometriosis [28,29]. Recent studies have also suggested that endometrial cells from women with endometriosis have an increased capacity for both proliferation and adhesion [30]. This loss of E-cadherin in ectopic endometriotic lesions would suggest a more invasive tissue type which would allow for the lesions to resemble a malignant phenotype and be able to migrate, attach and invade throughout the peritoneal cavity.

Tissue transglutaminase 2 (tTgase-2) is a ubiquitously expressed enzyme that is involved in several biological functions. It functions in the regulation of cell matrix interactions by cross-linking and binding the ECM proteins [31]. tTgase-2 has also been implicated in cell differentiation and growth, in growth factor activation pathways including the immunosuppressor transforming growth factor (TGF)-β [32,33], in cell spreading and adhesion and in programmed cell death [34,35]. Due to its GTPase activity, it is also thought to be involved in extracellular signaling [36]. In the ectopic endometrium of baboons, tTgase-2 was markedly increased when compared to the eutopic endometrium from animals with endometriosis. tTgase-2 has the ability to be both antiapoptotic and proapoptotic depending on which biological pathway is activated. A similar function could be envisioned for tTgase-2 in the peritoneal cavity, where it can protect the ectopic endometriotic lesions from undergoing apoptosis similar to that which has been reported for the survival of cancer cells [37,38].

Impact of endometriosis on endometrial development

There are many factors that contribute to the subfertility associated with endometriosis. In women it is difficult to assess whether the multitude of changes that have been identified by microarray analysis are a consequence of having the disease for an extended period of time or if the endometrium of women with disease is inherently defective. The dysregulation of the genetic profile of the eutopic endometrium during the window of receptivity has been suggested to result in decreased implantation success [39,40]. Using our baboon model of induced endometriosis, it is evident that the presence of the lesions directly affects the gene expression patterns of the eutopic endometrium as early as 1 month after onset of the disease. In addition, the presence of the lesions also has a progressive impact on the endometrium during the window of uterine receptivity. At the very onset of the disease process, the eutopic endometrium takes on an estrogenic phenotype and genotype which is characterized by the aberrant expression of c-fos, CYR61 and EMMPRIN [41–43]. Following the early onset of disease, c-fos, an estrogen-responsive gene, is highly

upregulated in addition to junD and JNK2 [44]. These genes are important for controlling cell cycle and cell fate by repressing or silencing gene expression. One of the targets of AP-1 transcription factors that are regulated by fos and jun is progesterone receptor (PR)A [45] which may have implications for hormone responsiveness of the eutopic endometrium throughout disease progression. With further manifestation of the disease process, an altered steroid hormone receptor profile imparts progesterone resistance to the eutopic endometrium and this is characterized by the suppression of genes associated with successful implantation, such as HOXA10 and calcitonin [41].

The co-ordinated changes that occur in the endometrium throughout the menstrual cycle are regulated by the ovarian steroid hormones estrogen and progesterone. Hormonal action is mediated through their interaction with their respective receptors on both endometrial stromal and epithelial cells. In baboons with endometriosis, the normal eutopic endometrial stromal expression of estrogen receptor (ER)α that is evident during the window of receptivity is suppressed [42]. The decrease in expression was seen primarily in the stromal cells 6 months after the induction of disease which is also coincident with the decrease in PR expression and responsiveness [42,43]. During progression of endometriosis, it has been reported that the eutopic endometrium becomes resistant to progesterone action and a number of progesterone-responsive genes are suppressed in women with disease [40,46,47]. In the baboon model of endometriosis, PRA immunolocalization in glandular epithelial cells is decreased but PRB remains unchanged. In stromal cells there was no difference in the immunolocalization of PRA or PRB but the ability of these cells to respond to PR stimulation was decreased [43]. This decrease was associated with a decrease in FKBP52, an immunophilin that regulates the action of progesterone [42,48].

We have also determined that HOXA10, a downstream target of PR which is also downregulated in FKBP52 null mice [49,50], was decreased in women and baboons with endometriosis [43]. In baboons, the decrease of HOXA10 expression resulted in a decrease of the downstream target gene integrin B3 (ITGB3) and an increase of empty spiracles homolog 2 (EMX2) [43]. The dysregulation of HOXA10 in endometriosis is a result of hypermethylation and strongly supports the concept that gene suppression in endometriosis may also be associated with epigenetic changes in the eutopic tissue [43,51]. HOXA10 has also been shown to be important in endometrial stromal cell decidualization and several studies have indicated that a defect in the decidualization process is evident in both baboons and humans with endometriosis [30,43].

FKBP52 is essential for embryo implantation and the loss of it is associated with decreased levels of HOXA10, Indian hedgehog (Ihh) and calcitonin (CALC) during the window of uterine receptivity [49,50,52]. Calcitonin, like HOXA 10, is also regulated by progesterone in the baboon endometrium [53].

Based on these data, we evaluated the localization of calcitonin and calcitonin-modulated proteins, E-cadherin and tTgase-2 in the eutopic endometrium during the window of receptivity in baboons with induced endometriosis. Calcitonin staining was decreased in both endometrial epithelial and stromal cells. In conjunction, E-cadherin staining was increased in endometrial epithelial cells and tTgase-2 staining was decreased in endometrial stromal cells compared to disease-free healthy controls [26]. These data further support the theory that during disease progression, the eutopic endometrium becomes progesterone resistant probably as a consequence of impaired PR function directly or indirectly related to the attenuated expression of critical chaperone proteins such as FKBP52 and Hic-5 [46].

These studies suggest that the subfertility that is associated with endometriosis is the result of several factors. The use of the baboon model of induced endometriosis has clearly established that ectopic endometrial lesions distinctly influence the eutopic endometrium and these changes sequentially result in an overall resistance to progesterone. In addition to the changes in gene expression, changes in the ultrastructural morphology of the eutopic endometrium during the window of uterine receptivity are also significantly altered, resulting in a phenotype that resembles the early estrogenic response and the later progesterone resistance that is manifested as a consequence of the disease [54]. Thus, it is evident that the presence of peritoneal disease results in an inherent endometrial defect with multiple etiologies, all of which may be detrimental to successful embryo implantation.

The aberrant dysregulation of the steroid receptors and their downstream targets, during the window of receptivity, not only affects the ability of the eutopic endometrium to respond to ovarian steroids but also blunts the response of the endometrium to the implanting embryo. resulting in implantation failure. This is clearly evident in our baboon model of simulated pregnancy in which, following the induction of endometriosis, the eutopic endometrium is unresponsive to human chorionic gonadotropin (hCG) stimulation [55]. The previously described morphological and molecular endometrial changes in all three major endometrial cell types, luminal, glandular and stromal, after *in vivo* infusion of hCG in disease-free animals were not observed in the majority of animals with endometriosis [55,56].

These studies demonstrate that the endometrial response to hCG in animals with endometriosis is compromised in multiple ways. Many of these transcripts are involved in the induction of a receptive endometrium. Secreted frizzled-related proteins (SFRP) are regulators of the Wnt signaling pathway, modulating embryogenesis, cell proliferation, differentiation, adhesion, and apoptosis [57,58]. SFRP4 expression is decreased in the secretory phase in both human and NHP endometrium, suggesting downregulation by progesterone [59,60]. Although no direct role for SFRP4 has been reported in the process of decidualization, we propose that the increase in SFRP4 induced by hCG in animals with endometriosis may alter stromal cell proliferation, and thus contribute to defective decidualization. Other factors which show altered responses to hCG, such as the ROS scavenger SOD2, are known to participate in decidualization and could clearly affect endometrial stromal cell differentiation during early pregnancy. SOD2 is upregulated by hCG in disease-free animals, but downregulated by hCG in animals with endometriosis. These data suggest that increased ROS scavenging is critical for

establishment and maintenance of pregnancy. Earlier studies in women showed increased levels of complement (C)3 in endometriotic tissues and recent studies demonstrate that C3 deficiency impairs early pregnancy in mice [61,62]. Since hCG may play a role in orchestrating the endometrial immune adaptation to pregnancy [56], the decrease in C3 together with several additional immunoregulatory factors including interleukin (IL)-1R2 and other members of the complement pathway as a consequence of endometriosis may result in an unfavorable immunological environment which could lead to the rejection of the fetal allograft.

There are a number of possible explanations for the aberrant endometrial response to hCG in animals with endometriosis. Both blood and peritoneal fluid from women with endometriosis contain elevated levels of proinflammatory cytokines [63,64]. These can alter expression of naturally occurring suppressors of cytokine signaling such as SOCS1 which can inhibit ERK 1/2 activation [65] which is the preferred signaling pathway through the luteinizing hormone/chorionic gonadotropin receptor (LHCGR) in endometrial epithelial cells [66]. Cytokines and other factors produced by ectopic endometrial lesions may therefore inhibit endometrial LHCGR signaling, via the ERK 1/2 pathway. Alternatively, the presence of endometriosis may inhibit the hCG-induced redistribution of LHCGR from the luminal and glandular epithelium to the stromal cells surrounding the spiral arteries that is seen during early pregnancy [67].

Decidualization itself is known to regulate LHCGR abundance [67]. Abnormal decidualization may therefore cause changes in LHCGR distribution since there is strong evidence that decidualization is defective in women and baboons with endometriosis [30,43]. Based on the altered expression of PR associated with endometriosis [42], we hypothesize that the altered responses to hCG may be due in part to decreased PR and the progesterone resistance that is associated with endometriosis. Furthermore, emerging evidence supports a widespread progesterone resistance in endometriosis [68] and in the baboon model of endometriosis, the blunted response to hCG was similar to those observed in disease-free animals treated with PR antagonist [69,70].

A number of genes are co-regulated in the endometrium by hCG and progesterone [56]. This co-regulation may explain why in *in vitro* fertilization (IVF) treatment protocols, where supraphysiological levels of progesterone are administered, the abnormal endometrial response to hCG seen in the presence of endometriosis could be overcome. Thus it is possible that endometrial implantation failure, caused by a deficiency of one component of the progesterone signaling pathway, can be overcome by high levels of progesterone. Huber and colleagues have also proposed that hCG has therapeutic potential in the suppression of endometriotic foci [71]. High doses of hCG may therefore enhance receptivity in two ways. First, by synergistically overcoming progesterone resistance directly within the endometrium and second, by diminishing the secretion of proinflammatory cytokines from endometriotic foci. Exogenous hCG may also exert a luteotropic effect to augment serum progesterone levels, overcoming endometriosis-associated infertility by providing

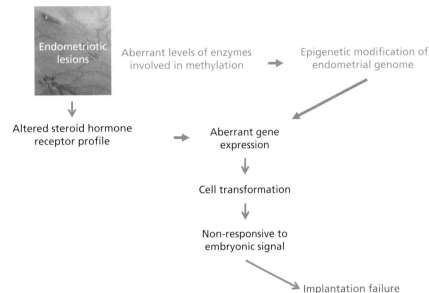

Figure 27.2 Endometriosis-associated infertility – a working hypothesis. The presence of endometriotic lesions alters the eutopic endometrium by altering the steroid hormone receptor expression profile and inducing epigenetic changes during the window of uterine receptivity. This altered environment leads to the development of progesterone resistance which in turn blunts the ability of the embryonic signal to modulate the estrogen- and progesterone-primed endometrium to facilitate embryo implantation.

critical luteal support necessary for the establishment and maintenance of pregnancy.

Conclusion

Induction of endometriosis results in altered responses to a major embryonic signal, hCG, in addition to the suppression of the progesterone-regulated genes during the window of uterine receptivity. These altered responses prevent the acquisition of the full endometrial molecular repertoire necessary for implantation. This attenuated response is, in part, a consequence of the progesterone resistance associated with endometriosis. We propose that the reduced fecundity associated with endometriosis has a multifactorial etiology, including abnormalities of differentiation, immunological and decidualization pathways, which ultimately create an endometrial environment that is unreceptive to an implanting blastocyst (Figure 27.2).

Acknowledgments

This research was supported by the Eunice Kennedy Shriver NICHD/NIH through co-operative agreement [U54 HD 40093 to ATF] as part of the Specialized Co-operative Centers Program in Reproduction and Infertility Research. I thank the various members of my laboratory for their contributions over many years to the work described in this chapter.

References

1. Eskenazi B, Warner ML. Epidemiology of endometriosis. Obstet Gynecol Clin North Am 1997;24:235–258.

2. Clement PB. The pathology of endometriosis: a survey of the many faces of a common disease emphasizing diagnostic pitfalls and unusual and newly appreciated aspects. Adv Anat Pathol 2007;14:241–260.

3. Batt RE, Smith RA. Embryologic theory of histogenesis of endometriosis in peritoneal pockets. Obstet Gynecol Clin North Am 1989;16:15–28.

4. Batt RE, Smith RA, Buck GM, Severino MF, Naples JD. Mullerianosis. Prog Clin Biol Res 1990;323:413–426.

5. Meyer R. Uber den Stand der Frage der Ademomyositis and Ademomyome serosepithelialis und Adenomyometritis sarcomatosa. Zentrakbl Gynakol 1919; 43:745–750.

6. Sampson J. Peritoneal endometriosis due to menstrual dissemination of endometrial tissue into the pelvic cavity. Am J Obstet Gynecol 1927;14:422–469.

7. Blumenkrantz MJ, Gallagher N, Bashore RA, Tenckhoff H. Retrograde menstruation in women undergoing chronic peritoneal dialysis. Obstet Gynecol 1981;57:667–670.

8. Verkauf BS. Incidence, symptoms, and signs of endometriosis in fertile and infertile women. J FLA Med Assoc 1987;74:671–675.

9. Sinaii N, Cleary SD, Ballweg ML, Nieman LK, Stratton P. High rates of autoimmune and endocrine disorders, fibromyalgia, chronic fatigue syndrome and atopic diseases among women with endometriosis: a survey analysis. Hum Reprod 2002;17:2715–2724.

10. Valle RF. Endometriosis: current concepts and therapy. Int J Gynaecol Obstet 2002;78:107–119.

11. Story L, Kennedy S. Animal studies in endometriosis: a review. Ilar J 2004;45:132–138.

12. Tirado-Gonzalez I, Barrientos G, Tariverdian N et al. Endometriosis research: animal models for the study of a complex disease. J Reprod Immunol 2010;86(2):141–147.

13. Hendrickx A. Reproduction: methods. In: Hendrickx A (ed) Embryology of the Baboon. Chicago: University of Chicago Press, 1971, pp.1–44.

14. Folse D, Stout L. Endometriosis in the baboon. Lab Anim Sci 1978;28:217–219.

15. Merrill J. Spontaneous endometriosis in the Kenya baboon. Am J Obstet Gynecol 1968;101:569–570.

16. D'Hooghe TM. Clinical relevance of the baboon as a model for the study of endometriosis. Fertil Steril 1997;68:613–625.

17. Fazleabas AT, Brudney A, Gurates B, Chai D, Bulun S. A modified baboon model for endometriosis. Ann N Y Acad Sci 2002;955:308–317.

18. Hastings JM, Fazleabas AT. A baboon model for endometriosis: implications for fertility. Reprod Biol Endocrinol 2007;4 Suppl 1:S7.

19. Debrock S, Perre SV, Meuleman C, Moerman P, Hill JA, D'Hooghe TM. In-vitro adhesion of endometrium to autologous peritoneal membranes: effect of the cycle phase and the stage of endometriosis. Hum Reprod 2002;17:2523–2528.

20. Witz CA, Montoya-Rodriguez IA, Schenken RS. Whole explants of peritoneum and endometrium: a novel model of the early endometriosis lesion. Fertil Steril 1998;71:56–60.

21. Braundmeier AG, Fazleabas AT, Lessey BA, Guo H, Toole BP, Nowak RA. Extracellular matrix metalloproteinase inducer regulates metalloproteinases in human uterine endometrium. J Clin Endocrinol Metab 2006;91:2358–2365.

22. McLaren J, Prentice A, Charnock-Jones DS, Smith SK. Vascular endothelial growth factor (VEGF) concentrations are elevated in peritoneal fluid of women with endometriosis. Hum Reprod 1996;11:220–223.

23. Mahnke JL, Dawood MY, Huang JC. Vascular endothelial growth factor and interleukin-6 in peritoneal fluid of women with endometriosis. Fertil Steril 2000;73:166–170.

24. Absenger Y, Hess-Stump H, Kreft B et al. Cyr61, a deregulated gene in endometriosis. Mol Hum Reprod 2004;10:399–407.

25. Gashaw I, Hastings JM, Jackson KS, Winterhager E, Fazleabas AT. Induced endometriosis in the baboon (Papio anubis) increases the expression of the proangiogenic factor CYR61 (CCN1) in eutopic and ectopic endometrium. Biol Reprod 2006;74:1060–1066.

26. Jackson KS, Hastings J, Mavrogianis P, Bagchi I, Fazleabas AT. Alterations in the calcitonin and calcitonin modulated proteins, E-cadherin and the enzyme tissue transglutaminase II during the window of implantation in a baboon model of endometriosis. J Endometriosis 2009;1:57–67.

27. Starzinski-Powitz A, Gaetie R, Zeitvogel A et al. Tracing cellular and molecular mechanisms involved in endometriosis. Hum Reprod Update 1998;4:724–729.

28. Poncelet C, Leblanc M, Walker-Combrouze F et al. Expression of cadherins and CD44 in human endometrium and peritoneal endometriosis. Acta Obstet Gynecol Scand 2002;3:195–203.

29. Gaetja R, Kotzian S, Herrmann G, Baumann R, Starzinsi-Powitz A. Nonmalignant epithelial cells, potentially invasive in human endometriosis, lack the tumor suppressor molecule E. Cadherin. Am J Pathol 1997;150:309–315.

30. Klemmt P, Carver J, Koninckx P, Mcveigh E, Mardon H. Endometrial cells from women with endometriosis have increased adhesion and proliferative capacity in response to extracellular matrix components: toward a mechanistic model for endometriosis progression. Hum Reprod 2007;22:3139–3147.

31. Martinez J, Chalupowicz D, Roush R, Sheth A, Barsigian C. Transglutaminase-mediated processing of fibronectin by endothelial cell monolayers. Biochemistry 1994;33:2538–2545.

32. Kojima S, Nara K, Rifkin DB. Requirement for transglutaminase in the activation of latent transforming growth factor-beta in bovine endothelial cells. J Cell Biol 1993;121:439–448.

33. Nunes I, Gleizes P, Metz C, Rifkin D. Latent transforming growth factor-beta binding protein domains involved in activation and transglutaminase-dependent cross-linking of latent transforming growth factor-beta. J Cell Biol 1997;136:1151–1163.

34. Gentile V, Thomazy V, PIacentini M, Fesus L, Davies PJ. Expression of tissue transglutaminase in Balb-C 3T3 fibroblasts: effects on cellular morphology and adhesion. J Cell Biol 1992;119:463–474.

35. Fesus L, Tomazy V, Falus A. Induction and activation of tissue transglutaminase during programmed cell death. FEBS Lett 1987;224:104–108.

36. Nakaoka H, Perez D, Baek K et al. Gh: a GTP-binding protein with transglutaminase activity and receptor signaling function. Science 1994;264:1593–1596.

37. Hwang J, Mangala L, Fok J et al. Clinical and biological significance of tissue transglutaminase in ovarian carcinoma. Cancer Res 2008;68:5849–5858.

38. Singer C, Hudelist G, Walter I et al. Tissue array-based expression of transglutaminase-2 in human breast and ovarian cancer. Clin Exp Metastasis 2006;2:33–39.

39. Ayers JW, Birenbaum DL, Menon KM. Luteal phase dysfunction in endometriosis: elevated progesterone levels in peripheral and ovarian veins during the follicular phase. Fertil Steril 1987;47:925–929.

40. Burney RO, Talbi S, Hamilton AE et al. Gene expression analysis of endometrium reveals progesterone resistance and candidate susceptibility genes in women with endometriosis. Endocrinology 2007;148:3814–3826.

41. Fazleabas AT. Progesterone resistance in a baboon model of endometriosis. Semin Reprod Med 2010;28:75–80.

42. Jackson KS, Brudney A, Hastings JM, Mavrogianis PA, Kim JJ, Fazleabas AT. The altered distribution of the steroid hormone receptors and the chaperone immunophilin FKBP52 in a baboon model of endometriosis is associated with progesterone resistance during the window of uterine receptivity. Reprod Sci 2007;14:137–150.

43. Kim JJ, Taylor HS, Lu Z, Ladhani O et al. Altered expression of HOXA10 in endometriosis: potential role in decidualization. Mol Hum Reprod 2007;13:323–332.

44. Hastings JM, Jackson KS, Mavrogianis PA, Fazleabas AT. The estrogen early response gene FOS is altered in a baboon model of endometriosis. Biol Reprod 2006;75:176–182.

45. Shemshedini L, Knauthe R, Sassone-Corsi P, Pornon A, Gronemeyer H. Cell-specific inhibitory and stimulatory effects of Fos and Jun on transcription activation by nuclear receptors. EMBO J 1991;10:3839–3849.

46. Aghajanova L, Velarde M, Giudice LC. The progesterone receptor coactivator Hic-5 is involved in the pathophysiology of endometriosis. Endocrinology 2009;150:3863–3870.

47. Kao LC, Germeyer A, Tulac S et al. Expression profiling of endometrium from women with endometriosis reveals candidate genes for disease-based implantation failure and infertility. Endocrinology 2003;144:2870–2881.

48. Hirota Y, Tranguch S, Daikoku T et al. Deficiency of immunophilin FKBP52 promotes endometriosis. Am J Pathol 2008;173:1747–1757.

49. Tranguch S, Cheung-Flynn J, Daikoku T et al. Cochaperone immunophilin FKBP52 is critical to uterine receptivity for embryo implantation. Proc Natl Acad Sci USA 2005;102:14326–14331.

50. Tranguch S, Wang H, Daikoku T, Xie H, Smith DF, Dey SK. FKBP52 deficiency-conferred uterine progesterone resistance is genetic background and pregnancy stage specific. J Clin Invest 2007;117:1824–1834.

51. Gui Y, Zhang J, Yuan L, Lessey BA. Regulation of HOXA-10 and its expression in normal and abnormal endometrium. Mol Hum Reprod 1999;5:866–873.

52. Yang Z, Wolf IM, Chen H et al. FKBP52 is essential to uterine reproductive physiology controlled by the progesterone receptor A isoform. Mol Endocrinol 2006;20:2682–2694.

53. Kumar S, Brudney A, Cheon YP, Fazleabas AT, Bagchi IC. Progesterone induces calcitonin expression in the baboon endometrium within the window of uterine receptivity. Biol Reprod 2003;68:1318–1323.

54. Jones CJ, Denton J, Fazleabas AT. Morphological and glycosylation changes associated with the endometrium and ectopic lesions in a baboon model of endometriosis. Hum Reprod 2006;21:3068–3080.

55. Sherwin JR, Hastings JM, Jackson KS et al. The endometrial response to chorionic gonadotropin is blunted in a baboon model of endometriosis. Endocrinology 2010;151(10):4982–4993.

56. Sherwin JR, Sharkey AM, Cameo P et al. Identification of novel genes regulated by chorionic gonadotropin in baboon endometrium during the window of implantation. Endocrinology 2007;148:618–626.

57. Nelson WJ, Nusse R. Convergence of Wnt, β-catenin, and cadherin pathways. Science 2004;303:1483–1487.

58. Jones SE, Jomary C. Secreted Frizzled-related proteins: searching for relationships and patterns. Bioessays 2002;24:811–820.

59. Abu-Jawdeh G, Comella N, Tomita Y et al. Differential expression of frpHE: a novel human stromal protein of the secreted frizzled gene family, during the endometrial cycle and malignancy. Lab Invest 1999;79:439–447.

60. Ace CI, Okulicz WC. Microarray profiling of progesterone-regulated endometrial genes during the rhesus monkey secretory phase. Reprod Biol Endocrinol 2004;2:54.

61. Isaacson KB, Galman M, Coutifaris C, Lyttle CR. Endometrial synthesis and secretion of complement component-3 by patients with and without endometriosis. Fertil Steril 1990;53:836–841.

62. Chow WN, Lee YL, Wong PC, Chung MK, Lee KF, Yeung WS. Complement 3 deficiency impairs early pregnancy in mice. Mol Reprod Dev 2009;76:647–655.

63. Pizzo A, Salmeri FM, Ardita FV, Sofo V, Tripepi M, Marsico S. Behaviour of cytokine levels in serum and peritoneal fluid of women with endometriosis. Gynecol Obstet Invest 2002;54:82–87.

64. Kalu E, Sumar N, Giannopoulos T et al. Cytokine profiles in serum and peritoneal fluid from infertile women with and without endometriosis. J Obstet Gynaecol Res 2007;33:490–495.

65. Yan L, Tang Q, Shen D et al. SOCS-1 inhibits TNF-alpha-induced cardiomyocyte apoptosis via ERK1/2 pathway activation. Inflammation 2008;31:180–188.

66. Banerjee P, Sapru K, Strakova Z, Fazleabas AT. Chorionic gonadotropin regulates prostaglandin E synthase via a phosphatidylinositol 3-kinase-extracellular regulatory kinase pathway in a human endometrial epithelial cell line: implications for endometrial responses for embryo implantation. Endocrinology 2009;150:4326–4337.

67. Cameo P, Szmidt M, Strakova Z et al. Decidualization regulates the expression of the endometrial chorionic gonadotropin receptor in the primate. Biol Reprod 2006;75:681–689.

68. Bulun SE. Endometriosis. N Engl J Med 2009;360:268–279.

69. Banaszak S, Brudney A, Donnelly K, Chai D, Chwalisz K, Fazleabas AT. Modulation of the action of chorionic gonadotropin in the baboon (Papio anubis) uterus by a progesterone receptor antagonist (ZK 137.316). Biol Reprod 2000;63:820–825.

70. Wang C, Mavrogianis PA, Fazleabas AT. Endometriosis is associated with progesterone resistance in the baboon (Papio anubis) oviduct: evidence based on the localization of oviductal glycoprotein 1 (OVGP1). Biol Reprod 2009;80:272–278.

71. Huber AV, Saleh L, Prast J, Haslinger P, Knofler M. Human chorionic gonadotrophin attenuates NF-kappaB activation and cytokine expression of endometriotic stromal cells. Mol Hum Reprod 2007;13:595–604.

6 Diagnosis of Endometriosis

28 Surgical Historical Overview

Ayman Al-Talib and Togas Tulandi

Department of Obstetrics and Gynecology, McGill University, Montreal, Canada

Introduction

A German physician, Daniel Shroen, first described endometriosis in 1690. In his book *Disputatio Inauguralis Medica de Ulceribus Ulceri* [1], he illustrated endometriosis as ulcers distributed throughout the peritoneum of the bladder, the intestines, the broad ligament, and the outside of the uterus and the cervix. Subsequently, endometriosis was associated with adhesion formation, infertility, and recurrent miscarriage [2]. In the late 18th century, it was also called adenomyosis externa where "The glands resemble in every particular those found in the mucosa lining of the body of the uterus" [3,4].

In the 1890s Russell reported the first ovarian endometriosis as "aberrant portions of the Mullerian duct found in an ovary" [4]. In 1921, Sampson described the retrograde menstruation theory as pathogenesis of endometriosis [5]. Endometriosis was then diagnosed at laparotomy and by pathological examination. In this chapter, we review the surgical history of endometriosis.

Laparotomy

Traditionally, visualization of the abdominal cavity could only be achieved by laparotomy, and radical surgery was the treatment of choice for endometriosis [6]. The development of endoscopic instruments allowed visualization of the abdominal cavity with a less invasive technique. This has increased further understanding of the disease and improved its treatment.

Culdoscopy

In an attempt to gain access into the abdominal cavity without laparotomy, physicians devised several endoscopic instru-

ments. The first endoscopic instrument in gynecology was a culdoscope, and the procedure was named culdoscopy. The culdoscope was introduced into the abdominal cavity via a puncture in the posterior vaginal wall. It is also called transvaginal pelviscopy, transvaginal peritoneoscopy or transvaginal celioscopy.

In 1891, von Ott performed culdoscopy by placing the patient in the Trendelenburg position and with the aid of a mirror and artificial forehead light (Fig. 28.1) [7]. Decker and Cherry modified and popularized the method, and it was used for about 20 years [8]. They used a knee–chest position (Fig. 28.2). In 1956, the fiberoptic culdoscope was invented [9].

A modification of culdoscopy is transhydrolaparoscopy. Gordt and colleagues popularized this technique in 1998 [10]. They perform the procedure in the Trendelenburg position and physiological saline is infused through a small trocar inserted into the posterior cul-de-sac. Endometriosis on the ovary or in the pouch of Douglas can be seen and vaporized (Plate 28.1). The disadvantage of this technique is the inability to inspect the entire pelvis and abdominal cavity. As a result, most gynecological surgeons prefer conventional laparoscopy. Furthermore, laparoscopy allows excision of the endometriosis.

Laparoscopy

Laparoscopy is considered the gold standard in the diagnosis and treatment of endometriosis. Palmer first introduced modern laparoscopy [11]. He used a transabdominal approach with the patient in the Trendelenburg position and after inducing a pneumoperitoneum. The use of laparoscopy became popular in the late 1960s mainly for diagnostic purposes and then for tubal sterilization [12].

The use of laparoscopy has allowed detailed descriptions of different types of endometriosis lesions and their association

Endometriosis: Science and Practice, First Edition. Edited by Linda C. Giudice, Johannes L.H. Evers and David L. Healy.
© 2012 Blackwell Publishing Ltd. Published 2012 by Blackwell Publishing Ltd.

295

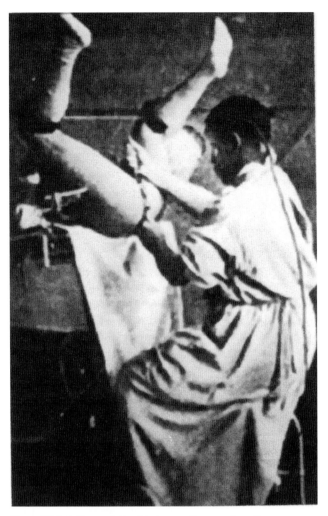

Figure 28.1 Culdoscopy in Trendelenburg position as performed by von Ott in 1891.

with pelvic pain and infertility. The typical lesion of endometriosis is the "powder burn lesion" which are bluish black. In 1979, the American Fertility Society classified endometriosis into stage I (minimal), II (mild), III (moderate), and IV (severe). The classification was based on the amount of endometriosis and adhesions [13].

Several authors compared laparotomy to laparoscopy for diagnosis and treatment of different stages of endometriosis. In a retrospective study, Milingos *et al* studied 102 patients with extensive endometriosis and endometrioma. Seventy patients underwent laparotomy and 32 were treated by laparoscopy. They found a significant reduction in blood loss, shorter hospital stay and faster recovery time in the laparoscopy group [14]. In a randomized trial comparing laparoscopy and laparotomy in 32 patients, Valerios *et al* found a significant decrease in postoperative pain and faster recovery in the laparoscopy group [15]. Crosignani *et al* compared a total of 216 patients operated by laparoscopy (n = 67) or laparotomy (n = 149) for severe endometriosis during a 5-year period with a median follow-up of 24 months. They reported that the efficacy of laparoscopy and laparotomy was similar [16].

Subtle appearances of endometriosis

In the mid 1980s, Jansen described non-pigmented endometriosis [17]. Subsequently, other authors also reported non-typical endometriosis (Plate 28.2). Today, it is known that endometriosis lesions can be pink, clear, red, white or puckered black. Stripling reported that 106 of 109 patients (97%) harbored all types of lesions [18]. The ability to detect such lesions increased with experience. Subtle lesions were documented at laparoscopy in

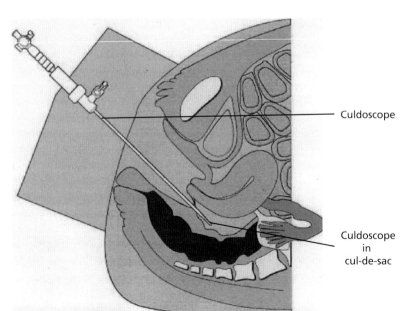

Culdoscope

Culdoscope in cul-de-sac

Figure 28.2 Culdoscopy in knee-to-chest position popularized by Decker and Cherry.

32% of patients in the first 5 months and in 72% of patients in the last 5 months of the study [18].

Differentiation between normal peritoneum and tissue harboring endometriosis can be further achieved with the use of a special filter to decrease the light illuminating the tissue (Plate 28.3). Peritoneal lesions exposed to small amounts of colored fluorescent light are seen more easily [19]. Buchewitz and colleagues performed a prospective analysis of 83 patients undergoing laparoscopy for suspected endometriosis using this type of filter. They found that the detection rate of non-pigmented endometriosis increased from 65% to 92% (1.42-fold increase) [20]. Treatment could be administered accordingly (Plate 28.4).

Endometrioma

Sampson first used the term "chocolate cyst" for ovarian endometrioma [5]. Several treatment modalities have been advocated.

Aspiration of endometrioma

Aspiration of endometrioma can be performed under ultrasound or laparoscopic guidance. The procedure is associated with high rates of recurrence (28.5–100%) and could lead to adhesion and infection. Abulghar et al aspirated endometriotic cysts transvaginally under ultrasound guidance in 21 women. Reaccumulation of the cyst at 12-month follow-up was 8.5% [21]. Chan et al aspirated eight endometriomas in six women. Recurrence rate was 83.3% within 3 months after aspiration [22]. In a study of 47 patients, the recurrence rate was 31.8% [23]. Muzii et al found that compared to control women (n = 42), previous transvaginal aspiration of the cyst (n = 13) was associated with a significantly higher degree of adhesions [24]. Accordingly, transvaginal aspiration of ovarian endometrioma is associated with a high degree of recurrence and intra-abdominal adhesion formation.

Sclerotherapy

Transvaginal sclerotherapy is widely used in Japan. It can be done by instilling ethanol 50% into the endometriotic cyst wall for 5 min, leading to tissue dehydration. However, leakage of ethanol outside the ovary could lead to adhesion formation. Noma et al compared 83 women who underwent transvaginal ethanol sclerotherapy and 30 others who underwent laparoscopic cystectomy for ovarian endometriomas. The recurrence rate of sclerotherapy was 14.9% and for laparoscopic cystectomy was 3.8%. The time of instillation of sclerotherapy appears to be important. The recurrence rates were 62.5% after instillation of less than 10 min and 9.1% after ≥10 min [25].

Koike et al compared clinical pregnancy of 45 infertile women after transvaginal ethanol sclerotherapy for ovarian endometriotic cyst with another 65 infertile women without ovarian cyst. The found no differences in the rates of pregnancy, abortion and term delivery between the two groups of women [26].

Other sclerosing agents are tetracycline and methotrexate. In 32 patients treated with these substances, the recurrence rate was 46.87% at 12 months follow-up [27]. Mesogiti et al used a single instillation of methotrexate in 26 women and 84.6% of the cysts resolved. However, they included postmenopausal women and those with simple ovarian cysts [28].

Laparoscopic treatment

Some authors have advocated laparoscopic fenestration and ablation of the cyst wall. The chocolate cyst was first drained and the "cyst wall" was then vaporized with either laser or electrocautery. Others excised the entire cyst wall by stripping it from the ovarian tissue. Saleh and Tulandi found that the recurrence rate in the excision group was 6.2% and in the fenestration group 18.8% [29]. In a randomized study of 64 women with endometrioma, Berreta et al compared laparoscopic cystectomy with fenestration and coagulation. The 24-month cumulative recurrence rates of dysmenorrhea, deep dyspareunia, and non-menstrual pelvic pain were lower in the cystectomy group than in the fenestration and coagulation group [30].

Alborzi et al reported similar findings [31]. In a systematic review of four studies including 212 patients, endometrioma recurrence after fenestration and ablation was 18.4%, and after cystectomy was 6.4% [31]. Therefore, fenestration and ablation of ovarian endometrioma is associated with a higher recurrence rate than cystectomy [32].

Peritoneal endometriosis

Surgical treatment of endometriosis can be done by vaporizing the lesions with laser or electrocautery, or by excision. The popularity of laser has decreased over time. Indeed, studies comparing these modalities found no difference in the clinical outcome [33–36]. Compared to expectant management, laparoscopic treatment of minimal and mild endometriosis increases fecundity [37]. In a randomized trial, Marcoux et al reported cumulative probability of pregnancy of 30.7% in the treated group and 17.7% in the non-treated group [37].

Conclusion

Endometriosis is still a poorly understood condition [38]. With the development of endoscopic technologies, we are now able to detect and treat endometriosis with minimally invasive techniques. Indeed, operative laparoscopy is considered the most appropriate surgical approach to all stages of endometriosis [39]. The new development in endoscopic surgery is the use of robotic assistance (see Chapter 43). Robotic surgery facilitates laparoscopic suturing, and its clinical value awaits more experience and randomized trials to determine its efficacy in the outcome of endometriosis treatment.

References

1. Shroen D. Disputatio inauguralis medica de ulceribus uteri. Jena: Krebs, 1690:6–17.

2. Benagiano G, Brosens I. The history of endometriosis: identifying the disease. Hum Reprod 1991;6:963–968.

3. Cullen T. Adeno-myoma uteri diffusum benignum. Johns Hopkins Hosp Rep 1896;6:133–154.

4. Russell W. Aberrant portions of the müllerian duct found in an ovary. Ovarian cysts of müllerian origin. Bull Johns Hopkins Hosp 1899;10:8–10.

5. Sampson J. Perforating hemorrhagic (chocolate) cysts of the ovary. Arch Surg 1921;3:245–323.

6. Nezhat C, Crowgey S, Garrison C. Surgical treatment of endometriosis via laser laparoscopy. Fertil Steril 1986;45:778–783.

7. Von Ott D. Die Beleuchtung der Bauchhohle (Ventroskopie) als Methode bei Vaginaler Coeliotomie. Abl Gynakol 1902;231:817–823.

8. Decker A, Cherry T. A new method in diagnosis of pelvic disease – preliminary report. Am J Surg 1944;64:40–44.

9. Clyman M. A new panculdoscope – diagnostic, photographic, and operative aspects. Obstet Gynecol 1963;21:343–348.

10. Gordts S, Campo R, Rombauts L, Brosens I. Transvaginal hydrolaparoscopy as an outpatient procedure for infertility investigation. Hum Reprod 1998;13:99–103.

11. Palmer R. Safety in laparoscopy. J Reprod Med 1974;13:1–5.

12. Paulson J, Ross J, El-Sahwi S. Development of flexible culdoscopy. Am Ass Gynecol Laparosc 1999;6:487–490.

13. American Fertility Society. Classification of endometriosis. Fertil Steril 1979;32:631–634.

14. Milingos S, Loutradis D, Kallipolitis G et al. Comparison of laparoscopy with laparotomy for the treatment of extensive endometriosis with large endometriomata. J Gynecol Surg 1999;15:131–136.

15. Mais V, Ajossa S, Guerriero S et al. Laparoscopic management of endometriomas: a randomized trial versus laparotomy. J Gynecol Surg 1996;12:41–46.

16. Crosignani P, Vercellini P, Biffignandi F et al. Laparoscopy versus laparotomy in conservative surgical treatment for severe endometriosis. Fertil Steril 1996;66:706–711.

17. Jansen R, Russell P. Nonpigmented endometriosis: clinical, laparoscopic, and pathologic definition. Am J Obstet Gynecol 1986;155:1154–1159.

18. Stripling M, Martin D, Chatman D et al. Subtle appearance of pelvic endometriosis. Fertil Steril 1988;49:427–431.

19. Palter S. V-4 A new autoflourescence-based endoscopic system for the detection of surface pathology including endometriosis. Fertil Steril 2006;86:516–517.

20. Buchweitz O, Staebler A, Tio J, Kiesel L. Detection of peritoneal endometriotic lesions by autofluorescence laparoscopy. Am J Obstet Gynecol 2006;195:949–954.

21. Aboulghar M, Mansour R, Serour G, Rizk B. Ultrasonic transvaginal aspiration of endometriotic cysts: an optional line of treatment in selected cases of endometriosis. Hum Reprod 1991;1408–1410.

22. Chan L, So W, Lao T. Rapid recurrence of endometrioma after transvaginal ultrasound-guided aspiration. Eur J Obstet Gynecol 2003;109:196–198.

23. Mittal S, Kumar S, Kumar A, Verma A. Ultrasound guided aspiration of endometrioma – a new therapeutic modality to improve reproductive outcome. Int J Gynecol Obstet 1999;65:17–23.

24. Muzii L, Marana R, Caruana P, Catalano G, Mancuso S. Laparoscopic findings after transvaginal ultrasound-guided aspiration of ovarian endometriomas. Hum Reprod 1995;10:2902–2903.

25. Noma J, Yoshida N. Efficacy of ethanol sclerotherapy for ovarian endometriomas. Int J Gynecol Obstet 2001;72:35–39.

26. Koike T, Minakami H, Motoyama M, Ogawa S, Fujiwara H, Sato I. Reproductive performance after ultrasound-guided transvaginal ethanol sclerotherapy for ovarian endometriotic cysts. Eur J Obstet Gynecol 2002;105:39–43.

27. Chang C, Lee H, Tsai H, Lo H. Sclerotherapy – an adjuvant therapy to endometriosis. Int J Gynecol Obstet 1997;59:31–34.

28. Mesogitis S, Daskalakis G, Pilalis A et al. Management of ovarian cysts with aspiration and methotrexate injection. Radiology 2005;235(2):668–673.

29. Saleh A, Tulandi T. Reoperation after laparoscopic treatment of ovarian endometriomas by excision and by fenestration. Fertil Steril 1999;72:322–324.

30. Beretta P, Franchi M, Ghezzi F, Busacca M, Zupi E, Bolis P. Randomized clinical trial of two laparoscopic treatments of endometriomas: cystectomy versus drainage and coagulation. Fertil Steril 1998;70:1176–1180.

31. Alborzi S, Momtahan M, Parsanezhad M, Dehbashi S, Zolghadri J. A prospective, randomized study comparing laparoscopic ovarian cystectomy versus fenestration and coagulation in patients with endometriomas. Fertil Steril 2004;82:1633–1637.

32. Vercellini P, Chapron C, de Giorgi O, Consonni D, Frontino G, Crosignani P. Coagulation or excision of ovarian endometriomas? Am J Obstet Gynecol 2003;188:606–610.

33. Daniell J, McTavish G, Kurtz B, Tallab F. Laparoscopic use of argon beam coagulator in the management of endometriosis. J Am Ass Gynecol Laparosc 1994;1:S9.

34. Robbins M. Excision of endometriosis with laparosonic coagulating shears. Am Ass Gynecol Laparosc 1999;6:199–203.

35. Badawy S, Choe J, Cohn G, Refaie A, Stefanu C, Cuenca V. Argon laser laparoscopy for treatment of pelvic endometriosis associated with infertility and pelvic pain. J Gynecol Surg 1991;7:27–32.

36. Sutton C, Jones K. Laser laparoscopy for endometriosis and endometriotic cysts. Surg Endosc 2002;16:1513–1517.

37. Marcoux S, Maheux R, Berube S. Laparoscopic surgery in infertile women with minimal or mild endometriosis. N Engl J Med 1997;337:217–222.

38. Tulandi T, Redwine D. Endometriosis: Advances and Controversies. Oxford: Informa Healthcare, 2003.

39. Bateman B, Kolp L, Mills S. Endoscopic versus laparotomy management of endometriomas. Fertil Steril 1994;62:690–695.

29 Diagnosis of Endometriosis: Imaging

Gerard A. J. Dunselman[1] and Regina G. H. Beets-Tan[2]
[1]Department of Gynaecology and
[2]Department of Radiology, Maastricht University Medical
Center, Maastricht, The Netherlands

Introduction

Endometriosis is a chronic disorder characterized by the presence of functional endometrial tissue outside the uterus. It affects 10–15% of women of reproductive age and has a strong social and professional impact on the life of patients because of its association with dyspareunia, dysmenorrhea, pelvic pain and subfertility [1,2].

Endometriosis presents as different clinical entities: ovarian endometriosis (endometrioma) and adenomyotic nodules, deep invasive lesions which can infiltrate different organs in the pelvic area. The majority of the patients, however, present with peritoneal endometriosis, lesions on and below the peritoneal surface. These lesions can be found during laparoscopy for different indications (subfertility, pain, sterilization) in a high proportion of women [3].

In this chapter the value of imaging in the course of diagnosing endometriosis will be dealt with in the three different localizations of endometriosis: peritoneal disease, ovarian endometriomas and deeply infiltrating endometriosis.

Peritoneal disease

The favored theory of the pathogenesis of peritoneal endometriosis is retrograde menstruation followed by implantation of endometrial tissue at ectopic locations. In the process of developing endometriosis, menstrual endometrium leaves the uterine cavity during menstruation and, via the fallopian tubes, enters the abdominal cavity. Thereafter, a conjunction of several environmental and genetic factors allows fragments of shed endometrium to adhere to the submesothelial extracellular matrix, invade the extracellular matrix, survive, grow, escape the immune surveillance and infiltrate other tissues [1,4–6]. One important event that allows the lesions to stabilize and survive at ectopic locations consists of the acquisition of blood and nutrient supply via neo-angiogenesis, which is extremely active in early endometriotic lesions [1,5,7–10].

One of the major problems associated with diagnosing peritoneal endometriosis is represented by the poor sensitivity of current non-invasive diagnostic tools. The diagnosis of endometriosis is suspected based on the patient history (dyspareunia, dysmenorrhea, pelvic pain and subfertility) and the presence of typical signs during gynecological examination. If these typical signs are not present, there is currently no diagnostic test available to increase the likelihood that a given patient has or does not have peritoneal endometriosis.

The gold standard for detecting peritoneal disease is laparoscopy and/or histopathology. Embarking on a laparoscopic investigation carries risks of morbidity, and it is costly. As a consequence, endometriosis is often diagnosed several years after occurrence of the first complaints (8–11 years on average) because (i) laparoscopy is not the primary diagnostic choice and (ii) endometriosis is difficult to diagnose since its symptoms present wide overlaps with other gynecological, gastrointestinal and urogenital disturbances. Moreover, in many adolescents dysmenorrhea is treated with oral contraceptives, without establishing a definitive diagnosis. When women want to get pregnant, oral contraception is stopped, dysmenorrhea recurs and the diagnosis is finally made when they undergo laparoscopy for pain or subfertility.

To reach a definitive diagnosis, laparoscopy is the only diagnostic tool available. The added advantage of performing a laparoscopy is the possibility of surgically treating the disease at the same time. However, based on current guidelines, there remains a place for the hormonal treatment of symptoms suggestive of endometriosis without a definitive diagnosis [11]. So the paradox is there: we start adolescents on oral contraceptives to decrease the dysmenorrhea possibly related to endometriosis without making a definitive diagnosis, while with this regimen we delay the diagnosis of endometriosis by several

Endometriosis: Science and Practice, First Edition. Edited by Linda C. Giudice, Johannes L.H. Evers and David L. Healy.
© 2012 Blackwell Publishing Ltd. Published 2012 by Blackwell Publishing Ltd.

Table 29.1 Methodological quality of studies analyzed.

Reference	Consecutive patients	Blinding	Diagnostic criteria	Technical details	Reference standard	Quality
Arrive et al 1989 [18]	Yes	Yes	Yes	Yes	Visual	Moderate
Ascher et al 1995 [15]	Not stated	Yes	Yes	Yes	Visual	Poor
Carbognin et al 2006 [19]	Yes	Not stated	Yes	Yes	Visual	Moderate
Ha et al 1994 [13]	Not stated	Yes	Yes	Yes	Histology	Moderate
Stratton et al 2003 [16]	Yes	Yes	Yes	Yes	Histology	Good
Takahashi et al 1994 [14]	Yes	Not stated	Yes	Yes	Histology	Moderate
Zanardi et al 2003 [20]	Yes	Not stated	Yes	Yes	r-AFS	Moderate

rAFS, revised American Fertility Society classification system [12].

years. During this time, it is not known whether or not the endometriosis becomes more serious and develops into adhesive disease, eventually hampering fertility. This treatment of symptoms without a definitive diagnosis, however, should be reserved for those women who do not show signs of more advanced disease, either by gynecological examination or by ultrasound. A point of concern is that adolescents and women in their 20s who do have positive signs of more advanced disease are also hormonally treated without a prior laparoscopy. During that laparoscopy, the disease could have been diagnosed and treated at the same time.

If we only consider the group of women with clinical symptoms but without clinical signs of endometriosis, it would be advantageous to have a non-invasive diagnostic test to include or exclude peritoneal endometriosis. Imaging could be one of these diagnostic tools.

Magnetic resonance imaging (MRI) has been extensively investigated in assessing the extent of disease in deep invasive and ovarian endometriosis. The use of MRI has to a lesser extent been studied to detect peritoneal implants of endometriosis. To evaluate the role of conventional MRI in the diagnosis of superficial peritoneal disease, the literature was searched. Prospective trials that involved women with suspected superficial peritoneal disease were included. Prospective trials that involved women with suspected deep invasive endometriosis or endometriomas were excluded. Studies involving women with known endometriosis were excluded. Reviews, cases series, case reports and descriptions of response to treatment were excluded. All patients should have undergone a laparoscopy to prove or reject the diagnosis of endometriosis. The MRI should have been used preoperatively as a diagnostic test. Studies before 1985 were not included because of technical advances made in the field of MRI after that time. The selected papers were assessed for methodological quality using the criteria below. To be considered of good quality, eligible women must have been recruited consecutively, and the following must have been described:

- the criteria used for a radiological diagnosis of endometriosis
- the type of MRI machine
- whether it had a magnet strength >1 tesla

- whether T1-weighted, fat suppression (FS) sequences were used
- whether the revised American Fertility Society (rAFS) classification system [12] or histological confirmation was used as the reference standard.

Blinding was ideal when it was clearly stated in the paper that the reporting radiologist was unaware of the surgical findings; preferably the surgeon was also blinded to the MRI findings (double blind). When one criterion was missing, the study was said to be of moderate quality; if two or more criteria were missing, the study was said to be of poor quality. The studies were analyzed in terms of how accurately MRI diagnosed both the number of patients with endometriosis and the number of lesions present. If the data were available to construct 2 × 2 tables, these were used to calculate the sensitivity, specificity, and likelihood ratios (LR) of a positive/negative test (LR+ and LR−) for each study.

For conventional MRI and peritoneal endometriosis, the search revealed a total of 62 citations/abstracts. After excluding reviews, case series, case reports, studies on deep invasive endometriosis and endometriomas, seven studies were identified that met the criteria (Table 29.1). Table 29.1 shows the overall quality of the studies included. The recruitment of patients, the blinding and the way in which endometriosis was diagnosed were not uniformly stated. Lesions were diagnosed when there were abnormal, hyperintense foci without mass formation on conventional or fat-suppressed T1-weighted images [13].

Takahashi and co-workers [14] used identical T1- and T2-weighted sequences, although the resolution was not mentioned. Ha and co-workers [13] used spin echo (SE) sagittal and axial T2, axial and coronal T1, and axial FatSat sequences for peritoneal lesions. The matrix size was 256 square with a 32 cm field of view, and the slice/gap thickness was 5/2.5 mm. The minimum voxel size therefore was $320/256*5 = 6.25$ mm³, and these authors commented that the smallest lesion detected was 3 mm in diameter (15 mm³). Ascher and co-workers [15] conducted a similar study, with the addition of either an antiperistaltic agent or fasting prior to the scan. The slice/gap thickness varied between 5–7 mm/<2 mm, with a 28–35 cm field of view, matrix size of 192–256*256, and minimum resolution of $280/256*5 = 5.46$ mm³. They also report the use of a body coil

Table 29.2 Number of patients correctly diagnosed by conventional MRI.

Reference	Sensitivity	Specificity	LR+	LR−
Arrive *et al* 1989 [18]	0.64	0.60	1.6	0.6
Ascher *et al* 1995 [15]	0.86	0.50	1.72	0.28
Carbognin *et al* 2006 [19]	Not stated	Not stated		
Ha *et al* 1994 [13]	0.76	1.00		0.24
Stratton *et al* 2003 [16]	0.69	0.75	2.76	0.41
Takahashi *et al* 1994 [14]	0.89	0.71	3.07	0.16
Zanardi *et al* 2003 [20]	1.00	0.00		

LR+, likelihood ratio of a positive test; LR−, likelihood ratio of a negative test.

Table 29.3 Number of (peritoneal) lesions correctly diagnosed by conventional MRI.

Reference	Sensitivity	Specificity	LR+	LR−
Arrive *et al* 1989 [18]	0.13	Not stated		
Ascher *et al* 1995 [15]	Not stated	Not stated		
Carbognin *et al* 2006 [19]	0.56	0.50	1.12	0.88
Ha *et al* 1994 [13]	0.61	0.87	4.69	0.45
Stratton *et al* 2003 [16]	0.18	Not stated		
Takahashi *et al* 1994 [14]	0.61	Not stated		
Zanardi *et al* 2003 [20]	0.77	Not stated		

LR+, likelihood ratio of a positive test; LR−, likelihood ratio of a negative test.

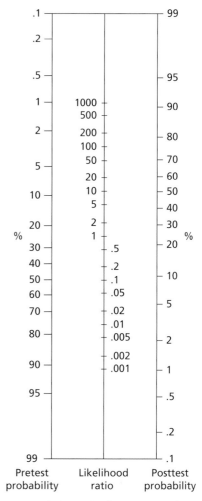

Figure 29.1 Nomogram for interpreting diagnostic test results: turning pretest probability of disease into post-test probability using the likelihood ratio (LR).

instead of a more sensitive phased-array coil. Stratton and co-workers [16] used a phased-array body or pelvis coil, T1 FatSat, and T2-weighted sequences, with axial and sagittal pre- and postcontrast images. Five millimeter contiguous slices were used throughout, and all the images had a minimum resolution of 6.8 mm³.

The studies reviewed show a wide variety in methodology, patient inclusion, techniques used, radiological and laparoscopic reporting.

Tables 29.2 and 29.3 show the results calculated from the studies for the sensitivity, specificity, LR+ and LR− where possible. The use of the LR+ and LR− to evaluate diagnostic tests has a major benefit since it is independent of the prevalence of the disease. This is in contrast to the use of the positive predictive and negative predictive value of a given test. The interpretation of the values for the LR+ and LR− is easily visualized using the nomogram for interpreting diagnostic test results (Fig. 29.1). In this nomogram, a straight line drawn from a patient's pretest probability of disease (which is estimated from experience, local data or published literature) through the LR for the test result that may be used will point to the post-test probability of disease [17].

Applying the values for LR+ in the nomogram, with a prevalence between 10% and 15%, will lead to a post-test probability between 30% and 40%. In other words, the conventional MRI cannot be used to diagnose endometriosis. Along the same lines, the values of the LR− show that conventional MRI is not

able to exclude the disease. The poor diagnostic accuracy of MRI for superficial peritoneal endometriosis is most probably related to the small implants that are difficult to detect on conventional MRI with large voxel volumes. Furthermore, a curved peritoneal viscera which may have implants on the surface is difficult to evaluate with the more rigid axial, sagittal or coronal MR planes. Moreover, the different types of lesions contain different amounts of endometriotic components, blood and fibrosis, resulting in large variations in MR signal features which lead to confounding images where structures such as blood vessels, adhesions and the sequelae of previous surgery can be easily mistaken for implants.

In conclusion, there is insufficient evidence from the literature reviewed here to suggest that conventional MR techniques are useful to diagnose or exclude peritoneal endometriosis.

An alternative might be the use of dynamic contrast-enhanced MRI (DCEMRI). As stated above, angiogenesis plays an important role in the development and maintenance of peritoneal lesions. The role of angiogenesis in the development of endometriosis has been studied intensively by our research group in the past few years. These and other studies are described in Chapter 19.

We used different model systems, such as the chick embryo chorioallantoic membrane (CAM) [6,8,21] and the nude mouse model [10]. Both the CAM and the mouse model systems have indicated that angiogenesis is a crucial and extremely active event in the establishment of endometriotic lesions. As proof of this, the formation of lesions in these models can be specifically inhibited by treatment with angiostatic compounds (anti-hVEGF antibody, TNP-470, endostatin, and anginex) [7–10]. This clearly indicates that angiogenesis occurs during endometriosis onset and that it is necessary for the establishment of the disease and the lesions at ectopic locations.

Our radiology research group has extensively focused on DCE MRI and has shown that with high molecular weight contrast agent, it is an excellent tool to visualize neo-angiogenesis [22–24]. The major advantage of the use of macromolecular contrast agents is that these are blood pool contrast agents that remain longer intravascularly and provide a higher MRI contrast (higher relaxivity) compared to conventional low molecular weight contrast agents. In addition, the long retention in the blood allows the acquisition of images with ultra-high resolution, suitable for visualizing small, highly vascularized spots. Furthermore, these contrast agents have a diminished permeability in healthy blood vessels, increasing the image intensity in the lesions compared to other "healthy" locations. We have extensively used DCE MRI with high molecular weight contrast agents to visualize angiogenesis in several animal models of cancer [25–28] and also in patients [29].

This technique has not yet been applied in endometriosis patients. If DCE MRI could detect peritoneal lesions, the following four groups of patients would benefit from such a non-invasive diagnostic tool.

• Women with endometriosis symptoms. A non-invasive test would increase the *a priori* probability of peritoneal endometriosis and avoid hormonal treatment for women with suspected endometriosis without the disease. DCE MRI may provide information of the extent and localization of the disease. This will allow selection of patients who need further invasive treatment, allow guidance of this invasive procedure and thus avoidance of laparoscopy in cases of absence of disease.

• Adolescents and young women with pelvic pain. DCE MRI will select those adolescents with a high probability of having peritoneal endometriosis. This will allow early diagnosis and surgical treatment of the peritoneal lesions by performing a laparoscopy in selected patients. An early diagnosis will be beneficial because it will avoid the complications associated with advanced stage disease, such as reduced fertility, reduced functionality of some organs and reduced efficacy of hormonal drugs.

• Women with recurrence of symptoms after a surgical treatment. In these cases, it is extremely difficult to distinguish between recurrent disease and postsurgery adhesions without a laparoscopy. DCE MRI could prevent the use of laparoscopy in this group of patients. The assumption is that DCE MRI will correctly

distinguish recurrent disease from fibrosis. Recurrent endometriosis will be accompanied by neo-angiogenesis, whereas fibrosis and adhesions will not.

• Asymptomatic women with infertility have a high prevalence of peritoneal endometriosis, which escapes the traditional non-invasive way of diagnosing the disease. It would be useful to develop a non-invasive diagnostic test to select those infertile women eligible for laparoscopy also for surgical treatment of endometriosis, which will improve their chances of becoming pregnant [30].

Ovarian endometriosis

Ovarian endometriosis is either superficial peritoneal endometriosis on the ovarian surface (see above) or represents an endometrioma, a pseudocyst formed by invagination of the ovarian cortex sealed off by adhesions. The adhesions are mostly very dense and result in close proximity of the ovarian endometrioma with adjacent structures like the rectosigmoid bowel and the ureters. In most women with endometrioma, this is not an isolated ovarian disease but rather constitutes an extensive problem involving other organs as well [31]. Preoperative diagnosis by ultrasound or MRI would be advantageous to select the patients who require less traumatic, fertility-preserving surgery by experienced pelvic surgeons, as is the case in women with endometriomata. It is therefore mandatory to be able to predict the nature of an adnexal mass before surgery is performed. Besides that, the finding of an adnexal mass that has a high suspicion of being an endometrioma should prompt the investigator to examine the patient again to find out if she has deep invasive endometriosis as well. Too often, the ultrasound focus in women with an adnexal mass, especially in subfertility patients, is on the ultrasound findings and less on proper pelvic examination, i.e. inspection of the vaginal posterior fornix and palpation of the cul-de-sac in search of the typical nodularities that lead to the diagnosis of deep infiltrating endometriosis.

Patients with endometriomata present either during subfertility work-up or with lower abdominal pain, or are asymptomatic. In asymptomatic women, the adnexal mass is found during imaging (ultrasound, computed tomography (CT) scan, MRI) for other indications. In women with adnexal masses, transvaginal ultrasound has become a primary diagnostic tool in ovarian endometriosis. This leads to the question: how accurate is the use of transvaginal ultrasound in the diagnosis of endometriomata? On gray-scale ultrasound, characteristic features of endometriomata are the presence of diffuse, low-level internal echos and hyperechoic foci in the wall [32]. In a series of 252 adnexal masses, sonograms were evaluated by two independent reviewers. Diffuse low-level internal echos were present in 38 (95%) endometriomata and in 40 (19%) non-endometriomata (LR+, 5). To exclude other hemorrhagic cysts (for example, bleeding in a corpus luteum cyst or follicular cyst), it is worth performing a repeat ultrasound. If other signs of malignancy are present

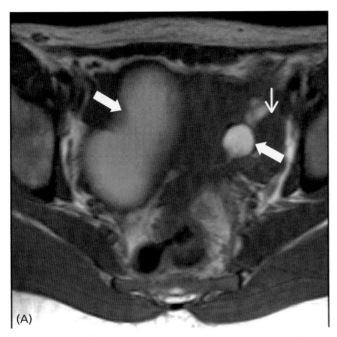 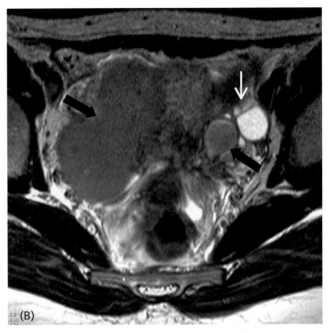

Figure 29.2 (A) Axial T1-weighted and (B) T2-weighted FSE MR images of a patient with deep infiltrating endometriosis. The MR images show typical "shading" features, characteristic for endometrioma. While an endometrioma is hyperintense on T1 (*thick white arrows in A*), it is isointense on T2 (*thick black arrows in B*), due to chronic blood degradation products and high concentration of protein in endometrioma. Note, however, the normal isointense signal on the T1-weighted image (*thin white arrow in A*) and hyperintense signal on T2-weighted image of a follicular ovarian cyst (*thin white arrow in B*).

(i.e. papillary formations of the cyst wall), appropriate diagnostic and therapeutic steps should be taken.

In 2002, the first and, currently, last comprehensive systematic review on the accuracy of ultrasound in the diagnosis of endometriosis was published by Moore and co-workers [33]. Interestingly while searching the literature on all types of endometriosis, the papers they could identify that met their strict criteria (prospective study, both ultrasound and laparoscopy or laparotomy) only concerned patients with ovarian endometriosis. In this review, the authors aimed to answer two questions: (i) can endometriosis be detected at all? and (ii) can an endometrioma be distinguished from other adnexal masses? Of the 67 selected papers, only seven could be included for analysis. In short, these studies showed that gray-scale transvaginal ultrasound can both rule in and rule out the diagnosis of ovarian endometriomata (LR+, 7.6–29.8; LR−, 0.1–0.4).

In view of the above, transvaginal ultrasound is the imaging method of choice if an adnexal mass is found with or without symptoms to make or exclude the diagnosis of an endometrioma pior to laparoscopy. If doubt remains on the exact nature of the mass or if by pelvic examination the suspicion arises of more extensive disease, an MRI can be helpful. The same applies if the patient's history in cases of an endometrioma points to other organ involvement, such as dyschezia, dysuria or flank pain.

On MRI, typical features of endometriomas include high signal on T1-weighted and isointense signal on T2-weighted sequences persisting on subsequent FS T1-weighted images [34]. Fat suppression is mandatory, as it helps to differentiate endometriomas from cystic teratomas [35] and to visualize more and smaller endometriomas than without FS techniques [34]. Gradual variation of signal intensity on T2-weighted images has been described as "shading" and is due to chronic bleeding with accumulation of high concentrations of iron and protein in endometriomas [36,37] (Fig. 29.2).

Deep invasive endometriosis

Women with deep invasive endometriosis present with the classic symptoms of the disease: dysmenorrhea, dyspareunia and pelvic pain. On top of that, due to the localization next to the rectosigmoid bowel, dyschezia is frequently present. If infiltrating endometriosis results in ureteral obstruction, most of the time no symptoms are encountered. In some women with endometriosis in the vesicouterine space, cyclical micturition problems may be the presenting complaint. In all these women, careful physical examination will reveal endometriosis in the rectovaginal space, posterior cul-de-sac or higher, easily accessible to the palpating finger and most of the time readily visible on speculum examination if properly performed. A properly performed speculum examination should include scrutinizing the posterior and lateral fornices to try to visualize any irregularities or nodularities suspicious of vaginal wall endometriosis. In many cases, transvaginal biopsy of the lesion in the vaginal wall can be performed to obtain tissue for a histological diagnosis. In these women, imaging is not needed in order to obtain a diagnosis of

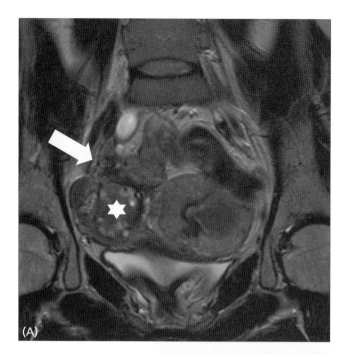

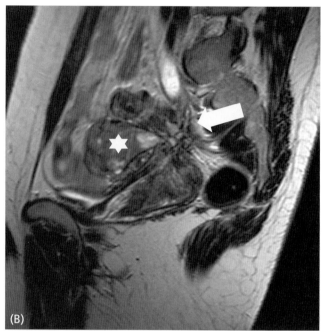

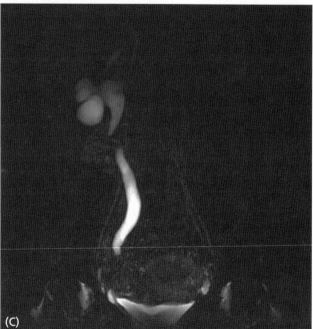

Figure 29.3 MRI of the pelvis provides detailed information of the DIE and its extent. The lesion (thick white arrow in A and B) extends to the right ureter and causes hydroureter. The lesion also invades the right adnexa, which contains endometrioma (*asterisk*). This pelvic MRI combined with the large field of view of a MRU provides information on the presence of hydroureter and hydronephrosis as well as the extent of the lesion that causes this obstruction. In this way, MRI represents the ideal "one stop shop" examination for patients with DIE. (C) MR urography (MRU), a heaviliy T2-weighted MRI of the same patient, that is performed in addition to the standard MRI. It shows the right-sided hydroureter and hydronephrosis due to obstruction by the DIE lesion. The advantage of MRU over IVU is that it only adds a few seconds to a standard pelvic MRI and contrast is not required.

endometriosis. Physical examination, however, cannot assess the true extent of disease, since it is far from perfect [38]. Detailed and adequate preoperative assessment of disease extent is helpful in planning laparoscopic surgery and assessing the need for bowel, bladder or ureter surgery. In this way, patients and doctors are better prepared for this sometimes extensive surgical procedure.

The accuracy of transvaginal ultrasound and MRI has been extensively described and studied. In order to ascertain the value

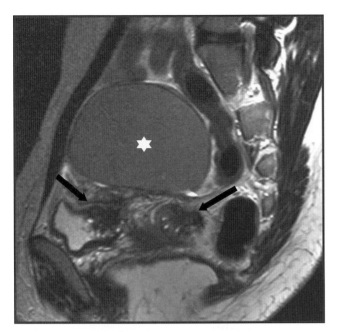

Figure 29.4 Sagittal T2-weighted FSE image of a patient with endometrioma co-existing with DIE of the bladder and in the posterior cul-de-sac. Ovarian endometriosis (*asterisk*) co-exists with DIE lesions of the bladder and the posterior cul-de-sac (*black arrows*). The DIE lesion is typically hypointense with small hyperintense spots within the lesion. The bladder detrusor muscle is fully penetrated by the lesion.

An advantage of pelvic MRI is that the relationship of the DIE to the rectosigmoid bowel is visualized in detail and also its relation to the ureters (MR urography, MRU). MRU as an adjunct to the standard MR pelvis provides additional information on the extent of deep lesions to the ureters. In contrast to the indirect information of an intravenous urography (IVU) of a lesion obstructing the ureter, MRI of the pelvis combined with MRU provides detailed information of the DIE causing the hydroureter [46,47] and the extent of the DIE into other pelvis structures. Furthermore, the large field of view of the MRU provides information on the presence of hydronephrosis. In this way, MRI represents the ideal "one stop shop" for examination of patients with DIE (Fig. 29.3).

Bladder endometriosis can be visualized equally well by TVUS and by MRI [48]. In a study using MRI in 195 patients with clinical suspicion of endometriosis, a sensitivity of 88% (14/16), a specificity of 99% (177/179) and a diagnostic accuracy of 98% (191/195) for the diagnosis of bladder endometriosis were reported [49] (Fig. 29.4).

Magnetic resonance imaging technique

Magnetic resonance imaging can be performed with a 1.5 or 3 tesla MR machine using a body phased array coil. MRI should not be scheduled earlier than day 8 of the menstrual cycle, because the hyperintensity of blood on T1-weighted sequences can cause confounding images, mistaking subacute bleeding degradation products for endometriotic implants. Bowel preparation is not necessary. Spasmolytics are not routinely given. When the small bowel descends very low in the pelvis, movements of the bowel loops can reduce image quality and IV spasmolytics may then be helpful.

Axial T1-weighted plus T2-weighted sequences in three planes (sagittal, axial and coronal) are part of the standard MR protocol. It is important to angle the plane perpendicular and parallel to the deep endometriotic lesions in the posterior pouch of Douglas as this angulation will be crucial for accurate assessment of rectal bowel wall invasion (Fig. 29.5). The exam is finalized with a MRU, a T2-weighted single-shot fast spin echo (FSE) sequence, on which fluid is visualized as strongly hyperintense while the background tissues are hardly visible due to the heavily T2-weighted images. A maximum-intensity projection (MIP) superimposing all structures that contain fluid allows for a full view of the urinary system, mimicking IVU images (see Fig. 29.3C). Gadolinium contrast is not necessary for the evaluation of DIE. The enhancement of pelvic organs and vessels as well as the fibrotic lesions on contrast-enhanced MRI hampers a clear delineation of the lesions and makes evaluation of their extent more difficult. The contrast between the hyperintense fat tissue and the hypointense fibrotic components of DIE is the strength of T2-weighted FSE sequences for accurately delineating DIE lesions. Therefore, T2-weighted FSE sequences in multiple planes are the preferred standard sequence in a standard MR endometriosis protocol.

of reports on the accuracy of diagnostic tests, some major issues have to be addressed. Patients studied should be either randomly or consecutively selected. If only women with a very high suspicion of deep invasive endometriosis are included in the study, the test results have to be regarded with caution. All women tested should have both the tests under study and the gold standard test. Are the investigators/performers of the test blinded to the results of the clinical exam and/or history of the patient? Is the examiner who performs the gold standard test unaware of the test result? So far there has been no systematic (Cochrane) review on the value of transvaginal sonography or MRI in the detection and staging of deeply infiltrating endometriosis.

Studies that report on the use of transvaginal ultrasound (TVUS) in detecting the extent of disease in deep infiltrating endometriosis (DIE) show positive LR values that indicate that TVUS is a good test to confirm rectal involvement in DIE (LR+ between 8 and 48) [39–42]. Likewise, negative LRs indicate that TVUS is a good test to exclude rectal involvement (LR− between 0.02 and 0.1) [39–44]. Studies reporting on the value of MRI in predicting the extent of disease in DIE are either prospectively [43] or retrospectively [44,45] conducted. Only one study included women with surgically proven endometriosis [45]. Positive LR ranged from 12.0 to 41.7. This indicates that MRI is a good test to predict whether DIE actually infiltrates the bowel wall. The negative LR ranged from 0.1 to 0.2, indicating a moderate test for excluding the presence of rectal infiltration.

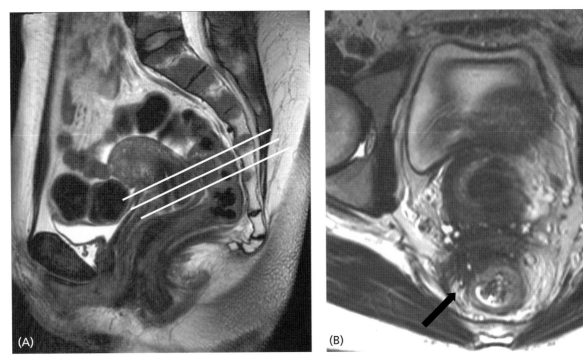

Figure 29.5 Sagittal (A) and axial (A) MR image of a patient with DIE infiltrating the anterior rectal wall. It is important to angle the axial plane perpendicular to the lesion axis (A). In this way, the bowel wall is sectioned perpendicularly to the bowel axis and true muscular invasion of the bowel wall can be more accurately assessed (*black arrow in B*).

Conclusion

Endometriosis is suspected based on the history. This suspicion is heightened by careful physical examination. Final visual diagnosis is made by the laparoscopist or the pathologist on biopsies taken during laparoscopy. Between the suspicion and the definitive diagnosis, imaging is mandatory. The first step in imaging is ultrasound which is readily available in most institutions and inexpensive. The burden of the investigation on the patient is not extraordinary. Transvaginal ultrasound is an accurate tool for predicting the presence of ovarian endometriomata and bladder endometriosis. In experienced hands, it is also accurate for predicting rectal wall involvement in deeply infiltrating endometriosis. One has to be aware that ovarian endometriosis rarely occurs alone and most of the time it is part of an adhesive disease, infiltrating the adjacent organs. The ultrasound finding of an ovarian endometrioma should prompt the investigator to carefully examine the patient again in search of deeply infiltrating disease. MRI has the advantage of being able to visualize the full spectrum of organ involvement in deeply infiltrating disease, i.e. rectosigmoid, bladder, ureters, and uterus.

Peritoneal disease so far has escaped all morphological imaging techniques, ultrasound or MRI. Eventually, the addition of functional information to the morphology of dynamic contrast-enhanced MRI might visualize the highly angiogenic early peritoneal lesions although further studies need to be performed to confirm its potential.

References

1. Groothuis PG, Nap AW, Winterhager E, Grummer R. Vascular development in endometriosis. Angiogenesis 2005;7:1–10.
2. Vigano P, Parazzini F, Somigliana E, Vercellini P. Endometriosis: epidemiology and aetiological factors. Best Pract Res Clin Obstet Gynaecol 2004;18(2):177–200.
3. Balasch J, Creus M, Fabregues F et al. Visible and non-visible endometriosis at laparoscopy in fertile and infertile women and in patients with chronic pelvic pain: a prospective study. Hum Reprod 1996;11(2):387–391.
4. Dunselman GA, Groothuis PG, de Goeij AF, Evers JL. The mesothelium, Teflon or Velcro? Mesothelium in endometriosis pathogenesis. Hum Reprod 2001;16(4):605–607.
5. Nap AW, Groothuis PG, Demir AY, Evers JL, Dunselman GA. Pathogenesis of endometriosis. Best Pract Res Clin Obstet Gynaecol 2004;18(2):233–244.
6. Nap AW, Groothuis PG, Demir AY et al. Tissue integrity is essential for ectopic implantation of human endometrium in the chicken chorioallantoic membrane. Hum Reprod 2003;18(1):30–34.
7. Van LA, Donnez J, Defrere S, Dunselman GA, Groothuis PG. Antiangiogenic and vascular-disrupting agents in endometriosis: pitfalls and promises. Mol Hum Reprod 2008;14(5):259–268.
8. Maas JW, Groothuis PG, Dunselman GA, de Goeij AF, Struijker-Boudier HA, Evers JL. Development of endometriosis-like lesions after transplantation of human endometrial fragments onto the chick embryo chorioallantoic membrane. Hum Reprod 2001;16(4):627–631.

9. Nap AW, Dunselman GA, Griffioen AW, Mayo KH, Evers JL, Groothuis PG. Angiostatic agents prevent the development of endometriosis-like lesions in the chicken chorioallantoic membrane. Fertil Steril 2005;83(3):793–795.

10. Nap AW, Griffioen AW, Dunselman GA et al. Antiangiogenesis therapy for endometriosis. J Clin Endocrinol Metab 2004;89(3): 1089–1095.

11. Kennedy S, Bergqvist A, Chapron C et al. ESHRE guideline for the diagnosis and treatment of endometriosis. Hum Reprod 2005;20(10):2698–2704.

12. American Fertility Society. Revised classification of endometriosis: 1985. Fertil Steril 1985;43(3):351–352.

13. Ha HK, Lim YT, Kim HS, Suh TS, Song HH, Kim SJ. Diagnosis of pelvic endometriosis: fat-suppressed T1-weighted vs conventional MR images. Am J Roentgenol 1994;163(1):127–131.

14. Takahashi K, Okada S, Ozaki T, Kitao M, Sugimura K. Diagnosis of pelvic endometriosis by magnetic resonance imaging using "fat-saturation" technique. Fertil Steril 1994;62(5):973–977.

15. Ascher SM, Agrawal R, Bis KG et al. Endometriosis: appearance and detection with conventional and contrast-enhanced fat-suppressed spin-echo techniques. J Magn Reson Imaging 1995;5(3):251–257.

16. Stratton P, Winkel C, Premkumar A et al. Diagnostic accuracy of laparoscopy, magnetic resonance imaging, and histopathologic examination for the detection of endometriosis. Fertil Steril 2003;79(5):1078–1085.

17. Fagan TJ. Letter: Nomogram for Bayes theorem. N Engl J Med 1975;293(5):257.

18. Arrive L, Hricak H, Martin MC. Pelvic endometriosis: MR imaging. Radiology 1989;171(3):687–692.

19. Carbognin G, Girardi V, Pinali L, Raffaelli R, Bergamini V, Pozzi MR. Assessment of pelvic endometriosis: correlation of US and MRI with laparoscopic findings. Radiol Med (Torino) 2006;111(5):687–701.

20. Zanardi R, Del FC, Zuiani C, Bazzocchi M. Staging of pelvic endometriosis based on MRI findings versus laparoscopic classification according to the American Fertility Society. Abdom Imaging 2003;28(5):733–742.

21. Maas JW, Le Noble FA, Dunselman GA, de Goeij AF, Struyker Boudier HA, Evers JL. The chick embryo chorioallantoic membrane as a model to investigate the angiogenic properties of human endometrium. Gynecol Obstet Invest 1999;48(2):108–112.

22. Aerts HJ, van Riel NA, Backes WH. System identification theory in pharmacokinetic modeling of dynamic contrast-enhanced MRI: influence of contrast injection. Magn Reson Med 2008;59(5):1111–1119.

23. De Lussanet QG, Backes WH et al. Dynamic contrast-enhanced magnetic resonance imaging of radiation therapy-induced microcirculation changes in rectal cancer. Int J Radiat Oncol Biol Phys 2005;63(5):1309–1315.

24. De Lussanet QG, Langereis S, Beets-Tan RG et al. Dynamic contrast-enhanced MR imaging kinetic parameters and molecular weight of dendritic contrast agents in tumor angiogenesis in mice. Radiology 2005;235(1):65–72.

25. De Lussanet QG, Backes WH, Griffioen AW et al. Dynamic contrast-enhanced magnetic resonance imaging of radiation therapy-induced microcirculation changes in rectal cancer. Int J Radiat Oncol Biol Phys 2005;63(5):1309–1315.

26. De Lussanet QG, Langereis S, Beets-Tan RG et al. Dynamic contrast-enhanced MR imaging kinetic parameters and molecular weight of dendritic contrast agents in tumor angiogenesis in mice. Radiology 2005;235(1):65–72.

27. De Lussanet QG, van Golde JC, Beets-Tan RG et al. Dynamic contrast-enhanced MRI of muscle perfusion combined with MR angiography of collateral artery growth in a femoral artery ligation model. NMR Biomed 2007;20(8):717–725.

28. De Lussanet QG, van Golde JC, Beets-Tan RG et al. Magnetic resonance angiography of collateral vessel growth in a rabbit femoral artery ligation model. NMR Biomed 2006;19(1):77–83.

29. Lahaye MJ, Engelen SM, Kessels AG et al. USPIO-enhanced MR imaging for nodal staging in patients with primary rectal cancer: predictive criteria. Radiology 2008;246(3):804–811.

30. Marcoux S, Maheux R, Berube S. Laparoscopic surgery in infertile women with minimal or mild endometriosis. Canadian Collaborative Group on Endometriosis. N Engl J Med 1997;337(4):217–222.

31. Redwine DB. Ovarian endometriosis: a marker for more extensive pelvic and intestinal disease. Fertil Steril 1999;72(2):310–315.

32. Patel MD, Feldstein VA, Chen DC, Lipson SD, Filly RA. Endometriomas: diagnostic performance of US. Radiology 1999;210(3):739–745.

33. Moore J, Copley S, Morris J, Lindsell D, Golding S, Kennedy S. A systematic review of the accuracy of ultrasound in the diagnosis of endometriosis. Ultrasound Obstet Gynecol 2002;20(6):630–634.

34. Sugimura K, Okizuka H, Imaoka I et al. Pelvic endometriosis: detection and diagnosis with chemical shift MR imaging. Radiology 1993;188(2):435–438.

35. Yamashita Y, Torashima M, Hatanaka Y et al. Value of phase-shift gradient-echo MR imaging in the differentiation of pelvic lesions with high signal intensity at T1-weighted imaging. Radiology 1994;191(3):759–764.

36. Togashi K, Nishimura K, Kimura I et al. Endometrial cysts: diagnosis with MR imaging. Radiology 1991;180(1):73–78.

37. Woodward PJ, Sohaey R, Mezzetti TP, Jr. Endometriosis: radiologic-pathologic correlation. Radiographics 2001;21(1):193–216.

38. Chapron C, Dubuisson JB, Pansini V et al. Routine clinical examination is not sufficient for diagnosing and locating deeply infiltrating endometriosis. J Am Assoc Gynecol Laparosc 2002;9(2):115–119.

39. Menada MV, Remorgida V, Abbamonte LH, Fulcheri E, Ragni N, Ferrero S. Transvaginal ultrasonography combined with water-contrast in the rectum in the diagnosis of rectovaginal endometriosis infiltrating the bowel. Fertil Steril 2008;89(3):699–700.

40. Guerriero S, Ajossa S, Gerada M, Virgilio B, Angioni S, Melis GB. Diagnostic value of transvaginal 'tenderness-guided' ultrasonography for the prediction of location of deep endometriosis. Hum Reprod 2008;23(11):2452–2457.

41. Hudelist G, Oberwinkler KH, Singer CF et al. Combination of transvaginal sonography and clinical examination for preoperative diagnosis of pelvic endometriosis. Hum Reprod 2009;24(5):1018–1024.

42. Piketty M, Chopin N, Dousset B et al. Preoperative work-up for patients with deeply infiltrating endometriosis: transvaginal

ultrasonography must definitely be the first-line imaging examination. Hum Reprod 2009;24(3):602–607.

43. Abrao MS, Goncalves MO, Dias JA Jr, Podgaec S, Chamie LP, Blasbalg R. Comparison between clinical examination, transvaginal sonography and magnetic resonance imaging for the diagnosis of deep endometriosis. Hum Reprod 2007;22(12):3092–3097.

44. Bazot M, Malzy P, Cortez A, Roseau G, Amouyal P, Darai E. Accuracy of transvaginal sonography and rectal endoscopic sonography in the diagnosis of deep infiltrating endometriosis. Ultrasound Obstet Gynecol 2007;30(7):994–1001.

45. Chapron C, Vieira M, Chopin N et al. Accuracy of rectal endoscopic ultrasonography and magnetic resonance imaging in the diagnosis of rectal involvement for patients presenting with deeply infiltrating endometriosis. Ultrasound Obstet Gynecol 2004;24(2):175–179.

46. Deprest J, Marchal G, Brosens I. Obstructive uropathy secondary to endometriosis. N Engl J Med 1997;337(16):1174–1175.

47. De Graaff AA, Beets-Tan RG, Beets GL, van de Beek CK, Dunselman GA. [Loss of renal function due to deep infiltrating endometriosis; a complicated consideration in women who wish to have children]. Ned Tijdschr Geneeskd 2009;153:B430.

48. Vercellini P, Frontino G, Pisacreta A, De GO, Cattaneo M, Crosignani PG. The pathogenesis of bladder detrusor endometriosis. Am J Obstet Gynecol 2002;187(3):538–542.

49. Bazot M, Darai E, Hourani R et al. Deep pelvic endometriosis: MR imaging for diagnosis and prediction of extension of disease. Radiology 2004;232(2):379–389.

30 Diagnosis of Endometriosis: Biomarkers

Beata E. Seeber[1] and Kurt T. Barnhart[2]

[1]Department of Gynecologic Endocrinology and Reproductive Medicine, Medical University Innsbruck, Innsbruck, Austria
[2]Division of Reproductive Endocrinology and Infertility, Department of Obstetrics and Gynecology, University of Pennsylvania, Philadelphia, PA, USA

Introduction

There is a great need for biomarkers that can serve as surrogates for important clinical endpoints such as endometriosis. A biomarker is a molecule produced by an affected individual that signals a specific exposure or disease state. A biomarker can be used for early diagnosis of a disease, identification of individuals for disease prevention, as a potential drug target, or as a potential marker for a drug response [1,2]. The identification and development of a biomarker have distinct phases [1,3–5]. The first phase is a preclinical exploration to identify promising markers. The second phase is the establishment of a clinical assay to be used on a larger scale. Phase III is testing the utility of the biomarker often with a longitudinal or retrospective cohort [1,3,4]. The goal is to verify that the marker detects disease, preferably early in the course of the disease. Phase IV is validation of the biomarker, usually in a prospective screening to identify the extent or characteristics of a disease when detected by tests. Some have suggested Phase V [4], which is to assess the impact of screening on reducing the burden of disease in a population, such as in the use of a cancer control.

What makes a good biomarker?

There are desirable characteristics for biomarkers to be used for diagnostic purposes. A general recommendation is that the validation effort concentrate on those biomarkers that are directly involved in the causal pathway of disease, since the closer to the causal pathway the biomarker is, the more precisely it will predict disease. A biomarker should be easily obtainable and have an assay that will obtain a rapid result in a disease process where non-invasive or early detection is of clinical benefit.

The definition of a biomarker should be straightforward but can mean different things depending on one's focus. One use of a biomarker is to screen for disease. Often, a biomarker is desirable to identify or predict the onset of disease, or detect disease prior to late-stage progression. Alternatively, a biomarker can be used to detect recurrence of a disease. A biomarker is not of value if it only detects late-stage disease that can already be identified by examination, imaging modality, or other clinical tests.

Characteristics of a biomarker for endometriosis

Identification of biomarkers for early non-invasive diagnosis and for following the progression of endometriosis has been identified as a priority for investigation [6]. The identification of a biomarker for endometriosis has similarities to, but also differs from classic biomarker development. To date, the goal of a biomarker for endometriosis has been the development of a non-invasive diagnostic test. The identification of a biomarker for endometriosis, however, has not been a concerted effort and has been complicated by multiple study designs and a variety of perspectives regarding utility of a marker. Complicating development is a lack of understanding of the disease process and progression of endometriosis. Factors that contribute to our lack of understanding are great heterogeneity in the presenting symptoms, the relative lack of correlation between severity of diseases and symptoms, deficiencies in understanding of the pathophysiology, and an incomplete understanding of the associated infertility and pain. Moreover, many patients suffer from co-morbidities, such as adenomyosis, irritable bowel syndrome, interstitial cystitis, and chronic pelvic pain, that can confound the symptomatology and accuracy of a potential biomarker.

Endometriosis: Science and Practice, First Edition. Edited by Linda C. Giudice, Johannes L.H. Evers and David L. Healy.
© 2012 Blackwell Publishing Ltd. Published 2012 by Blackwell Publishing Ltd.

A second controversy in the development of a biomarker for endometriosis is whether a developed biomarker or screening test should optimize sensitivity or specificity. A screening test has test characteristics which include sensitivity, specificity, predictive value and accuracy. The use of the area under a receiver operating characteristic (ROC) curve is a measure of the trade-off of sensitivity and specificity but may not be applicable to a clinical situation as it does not represent optimization of either test characteristic [7]. The choice of which test characteristic to optimize often depends on the clinical setting. Of note, optimization of sensitivity comes at the expense of specificity (and vice versa). While there is consensus regarding the need for a non-invasive test, some have proposed the test to replace surgical diagnosis while others have proposed that it should be used in conjunction with laparoscopy. For example, it has been proposed that the greatest need is for non-invasive detection of minimal-to-mild endometriosis, given that moderate-to-severe forms of the disease are more likely to be identified by clinical examination and/or imaging [8]. In this case, anyone with a positive test could undergo laparoscopy and few women with endometriosis would be missed (few false-negative tests). This would maximize those identified and treated. A possible alternative priority would be to optimize specificity, i.e. targeting only women with disease, and avoid overtreatment of those without disease. This situation may be more applicable to treatment with a high side-effect profile, complication rate, or contraindication in reproductive-age women. One example would be to avoid undesired *and unnecessary* medical treatment of women that may postpone or detrimentally affect potential fertility. In this case, one would prefer to only treat women with a high likelihood of endometriosis and avoid false-positive results.

The accuracy and predictive value of a biomarker are also of paramount importance. Predictive value is often difficult to interpret from small studies, because it is dependent not only on sensitivity and specificity, but also on the prevalence of the disease in the population. A sample of convenience, or a case control study, makes interpretation of predictive value particularly difficult because the true prevalence of the disease is not known. Accuracy is a concept related to predictive value. Some have suggested it is better to classify a small percentage of the population with an accurate test than to classify a large percentage with a concomitant increase in the numbers of false-positive and false-negative results [9]. Women with intermediate results (not classified by the test) may benefit from standard diagnostic procedures such as laparoscopy, rather than the implementation of therapy in women who may have false results.

Need for standardization

The field of biomarker identification is rapidly evolving. The quality of reporting of studies of diagnostic accuracy is less than optimal in general, and the field of endometriosis is not an exception. Complete and accurate reporting is necessary to enable readers to assess the potential for bias in the study and to evaluate the generalizability of the results. A group of scientists and editors has developed the STARD (Standards for Reporting of Diagnostic Accuracy) statement to improve reporting the quality of studies of diagnostic accuracy [10]. Future studies for biomarkers should use these standards. The goal of these guidelines is to encourage transparent and complete reporting so that the relevant information will be available to others to help them to judge the usefulness of the data and understand the context in which the conclusions apply [10].

This chapter reviews the extensive, yet uncoordinated effort of identification of a biomarker for endometriosis.

Tumor markers (CA-125 and CA-19–9) and soluble intracellular adhesion molecule-1

CA-125

The tumor marker CA-125 has been traditionally used to monitor the course of ovarian cancer and its response to treatment. The association between an increased serum CA-125 concentration and the presence of severe endometriosis has been known for over 20 years, with the first reports published in the mid 1980s [11,12]. Subsequent studies evaluating the diagnostic performance of this potential marker of endometriosis reported high specificities between approximately 80% and 95%, but with much lower sensitivities, rarely above 50% [13–15]. The diagnostic performance of CA-125 is further complicated by the fact that endometriosis has varying degrees of severity and chronicity, while CA-125 is elevated mostly in advanced disease. As previously discussed, a biomarker that could identify early-stage disease would be most useful clinically since advanced disease, with its associated pelvic adhesions and endometrioma formation, is in most cases detectable by bimanual pelvic exam or ultrasound. An additional problem with CA-125 is that it is not a marker specific to endometriosis, and thus an elevated level cannot differentiate among a host of other disorders such as uterine leiomyoma, pelvic inflammatory disease, and benign and malignant ovarian tumors.

In a large meta-analysis of 23 studies that had compared serum CA-125 levels and laparoscopically confirmed endometriosis, Mol and colleagues [16] analyzed the performance of CA-125 in the discrimination between endometriosis and healthy controls, as well as its ability to differentiate between mild (stage I/II) and severe (stage III/IV) endometriosis. Most studies included used a CA-125 cut-off level of 35 IU/mL, but there were several whose cut-off was as low as 20 IU/mL and one with 85 IU/mL. The authors excluded studies in which patients had a pelvic mass at ultrasonography, presumably eliminating those with a suspicion of endometrioma in whom a diagnosis of endometriosis was already highly suspected. They calculated summary ROC curves for a single CA-125 measurement's ability to predict any type of endometriosis or stage III and IV disease. For any stage endometriosis, the diagnostic performance was low: 90% specificity with only 28% sensitivity. Increasing sensitivity to 50% resulted in a corresponding 72% specificity. CA-125 was a somewhat better predictor of stage III and IV disease, with a specificity of 89% and sensitivity of

47%, but there was a very wide range of values in the single studies (sensitivity between 0% and 1% and specificity between 44% and 95%) and large differences in disease prevalence. This heterogeneity among the studies makes it difficult to accurately estimate a likelihood ratio of disease (the probability that a positive test is a true positive) for a single patient and difficult for the treating physician to use these results for clinical decision making.

Some additional, more recent studies which have evaluated CA-125 for the diagnosis of endometriosis have reached the same conclusion. These are summarized in Tables 30.1–30.4.

Appropriate CA-125 cut-off

Subsequent studies have confirmed the limited usefulness of CA-125 alone in making the diagnosis of endometriosis. Several have questioned whether the adopted cut-off of 35 IU/mL is the appropriate one. Kitawaki *et al* [17] evaluated preoperative CA-125 levels in a cohort of almost 800 patients and found that although mean concentrations were higher in women with

endometriosis and even higher in those with an endometrioma, there was considerable overlap between diseased and control subjects. The authors proposed a combined use of two cut-off values, 20 and 30 IU/mL, to simultaneously maximize specificity and sensitivity. In other words, a value of less than 20 IU/mL allows one to rule out endometriosis with a probability of 78% (negative predictive value (NPV)). Conversely, a patient with a serum concentration of greater than 30 IU/mL has a 92.9% probability of having endometriosis (positive predictive value (PPV)). Values in between (20–30 IU/mL) are indiscriminate and would necessitate further diagnostic testing with presumably the gold standard of laparoscopy. Although interesting, one must remember that predictive values depend on the prevalence of a disease in a population and these suggested diagnostic cut-offs would need to be validated in individual centers prior to clinical application.

Another group proposed using 20 IU/mL as the diagnostic cut-off, since this yielded a high specificity of 98% with a sensitivity of 30.4%, a PPV of 97.8% and NPV of 33.5% [18]. Xavier *et al*

Table 30.1 Cytokine panels for the diagnosis of endometriosis.

Tested cytokine panel in serum	Diagnostic panel (cut-off)	# Cases and endometriosis stage	# Controls and description	Sensitivity/ specificity	PPV/NPV	LR+/LR−	Reference
IL-1β, IL-6, IL-8, IL-12, IL-13, TNF-α	IL-6 (2 pg/mL)	20 (stage not specified)	15 (11 tubal surgery + 4 idiopathic infert)	90%/67%	Not reported	2.7/0.14	[33]
IL-6, CA-125, CA-19–9	CA-125 (31.0 IU/mL), IL-6 (3.9 pg/mL), CA-19–9 (36.4 IU/mL)	45 (14 stage I/II, 31 stage III/IV)	35 (12 dermoids, 6 PID, 9 cysts, 2 myomas, 5 normal pelvis)	42%/71%	66%/49%	Not reported	[34]
IL-6, CA-125	IL-6 (25.75 pg/mL)	47 (11 stage I/II, 36 stage III/IV)	38 Controls (no pathology, tubal sterilization); 13 myoma; 21 ovarian pathology	75%/83.3%	65.8%/88.6%	Not reported	[50]
IL-6, TNF-α, MIF, MCP-1, IFN-γ, leptin, CA-125	CA-125 (20 IU/mL), MCP-1 (76.4 pg/mL)	63 (22 stage II, 17 stage III, 24 stage IV)	78 (27 BTL/no pathology, 36 pain/infertility no pathology, 7 myoma, 4 ovarian cyst, 4 hydrosalpinx)	95%/44%		Not reported	[53]
IL-6, TNF-α, MIF, MCP-1, IFN-γ, leptin, CA-125	CA-125 (20 IU/mL), MCP-1 (152.7 pg/mL), leptin (3.14 ng/mL)	63 (22 stage II, 17 stage III, 24 stage IV)	78 (27 BTL/no pathology, 36 pain/infertility no pathology, 7 myoma, 4 ovarian cyst, 4 hydrosalpinx)	49%/94%		Not reported	[53]
IL-6, TNF-α, MIF, MCP-1, IFN-γ, leptin, CA-125	CA-125 (20 IU/mL), MCP-1 (152.7 pg/mL), leptin (29.1 ng/mL), MIF (14.7 ng/mL)	63 (22 stage II, 17 stage III, 24 stage IV)	78 (27 BTL/no pathology, 36 pain/infertility no pathology, 7 myoma, 4 ovarian cyst, 4 hydrosalpinx)	100%/40%		Not reported	[53]
IL-2, IL-6, IL-8, IL-15, MCP-1, IFN-γ, VEGF, TNF-α, GM-CSF	IL-6 (cut-off 1.03 pg/mL) IL-6 (cut-off 1.9 pg/mL)	68 (32 stage I/II, 36 stage III/IV)	70 (infertile, no pelvic pathology)	81%/51% 71%/66%	Not reported Not reported	1.38/0.38 2.06/0.45	[54]
IL-6, IL-8, TNF-α, CA-125, CA-19–9, hsCRP		201 (132 stage I/II, 69 stage III/IV)	93 (infertile, no pelvic pathology)				[55]

BTL, bilateral tubal ligation; GM-CSF, granulocyte macrophage-colony stimulating factor; hsCRP, high-sensitivity C-reactive protein; IFN, interferon; IL, interleukin; LR, likelihood ratio; MCP, macrophage chemotactic protein; MIF, migration inhibitory factor; NPV, negative predictive value; PID, pelvic inflammatory disease; PPV, positive predictive value; TNF, tumor necrosis factor; VEGF, vascular endothelial growth factor.

Table 30.2 Non-cytokine potential biomarkers for the diagnosis of endometriosis.

Tested biomarkers in serum	Biomarkers used for diagnosis (cut-off)	# Cases and endometriosis stage	# Controls and description	Sensitivity/ specificity	PPV/NPV	LR+/LR−	Reference
CCR1 mRNA	CCR1 mRNA (no cut-off provided)	83 (no information on stage)	51 (subserosal myoma, tubal ligation, pelvic pain)	90%/74%	82%/85%	Not reported	[58]
CCR1 mRNA, MCP-1, CA-125	CCR1/HPRT (1.16), MCP-1 (140 pg/mL), CA-125 (50 IU/mL)	102 (23 stage I, 14 stage II, 34 stage III, 31 stage IV)	49 (subserosal myoma, tubal ligation)	92.2%/81.6% 27.5%/100%	92.3%/83.3%	5.017/0.096	[60]
Differential WBC, NLR, CA-125	NLR (55.7), CA-125 (35 IU/mL) CA-125 (35 IU/mL)	231 (38 stage I/II, 193 stage III/IV)	384 (presumed healthy women, no surgical evaluation)	69.3%/83.9% 55.8%/92.8%	Not reported Not reported	Not reported Not reported	[61]
ccf nDNA, ccf mtDNA	ccf nDNA in plasma	19 (5 stage I, 8 stage II, 6 stage IV)	15 (presumed healthy women, no surgical evaluation)	70%/87%	Not reported	Not reported	[62]
Urocortin, CA-125	Urocortin (33 pg/mL) CA-125 (36 IU/mL)	40 (33 stage III, 7 stage IV)	40 (benign ovarian cysts)	88%/90% 65%/90%	Not reported	8.8/0.14 6.5/0.39	[56]
Follistatin, CA-125	Follistatin (1433 pg/mL) Follistatin (1025 pg/mL) CA-125 (42 IU/mL)	52 stage III/IV 52 stage III/IV	52 (benign cysts) 38 (11 stage I/II, 27 healthy controls)	92%/92% 100%/96% 44%/90%	Not reported	12/0.08 25/0 5/0.62	[57]

ccf, circulating cell free; CCR, cognate chemokine receptor; HPRT, hypoxanthine-guanine phosphoribosyl transferase; LR, likelihood ratio; MCP, macrophage chemotactic protein; mtDNA, mitochondrial DNA; nDNA, nuclear DNA; NLR, neutrophil/lymphocyte ratio; NPV, negative predictive value; PPV, positive predictive value; WBC, white blood cell.

Table 30.3 CA-125 for the diagnosis of endometriosis.

Tested biomarkers including CA-125	Diagnostics using CA-125 alone	# Cases and endometriosis stage	# Controls and description	Sensitivity/ specificity	PPV/NPV	LR+/LR−	Reference
IL-6, CA-125, CA-19–9	CA-125 at 31.0 IU/mL	45 (14 stage I/II, 31 stage III/IV)	35 (12 dermoids, 6 PID, 9 cysts, 2 myomas, 5 normal pelvis)	27%/94%	86%/50%	Not reported	[34]
IL-6, CA-125	CA-125 at 35 IU/mL	47 (11 stage I/II, 36 stage III/IV)	38 (no pathology, tubal sterilization)	47.2%/97.5%	89.0%/81.1%	Not reported	[50]

IL, interleukin; LR, likelihood ratio; NPV, negative predictive value; PID, pelvic inflammatory disease; PPV, positive predictive value.

[19] concluded that a CA-125 cut-off value of 22.6 IU/mL had a specificity comparable to that of most studies of 92.3% with a sensitivity of 72.0% and proposed a re-evaluation of the usefulness of the 35 IU/mL in clinical use. Importantly, the recommendations of this latter study need to be validated in light of its very small number of subjects.

CA-125 as marker of disease recurrence

As described above, CA-125 appears to have limited value alone as a diagnostic marker of endometriosis. However, its use as a predictor of disease recurrence has not been extensively studied. In a longitudinal study evaluating serial CA-125 measurements over 12 months postoperatively in women with endometriosis, the investigators found that the women whose CA-125 dropped to below 16 IU/mL after surgery were more successful at achieving pregnancy within 1 year [20]. However, only 46% of the study's 123 subjects with endometriosis had a preoperative value greater than 16 IU/mL, underscoring once again the limited sensitivity of CA-125 concentration for diagnosis. Nonetheless, if CA-125 is confirmed to aid in predicting the success rate of endometriosis-related infertility, it could be of great value in the postoperative management of women with this condition. Those with rising CA-125 concentrations might be counseled towards more aggressive treatment with assisted reproductive procedures.

Table 30.4 Potential biomarkers in endometrium for the diagnosis of endometriosis.

Tested biomarkers in endometrium	Biomarkers used for diagnosis	# Cases and endometriosis stage	# Controls and description	Sensitivity/ specificity	PPV/NPV	LR+/LR−	Reference
Leukocytes: CD3+, CD16+, CD3−HLADR−, CD3−CD45RA−, CD3+CD16−, CD3+CD56−, CD56−CD16+, CD16b+	CD3+, CD16+, CD3−HLADR−, CD3−CD45RA−, CD3+CD16−, CD3+CD56−, CD56−CD16+, CD16b+ and serum CA125 (12.8 IU/mL) plus menses length, gravidity and histological dating) CA-125 (35 IU/mL)	173 (stages not specified)	195 (infertility, pain, fibroids, menorrhagia, cysts)	61%/95% 20%/92%	91%/75%	Not reported	[69]
Aromatase P450 via PCR and immunostaining	Aromatase P450 (H-score 20)	84 (stages not specified)	21 (normally cycling, free of gynecological pathology)	91%/100%	100%/72%	Not reported	[71]
Aromatase P450 mRNA via PCR	Aromatase P450 mRNA	34 (28 stage I/II, 6 stage III/IV)	26 (infertility, pain, tubal sterilization)	82%/57%	76%/67%	Not reported	[72]

A particularly difficult clinical scenario occurs when a women who has already been surgically treated for endometriosis returns with recurrent symptoms and the clinician needs to determine if she has developed recurrent disease. A non-invasive test of recurrence would be very useful in such an instance, but it is not entirely clear whether CA-125 concentrations can be helpful in this context. Consistent with many previous studies of CA-125 in initial diagnosis, Fedele *et al* [21] found that on follow-up laparoscopy, patients with stages I and II endometriosis had serum CA-125 levels not significantly higher than those in patients with negative findings, whereas those with stages III and IV endometriosis presented with significantly higher levels than the disease-free women. In this study, the sensitivity of serum CA-125 measurements in the diagnosis of endometriosis recurrence was 14.8%, the specificity was 100%, and the predictive values of normal (less than 35 IU/mL) and elevated levels were 27% and 100%, respectively.

Another group followed a cohort of women who had been diagnosed with endometriosis, performing a second-look laparoscopy and CA-125 measurement on 24 study subjects [22]. They found that the 15 women whose CA-125 levels were greater than 35 IU/mL all had evidence of recurrent disease during surgery, while the remaining nine with CA-125 levels below this cut-off were all disease free, a PPV of 100% in this small subset of subjects. Although these findings appear very promising, the authors reported a lack of correlation between CA-125 levels and the American Fertility Society (AFS) score of disease severity. An additional 10 patients who had received adjuvant danazol therapy after initial laparoscopy underwent second-look laparoscopy. The researchers found that although in all these patients the CA-125 had decreased to normal (<35 IU/mL), all had evidence of endometriosis on subsequent laparoscopy, albeit a reduced burden of disease and lower AFS score.

Based on the existing evidence, serum CA-125 concentration alone does not have adequate sensitivity or specificity to be used to diagnose endometriosis. Although women with advanced stage III or IV disease have, on average, higher CA-125 levels than those with mild disease and disease-free women, there is no cut-off that can confirm disease presence or stage. Complicating things further is the fact that elevated CA-125 concentrations are seen in other conditions, such as uterine leiomyoma, pelvic inflammatory disease and benign and malignant ovarian neoplasms. Conversely, women with milder disease may have no elevation in CA-125 concentration, which may also be the case in some women with severe disease. Although preliminary reports of the use of CA-125 as an indicator of the presence of disease recurrence have shown some promise, these studies are limited by small subject numbers, uncertainty about whether an absolute cut-off or a drop of CA-125 pre- to postsurgically should be employed, and the unpredictability of CA-125 levels in medically treated endometriosis. Until future studies are able to address these issues, CA-125 alone does not have a defined role in the evaluation of suspected recurrent endometriosis.

CA-19–9

Another tumor marker that has been evaluated in endometriosis is carbohydrate antigen 19–9 (CA-19–9), a marker associated with colorectal and pancreatic carcinoma. One of the first reports of this marker's association with endometriosis was published by Matalliotakis *et al* [23]. Since that time, several studies have assessed the diagnostic properties of CA-19–9, comparing them to those of the better studied tumor marker, CA-125.

In one study, serum CA-19–9 concentrations were evaluated in 101 women with endometriosis and compared to those in 22 endometriosis-free subjects [24]. The mean CA-19–9 was higher in women with endometriosis compared to the control group, and concentration correlated positively with disease stage. Using 37.0 IU/mL as the cut-off, the authors reported an elevated level in 34/101 (33.7%) women with endometriosis compared to none (0%) of the control group. Moreover, only women with stage III and IV disease had CA-19–9 greater than 37.0 IU/mL, with 34/63 (54%) having serum concentrations above the cut-off. However, with a maximal specificity of 100%, the calculated sensitivity was only 34%, prompting the authors to conclude that CA-19–9 does not outperform CA-125 in diagnosing endometriosis.

A more recent study likewise reported higher serum CA-19–9 concentrations in 101 women with endometriosis compared to 78 controls, with the significant difference seen between stage III/IV disease and controls [25]. A positive correlation was also reported between CA-19–9 and disease stage. However, using the commonly accepted cut-off of 37.0 IU/mL, the sensitivity was for CA-19–9 was 89% and specificity 52%, values similar to those for CA-125 in this series. These results are in contradiction to previous studies which have reported high specificity and low sensitivity for this tumor marker [24,25]. Nonetheless, consistent with previous reports, the predictive value of CA-19–9 was only high for the ability to predict severe stage III and IV disease, a fact that limits this marker's use for broad application.

Similar to the situation with CA-125, the appropriate cut-off value for CA-19–9 in the diagnosis of endometriosis has been questioned [19]. Outside this very small series of subjects which suggested a cut-off for CA-19–9 as low as 5.4 IU/mL to improve test sensitivity, no large-scale studies have been performed with this potential marker. Due to the contradictory reports, unclear optimal cut-offs and the inability to diagnose early stage disease, CA-19–9 does not appear to be a good marker on its own for endometriosis.

Summary

In conclusion, neither CA-125 nor CA-19–9 alone, nor the two markers in combination, have adequate diagnostic performance to diagnose endometriosis. It has not been clearly established what cut-off values for these markers should be used in the diagnosis of endometriosis and whether the values commonly used for other diseases, especially cancer, also apply to endometriosis. Either way, varying the cut-offs used to define "normal" on these tests may slightly improve the test's sensitivity or specificity, but rarely both. Studies have consistently shown elevated tumor marker levels in women with stage III and IV disease, almost all of whom by definition have a unilateral or bilateral endometrioma or severe adhesive disease. These entities can be felt on physical exam or seen on ultrasound, obviating the need for a blood test for the disease. More research is needed to determine whether CA-125 levels could be used postoperatively to diagnose disease recurrence, with the caveat that women with surgically treated endometriosis who never had an elevation in their CA-125 would not be expected to show any change after surgery, and would not benefit from postoperative testing of their CA-125 levels. Thus, an evaluation of the CA-125 or CA-19–9 levels in a woman with symptoms suspicious for endometriosis, or one with otherwise unexplained infertility, does not aid in ruling in or ruling out this disease.

Recent investigations have combined these tumor markers with other potential biomarkers as part of multi-marker panels, hoping to improve the diagnostic performance. These studies will be discussed in more detail below.

Soluble intracellular adhesion molecule-1

The soluble intracellular adhesion molecule (sICAM)-1 has been shown by Vigano et al to be secreted from the endometrium and endometriotic implants [26]. Although follow-up evaluations of this polypeptide in endometriosis reported an increase in serum concentrations in women with endometriosis, only one study directly evaluated sICAM-1 for its diagnostic properties and deserves brief mention [27]. In a series of 120 women undergoing laparoscopy, the authors did not see statistically significant differences in sICAM-1 levels between all women with endometriosis and controls. However, they did report that the women with severe disease characterized by deep peritoneal lesions (n = 21) had significantly elevated sICAM-1 levels compared to those with other forms of endometriosis and controls. The authors thus report sensitivity and specificity only for the presence of deep infiltrating lesions as 19% and 97%, respectively. In comparison, CA-125 measurement in this same study population again for deep peritoneal lesions had a sensitivity of 14% and specificity of 92%. The sensitivity and specificity of both markers used together were reported as 28% and 92%.

It appears from these studies that sICAM-1 may play a role in the pathophysiology of endometriosis but, according to the results of these studies, does not form the basis for a non-invasive diagnostic test of the disease. Certainly, a test that picks out only one subset of the disease and is not able to differentiate this from other forms or controls cannot be a reliable test for the disease.

Cytokines

Why use cytokines as potential biomarkers?

Cytokines are proteins that play an integral role in regulating cell proliferation, immune cell activation, motility, cell adhesion and chemotaxis. They are secreted into the extracellular environment by leukocytes, macrophages or other inflammatory cells. Because endometriosis is characterized by the presence of ectopic implants of endometrial glands and stroma, it has been widely believed since the theory's inception by Sampson [28] that endometriosis results from the implantation of endometrial-derived cells arriving in the peritoneal cavity via retrograde menstruation. An important concept has emerged, namely that endometriosis induces a local inflammatory process in the peritoneal cavity. Why endometriosis develops in some women but not in others, despite the nearly universal presence of retrograde menstruation, may be in part explained by an alteration in the function of the immune cells in the peritoneal environment of those affected [29,30]. This immune system in the peritoneal cavity consists of a complicated interplay of different cell types and their secretory products, or cytokines, that interact by autocrine and paracrine systems. Macrophages, principal secretors of cytokines, appear to play a central role in the immunobiology of endometriosis and their increased presence in the peritoneal cavity of women with endometriosis confirms the presence of a local inflammatory process.

Thus, alterations or elevations in cytokine concentrations may reflect the immune system's response to initial disease. Alternatively, if chronically present, they may be a sign of a derangement in the organism's normal ability to resist or fight the localized disease process. Based on this fact that endometriosis induces this local, and likely also some degree of systemic, inflammatory process, numerous studies have focused on finding differences in markers of inflammation between women with and without endometriosis. That differences in certain cytokines have been found between diseased and healthy women is not unexpected and is summarized briefly below.

Interleukin (IL)-6 was found to be elevated in the peritoneal fluid and serum of women with endometriosis [31–34]. Concentrations of IL-8 have also been found to be higher in the peritoneal fluid of women with endometriosis, and in one of these studies [35] also in the serum [36–38]. However, another study looking at IL-8 levels was unable to demonstrate differences [33]. Tumor necrosis factor (TNF)-α, a cytokine secreted by activated macrophages, has also been shown to have higher levels in women with endometriosis in some studies [33,35,39], but not in others [40]. Other members of the interleukin family that have been evaluated in fewer studies, but have shown elevated levels, include IL-16 and IL-18 [41,42]. In addition, levels of macrophage migration inhibitory factor (MIF), macrophage chemotactic protein-1 (MCP-1), Regulated on Activation Normal T-cell Expressed and Secreted (RANTES), and epithelial neutrophil-activating peptide-78 (ENA-78) have been noted by some studies to be higher in those with endometriosis, while interferon (IFN)-γ levels have been found to be lower in those with the disease [35,43–49].

Despite the numerous findings of different *mean* concentrations of cytokines between women with and without endometriosis, confirming the pathophysiology of disease, these cannot serve as diagnostic tests. In fact, very few studies have directly examined the diagnostic properties of cytokines in endometriosis, and all have done so as part of multi-marker panels. These research studies and the success of their studied markers in diagnosing endometriosis will now be discussed in detail.

Cytokines as part of multi-marker panels for diagnosis

Many investigators have undertaken the study of multiple potential markers simultaneously in the hope of finding a multi-marker diagnostic panel. In many of these investigations, only a few of the markers studied proved to be worthwhile.

Bedaiwy *et al* [33] was one of the first researchers to measure the concentrations of more than one or two cytokines at a time, and to analyze directly the predictive value of a multi-marker panel for the non-invasive diagnosis of endometriosis. Of 91 women surgically evaluated for pain or infertility or undergoing tubal ligation or tubal reversal surgery (after the exclusion of women with bloody peritoneal fluid), 56 were diagnosed with endometriosis, 34 with stage I and II and 22 with stage III and IV disease. The researchers measured concentrations of a panel of markers including serum and peritoneal fluid (PF), IL-1β, IL-6, IL-8, IL-12, IL-13, and TNF-α in the subjects with endometriosis, comparing them to those of the 35 disease-free women, eight of whom had idiopathic infertility and 27 were presumably fertile and symptom free, undergoing elective tubal surgery. Of the serum markers, only IL-6 could be used to discriminate between patients with and without endometriosis. A threshold of 2 pg/mL of serum IL-6 had a sensitivity of 90% and specificity of 67%, with a positive likelihood ratio of 2.7 and negative likelihood ratio of 0.14. None of the other markers measured in serum was discriminatory for endometriosis. However, a closer review of this study showed that the investigators admitted to not being able to obtain sufficient serum to measure all the cytokines in all subjects, and the promising results reported are based on the comparison of only 20 subjects in the endometriosis group to 11 control subjects and to four subjects with idiopathic infertility. These small numbers severely limit the power of this study and need to be validated in larger study groups.

Another research group evaluated IL-6 in combination with the two tumor markers CA-125 and CA-19–9 as a diagnostic panel for endometriosis [34]. They compared serum levels between 45 women with and 35 without endometriosis. The endometriosis group was dominated by moderate-to-severe disease (n = 31 with stage III/IV, n = 14 with stage I/II), including 31 women with an endometrioma. The control group was a heterogenous one with the diagnoses of benign ovarian and paraovarian cysts, but also containing six cases of pelvic inflammatory disease (PID). Of the three potential markers, only mean CA-125 concentration was significantly higher in the endometriosis group, while no differences existed in CA-19–9 or IL-6 levels. When the diagnostic properties of the markers were evaluated, the combined panel using cut-offs of 31.0 IU/mL, 3.9 pg/mL, and 36.4 IU/mL for CA-125, IL-6, and CA-19–9 respectively yielded a sensitivity of 42% and specificity of 71%. Using all three markers did not improved the diagnostic properties compared to using CA-125 alone, which had an individual sensitivity of 27% and specificity of 97% at a cut-off of 35.0 IU/mL, with PPV of 92% and NPV of 51%.

Thus, this study was not able to demonstrate that a panel of the three markers studied improved diagnostic ability beyond that of CA-125, which alone had limited diagnostic potential. Certainly, the inclusion of such varied diagnoses in the control group, including women with PID, may have resulted in a regression towards the mean and an underestimation of differences between women with endometriosis and controls. The fact that so many women in the endometriosis group had stage III disease and endometriomas invites the question of whether these really were patients in whom the diagnosis was in question. On the other hand, if a test is to be used for diagnosis in suspected cases with gynecological problems, then the cohort of sequential, symptomatic patients evaluated here is exactly the type of "real-world" scenario for which a non-invasive diagnostic test is needed.

In a subsequent study, Martinez *et al* [50] re-examined the utility of IL-6 measurement in the diagnosis of endometriosis, comparing it to CA-125. These authors were careful to separate endometriosis subjects by severity of disease (minimal-to-mild versus moderate-to-severe endometriosis), and compared them to a pathology-free control group, a group with uterine myoma and a group with non-endometriosis ovarian pathology. Interestingly, the group with minimal-to-mild endometriosis had the highest serum concentrations of IL-6 among the groups, exceeding even those of the women with moderate-to-severe endometriosis. In the same women, CA-125 concentrations were more than three-fold higher in the women with moderate-to-severe disease than in the remaining groups, in which no inter-group differences were otherwise seen. The optimal serum IL-6 threshold using ROC curve for the diagnosis of minimal-to-mild endometriosis was 25.74 pg/mL in this study, corresponding to a sensitivity of 75.0%, specificity of 83.3%, PPV of 65.8% and NPV of 88.6%. The combination of IL-6 and CA-125 did not offer any additional value over each marker alone for the diagnosis of endometriosis.

The results of this study by Martinez *et al* [50] are particularly interesting because IL-6 was shown to be a marker for early-stage endometriosis, and was not affected by other pelvic pathologies, including uterine myoma or benign ovarian cysts. As previously discussed, such a marker would be most useful in the clinical setting, when ultrasound is not helpful. However, this study's findings diverge from other reports in small numbers of women in which IL-6 was only elevated in women with endometriomas [51] or showed no value for diagnosis [34,52]. In addition, the IL-6 levels used as a cut-off were five- to even 10-fold higher than those previously reported by other investigators, calling into question the interobserver reliability and reproducibility of using commercially available kits. This fact illustrates yet another limitation to the application of these markers for diagnosis outside the research setting: if the cut-off values have not been validated across testing sites, then they cannot be applied to individuals in the clinical setting.

Three additional studies have evaluated panels of cytokines for the diagnosis of endometriosis. One of these, Seeber *et al* [53], applied classification tree analysis to determine the diagnostic performance of six markers jointly: IL-6, TNF-α, MCP-1, MIF, leptin and CA-125. Analyzed singly, all markers, including CA-125, had poor diagnostic performance. Although they were unable to create a diagnostic algorithm that maximized both sensitivity and specificity simultaneously with a multi-marker panel, they were able to create two separate classification trees, each maximizing one of these parameters. As such, CA-125, MCP-1 and leptin had a sensitivity of 95% and specificity of 44% on the first classification tree, and a sensitivity of 49% and specificity of 94% on the second tree with different cut-offs. This two-tiered algorithm was able to diagnose 64 of the study's 141 subjects (45%) with a combined accuracy of 89%. According to the authors, the remaining subjects would receive a status of "no diagnosis" and would need further evaluation, likely diagnosis with laparoscopy. Alternatively, by expanding the diagnostic panel to four markers (CA-125, MCP-1, MIF, leptin), the sensitivity of the first classification tree improved to 100% with a specificity of 40%. In the revised two-tiered algorithm, 31/63 (49%) women with endometriosis would be diagnosed with complete accuracy and an additional 36/78 (46%) of control women would be deemed disease free, albeit with a 86% accuracy and five false positives. Again, those unable to be diagnosed by the combined classification trees would need to undergo further evaluation with traditional methods.

Although the statistical approach taken by Seeber and colleagues is a novel and interesting one, the diagnostic algorithm they describe was only able to provide a diagnosis in a portion of the study's participants, and that not always with complete accuracy. In addition, the authors' exclusion of women with stage I disease was unfortunate since, as discussed previously, this is the group for whom a diagnostic test would be of most value and most use.

In the second study [54], a nine-protein array system using cytokine-specific antibody-coated beads was used to quantify cytokine concentrations in samples from 68 women with endometriosis (32 stage I/II, 36 stage III/IV) and 70 controls. Of the cytokines evaluated (IL-2, IL-6, IL-8, IL-15, MCP-1, vascular endothelial growth factor (VEGF), TNF-α, INF-γ and granulocyte macrophage colony stimulating factor (GM-CSF)), only IL-6, MCP-1 and INF-γ had mean serum concentrations that were higher in the endometriosis group compared to controls. When all measured cytokines were evaluated for their ability to discriminate between endometriosis and non-endometriosis using multivariate regression analysis, IL-6 provided the best results. With a cut-off of 1.03 pg/mL, IL-6 had a sensitivity of 81%, a specificity of 51%, a LR+ of 1.38 and LR- of 0.38. Setting the cut-off point at 1.9 pg/mL, the sensitivity decreased to 71% with a concomitant rise in specificity to 66%. Combining IL-6 with MCP-1 and INF-γ, the other markers that showed a difference in means between groups did not improve the discrimination between disease and control subjects over that of IL-6 alone. This study did not see a correlation between serum IL-6 levels and stage of the disease, unlike that described by a previous study [50].

The largest study published to date comparing serum concentrations of multiple markers was conducted in 294 infertile women, 201 of whom had endometriosis and 93 a surgically normal pelvis [55]. Mihalyi *et al* compared serum concentrations of six markers, IL-6, IL-8, TNF-α, CA-125, CA-19–9, high-sensitivity C-reactive protein (hsCRP), between the two groups and used sophisticated statistical modeling to evaluate whether these markers in combination could prove to be accurate for the diagnosis of endometriosis. They performed multiple subgroup analyses based on disease stage, each time finding the combination of markers with the best diagnostic performance.

These investigators were also the first to account for the time in the menstrual cycle at which serum was collected, reporting differences in the optimal diagnostic panel depending on whether the specimen was collected in the secretory, proliferative or menstrual phase. The multiple permutations of disease stage and cycle phase resulted in an extensive list of combinations of markers yielding the best sensitivity and specificity. These are detailed in the publication [55]. At best, moderate-to-severe endometriosis could be diagnosed during the secretory phase with a sensitivity of 100% and specificity of 84% using IL-6, TNF-α and CA-125. Minimal-to-mild disease was detected with a sensitivity of 87% and specificity of 71% during the secretory phase with IL-6 and TNF-α. When least squares support vector machines were applied to the data, minimal-to-mild endometriosis could be diagnosed with a sensitivity of 93.6% at the cost of a lower specificity of 60.5%.

This study by Mihalyi and colleagues [55] is certainly novel in its advanced statistical approach to the question of which of a panel of preselected serum markers best predicts the presence of endometriosis. However, the authors did not present any clinically utilizable cut-offs for the management of women with possible endometriosis. Their model performed best for the discrimination between moderate-to-severe disease versus controls, reiterating that the diagnosis of stage I/II (minimal-to-mild disease) remains a challenge. Mihalyi *et al* focused on maximizing sensitivity in their diagnostic test, arguing that a relatively high false-positive rate (low specificity) is acceptable, even if it results in a false indication for laparoscopic evaluation. The justification is that laparoscopy in this group of women, with presumed pain and/or infertility, would be useful to rule out other pelvic pathology and to evaluate tubal patency. One must keep in mind, however, that the point of diagnosing endometriosis non-invasively is not to then perform surgery (whether correctly indicated or not) but to manage the patient regarding her symptoms or infertility appropriately. As such, one can definitely propose the alternative argument that maximizing specificity is the goal of a diagnostic test of endometriosis.

Other protein markers

Two studies that have evaluated serum or plasma proteins for the diagnosis of endometriosis will be briefly reviewed. The first examined plasma levels of urocortin, a neuropeptide and member of the corticotropin-releasing hormone family that is produced by the human endometrium [56]. This protein has been shown to influence key events in the development of endometriosis, such as endometrial growth and differentiation, endometrial adhesion and angiogenesis and, speculatively, its secretion may be part of the host response against ectopic endometrium implantation. The researchers focused on using urocortin to be able to distinguish endometriomas from other benign cysts in 40 women of each group. They found that plasma urocortin levels were twice as high in the ovarian endometrioma group compared to the

benign cyst group. The sensitivity and specificity were an impressive 88% and 90%, respectively. In the same cohort of patients, the corresponding results for CA-125 were 65% and 90%. The discrimination of endometriomas from other benign cysts can in most cases be accomplished with ultrasonography, but measuring serum urocortin levels appears promising as an additional diagnostic marker. However, further studies looking at this protein in non-ovarian endometriosis (stage I/II disease) would be needed before applying these findings in clinical practice.

Members of this group of researchers reported on another candidate protein, the activin-binding protein follistatin, which is produced by several tissues including endometrium and endometriotic implants [57]. They found that follistatin was increased in women with endometriosis compared with controls, and was especially high in those with an endometrioma (stage III/IV disease). In fact, follistatin levels above the predetermined cut-off were able to detect all 52 cases of endometrioma in this study with 100% sensitivity versus a mixed group of stage I/II and healthy controls. Problematic, however, was that follistatin levels overlapped between women with stage I/II disease, non-endometriotic ovarian cysts and healthy controls and was unable to distinguish among these women. Thus, although promising, the authors conclude that future investigations should evaluate the diagnostic accuracy of follistatin for non-ovarian endometriosis and early-stage disease. These are conditions for which a serum marker is most necessary.

Other blood-based markers

Over the years, several researchers have tested novel potential diagnostic markers in serum, some focusing on proteins (other than above) and mRNA and DNA expression. Agic and colleagues studied the cognate chemokine receptor (CCR) 1 which is a G-protein-coupled chemokine receptor expressed on the surface of neutrophils/mononuclear leukocytes with a high affinity for RANTES [58]. RANTES has been previously shown to be a mediator of peritoneal inflammation by recruiting different leukocytes to endometriotic inflammatory sites [59]. Eighty-three women with endometriosis diagnosed with laparoscopy were compared to 51 age-matched controls based on the ratio of CCR1 to hypoxanthine-guanine phosphoribosyl transferase (HPRT), the latter being a housekeeping gene. The researchers found that this ratio was significantly higher in the endometriosis group compared to disease-free women, but was also nearly equally elevated in a small group of pregnant women. In another four women with PID, the values were twice that of the endometriosis group.

In terms of its diagnostic properties in distinguishing endometriosis from non-endometriosis, this method showed a sensitivity of 90%, a specificity of 74%, a NPV of 85% and a PPV of 82%. One must keep in mind, however, that other conditions such as acute inflammatory disease, pregnancy, and malignancy must be ruled out prior to testing since these conditions were associated with an elevation of the CCR1/HPRT ratio. Although the authors state that these conditions may be easily diagnosed with standard laboratory testing (hCG, C-reactive protein, etc.) and/or sonography, one might argue that this is certainly not always the case and the inclusion of these patients would increase the number of presumed diagnoses of endometriosis, raising the false-positive rate and reducing both the specificity and PPV of the test. In addition, real-time polymerase chain reaction (PCR) is needed to perform the measurements described, making this a labor-intensive test requiring highly trained laboratory personnel, and not easily performed in the clinical setting. Still, it is an interesting and novel approach to the potential non-invasive diagnosis of endometriosis, and one which the authors further evaluated in a subsequent study.

In a follow-up study, Agic et al [60] evaluated the performance of the previously studied CCR1 mRNA in peripheral blood leukocytes in combination with MCP1 and CA-125. At the cut-offs specified by the authors for the three markers, the diagnostic success was a sensitivity of 92.2% and specificity of 81.6%, a PPV of 92.3% and NPV of 83.3%. These results appeared to be similar for the diagnosis of all stages of endometriosis. The diagnostic properties of this triple marker test were not much better over using CCR1 alone, as evaluated in the previous study discussed. Accordingly, CCR1 measurement contributed most to this test, with MCP-1 used alone showing a sensitivity of only 36.3% and specificity of 95.9% and CA-125 alone at a cut-off of 50 IU/mL a sensitivity of 27.5% and specificity of 100% (only 28/102 endometriosis patients had a CA-125 above the cut-off).

The authors illustrate the results of using their diagnostic test in practice with two useful examples. In the test-positive case, a woman has a pretest odds of having endometriosis of 1/10 to 1/15 based on the prevalence of endometriosis alone and a positive test using the triple panel (LR+ of 5.017) increases the post-test probability to 1/2 to 5/7 (50–72%). In the test-negative case, they present a woman with infertility with a proven pretest probability of 30% of having endometriosis, in whom the negative test (LR- of 0.096) decreases the odds by a factor of 10, making her post-test probability of endometriosis only 3.3%. The corresponding decrease in odds for the woman in the first example, had she tested negative, would be a decrease from approximately 10% to 1% probability of endometriosis. These results certainly seem relevant and potentially clinically useful, though one must again remember that the testing of CCR1 mRNA in peripheral blood leukocytes is rather cumbersome and complicated. Of even greater utility would be a test in which the pretest probability could be more precisely specified by a patient's symptoms and findings on physical examination, improving the diagnostic precision of the test and its post-test probability.

Another group tested the clinical value of parameters of the differential white blood cell (WBC) count including the absolute neutrophil/lymphocyte ratio (NLR), in conjunction with CA-125, for the diagnosis of endometriosis [61]. NLR has been previously evaluated in other disease states, including chronic inflammation and cancer, as a possible prognostic indicator. In this large study of 231 women with endometriosis, 145 with benign tumors, and 384 presumed healthy controls (not surgically evaluated), the authors evaluated the ability of each potential marker alone as well as a combination of NLR and CA-125 to differentiate between endometriosis and controls. NLR had a sensitivity of 59.7% and specificity of 60.1% while CA-125 (cut-off 35 IU/mL) had a sensitivity of 55.8% and specificity of 92.8%. Absolute neutrophil count alone had the highest sensitivity (68.4%) but a low specificity of only 45.4%. The combined factor of CA-125 and NLR calculated by multiplying these two factors fared a bit better, with a sensitivity of 69.3% and specificity of 83.9%. No statistical differences were observed in the WBC parameters between women with stage I/II and stage III/IV disease, beyond a slightly higher NLR in the latter group. Of the only 38 women with stage I/II endometriosis, 25 (65.8%) had a NLR value exceeding the cut-off. In addition, when comparing mean levels of these parameters, only NLR showed a difference between the benign tumor and healthy control groups, while CA-125 and the CA-125'NLR combined factor did not differentiate between these two non-endometriosis groups.

Although this large retrospective study is interesting in its concept, it has some significant limitations. First, the control group was not surgically evaluated and thus endometriosis cannot be definitively excluded, as it can also be symptom free. Second, although WBC parameters were measured, there was no clinical information about the patients reported; thus, one cannot exclude the possibility that the participants had concurrent illness or acute inflammatory processes influencing the WBC and NLR. Third, of the subjects with endometriosis, fewer than 20% had minimal-to-mild endometriosis, limiting the conclusions regarding the diagnostic ability of the markers for stage I/II disease. As previously discussed, this group of patients is the one for whom a non-invasive diagnostic test would be of most use. Finally, it is important to note that the non-endometriosis tumor group consisting of subjects with benign ovarian neoplasms could not be differentiated from the presumably disease-free control group. Thus, this blood test would need to be supplemented by an ultrasound to visualize and diagnose these ovarian cysts, during which (one might argue) the endometriomas necessary for the diagnosis of stage IV and possibly stage III disease would inevitably also be seen. Does the WBC differential and CA-125 then really add value? Because of the skew in diagnosis towards severe disease, the authors could not provide accurate predictive values for their test, but they also failed to report the likelihood ratios.

Zachariah and colleagues took yet another approach to the non-invasive diagnosis of endometriosis by examining the cell-free DNA in the plasma and in serum of women with endometriosis [62]. Increased concentration of circulating cell-free (ccf) DNA have been reported in inflammatory conditions such as systemic lupus erythematosus and rheumatoid arthritis and it is believed to be a marker of apoptosis and necrosis. The detection of ccf DNA is accomplished with real-time PCR, using specific probes for determining both mitochondrial DNA (mtDNA) and nuclear DNA (nDNA). DNA was extracted from 19 cases of surgically confirmed endometriosis and compared to that of a control group of 15 asymptomatic reproductive-age women who were presumably endometriosis free but who were not surgically evaluated. The authors found that the mean concentration of plasma ccf nDNA was significantly higher in the women with stage I and II endometriosis (n = 13) compared to the control group. Using a cut-off of 416 ccf nDNA in plasma provided a sensitivity of 70% and specificity of 87% to discriminate between stage I/II and controls. The authors stated that due to the small sample of stage IV endometriosis (only six subjects), they did not include these subjects in the diagnostic analyses. They found no differences in the serum ccf DNA (nDNA and mtDNA) nor in plasma ccf mtDNA.

This study was innovative in its idea of studying a marker not previously investigated in endometriosis. An additional strength of the study was that the authors reported the diagnostic properties of this potential marker in stage I/II disease, the group of patients who would most benefit from a non-invasive diagnostic test. However, the study has several weaknesses: it is small, the control group was not surgically evaluated, there are no demographic or clinical data provided, and it did not report results for moderate-to-severe endometriosis. In terms of clinical application, the method of detection of ccf DNA is complicated and labor intensive. In addition, the test is not specific to endometriosis in that ccf DNA appears to be elevated in many inflammatory conditions, and thus the test would not be able to distinguish these from endometriosis. The authors did not evaluate whether the presence of pelvic pain or infertility influenced ccf DNA concentrations.

Peritoneal fluid markers

Peritoneal fluid (PF) bathes the pelvic organs and is often visualized in the cul-de-sac during surgery. It has been demonstrated that components of the immune system, especially macrophages, are present in high concentrations in the peritoneal fluid [63]. As such, PF is also rich in cytokines, growth factors and chemotactic factors and reflects activity of the peritoneal microenvironment. Recent theory states that the local inflammation induced by endometriosis in the pelvic cavity and mediated by factors in the PF induces a feedforward loop that propagates endometriotic lesion formation and persistence.

Many investigators have measured levels of tumor markers including CA-125 in the PF of women with endometriosis. Others have evaluated markers of inflammation, especially concentrations of cytokines, and have identified a host of these in the local peritoneal environment, including IL-4, IL-5, IL-8, IL-10, IL-12, IL-13, MCP-1 [64], and macrophage colony simulating factor (MCSF). These findings have improved our understanding of the pathophysiology of the disease process, but none has proven to be the basis of a diagnostic test of endometriosis.

An important point deserves mention. Peritoneal fluid is easily obtained during surgery and analyses of its contents could reveal interesting differences in the concentrations of substances that could be the basis for further investigations of these factors in the

serum. But, without surgery, the collection of PF for the potential diagnosis of endometriosis is *not* a feasible option. Although PF volume may increase at the time of ovulation and may be higher in endometriosis, it is rarely copious enough to be obtained via transvaginal peritoneal puncture. Thus, searching for biomarkers in PF violates one of the defining factors of a biomarker, namely that it be easily obtainable.

Endometrial markers

Nearly all theories explaining the development of endometriosis include the phenomenon of retrograde menstruation and transport of endometrial contents into the peritoneal cavity. Retrograde menstruation is more and more thought of as a necessary, but not definitive, reason for the development of ectopic endometrial lesions in the pelvis. What co-factors allow for the development of endometriosis in some women but not in others, despite a near-universal presence of retrograde menstruation, remains the topic of some debate. It is certainly possible that the shed endometrium in women with endometriosis is somehow aberrant and drives its own implantation as ectopic lesions or endometriosis. These theories have spurred many investigations into the possible differences between endometrium from women with endometriosis and healthy menstruating women. Most of these studies have been concerned with explaining the pathophysiology of the disease process [65–68], but a few have also evaluated the endometrium as a possible source of biomarkers. Endometrial glands and stroma can be obtained semi-invasively via endometrial pipelle biopsy in the office, with only mild-to-moderate discomfort to the patients. Thus, we believe that endometrial biopsy fits the criterion of being easily obtainable, and could serve as a source of biomarkers of endometriosis.

In 2003, Gagné *et al* [69] studied the proportion of specific subsets of leukocytes that made up the endometrium of women with endometriosis, comparing them to control women. This was a large study of 368 women: 173 with surgically confirmed endometriosis and 195 controls who were surgically confirmed to be free of endometriosis. Cytometry analysis was used to measure the proportion of several leukocyte subsets in the endometrial cells, namely CD3+, CD16+, CD3−HLADR−, CD3−CD45RA−, CD3+CD16−, CD3+CD56−, CD56−CD16+, and CD16b+. The study also included measurements of CA-125 in serum and collected clinical information such as gravidity, infertility, presence of pelvic pain or fibroids, and histological dating of the endometrial specimen as possible confounder variables. The final predictive model reported by the study included the proportion of the above listed leukocytes in conjunction with serum CA-125 (cut-off 12.8 IU/mL) and length of menses.

Based on the final model, the predictive probability of having endometriosis was calculated for each individual study participant and a threshold value of 0.61 was established. Thus, when the estimated probability exceeded this value of 0.61, the subject was assigned a positive result. The diagnostic performance of this model showed a sensitivity of 61% and specificity of 95% for predicting endometriosis, and outperformed CA-125 alone which had a sensitivity of 20% and specificity of 92% at a cut-off of 35 IU/mL. In addition, the researchers also assessed their model according to the severity of endometriosis. They showed that the diagnostic performance was exactly the same in the subgroup of women with minimal-to-mild endometriosis and in those with moderate-to-severe stages of the disease.

With its high PPV, this predictive test would provide a high probability that a test positive is a true positive, but of course could not diagnose all cases of endometriosis, and a negative test had a lower prediction for being a true negative. While the collection of material needed for study, serum and endometrium, is not complicated, the endometrial leukocyte preparation, staining, and flow cytometric analysis are complicated and labor intensive. There have been no further reports from these authors regarding how their model has subsequently performed, especially in a new study population.

Several investigators have studied endometrial aromatase P450, the enzyme that catalyzes the conversion of androstenedione and testosterone to estrone, as a promising marker for the presence of endometriosis. Aromatase P450 became a potential marker of interest when it was reported that the protein is expressed in endometriotic and adenomyotic tissues as well as in the eutopic endometrium of women with endometriosis, but not in normal endometrium [70]. Kitawaki *et al* [71] evaluated the clinical usefulness of examining endometrial biopsy specimens for the presence of aromatase P450 activity. They evaluated preoperatively obtained endometrial biopsy specimens in 105 women for the expression of aromatase P450 by reverse transcription PCR and immunohistochemical analysis. Using PCR, they confirmed their earlier findings that aromatase P450 transcripts were detected only in women with endometriosis, adenomyosis or leiomyoma and were absent in all 21 disease-free women.

However, the visualization of the transcripts on Southern blots did not allow for quantitative comparisons and thus immunohistochemical analyses were performed. The results confirmed the previous findings: immunostaining for aromatase P450 was detected in the specimens of subjects with the aforementioned diagnoses in both the proliferative and secretory phases of the cycle and none in the specimens from healthy women. The authors were able to semi-quantitatively compare the intensity and distribution between samples by H-score computed by accounting for the intensity of staining and the percentage of stained cells. The differences in H-scores and the construction of ROC curves allowed the investigators to report the sensitivity and specificity of this test as 91% and 100% respectively, with a PPV of 100% and NPV of 72%. No correlation was observed between the H-score and the severity of disease.

There are some limitations to this study. First, the control group consisted of only 21 subjects or only a quarter of the number in the diseased group, so that confirmation of lack of

aromatase would be needed in a larger healthy group. Since this was not a series of consecutive patients and the prevalence of disease of 80% in this sample is much higher that in the general population or even in a preoperative one, the positive and negative predictive values apply only to this study. The H-scores measured are only semi-quantitative and the study did not report intra- and interobserver consistency in applying the score. The authors did find that H-scores were higher in endometriosis patients, but also in those with adenomyosis and leiomyomas, thus making it impossible to distinguish between these entities with this test alone. Finally, the authors acknowledge themselves that the method of immunohistostaining is rather complicated to perform and is not an optimal diagnostic test to be used in the clinic.

A subsequent study by Dheenadayalu and colleagues used PCR to study aromatase expression in endometrium of women with and without endometriosis [72]. They collected intraoperative endometrial samples from 60 women undergoing laparoscopy for the indications of pain, infertility, and tubal ligation, 34 of whom ended up having endometriosis and 26 of whom were disease free. The researchers were successful in amplifying aromatase P450 RNA from 56 of the 60 samples. Twenty-three (82%) of the 28 women with stage I/II and five of six women with stage III/IV tested positive for endometrial aromatase expression. However, unlike in the previous study described, four of the 16 (25%) women without endometriosis or other pelvic pathology also had positive aromatase P450 mRNA expression. In addition, five of six (83%) of the remaining women in the endometriosis-free group who had fibroids or tubal disease also expressed endometrial aromatase P450. Thus, as a diagnostic test for endometriosis, aromatase P450 mRNA expression from the endometrium had a sensitivity of 82%, specificity of 57%, PPV 76% and NPV 67%.

Thus, despite the previous promising results on endometriosis, the study by Dheenadayalu [72] confirmed that aromatase P450 expression is not confined to the endometrium of women with endometriosis, but is also seen in those with other gynecological disorders, not all of which are detectable by ultrasonography. In addition, more than one-fourth of seemingly disease-free women with no pelvic pathology expressed endometrial aromatase. Whether these women are at risk of developing problems in the future based on these findings could not be answered by this study, but would require long-term longitudinal follow-up. Further complicating the picture... is the fact that a substantial number of women with endometriosis did not express P450 in the endometrium. This could be due to fluctuations during the course of the disease, or perhaps that aromatase P450 expression is only one of many possibly etiological factors contributing to the development of endometriosis. In the meantime, however, aromatase P450 expression cannot be used as a diagnostic test.

A discussion of potential biomarkers in endometrium would not be complete without mention of a series of studies in the 1980s and early 1990s that looked at autoimmunity to the endometrium in women with endometriosis. One of the first reports by Mathur *et al* [73] measured serum antibody titers to whole ovary, theca cells, granulosa cells and endometrium in a small series of 13 women with endometriosis and 15 normal control women. Using passive hemagglutination and immunofluorescence assays, they found higher antibody titers to endometrium as well as to ovary, granulosa cells and theca cells. A subsequent study used indirect immunofluorescence to test for the presence of anti-endometrium antibodies in the sera of 42 patients with infertility and found that positive antibodies predicted endometriosis [74]. A follow-up study testing the diagnostic performance of endometrial antibodies was undertaken and the results compared to those for CA-125 [75]. The antibodies outperformed CA-125 with a sensitivity of 83.1% and specificity of 78.8% compared to a sensitivity of 27.3% and specificity of 82.6% for CA-125. However, due to the complicated methodology with immunofluorescence and interobserver variations, the method of measuring endometrial antibodies in serum was never adopted as part of the diagnostic work-up for endometriosis.

Conclusion

The search for a biomarker to non-invasively diagnose endometriosis has spanned at least three decades and involved researchers from around the world. All have had their sights on a marker or panel of markers that would be easily obtained (i.e. from serum), give a rapid result and have a high sensitivity and specificity. Ideally, the biomarker would be measured in blood at room temperature, require no special handling of the blood, and involve an easy, commercially available assay with high reproducibility. It should be stable across ages, menstrual cycle phase, and time of collection, requiring no additional patient visits. Unfortunately, despite all the studies and the efforts spent, such a marker still does not exist.

Given the great variability in the disease, there will likely not be one single biomarker for endometriosis. Patterns of multiple markers or fingerprints will likely be required. Moreover, there will likely be different markers to maximize sensitivity or specificity of diagnosis. It is also possible that different subsets of biomarkers may be required for different stages or clinical classifications of endometriosis.

Many of the past efforts were hypothesis driven, testing potential markers because of their involvement in hormonal regulation, inflammatory response, or tissue implantation. In recent years, new non-biased approaches to the problem of finding a biomarker of endometriosis have emerged. These investigations scan protein profiles or gene expression matrices to discover ones that are differentially regulated in endometriosis. Such approaches may uncover associations between endometriosis and certain proteins or genes that have not been previously considered with the traditional approach. These studies will be discussed in more detail in Chapter 31 on proteomics approaches to biomarker discovery.

References

1. Bonassi S, Neri M, Puntoni R. Validation of biomarkers as early predictors of disease. Mutat Res 2001;480–481:349–358.
2. McMichael AJ, Hall AJ. The use of biological markers as predictive early-outcome measures in epidemiological research. In: Toniolo P, Boffetta P, Shuker DEG, Rothman N, Hulka B, Pearce N (eds) Application of Biomarkers in Cancer Epidemiology. Lyon: International Agency for Research on Cancer; 1997, pp. 281–289.
3. Hall JA, Brown R, Paul J. An exploration into study design for biomarker identification: issues and recommendations. Cancer Genom Proteom 2007;4:111–120.
4. Pepe MS, Etzioni R, Feng AZ et al. Phases of biomarker development for early detection of cancer. J Nat Cancer Inst 2001;93:1054–1061.
5. Rothman N, Stewart WF, Schulte PA. Incorporating biomarkers into cancer epidemiology: a matrix of biomarker and study design categories. Cancer Epidem Biomark Prevent 1995;4:301–311.
6. Rogers PA, D'Hooghe TM, Fazleabus A et al. Priorities for endometrioisis reseach: recommendation from an international consensus workshop. Reprod Sci 2009;16(4):335–346.
7. Hanley J, McNeil BJ. The meaning and use of the area under a receiver operating characteristic (ROC) curve. Radiology 1982;143:29–36.
8. D'Hooghe TM, Mihalyi AM, Simsa P et al. Why we need a noninvasive diagnostic test for minimal to mild endometriosis with a high sensitivity. Gynecol Obstet Invest 2006;62:136–138.
9. Seeber B, Sammel M, Fan X et al. Proteomic analysis of serum yields six candidate proteins that are unregulated in a subset of women with endometriosis. Fertil Steril 2010;93:2177–2144
10. Bossuyt PM, Reitsma JB, Bruns DE et al. The STARD statement for reporting studies of diagnostic accuracy: explanation and elaboration. Ann Intern Med 2003;138:1–12.
11. Pittaway DE, Fayez JA. The use of CA-125 in the diagnosis and management of endometriosis. Fertil Steril 1986;46:790–795.
12. Giudice LC, Jacobs A, Pineda J et al. Serum levels of CA-125 in patients with endometriosis: a preliminary report. Fertil Steril 1986; 45:876–878.
13. Moretuzzo RW, DiLauro S, Jenison E et al. Serum and peritoneal lavage fluid CA-125 levels in endometriosis. Fertil Steril 1988; 50:430–433.
14. Franchi M, Beretta P, Zanaboni F et al. Use of serum CA-125 measurement in patients with endometriosis. Fertil Steril 1993;4:149–152.
15. Barbati A, Cosmi EV, Spanziani R et al. Serum and peritoneal fluid CA-125 levels in patients with endometriosis. Fertil Steril 1994; 61:438–442.
16. Mol BW, Bayram N, Lijmer JG et al. The performance of CA-125 measurement in the detection of endometriosis: a metaanalysis. Fertil Steril 1998;70:1101–1108.
17. Kitawaki J, Ishihara H, Koshiba H et al. Usefulness and limits of CA-125 in diagnosis of endometriosis without associated ovarian endometriomas. Hum Reprod 2005;20:1999–2003.
18. Rose e Silva ACJS, Rosa e Silva JC, Ferriani RA. Serum Ca-125 in the diagnosis of endometriosis. Int J Gynecol Obstet 2007;96:206–207.

19. Xavier P, Beries J, Belo L et al. Are we employing the most effective CA 125 and CA-19–9 cut-off values to detect endometriosis? Eur J Obstet Gynecol Reprod Biol 2005;123:254–255.

20. Pittaway DE, Rondinone D, Miller KA, Barnes K. Clinical evaluation of CA-125 concentrations as a prognostic factor for pregnancy in infertile women with surgically treated endometriosis. Fertil Steril 1995;64:321–324.

21. Fedele L, Arciani L, Vercellini P et al. Serum CA 125 measurement sin the diagnosis of endometriosis recurrence. Obstet Gynecol 1988;72:19–22.

22. Chen FP, Soong YK, Lee N et al. The use of serum CA-125 as a marker for endometriosis in patients with dysmenorrheal for monitoring therapy and for recurrence of endometriosis. Acta Obstet Gynecol Scand 1998;77:665–670.

23. Matalliotakis I, Panidis D, Vlassis G et al. Unexpected increase of the CA-19–9 tumour marker in patients with endometriosis. Eur J Gynaecol Oncol 1998;19:498–500.

24. Harada T, Kubota T, Aso T. Usefulness of CA-19–9 versus CA 125 for the diagnosis of endometriosis. Fertil Steril 2002;78:733–739.

25. Kurdoglu Z, Gursoy R, Kurdoglu M et al. Comparison of the clinical value of CA-19–9 versus CA 125 for the diagnosis of endometriosis. Fertil Steril 2009;92:1761–1763.

26. Vigano P, Somigliana E, Gaffuri B, Santorsola R, Busacca M, Vignali M. Endometrial release of soluble intercellular adhesion molecule 1 and endometriosis: relationship to the extent of the disease. Obstet Gynecol 2000;95:115–118.

27. Somigliana E, Vigano P, Candiani M, Felicetta I, di Blasio AM, Vignali M. Use of serum-soluble intercellular adhesion molecule-1 as a new marker of endometriosis. Fertil Steril 2002;77:1028–1031.

28. Sampson JA. Peritoneal endometriosis due to the menstrual dissemination of endometrial tissue into the peritoneal cavity. Am J Obstet Gynecol 1927;14:422.

29. Wu MY, Ho HN. The role of cytokines in endometriosis. Am J Reprod Immun 2003;49:285–296.

30. Lebovic DI, Mueller MD, Taylor RN. Immunobiology of endometriosis. Fertil Steril 2001;75:1–10.

31. Shimoya K, Moriyama A, Ogata I et al. Increased concentrations of secretory leukocyte protease inhibitor in peritoneal fluid of women with endometriosis. Mol Hum Reprod 2000;6:829–834.

32. Cheong YC, Shelton JB, Laird SM et al. IL-1, IL-6 and TNF-alpha concentrations in the peritoneal fluid of women with pelvic adhesions. Hum Reprod 2002;17:69–75.

33. Bedaiwy MA, Falcone T, Sharma RK et al. Prediction of endometriosis with serum and peritoneal fluid markers: a prospective controlled trial. Hum Reprod 2002;17:426–431.

34. Somigliana E, Vigano P, Tirelli AS et al. Use of the concomitant serum dosage of CA 125, CA-19–9 and interleukin-6 to detect the presence of endometriosis. Results from a series of reproductive age women undergoing laparoscopic surgery for benign gynaecological conditions. Hum Reprod 2004;19:1871–1876.

35. Pizzo A, Salmeri FM, Ardita FV, Sofo V, Tripepi M, Marsico S. Behavior of cytokine levels in serum and peritoneal fluid of women with endometriosis. Gynecol Obstet Invest 2002;54:82–87.

36. Gomez-Torres MJ, Acien P, Campos A, Velasco I. Embryotoxicity of peritoneal fluid in women with endometriosis. Its relation with cytokines and lymphocyte populations. Hum Reprod 2002; 17:777–781.

37. Barcz E, Skopinska Rozewska E, Kaminski P, Demkow U, Bobrowska K, Marianowski L. Angiogenic activity and IL-8 concentrations in peritoneal fluid and sera in endometriosis. Int J Gynecol Obstet 2002;79:229–235.

38. Calhaz-Jorge C, Costa AP, Barata M, Santos MC, Palma-Carlos ML. Peritoneal fluid concentrations of interleukin-8 in patients with endometriosis depend on the severity of the disorder and are higher in the luteal phase. Hum Reprod 2003;18:593–597.

39. Harada T, Yoshioka H, Yoshida S et al. Increased interleukin-6 levels in peritoneal fluid of infertile patients with active endometriosis. Am J Obstet Gynecol 1997;176:593–597.

40. Vercellini P, de Benedetti F, Rossi E, Colombo A, Trespidi L, Crosignani PG. Tumor necrosis factor in plasma and peritoneal fluid of women with and without endometriosis. Gynecol Obstet Invest 1993; 36(1):39–41.

41. Koga K, Yutaka O, Yoshino O et al. Elevated interleukin-16 levels in the peritoneal fluid of women with endometriosis may be a mechanism for inflammatory reactions associated with endometriosis. Fertil Steril 2005;83:878–882.

42. Arici A, Matalliotakis I, Goumenou A, Koumantakis G, Vassiliadis S, Mahutte NG. Altered expression of interleukin-18 in the peritoneal fluid of women with endometriosis. Fertil Steril 2003;80: 889–894.

43. Morin M, Bellehumeur C, Therrialut M-J, Metz C, Maheux R, Akoum A. Elevated levels of macrophage migration inhibitory factor in the peripheral blood of women with endometriosis. Fertil Steril 2005;83:865–872.

44. Yih S, Katabuchi H, Araki M et al. Expression of monocyte chemoattractant protein-1 in peritoneal endometriotic cells. Virchows Arch 2001;438:70–77.

45. Arici A, Oral E, Attar E, Tazuke SI, Olive DL. Monocyte chemotactic protein-1 concentration in peritoneal fluid of women with endometriosis and its modulation of expression in mesothelial cells. Fertil Steril 1997;67(6):1065–1072.

46. Khorram O, Taylor RN, Ryan IP, Schall TJ, Landers DV. Peritoneal fluid concentrations of the cytokine RANTES correlate with the severity of endometriosis. Am J Obstet Gynecol 1993;169: 1545–1549.

47. Mueller MD, Mazzacchelli L, Buri C, Lebovic DI, Dreher E, Taylor R. Epithelial neutrophil-activating peptide 78 concentrations are elevated in the peritoneal fluid of women with endometriosis. Fertil Steril 2003;79(Suppl 1):815–820.

48. Hsu CC, Yang BC, Wu MH, Huang KE. Enhanced interleukin-4 expression in patients with endometriosis. Fertil Steril 1997; 67:1059–1064.

49. Ho HN, Wu MY, Chao KH et al. Decrease in interferon gamma production and impairment of T-lymphocyte proliferation in peritoneal fluid of women with endometriosis. Am J Obstet Gynecol 1996;175:1236–1241.

50. Martinez S, Garrido N, Coperias JL et al. Serum interleukin-6 levels are elevated in women with minimal-mild endometriosis. Hum Reprod 2007;22:836–842.

51. Iwabe T, Harada T, Sakamoto Y, Iba Y, Horie S, Mitsunari M, Terakawa N. Gonadotropin-releasing hormone agonist treatment reduced serum interleukin-6 concentrations in patients with ovarian endometriomas. Fertil Steril 2003;80:300–304.

52. D'Hooghe TM, Xiao L, Hill JA. Cytokine profiles in autologous peritoneal fluid and peripheral blood of women with deep and superficial endometriosis. Arch Gynecol Obstet 2001;265:40–44.

53. Seeber B, Sammel MD, Fan X et al. Panel of markers can accurately predict endometriosis in a subset of patients. Fertil Steril 2008;89:1073–1081.

54. Othman EE, Hornung D, Salem HT, Khalifa EA, El-Metwally TH, Al-Hendy A. Serum cytokines as biomarkers for nonsurgical prediction of endometriosis. Eur J Obstet Gynecol 2008; 137:240–246.

55. Mihalyi A, Gevaert O, Kyama CM et al. Non-invasive diagnosis of endometriosis based on a combined analysis of six plasma biomarkers. Hum Reprod 2010;25:654–664.

56. Florio P, Reis FM, Torres PB et al. Plasma urocortin levels in the diagnosis of ovarian endometriosis. Obstet Gynecol 2007;110:594–600.

57. Florio P, Reis FM, Torres PB et al. High serum follistatin levels in women with ovarian endometriosis. Hum Reprod 2009;24: 2600–2606.

58. Agic A, Xu H, Rehbein M, Wolfler MM, Ebert AD, Hornung D. Cognate chemokine receptor 1 messenger ribonucleic acid expression in peripheral blood as a diagnostic test for endometriosis. Fertil Steril 2007;87:982–984.

59. Rosse D, Zoltnik A. The biology of chemokines and their receptors. Ann Rev Immunol 2000;18:217–242.

60. Agic A, Djalali S, Wolfler MM, Halis G, Diedrich K, Hornung D. Combination of CCR1 mRNA, MCP1, and CA-125 measurements in peripheral blood as a diagnostic test for endometriosis. Reprod Sci 2008;15:906–911.

61. Cho S, Cho H, Nam A et al. Neutrophil-to-lymphocyte ratio as an adjunct to CA-125 for the diagnosis of endometriosis. Fertil Steril 2008;90:2073–2079.

62. Zachariah R, Schmid S, Radpour R et al. Circulating cell-free DNA as a potential biomarker for minimal and mild endometriosis. Reprod Biomed Online 2009;18:407–411.

63. Taylor RN, Ryan IP, Moore ES, Hornung D, Shifren JL, Tseng JF. Angiogenesis and macrophage activation in endometriosis. Ann N Y Acad Sci 1997;26:194–207.

64. Bedaiwy MA, Falcone T. Laboratory testing for endometriosis. Clin Chim Acta 2004;340:41–56.

65. Rombauts L, Donoghue J, Cann L, Jones RL, Healy DL. Activin-A secretion is increased in the eutopic endometrium from women with endometriosis. Aust N Z J Obstet Gynaecol 2006; 46:148–153.

66. Luo Q, Ning W, Wu Y et al. Altered expression of interleukin-18 in the ectopic and eutopic endometrium of women with endometriosis. J Reprod Immunol 2006;72:108–117.

67. Sha G, Zhang Y, Zhang C et al. Elevated levels of gremlin-1 in eutopic endometrium and peripheral serum in patients with endometriosis. Fertil Steril 2009;91:350–358.

68. Wei Q, St Clair JB, Fu T, Stratton P, Nieman LK. Reduced expression of biomarkers associated with the implantation window in women with endometriosis. Fertil Steril 2009;91:1686–1691.

69. Gagné D, Rivard M, Page M et al. Development of a nonsurgical diagnostic tool for endometriosis based on the detection of endometrial leukocyte subsets and serum CA-125. Fertil Steril 2003; 80:876–885.

70. Kitawaki J, Noguchi T, Amatsu T et al. Expression of aromatase cytochrome P450 protein and messenger ribonucleic acid in human endometriotic and adenomyotic tissues but not in normal endometrium. Biol Reprod 1997;57:514–519.

71. Kitawaki J, Kusuki I, Koshiba H, Tsukamoto K, Fushiki S, Honjo H. Detection of aromatase cytochrome P-450 in endometrial biopsy specimens as a diagnostic test for endometriosis. Fertil Steril 1999;72:1100–1106.

72. Dheenadayalu K, Mak I, Gordts S et al. Aromatase P450 messenger RNA expression in eutopic endometrium is not a specific marker for pelvic endometriosis. Fertil Steril 2002;78:825–829.

73. Mathur S, Peress MR, Williamson HO et al. Autoimmunity to endometrium and ovary in endometriosis. Clin Exp Immunol 1982;50:259–266.

74. Wild RA, Shivers CA. Antiendometrial antibodies in patients with endometriosis. Am J Reprod Microbiol 1985;8:84–86.

75. Wild RA, Hirisave V, Bianco A, Podczaski ES. Demers LM. Endometrial antibodies versus CA-125 for the detection of endometriosis. Fertil Steril 1991;55:90–94.

31 Diagnosis of Endometriosis: Proteomics

Andrew N. Stephens[1], Luk J.F. Rombauts[2,3] and Lois A. Salamonsen[1]

[1]Prince Henry's Institute of Medical Research, Melbourne, Australia
[2]Department of Obstetrics and Gynaecology, Monash University, Melbourne, Australia
[3]Monash IVF, Melbourne, Australia

Introduction

The term "proteomics" is applied to the large-scale (global) study of proteins. In recent years, advances in technology have enabled not only the qualitative examination of the total protein profile of a tissue or fluid, but also the identification and quantitative analysis of differences between samples such as between diseased and healthy states. To date, the proteomic techniques applied to endometriosis have enabled the resolution of up to 2000 proteins from a sample; however, when applied to complex mixtures of proteins (such as tissue extracts), it is the abundant structural proteins that dominate. The development and application of prefractionation techniques that selectively remove abundant proteins from samples, along with recent advances in mass spectrometry, are now enabling identification and quantitation of the proteins of lower abundance such as those important for cell regulatory functions.

Genomics was the first of the global analysis techniques to be widely applied and has provided useful information regarding changes in transcription between women with and without endometriosis (Chapter 32, this volume). Whilst complementary to genomics, proteomics has the potential to provide considerably more information about the disease and to identify relevant targets for diagnosis. Not all changes in gene expression are reflected by the proteins they encode: neither differences in mRNA stability, levels of protein production, nor the numerous splice and post-translationally modified isoforms that can occur are reflected by a static genome. In addition, post-translational modifications resulting from enzymatic alterations – glycosylation, phosphorylation, proteolytic cleavage and so on – are extensively employed to regulate localization, activity and degradation of many proteins. More than 50% of all proteins in human serum are glycosylated [1], leading to altered bio-activities; it is not known how many proteolytically cleaved forms, for example, might exist. It is therefore necessary to study proteins directly: proteomics can provide considerable insights into cellular function and indications as to whether changes associated with any disease state are likely to be critical in terms of function.

Proteomics has been enabled by the integration of a number of disciplines, particularly the large-scale sequencing of genomes, protein separation science including sophisticated protein fractionation techniques, mass spectrometry and bio-informatics [2]. Nevertheless, difficulties continue to hamper the effective application of proteomics to the identification of novel disease-specific markers. These include the vast dynamic range of proteins in biological samples, from abundant structural or house-keeping proteins to the much less abundant regulatory proteins (more than 10^6-fold range); difficulties associated with the analysis of post-translational modifications (now being addressed by the application of glycomics [3], phosphoproteomics, metabolomics and degradomics); and the considerable developmental, temporal and biological heterogeneity inherent to endometrial tissue. The endometrium is a classic example of a constantly remodeling tissue, analysis of which is often confounded by widely used hormone treatment such as steroidal contraceptives, drug administration or the presence of disease.

Proteomics is now beginning to impact on clinical diagnosis and drug discovery. The greatest emphasis to date has been on the search for sensitive and discriminatory biomarkers for early cancer detection, for disease classification, for monitoring response to therapy and recurrence of disease and for assessing prognosis. Advances in multiplex immunoassays are also enabling diagnosis using multiple targets discovered by proteomics, as well as the generation of multiple marker profiles that offer greater diagnostic and prognostic efficacy compared to individual markers alone. Such protein-array platforms must continue to move into clinical laboratories that have traditionally focused on the analysis of single biochemical entities for diagnosis. It is unlikely that a single

Endometriosis: Science and Practice, First Edition. Edited by Linda C. Giudice, Johannes L.H. Evers and David L. Healy.
© 2012 Blackwell Publishing Ltd. Published 2012 by Blackwell Publishing Ltd.

marker will be sufficient for diagnosis of such an enigmatic disease as endometriosis.

Proteomic approaches to provide markers for diagnosis

Despite considerable effort, the 'omics' have yet to deliver in terms of a diagnostic test for endometriosis, although they are providing a greater understanding of the molecular events and pathways leading to development of the disease and its maintenance. While proteomic techniques have evolved alongside genomics, they have been slower to make a similar impact – mainly due to the greater complexity and dynamic nature of the proteome. Nevertheless, rapid technological advances as detailed later in this chapter are likely to provide important leads in the near future.

To date, two proteomic technologies have been most commonly applied to the study of endometriosis. In surface-enhanced laser desorption/ionization time of flight mass spectrometry (SELDI-TOF-MS), proteins are captured from a complex mixture on a chip-style protein array; these arrays have different chromatographic surface chemistries, facilitating the capture of specific protein subsets (for example, anion or cation exchange chips). The captured proteins may then be directly analyzed by mass spectrometry, and comparisons made between spectra to identify changes in protein abundance between samples. While SELDI-TOF-MS allows the very rapid, high-throughput analysis of patterns of small proteins in samples, it does not enable their identification. By contrast, two-dimensional polyacrylamide gel electrophoresis (2D PAGE) separates proteins in a complex mixture according to both their isoelectric point (pI) and molecular weight, effectively generating a protein array that can be used for comparison between samples. Typically, the protein spots that show altered abundance between samples are excised from the gel and identified using mass spectrometry (MS).

Recent proteomic analyses utilizing these techniques have included comparisons of eutopic tissue from women without or with endometriosis in the midproliferative [4] or midsecretory phases of the menstrual cycle [4–7], comparison of ectopic lesions with eutopic endometrium [8,9] or normal peritoneum [10], analysis of peritoneal fluid [8,11,12], uterine fluid [13,14], and serum/plasma [7,15–17]. The proteins discovered in relationship to endometriosis have been recently summarized [8] and will not be listed again here.

Application of surface-enhanced laser desorption/ionization time of flight mass spectrometry

Surface-enhanced laser desorption/ionization time of flight mass spectrometry has been applied to analysis of both serum/plasma [15,17] and eutopic biopsies [18,19] from endometriosis patients. Seeber and colleagues used SELDI-TOF-MS to identify a serum-based pattern of markers that might aid in developing a non-invasive, serum-based diagnostic test for endometriosis. Using cation exchange arrays, 169 different peaks between 1 and 9 kDa in size were identified in the combined spectra from 197 patients; of these, 57

achieved the diagnostic targets of either >90% specificity and >20% sensitivity, or >90% sensitivity and >20% specificity, for the diagnosis of endometriosis in a test group. Building upon earlier work (which highlighted the diagnostic potential of CA-125, interleukin (IL)-6, tumor necrosis factor (TNF)-α, macrophage migration inhibitory factor (MMIF), macrophage chemotactic protein (MCP)-1, interferon (IFN)-γ and leptin [16]), sequential analysis of the serum-based proteomic pattern combined with the best performing markers from the previous study (MCP-1, MMIF, leptin, CA-125) improved the effective diagnostic performance. Overall, 73% of subjects would have been diagnosed using a two-step approach with 94% accuracy. However, the group tested included only patients with stage II/IV endometriosis, and it is not clear whether the test would also have detected early-stage disease. An earlier study on plasma [15] also identified similarly discriminatory spectral patterns, specifically with respect to 20 protein peaks, between endometriosis and control patients; again, however, no protein identities were obtained.

Tissue analysis by SELDI-TOF-MS is also feasible. In a preliminary study using eutopic endometrium from normal women and women with mild endometriosis, along with peritoneal lesions and normal peritoneal biopsies, Kyama et al [10] demonstrated that endometrial proteins of 2.8–12.3 kDa were present in decreased abundance in women with endometriosis. As might have been expected, greater differences were found between peritoneal lesions and normal peritoneum, with a cluster of proteins at ~23 kDa identified as transgelin being at markedly increased abundance in lesions. Apolipoprotein A1, a potent anti-inflammatory molecule, was also initially detected as a 28 kDa peak by SELDI-TOF-MS analysis of endometrial biopsy material and subsequently unambiguously identified by tandem MS [18]. Transgelin was also shown to be regulated by human chorionic gonadotropin in normal eutopic endometrium but not in that from women with endometriosis [18].

Application of gel-based proteomics

Two-dimensional PAGE has undergone considerable development since its early use in the 1980s [20], with the advent of sensitive protein-staining techniques and improved reproducibility, particularly resulting from technological changes in the first dimension separation. 2D PAGE has recently been applied to both tissue biopsies and fluids (serum, peritoneal and uterine aspirate) in the context of endometriosis. An early comparison of silver-stained gels of eutopic biopsies, and of serum from women without and with endometriosis, defined a cohort of proteins that differed in both serum and tissue including cytoskeletal proteins, regulators of cell cycle and those with immunological function [7]. Fowler et al [4] likewise used silver-stained 2D PAGE and MS to identify differences in the proteome of eutopic endometrium in both the proliferative and secretory phases of women without and with endometriosis. Proteins identified as aberrant in women with endometriosis included secretory proteins (such as apolipoprotein A2), redox regulators (peroxiredoxin (PRDX)2), chaperonins (heat shock protein 90, annexin A2) and proteins associated with DNA metabolism and catabolism, all of which could contribute to the pathogenesis of endometriosis.

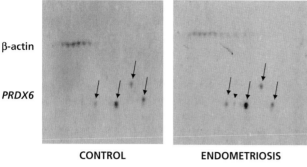

Figure 31.1 Two-dimensional Western blot demonstrates multiple charge and size isoforms of peroxiredoxin 6. Reproduced from Stephens *et al* [6] with permission from the American Chemical Society.

More recently, the application of 2D-differential in-gel electrophoresis (DIGE), one of the most sensitive methods available at present to analyze eutopic midsecretory phase tissue, identified and validated vimentin (VIM), PRDX6 and ribonuclease/angiogenin inhibitor 1 (RNH1) as proteins decreased in endometrium from women with endometriosis compared with normal women [6]. Importantly, and emphasizing the power of proteomics, 2D Western blot demonstrated multiple charge and size isoforms for VIM and PDRX6 while an additional PDRX6 isoform was observed in women with endometriosis that was below the level of detection in women without the disease (Fig. 31.1). Notably, specific isoforms of proteins may have very different biological activities and/or clearance rates [21,22], that can provide functional changes when they are altered in pathological conditions. Furthermore, unique isoforms may provide excellent candidates for diagnostic purposes, providing enhanced discrimination. Stephens and colleagues [6] also noted low correlation between the protein changes and published gene array data, highlighting extensive post-translational modification as observed previously in normal endometrium at different cycle stages [23].

The protein components of peritoneal fluid (PF) in women without and with endometriosis have also been extensively analyzed using 2D PAGE, silver stain and mass spectrometry [8,11,12]. Proteins in PF did not change with time of cycle. However, of some 450 protein spots, 98 were consistently present in the samples and 11 were increased in women with endometriosis while two were decreased [11]. Several protein isoforms differed between women with American Society for Reproductive Medicine (ASRM) stage I/II and those with ASRM stage III/IV disease [8]. Subsequently, when peritoneal fluids of women with endometriosis who were either infertile or fertile were compared with infertile controls, nine isoprotein spots were more intense in fluid from infertile women with endometriosis compared to controls. Most of these proteins are involved in the immune response, consistent with our understanding of the disease [12].

Endometrial fluid aspirate or endometrial lavage offers opportunity for less invasive sampling than peritoneal fluid and it may be anticipated that its composition will reflect the secretory status of the eutopic endometrium. However, 2D PAGE

demonstrated that >90% of the total protein in lavage fluid comprises proteins transudated from serum; immmunodepletion was therefore required to remove the most abundant of these and enabled analysis of the lower abundance proteins [24]. Ametzazurra *et al* [13] analyzed immunodepleted aspirates from women with early (stages I/II) or advanced (stages III/IV) endometriosis and from those without evidence of the disease, and identified 31 proteins with statistically significant differences in spot intensity. Subsequent *in silico* functional analysis using Ingenuity Pathways Analysis software and Western blot analyses provided further insight. Amongst the differentially produced proteins, there was a high representation of cytoskeletal proteins, proteins associated with signal transduction and cell cycle regulation, and cellular redox state. This is in accordance with findings in tissue homogenates [4,6]. In addition the secreted protein glycodelin precursor, a well-established product of endometrial epithelium with contraceptive and immunosuppressive properties [25], was decreased in association with early-stage endometriosis consistent with its reduced gene expression [26] and protein levels in tissue [4].

This study and others [14,24,27] support the feasibility of using endometrial aspirate for diagnosis of endometrial diseases, including endometriosis. However, the differentially produced proteins need to be fully validated to ensure they are endometrial products (particularly from the secretory epithelium), to establish their specificity and sensitivity for detection of endometriosis and to define their potential to differentiate between subsets of the disease in large cohorts of women.

The emerging technologies, such as iTRAQ (see below), have not yet been applied to endometriosis and are likely to provide further advances in terms of identifying targets for diagnosis.

It is clear that no proteomics technique yet applied has proven useful for the diagnosis of endometriosis in a normal clinical setting: most studies were based on very small sample sizes and in most cases, the findings were not further validated (for example, by determining their levels in the tissues by alternative means such as Western blot or immunohistochemistry). Most of the potential known candidates for a diagnostic test in serum or peritoneal fluid have been derived from our understanding of the biology of the disease and focused on cytokines, chemokines and growth factors involved in processes such as tissue remodeling, inflammation, the immune response and angiogenesis. These have individually been shown to differ in peritoneal fluid and tested for their efficacy in serum tests for endometriosis [16,28,29]. Some markers differ with respect to the stage of endometriosis [8] while others differ with the cycle and with infertility [12]. While other potentially new markers in serum have been detected by SELDI [17], since this technique does not lend itself to easy protein identification, other approaches are required.

Biological pathway analysis of proteomic data can provide additional and considerable information regarding possible molecular disturbances that either initiate or maintain the disease. GeneGO or similar bio-informatic tools have been applied to data in a number of studies [6]. These are discussed in detail later in this chapter.

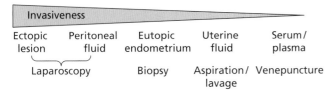

Figure 31.2 Sampling for diagnosis of endometriosis. Diagrammatic representation of the extent of invasiveness of the different sampling techniques applied for testing for endometriosis. Excision of ectopic lesions is the most invasive and venepuncture the least invasive.

Issues to be considered

Sampling

For diagnosis of any disease, sampling is an important consideration and this holds also for diagnosis of endometriosis for which visualization at laparoscopy and examination of a biopsy by a pathologist is the gold standard. While there is a need for non-invasive detection of minimal-to-mild endometriosis [30], it must be noted that at least 50% of these forms resolve spontaneously. Although the moderate-to-severe forms are more likely to be identified by clinical examination, diagnosis cannot reliably be based on symptoms alone. Sampling can take a number of forms (for example, different tissue and fluid types). Figure 31.2 shows the spectrum of sampling modalities that could be applied along a scale of invasiveness of the patient: clearly, either serum/plasma or uterine fluid would be the preferred fluid for analysis. Uterine fluid bathes the eutopic endometrium, which is known to present a different genomic profile in women with endometriosis compared with women free of disease [26], and is hence more likely than serum to contain proteins that could indicate presence of disease. Peritoneal fluid bathes the endometriotic lesions, but could be confounded by secretions by other tissues within the peritoneal cavity and from the abundant leukocytes. In addition, the effect of the sampling procedure on biomarkers must be considered: for tissues, the surgical sampling technique (scissor, laser, etc.) is important and for fluids, samples must be gently centrifuged to remove cellular material (including leukocytes) before freezing.

While fluids are optimal for diagnosis, for the initial identification of markers it may be necessary to analyze the proteome or at least the secreted proteome of tissue. Although it would be ideal to work with ectopic lesions from different sites, the variability of the cellular composition of these, coupled with the need for sufficient total protein for proteomic analysis, make this extremely difficult if not impossible. Indeed, while some lesions have clearly defined endometrial tissue including stroma and glands (Plate 31.1A), in other instances there are only clusters of a few cells and a single gland [31] (Plate 31.1B). Laser capture of endometriotic glands from lesions containing sufficient material (Plate 31.1C) has proven to be useful for gene array analysis following amplification of the RNA [32], although the results may be indicative only of those

substantial lesions containing numbers of glands but not representative of others containing much less glandular tissue. There is insufficient material for satisfactory proteomic analysis of laser-captured tissue using current technologies. Indeed, in our hands, DIGE resolved 533 proteins in captured tissue (both stroma and glands, separated from surrounding peritoneal tissue) from ectopic endometrium. These were labeled with saturation dyes as is essential for such low protein concentrations. Fifty-three of these proteins were differentially produced, but attempts to identify them by mass spectrometry were unsuccessful due to both the very low amount of protein and difficulties in spectral analysis caused by the additional mass of the saturation dye label (unpublished data).

Classification of endometriosis

There are considerable difficulties in classifying endometriosis, partly due to a lack of adequate classification systems. The current American Fertility Society (AFS) classifications [33,34] are the gold standards but are restricted to a limited number of criteria and do not predict pain or fertility status or the outcome of treatment. A newer "endometriosis fertility index" [35] provides a clinical tool that predicts pregnancy rates in endometriosis patients who attempt non-IVF conception but it must be used in patients who have already had surgical staging of their disease. It is now clear from transcriptomic studies that ovarian endometriosis and peritoneal disease are different disorders [36], and that rectovaginal disease differs from both of these as it does not affect gene expression in eutopic endometrium [37].

Careful consideration must be given to the choice of material for discovery of markers, taking such issues into account. For example, is it better to use material from women with most extreme disease (stage III/IV) than from those with mild disease? Are these similar or quite different in their proteome? In addition, it must not be forgotten that the endometrium is highly dynamic and that both eutopic and ectopic endometrium change with cycle stage. Both also contain a multiplicity of cell types, with differing extents of differentiation. It is well recognized that endometriosis is an inflammatory condition and that most lesions contain an abundance of leukocytes: hence leukocyte numbers and their activation status need also to be taken into account.

Looking to the future: emerging proteomics technologies

To date, 2D PAGE and SELDI-TOF-MS have proven the mainstay technologies for proteomic investigations into the pathology of endometriosis. Despite considerable efforts, however, no biomarkers have yet been identified that are suitable as non-invasive, accurate and viable diagnostic and prognostic tools for the treatment and clinical management of endometriosis. The underlying complexity of the proteome, coupled with the dynamic and heterogeneous nature of endometrial tissue, has proven the major barrier for existing technologies. New and emerging techniques are becoming available for better sample fractionation,

Table 31.1 New proteomic techniques applicable to endometriosis research.

Technique		Overview	Application/use	References
	Differential in-gel electrophoresis (DIGE)	Fluorescent labeling of intact proteins prior to separation by 2D PAGE. "Minimal" (lysine residues) or "saturation" (cysteine residues) labeling is possible. Other alternatives are available	Multiplexed comparative analysis by 2D PAGE	[63,64,66,98]
	Isotopic peptide labeling (iTRAQ and iCAT)	Labelling and multiplexing of up to 8 different samples prior to fractionation and subsequent MS/MS analysis	Multiplexed quantitative analysis and protein identification by MS/MS	[76,99]
Comparative proteomics	Isotope-coded protein labeling (ICPL)	Similar to iTRAQ, but labeling is performed on intact proteins prior to fractionation and/or digestion	Label proteins prior to digestion and direct analysis by MS/MS	[77,78]
	Stable isotope labeling with amino acids in cell culture (SILAC)	Incorporation of light or heavy amino acids into proteins during cell culture	Multiplexed quantitative analysis and protein identification by MS/MS	[100]
	Label-free	Comparative peptide abundance based on peak intensity or spectral counting; requires measurement of several replicate samples	Direct peptide analysis by MS/MS	[83,101]
	Immunoaffinity depletion resins	Depletion of abundant proteins (typically applied to plasma), e.g. IgY (Beckman), MARS (Agilent), ProteoPrep (SIGMA); others are available	Enrichment of lower abundance proteins prior to analysis	[51,94]
	Phosphopeptides	Enrichment of phosphorylated peptides on immobilized metal ion affinity chromatography (IMAC) or TiO_2 resin	Specific analysis of phosphorylated peptides	[45,46]
	Glycopeptides	Enrichment of glycosylated peptides on immobilized lectin affinity resin. Specificity conferred by lectin type	Enrichment and analysis of modified peptides/sugar groups	[102]
Fractionation technologies	Size exclusion/affinity nanoparticles	Hydrogel core-shell nanoparticles bind and concentrate low molecular mass peptides/proteins whilst removing larger, abundant proteins	Enrichment of low molecular mass components from biological samples	[52]
	Array technologies	Specific binding of protein subsets based on array surface affinity. Protein, antibody, carbohydrate arrays are available	Rapid screening of protein subsets	[103,104]
	Combinatorial peptide ligand libraries	Hexapeptides coupled to beads for protein affinity capture from complex mixtures. Alternative is hexapeptide-specific antibodies to capture proteins	Enrichment of protein subsets via affinity for short peptide sequences	[50,51]
	Multiplexed assay technologies	Analysis of multiple analytes in a single ELISA assay format. Theoretically up to 100 analytes per assay is possible; in practice, 42-plex kits are available.	Validation of multiple analytes simultaneously by immunoassay	[92,105]
Validation	Multiple reaction monitoring (MRM)	Quantitative detection and validation of candidate biomarkers by mass spectrometry. Multiple analytes can be analysed in a single experiment.	Validation of multiple analytes simultaneously, without use of antibodies	[94]
	MALDI Tissue Imaging	Direct visualization of protein and peptide patterns in tissue by mass spectrometry. Allows "histology without antibodies". Protein, lipid, small metabolite analyses have all been described.	Discovery of novel biomarkers; classification and localization of known markers	[97,106,107]

2D PAGE, two-dimensional polyacrylamide gel electrophoresis; MS, mass spectrometry.

protein labeling and analysis, more powerful bio-informatics tools and independent validation methods; however, these remain largely unapplied to endometriosis proteome research to date. A number of these are summarized in Table 31.1; whilst not exhaustive, these represent some of the newest techniques that could be applied to future endometriosis research. Their use is clearly warranted, and promises to considerably enhance our ability to identify and develop appropriate diagnostic markers for the clinical diagnosis of endometriosis.

New techniques for sample fractionation: unraveling the complexity of the proteome

Sample complexity is a major limitation for proteomic technologies, and thus fractionation is a standard procedure undertaken in any proteomic analysis. The number of proteins present in a sample (including their various splice and post-translationally modified isoforms) and their dynamic expression range dictate the level of fractionation required; this is especially true for a heterogeneous and highly dynamic tissue such as endometrium. Low-abundance proteins including cytokines, growth factors, receptors or signal transduction molecules are often poorly represented in proteomic studies, due to both "masking" by abundant house-keeping proteins and the loading capacity constraints inherent in analysis techniques [38]. Indeed, many a "hit parade" of commonly identified proteins [39,40] has appeared in proteomic studies of endometriosis to date. Targeting specific protein subsets through fractionation – for example, specific post-translational modifications (PTMs) or small and low-abundance proteins – is likely to provide the way forward for the identification of novel, endometriosis-specific biomarkers.

Immunoaffinity depletion

A wide array of chromatographic supports is commercially available for application to proteomic research, according to the type of fractionation or enrichment required (see [38] for a review). In particular, affinity depletion is now considered *de rigueur* for the analysis of serum or plasma samples, where over 99% of the protein present is contributed by only 20 different protein species [41]. Various techniques for plasma depletion are available (reviewed in [42]). Nevertheless, few studies to date have taken advantage of even the least effective of these available technologies [7,43], and none has employed newer immunodepletion techniques capable of removing up to 58 of the most abundant proteins prior to analysis [42]. Clearly, endometriosis research is experiencing a substantial lag behind the rest of the proteomic field in this area.

Post-translational modifications

Post-translational modification of the proteins present in endometrial tissue has recently been shown to be an important feature of endometriosis and endometrial biology in general [6,23]. Accordingly, the dynamic changes induced by the phosphorylation or glycosylation of proteins should prove of interest in future studies of endometriosis. Phosphorylation plays

a key role in most intracellular processes, and is currently one of the best understood PTMs [44,45]. The tightly controlled, dynamic and reversible nature of phosphorylation makes it an interesting research area; in addition, the kinases and phosphorylases that control phosphorylation are often considered to be excellent choices for the development of new therapeutics. The anticancer drug Gleevac, for example, is a protein tyrosine kinase inhibitor [46]. Substantial progress has been made in recent years in the proteomic analysis of dynamic phosphorylation events [46]. Typically, one or both of immobilized metal ion affinity chromatography (IMAC) and TiO_2 affinity media are used to capture phosphorylated peptidases from complex samples prior to analysis by mass spectrometry. The enrichment achieved using these complementary methods is essential for increased signal intensity and efficient characterization during analysis. Additional techniques for phosphopeptide capture, identification and analysis have been reviewed recently [45].

Similar to phosphorylation, glycosylation is estimated to occur on 50–70% of all proteins, making it one of the most common PTMs known [47]. An important feature of structural, signaling and recognition pathways [48], the analysis of glycan structures and their attachment sites has lead to the term "glycomics" which has become a research field in its own right. Typically, lectin affinity chromatography combining single or multiple lectins is used to capture and enrich glycosylated peptides and proteins from samples. Affinity for different lectins can be used to demonstrate the type of carbohydrate modification on a protein; subsequent MS analysis can determine the structure and location of the modification, and even comparatively analyze the carbohydrate structures themselves to uncover disease-related alterations. Used as a depletion tool, carbohydrate affinity supports have enabled the proteomic identification of proteins at low ng/ml concentrations from plasma [49]; used as an enrichment tool, lectin affinity media can be applied to examine particular subsets of proteins based on their specific sugar modifications [47].

Emerging affinity capture techniques

Of note are two emerging technologies: the use of combinatorial peptide libraries or core-shell nanoparticle technologies. Combinatorial peptide libraries can be applied to capture and concentrate low-abundance proteins from samples [50]. Small hexapeptides coupled to beads are mixed with a sample; proteins with affinity for the hexapeptides used are captured and subsequently purified and eluted for further analysis. An attractive notion is that a combinatorial library has almost limitless permutations, thereby enabling access to the "deep proteome" for enrichment prior to analysis [50]. An alternative is the use of hexapeptide-specific antibodies – "triple X proteomic antibodies" – to enrich signature peptides [51]. Each of these technologies remains largely untested, but promises to provide an additional avenue for the capture of low-abundance protein biomarkers.

A similar approach, but using entirely unrelated technology, is the recent application of hydrogel nanoparticles to capture small and low-abundance proteins from complex mixtures [52]. In this case, nanoparticles are synthesized with an "affinity core" surrounded by a porous shell. Proteins larger than the pore size of the shell are excluded, whilst proteins small enough to move through the pores are tightly bound in the core. In practice, these dual size exclusion/affinity nanoparticles (abbreviated to SEAN) effectively remove highly abundant proteins and concentrate very low-abundance proteins for analysis. SEAN have several advantages over other technologies; they may be easily produced in most laboratories, are far cheaper than any other fractionation technique currently available and offer substantial and rapid concentration of low-abundance proteins. Our laboratory has employed SEAN to capture and concentrate cytokines and growth factors from biological samples, and subsequently confirmed their presence at low pg/ml concentrations in the source material. This technology promises to be an important tool in the detection and identification of low-abundance biomarkers of endometriosis.

Microarray technologies

Advances in robotic technologies have led to the development of microarray formats for use in the analysis of specific protein subsets. These include protein arrays for targeting specific functional groups (for example, enzyme specificity or subcellular localizations); protein or peptide interaction arrays to determine binding partners (see [53] for a recent review); antibody (or "reverse protein") arrays to identify specific antigens or dissect signaling pathways [54]; and many others [55,56]. Similar approaches employ glycan arrays for the specific capture and analysis of interactions between carbohydrates and macromolecules [57,58]; their use in functional "immunomics" has also been proposed [59]. Array technologies are an emerging area, and require further development and validation before integration into routine applications; nevertheless, they represent an area of new technological direction that could have considerable impact on future endometriosis research.

New labeling techniques for the detection and comparative analysis of the proteome

As detailed above, several studies of endometriosis have utilized 2D PAGE to compare tissue [4,7,60], peritoneal fluid or serum [11,61,62], either between patients or between eutopic and ectopic implants from the same patient, in an effort to identify proteomic changes specific to endometriosis. Surprisingly, techniques such as silver staining have been the most commonly used for the visualization and quantitation of protein abundance – despite myriad newer labeling and staining technologies that offer greater sensitivity and better linear dynamic range for analysis. In particular, DIGE is now one of the most common techniques for performing comparisons by 2D PAGE, and has been extensively reviewed [63–66]. By labeling proteins with different fluorescent cyanine dyes (Cy2, Cy3 or Cy5 – GE Healthcare), DIGE allows up to three samples to be co-separated in the same 2D PAGE experiment, eliminating the need to perform multiple technical replicates, greatly improving reproducibility and reducing the time

associated with postexperimental data analysis. Whilst common in many other fields of proteomic research, to date only a single study has applied DIGE to examine endometriosis-specific changes in ectopic versus eutopic endometrium [6]. With claimed linear detection over 4–5 orders of magnitude and the ability to directly visualize and quantitatively analyze proteins without staining, the use of DIGE should become more widely applied in endometriosis research using 2D PAGE.

Inherent limitations to the 2D PAGE approach include its limited mass range and poor resolution of certain classes of proteins – for example, hydrophobic, membrane or very small proteins [67–70] – as well as the common identification of multiple proteins from a single spot that hampers unambiguous quantitative analyses [71]. A number of studies (also detailed above) have employed SELDI-TOF-MS either on patient serum [15–17,43,72,73] or tissue samples [18,19] to identify diagnostic patterns. SELDI-TOF-MS is also limited by its effective size range (suitable for small proteins only) and the inability to identify peaks of interest. Generally, this requires extensive postanalysis experimentation, although the recent development of SELDI "interface" technology now permits further characterization of protein peaks using higher resolution mass spectrometers [74]. New MS technologies with increased resolution, sensitivity and accuracy have therefore come to prominence recently for quantitative MS-based analyses (reviewed in [75]). In combination with fractionation strategies, these technologies provide a complementary set of data that cannot be accessed by 2D PAGE or SELDI-TOF-MS and offer researchers a series of alternatives for the direct mass spectrometric analysis of biological samples.

Myriad labeling strategies are now available for direct mass spectrometric analyses, of which the most extensively applied has been isobaric tags for relative and absolute quantitation (iTRAQ – Applied Biosystems). In this system, isobaric mass tags are added to a protein solution; up to eight different samples may be combined prior to sample fractionation and analysis. Both protein identities and quantitative information are obtained from the MS and MS/MS spectrum in a single experiment, rapidly producing very large datasets. Although less widely used, similar alternatives include isotope-coded affinity tags (iCAT: for thiol group labeling) [76] or isotope-coded protein labeling (ICPL: for intact protein labeling) [77,78], isobaric peptide termini labeling (iPTL) [79], and various single or dual stable isotope coding systems (DSIC) [80] (see Table 31.1). Stable isotope labeling by amino acids in cell culture (SILAC) is also an option, where cells are cultured in the presence of heavy or light amino acids; provided the cells can be maintained for six or more doublings, the incorporation of amino acids in different cultures should be identical and this allows a direct and unbiased comparison by mass spectrometry of the extracted proteins. Despite the plethora of techniques now available, only a single study to date has employed iTRAQ and ICAT to analyze differences present in endometriotic tissue [81].

The advent of very high mass accuracy and resolution instrumentation is now also seeing a shift towards "label-free" proteomics. In this instance, spectral counting or peptide intensities are compared across multiple spectra to identify those peptides showing differences in abundance between treatment groups. Whilst requiring multiple technical replicates, label-free quantitative analyses typically use smaller amounts of protein (an important consideration where clinical samples are involved), and do not require expensive labeling reagents. Still in its infancy, label-free proteomics is an emerging technology and offers a viable alternative to labeling strategies [82,83].

Whilst all these new techniques provide excellent ways to investigate the proteome, none is mutually exclusive; indeed, several studies have now shown that the use of several techniques to perform an analysis provides complementary, rather than redundant data [14,84–86]. The choice of technique is therefore dictated by the question to be asked, the research budget, and the outcome desired.

New analysis tools for data mining

With the advent of high-throughput proteomic experiments, large datasets are generated that hold enormous amounts of data. New bio-informatics tools have developed alongside the new proteomics technologies in an effort to more fully exploit emerging technological abilities; nevertheless, data analysis remains one of the greatest bottlenecks in proteomics research. New and emerging algorithms for data interpretation, quantitative analyses, post-translational modification analysis and other aspects are beyond the scope of this chapter; they were extensively reviewed in the January 2008 issue of the *Journal of Proteome Research*. With respect to protein classification and analysis, the best known functional database is the Gene Ontology (GO) [87], which provides standardized functional annotations for all known proteins; GO classification is used in databases such as UniProt (www.uniprot.org), the mainstay of proteomic analyses. GO has been commonly used in endometriosis research for the limited analysis and interpretation of gene expression [88–90] and proteomic data [12,13].

Of greater interest are manually curated protein interaction databases – for example, Ingenuity Pathways Analysis™ (www.ingenuity.com) and GeneGO™ (www.genego.com). These databases have been constructed based on published literature, and contain information concerning known canonical pathways, published protein interactions and their functions. By uploading gene or protein expression data, the researcher can generate statistically validated protein interaction maps to aid in identifying key networks over-represented within their dataset. Such an approach is particularly important for proteomic analyses of endometriosis; changes identified by proteomics tend to focus on abundant proteins, whereas the effectors of those changes may be low-abundance regulatory molecules that are not typically identified. By conducting pathway profiling analyses, it is possible to determine key nodes of interaction that may play roles in the pathogenesis of endometriosis. Surprisingly, pathway profiling has not yet been applied to endometriosis research, with only a single publication using GeneGO to highlight key nodes of interaction that appear to be altered in ectopic endometrium

from endometriosis patients [6]. Pathway profiling is clearly a tool that has immediate application for endometriosis research.

New technologies for the validation of protein abundance changes

Following the identification of potential biomarkers of disease, it is essential to independently test their validity and this often requires the use of multiple strategies, especially for endometrial tissue [6]. As discussed above, enzyme-linked immunosorbent assay (ELISA), Western blot, immunohistochemical staining and real-time polymerase chain reaction (PCR) have been extensively applied in this context; however, new technologies are significantly improving the speed and accuracy of validation studies. The use of novel, multiplexed ELISA-based technology is now widespread, with the Luminex™ and AlphaScreen™ technologies (or branded variants thereof; reviewed in [91,92]) most commonly applied. Each employs an ELISA-based assay system using capture antibodies immobilized on beads, with fluorescent detection and quantitation of the analyte of interest. These technologies allow the analysis of multiple analytes in a single assay; for example, the simultaneous analysis of up to 42 different cytokines in a single assay is now common [93]. These multiplexed assay technologies provide an important tool for the analysis of biomarker patterns, and will be crucial to deciphering the diagnostic patterns required for the development of effective clinical tools.

A major limitation to validation studies has been the availability of suitable antibodies, without which independent validation of protein abundance changes is often not possible. Efforts such as the Human Protein Atlas (www.proteinatlas.org), raising antibodies against as many human proteins as possible, provide an important resource for endometriosis research. Nevertheless, it is not always possible to develop antibodies with suitable specificity, especially within time and budget constraints. New, targeted mass spectrometry-based assays are now becoming more widely used in validation studies. Selected reaction monitoring (SRM; also referred to as multiple reaction monitoring, MRM) involves the detection and quantitation of specific peptides, with known fragmentation properties, in a complex sample [94]. With the theoretical ability to multiplex large numbers of analytes in a single sample, SRM provides one potential alternative for validation where traditional ELISA-based assays are not possible. The methods and technologies involved in the application of SRM have been recently reviewed [94–96].

An exciting development which spans both discovery and validation is the use of MALDI imaging mass spectrometry (IMS) for the direct analysis of tissue samples (reviewed in [97]). In IMS, proteins are ionized directly from the surface of a tissue sample by mass spectrometry, generating a characteristic pattern derived from hundreds or thousands of individual proteins. The proteins contributing to this pattern may then be further analyzed by MS/MS, allowing their identification. The result is an effective histological map of the tissue, containing information including the expression pattern, localization and identification of thousands of proteins present; peptides, lipids and other small molecules may be analyzed simultaneously. Used as a validation tool, IMS can generate histological data for a tissue in the absence of antibodies, as long as the mass of the protein of interest is known. As a discovery tool, expression analysis can be performed to identify, quantitate and localize novel proteins in a single experiment. The clinical applications of IMS are currently focused on tumor biology; mapping tumor margins, typing unknown tumors, and monitoring drug metabolism or effects [97]. MALDI IMS represents an exciting new technology that could easily be applied to endometriosis research, facilitating better classification of endometriotic lesions and their surrounding margins, characterization of underlying pathogenic pathways and the discovery and classification of novel markers of disease.

Conclusion

The application of proteomic technologies has not yet provided widely applicable clinical tools for diagnosis of early-mid or mid-late stage endometriosis for a number of reasons. These include the complexity of proteins and their post-translationally modified forms, the heterogeneity of endometrial tissue between individual women, the time of the cycle when sampling is performed, and the vast dynamic range of protein abundance. The rapidly emerging new technologies for protein detection, coupled with prefractionation techniques and developments in bio-informatics, are now enabling much deeper penetration of the proteome of both tissues and biological fluids. It is thus anticipated that meticulous application of these new techniques to the most appropriate samples will provide that "holy grail" – a reliable, minimally invasive and high-throughput diagnostic for endometriosis.

Acknowledgments
LAS is a Senior Principal Research Fellow of the National Health and Medical Research Council of Australia (NHMRC, #388901). ANS is the Ovarian Cancer Research Foundation Fellow. Research in the authors' laboratories is funded by an NHMRC Program grant (#494802) and the Victorian Government's Operational Infrastructure Support Program.

References

1. Apweiler R, Hermjakob H, Sharon N. On the frequency of protein glycosylation, as deduced from analysis of the SWISS-PROT database. Biochim Biophys Acta 1999;1473:4–8.
2. Tyers M, Mann M. From genomics to proteomics. Nature 2003;422:193–197.
3. Taylor AD, Hancock WS, Hincapie M et al. Towards an integrated proteomic and glycomic approach to finding cancer biomarkers. Genome Med 2009;1:57.
4. Fowler PA, Tattum J, Bhattacharya S et al. An investigation of the effects of endometriosis on the proteome of human eutopic endometrium: a heterogeneous tissue with a complex disease. Proteomics 2007;7:130–142.
5. Have TR, Joffe MM, Lynch KG et al. Causal mediation analyses with rank preserving models. Biometrics 2007;63:926–934.
6. Stephens A, Hannan N, Rainczuk A et al. Post-translational modifications and protein-specific isoforms in endometriosis revealed by 2D DIGE. J Proteome Res 2010;9(5):2438–2449.
7. Zhang H, Niu Y, Feng J et al. Use of proteomic analysis of endometriosis to identify different protein expression in patients with endometriosis versus normal controls. Fertil Steril 2006;86:274–282.
8. Ferrero S, Gillott DJ, Remorgida V et al. Proteomics technologies in endometriosis. Expert Rev Proteomics 2008;5:705–714.
9. Kyama CM, Overbergh L, Mihalyi A et al. Endometrial and peritoneal expression of aromatase, cytokines, and adhesion factors in women with endometriosis. Fertil Steril 2008;89:301–310.
10. Kyama CM, Overbergh L, Debrock S et al. Increased peritoneal and endometrial gene expression of biologically relevant cytokines and growth factors during the menstrual phase in women with endometriosis. Fertil Steril 2006;85:1667–1675.
11. Ferrero S, Gillott DJ, Remorgida V et al. Proteomic analysis of peritoneal fluid in women with endometriosis. J Proteome Res 2007;6:3402–3411.
12. Ferrero S, Gillott DJ, Remorgida V et al. Proteomic analysis of peritoneal fluid in fertile and infertile women with endometriosis. J Reprod Med 2009;54:32–40.
13. Ametzazurra A, Matorras R, Garcia-Velasco JA et al. Endometrial fluid is a specific and non-invasive biological sample for protein biomarker identification in endometriosis. Hum Reprod 2009;24:954–965.
14. Casado-Vela J, Rodriguez-Suarez E, Iloro I et al. Comprehensive proteomic analysis of human endometrial fluid aspirate. J Proteome Res 2009;8:4622–4632.
15. Liu H, Lang J, Zhou Q et al. Detection of endometriosis with the use of plasma protein profiling by surface-enhanced laser desorption/ionization time-of-flight mass spectrometry. Fertil Steril 2007;87:988–990.
16. Seeber B, Sammel MD, Fan X et al. Panel of markers can accurately predict endometriosis in a subset of patients. Fertil Steril 2008;89:1073–1081.
17. Seeber B, Sammel MD, Fan X et al. Proteomic analysis of serum yields six candidate proteins that are differentially regulated in a subset of women with endometriosis. Fertil Steril 2009;93(7):2137–2144.
18. Brosens JJ, Hodgetts A, Feroze-Zaidi F et al. Proteomic analysis of endometrium from fertile and infertile patients suggests a role for apolipoprotein A-I in embryo implantation failure and endometriosis. Mol Hum Reprod 2010;16(4):273–285.
19. Kyama CM, T'Jampens D, Mihalyi A et al. ProteinChip technology is a useful method in the pathogenesis and diagnosis of endometriosis: a preliminary study. Fertil Steril 2006;86:203–209.
20. O'Farrell PH. High resolution two-dimensional electrophoresis of proteins. J Biol Chem 1975;250:4007–4021.
21. Baumann GP. Growth hormone isoforms. Growth Horm IGF Res 2009;19:333–340.
22. Makanji Y, Harrison CA, Stanton PG et al. Inhibin A and B in vitro bioactivities are modified by their degree of glycosylation and their affinities to betaglycan. Endocrinology 2007;148:2309–2316.

23. Chen J, Hannan N, Mak Y et al. Proteomic characterization of mid-proliferative and mid-secretory human endometrium. J Proteome Res 2009;8:2032–2044.

24. Hannan NJ, Stoikos CJ, Stephens AN et al. Depletion of high-abundance serum proteins from human uterine lavages enhances detection of lower-abundance proteins. J Proteome Res 2009;8: 1099–1103.

25. Seppala M, Koistinen H, Mandelin E et al. [Importance of uterus and sperm glycodelins in the regulation of reproduction]. Duodecim 1998;114:761–767.

26. Kao LC, Germeyer A, Tulac S et al. Expression profiling of endometrium from women with endometriosis reveals candidate genes for disease-based implantation failure and infertility. Endocrinology 2003;144:2870–2881.

27. Hannan NJ, Stephens AN, Rainczuk A et al. Proteomic analysis of the human endometrial secretome reveals differences between receptive and non-receptive states in fertile and infertile women. Hum Reprod 2010;9(12):6256–6264.

28. Bohler HC, Gercel-Taylor C, Lessey BA et al. Endometriosis markers: immunologic alterations as diagnostic indicators for endometriosis. Reprod Sci 2007;14:595–604.

29. Mihalyi A, Gevaert O, Kyama CM et al. Non-invasive diagnosis of endometriosis based on a combined analysis of six plasma biomarkers. Hum Reprod 2010;25:654–664.

30. Rogers PA, D'Hooghe TM, Fazleabas A et al. Priorities for endometriosis research: recommendations from an international consensus workshop. Reprod Sci 2009;16:335–346.

31. Clement PB. The pathology of endometriosis: a survey of the many faces of a common disease emphasizing diagnostic pitfalls and unusual and newly appreciated aspects. Adv Anat Pathol 2007;14:241–260.

32. Chand AL, Murray AS, Jones RL et al. Laser capture microdissection and cDNA array analysis of endometrium identify CCL16 and CCL21 as epithelial-derived inflammatory mediators associated with endometriosis. Reprod Biol Endocrinol 2007;5:18.

33. American Fertility Society. Revised classification of endometriosis: 1985. Fertil Steril 1985;43:351–352.

34. American Society for Reproductive Medicine. Revised classification of endometriosis: 1996. Fertil Steril 1996;67:817–821.

35. Adamson GD, Pasta DJ. Endometriosis fertility index: the new, validated endometriosis staging system. Fertil Steril 2010;94(5):1609–1615.

36. Wu Y, Kajdacsy-Balla A, Strawn E et al. Transcriptional characterizations of differences between eutopic and ectopic endometrium. Endocrinology 2006;147:232–246.

37. Matsuzaki S, Canis M, Pouly J et al. Endometrial dysfunction in endometriosis – biochemical aspects. In: Rombauts L et al (eds.) Endometriosis. Oxford: Blackwell; 2008, pp. 89–100.

38. Nice EC, Rothacker J, Weinstock J et al. Use of multidimensional separation protocols for the purification of trace components in complex biological samples for proteomics analysis. J Chromatogr A 2007;1168:190–210; discussion 189.

39. Wang P, Bouwman FG, Mariman EC. Generally detected proteins in comparative proteomics – a matter of cellular stress response? Proteomics 2009;9:2955–2966.

40. Petrak J, Ivanek R, Toman O et al. Deja vu in proteomics. A hit parade of repeatedly identified differentially expressed proteins. Proteomics 2008;8:1744–1749.

41. Tirumalai RS, Chan KC, Prieto DA et al. Characterization of the low molecular weight human serum proteome. Mol Cell Proteomics 2003;2:1096–1103.

42. Pernemalm M, Lewensohn R, Lehtio J. Affinity prefractionation for MS-based plasma proteomics. Proteomics 2009;9:1420–1427.

43. Wang L, Zheng W, Yu JK et al. Artificial neural networks combined with surface-enhanced laser desorption/ionization mass spectra distinguish endometriosis from healthy population. Fertil Steril 2007;88:1700–1702.

44. Graves JD, Krebs EG. Protein phosphorylation and signal transduction. Pharmacol Ther 1999;82:111–121.

45. Thingholm TE, Jensen ON, Larsen MR. Analytical strategies for phosphoproteomics. Proteomics 2009;9:1451–1468.

46. Lemeer S, Heck AJ. The phosphoproteomics data explosion. Curr Opin Chem Biol 2009;13:414–420.

47. An HJ, Froehlich JW, Lebrilla CB. Determination of glycosylation sites and site-specific heterogeneity in glycoproteins. Curr Opin Chem Biol 2009;13:421–426.

48. Dennis JW, Granovsky M, Warren CE. Protein glycosylation in development and disease. Bioessays 1999;21:412–421.

49. Yang Z, Harris LE, Palmer-Toy DE et al. Multilectin affinity chromatography for characterization of multiple glycoprotein biomarker candidates in serum from breast cancer patients. Clin Chem 2006;52:1897–1905.

50. Boschetti E, Righetti PG. The art of observing rare protein species in proteomes with peptide ligand libraries. Proteomics 2009;9:1492–1510.

51. Poetz O, Hoeppe S, Templin MF et al. Proteome wide screening using peptide affinity capture. Proteomics 2009;9:1518–1523.

52. Rainczuk A, Meehan K, Steer DL et al. An optimized procedure for the capture, fractionation and proteomic analysis of proteins using hydrogel nanoparticles. Proteomics 2010;10:332–336.

53. Wolf-Yadlin A, Sevecka M, MacBeath G. Dissecting protein function and signaling using protein microarrays. Curr Opin Chem Biol 2009;13:398–405.

54. Voshol H, Ehrat M, Traenkle J et al. Antibody-based proteomics: analysis of signaling networks using reverse protein arrays. FEBS J 2009;276:6871–6879.

55. Joos T, Bachmann J. Protein microarrays: potentials and limitations. Front Biosci 2009;14:4376–4385.

56. Hartmann M, Roeraade J, Stoll D et al. Protein microarrays for diagnostic assays. Anal Bioanal Chem 2009;393:1407–1416.

57. Hsu KL, Mahal LK. Sweet tasting chips: microarray-based analysis of glycans. Curr Opin Chem Biol 2009;13:427–432.

58. Oyelaran O, Gildersleeve JC. Glycan arrays: recent advances and future challenges. Curr Opin Chem Biol 2009;13:406–413.

59. Prechl J, Papp K, Erdei A. Antigen microarrays: descriptive chemistry or functional immunomics? Trends Immunol 2010;31(4): 133–137.

60. Hou Z, Zhou J, Ma X et al. Role of interleukin-1 receptor type II in the pathogenesis of endometriosis. Fertil Steril 2008;89:42–51.

61. Ferrero S, Gillott DJ, Remorgida V et al. GnRH analogue remarkably down-regulates inflammatory proteins in peritoneal fluid proteome of women with endometriosis. J Reprod Med 2009;54:223–231.

62. Ferrero S, Gillott DJ, Remorgida V et al. Haptoglobin beta chain isoforms in the plasma and peritoneal fluid of women with endometriosis. Fertil Steril 2005;83:1536–1543.

63. Marouga R, David S, Hawkins E. The development of the DIGE system: 2D fluorescence difference gel analysis technology. Anal Bioanal Chem 2005;382:669–678.

64. Friedman DB. Quantitative proteomics for two-dimensional gels using difference gel electrophoresis. Methods Mol Biol 2007;367:219–239.

65. Wheelock AM, Morin D, Bartosiewicz M et al. Use of a fluorescent internal protein standard to achieve quantitative two-dimensional gel electrophoresis. Proteomics 2006;6:1385–1398.

66. Timms JF, Cramer R. Difference gel electrophoresis. Proteomics 2008;8:4886–4897.

67. Friedman DB, Hoving S, Westermeier R. Isoelectric focusing and two-dimensional gel electrophoresis. Methods Enzymol 2009;463:515–540.

68. Westermeier R, Schickle H. The current state of the art in high-resolution two-dimensional electrophoresis. Arch Physiol Biochem 2009;115:279–285.

69. Gorg A, Drews O, Luck C et al. 2-DE with IPGs. Electrophoresis 2009;30 Suppl 1:S122–132.

70. Gorg A, Weiss W, Dunn MJ. Current two-dimensional electrophoresis technology for proteomics. Proteomics 2004;4:3665–3685.

71. Hunsucker SW, Duncan MW. Is protein overlap in two-dimensional gels a serious practical problem? Proteomics 2006;6:1374–1375.

72. Wang L, Zheng W, Mu L et al. Identifying biomarkers of endometriosis using serum protein fingerprinting and artificial neural networks. Int J Gynaecol Obstet 2008;101:253–258.

73. Jing J, Qiao Y, Suginami H et al. Two novel serum biomarkers for endometriosis screened by surface-enhanced laser desorption/ionization time-of-flight mass spectrometry and their change afterlaparoscopic removal of endometriosis. Fertil Steril 2009;92:1221–1227.

74. Peng J, Stanley AJ, Cairns D et al. Using the protein chip interface with quadrupole time-of-flight mass spectrometry to directly identify peaks in SELDI profiles – initial evaluation using low molecular weight serum peaks. Proteomics 2009;9:492–498.

75. Mann M and Kelleher NL. Precision proteomics: the case for high resolution and high mass accuracy. Proc Natl Acad Sci USA 2008;105:18132–18138.

76. Gygi SP, Rist B, Gerber SA et al. Quantitative analysis of complex protein mixtures using isotope-coded affinity tags. Nat Biotechnol 1999;17:994–999.

77. Kellermann J. ICPL – isotope-coded protein label. Methods Mol Biol 2008;424:113–123.

78. Turtoi A, Mazzucchelli GD, de Pauw E. Isotope coded protein label quantification of serum proteins – comparison with the label-free LC-MS and validation using the MRM approach. Talanta 2010;80:1487–1495.

79. Koehler CJ, Strozynski M, Kozielski F et al. Isobaric peptide termini labeling for MS/MS-based quantitative proteomics. J Proteome Res 2009;8:4333–4341.

80. Wang H, Wong CH, Chin A et al. Quantitative serum proteomics using dual stable isotope coding and nano LC-MS/MSMS. J Proteome Res 2009;8:5412–5422.

81. DeSouza L, Diehl G, Yang EC et al. Proteomic analysis of the proliferative and secretory phases of the human endometrium: protein identification and differential protein expression. Proteomics 2005;5:270–281.

82. Matthiesen R, Carvalho AS. Methods and algorithms for relative quantitative proteomics by mass spectrometry. Methods Mol Biol 2010;593:187–204.

83. Zhu W, Smith JW, Huang CM. Mass spectrometry-based label-free quantitative proteomics. J Biomed Biotechnol 2010;2010:840518.

84. Patel VJ, Thalassinos K, Slade SE et al. A comparison of labeling and label-free mass spectrometry-based proteomics approaches. J Proteome Res 2009;8:3752–3759.

85. Chenau J, Michelland S, de Fraipont F et al. The cell line secretome, a suitable tool for investigating proteins released in vivo by tumors: application to the study of p53-modulated proteins secreted in lung cancer cells. J Proteome Res 2009;8:4579–4591.

86. Thon JN, Schubert P, Duguay M et al. Comprehensive proteomic analysis of protein changes during platelet storage requires complementary proteomic approaches. Transfusion 2008;48:425–435.

87. Dimmer EC, Huntley RP, Barrell DG et al. The Gene Ontology – providing a functional role in proteomic studies. Proteomics 2008 July 17; epub ahead of print.

88. Wren JD, Wu Y, Guo SW. A system-wide analysis of differentially expressed genes in ectopic and eutopic endometrium. Hum Reprod 2007;22:2093–2102.

89. Taylor RN, Lundeen SG, Giudice LC. Emerging role of genomics in endometriosis research. Fertil Steril 2002;78:694–698.

90. Burney RO, Talbi S, Hamilton AE et al. Gene expression analysis of endometrium reveals progesterone resistance and candidate susceptibility genes in women with endometriosis. Endocrinology 2007;148:3814–3826.

91. Vignali DA. Multiplexed particle-based flow cytometric assays. J Immunol Methods 2000;243:243–255.

92. Taouji S, Dahan S, Bosse R et al. Current screens based on the AlphaScreen technology for deciphering cell signalling pathways. Curr Genomics 2009;10:93–101.

93. Richens JL, Urbanowicz RA, Metcalf R et al. Quantitative validation and comparison of multiplex cytokine kits. J Biomol Screen 2010;15(5):562–568.

94. Huttenhain R, Malmstrom J, Picotti P et al. Perspectives of targeted mass spectrometry for protein biomarker verification. Curr Opin Chem Biol 2009;13:518–525.

95. Schmidt A, Claassen M, Aebersold R. Directed mass spectrometry: towards hypothesis-driven proteomics. Curr Opin Chem Biol 2009;13:510–517.

96. Pan S, Aebersold R, Chen R et al. Mass spectrometry based targeted protein quantification: methods and applications. J Proteome Res 2009;8:787–797.

97. Walch A, Rauser S, Deininger SO et al. MALDI imaging mass spectrometry for direct tissue analysis: a new frontier for molecular histology. Histochem Cell Biol 2008;130:421–434.

98. Tsolakos N, Techanukul T, Wallington A et al. Comparison of two combinations of cyanine dyes for prelabelling and gel electrophoresis. Proteomics 2009;9:1727–1730.

99. Ross PL, Huang YN, Marchese JN et al. Multiplexed protein quantitation in Saccharomyces cerevisiae using amine-reactive isobaric tagging reagents. Mol Cell Proteomics 2004;3:1154–1169.

100. Ong SE, Blagoev B, Kratchmarova I et al. Stable isotope labeling by amino acids in cell culture, SILAC, as a simple and accurate approach to expression proteomics. Mol Cell Proteomics 2002;1:376–386.

101. America AH, Cordewener JH. Comparative LC-MS: a landscape of peaks and valleys. Proteomics 2008;8:731–749.

102. Domon B. Glycosylation as means of reducing sample complexity to enable quantitative proteomics. Proteomics 2009;9:1488–1491.

103. Wingren C, James P, Borrebaeck CA. Strategy for surveying the proteome using affinity proteomics and mass spectrometry. Proteomics 2009;9:1511–1517.

104. Wingren C, Borrebaeck CA. Antibody-based microarrays. Methods Mol Biol 2009;509:57–84.

105. Dunbar SA. Applications of Luminex xMAP technology for rapid, high-throughput multiplexed nucleic acid detection. Clin Chim Acta 2006;363:71–82.

106. Franck J, Arafah K, Elayed M et al. MALDI imaging mass spectrometry: state of the art technology in clinical proteomics. Mol Cell Proteomics 2009;8:2023–2033.

107. Hardesty WM, Caprioli RM. In situ molecular imaging of proteins in tissues using mass spectrometry. Anal Bioanal Chem 2008; 391:899–903.

32 Diagnosis of Endometriosis: Transcriptomics

Richard O. Burney[1] and Linda C. Giudice[2]

[1]Division of Reproductive Endocrinology and Infertility, Department of Obstetrics and Gynecology, Madigan Healthcare System, Tacoma, WA, USA

[2]Department of Obstetrics, Gynecology and Reproductive Sciences, University of California, San Francisco, CA, USA

Introduction

Although the clinical sequelae of endometriosis are well described, the pathogenesis remains to be elucidated. Originally popularized by Sampson in the 1920s, the theory of retrograde menstruation gained strong support 60 years later via laparoscopic studies demonstrating endometrial cells in the peritoneal cavity post menstruation [1,2]. The endometrial origin of endometriotic lesions has been observed surgically and confirmed by molecular studies [3]. An innate or acquired abnormality within the endometrium may predispose to the implantation, proliferation, neo-angiogenesis and survival of endometriotic lesions in the pelvis [4]. The histological impression of endometrial glands and stroma via surgically obtained biopsy remains the gold standard for diagnosis of endometriosis. However, this procedure carries associated surgical risk, is time consuming for the patient, and involves significant cost to the healthcare system [5,6]. The inordinately long interval between onset of symptoms and definitive surgical diagnosis highlights the pressing need for a relatively less invasive means of diagnosing the condition [7–9].

The era of transcriptomics has ushered in exciting possibilities with respect to the molecular diagnosis of disease, particularly multifactorial conditions that elude a genomic approach. Also known as gene expression profiling, transcriptomics refers to the study of transcript (mRNA) levels in a given cell population or tissue. Transcervical access to the endometrium allows a relatively non-invasive approach to tissue for purposes of molecular interrogation. The utility of endometrial gene expression profiling in the diagnosis of this disorder is predicated on documentation of a difference in mRNA signatures of women with versus without endometriosis. In this chapter, we shall review the evidence substantiating these differences and the prospect for a eutopic endometrial transcriptomic approach to the diagnosis of this enigmatic condition.

Transcriptomic platforms

It should be emphasized that gene expression profiling of the endometrium provides a cross-sectional perspective of transcript abundance in the tissue at a given point in time. Whether differential expression of genes in the endometrium is a cause and/or a consequence of endometriosis, an often debated topic in the interpretation of endometrial gene expression, is immaterial to the utility of transcriptomic profiling in the diagnostic sense. The consistent differential expression between women with versus without disease is the critical element.

A number of methods have been developed for the measurement of transcript abundance and have been used to investigate gene expression in human endometrium [10]. Oligonucleotide spotted arrays spotted on gene chips were the first platform to allow simultaneous interrogation of mRNA expression of large numbers of genes. Quantitative real-time polymerase chain reaction (Q-RT-PCR) emerged as a sensitive method for the quantification of transcripts. RNA-Seq is a recently developed approach to transcriptome profiling that uses deep-sequencing technologies. Microarray technology is a method of gene expression profiling that measures the relative activity of previously identified target genes.

Importantly, relatively small changes in mRNA expression can produce large changes in the total amount of corresponding protein. Due to post-transcriptional events such as mRNA degradation, microRNA silencing and alternative splicing, the mRNA level may not accurately reflect the corresponding protein level.

Unique caveats in endometrium and endometriosis

Cyclic variation and cellular constituents of human endometrium

The endometrium presents several unique caveats to the interpretation of gene expression profiling. By nature, the endometrium evidences remarkable cyclic variation and is a unique tissue in this regard. The sex steroid dependence and regenerative capacity of the endometrium are hallmark features. The cyclic variation in the endometrium presents a significant challenge with regard to transcriptomic profiling, highlighting the importance of phase-specific delineation of results, although an ideal diagnostic would theoretically be phase independent. Stromal, glandular, epithelial, endothelial and immune cell fractions underscore the heterogeneity of the endometrium. While the dissection of compartments is important to investigations of pathophysiology, it is less relevant and indeed impractical in a diagnostic sense, except if the tissue sample presents heterogeneous populations of cells that affect the read-out of the test. Thus, documentation of gene expression differences in whole-tissue specimens is most relevant to diagnostic biomarker development.

Disease heterogeneity

Endometriosis is a clinically heterogeneous disease, which can be asymptomatic, and a well-described discrepancy exists between severity of disease and symptoms [11]. The presence of endometrial tissue in the pelvis transiently does not appear to be necessarily pathological. Subtle endometriosis may be a condition occurring intermittently in women [12]. An anatomical subclassification of disease has been advocated, and eutopic endometrium may be different among patients with peritoneal, ovarian and rectovaginal disease [13]. Furthermore, the eutopic endometrial transcriptome in women with endometriosis may have shared patterns of dysregulation with other inflammatory conditions such as hydrosalpinx [14] or other estrogen-dependent diseases such as leiomyomata, endometrial polyps or adenomyosis [15,16]. These caveats represent potential confounders that must be addressed during development of an endometrial-based diagnostic approach and underscore the importance in clinical trials of subject annotation.

Numerous microarray studies in endometriosis have been reported, and these can be largely categorized into two designs. The first compares gene expression profiles in paired ectopic (from endometriotic lesions) and eutopic endometrium collected from the same individual. The second study design compares eutopic endometrium from women with versus without endometriosis. This design is most relevant to the identification of altered transcriptomic profiles for diagnostic purposes, and we focus this review on studies employing the latter approach.

Global gene expression profiling of eutopic endometrium

Increasing evidence supports endometriosis as a polygenic and multifactorial disease, indicating that multiple distinct pathways could be involved in its pathogenesis. Perhaps the most compelling evidence for a multifactorial etiology is the absence of highly significant linkage to any single locus in a well-powered genome-wide linkage analysis study [17]. Furthermore, many sentinel features of endometriosis, such as inflammation and neo-angiogenesis, are shared with other diseases, rendering it unlikely that a single biochemical marker, particularly a serum-based assay, will yield sufficient sensitivity and specificity to be used in clinical practice. Because of this complexity, endometriosis is ideally suited as a target for genome-wide scanning for biomarker panel development. In recent years, the human genome sequencing project ushered in the era of functional genomics. Global gene profiling studies have galvanized the search for a relatively non-invasive diagnostic approach [18].

In 2003, the first global gene expression study of eutopic endometrium from women with versus without endometriosis was reported [19]. This study used high-density microarray chip technology to evaluate whole endometrium from eight women with revised American Fertility Society (rAFS) stage I/III endometriosis and compared the gene expression profiles with those of 12 women surgically confirmed to be free of disease. All endometrial samples were obtained by Pipelle catheter during the midsecretory (MSE; cycle day 19–23) phase of the menstrual cycle, also known as the window of implantation. A total of 206 genes demonstrated at least a two-fold difference in endometrial expression between the two groups, including genes involved in regulating apoptosis, immune function, extracellular matrix (ECM) components, and transcription factors. Among the downregulated genes were glycodelin, osteopontin and mucin-1, genes known to be important in embryonic implantation. Importantly, this study demonstrated impressive molecular differences in the endometrium of women with endometriosis, compared to those without disease, and established the exciting possibility that these differences could be leveraged in the design of an endometrial biomarker for the non-surgical diagnosis of the condition.

Using laser capture microdissection and cDNA microarray analysis, Matsuzaki and colleagues determined cell compartment-specific differences in gene expression in eutopic late proliferative (PE; cycle day 8–14), early secretory (ESE; cycle day 15–18), MSE, and late secretory (LSE; cycle day 24–28) endometrium of women with versus without deep endometriosis [20]. Although the stage of disease was not specified, women with endometriosis had deep infiltrative disease defined by a lesional depth >5 mm below the peritoneal surface. This study demonstrated upregulation in LSE of uPAR in epithelial cells and KSR (a MAPK scaffold of the Ras pathway), and PI3K p85 regulatory subunit a in stromal cells. Relatively fewer differentially expressed genes were identified as

Table 32.1 Gene expression profiling studies comparing eutopic endometrium from women with versus without endometriosis.

Authors	Date	Cycle phase	NL (n)	Endo (n) (rAFS)	Array EM	Reference	DE
Kao *et al*	2003	MSE	8	12 (II/III)	Whole	Affy Hu95A[1]	206
Matsuzaki *et al*	2005	PE	3	3 (Unknown)	LCM	Clontech 1.2 cDNA[2]	12
Matsuzaki *et al*	2005	ESE	3	3 (Unknown)	LCM	Clontech 1.2 cDNA	90
Matsuzaki *et al*	2005	MSE	3	3 (Unknown)	LCM	Clontech 1.2 cDNA	26
Matsuzaki *et al*	2005	LSE	3	3 (Unknown)	LCM	Clontech 1.2 cDNA	28
Burney *et al*	2007	PE	5	6 (III/IV)	Whole	Affy Hu 133 2.0[3]	38
Burney *et al*	2007	ESE	3	6 (III/IV)	Whole	Affy Hu 133 2.0	734
Burney *et al*	2007	MSE	9	8 (III/IV)	Whole	Affy Hu 133 2.0	26
Sherwin *et al*	2008	LSE	6	8 (I/IV)	Whole	Custom array[4]	9

[1]Affymetrix Human 95A gene chip with 12,500 genes represented.

[2]Clontech Human 1.2 cDNA chip with 1176 genes represented.

[3]Affymetrix Human 133 Plus 2.0 gene chip with 42,203 genes represented.

[4]Custom-made array with 22,000 genes represented.

Phase designations: PE, proliferative; ESE, early secretory; MSE, mid secretory.

DE, differentially expressed genes, defined as ≥2-fold change in expression; EM, endometrium; Endo, endometriosis (rAFS stage of disease); LCM, laser capture microdissected tissue; NL, normal/without endometriosis.

compared to other eutopic-eutopic studies, and this may reflect the use of a chip with fewer genes represented (Table 32.1). The involvement of two important signaling pathways, RAS/RAF/MAPK and PI3K, is strikingly similar to results in ectopic lesions of deep endometriosis versus ovarian endometriomas and peritoneal disease [21]. The data overall suggest a common dysregulation of signaling in eutopic and ectopic endometrium in women with endometriosis among pathways that participate in cell cycle regulation and cell survival, and add further evidence that eutopic endometrium from endometriosis patients may be different from that of women without endometriosis.

Subsequently, global analysis of the endometrial transcriptome across the menstrual cycle was performed [3]. This study compared whole-tissue transcript profiles obtained via Pipelle catheter during the proliferative, early secretory and midsecretory phases. Because endometriosis is a visually heterogeneous condition and studies have documented inaccuracy in its visual diagnosis, particularly in cases of minimal/mild stages [22], this study sought to improve the fidelity of the study cohort by including only women with surgically documented and histologically validated moderate-to-severe-stage (r-AFS stage III/IV) endometriosis. Of note in this study was the marked persistence of estrogen-regulated genes in ESE from women with disease at a time when progesterone action should downregulate these genes. In the proliferative-secretory transition, the fingerprint of persistent cellular mitosis and minimal responsiveness of classically progesterone-regulated genes in ESE extended to MSE. Principal component analysis revealed that ESE specimens from women with disease clustered closer to PE specimens than ESE from women without disease, confirming the observed attenuation of progesterone action. Many genes known to be progesterone regulated were differentially expressed in the secretory endometrium of women in the disease cohort.

This study highlighted the power of modern bio-informatic approaches in the identification of biological phenomena in a high-content dataset. In this case, progesterone resistance was evident in the secretory endometrium of women with endometriosis. Finally, this study confirmed the finding of transcriptomic differences in the endometrium of women with versus without endometriosis and highlighted candidates for biomarker development.

A pairwise eutopic comparison of the transcriptome in LSE from women with versus without endometriosis was recently reported [23]. The authors found a limited number of genes dysregulated during this period of progesterone withdrawal. Furthermore, they concluded that relative to other cycle phases, late secretory endometrium was uninformative from a diagnostic perspective.

Diagnostic DNA microarray with disease-relevant biomarkers

Much like casting a net over the entire genome in anticipation of retrieving key targets, global gene expression analysis using DNA microarray technology allows identification of candidate biomarkers in the form of differentially expressed genes in the endometrium of women with versus without endometriosis. DNA microarray-based approaches for tissue-based biomarker discovery have been applied to the diagnosis of chronic diseases such as diabetes [24], arthritis [25] and cardiovascular disease [26].

Like endometriosis, inflammatory bowel disease is characterized as a chronic inflammatory condition [27]. Using biomarker genes selected from differential gene expression profiling using DNA microarray, Crohn's disease and ulcerative colitis can be diagnosed. Specifically, von Stein and colleagues designed a diagnostic oligonucleotide spotted chip for these diseases based on the sequences of up- and downregulated genes selected from Affymetrix GeneChip experiments. Twenty-five sequences were identified as genes relevant to inflammatory bowel disease, resulting in a sensitivity of 84% and a specificity of 100%. Likewise, 36 genes were demonstrated to be Crohn specific, resulting in a diagnostic sensitivity of 89% and a specificity of 80% [28].

Conclusion

Properties of an ideal biomarker include simplicity, reproducibility, minimal or non-invasiveness, and specificity. A serum biomarker, though attractive, remains elusive, although a panel of biomarkers with appropriate classifier algorithms shows promise. Serological markers such as CA-125 and antinuclear antibody (ANA) titer lack sufficient specificity to be useful in diagnosing endometriosis. Serological markers may be affected by other local or systemic inflammatory conditions, and therefore endometrial markers would seem likely to have improved specificity. Though more invasive than serology, endometrial tissue is accessible via Pipelle biopsy in the office setting. An endometrial diagnostic assay is preferably obtained in the proliferative phase, as this avoids interruption of an unanticipated pregnancy that would be undetectable by current pregnancy tests in the secretory phase. This diagnostic assay is predicated on reliable differential expression of a biomarker between women with and without endometriosis during the proliferative phase of the menstrual cycle.

References

1. Sampson JA. Peritoneal endometriosis due to menstrual dissemination of endometrial tissue into the peritoneal cavity. Am J Obstet Gynecol 1927;14:442–469.
2. Halme J, Hammond MG, Hulka JF, Raj SG, Talbert LM. Retrograde menstruation in healthy women and in patients with endometriosis. Obstet Gynecol 1984;64:151–154.
3. Burney RO, Talbi S, Hamilton AE et al. Gene expression analysis of endometrium reveals progesterone resistance and candidate genetic loci in women with endometriosis. Endocrinology 2007;148:3814–3826.
4. Giudice LC, Kao LC. Endometriosis. Lancet 2004;364:1789–1799.
5. Davis L, Gangar KF, Drummond M. The economic burden of intractable gynecological pain. J Obstet Gynecol 1992;33:S54–56.
6. Zhao SZ, Wong JM, Davis MB, Gersh GE, Johnson KE. The cost of inpatient endometriosis treatment: an analysis based on the Healthcare Cost and Utilization Project Nationwide Inpatient Sample. Am J Manag Care 1998;4:1127–1134.
7. Matsuzaki S, Canis M, Pouly JL, Rabischong B, Botchorishvili R, Mage G. Relationship between delay of surgical diagnosis and severity of disease in patients with symptomatic deep infiltrating endometriosis. Fertil Steril 2006;5:1314–1316.
8. Ballard K, Lowton K, Wright J. What's the delay? A qualitative study of women's experiences of reaching a diagnosis of endometriosis. Fertil Steril 2006;5:1296–1301.
9. Stratton P. The tangled web of reasons for the delay in diagnosis of endometriosis in women with chronic pelvic pain: will the suffering end? Fertil Steril 2006;5:1302–1304.
10. Giudice LC. Elucidating endometrial function in the post-genomic era. Hum Reprod Update 2003;9(3):223–235.
11. Giudice LC. Clinical practice. Endometriosis. N Engl J Med 2010;362(25):2389–2398.
12. Harrison RF, Barry-Kinsella C. Efficacy of medroxyprogesterone treatment in infertile women with endometriosis: a prospective, randomized, placebo-controlled study. Fertil Steril 2000;74:24–30.
13. Nisolle M, Donnez J. Peritoneal endometriosis, ovarian endometriosis, and adenomyotic nodules of the rectovaginal septum are three different entities. Fertil Steril 1997;68:585–596.
14. Daftary GS, Taylor HS. Hydrosalpinx fluid diminishes endometrial cell HOXA10 expression. Fertil Steril 2002;78:577–580.
15. Kitawaki J, Koshiba H, Ishihara H, Kusuki I, Tsukamoto K, Honjo H. Progesterone induction of 17 beta-hydroxysteroid dehydrogenase type 2 during the secretory phase occurs in the endometrium of estrogendependent benign diseases but not in normal endometrium. J Clin Endocrinol Metab 2000;85:3292–3296.
16. Rackow BW, Taylor HS. Submucosal uterine leiomyomas have a global effect on molecular determinants of endometrial receptivity. Fertil Steril 2010;93:2027–2034.
17. Treloar SA, Wicks J, Nyholt DR et al. Genomewide linkage study in 1,176 affected sister pair families identifies a significant susceptibility locus for endometriosis on chromosome 10q26. Am J Hum Genet 2005;77:365–376.
18. Taylor RN, Lundeen SG, Giudice LC. Emerging role of genomics in endometriosis research. Fertil Steril 2002;78:694–698.
19. Kao LC, Germeyer A, Tulac S et al. Expression profiling of endometrium from women with endometriosis reveals candidate genes for disease-based implantation failure and infertility. Endocrinology 2003;144:2870–2881.
20. Matsuzaki S, Canis M, Vaurs-Barrière C, Boespflug-Tanguy O, Dastugue B, Mage G. DNA microarray analysis of gene expression in eutopic endometrium from patients with deep endometriosis using laser capture microdissection. Fertil Steril 2005;84:1180–1190.
21. Giudice LC, Talbi S, Hamilton A, Lessey BA. Transcriptomics. In: Aplin J, Fazleabas A, Glasser S (eds) The Endometrium: Molecular, Cellular and Clinical Perspectives, 2nd edn. London: Informa Healthcare; 2008, pp.193–222.
22. Marchino GL, Gennarelli G, Enria R, Bongioanni F, Lipari G, Massobrio M. Diagnosis of pelvic endometriosis with use of macroscopic versus histologic findings. Fertil Steril 2005;82:12–15.
23. Sherwin JRA, Sharkey AM, Mihalyi A et al. Global gene analysis of late secretory phase, eutopic endometrium does not provide the basis for a minimally invasive test of endometriosis. Hum Reprod 2008;23:1063–1068.
24. Baelde HJ, Eikmans M, Doran PP, Lappin DW, de Heer E, Bruijn JA. Gene expression profiling in glomeruli from human

kidneys with diabetic nephropathy. Am J Kidney Dis 2004;43:636–650.

25. Barnes MG, Aronow BJ, Luyrink LK et al. Gene expression in juvenile arthritis and spondyloarthropathy: pro-angiogenic ELR+ chemokine genes relate to course of arthritis. Rheumatology 2004;43:973–979.

26. Ma J, Liew CC. Gene profiling identifies secreted protein transcripts from peripheral blood cells in coronary artery disease. J Mol Cell Cardiol 2003;35:993–998.

27. Hugot JP, Thomas G. Genome-wide scanning in inflammatory bowel diseases. Dig Dis 1998;16:364–369.

28. von Stein P, Lofberg R, Kuznetsov NV et al. Multigene analysis can discriminate between ulcerative colitis, Crohn's disease, and irritable bowel syndrome. Gastroenterol 2008;134:1869–1881.

7 Medical Therapies for Pain

33 Medical Therapies: Randomized Controlled Trials/Traditional Medical Therapies

Neil P. Johnson

Department of Obstetrics and Gynaecology, University of Auckland, and Fertility Plus, Green Lane Clinical Centre, Auckland, New Zealand

Introduction

Traditional medical therapies for women with endometriosis are amongst the most rigorously researched treatments in the field of gynaecology. There are many randomized controlled trials (RCTs) and systematic reviews of RCTs which were, again, amongst the first systematic reviews of trials to be conducted in gynecology.

Why is it important to have so-called "level 1 evidence" from RCTs? For endometriosis, as much as any other condition, the key outcomes of paramount importance to patients are subjective, such as pain and quality of life. Thus it is crucial to have the most robust trial design to minimize bias. Hence, not only is it imperative to have truly randomized trials where treatment allocation is adequately concealed prior to randomization, but the best trials also include blinding (masking), where patients, caregivers and outcome assessors are all unaware of the treatment being administered, in order to optimize the reliability of trial results. Reassuringly, it is becoming apparent that the quality of RCTs in gynecology is steadily improving [1].

The importance of registering clinical trials has been emphasized by Guo *et al*, as genuine advances, proven to be effective in RCTs, occur very rarely [2].

Outcomes of importance to women suffering from endometriosis are the most important to study, including quality of life and pain, with impacts on the stage of disease and objective evidence of recurrence (gauged through laparoscopy with disease staging, imaging or perhaps measurement of CA-125 as a marker of disease activity) being of secondary importance.

Sources of randomized controlled trial evidence for medical therapies for endometriosis

Useful resources that are updated periodically with the intention of accumulating the latest best evidence, rather than being published once only, are the Cochrane Database of Systematic Reviews of RCTs (www.Cochrane.org), the Clinical Evidence series [3], the European Society of Human Reproduction and Embryology (ESHRE) guidelines (http://guidelines.endometriosis.org/), American Society of Reproductive Medicine (ASRM) guidelines (www.asrmshopping.org/guidelines.html) and the Royal College of Obstetricians and Gynaecologists (RCOG) Green Top guidelines (www.rcog.org.uk/resources/Public/pdf/endometriosis_gt_24_2006.pdf). Other helpful evidence-based guidelines, laying appropriate heavy emphasis on evidence from randomized trials, are from Medicine 1000 on-ine reviews, in which we are attempting to report on all new RCTs published in the field of endometriosis (www.MedicineF1000). The World Endometriosis Society intends to hold a consensus meeting on the management of endometriosis at the Montpelier World Congress on Endometriosis in 2011 to attempt to attain an international consensus that reflects the global view on endometriosis treatments.

Of Cochrane systematic reviews published in 2009, Issue 1 (see Tables 33.1 and 33.2), 12 reviews assessed interventions for women with endometriosis – these included 72 RCTs reporting on 6806 women. Seven of these 12 reviews examined purely medical therapies for pain symptoms (with two reviews examining surgical interventions and three examining interventions for infertility).

Endometriosis: Science and Practice, First Edition. Edited by Linda C. Giudice, Johannes L.H. Evers and David L. Healy.
© 2012 Blackwell Publishing Ltd. Published 2012 by Blackwell Publishing Ltd.

Table 33.1 Cochrane reviews of treatments for endometriosis.

Review title	Author (year of most recent update)	No. of RCTS/ women	Main outcomes	Conclusions	Research recommendations	Linked to recommendations in ESHRE guidelines with strength and level of evidence
Non-steroidal anti-inflammatory drugs for pain in women with endometriosis [4]	Allen et al	1/24	Relief of pain, adverse events	There is inconclusive evidence to show whether NSAIDs (naproxen) are effective in managing pain caused by endometriosis. Women using NSAIDs need to be aware of the possibility that these drugs may cause unintended effects	Further research is required	No ESHRE recommendation
Progestagens and antiprogestagens for pain associated with endometriosis [8]	Prentice et al (2000)	7/576	Pain relief Adverse events	The limited available data suggest that both continuous progestagens and antiprogestagens are effective therapies in the treatment of painful symptoms associated with endometriosis	More research required	A, level 1a Suppression of ovarian function for 6 months reduces endometriosis-associated pain. The hormonal drugs investigated (COC, danazol, gestrinone, MPA and GnRHa) are equally effective but their side-effects and cost profiles differ
Danazol for pelvic pain associated with endometriosis [9]	Selak et al (2007)	5/370	Relief of pain Adverse effects	Danazol is effective in treating the symptoms and signs of endometriosis. However, its use is limited by the occurrence of androgenic side-effects	Further research is unlikely	A, level 1a Suppression of ovarian function for 6 months reduces endometriosis-associated pain. The hormonal drugs investigated (COC, danazol, gestrinone, MPA and GnRHa) are equally effective but their side-effects and cost profiles differ
Modern combined oral contraceptives for pain associated with endometriosis [10]	Davis et al (2007)	1/57	Relief of pain	Adverse effects	The limited data suggest that there is no evidence of a difference in outcomes between the oral contraceptive pill (OCP) and GnRHa in treating endometriosis-associated pain	Further research is required
Pre- and postoperative medical therapy for endometriosis surgery [27]	Yap et al (2004)	11/946	Pain scores AFS scores Patient satisfaction Pregnancy. Adverse events	There is insufficient evidence from the studies identified to conclude that hormonal suppression in association with surgery for endometriosis is associated with a significant benefit with regard to any of the outcomes identified. There may be a benefit	More research required	A, Level 1b Treatment with danazol or a GnRHa after surgery does not improve fertility compared with expectant management Treatment with danazol or GnRHa for 6 months after surgery reduced endometriosis-associated pain and delays recurrences at 12 and 24 months

Review	Author (year)	Studies/participants	Outcome measures	Findings	Research recommendation	ESHRE recommendation
Gonadotropin-releasing hormone analogs (GnRHa) for endometriosis: bone mineral density [30]	Sagsveen et al (2003)	15/910	Bone mineral density (BMD)	Both danazol and progesterone + estrogen add-back have been shown to be protective of BMD, while on treatment and up to 6 and 12 months later. However, by 24 months of follow-up there was no difference in BMD in those women who had HRT add-back. The significant side-effects associated with danazol limit its use	Future research should consider the dose regimens of estrogen and progesterone add-back therapy, the length of treatment and duration of response. Alternatives to HRT should also be investigated further, particularly calcium-regulating agents	No ESHRE recommendation
LNG-IUS for symptomatic endometriosis following surgery [35]	Abou-Setta et al (2006)	1/40	LNG-IUS for symptomatic endometriosis following surgery	One small study has shown that postoperative use of the LNG-IUS reduces the recurrence of painful periods in women who have had surgery for endometriosis	Further research is required	No ESHRE recommendation
Laparoscopic surgery for pelvic pain associated with endometriosis [36]	Jacobson et al (2001)	1/74	Pain relief; Adverse events	The combined surgical approach of laparoscopic laser ablation, adhesiolysis and uterine nerve ablation is likely to be a beneficial treatment for pelvic pain associated with minimal, mild and moderate endometriosis	More research required	A, level 1b; Ablation of endometriotic lesions and LUNA in minimal-moderate disease reduces pain at 6 months compared to diagnostic laparoscopy
Excisional surgery versus ablative surgery for ovarian endometriomata [37]	Hart et al (2008)	2/164	Pregnancy; Relief of pain and recurrence of cyst	Some evidence that excisional surgery for endometriomata provides for a more favorable outcome	More research required in women undergoing ART	A, Level 1b; Laparoscopic cystectomy for ovarian endometrioma >4 cm improves fertility compared to drainage and coagulation. Drainage and coagulation are associated with ↑ risk of recurrence
Long-term pituitary downregulation before IVF for women with endometriosis [38]	Sallam et al (2006)	3/165	Pregnancy outcomes	The administration of GnRH agonists for a period of 3–6 months prior to IVF or ICSI in women with endometriosis increases the odds of clinical pregnancy four-fold	More research required	A, Level 1b; Prolonged treatment with a GnRHa before IVF in moderate-severe endometriosis should be considered and discussed with patients because improved pregnancy rates have been reported
Ovulation suppression for endometriosis [39]	Hughes et al (2007)	23/3043	Pregnancy; Adverse effects	There is no evidence of benefit in the use of ovulation suppression in subfertile women with endometriosis who wish to conceive	No further research is indicated	A, level 1a; Suppression of ovarian function to improve infertility in minimal-mild endometriosis is not effective and should not be offered for this indication alone. There is no evidence of its effectiveness in more severe disease
Laparoscopic surgery for subfertility associated with endometriosis [40]	Jacobson et al (2009)	2/437	Pregnancy; Adverse events	The use of laparoscopic surgery in the treatment of minimal and mild endometriosis may improve success rates	More research required	A, level 1a; Ablation of endometriotic lesions plus adhesiolysis to improve fertility in minimal-mild endometriosis is effective compared to diagnostic laparoscopy alone

ART, assisted reproductive technologies; COC, combined oral contraceptive; ESHRE, European Society of Human Reproduction and Embryology; GnRH, gonadotropin releasing hormone; HRT, hormone replacement therapy; ICSI, intracytoplasmic sperm injection; IVF, in vitro fertilization; LNG-IUS, levonorgestrel-releasing intrauterine system; LUNA, laparoscopic uterine nerve ablation; MPA, medroxyprogesterone acetate; NSAID, non-steroidal anti-inflammatory drug.

Key to Table 33.1

	Grades of recommendations
A	Requires at least one randomized controlled trial as part of a body of literature of overall good quality and consistency addressing the specific recommendation. (Evidence levels 1a, 1b)
B	Requires the availability of well-controlled clinical studies but no randomized clinical trials on the topic of recommendations. (Evidence levels 2a, 2b, 3)
C	Requires evidence obtained from expert committee reports or opinions and/or clinical experiences of respected authorities. Indicates an absence of directly applicable clinical studies of good quality. (Evidence level 4)
GPP	Recommended best practice based on the clinical experience of the guideline development group.
Level	**Hierarchy of evidence**
1a	Systematic review and meta-analysis of randomized controlled trials (RCTs)
1b	At least one RCT
2a	At least one well-designed controlled study without randomization
2b	At least one other type of well-designed quasi-experimental study
3	Well-designed, non-experimental, descriptive studies, such as comparative studies, correlation studies or case studies

Table 33.2 Summary of research conclusions from systematic reviews in the ESHRE guidelines.

Effectiveness demonstrated and no further research is indicated	2007 Danazol for pelvic pain associated with endometriosis 2002 Gonadotropin-releasing hormone analogs for endometriosis: bone mineral density
Likely to be effective but further research indicated	2000 Progestagens and antiprogestagens for pain associated with endometriosis 2002 Laparoscopic surgery for subfertility associated with endometriosis 2001 Laparoscopic surgery for pelvic pain associated with endometriosis 2006 LNG-IUS for symptomatic endometriosis following surgery 2006 Long-term pituitary downregulation before IVF for women with endometriosis 2006 Excisional surgery versus ablative surgery for ovarian endometriomata
Inconclusive and further studies required	2004 Pre- and postoperative medical therapy for endometriosis surgery 2005 Non-steroidal anti-inflammatory drugs for pain in women with endometriosis 2007 Modern combined oral contraceptives for pain associated with endometriosis
Inconclusive results but further studies unlikely	2007 Ovulation suppression for endometriosis

Inevitably, even with systematic reviews of RCTs that are updated on an ongoing basis, there will be RCTs published recently – or unpublished – that may sway the evidence base, but these may not yet have been included in a systematic review. Thus it is important to maintain vigilance in the literature and gray literature for interventions proven to be effective in recent trials that may not yet have been accepted into consensus best practice.

Randomized controlled trial evidence for interventions

Non-hormonal medical treatments

Non-steroidal anti-inflammatory drugs

A systematic review [4] included one small cross-over RCT (24 women with mild-to-severe endometriosis) comparing non-steroidal anti-inflammatory drugs (naproxen) with placebo. The RCT was underpowered to show a significant difference for pain relief (odds ratio (OR) 3.3, 95% confidence interval (CI) 0.6–17.7) [4].

One RCT assessed the efficacy of the cyclo-oxygenase (COX)-2 inhibitor rofecoxib, but rofecoxib has been withdrawn worldwide owing to cardiovascular side-effects.

Pentoxifylline

Recent RCTs have assessed the value of pentoxifylline, a tumor necrosis factor (TNF)-α inhibitor, believed to function through an immunomodulating mechanism, amongst women who had undergone laparoscopic surgery for endometriosis. One small RCT (34 women) suggested that visual analog pain scores (VAS) were significantly improved at 2 and 3 months in women receiving pentoxifylline versus placebo [5]. Another RCT (104 women) did not show a significant fertility benefit in women treated with pentoxifylline [6]. Clearly more research is required.

Hormonal medical treatments

Most of the RCT evidence suggests that medical hormonal treatments, in the form of either the combined oral contraceptive pill (OCP), progestins, gestrinone, danazol and gonadotropin-releasing hormone analogs (GnRHa), are effective at treating pain related to endometriosis, but that all have side-effects, and there is no clear and consistent evidence of benefit of one agent over another.

Hormonal treatments versus placebo

Four systematic reviews of RCTs [7–10] assessing 6 months of continuous ovulation suppression (using OCP, danazol, gestrinone, GnRHa, or medroxyprogesterone acetate) found that all treatments reduced severe and moderate pain, and were similarly effective. Two additional RCTs [11,12], one subsequent RCT [13], and six further RCTs [14–19] assessing danazol, gestrinone or GnRHa were consistent with the systematic review findings. Three RCTs (155 women) identified by the reviews [8–10] found that danazol, GnRHa and medroxyprogesterone acetate all significantly reduced pain at

3–6 months compared with placebo. One RCT (22 women) identified by the second review [9] found no significant difference between dydrogesterone 40 or 60 mg versus placebo in the proportion of women who had pain relief, but it may have been underpowered to detect a clinically important difference. A subsequent RCT of 96 women showed significant benefit of OCP versus placebo for treating dysmenorrhea [20]. A further RCT of 217 women showed that OCP, whether given cyclically or continuously, reduces the chance of endometrioma recurrence after surgical removal [21].

These systematic reviews [7–10] also demonstrated that adverse effects of hormonal treatments are common, and include hot flushes and bone loss with GnRHa or gestrinone and androgenic adverse effects with danazol.

Comparison of hormonal treatments

Oral contraceptive pill versus progestins

One RCT (90 women with rectovaginal endometriosis and persistent pain after conservative surgery) showed a similar reduction in visual analog scores (VAS) for ethinylestradiol 0.01 mg plus cyproterone acetate 3 mg daily compared to norethindrone acetate 2.5 mg daily for dysmenorrhea (mean reduction of VAS 63.7 [standard deviation (SD) 23.3] versus 72.8 [22.5]), non-menstrual pelvic pain (27.5 [31.2] versus 43.0 [21.7]), dysmenorrhea (35.6 [28.3] versus 37.6 [22.2]), and dyschezia (42.9 [22.0] versus 45.7 [21.8]) [14].

Oral contraceptive pill versus gonadotropin-releasing hormone agonist

One RCT [22] of 57 women with laparoscopically diagnosed endometriosis and moderate or severe pain found that the GnRHa goserelin (3.6 mg subcutaneous depot formulation monthly for 6 months of treatment) was significantly more effective for relief of dysmenorrhea than OCP (21/24 [88%] with goserelin versus 0/25 [0%] with OCP; OR 33.1, 95% CI 10.8–101.0). After 6 months of follow-up without treatment, all women improved (24/24 [100%] with goserelin versus 25/25 [100%] with OCP). There was no significant difference between OCP and goserelin in the relief of dyspareunia or non-menstrual pain at the end of 6 months of treatment (OR 0.93, 95% CI 0.25–3.53) [22]. One additional RCT (102 women) compared OCP for 12 months versus OCP for 4 months followed by GnRHa for 8 months [11]. It found no significant difference in the proportion of women with pain (either menstrual or non-menstrual) at 12 months (menstrual pain 14/47 [29.8%] with OCP versus 16/55 [29.1%] with OCP followed by GnRHa; non-menstrual pain 15/47 [31.9%] with OCP versus 17/55 [30.9%] with OCP for 4 months followed by GnRHa; reported as non-significant, CI not reported). One subsequent RCT found that GnRHa (with and without add-back estrogen/progestin) for 12 months significantly reduced dysmenorrhea, pelvic pain, and dyspareunia compared with OCP for 12 months (133 women, pain measured on VAS after 6 months follow-up [range not reported]; dysmenorrhea: 3.1 with leuprolide acetate plus norethindrone versus 3.4 with leuprolide acetate versus 4.9 with estroprogestin; P=0.01; pelvic pain: 3.7 with leuprolide acetate plus norethindrone versus 3.2 with leuprolide

acetate versus 5.9 with estroprogestin; P=0.01; dyspareunia: 2.7 with leuprolide acetate plus norethindrone versus 2.2 versus leuprolide acetate versus 3.9 with estroprogestin; P=0.01 for leuprolide acetate plus norethindrone versus estroprogestin) [13].

Progestin versus gonadotropin-releasing hormone agonist

One RCT of 253 women found no significant difference in relief of pain symptoms for dienogest versus the intranasal GnRHa, buserelin acetate [23].

Danazol versus gestrinone

One RCT (269 women), comparing danazol 200 mg daily versus gestrinone 2.5 mg twice weekly [24] found no significant difference in dysmenorrhea over 6 months of treatment between danazol and gestrinone (reported as non-significant, results presented graphically), although both groups significantly improved from baseline (P>0.001).

Danazol versus gonadotropin-releasing hormone agonist

The first systematic review identified 15 RCTs (1299 women) comparing GnRHa versus danazol [7]. After 6 months of treatment, the review found no significant difference in menstrual pain (five RCTs, 386 women; relative risk [RR] 1.09, 95% CI 0.99–1.20), dyspareunia (six RCTs, 476 women; RR 0.98, 95% CI 0.93–1.02), or resolution of endometrial deposits (three RCTs, 426 women; RR 0.84, 95% CI 0.56–1.26) [7]. A further RCT (59 women) found no significant differences in the improvement of total symptom severity score (TSSS) that included pelvic pain, dysmenorrhea and dyspareunia after 180 days of treatment for the GnRHa nafarelin (mean reduction in TSSS 4.2 [SD 2.4]) compared to danazol (mean reduction in TSSS 4.6 [SD 1.7]) (P=0.502) [15].

Gestrinone versus gonadotropin-releasing hormone agonist

One RCT identified by the second systematic review [8] found that gestrinone modestly, but significantly, reduced dyspareunia after 6 months' treatment compared with GnRHa (measured on VAS [range 0–10]: weighted mean difference [WMD] −1.16, 95% CI −2.08 to −0.24). GnRHa significantly reduced dysmenorrhea compared with gestrinone (WMD 0.82, 95% CI 0.15–1.49). The RCT found no significant difference in non-menstrual pain between gestrinone and GnRHa (WMD −0.41, 95% CI −1.76 to +0.94). It found that gestrinone significantly reduced dysmenorrhea, dyspareunia, and non-menstrual pain compared with GnRHa after 6 months follow-up (dysmenorrhea WMD −3.00, 95% CI −4.79 to −1.21; dyspareunia WMD −2.34, 95% CI −3.60 to −1.02; non-menstrual pain WMD −2.30, 95% CI −3.70 to −0.90).

Medroxyprogesterone acetate versus oral contraceptive pill plus danazol

One RCT (80 women) identified by the second review [8] compared medroxyprogesterone acetate (150 mg every 3 months) versus OCP plus danazol 50 mg daily. It found that medroxyprogesterone acetate was more effective at reducing dysmenorrhea, but not dyspareunia or non-menstrual pain (CI not reported).

Medroxyprogesterone acetate versus gonadotropin-releasing hormone agonist

One RCT (double blind, 48 women with endometriosis treated for 6 months and followed for 1 year after allocation) compared medroxyprogesterone acetate versus GnRHa [12]. It found that both treatments significantly improved symptoms attributable to endometriosis, sleep disturbances, and anxiety–depression scores from baseline measurements ($P > 0.05$ for all outcomes). It found no significant difference between treatments (reported as non-significant, CI not reported). Two further RCTs assessed the efficacy of subcutaneous depot medroxyprogesterone acetate versus the GnRHa leuprolide acetate (both 3-monthly injections) in a North American population (274 women) [16] and a population from Europe, Asia, Latin America and New Zealand (300 women) [17]. These two equivalence trials both found equivalent reductions in all pelvic pain symptoms (that included dysmenorrhea, dyspareunia and pelvic pain) at 12-month follow-up after 6 months of therapy [16,17].

Levonorgestrel-releasing intrauterine system versus gonadotropin-releasing hormone agonist

One RCT (82 women) showed similar efficacy for the levonorgestrel-releasing intrauterine system (LNG-IUS) versus the depot GnRHa leuprolelin in reduction of VAS for chronic pelvic pain (post-treatment change in VAS scores not specified, P-value for the difference in VAS change >0.999) [18].

Medroxyprogesterone acetate versus danazol

One RCT identified by the second review [8] compared three treatments: medroxyprogesterone acetate, danazol, and placebo. The RCT found no significant difference in pelvic pain and total symptoms between medroxyprogesterone acetate and danazol after 6 months of treatment (34 people, four-point verbal rating scale; pelvic pain WMD +0.10, 95% CI –0.26 to +0.46; sum of all symptoms WMD +0.50, 95% CI –1.10 to +2.10). The RCT found that medroxyprogesterone acetate reduced total symptoms compared with danazol, but it found no significant difference in pelvic pain after 6 months' follow-up (four-point verbal rating scale, pelvic pain WMD +0.23, 95% CI –0.11 to +0.57; total symptoms WMD –3.40, 95% CI –4.83 to –1.97) [8].

Implanon versus medroxyprogesterone acetate

One RCT of 41 women found no significant difference in improving pain scores for these two treatments [25].

Adverse effects

These systematic reviews [7–10] also demonstrated differences in adverse effects of hormonal treatments. Two RCTs found that OCP reduced bone mineral density loss, hot flushes, insomnia, and vaginal dryness compared with GnRHa. One RCT found that danazol increased withdrawal because of adverse effects compared with GnRHa. One RCT identified by a systematic review found that GnRHa plus add-back estrogen or estrogen/progestin reduced short-term loss in bone mineral density compared with GnRHa alone.

Medical hormonal treatment versus surgical treatment

Laparoscopic removal versus gonadotropin-releasing hormone agonist hormonal treatment

One RCT (35 women with minimal-to-moderate endometriosis) assessed primarily treatment costs of laparoscopic ablation or excision with helium thermal coagulator versus 6 months of treatment with the GnRHa Zoladex [26]. This RCT found that the women who were symptom free 12 months after their treatment included nine out of 17 treated surgically and three out of 18 treated with GnRHa [26].

Medical treatment as an adjunct to surgery

There is little evidence to support routine preoperative or postoperative medical treatment as an adjunct to surgery, when outcomes of relevance to patients, including pain, are considered.

Preoperative hormonal treatment

One systematic review [27] and one additional RCT [28] provided RCT evidence. The systematic review (search date 2003) found that hormonal treatment before surgery significantly improved American Fertility Society (AFS) scores compared with no presurgical hormone treatment (one RCT, 80 people; WMD –9.60, 95% CI –11.42 to –7.78). However, the RCT did not report on pain outcomes, which are of much greater relevance to women [27]. The additional RCT (48 women with moderate or severe endometriosis) compared 3 months GnRHa treatment using goserelin before surgery with no preoperative hormonal treatment, and found similar symptoms in both groups at 6 months after surgery [28]. It also found no significant difference in the proportion of women whose surgery was rated as "moderately" or "very" difficult (14/20 [70%] with goserelin before surgery versus 20/27 [74%] with no treatment before surgery; RR 0.94, 95% CI 0.60–1.50).

Pre- and postoperative hormonal treatment

Hormonal treatment before surgery versus hormonal treatment after surgery

One systematic review [27] reported on one RCT comparing 6 months of nafarelin before surgery versus surgery followed by 6 months of nafarelin [29]. It found that 6 months of nafarelin 200 5g before surgery significantly reduced symptom scores compared with 6 months of nafarelin 200 5g after surgery (75 women with moderate or severe endometriosis; mean AFS score: 0 with nafarelin before surgery versus 6 with nafarelin after surgery; $P = 0.007$) [29]. It found no significant difference in ease of surgery as assessed by the surgeon (proportion of women judged easy to treat: 14/25 [56%] with nafarelin before surgery versus 10/28 [36%] with no treatment before surgery; RR 1.60, 95% CI 0.86–2.90) [29]. It also found no significant difference in pelvic pain between hormonal treatment before and after surgery (RR 1.01, 95% CI 0.49–2.07) [29].

Hormonal treatment before and after surgery versus hormonal treatment after surgery

One systematic review [27] reported on one RCT [29] comparing 6 months of intramuscular triptorelin 3.75 mg before and after surgery versus intramuscular triptorelin 3.75 mg after surgery. It found no significant difference in AFS scores between groups (25 people with ovarian endometrioma >3 cm unilateral/bilateral; total AFS score: WMD +3.49, 95% CI −5.10 to +12.08; implant AFS score: WMD −0.37, 95% CI −1.17 to +0.43; adhesion AFS score: WMD +0.55, 95% CI −7.16 to +8.26). However, the RCT did not report on pain outcomes [29].

In an additional RCT, adverse events were reported frequently both in women receiving GnRHa before surgery and in women receiving no treatment (AR (absolute risk) for at least one adverse event: 18/21 [86%] with GnRHa versus 21/27 [78%] with no treatment; RR 1.1, 95% CI 0.8–1.4) [28]. The most frequently reported adverse effects were hot flushes and headaches, and these happened only in women receiving GnRHa (hot flushes: 13/21 [62%]; headaches: 6/21 [29%]). The RCT identified by the review [27] found that nafarelin was associated with hot flushes (96% with nafarelin before surgery versus 92% with nafarelin after surgery), vaginal dryness (43% with nafarelin before surgery versus 32% with nafarelin after surgery), and decreased libido (36% with nafarelin before surgery versus 36% with nafarelin after surgery) [29].

Postoperative hormonal treatments

One systematic review [27], one subsequent[31] and three additional RCTs [32–34] investigated hormonal treatment after surgery. The review (search date 2003, eight RCTs, 811 people) found that hormonal treatment after surgery significantly improved AFS scores compared with surgery alone or surgery plus placebo (search date 2003; WMD −2.30, 95% CI −4.02 to −0.58) [27]. The review found no significant difference in pain between groups at 12 or 24 months (12 months, three RCTs, 332 people: RR 0.76, 95% CI 0.52–1.10; 24 months, three RCTs, 312 people: RR 0.70, 95% CI 0.47–1.03), although no separate meta-analyses were performed for different drugs or treatment lengths.

The systematic review did not perform meta-analyses of adverse effects [27], although the side-effects of medical interventions have been described above.

Future clinical trials

Although the evidence base of RCTs for traditional medical therapies is extensive, there is always scope for further research. Despite proven effectiveness, the problem rests with the side-effects, extensively highlighted above, from the traditional hormonal medical treatments.

Recently it has been highlighted that, although many animal and *in vitro* studies have shown positive results, very few have gone on to even become phase II/III clinical trials, let alone be proven to be effective [2]. Of 25 registered clinical trials on endo-metriosis, listed as completed, only three have been published, whilst the remainder, a staggering 80%, remain unpublished [2]. Thus much more energy and work are required in this area.

Recently reported trials of newer treatments, including pentoxifylline, raloxifene and infliximab (an anti-tumor necrosis factor monoclonal antibody), have not lived up to the promise, in terms of effectiveness, that therapeutic rationale and animal studies had suggested [2]. It is often the case, however, that genuine clinical advances occur only very slowly and require much clinical research effort to demonstrate effectiveness of innovative treatments.

Randomized trials should also ideally be blinded to all concerned, particularly as the main outcomes of importance are subjective. Trials should focus their primary outcomes on the outcomes of most importance to women with endometriosis, including quality of life (very rarely reported in trials to date) and pain relief.

Whilst the "breakthrough" in curing the enigma that is endometriosis is likely to come in the form of a medical rather than surgical intervention, such a breakthrough remains elusive at present.

References

1. Selman TJ, Johnson NP, Zamora J, Khan KS. Gynaecologic surgery from uncertainty to science: evolution of randomized controlled trials. Hum Reprod 2008;23:827–831.
2. Guo SW, Hummelshoj L, Olive D et al. A call for more transparency of registered clinical trials on endometriosis. Hum Reprod 2009;24:1247–1254.
3. Johnson N, Farquhar C. Endometriosis. Clin Evid 2006;15:2449–2464.
4. Allen C, Hopwell S, Prentice A. Non-steroidal anti-inflammatory drugs for pain in women with endometriosis. Cochrane Database Syst Rev 2009;2:CD004753.
5. Kamencic H, Thiel JA. Pentoxifylline after conservative surgery for endometriosis: a randomized, controlled trial. J Minim Invasive Gynecol 2008;15:62–66.
6. Creus M, Fabregues F, Carmona F et al. Combined laparoscopic surgery and pentoxifylline therapy for treatment of endometriosis-associated infertility: a preliminary trial. Hum Reprod 2008;23:1910–1916.
7. Prentice A, Deary AJ, Goldbeck-Wood S et al. Gonadotrophin releasing hormone analogues for pain associated with endometriosis. Cochrane Library, Issue 1. Oxford: Update Software; 2005.
8. Prentice A, Deary AJ, Bland E. Progestagens and antiprogestagens for pain associated with endometriosis. Cochrane Database Syst Rev 2000;2:CD002122.
9. Selak V, Farquhar C, Prentice A et al. Danazol for pelvic pain associated with endometriosis. Cochrane Database Syst Rev 2007;4;CD000068.
10. Davis LJ, Kennedy SS, Moore J, Prentice A. Oral contraceptives for pain associated with endometriosis. Cochrane Database Syst Rev 2007;3:CD001019.
11. Parazzini F, Di Cintio E, Chatenoud L et al. Estroprogestin vs. gonadotrophin agonists plus estroprogestin in the treatment of endome-

triosis-related pelvic pain: a randomized trial. Eur J Obstet Gynecol Reprod Biol 2000;88:11–14.

12. Bergqvist A, Theorell T. Changes in quality of life after hormonal treatment of endometriosis. Acta Obstet Gynecol Scand 2001;80:628–637.

13. Zupi E, Marconi D, Sdracia M et al. Add-back therapy in the treatment of endometriosis-associated pain. Fertil Steril 2004;82:1303–1308.

14. Vercellini P, Pietropaolo G, de Giorgi O et al. Treatment of symptomatic rectovaginal endometriosis with an estrogen-progestogen combination versus low-dose norethindrone acetate. Fertil Steril 2005;84:1375–1387.

15. Cheng MH, Yu BKJ, Chang SP et al. A randomized, parallel, comparative study of the efficacy and safety of nafarelin versus danazol in the treatment of endometriosis in Taiwan. J Chin Med Assoc 2005;68:307–314.

16. Schlaff WD, Carson SA, Luciano A et al. Subcutaneous injection of depot medroxyprogesterone acetate compared with leuprolide acetate in the treatment of endometriosis-associated pain. Fertil Steril 2005;85:314–325.

17. Crosignani PG, Luciano A, Ray A et al. Subcutaneous depot medroxyprogesterone acetate versus leuprolide acetate in the treatment of endometriosis-associated pain. Hum Reprod 2005;21:248–256.

18. Petta CA, Ferriani RA, Abrao MS et al. Randomized clinical trial of a levonorgestrel-releasing intrauterine system and a depot GnRH analogue for the treatment of chronic pelvic pain in women with endometriosis. Hum Reprod 2005;20:1993–1998.

19. Cheung TH, Lo KW, Yim SF et al. Dose effects of progesterone in add-back therapy during GnRHa treatment. J Reprod Med 2005;50:35–40.

20. Harada T, Momoeda M, Taketani Y et al. Low-dose oral contraceptive pill for dysmenorrhoea associated with endometriosis: a placebo-controlled, double-blind, randomized trial. Fertil Steril 2008;90:1583–1588.

21. Serrachioli R, Mabrouk M, Frasca C et al. Long-term cyclic and continuous oral contraceptive therapy and endometrioma recurrence: a randomized controlled trial. Fertil Steril 2010;93:52–56.

22. Vercellini P, Trespidi L, Colombo A et al. A gonadotropin-releasing hormone agonist versus a low-dose oral contraceptive for pelvic pain associated with endometriosis. Fertil Steril 1993;60:75–79.

23. Harada T, Momoeda M, Taketani Y et al. Dienogest is as effective as intranasal buserelin acetate for the relief of pain symptoms associated with endometriosis – a randomized, double-blind, multicenter, controlled trial. Fertil Steril 2009;91:675–681.

24. Bromham DR, Bookere MW, Rose GR et al. Updating the clinical experience in endometriosis—the European perspective. Br J Obstet Gynaecol 1995;102(suppl):12–16.

25. Walch K, Unfried G, Huber J et al. Implanon versus medrocyprogesterone acetate: effects on pain scores in patients with symptomatic endometriosis – a pilot study. Contraception 2009;79:29–34.

26. Lalchandani S, Baxter A, Phillips K. Is helium thermal coagulator therapy for the treatment of women with minimal to moderate endo-

metriosis cost-effective? A prospective randomized controlled trial. Gynecol Surg 2005;2:255–285.

27. Yap C, Furness S, Farquhar C. Pre and post operative medical therapy for endometriosis surgery. Cochrane Database Syst Rev 2004;3:CD003678.

28. Shaw R, Garry R, McMillan L et al. A prospective randomized open study comparing goserelin (Zoladex) plus surgery and surgery alone in the management of ovarian endometriomas. Gynaecol Endosc 2001;10:151–157.

29. Audebert A, Descampes P, Marret H et al. Pre or post operative medical treatment with nafarelin in Stage III–IV endometriosis: a French multicentred study. Eur J Obstet Gynecol Reprod Biol 1998;79:145–148.

30. Sagsveen M, Farmer JE, Prentice A et al. Gonadotrophin-releasing hormone analogues for endometriosis: bone mineral density. Cochrane Database Syst Rev 2003;4:CD001297.

31. Wong AYK, Tang L. An open and randomized study comparing the efficacy of standard danazol and modified triptorelin regimens for postoperative disease management of moderate to severe endometriosis. Fertil Steril 2004;81:1522–1527.

32. Morgante G. Low-dose danazol after combined surgical and medical therapy reduces the incidence of pelvic pain in women with moderate and severe endometriosis. Hum Reprod 1999;14:2371–2374.

33. Vercellini P, de Giorgi O, Mosconi P et al. Cyproterone acetate versus a continuous monophasic oral contraceptive in the treatment of recurrent pelvic pain after conservative surgery for symptomatic endometriosis. Fertil Steril 2002;77:52–61.

34. Vercellini P, Frontino G, de Giorgi O et al. Comparison levonorgestrel-releasing intrauterine device versus expectant management after conservative surgery for symptomatic endometriosis: a pilot study. Fertil Steril 2003;80:305–309.

35. Abou-Setta AM, Al-Inany HG, Farquhar C. Levonorgestrel-releasing intrauterine device (LNG-IUD) for symptomatic endometriosis following surgery. Cochrane Database Syst Rev 2006;4:CD005072.

36. Jacobson TZ, Barlow D, Garry R, Koninckx PR. Laparoscopic surgery for pelvic pain associated with endometriosis. Cochrane Database Syst Rev 2001;4:CD001300.

37. Hart RJ, Hickey M, Maouris P, Buckett W. Excisional surgery versus ablative surgery for ovarian endometriomata. Cochrane Database Syst Rev 2008;2:CD004992.

38. Sallam HN, Garcia-Velasco JA, Dias S, Arici A. Long-term pituitary down-regulation before in vitro fertilization (IVF) for women with endometriosis. Cochrane Database Syst REv 2006;1:CD004635.

39. Hughes E, Brown J, Collins JJ, Farquhar C, Fedorkow DM, Vanderkerchove P. Ovulation suppression for endometriosis. Cochrane Database Syst Rev 2007;3:CD000155.

40. Jacobson TZ, Duffy JMN, Barlow D, Farquhar C, Koninckx PR, Olive D. Laparoscopic surgery for subfertility associated with endometriosis. Cochrane Database Syst Rev 2009;3:CD001398.

34 Medical Therapies: Progestins

Andrew Horne and Hilary O.D. Critchley
MRC Centre for Reproductive Health, University of Edinburgh, Edinburgh, UK

Introduction

Progestins have been used successfully as therapy for endometriosis for approximately 50 years due to their safety, good side-effect profile and cost effectiveness [1,2]. Currently, continuous use of a low-dose monophasic combined oral contraceptive is probably the preferred treatment option for painful symptoms of endometriosis to prevent the effects of estrogen deprivation in women for whom a long period of therapy is anticipated. However, progestins should be considered when it is necessary to avoid the subjective and metabolic effects of estrogen, or in women who do not want to use contraception for cultural or religious reasons.

Mode of action

The precise mechanism by which progestins decrease the painful symptoms of endometriosis is not known due to a lack of basic understanding regarding the relationship of endometriosis and pelvic pain. There is good evidence supporting the association of endometriosis with painful symptoms, such as dysmenorrhea and dyspareunia, but it is difficult to prove that endometriosis causes pain [3]. More than 80% of women with endometriosis have other pain-related diagnoses and women with and without endometriosis can have identical pain symptoms [4]. Nevertheless, there is clear evidence that "removal" of lesions, either surgically or using pharmacological treatments, decreases pain [5].

There are three commonly suggested mechanisms for endometriosis-associated pain: the effects of active bleeding from endometriotic lesions, the production of growth factors and proinflammatory cytokines by activated macrophages and other cells associated with endometriotic lesions, and irritation or direct invasion of pelvic nerves [6].

The known effects of progestins on endometriotic lesions are detailed below and suggested mechanisms by which progestins decrease the painful symptoms of endometriosis are presented.

Ovarian suppression

It is likely that many progestins effectively treat endometriosis-related painful symptoms due to their suppression of ovulation (variable depending of the type of progestin and doses used) and a consequent decrease in active bleeding from the lesion sites [7].

Effects on endometrial morphology

Treatment with progestins changes endometrial morphology and this is likely to affect all three proposed mechanisms for endometriosis-related pain. Progestins can cause marked endometrial decidualization (such as the levonorgestrel intrauterine system delivering high-dose progestin) or atrophy (such as oral norethisterone) of both the eutopic endometrium and endometriotic lesions [8,9]. It is probable that this response is mediated by an as yet undetermined local mechanism rather than as a consequence of steroid hormone ligand-receptor binding [8,10].

Local modulation of the immune response

Progestins have been reported to modulate immune responses via suppression of interleukin (IL)-8 production in lymphocytes and increased nitric oxide production [11,12]. Progestins also reduce tumor necrosis factor (TNF)-α-induced nuclear factor-κ-B (NFκB) activation, preventing proliferation of endometriotic stromal cells [13].

Effects on angiogenesis

Progestins have also been suggested to work by inhibiting angiogenesis required for growth and development of endometriotic lesions [14,15]. Progesterone alone is proangiogenic, although this can be moderated by pretreatment with estrogen (reviewed in [16]). In a mouse model of endometriosis, the transcription of basic fibroblast growth factor (bFGF) can be suppressed by treatment with progesterone and dihydrodydrogesterone, and vascular endothelial growth factor (VEGFA) and cysteine-rich angiogenic inducer (CYR61) are suppressed by treatment with dihydrodydrogesterone and dydrogesterone [17].

Progesterone receptor expression and progesterone resistance

Emerging evidence for progesterone resistance in the endometrium of women with endometriosis may explain why progestins are effective in reducing pelvic pain but ineffective in improving pregnancy rates [10,18]. This may be explained by the extremely low progesterone receptor (PR) levels observed in ectopic and eutopic endometrium of women with endometriosis: PR-B is undetectable, and PR-A is markedly reduced [12,19]. In addition, a number of progesterone-regulated genes, for example IL-15, proline-rich protein, B61, Dickkopf-1, glycodelin, N-acetylglucos-amine-6-O-sulfotransferase, and G0S2, have been noted to be dysregulated in midsecretory (when progesterone levels are highest) eutopic endometrium of women with endometriosis compared to normal endometrium [20].

Evidence base for treating endometriosis with progestins

There is a paucity of good -quality comparable data relating to the use of progestins in the treatment of painful symptoms associated with endometriosis. Studies vary considerably in their protocols, inclusion and exclusion criteria, as well as in the drugs and doses administered. Nevertheless, a Cochrane systematic review of the literature concerning use of progestins for the treatment of painful symptoms due to endometriosis suggests that progestins are just as effective as other medical treatments of endometriosis [21]. A systematic review of medical treatment options for endometriosis that have been investigated in prospective randomized studies has shown that the progestins have the best clinical profile and a good cost-effectiveness balance [2]. Progestins administered to ovulating women in the luteal phase are not effective [21].

When the European Society for Human Reproduction and Embryology (ESHRE) published guidelines for treatment of endometriosis in 2005, the guideline group concluded that suppression of ovarian function for 6 months reduced endometriosis-associated pain [22]. In the review of the literature for this guideline exercise, data were included on the use of progestins, gestrinone and medroxyprogesterone acetate, and the conclusion after analysis of available data was that these compounds were equally effective as combined oral contraceptives and gonadotropin-releasing hormone (GnRH) agonists. At that time the guideline group were unable to make recommendations about other progestins or other routes of administration. The

ESHRE guidelines on endometriosis are currently being reviewed and updated. The American Society for Reproductive Medicine (ASRM) commented in their guideline published in 2008 that few studies had evaluated progestins alone for the treatment of endometriosis [6].

Route of administration

Progestins are available in many forms, including oral preparations, injections, subdermal implants and intrauterine systems. All of these routes of delivery have been studied for their effects on the painful symptoms of endometriosis, and are currently used as treatments in clinical practice.

Oral preparations

Norethisterone (norethindrone) acetate

Norethisterone (norethindrone) acetate (NA) (suggested dose 2.5 mg daily continuously) has been approved by the US Food and Drug Administration and Italian Ministry of Health for continuous administration to treat endometriosis. This is likely based on evidence of pain relief from two studies observing treatment over 6 months, one using increasing doses (5–20 mg) of NA alone (without placebo) until amenorrhea was achieved, and one comparing NA 10 mg daily to dienogest 2 mg daily [23,24]. NA's advantages for the long-term treatment of endometriosis include good control of uterine bleeding compared to other medical treatments, a positive effect on calcium metabolism and lack of negative effects on lipoprotein profiles [25]. Furthermore, a small study has recently shown that NA 2.5 mg daily may effectively relieve pain and gastrointestinal symptoms in women with colorectal endometriosis, particularly when the latter symptoms are related to the menstrual cycle [26]. There are also emerging data to support use of NA as an alternative to surgery for symptomatic rectovaginal endometriosis (reviewed in [27]). A recent randomized controlled trial compared the efficacy and tolerability of the aromatase inhibitor letrozole 2.5 mg daily combined with NA 2.5 mg daily versus NA 2.5 mg daily alone in treating painful symptoms due to rectovaginal endometriosis [28]. The combination drug regimen was more effective in reducing pain and deep dyspareunia than NA alone. However, letrozole caused a higher incidence of adverse effects, cost more and did not improve patients' satisfaction or influence recurrence of pain.

Medroxyprogesterone acetate

Medroxyprogesterone acetate (MPA) (suggested dose 15–50 mg daily continuously, optimum dosage not determined) has been studied in two randomized controlled trials, one comparing MPA 50 mg daily against placebo for 3 months and one comparing MPA 15 mg daily against the GnRH agonist nasal nafarelin 1 spray twice daily [29,30]. This demonstrated greater efficacy of MPA than placebo at alleviating pain and improving quality of life, but that administration of MPA was no better than the GnRH agonist.

The disadvantage of medroxyprogesterone in the long-term treatment of endometriosis is breakthrough bleeding [7].

Cyproterone acetate

Cyproterone acetate (CA) is an antiandrogen with weak progestational activity [31]. CA (suggested dose 10–12.5 mg daily continuously) has been studied in one randomized controlled trial when CA 12.5 mg daily was compared with the combined oral contraceptive desogestrel 0.15 mg/ethinylestradiol 0.02 mg for treatment of endometriosis [32]. Pain, sexual satisfaction and quality of life were substantially improved after 6 months' treatment in both groups but no major between-group differences were observed. The disadvantage of cyproterone is its side-effect profile: it is associated with depression, markedly decreased libido, hot flushes and vaginal dryness.

Dienogest

Good efficacy and tolerability of dienogest (suggested dose 2 mg daily continuously) in patients with endometriosis have been demonstrated in two randomized controlled trials over 24 weeks, one comparing dienogest 2 mg daily with the GnRH agonist buserilin acetate 0.9 mg daily intranasally and the other with leuprolide acetate 3.75 mg depot intramuscular injection every 4 weeks [33,34]. In both studies, dienogest had a substantially lower incidence of hot flushes and minimal change in bone mineral density and bone metabolism compared to the GnRH agonist. High-dose dienogest (20 mg daily) has also been reported in a pilot study to be effective in preventing progression of disease after surgical excision but further large-scale studies are required to confirm this finding [35].

Depot injections

Depot medroxyprogesterone acetate (DMPA) (150 mg intramuscular injection or 104 mg subcutaneously every 3 months) has been studied in a three randomized controlled trials [36–38]. The first study compared the intramuscular preparation against a combination of a monophasic combined oral contraceptive and danazol 50 mg/day and concluded that DMPA offers good analgesia with tolerable side-effects [38]. Patients on the progestin experienced a higher incidence of bloating and spotting but benefited from a greater incidence of amenorrhea. The second two studies compared subcutaneous DMPA 104 mg to the GnRH agonist leuprorelin 11.25 mg [36,37]. Both studies showed that DMPA was statistically equivalent to leuprorelin in reducing pain, and improving productivity and quality of life. A more recent randomized controlled trial investigated the optimal interval of injections of intramuscular DMPA (150 mg) in the long-term treatment of endometriosis-associated pain and confirmed that the optimum interval for administration was 3 months [39]. DMPA, however, has a number of disadvantages precluding its long-term use. Prolonged delay in the resumption of ovulation is a contraindication to the use of DMPA in women desiring pregnancy in the near future. Breakthrough bleeding can be significant. Furthermore, there are data to suggest that long-term users of DMPA may develop bone demineralization secondary to hypoestrogenism although the site specificity of the bone density deficit suggests that estrogen deficiency may not be the only route through which DMPA acts on the skeleton [40,41].

Subdermal implants

The single-rod 68 mg etonorgestrel-containing contraceptive implant (Implanon®; lifespan 3 years) has been shown to be comparable in efficacy up to 12 months in the treatment of pain (as measured by a visual analog scale score) in women with endometriosis to DMPA in a recent randomized controlled trial [42]. Thus, Implanon® may become an additional effective, safe and well-tolerated treatment option for women with endometriosis who need highly effective long-term contraception. Further clinical research is required in a larger population to determine the long-term effects of this treatment.

Intrauterine systems

The benefit of delivering levonorgestrel via an intrauterine route is that it can be administered at a high dose to the endometrium with few adverse effects (inducing glandular atrophy, decidual transformation of the stroma, a reduction in endometrial cell proliferation and an increase in apoptotic activity) [43]. The precise mechanism of action of the levonorgestrel intrauterine system (LNG-IUS) in endometriosis is unclear. However, antiproliferative changes (indicated by changes in the expression of proliferating cell nuclear antigen, Fas) in the ectopic endometrium of patients with pelvic pain and endometriosis treated with the LNG-IUS have been demonstrated [44,45]. Nonetheless, the intrauterine system releasing 0.02 mg/day of levonorgestrel (Mirena®) has been shown in a randomized controlled trial to have similar efficacy to a depot GnRH agonist in the control of endometriosis-related pain over a period of 6 months [46]. Other observational studies have reported similar positive effects on painful symptoms of endometriosis [27,47].

The LNG-IUS has also been suggested in a small study to be effective in relieving pelvic pain symptoms attributed to rectovaginal endometriosis [48] and in reducing the risk of recurrence of dysmenorrhea after conservative surgery [49]. Further trials are needed, however, to verify whether the good results observed are maintained during an entire 5-year period and to compare the effects of the LNG-IUS with those of other treatment options. The advantages of the LNG-IUS include the avoidance of the need for repeated administration, provision of highly reliable contraception and few hypoestrogenic side-effects. In addition, although the LNG-IUS is costly at the outset, the fact that it has long-term effects could mean that final costs are less than that of other medications. The major disadvantage of the LNG-IUS, like all progestins, is the unscheduled bleeding disturbances associated with it.

Table 34.1 Progestins used to treat endometriosis.

Progestin	Route	Efficacy in randomized controlled trial (RCT)	Dose	Specific advantages	Specific disadvantages
Norethisterone acetate (NA)	Oral	Not evaluated in RCT	2.5 mg daily	Good control of uterine bleeding Cheap Bone-sparing effect	Daily preparation Not contraceptive
Cyproterone acetate (CA)	Oral	Equivalent to desogestrel 0.15 mg /ethinylestradiol 0.02 mg	10–12.5 mg daily	Positive effect on acne and hirsuitism	Daily preparation Not contraceptive
Medroxyprogesterone acetate (MPA)	Oral	Equivalent to nasal nafarelin	15–50 mg daily	None identified	Unscheduled uterine bleeding Daily preparation Not contraceptive
	Intramuscular injection	Equivalent to ethinylestradiol 0.02 mg/ desogestrel 0.15 mg and danazol	150 mg every 3 months	Three-monthly administration Contraceptive Amenorrhea	Weight gain Unscheduled uterine bleeding
	Subcutaneous injection	Equivalent to leuprorelin 11.25 mg	104 mg every 3 months	Three-monthly administration Contraceptive Reportedly better side-effect profile than intramuscular preparation	None identified
Dienogest	Oral	Equivalent to buserilin acetate 900 μg daily intranasally and leuprolide acetate 3.75 mg depot intramuscular injection every 4 weeks	2 mg daily	Good control of uterine bleeding Bone-sparing effect	Daily preparation Not contraceptive
Etonorgestrel	Subcutaneous implant	Equivalent to depot medroxyprogesterone acetate 150 mg intramuscular injection every 3 months	168 mg every 3 years	Three-yearly administration Contraceptive	Unscheduled uterine bleeding
Levonorgestrel	Intrauterine system	Equivalent to leuprolide acetate 3.75 mg depot intramuscular injection every 4 weeks	52 mg every 5 years	Five-yearly administration Contraceptive	Unscheduled uterine bleeding

Side-effects of progestins

Unscheduled uterine bleeding is the most common side-effect of treatment with progestins [50]. Thus, it is very important to counsel women appropriately about likely bleeding side-effects prior to starting with this class of compound. A variety of treatment options have been explored, but none appear as reliable as time in reducing the extent of bleeding [51]. Other progestogenic side-effects include weight gain, mood changes, bloating, fatigue, depression, and nausea. Concern has also been raised that variations in serum lipid pattern observed with higher dose progestins may increase long-term atherogenic risk [24] but this concern has yet to be formally addressed due to the difficulties in designing long-term disease susceptibility studies.

Conclusion

In clinical studies, progestins have been shown to be as efficacious as other hormonal regimes for the treatment of endometriosis-related pain. The specific advantages and disadvantages of each preparation are detailed in Table 34.1. However, the exact mechanism by which progestins decrease endometriosis-associated pain is not known. Studies directed at understanding the precise effects of progestins on nociceptive, inflammatory and neuropathic pain in endometriosis are required to further knowledge of the pathophysiology and improve the treatment of endometriosis.

References

1. Vercellini P, Fedele L, Pietropaolo G, Frontino G, Somigliana E, Crosignani PG. Progestogens for endometriosis: forward to the past. Hum Reprod Update 2003;9(4):387–396.

2. Schroder AK, Diedrich K, Ludwig M. Medical management of endometriosis: a systematic review. IDrugs 2004;7(5):451–463.

3. Whiteside JL, Falcone T. Endometriosis-related pelvic pain: what is the evidence? Clin Obstet Gynecol 2003;46(4):824–830.

4. Howard FM. Endometriosis and mechanisms of pelvic pain. J Minim Invasive Gynecol 2009;16(5):540–550.

5. Fauconnier A, Chapron C. Endometriosis and pelvic pain: epidemiological evidence of the relationship and implications. Hum Reprod Update 2005;11(6):595–606.

6. American Society for Reproductive Medicine Practice Committee. Treatment of pelvic pain associated with endometriosis. Fertil Steril 2006;90(5 Suppl):S260–269.

7. Luciano AA, Turksoy RN, Carleo J. Evaluation of oral medroxyprogesterone acetate in the treatment of endometriosis. Obstet Gynecol 1988;72(3 Pt 1):323–327.

8. Guttinger A, Critchley HO. Endometrial effects of intrauterine levonorgestrel. Contraception 2007;75(6 Suppl):S93–98.

9. Schweppe KW. Current place of progestins in the treatment of endometriosis-related complaints. Gynecol Endocrinol 2001;15 (Suppl 6):22–28.

10. Bulun SE. Endometriosis. N Engl J Med 2009;360(3):268–279.

11. Raghupathy R, Al Mutawa E, Makhseed M, Azizieh F, Szekeres-Bartho J. Modulation of cytokine production by dydrogesterone in lymphocytes from women with recurrent miscarriage. Br J Obstet Gynaecol 2005 112(8):1096–101.

12. Schweppe KW. The place of dydrogesterone in the treatment of endometriosis and adenomyosis. Maturitas 2009;65(Suppl 1):S23–27.

13. Horie S, Harada T, Mitsunari M, Taniguchi F, Iwabe T, Terakawa N. Progesterone and progestational compounds attenuate tumor necrosis factor alpha-induced interleukin-8 production via nuclear factor kappa B inactivation in endometriotic stromal cells. Fertil Steril 2005;83(5):1530–1535.

14. Blei F, Wilson EL, Mignatti P, Rifkin DB. Mechanism of action of angiostatic steroids: suppression of plasminogen activator activity via stimulation of plasminogen activator inhibitor synthesis. J Cell Physiol 1993;155(3):568–578.

15. Smith OP, Critchley HO. Progestogen only contraception and endometrial break through bleeding. Angiogenesis 2005;8(2):117–126.

16. Rogers PA, Donoghue JF, Walter LM, Girling JE. Endometrial angiogenesis, vascular maturation, and lymphangiogenesis. Reprod Sci 2009;16(2):147–151.

17. Mönckedieck V, Sannecke C, Husen B et al. Progestins inhibit expression of MMPs and of angiogenic factors in human ectopic endometrial lesions in a mouse model. Mol Hum Reprod 2009;15(10):633–643.

18. Aghajanova L, Velarde MC, Giudice LC. Altered gene expression profiling in endometrium: evidence for progesterone resistance. Semin Reprod Med 2010;28(1):51–58.

19. Attia GR, Zeitoun K, Edwards D, Johns A, Carr BR, Bulun SE. Progesterone receptor isoform A but not B is expressed in endometriosis. J Clin Endocrinol Metab 2000;85:2897–2902.

20. Kao LC, Germeyer A, Tulac S et al. Expression profiling of endometrium from women with endometriosis reveals candidate genes for disease-based implantation failure and infertility. Endocrinology 2003;144(7):2870–2881.

21. Prentice A, Deary AJ, Bland E. Progestagens and anti-progestagens for pain associated with endometriosis. Cochrane Database Syst Rev 2000;2:CD002122.

22. Kennedy S, Bergqvist A, Chapron C et al, ESHRE Special Interest Group for Endometriosis and Endometrium Guideline Development Group. ESHRE guideline for the diagnosis and treatment of endometriosis. Hum Reprod 2005;20(10):2698–2704.

23. Moore C, Kohler G, Muller A. The treatment of endometriosis with dienogest. Drugs Today 1999;35(Suppl C):41–52.

24. Muneyyirci-Delale O, Karacan M. Effect of norethindrone acetate in the treatment of symptomatic endometriosis. Int J Fertil Womens Med 1998;43(1):24–27.

25. Riis BJ, Lehmann HJ, Christiansen C. Norethisterone acetate in combination with estrogen: effects on the skeleton and other organs: a review. Am J Obstet Gynecol 2002;187:1101–1106.

26. Ferrero S, Camerini G, Ragni N, Venturini PL, Biscaldi E, Remorgida V. Norethisterone acetate in the treatment of colorectal endometriosis: a pilot study. Hum Reprod 2010;25(1):94–100.

27. Vercellini P, Somigliana E, Viganò P, Abbiati A, Barbara G, Crosignani PG. Endometriosis: current therapies and new pharmacological developments. Drugs 2009;69(6):649–675.

28. Ferrero S, Camerini G, Seracchioli R, Ragni N, Venturini PL, Remorgida V. Letrozole combined with norethisterone acetate compared with norethisterone acetate alone in the treatment of pain symptoms caused by endometriosis. Hum Reprod 2009;24(12):3033–3041.

29. Bergqvist A, Theorell T. Changes in quality of life after hormonal treatment of endometriosis. Acta Obstet Gynecol Scand 2001;80(7):628–637.

30. Harrison RF, Barry-Kinsella C. Efficacy of medroxyprogesterone treatment in infertile women with endometriosis: a prospective, randomized, placebo-controlled study. Fertil Steril 2000;74(1):24–30.

31. Neumann F, Kalmus J. Cyproterone acetate in the treatment of sexual disorders: pharmacological base and clinical experience. Exp Clin Endocrinol 1991;98(2):71–80.

32. Vercellini P, de Giorgi O, Mosconi P, Stellato G, Vicentini S, Crosignani PG. Cyproterone acetate versus a continuous monophasic oral contraceptive in the treatment of recurrent pelvic pain after conservative surgery for symptomatic endometriosis. Fertil Steril 2002;77(1):52–61.

33. Harada T, Momoeda M, Taketani Y et al. Dienogest is as effective as intranasal buserelin acetate for the relief of pain symptoms associated with endometriosis – a randomized, double-blind, multicenter, controlled trial. Fertil Steril 2009;91(3):675–681.

34. Strowitzki T, Marr J, Gerlinger C, Faustmann T, Seitz C. Dienogest is as effective as leuprolide acetate in treating the painful symptoms of endometriosis: a 24-week, randomized, multicentre, open-label trial. Hum Reprod 2010;25(3):633–641.

35. Schindler AE, Christensen B, Henkel A, Oettel M, Moore C. High-dose pilot study with the novel progestogen dienogestin patients with endometriosis. Gynecol Endocrinol 2006;22(1):9–17.

36. Crosignani PG, Luciano A, Ray A, Bergqvist A. Subcutaneous depot medroxyprogesterone acetate versus leuprolide acetate in the treatment of endometriosis-associated pain. Hum Reprod 2006;21(1):248–256.

37. Schlaff WD, Carson SA, Luciano A, Ross D, Bergqvist A. Subcutaneous injection of depot medroxyprogesterone acetate compared with leuprolide acetate in the treatment of endometriosis-associated pain. Fertil Steril 2006;85(2):314–325.

38. Vercellini P, de Giorgi O, Oldani S, Cortesi I, Panazza S, Crosignani PG. Depot medroxyprogesterone acetate versus an oral contraceptive combined with very-low-dose danazol for long-term treatment of pelvic pain associated with endometriosis. Am J Obstet Gynecol 1996;175:396–401.

39. Cheewadhanaraks S, Peeyananjarassri K, Choksuchat C, Dhanaworavibul K, Choobun T, Bunyapipat S. Interval of injections of intramuscular depot medroxyprogesterone acetate in the long-term treatment of endometriosis-associated pain: a randomized comparative trial. Gynecol Obstet Invest 2009;68(2):116–121.

40. Cundy T, Evans M, Roberts H, Wattie D, Ames R, Reid IR. Bone density in women receiving depot medroxyprogesterone acetate for contraception. BMJ 1991;303(6793):13–16.

41. Walsh JS, Eastell R, Peel NF. Depot medroxyprogesterone acetate use after peak bone mass is associated with increased bone turnover but no decrease in bone mineral density. Fertil Steril 2010;93(3):697–701.

42. Walch K, Unfried G, Huber J et al. Implanon versus medroxyprogesterone acetate: effects on pain scores in patients with symptomatic endometriosis – a pilot study. Contraception 2009;79(1):29–34.

43. Viganò P, Somigliana E, Vercellini P. Levonorgestrel-releasing intrauterine system for the treatment of endometriosis: biological and clinical evidence. Womens Health 2007;3(2):207–214.

44. Bahamondes L, Bahamondes MV, Monteiro I. Levonorgestrel-releasing intrauterine system: uses and controversies. Expert Rev Med Devices 2008;5(4):437–445.

45. Gomes MK, Rosa-e-Silva JC, Garcia SB et al. Effects of the levonorgestrel-releasing intrauterine system on cell proliferation, Fas expression and steroid receptors in endometriosis lesions and normal endometrium. Hum Reprod 2009;24(11):2736–2745.

46. Petta CA, Ferriani RA, Abrao MS et al. Randomized clinical trial of a levonorgestrel-releasing intrauterine system and a depot GnRH analogue for the treatment of chronic pelvic pain in women with endometriosis. Hum Reprod 2005;20(7):1993–1998.

47. Lockhat FB, Emembolu JO, Konje JC. The evaluation of the effectiveness of an intrauterine-administered progestogen (levonorgestrel) in the symptomatic treatment of endometriosis and in the staging of the disease. Hum Reprod 2004;19(1):179–184.

48. Fedele L, Bianchi S, Zanconato G, Portuese A, Raffaelli R. Use of a levonorgestrel-releasing intrauterine device in the treatment of rectovaginal endometriosis. Fertil Steril 2001;75(3):485–488.

49. Vercellini P, Frontino G, de Giorgi O, Aimi G, Zaina B, Crosignani PG. Comparison of a levonorgestrel-releasing intrauterine device versus expectant management after conservative surgery for symptomatic endometriosis: a pilot study. Fertil Steril 2003;80(2):305–309.

50. Porter C, Rees MC. Bleeding problems and progestogen-only contraception. J Fam Plann Reprod Health Care 2002;28(4):178–181.

51. Warner P, Guttinger A, Glasier AF et al. Randomized placebo-controlled trial of CDB-2914 in new users of a levonorgestrel-releasing intrauterine system shows only short-lived amelioration of unscheduled bleeding. Hum Reprod 2010;25(2):345–353.

35 Medical Therapies: Aromatase Inhibitors

Serdar E. Bulun[1], Erkut Attar[2], Bilgin Gurates[2], You-Hong Chen[1], Hideki Tokunaga[3], Diana Monsivais[1] and Mary Ellen Pavone[1]

[1]Division of Reproductive Biology Research, Department of Obstetrics and Gynecology, Northwestern University Feinberg School of Medicine, Chicago, IL, USA

[2]Division of Reproductive Endocrinology and Infertility, Department of Obstetrics and Gynecology, Istanbul University, Istanbul Medical School, Istanbul, Turkey

[3]Department of Obstetrics and Gynecology, Tohoku University School of Medicine, Sendai, Japan

Introduction

Because endometriosis is an estrogen-dependent disease, standard medical treatments aim at either inducing hypoestrogenism or antagonizing estrogen action. However, almost all of these treatment modalities fail to treat endometriosis-associated pain. Recently, the aromatase enzyme has been demonstrated locally in endometriotic implants and a molecular etiology of endometriosis has been proposed [1]. Aromatase (estrogen synthetase) is the key enzyme in the synthesis of estrogens and mediates the conversion of androstenedione and testosterone to estrone and estradiol, respectively.

In the human, aromatase is expressed in a number of cells including ovarian granulosa cells, placental syncytiotrophoblasts, and testicular Leydig cells, as well as various extraglandular sites including the brain, adipose fibroblasts and skin fibroblasts [2]. The aromatase enzyme complex is composed of two polypeptides. One of these is a specific cytochrome, P450 (the product of the CYP19 gene) [3], which will be referred as P450 aromatase in this text. The second is a flavoprotein, NADPH-cytochrome P450 reductase, which is ubiquitously distributed in most cells.

Aromatase is an excellent target for inhibition of estradiol synthesis because it is the last step in steroid biosynthesis; therefore, there are no important downstream enzymes to be affected. In addition, although aromatase is a P450 enzyme and shares common features with other enzymes in this class (such as liver metabolizing enzymes and steroidogenic enzymes), it has unique features for the aromatizing reaction, making it amenable to selective inhibition [4]. Because of the importance of estrogen in stimulating endometriotic tissues and the *in situ* presence of aromatase in these tissues, the inhibition of estrogen synthesis is a rational approach to treatment [1,5].

Aromatase enzyme and endometriosis

In the ovary, the biologically active estrogen estradiol is produced from cholesterol through six serial enzymatic conversions in two cell types that co-operate in a paracrine fashion. The rate-limiting two steps include the entry of cholesterol into the mitochondrion facilitated by the steroid acute response (StAR) protein in theca cells and conversion of androstenedione to estrone by aromatase in granulosa cells. This key enzyme catalyzes the final and rate-limiting step in estrogen biosynthesis. Since there is a single gene for aromatase which encodes a single protein, targeting the aromatase protein by specific inhibitors effectively eliminates estrogen synthesis.

The aromatase enzyme is localized in the endoplasmic reticulum of estrogen-producing cells [6,7]. Estrogen synthesis by aromatase occurs not only in the ovary but also in a number of tissues throughout the body. Recent studies indicate that the transcription of the aromatase gene is highly regulated [8–10]. Aromatase catalyzes the formation of estrogen in several human tissues under the control of alternatively used promoters. Transcription of the aromatase gene in human tissues is regulated by at least 10 distinct promoters (Fig. 35.1).

The first exon of the aromatase gene is transcribed into aromatase mRNA but not translated into protein. Each promoter is regulated by a distinct signaling pathway in a tissue- and hormone-specific manner and gives rise to aromatase species with variable first exons but an identical coding region. For example, the placenta utilizes alternate exon I.1, the testis alternate exon II (promoter II-specific exon), adipose tissue I.3 and I.4 and brain If. Enhancers that react with upstream elements of these alternate exons markedly stimulate the rate of transcription of the aromatase gene. Thus, each tissue can regulate the amount of aromatase transcribed in a highly specific manner [9].

Extraovarian endometriotic tissue and ovarian endometrioma-derived cells almost exclusively use promoter II, which is the

Endometriosis: Science and Practice, First Edition. Edited by Linda C. Giudice, Johannes L.H. Evers and David L. Healy.
© 2012 Blackwell Publishing Ltd. Published 2012 by Blackwell Publishing Ltd.

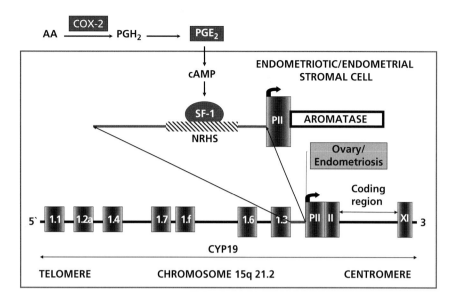

Figure 35.1 Molecular basis of extraovarian steroidogenesis in endometriotic tissues and endometrium of patients with endometriosis. Both endometriotic and endometrial stromal cells contain intact PGE_2 receptors that give rise to intracellular cAMP formation. cAMP induces binding of the transcription factor SF-1 to the proximal promoter II (PII) of the aromatase gene in endometriotic cells. SF-1 is primarily responsible for starting transcription of the aromatase gene. AA, arachidonic acid; cAMP, cyclic adenosine monophosphate; COX-2, cyclo-oxygenase-2; NRHS, nuclear receptor half site; PII, promoter II; PGE_2, prostaglandin E_2; PGG_2, prostaglandin G_2; SF1, steroidogenic factor-1.

prostaglandin E_2(PGE_2)/cyclic adenosine monophosphate (cAMP)-responsive proximal promoter, for aromatase expression *in vivo* [11–13]. Thus, aberrant aromatase expression in endometriosis is primarily mediated by promoter II (see Fig. 35.1).

Many molecular abnormalities have been demonstrated in endometriosis in contrast to eutopic endometrium of disease-free women. A clinically relevant abnormality is the presence of significant levels of StAR and aromatase activity in ectopic and eutopic endometrium of women with endometriosis. PGE_2 is the most potent inducer of StAR and aromatase in endometriotic stromal cells. A transcription factor, steroidogenic factor 1 (SF-1), is also aberrantly expressed and binds to steroidogenic promoters in endometriotic tissues. SF-1 mediates PGE_2-cAMP dependent co-activation of multiple steroidogenic genes, most notably StAR and aromatase [12] (see Fig. 35.1).

The enzyme cyclo-oxygenase-2 (COX-2) that catalyzes the key step in the conversion of arachidonic acid to PGE_2 is strikingly upregulated in stromal cells of endometriotic tissue and endometrium of the patients with endometriosis [14,15]. Additionally, the product of aromatase, estradiol, is a potent stimulator of COX-2 in uterine endothelial cells. Thus, a positive feedforward cycle involving StAR/aromatase, estradiol, COX-2 and PGE_2 favors continuous formation of estrogen and prostaglandin in endometriosis.

Expression of StAR, aromatase, and other steroidogenic genes enables endometriotic tissue to synthesize estradiol from cholesterol *de novo* [16,17]. However, StAR and/or aromatase expression is either absent or barely detectable in the endometrium of disease-free women. This implies that endometriotic aromatase is not solely dependent for substrate on adrenal or ovarian secretion.

Pharmacology of aromatase inhibitors

The aromatase inhibitors (AIs) are classified into type I (suicidal or non-competitive) inhibitors and type II (competitive) inhibitors [18,19] (Fig. 35.2). Both types of inhibitors compete

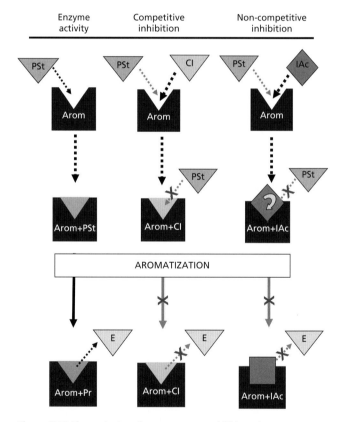

Figure 35.2 The mechanism of aromatase enzyme inhibitors. Arom, aromatase enzyme; Arom+CI, aromatase enzyme+competitive inhibitor; Arom+IAc, aromatase enzyme+ inactivator; Arom+Pr, aromatase enzyme+product; Arom+PSt, aromatase enzyme+precursor steroid; CI, competitive inhibitor; E, estrogen; IAc, inactivator; PSt, precursor steroid.

for binding to the active site. Once a type I inhibitor has bound, the enzyme initiates hydroxylation, which produces an unbreakable bond between the inhibitor and enzyme protein.

Enzyme activity is thus permanently blocked [20]. Exemestane is a type I (suicidal) inhibitor.

Type II inhibitors reversibly bind to the active enzyme site and no enzyme activity is triggered. The inhibitor can disassociate from the binding site, allowing renewed competition between the inhibitor and the substrate for binding to the site. As a result, continued activity requires constant presence of the inhibitor, and the effectiveness of competitive inhibitors depends on the affinities of the inhibitor and the substrate [20]. Anastrozole and letrozole are type II inhibitors.

Aromatase inhibitors were developed to act on sex steroid-dependent neoplasms by suppressing *in situ* estrogen production [21]. The first AI to be widely used in the treatment of metastatic breast cancer in postmenopausal women was the drug aminoglutethimide [22–26]. With further study of aminoglutethimide, multiple metabolic effects were demonstrated, including inhibition of 11β-hydroxylase, aldosterone synthase, and thyroxine synthesis as well as induction of enzymes metabolizing synthetic glucocorticoids and aminoglutethimide itself [27,28].

Eventually, increasing numbers of AIs have been introduced into clinical practice [29,30]. The second-generation AIs fadrozole and formestane have more specific effects on aromatase and less toxicity. In 1996, the third generation of AIs (exemestane, letrozole and anastrozole) was approved by the FDA. Anastrozole (Arimidex), letrozole (Femara) and exemestane (Aromasin) have been approved to treat advanced breast carcinoma in postmenopausal women [31–40].

Side-effects of aromatase inhibitors

The side-effect profile for AIs is reasonably benign, with mild headache, nausea, and diarrhea. Compared to gonadotropin releasing hormone (GnRH) analogs, hot flashes are milder and infrequent. There is a possible effect on the lipid profile, but more studies are needed to clarify this issue [41]. Long-term use of AIs carries the potential risk of osteoporosis and osteopenia. Most of the long-term data on bone fractures in breast cancer patients treated with AIs came from the ATAC (Anastrozole, Tamoxifen, Alone or in Combination) trial. Results from this trial after completion of adjuvant treatment of breast cancer for 5 years showed that the safety profile of anastrozole remains unchanged during the entire treatment period [42].

The overall fracture rate during 5 years of anastrozole treatment (7.1%) was significantly higher than that associated with tamoxifen (4.6%) treatment. Interestingly, the rate of spine fractures increased significantly, whereas no significant difference was found between anastrozole and tamoxifen treatments with respect to hip fractures [42]. We should point out here that tamoxifen is not an option for endometriosis treatment because it acts as an agonist in endometrium [43].

The LET+NEA (letrozole plus norethindrone acetate) pilot trial examined the risk of bone loss in premenopausal women. In this regimen, calcium citrate (1250 mg) and vitamin D (800 IU) were also given daily. Dual-energy x-ray absorptiometry (DEXA) scans for 10 individual patients showed that there was no bone density loss in nine of 10 subjects. Instead, a statistically significant overall improvement in hip bone density occurred ($P < 0.05$) [44].

The anastrozole plus an oral contraceptive pilot trial in the treatment of premenopausal patients with endometriosis showed no significant changes in bone density during 6 months of treatment [41]. On the other hand, a randomized controlled clinical trial using anastrozole plus the GnRH agonist goserelin showed significant bone loss after 6 months of treatment [45]. The observed bone mineral density (BMD) loss was significantly greater at 6 months in the goserelin plus anastrozole arm versus the goserelin only arm. This effect persisted even after cessation of treatment. However, none of the subjects became osteopenic or osteoporotic during the treatment and follow-up periods.

The regimens that combine AIs with add-back progestins or oral contraceptives do not appear to be associated with significant bone loss after 6 months of treatment and therefore may be suitable for long-term use [41,44].

Aromatase inhibitors in premenopausal women

Aromatase inhibitors inhibit estrogen production in at least four critical body sites: the brain, ovary, endometriosis, and the periphery (e.g. adipose tissue and skin) (Fig. 35.3). Both locally produced (brain and endometriosis) and circulating (ovary and periphery) estrogen make physiological and pathological impacts on target tissues (brain and endometriosis). Local estrogen production by brain aromatase is, in part, responsible for the suppression of follicle stimulating hormone (FSH) and luteinizing hormone (LH) secretion [46].

The amount of aromatase in the brain, endometriosis or periphery is small compared with overwhelming levels of aromatase in granulosa cells of the human Graafian follicle. Thus, it is likely that AIs inhibit aromatase activity in the brain, endometriosis and periphery totally, but only a part of aromatase activity is blocked in the ovary, thus accounting for the observations regarding bone mineral density and minimal hot flashes in women in clinical trials (above). Primate data support this interpretation [47].

Three early studies have examined estrogen levels in premenopausal women with breast cancer treated with aminoglutethimide [48–50]. These studies showed elevated gonadotropin concentrations indicating a partly compensated inhibition of ovarian estrogen synthesis. Studies using supratherapeutic levels of formestane also showed no significant impact on serum estradiol but elevated FSH and LH levels [51]. Vorozole, a third-generation AI, administered to premenopausal women suppressed plasma estradiol concentrations more efficiently, although a near-complete suppression could not be achieved as in the case of postmenopausal women [52]. However,

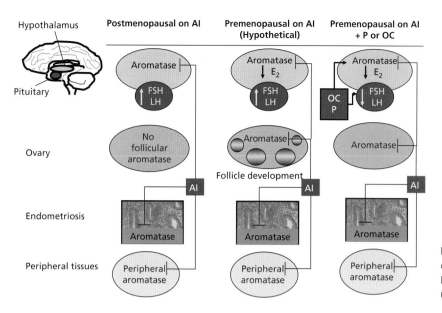

Figure 35.3 The effect of aromatase inhibitors in four critical body sites. AI, aromatase inhibitor; E$_2$, estradiol; FSH, follicle stimulating hormone; LH, luteinizing hormone; OC, oral contraceptive; P, progesterone.

AIs effectively suppress circulating estrogen concentrations in premenopausal women after the addition of a GnRH agonist [53].

The compensatory response to estradiol depletion in the hypothalamus results in higher serum FSH secretion and ovarian stimulation. Therefore, AIs increase follicular recruitment and may lead to ovarian stimulation and cyst formation [54]. By using their pharmacological effects on FSH secretion from the pituitary, third-generation AIs have been used in infertility treatment to induce ovulation. Clinical trials have shown that transient inhibition of aromatase activity in the early follicular phase results in moderate ovarian hyperstimulation similar to that seen with clomiphene citrate [55,56]. Additionally, letrozole reduces the gonadotropin dose required to induce follicular maturation especially in poor responders, and adjunctive use of letrozole may form an effective means of low-cost *in vitro* fertilization (IVF) protocols in these patients [57–59].

A group of premenopausal women with breast cancer were treated successfully with a combination of anastrozole and the GnRH agonist goserelin, without any evidence of ovarian stimulation [60]. Recent phase I studies have shown that the use of AIs with an oral contraceptive or progestin prevents ovarian stimulation and suppresss plasma estrogen concentrations to postmenopausal levels. Taken together, phase I studies on healthy premenopausal women and clinical approaches to ovulation induction and breast cancer treatment indicate that adjunctive therapy is recommended to suppress the ovaries when using AIs for the treatment of premenopausal women with endometriosis.

Aromatase inhibitors and endometriosis

Approximately half of the patients with chronic pain associated with endometriosis are refractory to currently available treatments that create a hypoestrogenic state including oral contraceptives

(OC), Depo-Provera, oral progestins and GnRH analogs [61–63]. The majority of these patients refuse to be treated with danazol because of its potential androgenic side-effects [64].

Conservative surgical removal of endometriosis provides some pain relief. Response to surgical treatment varies extensively and depends on many factors including the experience of the surgeon, previous attempts at treatment, use of adjuvant medical treatment and definition of the therapeutic endpoint [65–68]. Following conservative surgery, endometriosis often recurs at some point after surgery, and pain is usually more refractory to repeated surgical attempts. The immediate overall response of chronic pain to conservative surgery in an unselected population of women is approximately 50% [68]. The value of uterosacral nerve ablation or presacral nerve resection has not yet been clearly demonstrated, and the benefits of these adjunctive surgical approaches for endometriosis-associated pain remain controversial [65,66].

Currently, when no other medical options remain and minimally invasive surgery has failed, women resort to a total hysterectomy with or without bilateral salpingo-oopherectomy. Even after this invasive procedure, their pain may not be relieved [1,69,70]. The results of the five studies on the effect of hysterectomy on chronic pelvic pain of presumed uterine origin consistently demonstrated that 3–17% of operated women reported recurrence of pain 1 year after surgery [71].

Failure of current medical and surgical treatments to relieve pain prompted us and others to target the aromatase molecule in endometriosis using AIs. The rationale was that continued local estrogen production in endometriotic implants during other medical treatments (e.g. GnRH analogs) was, in part, responsible for resistance to these therapies. Anastrozole and letrozole have been successfully used to treat endometriosis [41,44,45,72–74]. Table 35.1 summarizes these clinical studies in endometriosis.

Table 35.1 The use of aromatase inhibitors in endometriosis: current clinical reports.

Year	Author	Study type	Indication	Medication	Length	Sample size	Outcome (6 mo)
1998	Takayama *et al*	Case report	Postmenopausal endometriosis not responding to surgical or medical treatment	A	9 months	1	Pain relief/reduced lesion size
2004	Razzi *et al*	Case report	Postmenopausal endometriosis not responding to surgical or medical treatment	L	9 months	1	Pain relief/reduced lesion size
2004	Ailawadi *et al*	Pilot prospective	Premenopausal endometriosis not responding surgical or medical treatment	L+NEA	6 months	10	90% pain relief/ 100% reduced lesion size
2004	Soysal *et al*	Randomized	Premenopausal endometriosis	A+GnRHa	6 months	80	100% pain relief
2004	Shippen *et al*	Case report	Premenopausal endometriosis not responding surgical or medical treatment	L+P	6 months	2	Pain relief/ reduced lesion size
2005	Amsterdam *et al*	Pilot prospective	Premenopausal endometriosis not responding surgical or medical treatment	A+OC	6 months	10	93% pain relief

A, anastrozole; A+GnRHa, anastrozole+gonadotropin releasing hormone analog; A+OC, anastrozole+oral contraceptive; L, letrozole; L+NEA, letrozole+norethindrone acetate; L+P, letrozole+progesterone.

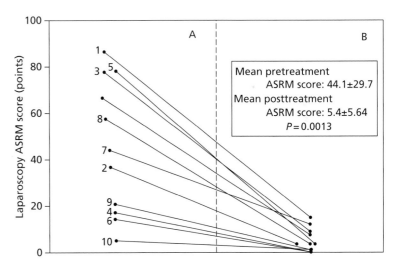

Figure 35.4 Pre- and post-treatment disease stages, based on ASRM endometriosis scores, for individual patients (n = 10). (A) Baseline: first-look laparoscopy 1 month before treatment. (B) One month post treatment: second-look laparoscopy 1 month after treatment. Determinations for each patient before and after treatment are interconnected.

Studies examining the combination of an aromatase inhibitor with a progestin or progesterone

A small phase II trial and a case report in which an aromatase inhibitor was administered together with a progestin and progesterone have been published. In the pilot trial, 10 premenopausal patients resistant to existing medical and surgical treatments of endometriosis were administered an AI (letrozole 2.5 mg) and a progestin (norethindrone acetate (NEA), 2.5 mg) daily for 6 months [44]. No control group was included. Endometriosis was evaluated by pretreatment and post-treatment laparoscopies, and pain scores determined by a visual analog scale [44]. Both pelvic pain scores and revised American Society for Reproductive Medicine (rASRM) laparoscopic scores decreased significantly (Fig. 35.4). Nine out of 10 patients responded to this regimen by decreased pelvic pain (Table 35.2). Side-effects were breakthrough bleeding, moodiness, sleepiness, and mild hot flashes. No

Table 35.2 Pain scores before and after treatment in two recent trials.

Regimen	L+NEA	A+OC	L+NEA	A+OC
Time	Baseline		6 months	
N	10	19	10	15
Mean	6.22	8.24	2.34	4.24
SD±	2.07	1.76	2.11	2.70

A+OC, anastrozole+oral contraceptive; L+NEA, letrozole+norethindrone acetate; N, number of patients; SD, standard deviation: $P < 0.01$ (L+NEA baseline versus 6 months); $P < 0.0001$(A+OC baseline versus 6 months).

significant bone loss was detected at the end of the 6-month therapy, and no evidence of ovarian enlargement was found by monthly bimanual examination during the therapy [44].

In a report by Shippen et al, an AI, anastrozole (1 mg/day), together with oral progesterone (200 mg/day) was given to two premenopausal sisters (24 and 26 years old) with advanced endometriosis for 6 months [72]. Both had their disease diagnosed by laparoscopy and failed to respond to oral contraceptives and nonsteroidal anti-inflammatory and analgesic medications. Neither patient could tolerate initial or repeated treatments with a GnRH agonist. Anastrozole and oral progesterone were given daily for 21 days followed by 7 days off, for a 28-day treatment cycle. Treatment resulted in a rapid, progressive reduction in symptoms over 3 months, with the maintenance of remission of symptoms for over 24 months post treatment in both cases. There was confirmation of absence of disease in one case by follow-up laparoscopy 15 months after treatment. Pregnancy was achieved in both cases after 24 months. Bone densitometries were in the mid-normal ranges 18 months after completion of treatment. Side-effects were minimal and well tolerated by both patients. Patients did not show ovarian hyperstimulation because of the additional progesterone.

In conclusion, in non-randomized trials the combination of an AI with a progestin or progesterone was successful in significantly decreasing pain and reducing the amount of visible endometriosis in patients who have not responded to or tolerated existing medical or surgical treatments. Side-effect profiles were favorable. No significant bone loss has been noted. These results were suggestive that the addition of a progestin (NEA) or progesterone in moderate doses to an AI suppresses gonadotropins sufficiently in the majority of premenopausal patients with endometriosis.

Use of an aromatase inhibitor together with a combination oral contraceptive

We published another prospective open label pilot study employing a novel regimen consisting of an AI plus a combination OC [41]. This trial recruited 19 subjects with endometriosis documented by laparoscopy or laparotomy. All subjects included in this study were premenopausal, had failed multiple other medical treatments for endometriosis, and had at least 6 months of pelvic pain. Patients were excluded if they were osteopenic, had a prior hysterectomy, hypercholesterolemia or hypertriglyceridemia. Fifteen of the 19

subjects completed this trial [41]. In this study, each subject was started on a daily regimen of anastrozole plus an oral contraceptive to be taken continuously for 6 months. Symptoms were evaluated via recording daily pain scores using the visual analog pain scale, and subjects kept a bleeding diary. A summary of the pain scores of the subjects for 6 months of therapy is shown in Table 35.2. A significant reduction in pain was noted at the end of the study. Pain scores fell starting at month 1 and continued to decrease with each subsequent month of treatment. There was a reduction in pelvic pain in 14 of 15 subjects who completed the study.

Use of AI+OC appears to be effective in controlling pain in premenopausal women with endometriosis. These results were particularly significant in light of the fact that the women in this study failed multiple other treatment modalities for endometriosis.

Combination of an aromatase inhibitor with a gonadotropin releasing hormone agonist

Soysal et al performed a randomized placebo-controlled trial to assess the clinical efficacy of anastrozole in conjunction with goserelin, compared to goserelin alone [45]. Eighty patients with severe endometriosis according to the rASRM (>40) criteria were enrolled in the study after conservative surgery [75]. A scale previously described by Biberoglu et al was used to obtain a total pelvic symptom score (TPSS) before the surgery [76]. The first group of subjects (n=40) received anastrozole 1 mg/day plus depot injections of 3.6 mg goserelin every 4 weeks, and the second group of subjects (n=40) received a placebo tablet in addition to the goserelin regimen for 24 weeks. Elemental Ca (600 mg/day) and vitamin D (800 IU/day) were also added to these treatment protocols. Exclusion criteria were further desire for child bearing, any treatment for endometriosis within the previous 3 months, concomitant disease that can be an established cause of chronic pelvic pain, osteopenia or osteoporosis, and any concomitant disease that can be a contraindication to goserelin or anastrozole. The primary outcome measures of this trial were the recurrence rate and the impact of allocated treatments on TPSS during the follow-up period of 24 months after the end of medical treatment. Thus, patients were evaluated at 24 weeks of medical treatment and at 6, 12, 18 and 24 months after the end of medical treatment.

Both treatment protocols proved to be effective in reducing the TPSS during the study period. However, the GnRH agonist plus AI regimen showed a more profound, stable and long-lasting effect on TPSS during the study period. It was found that the goserelin plus anastrozole regimen has a significantly longer time to recurrence than goserelin alone (>24 versus 17 months, respectively). At the end of the 24-month follow-up period, 54.7% of the subjects were free of pain recurrence in the GnRH agonist plus anastrozole arm versus 10.4% in the GnRH agonist only arm ($P < 0.0001$, Fig. 35.5). Additionally, the impact of treatment on TPSS and individual symptoms score reduction was statistically significant in favor of goserelin plus anastrozole. The effect of the combination treatment on TPSS was achieved at 6 months after the medical therapy and persisted until the end of

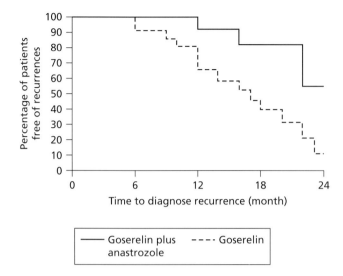

Figure 35.5 Kaplan–Meier curves for pain-free (recurrence-free) periods in patients treated with goserelin only versus goserelin plus anastrozole.

the 24-month follow-up period. Individual symptoms evaluated at 24 months from the completion of medical therapy were also significantly decreased ($P < 0.05$–0.0001). Based on these data, the authors concluded that a novel treatment regimen with an AI plus a GnRH analog following conservative surgery is effective to control recurrence and pain in patients with severe endometriosis.

Climacteric symptoms as a measure of life quality were not significantly different between anastrozole only versus anastrozole plus GnRH analog arms. Goserelin plus anastrozole treatment caused significantly higher bone loss at the spine compared with goserelin-only treatment after 6 months of treatment ($P < 0.01$). No significant difference between these groups, however, was observed at the 24-month follow-up.

Conclusion

The number of clinical trials employing AIs in the treatment of endometriosis strikingly increased after 2004. AIs appear to be the first breakthrough in the medical treatment of endometriosis since the introduction of GnRH agonists in the 1980s. A plausible mechanism of action of AIs has been uncovered and discussed briefly in this chapter; a broader discussion of mechanisms has been provided in other reviews [77]. Patients with endometriosis who do not respond to existing treatments appear to obtain significant pain relief from AIs. Most of the AI regimens consist of taking one or two tablets a day, and the side-effect profiles of the AI regimens (including a progestin or OC add-back) are more favorable compared to treatments using GnRH agonists or danazol. Thus, some of these regimens may potentially be administered over prolonged periods of time.

Aromatase inhibitors administered in combination with an ovarian suppressant comprise a promising and novel treatment of premenopausal endometriosis. The requirement for calcium,

vitamin D or bisphosphonate supplementation in premenopausal women needs further evaluation.

We predict that regimens including combinations of an AI with a progestin or OC will gain more popularity over the combination of an AI with a GnRH analog because the former are simpler, cheaper, associated with fewer side-effects, and may be administered for longer periods of time. Randomized clinical trials are needed to establish the efficacy and side-effects of these regimens. Lower doses of AIs may also be used potentially in the treatment of pain or infertility associated with endometriosis. The clinician should await future randomized trials before using AIs routinely for the treatment of endometriosis, as this class of drug is not approved by the US Food and Drug Administration or its equivalent elsewhere.

Acknowledgments

The work was carried out at the Division of Reproductive Biology Research, Department of Obstetrics and Gynecology, Northwestern University Feinberg School of Medicine with financial support from a NIH grant HD36891 and a grant from Friends of Prentice.

References

1. Zeitoun KM, Bulun SE. Aromatase: a key molecule in the pathophysiology of endometriosis and a therapeutic target. Fertil Steril 1999;72(6):961–969.

2. Simpson ER, Mahendroo MS, Means GD et al. Aromatase cytochrome P450, the enzyme responsible for estrogen biosynthesis. Endocrine Rev 1994;15:342–355.

3. Simpson ER, Clyne C, Rubin G et al. Aromatase – a brief overview. Annu Rev Physiol 2002;64:93–127.

4. Brodie A, Long B. Aromatase inhibition and inactivation. Clin Cancer Res 2001;7(12 Suppl):4343s–4349s; discussion 411s–412s.

5. Bulun SE, Zeitoun K, Takayama K et al. Estrogen production in endometriosis and use of aromatase inhibitors to treat endometriosis. Endocr Relat Cancer 1999;6(2):293–301.

6. Sebastian S, Takayama K, Shozu M, Bulun S. Cloning and characterization of a novel endothelial promoter of the human CYP19 (aromatase P450) gene that is up-regulated in breast cancer tissue. Mol Endocrinol 2002;16:2243–2254.

7. Simpson ER, Clyne C, Rubin G et al. Aromatase – a brief overview. Annu Rev Physiol 2002;64:93–127.

8. Simpson ER, Zhao Y, Agarwal VR et al. Aromatase expression in health and disease. Recent Prog Horm Res 1997;52:185–214.

9. Simpson ER, Mahendroo MS, Means GD, Kilgore MW, Corbin CJ, Mendelson CR. Tissue-specific regulation of aromatase cytochrome P450 expression. In: Schenkmon JB, Greim H (eds) Handbook of Experimental Pharmacology Cytochrome P450. Berlin: Springer-Verlag, 1993, pp. 611–625.

10. Simpson ER, Graham-Lorence S, Corbin CJ et al. Regulation of expression of the gene encoding aromatase cytochrome P450. In: Nunez J, Dumont JE (eds) Hormones and Cell Regulation. New Barnet, Herts: John Libby, 1992, pp. 49–55.

11. Noble LS, Takayama K, Putman JM et al. Prostaglandin E2 stimulates aromatase expression in endometriosis-derived stromal cells. J Clin Endocrinol Metab 1997;82:600–606.

12. Zeitoun K, Takayama K, Michael MD, Bulun SE. Stimulation of aromatase P450 promoter (II) activity in endometriosis and its inhibition in endometrium are regulated by competitive binding of SF-1 and COUP-TF to the same cis-acting element. Mol Endocrinol 1999;13:239–253.

13. Noble LS, Simpson ER, Johns A, Bulun SE. Aromatase expression in endometriosis. J Clin Endocrinol Metab 1996;81:174–179.

14. Wu M, Wang C, Lin C, Chen L, Chang W, Tsai S. Distinct regulation of cyclooxygenase-2 by interleukin-1{beta} in normal and endometriotic stromal cells. J Clin Endocrinol Metab 2005;90(1):286–295.

15. Ota H, Igarashi S, Sasaki M, Tanaka T. Distribution of cyclooxygenase-2 in eutopic and ectopic endometrium in endometriosis and adenomyosis. Hum Reprod 2001;16:561–566.

16. Bulun SE, Yang S, Fang Z et al. Role of aromatase in endometrial disease. J Steroid Biochem Mol Biol 2001;79:19–25.

17. Tsai SJ, Wu MH, Lin CC, Sun HS, Chan HM. Regulation of steroidogenic acute regulatory protein expression and progesterone production in endometriotic stromal cells. J Clin Endocrinol Metab 2001;86:5765–5773.

18. Goss PE, Strasser K. Aromatase inhibitors in the treatment and prevention of breast cancer. J Clin Oncol 2001;19(3):881–894.

19. Buzdar A, Howell A. Advances in aromatase inhibition: clinical efficacy and tolerability in the treatment of breast cancer. Clin Cancer Res 2001;7(9):2620–2635.

20. Buzdar AU, Robertson JF, Eiermann W, Nabholtz JM. An overview of the pharmacology and pharmacokinetics of the newer generation aromatase inhibitors anastrozole, letrozole, and exemestane. Cancer 2002;95(9):2006–2016.

21. De Jong PC, van de Ven J, Nortier HW et al. Inhibition of breast cancer tissue aromatase activity and estrogen concentrations by the third-generation aromatase inhibitor vorozole. Cancer Res 1997;57(11):2109–2111.

22. Santen RJ, Misbin RI. Aminoglutethimide: review of pharmacology and clinical use. Pharmacotherapy 1981;1(2):95–120.

23. Santen RJ. Suppression of estrogens with aminoglutethimide and hydrocortisone (medical adrenalectomy) as treatment of advanced breast carcinoma: a review. Breast Cancer Res Treat 1981;1(3):183–202.

24. Santen RJ, Santner S, Davis B, Veldhuis J, Samojlik E, Ruby E. Aminoglutethimide inhibits extraglandular estrogen production in postmenopausal women with breast carcinoma. J Clin Endocrinol Metab 1978;47(6):1257–1265.

25. Santen RJ, Lipton A, Harvey H, Wells SA. Use of aminoglutethimide and hydrocortisone as a "medical adrenalectomy" for treatment of breast carcinoma. Prog Clin Cancer 1982;8:245–265.

26. Santen RJ. Clinical use of aromatase inhibitors: current data and future perspectives. J Enzyme Inhib 1990;4(2):79–99.

27. Santen RJ, Manni A, Harvey H, Redmond C. Endocrine treatment of breast cancer in women. Endocrine Rev 1990;11:221–265.

28. Santen RJ. Recent progress in development of aromatase inhibitors. J Steroid Biochem Mol Biol 1990;37(6):1029–1035.

29. Dowsett M. Endocrine treatment of advanced breast cancer. Acta Oncol 1996;35(Suppl 5):68–72.

30. Dowsett M, Lonning PE. Anastrozole – a new generation in aromatase inhibition: clinical pharmacology. Oncology 1997;54(Suppl 2):11–14.

31. Buzdar AU, Jonat W, Howell A, Plourde PV. ARIMIDEX: a potent and selective aromatase inhibitor for the treatment of advanced breast cancer. J Steroid Biochem Mol Biol 1997;61(3–6):145–149.

32. Buzdar AU, Plourde PV, Hortobagyi GN. Aromatase inhibitors in metastatic breast cancer. Semin Oncol 1996;23(4 Suppl 9):28–32.

33. Buzdar AU, Hortobagyi G. Update on endocrine therapy for breast cancer. Clin Cancer Res 1998;4(3):527–534.

34. Dombernowsky P, Smith I, Falkson G et al. Letrozole, a new oral aromatase inhibitor for advanced breast cancer: double-blind randomized trial showing a dose effect and improved efficacy and tolerability compared with megestrol acetate. J Clin Oncol 1998;16(2):453–461.

35. Gershanovich M, Chaudri HA, Campos D et al. Letrozole, a new oral aromatase inhibitor: randomised trial comparing 2.5 mg daily, 0.5 mg daily and aminoglutethimide in postmenopausal women with advanced breast cancer. Letrozole International Trial Group (AR/BC3). Ann Oncol 1998;9(6):639–645.

36. Demers LM, Lipton A, Harvey HA et al. The efficacy of CGS 20267 in suppressing estrogen biosynthesis in patients with advanced stage breast cancer. J Steroid Biochem Mol Biol 1993;44(4–6):687–691.

37. Plourde PV, Dyroff M, Dukes M. Arimidex: a potent and selective fourth-generation aromatase inhibitor. Breast Cancer Res Treat 1994;30(1):103–111.

38. Dowsett M, Jones A, Johnston SR, Jacobs S, Trunet P, Smith IE. In vivo measurement of aromatase inhibition by letrozole (CGS 20267) in postmenopausal patients with breast cancer. Clin Cancer Res 1995;1(12):1511–1515.

39. Kleeberg UR, Dowsett M, Carrion RP et al. A randomised comparison of oestrogen suppression with anastrozole and formestane in postmenopausal patients with advanced breast cancer. Oncology 1997;54(Suppl 2):19–22.

40. Scott LJ, Wiseman LR. Exemestane. Drugs 1999;58(4):675–680; discussion 81–82.

41. Amsterdam LL, Gentry W, Jobanputra S, Wolf M, Rubin SD, Bulun SE. Anastrazole and oral contraceptives: a novel treatment for endometriosis. Fertil Steril 2005;84(2):300–304.

42. Buzdar AU. The ATAC (Arimidex, Tamoxifen, Alone or in Combination) trial: an update. Clin Breast Cancer 2004;5(Suppl 1):S6-S12.

43. Senkus-Konefka E, Konefka T, Jassem J. The effects of tamoxifen on the female genital tract. Cancer Treat Rev 2004;30(3):291–301.

44. Ailawadi RK, Jobanputra S, Kataria M, Gurates B, Bulun SE. Treatment of endometriosis and chronic pelvic pain with letrozole and norethindrone acetate: a pilot study. Fertil Steril 2004;81(2):290–296.

45. Soysal S, Soysal M, Ozer S, Gul N, Gezgin T. The effects of post-surgical administration of goserelin plus anastrozole compared to goserelin alone in patients with severe endometriosis: a prospective randomized trial. Hum Reprod 2004;19:160–167.

46. Sebastian S, Bulun SE. A highly complex organization of the regulatry region of the human CYP19 (aromatase) gene revealed by the human genome project. J Clin Endocrinol Metab 2001;86:4600–4602.

47. Moudgal NR, Shetty G, Selvaraj N, Bhatnagar AS. Use of a specific aromatase inhibitor for determining whether there is a role for oestrogen in follicle/oocyte maturation, ovulation and preimplantation embryo development. J Reprod Fertil 1996;50(Suppl):69–81.

48. Santen RJ, Samojlik E, Wells SA. Resistance of the ovary to blockade of aromatization with aminoglutethimide. J Clin Endocrinol Metab 1980;51(3):473–477.

49. Harris AL, Dowsett M, Jeffcoate SL, McKinna JA, Morgan M, Smith IE. Endocrine and therapeutic effects of aminoglutethimide in premenopausal patients with breast cancer. J Clin Endocrinol Metab 1982;55(4):718–722.

50. Wander HE, Blossey HC, Nagel GA. Aminoglutethimide in the treatment of premenopausal patients with metastatic breast cancer. Eur J Cancer Clin Oncol 1986;22(11):1371–1374.

51. Stein RC, Dowsett M, Hedley A et al. Treatment of advanced breast cancer in postmenopausal women with 4-hydroxyandrostenedione. Cancer Chemother Pharmacol 1990;26(1):75–78.

52. Wouters W, de Coster R, Krekels M et al. R 76713, a new specific nonsteroidal aromatase inhibitor. J Steroid Biochem 1989;32(6):781–788.

53. Stein RC, Dowsett M, Hedley A, Gazet JC, Ford HT, Coombes RC. The clinical and endocrine effects of 4-hydroxyandrostenedione alone and in combination with goserelin in premenopausal women with advanced breast cancer. Br J Cancer 1990;62(4):679–683.

54. Mitwally MF, Casper RF. Use of an aromatase inhibitor for induction of ovulation in patients with an inadequate response to clomiphene citrate. Fertil Steril 2001;75(2):305–309.

55. Cortinez A, de Carvalho I, Vantman D, Gabler F, Iniguez G, Vega M. Hormonal profile and endometrial morphology in letrozole-controlled ovarian hyperstimulation in ovulatory infertile patients. Fertil Steril 2005;83(1):110–115.

56. Fisher SA, Reid RL, van Vugt DA, Casper RF. A randomized double-blind comparison of the effects of clomiphene citrate and the aromatase inhibitor letrozole on ovulatory function in normal women. Fertil Steril 2002;78(2):280–285.

57. Mitwally MF, Casper RF. Aromatase inhibition improves ovarian response to follicle-stimulating hormone in poor responders. Fertil Steril 2002;77(4):776–780.

58. Mitwally MF, Casper RF. Aromatase inhibition reduces the dose of gonadotropin required for controlled ovarian hyperstimulation. J Soc Gynecol Invest 2004;11(6):406–415.

59. Goswami SK, Das T, Chattopadhyay R et al. A randomized single-blind controlled trial of letrozole as a low-cost IVF protocol in women with poor ovarian response: a preliminary report. Hum Reprod 2004;19(9):2031–2035.

60. Forward DP, Cheung KL, Jackson L, Robertson JF. Clinical and endocrine data for goserelin plus anastrozole as second-line endocrine therapy for premenopausal advanced breast cancer. Br J Cancer 2004;90(3):590–594.

61. Vercellini P, Trespidi L, Colombo A. A gonadotropin-releasing hormone agonist versus a low-dose oral contraceptive for pelvic pain associated with endometriosis. Fertil Steril 1993;60(1):75–79.

62. Waller KG, Shaw RW. Gonadotropin-releasing hormone analogues for the treatment of endometriosis: long-term follow-up. Fertil Steril 1993; 59(3):511–515.

63. Vercellini P, Trespidi L, de Giorgi O, Cortesi I, Parazzini F, Crosignani PG. Endometriosis and pelvic pain: relation to disease stage and localization. Fertil Steril 1996;65:299–304.

64. Kauppila A. Changing concepts of medical treatment of endometriosis. Acta Obstet Gynecol Scand 1993;72(5):324–336.

65. Vercellini P, Fedele L, Bianchi S, Candiani GB. Pelvic denervation for chronic pain associated with endometriosis: fact or fancy? Am J Obstet Gynecol 1991;165(3):745–749.

66. Wilson ML, Farquhar CM, Sinclair OJ, Johnson NP. Surgical interruption of pelvic nerve pathways for primary and secondary dysmenorrhoea. Cochrane Database Syst Rev 2000;2:CD001896.

67. Gambone JC, Mittman BS, Munro MG, Scialli AR, Winkel CA. Consensus statement for the management of chronic pelvic pain and endometriosis: proceedings of an expert-panel consensus process. Fertil Steril 2002;78(5):961–972.

68. Olive DL, Pritts EA. The treatment of endometriosis: a review of the evidence. Ann N Y Acad Sci 2002;955:360–372; discussion 89–93, 96–406.

69. Pierce SJ, Gazvani MR, Farquharson RG. Long-term use of gonadotropin-releasing hormone analogs and hormone replacement therapy in the management of endometriosis: a randomized trial with a 6-year follow-up. Fertil Steril 2000;74(5):964–968.

70. Martin DC, Ling FW. Endometriosis and pain. Clin Obstet Gynecol 1999;42(3):664–686.

71. Vercellini P, de Giorgi O, Pisacreta A, Pesole AP, Vicentini S, Crosignani PG. Surgical management of endometriosis. Baillière's Best Pract Res Clin Obstet Gynaecol 2000;14(3):501–523.

72. Shippen ER, West WJ Jr. Successful treatment of severe endometriosis in two premenopausal women with an aromatase inhibitor. Fertil Steril 2004;81(5):1395–1398.

73. Takayama K, Zeitoun K, Gunby RT, Sasano H, Carr BR, Bulun SE. Treatment of severe postmenopausal endometriosis with an aromatase inhibitor. Fertil Steril 1998;69:709–713.

74. Razzi S, Fava A, Sartini A, De Simone S, Cobellis L, Petraglia F. Treatment of severe recurrent endometriosis with an aromatase inhibitor in a young ovariectomised woman. Br J Obstet Gynaecol 2004;111(2):182–184.

75. American Society for Reproductive Medicine. Revised classification of endometriosis: 1996. Fertil Steril 1997;67(5):817–821.

76. Biberoglu KO, Behrman SJ. Dosage aspects of danazol therapy in endometriosis: short-term and long-term effectiveness. Am J Obstet Gynecol 1981;139(6):645–654.

77. Bulun SE, Imir G, Utsunomiya H, Thung S, Gurates B, Tamura M, Lin Z. Aromatase in endometriosis and uterine leiomyomata. J Steroid Biochem Mol Biol 2005;95(1–5):57–62.

36 Medical Therapies: Statins

Anna Sokalska and Antoni J. Duleba

Department of Obstetrics and Gynecology, University of California Davis, Sacramento, CA, USA

Introduction

Scope of the problem

Endometriosis is one of the most debilitating and yet poorly understood gynecological disorders. It is associated with a broad range of symptoms including dysmenorrhea, chronic intermenstrual pelvic pain, dyspareunia and infertility. The prevalence of endometriosis among women of reproductive age is in the range of 6–10% and the annual cost of healthcare and loss of productivity related to endometriosis in the United States has been estimated to be in the region of 22 billion dollars [1–4].

One of the great, if not the greatest, challenges related to endometriosis is the search for new effective long-term therapies, which would be safe and free of significant side-effects. Optimal therapies should not be focused only on isolated facets of the pathophysiology of endometriosis, but ideally should treat presumed causes as well as manifestations of this condition.

While the etiology of endometriosis remains debatable, the dominant concept invokes retrograde menstruation followed by ectopic implantation of endometrial glands and stroma. Other proposed concepts include coelomic metaplasia, immune dysfunction and environmental pollutants. It is most likely that the majority of cases of endometriosis involve multiple processes including attachment of endometrial tissues, invasion, growth of glands and stroma, local neo-angiogenesis and inflammation. Ideally, treatment of endometriosis would address several or even most of these processes.

This chapter will advance a hypothesis that statins may provide a novel and effective treatment of endometriosis, targeting most of its pathophysiological aspects. Specifically, we will: (i) briefly review currently available treatments of endometriosis and their limitations, (ii) summarize mechanisms of action of statins and their potential relation to treatment of endometriosis, (iii) describe key pathophysiological features of endometriosis with special emphasis on potential actions of statins, and finally (iv) present available evidence from *in vitro* and *in vivo* studies evaluating effects of statins on endometrial tissues and animal models of endometriosis.

Limitations of current therapies of endometriosis

Several well-established therapies address various individual features of endometriosis. Typical primary targets of these therapies are analgesic/anti-inflammatory effects, by using nonsteroidal anti-inflammatory agents (NSAIDs) or ovulation/estrogen suppression by using oral contraceptives (OCs), progestagens, danazol, and gonadotropin releasing hormone (GnRH) analogs. Unfortunately, these treatments have either modest effectiveness or are associated with significant side-effects. In particular, progestagens often cause premenstrual syndrome (PMS)-type effects and breakthrough bleedings. Furthermore, resistance to progesterone/progestagens is now recognized as a major concern [5]. Danazol use leads to profound hyperandrogenic symptomatology and is usually poorly tolerated. GnRH analogs induce a hypoestrogenic state associated with a broad range of menopausal-like symptoms and their long-term use may lead to serious long-term health issues such as osteoporosis.

More recently, several new therapies have been introduced, including the levonorgestrel intrauterine system (LNG-IUS) and aromatase inhibitors (AIs). The LNG-IUS was shown to lower pain score, reduce the size of rectovaginal nodules and improve American Fertility Society (AFS) staging of the disease. In spite of the good safety profile, to date, this system has been tested only on a small number of patients [6–8]. Aromatase inhibitors reduce estrogen biosynthesis including inhibition of aromatase activity within ectopic-endometriotic deposits and are used primarily as the adjunctive therapy to OC, progestagens and GnRH analogs in cases of resistant endometriosis. Patients with endometriosis using AIs may experience vasomotor symptoms, vaginal bleeding,

Endometriosis: Science and Practice, First Edition. Edited by Linda C. Giudice, Johannes L.H. Evers and David L. Healy.
© 2012 Blackwell Publishing Ltd. Published 2012 by Blackwell Publishing Ltd.

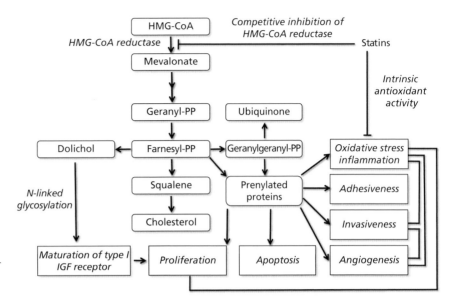

Figure 36.1 Outline of mevalonate pathway and the site of action of statins. HMG-CoA, 3-hydroxy-3-methyl-glutaryl-coenzyme A; IGF, insulin-like growth factor; PP, pyrophosphate.

joint and bone pain, decreased libido, depression, weight gain and insomnia [9]. Long-term therapy with AIs is associated with loss of bone density as well as potential adverse effects on lipid profile and cardiovascular disease risk [10,11].

Several experimental therapies are also being investigated and include progesterone antagonists, selective estrogen modulators (SERMs) and selective progesterone modulators (SPRMs), and selective estrogen receptor (ER)β agonists. However, data are still insufficient to recommend their usage outside clinical trials [2]. These new treatments are not free from adverse effects. Thus, for example, progesterone antagonists cause erratic vaginal bleeding, SERMs use is associated with menopausal symptoms, SPRMs cause endometrial changes requiring further investigations and selective ERβ agonists could lead to vaginal bleeding and endometrial thickening [2,12–15].

In addition to the above medical therapies, surgical resection or ablation of endometriotic lesions is often effective in reducing pain and possibly improving fertility. However, surgery for endometriosis is often technically challenging and is associated with significant intraoperative and long-term risks and complications. Unfortunately, surgery often provides only temporary relief followed by return of symptoms and the necessity for repeat operations; even after a second surgery, 14–20% of patients require a third procedure [16,17].

In summary, currently available therapies are often not effective and are associated with significant risks and side-effects. Furthermore, upon discontinuation of these therapies, symptoms of endometriosis frequently return.

Statins: overview of mechanisms of action and potential effects on endometriosis

Statins are cholesterol-lowering agents effective in treatment of hypercholesterolemia and cardiovascular disorders. However, growing evidence indicates that beneficial effects of statins therapy are also related to the cholesterol-independent actions including modulation of signal transduction pathways involved in regulation of cell proliferation and apoptosis, as well as antioxidant activity, which may also affect the cell growth and function.

The major mode of action of statins is due to their competitive inhibition of the key enzyme regulating the mevalonate pathway: 3-hydroxy-3-methylglutaryl-coenzyme A (HMG-CoA) reductase. Several van der Waals interactions contribute to tight binding between statins and the HMG-CoA reductase-binding pocket and part of the binding surface for CoA [18]. This binding is responsible for blocking access of the substrate, HMG-CoA, to the enzyme. The mevalonate pathway is composed of a series of reactions starting with acetyl-coenzyme A (acetyl-CoA) and involving the formation of farnesyl pyrophosphate (FPP), the substrate for several biologically important agents including cholesterol, isoprenylated proteins, coenzyme Q (ubiquinone), and dolichol [19]. Among the most crucial to cellular function appear to be components of the pathway leading to isoprenylation of proteins: FPP and geranylgeranyl-pyrophosphate (GGPP) (Fig. 36.1).

Isoprenylation consists of attachment of FPP (farnesylation) or GGPP (geranylgeranylation) to the carboxyl terminus of proteins [20]. Geranylgeranylation is a process whereby geranylgeranyl-transferase I or II (GGTase I or GGTase II) attaches the geranylgeranyl moiety from GGPP to the free sulfhydryl of cysteine at the carboxyl terminus of the protein substrate in CAAX box (where A is aliphatic and X is leucine). Farnesylation is a similar process carried out by farnesyltransferase (FTase), which recognizes the CAAX box (where A is aliphatic and X is serine or methionine) [20]. This post-translational modification is important to membrane attachment and the function of several families of proteins including Ras and Ras-related GTP binding proteins (small GTPases), subunits of trimeric G proteins and protein kinases [20]. The functions of these proteins depend on association with the cytoplasmic leaflet of the cellular membrane: farnesylation of Ras and geranylgeranylation of Rho, Rac and Cdc42.

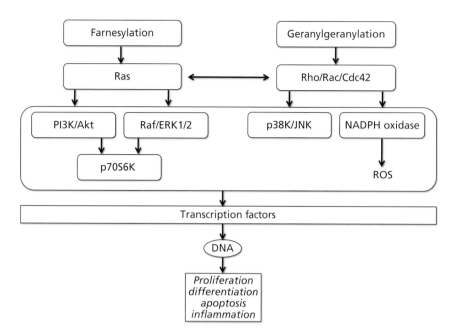

Figure 36.2 Proposed mechanisms of action of mevalonate pathway metabolites on endometriotic tissue in relation to modification of isoprenylation. DNA, deoxyribonucleic acid; ERK1/2, extracellular signal-regulated kinase 1 and 2; JNK, c-Jun N-terminal kinase; NADPH oxidase, nicotinamide adenine dinucleotide phosphate oxidase; PI3K/Akt, phosphoinositide 3-kinase/serine-threonine protein kinase Akt; p38K, p38 mitogen-activated protein kinase; p70S6K, p70 ribosomal protein S6 kinase; Raf, Raf kinase; Ras, Rho, Rac, Cdc42, small GTPases; ROS, reactive oxygen species.

Statins can impair both geranylgeranylation and farnesylation by depletion of GGPP and FPP and hence may affect several signal transduction steps relevant to regulation of proliferation and apoptosis. The most important pathways regulating proliferation, which may be affected by isoprenylation, include mitogen-activated protein kinase (MAPK) pathways: (i) Ras-Raf-Erk1/2, (ii) P38 kinase (p38K) and (iii) c-Jun N-terminal protein kinase (JNK). The Ras-Raf-Erk1/2 pathway may be stimulated by agents such as insulin or insulin-like growth factor I (IGF-I) via activation of the tyrosine kinase system. P38 and JNK pathways may be also activated by insulin/IGF-I as well as by other stimuli such as oxidative stress.

Apoptosis is largely regulated via the phosphatidylinositol 3'-kinase/protein kinase B (PI3 kinase/PKB) pathway. Finally, p70S6 kinase (p70S6K) is particularly important to proliferation and may be affected by both PI3K and MAPK.

Key steps required for activation of the above pathways include isoprenylation of Ras, Rho, Rac and Cdc42. Since these small GTPases modulate function of cells, proliferation and apoptosis, any interference with isoprenylation may have profound effects (Fig. 36.2).

Another aspect of the actions of statins pertains to their effects on oxidative stress. Reactive oxygen species (ROS) play a major role in regulation of cellular functions including proliferation and gene expression [21]. Proliferation of endometrial stroma is stimulated by moderate oxidative stress, but inhibited by a broad range of antioxidants [22].

Statins may affect oxidative stress via several mechanisms including their intrinsic antioxidant activity, modulation of the synthesis of the antioxidant coenzyme Q, and isoprenylation-related changes in the activity of nicotinamide adenine dinucleotide phosphate (NADPH) oxidase, an important cellular source of ROS. Most evidence supports the concept that the predominant effect of statins is reduction of oxidative stress. This subject is presented in greater detail in the section entitled Statins: effects on inflammation, immune responses and oxidative stress, below.

All the above mechanisms of action of statins are highly relevant to endometriosis. Formation of endometriotic implants requires ectopic attachment and proliferation of endometrial stroma and glands. Prominent features of endometriosis include inflammatory reaction, increased oxidative stress and intense angiogenesis surrounding the implants [23].

The rationale for proposing statins as a promising treatment of endometriosis is based on several considerations. First, statins inhibit HMG-CoA reductase, a rate-limiting step of the mevalonate pathway. The inhibition of HMG-CoA reductase depletes downstream products of the mevalonate pathway, especially isoprenyls [24] which in turn decreases activity of small GTPases such as Ras and Rho, resulting in diminution of signaling of important growth-regulating pathways [25]. Second, inhibition of HMG-CoA reductase may reduce another downstream product, dolichol, which is required for maturation of IGF-I receptors, and hence may decrease the mitogenic effect of IGF-I on endometrial stromal cells. Third, statins can interfere with angiogenesis, which is necessary for the development of endometriotic implants. In addition, statins possess anti-inflammatory and immunomodulatory properties, which may reduce the inflammatory reaction associated with endometriosis.

The hypothesis that statins may be used in the treatment of endometriosis is also supported by the evidence that in several tissues, such as vascular smooth muscle, products of the mevalonate pathway have been shown to facilitate isoprenylation of small GPTases and thus activate signal transduction pathways promoting growth while inhibition of the mevalonate pathway by statins decreases growth and exerts antioxidant effects [24,26].

The safety of statins is another highly pertinent issue. While, overall, their safety profile is excellent, the use of statins is associated with some risks and side-effects. Among the most important risks are those related to their proapoptotic and cytotoxic activity, including rhabdomyolysis and liver cytolysis [27–29]. The molecular basis of these side-effects remains unclear. It has been postulated that the cytotoxic effect of statins is caused by reduced activity of small GTPases and reduced synthesis of the side chain of coenzyme Q [28]. Coenzyme Q is an antioxidant serving as an electron transporter in the mitochondria which plays a crucial role in mitochondrial respiration and adenosine triphosphate (ATP) synthesis. Decreased intracellular levels of coenzyme Q have been linked to impaired metabolism of muscles and their myolysis [27,28]. However, clinical trials evaluating coenzyme Q supplementation during statin therapy indicate that administration of coenzyme Q does not fully prevent the toxicity of statins and may be beneficial only for a small subgroup of patients [27,28].

Use of statins is also associated with potential risk of teratogenicity and at present these drugs are listed as category X medications. The evidence for teratogenicity of statins is limited to theoretical considerations and conflicting findings from a small series of cases; nevertheless, the use of statins should be avoided in sexually active women not using reliable contraception [30–32].

In summary, the available evidence supports the concept that statins exert antiproliferative, proapoptotic, antioxidant, immunomodulatory and anti-inflammatory properties, all of which may be beneficial in the treatment of endometriosis. The following sections of this chapter will address these issues in greater detail.

Pathophysiology of endometriosis and mechanisms of action of statins

The series of events leading to development of symptomatic endometriosis involves multiple processes including adhesion of endometrial tissues to intraperitoneal structures, invasiveness, angiogenesis, growth of endometrial stroma and glands, stimulation by systemic and local estrogens, as well as inflammation, oxidative stress and immune dysfunction. The following text will summarize these processes in relation to proven or potential actions of statins (Figs 36.3, 36.4).

Increased endometriotic cell adhesiveness

The establishment of endometriotic implants requires a complex interaction between endometriotic tissue and host peritoneum. One of the key processes is the adhesiveness of endometriotic cells to the mesothelium [33,34], a process depending on the presence of integrins on the surface of endometrial cells [35,36]. Integrins are adhesive molecules that play a major role in the formation of cell-to-cell and cell-to-extracellular matrix (ECM) attachments; integrins also function as intra- and extracellular signal-transducing receptors [37–40]. *In vitro* studies indicate that eutopic and ectopic endometrial stromal cells derived from women with endometriosis exhibit an aberrant integrin

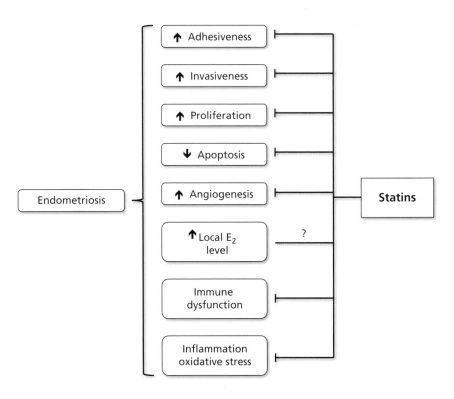

Figure 36.3 Proposed role of statins in treatment of endometriosis. E_2, estradiol; "?" denotes potential effect.

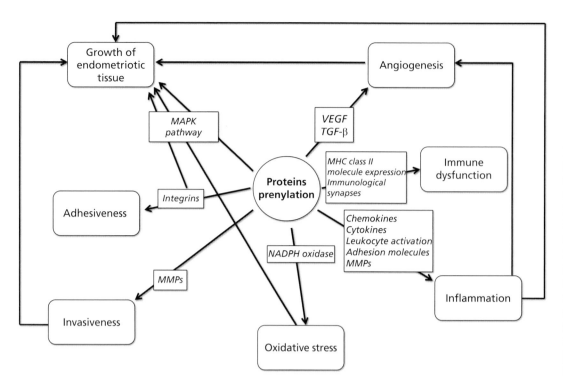

Figure 36.4 Proposed mechanisms of action of statins in relation to modification of isoprenylation. MAPK, mitogen-activated protein kinase; MHC, major histocompatibility complex; MMPs, matrix metaloproteinases; NADPH oxidase, nicotinamide adenine dinucleotide phosphate oxidase; TGF-β, transforming growth factor β; VEGF, vascular endothelial growth factor.

expression profile and increased adhesion capacity after exposure to specific ECM components when compared to cells obtained from healthy controls [41]. These findings are supported by observations that menstrual-phase endometrial mRNA levels of integrin αvβ3 are elevated in patients with endometriosis when compared to control subjects [42]. Furthermore, transcripts of several integrins (β1, β3, αv) were detected in xenografts in a nude mouse model of endometriosis [43].

CD44 is another molecule that plays a role in the attachment of endometrial cells to the peritoneum [44]. Its principal ligand, hyaluronic acid (HA), is produced by many cell types. HA promotes actin stress fiber formation [45]. The binding capacity of HA is partially regulated by the specific CD44 splice variant and probably also by the degree of CD44 glycosylation. As presented by Griffith *et al*, menstrual endometrial stromal cells derived from women with endometriosis exhibit an increased rate of adherence to peritoneal mesothelium and elevated expression of several isoforms of CD44 (v6, v7, v8, v9) when compared to healthy controls. This different pattern of splice variants of CD44 as well as additional glycosylation sites on the variants may contribute to increased adhesiveness of the endometrial cells [46].

Statins: effects on cell-cell and cell-extracellular matrix interactions and cell morphology

Statins, by interfering with the isoprenylation (farnesylation and geranylgeranylation), cause the alteration of the actin cytoskeleton [47]. Small GPTases: Rho, Rac and Cdc42 play an important role

in maintenance and rearrangement of the cytoskeleton, and cellular polarity [48–51]. In particular, Rho activation is involved in signaling pathways stimulating actin stress fiber formation [52] while Rac plays a role in the generation of lamellipodia and Cdc42 is important in the formation of actin spikes and filopodia [53]. The active (prenylated) form of Rho also seems to be responsible for integrin β activation [54]. Statins reduce GGPP and hence decrease geranylgeranylation of Rho, Rac and Cdc42 leading to an accumulation of these proteins in their inactive form in the cytoplasm and causing detrimental changes in the cell cytoskeleton leading to loss of attachment and deterioration of integrin-mediated signaling. Statins have been shown to reduce expression of integrins [55] and/or prevent their conformational activation without significant change in their total level [54].

Statins and endometrium: disruption of the cell morphology and endometrial-peritoneal interactions

Statins were shown to decrease endometrial stromal cell adhesiveness to collagen fibers in a three-dimensional (3-D) matrix [56]. Untreated endometriotic stromal cells, isolated from endometrial cysts, cultured in 3-D collagen gels developed dendritic morphology, adhered to collagen fibers and formed tissue-like structures. In contrast, simvastatin-treated cells did not adhere to collagen and cells became round or polygonal. These observations indicate that statins may suppress formation of endometriotic lesions, in part, by disrupting the interaction between endometrial cells and extracellular matrix components.

Increased endometriotic cell invasiveness

Formation of endometriotic implants requires increased invasive potential of the endometriotic cells. Invasion may be enhanced by excessive expression of matrix metalloproteinases (MMPs) leading to local destruction of the extracellular matrix and hence establishment of the disease [57]. Several MMPs are inappropriately expressed in the endometrium of women with endometriosis [58] and are upregulated by tumor necrosis factor (TNF)-α and interleukin (IL)-1. The endometrium of women with endometriosis compared to healthy controls is characterized by increased mRNA levels of MMP-2 and MMP-3 and decreased mRNA expression of tissue inhibitor of metalloproteinase 2 (TIMP-2) [58,59]. These features of endometrial cells favor implantation of endometriotic tissue in the peritoneal cavity. Additionally, the continuous expression of several MMPs, especially MMP-3, MMP-7, MMP-2, and decreased expression of TIMP-2 in endometriotic lesions play a role in the establishment of endometriosis [44,58,60].

While the role of autoantibodies in endometriosis is still not well understood, it has been shown that a hemopexin domain expressed by MMPs, except MMP-7, can be recognized and bound by T-like autoantibodies in women with endometriosis, leading to dysregulation of MMPs and TIMPs in ectopic lesions [61]. Reduced sensitivity of MMPs to progesterone in the endometrium of women with endometriosis, combined with all the mechanisms listed above, is likely to contribute to the invasive potential of refluxed endometrial tissues [57].

Statins: effects on matrix metalloproteinases

Many studies on the pathogenesis and treatment of cardiovascular diseases have shown that statins modulate MMPs expression and/or activity [62,63]. Thus, for example, statins reduce MMPs secretion and activity and increase TIMP-1, as demonstrated by their plaque-stabilizing effect [64] and reduction of abdominal aortic aneurysm progression [62]. Furthermore, Porter *et al* found that statins inhibit MMPs and block migration through a matrix barrier of cultured human saphenous vein smooth muscle cells, preventing vein graft stenosis [65]. Statins were also studied as a new therapeutic strategy for human immunodeficiency virus (HIV). An imbalance between MMPs and TIMPs might contribute to HIV-associated pathology by inducing extracellular matrix remodeling; this process may be inhibited by statins [66]. The effects of statins on MMPs are likely mediated by the reduction of protein isoprenylation [67,68].

Statins and endometrium: inhibition of matrix metalloproteinases

Since development of endometriosis requires ectopic attachment of endometrial tissue by a process involving MMPs, statins may interfere with this process in several ways. First, MMP-9 production may be affected by modulation of isoprenylation [67]. Second, statins may decrease MMP-9 production by monocytes via activation of the nuclear receptor transcription factor peroxisome proliferator-activated receptor-γ (PPARγ) [69].

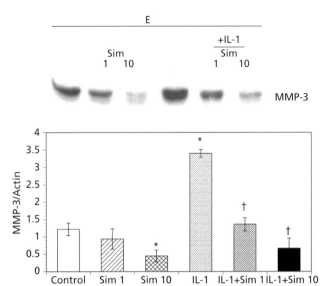

Figure 36.5 Western analysis of expression and regulation of MMP-3 protein in human endometrial stromal cells isolated from proliferative phase endometrial biopsies (n = 5). Cells were cultured for 48 h in the presence of estradiol (E, 1 nM), followed by an additional 24 h with E alone or E plus simvastatin (Sim) at 1 or 10 μM. Some cultures were also exposed to IL-1α during the last 6 h of culture. A representative experiment is shown in *top panel*. Densitometric analysis of all studies is shown in *bottom panel*. *, means significantly different from control; †, means significantly different from IL-1α. Reproduced from Bruner-Tran *et al* [71] with permission from the Endocrine Society.

Recently, Bruner-Tran *et al* have shown that simvastatin inhibits expression of MMP-3 in human endometrial stroma [70,71] (Fig. 36.5). Cells were cultured in the presence of estradiol (E$_2$; 1 nM). In addition, the cells were treated with simvastatin (1 and 10 μM), medroxyprogesterone acetate (MPA; 50 pM) and/or IL-1α (200 ng/mL). Collected media were tested by Western analysis for expression of MMP-3. Endometrial stromal cells expressed abundant levels of MMP-3 following treatment with E$_2$, but minimal levels in cultures also supplemented with simvastatin or MPA. IL-1α induced a profound increase in MMP-3 secretion from cells pretreated with E$_2$ alone; however, the addition of either simvastatin or MPA abrogated this effect. Cultures containing both simvastatin and MPA were the most resistant to MMP-3 induction by IL-1α. These findings indicate that statins inhibit both basal and Il-1α-induced MMP levels by mechanisms independent of and complementary to MPA.

Endometriosis and angiogenesis

The establishment of a blood supply through angiogenesis represents another important step in the development of the endometriotic lesions following implantation of endometrial fragments. Angiogenesis is an integral component of the pathogenesis of endometriosis and human endometrium is highly angiogenic [72]. Studies on a nude mouse model of endometriosis showed that murine-derived neovascularization of transplanted human endometrium begins after 24 h and continues up to the fifth or even the eighth day after transplantation [71,73]. It has been proposed that endometrial implants send angiogenic signals to the murine vessels leading to destabilization of the vessels, guided migration of the endothelial cells and induction of the growth of blood vessels into endometrial tissue [74]. Integrins (αvβ3, αvβ5, α1β1, α5β1) mediate interactions between the cells and the ECM at the time of invasion and development of vascularization [75,76]. Several studies have reported that endometriosis is associated with an increased level of inducers of angiogenesis such as vascular endothelial growth factor (VEGF) and transforming growth factor (TGF)-β [44,77]. Activated peritoneal macrophages, T-cells, endometrium and endometriotic implants have the capacity to secrete VEGF, while TGF-β is predominantly produced by endometrial stroma, platelets, activated lymphocytes and macrophages [61,78].

Vascular endothelial growth factor promotes endothelial cell proliferation, migration, differentiation and capillary formation and it may play an important role in the progression of endometriosis [79]. TGF-β stimulates endometrial stromal cells to produce urokinase-type plasminogen activator (uPA) and plasminogen activator inhibitor 1 (PAI-1) playing the role in endothelial cells migration [72]. TGF-β also stabilizes the vessel wall, by stimulating binding of the endothelial cells to the pericytes [80].

Cyclooxygenase-2 (COX-2) is also a potent angiogenic factor. Its elevated expression in endometriosis [81] may be related to the inflammatory response. COX-2 stimulates VEGF production by fibroblasts and, via prostaglandin-cAMP-PKA-dependent activation of small GTPase, promotes integrin αvβ3-mediated adhesion and migration of endothelial cells [75].

Statins: effects on angiogenesis

The effects of statins on angiogenesis are complex and appear to be tissue specific as well as dependent on the dose of statin [82]. Weis *et al* and Skaletz-Rorowski *et al* demonstrated that low doses of statins have a proangiogenic effect via the serine/threonine protein kinase Akt activation, upregulation of endothelial nitric oxide synthase (eNOS) expression and increased nitric oxide production, whereas high doses promote decreased protein isoprenylation, inhibit capillary tube formation and decrease VEGF production, inducing angiostatic effects [82–84]. The higher affinity of mevalonate-derived intermediates for enzymes involved in the synthesis of non-sterol products of the mevalonate pathway required for cellular house-keeping functions (prenyl groups, ubiquinone and dolichol), rather than for biosynthesis of cholesterol, seems to be responsible for the biphasic effect of statins on angiogenesis. At low doses, statins affect mainly cholesterol synthesis, with no significant negative effect on non-sterol products essential for cellular processes. However, at high doses, statins inhibit multiple pathways and ultimately induce apoptosis of endothelial cells [84,85].

It has been proposed that statins, in addition to stimulation of nitric oxide production [86], also prevent its biodegradation by free radicals. Proangiogenic effects of statins can also be explained by upregulation of hypoxia inducible factor (HIF-1α), a stimulator of VEGF expression [87]. Furthermore, specific actions of statins on blood vessel formation in primary invasive tumors or metastases depend on statin doses and also on tumor cell type [82].

The studies of Park *et al* confirmed the role of protein isoprenylation in angiogenesis and demonstrated that statins inhibit the VEGF-stimulated phosphorylation of the VEGF receptor, thus preventing the progression of atherosclerosis by inhibition of plaque angiogenesis [88]. Zhang *et al* have shown that statins markedly reverse angiotensin II-stimulated angiogenesis and MMPs secretion [89]. The antiangiogenic effect of statins is also related to reduction of COX-2 and MMP-9 expression and activity [63].

Statins and endometrium: inhibition of angiogenesis

Initial *in vitro* studies on the effects of statins on angiogenesis in endometrial tissues are encouraging and indicate an inhibitory effect of statins on this process [90]. Growth of human endometrial biopsy tissues in a three-dimensional culture in a fibrin matrix was observed during the first week of culture, while new vessel formation was noticed after 2–3 weeks. Lovastatin at 5 and 10 μM induced a concentration-dependent inhibitory effect on endometrial cell growth and on angiogenesis. However, at 1 μM concentration, lovastatin inhibited only angiogenesis, with no demonstrable effect on cell proliferation. The proposed mechanism of diminished blood vessel formation is related to statin-induced inhibition of expression of VEGF [90]. The authors of this study suggested that administration of statins during menstrual bleeding and for a few days afterwards may prevent endometrial tissue attachment to the peritoneum and inhibit endometriotic implant-related angiogenesis, with no deleterious effects on physiological angiogenesis in the corpus luteum and during trophoblast implantation.

In a related study, Sharma *et al* demonstrated an *in vitro* inhibitory effect of atorvastatin on both mRNA expression and protein level of COX-2 and VEGF in endometrial-endometriotic cell cultures [91].

The angiostatic effect of statins has been confirmed by *in vivo* studies using a nude mouse model of endometriosis. The authors observed significantly reduced vascularization of endometrial implants after simvastatin treatment [71].

Growth of endometrial tissue

Endometriosis is characterized by inappropriate invasiveness and excessive growth of tissues. The growth of endometriotic tissue may be viewed as the net effect of the increased proliferation and decreased apoptosis ratio. As demonstrated by Klemmt *et al*, DNA synthesis in the endometrial stromal cells derived from patients with endometriosis is significantly elevated in response to specific ECM components (fibronectin, laminin, vitronectin, tanescin-C), suggesting that excessive proliferation starts just after the endometrial stromal cells attach to the soluble and insoluble forms of ECM present in the peritoneal cavity [41]. This process is probably mediated by integrins, cell-to-cell and cell-to-ECM adhesion molecules functioning as signal-transducing receptors in the mitogen-activated protein (MAP) kinase pathway [39,40,92].

Excessive proliferation may also be induced by a broad range of cytokines and growth factors secreted by immunocompetent cells. Thus, hepatocyte growth factor (HGF), produced by peritoneal macrophages, increases *in vitro* growth of endometrial epithelial and stromal cells [93]. Monocyte chemotactic protein (MCP)-1 has also been shown to stimulate endometrial cell proliferation both directly and by stimulation of macrophages to secrete various growth factors (e.g. VEGF, TGF-β, epidermal growth factor (EGF)) and cytokines (e.g. IL-1, IL-6, IL-8, IL-12, RANTES, TNF-α) [94].

Another potentially relevant contributor to growth of endometriotic lesions is IGF-I. Both endometrial stroma and glands express type I and type II IGF receptors [95] and the expression of these receptors may be stimulated by estrogen. Estradiol also increases the sensitivity of cells to IGF by decreasing expression of IGF binding protein (IGFBP)-3 [96]. IGF-I and IGF-II are mitogenic factors for endometrial stromal cells in culture while antibodies blocking IGF-I receptor induce partial inhibition of endometrial stromal cell proliferation [97].

Excessive growth of endometriotic tissue is also related to resistance to apoptosis. As demonstrated by Gebel *et al*, both eutopic and ectopic endometrium from women with endometriosis, independently of the cycle phase, exhibits decreased levels of spontaneous apoptosis when compared to the endometrium of healthy controls [98]. Furthermore, Dmowski *et al* observed decreased spontaneous apoptosis in endometrial glandular cells from patients with endometriosis, especially during the late secretory and early proliferative phases [99]. This increased ability of endometrial cells to survive contributes to the development of the disease.

One of the proposed mechanisms of decreased endometriotic cell death is the secretion of proteins that interfere with recognition of the implant. Increase in the level of the soluble form of Fas ligand (FasL), interfering with the scavenging activity of immune cells, was detected in the peritoneal fluid of women with endometriosis [100]. It was suggested that stromal cells stimulated by TGF-β and platelet-derived growth factor (PDGF), express FasL and induce apoptosis of Fas-bearing immune cells [101,102]. Integrin-mediated endometrial cell attachment to the ECM components (laminin, fibronectin and collagen IV) also upregulates FasL expression, leading to immune cell apoptosis [103]. Furthermore, B-cell lymphoma/leukemia-2 gene (Bcl-2), the proto-oncogene that blocks cell death without promoting cell proliferation, is overexpressed in the eutopic endometrium of women with endometriosis, leading to decreased apoptosis [104,105].

In summary, molecular mechanisms of increased proliferation and reduced apoptosis of endometrial cells from women with endometriosis invoke constitutive activation of the nuclear factor-κ-B (NF-κB) [106, 107] and one of the MAPK pathways: extracellular signal-regulated kinase (ERK1/2) [108].

Statins: effects on growth of mesenchymal tissues
As noted above, the mevalonate pathway can affect several key signal transduction steps relevant to regulation of tissue growth by modulation of isoprenylation of several small GTPases. The most important pathways regulating proliferation include mitogen-activated protein kinase (MAPK) pathways, which are stimulated by growth factors such as IGF-I, as well as by other stimuli including moderate oxidative stress.

Another aspect of tissue growth regulation involves modulation of apoptosis; this process is largely controlled via the PI3 kinase/PKB pathway. Key steps required for activation of the above pathways include isoprenylation of several small GTPases. Consistent with these concepts, inhibition of HMG-CoA reductase by statins decreases proliferation of several cell types including vascular smooth muscle, hepatocytes, mesangial cells, ovarian theca-interstitial cells and several cancer cells [24,47, 109–113]. In these tissues, statin-induced inhibition of proliferation is partly reversed by the intermediate products of the mevalonate pathway including mevalonic acid, FPP and GGPP, but not by squalene or cholesterol, indicating a key role of isoprenylation. Recently, Acquavella *et al* demonstrated that statins increase *in vitro* liver sinusoid endothelial cell apoptosis induced by Fas and TNF-α [114]. The authors suggested that in some clinical conditions associated with the elevated level of apoptosis-related molecules, like soluble FasL and TNF-α, statins can sensitize the endothelial cells to undergo apoptosis. It was also shown that statin-induced apoptosis is mediated by p53 protein and Bax, a Bcl-2 family member [115].

The above mechanisms, however, are not ubiquitous and depend on the cell type. Hence, for example, the statin-induced proliferation of endothelial progenitor cells [116]. Such a range of responses to statins underscores the complexity of the interactions between pathways regulating proliferation and apoptosis. The difference in responses to statins may be, at least in part, due to distinctly different effects of individual small GTPases: for example, two forms of Ras, K-Ras and H-Ras, exert opposite effects on cell sensitivity to apoptosis. Such effects may be related to differential activation of PI3K/PKB and MAPK pathways by K-Ras and H-Ras [117].

Statins and endometrium: inhibition of endometrial stromal growth
Endometriosis is associated with abnormal activation of the MAPK and/or PI3K/PKB pathways, leading to excessive growth of endometriotic implants [118]. Statins may reverse or at least reduce this growth. The inhibitory effect of statins on endometrial stromal cell proliferation was observed in several *in vitro* studies. Piotrowski *et al* have shown that statins exert a potent, concentration-dependent, inhibition of proliferation of endometrial stromal cells; this effect was observed irrespective of the supply of cholesterol. This action of statins was, at least in part, due to decreased production of mevalonate and was associated with decreased activity of the MAPK pathway, possibly via decreased isoprenylation of Ras. In addition, statins induce apoptosis [119]. Comparable findings were also reported by Esfandiari *et al* [90] who demonstrated a concentration-dependent inhibitory effect of lovastatin on cell

growth in an experimental model of endometriosis-like tissue. The above studies carried out on eutopic endometrial cells were recently verified on ectopic-endometriotic tissues, whereby simvastatin inhibited proliferation of cells collected from endometriomas [56].

Another potentially important element in action of statins on growth of endometriotic tissue is related to IGFBP-1. Sharma *et al* observed that atorvastatin increased the level of IGFBP-1 in endometrial-endometriotic cell cultures treated with lipopolysaccharide (LPS). Increased IGFBP-1 level suggests reduced capacity of cells for proliferation and increased differentiation [91].

Estrogens in endometriotic lesions

Endometriosis is an estrogen-dependent disease. The key enzyme in estrogen biosynthesis, aromatase (CYP19), is present in eutopic and ectopic endometrium of women with endometriosis, but is absent in the endometrium of disease-free women [42,120]. Aromatase catalyzes conversions of androstenedione to estrone and testosterone to estradiol. The COX-2–prostaglandin E$_2$ (PGE$_2$) pathway stimulates aromatase activity in the endometriotic implants, increasing local estradiol concentration, which, in turn, by a positive feedback, upregulates PGE$_2$ production. Increased concentration of PGE$_2$ seems to be responsible for increased intracellular 3'-5'-cyclic adenosine monophosphate (cAMP) level, which in turn stimulates aromatase promoter II and initiates transcription [120,121].

Another mechanism regulating endometrial aromatase activity has been described by Bukulmez *et al* who demonstrated that androstenedione, via its conversion to estrone and subsequently to estradiol, enhances recruitment of steroidogenic transcription factor (SF)-1 to the CYP19 IIa promoter and stimulates *in vitro* endometrial aromatase expression [122]. The upregulation of SF-1 mRNA is blocked by estrogen receptor antagonist, indicating that this effect of estradiol is due to direct actions on estrogen receptors (ER). Such positive feedback mechanisms of estrogen on its own production may play an important role in the pathophysiology of endometriosis.

This positive feedback may be enhanced by progesterone resistance, which is commonly observed in women with endometriosis [5,123] and may be due to increased expression of ERβ and decreased ERα/ERβ ratio [5]. Under physiological conditions, progesterone downregulates ER level and hence reduces estrogenic effects; however, in the presence of progesterone resistance, high ER level may increase tissue responsiveness to estrogens and lead to stimulation of aromatase activity. Progesterone resistance may also have other important consequences, for example, conversion of estradiol to a weaker estrogen: estrone is catalyzed in response to progesterone by 17β-hydroxysteroid dehydrogenase 2, normally expressed in the endometrium of healthy women. The resistance to progesterone leads to reduction of this enzyme activity in endometriotic cells and a consequent increase of estradiol in endometriotic lesions [124,125].

Ultimately, excessive local estrogen production and decreased estradiol metabolism to estrone promote inflammation and growth of endometriotic tissue [120,125,126] (Fig. 36.6).

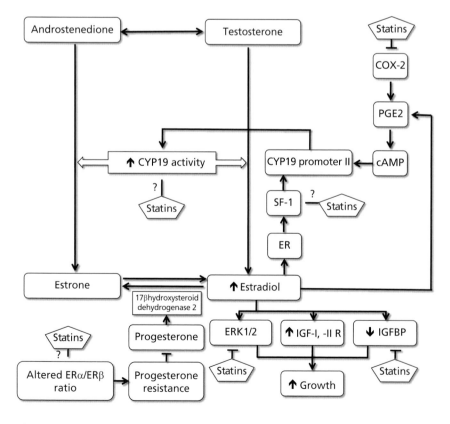

Figure 36.6 Proposed mechanisms regulating estradiol production and function in endometriotic implants in relation to postulated sites of action of statins. cAMP, 3'-5', cyclic adenosine monophosphate; COX-2, cyclooxygenase-2; CYP19, aromatase; ER, estrogen receptor; ERK1/2, extracellular signal-regulated kinase 1 and 2; IGF, insulin-like growth factor; IGFBP, insulin-like growth factor binding protein; PGE$_2$, prostaglandin E$_2$; SF-1, steroidogenic factor 1; "?" denotes potential site of action.

Possible effects of statins on local estrogen production and responsiveness

To date, the effects of statins on endometrial/endometriotic tissue responsiveness and local aromatase activity are not known. However, statins are known to modulate a number of transcription factors [127,128] and their effects on aromatase as well as factors relevant to regulation of aromatase activity, such as SF-1, are plausible and should be tested. Statins may also affect tissue sensitivity to estrogen by alteration of estrogen (ER) and progesterone (PR) receptors.

Indeed, in several tissues statins have been shown to alter ERα levels; thus, for example, simvastatin increases ERα protein level in murine bone marrow stromal cells [129]. In patients with breast cancer receiving lipophilic statins for 1 year or more, there were fewer ER/PR-negative tumors. Moreover, tumors in these patients were of lower grade and stage [130]. This effect of statins on steroid receptor expression may be related to interruption of two pathways known to decrease ER expression (MAPK and NF-κB) [130].

In another study, statins inhibited histone deacetylase (HDAC) in human cancer cells [131]; this finding is relevant since some inhibitors of HDAC have been shown to reactivate ERα in ER-negative breast cancer cells [132]. On the other hand, Eaton *et al* demonstrated that obese women using hydrophobic statins have an increased risk of PR-negative breast cancer compared to non-users [133].

Statins may also affect local estrogen production by interaction with the COX-2–PGE$_2$ pathway although the evidence in support of this concept is indirect. In a rat model of endometriosis, Machado *et al* have shown that selective COX-2 inhibitors decreased PGE$_2$ level, induced antiangiogenic effects and suppressed the growth of endometriotic tissue [134]. Furthermore, statin (atorvastatin) inhibited LPS-induced COX-2 gene expression in endometrial-endometriotic stromal cells; however, estradiol levels in culture medium were not significantly altered [91]. Inhibitory effects of statins on COX-2 were also shown in other tissues such as in endothelial cells or plaque macrophages [63,135] (see Fig. 36.6).

Endometriosis: inflammation, immune dysfunction and oxidative stress

Although the etiology of endometriosis is still not well understood, there is substantial evidence that retrograde menstruation plays a major role in increasing the level of mediators of inflammation in the peritoneal cavity [136]. This distorted intraperitoneal inflammatory microenvironment favors development of endometriosis. Specifically, endometriosis is associated with increased concentrations of activated macrophages and changes in the cytokine network including IL-8, TNF-α, MCP-1, TGF-β, regulated on activation normal T-cell expressed and secreted (RANTES), macrophage colony-stimulating factor (MCSF), interferon (INF)-γ and several other proinflammatory chemoattractant cytokines (e.g. IL-1, IL-4, IL-5, IL-6, IL-10, IL-13, IL-15) [61,137,138]. Menstrual endometrium and macroscopically normal peritoneum of women with endometriosis

demonstrate increased mRNA levels of inflammatory cytokines (TNF-α, IL-6, IL-8) compared to healthy controls [59]. Significant elevation of IL-1β and RANTES mRNA levels was also observed in the luteal-phase endometrium of subjects with endometriosis when compared to disease-free women [42].

Changes in cytokine levels and immune-related cell number in the peritoneal fluid of women with endometriosis are accompanied by elevation of C-reactive protein (CRP), serum amyloid A (SAA), TNF-α, IL-6, IL-8 and MCP-1 in peripheral blood, suggesting that endometriosis is associated with subclinical systemic inflammation [139,140].

Another important consideration relates to the association of endometriosis with impaired immune recognition and clearance of ectopic endometrial cells, suppressed cytotoxicity of natural killer (NK) cells, as well as autoimmune activation of B-cells accompanied by increased production of antinuclear autoantibodies (ANA) [61,141–143]. Activated macrophages in patients with endometriosis also promote growth and vascularization of lesions [144]. A defective immune response in women with endometriosis allows for the survival of the ectopic endometrial tissue and establishment of the disease [101].

Systemic inflammation may be induced by oxidative stress, another important component of endometriosis [23,145]. Leukocytes attracted to the peritoneal cavity and endometriotic lesions are activated by the above listed chemokines and are an important source of ROS. ROS production is also upregulated in endometriotic cells [145]. Furthermore, it appears that endometriosis is associated with depletion of antioxidant capacity. Intraperitoneal levels of vitamin E are decreased, likely due to its consumption by oxidation reactions [146]. These observations are also in accord with the findings of Ota *et al*, who demonstrated elevated levels of several enzymes involved in the generation and metabolism of ROS in endometrial tissues and endometrial implants from women with endometriosis [147–150]. Moreover, Foyouzi *et al* and Ngo *et al* found that proliferation of endometrial stroma is stimulated by moderate oxidative stress and inhibited by antioxidants [22,145]. The proposed mechanism is related to the stimulatory effect of ROS on the MAP kinase ERK1/2 pathway [145]. These findings are consistent with the notion that ROS at lower concentrations may serve as a second messenger system modulating enzymes and intracellular signaling molecules [21].

Statins: effects on inflammation, immune responses and oxidative stress

Extensive evidence from various biological systems demonstrates that statins reduce inflammation, modulate immune responses and exert antioxidant effects. Anti-inflammatory effects of statins are manifested by lowering CRP level and suppressing proinflammatory agents such as TNF-α and interleukins [151]. *In vitro* studies have shown that statins reduce oxidized low-density lipoprotein (oxLDL)-induced secretion of IL-8 and decrease production of MCP-1 by endothelial cells [152].

As immunomodulators, statins may exert beneficial effects on autoimmune diseases [153]. Increased major histocompatibility complex (MHC) class II molecule expression occurs in several autoimmune diseases. Statins have been shown to alter the function of antigen-presenting cells (APCs) by inhibiting INF-γ-inducible expression of the MHC class II transactivator (CIITA) and by preventing cytokine-induced maturation of APCs [154–156]. MHC class II molecule expression could also be affected by statins via reduced cholesterol level and altered integrity of cell membrane lipid rafts but this still needs to be verified [157,158].

Another mechanism of action of statins on immune response involves changing the expression of leukocyte and endothelial cell adhesion molecules (i.e. ICAM, VCAM) as well as reducing leukocyte proliferation, extravasation, infiltration of the target tissue and phagocytosis. Decreased cell adhesion molecules caused by statins could be related to inhibition of TNF-α-induced activation of NF-κB and enhanced expression of PPARα [159]. Furthermore, it has also been suggested that statins could directly bind the β2 integrin leukocyte function antigen (LFA)-1, resulting in reduced adhesion and stimulation of leukocytes [160]. Leukocyte motility and migration are also affected [67].

Effects of statins on immune function, in large measure, are related to reduction of protein isoprenylation [67]. Statin-induced reduction in activity of small GTPases may alter the formation of the immunological synapses between T-cells and APCs and decrease T-cell proliferation. Moreover, statins can modulate disease progression through alteration of T-cell phenotype. Current, but still controversial concepts propose that statins induce a shift in T-cell phenotype, from Th1 to Th2, causing a strong attenuation of the Th1-type immune response (IL-2, IL-12, INF-γ, TNF) and increased secretion of anti-inflammatory Th2-type cytokines (IL-4, I-5, IL-10) [67].

In addition to modulation of isoprenylation, statins may affect immune responses through other mechanisms such as cellular lipid raft structure distortion which seems to be responsible for the inhibition of NK cell cytotoxity and inhibition of Fcγ-receptor-mediated activation of ERK and p38 MAPK in monocytes, resulting in decreased cytokine release [161,162].

Statins may also have a significant effect on the level of oxidative stress. A broad range of non-phagocytic cells produce superoxide anions and other ROS in response to extracellular stimuli such as PDGF or EGF [163,164]. The mevalonate pathway may modulate oxidative stress by reduction of the synthesis of an antioxidant, coenzyme Q, upregulation of expression and activity of catalase (CAT; an enzyme metabolizing hydrogen peroxide into water and molecular oxygen) and isoprenylation-related changes (inhibition of Rac1 isoprenylation) of the activity of NADPH oxidase, an important source of ROS [165].

Coenzyme Q, a product of FPP via polyprenyl-pyrophosphate, plays a central role in the mitochondrial respiratory chain and is involved in a number of cellular functions including modulation of the plasma membrane redox state, regulation of mitochondrial permeability, activation of mitochondrial uncoupling proteins, and control of tyrosine kinase [166,167]. Coenzyme Q is able to prevent lipid peroxidation in most intracellular membranes and as an antioxidant, it may be more efficient than vitamin E [168,169]. Reduction of the level of coenzyme Q by statins may play a role in statin-induced liver and muscle cytolysis as discussed above.

Statins may also affect oxidative stress by inhibition of the mevalonate pathway and decreasing the activity of a small GTPase, Rac, which is essential for generation of ROS by NADPH oxidase [165]. The assembly of NADPH oxidase requires the presence of Rac at the plasma membrane (i.e. isoprenylation of Rac). Two components of NADPH oxidase, p47phox and p67phox, are cytosolic proteins which complex with Rac1 in order to induce NADPH oxidase activity [170]. These proteins combine with membrane-bound p22phox and gp91phox (or its homologs Nox1, 3, 4 or 5).

Studies on vascular smooth muscle, cardiac muscle and ovarian theca-interstitial cells confirmed the role of statins in reducing oxidative stress level in association with inhibition of isoprenylation [165,171,172]. Thus, for example, Wassmann *et al* reported that atorvastatin decreased oxidative stress, and that this effect was reversed by the addition of mevalonate but not cell- and mitochondrion-permeable cholesterol (25-hydroxycholesterol), indicating the importance of isoprenylation rather than cholesterol synthesis in the regulation of oxidative stress [165]. Atorvastatin reduced oxidative stress by inhibiting vascular mRNA expression of p22phox and Nox1, as well as increasing catalase expression. This was accompanied by reduced translocation of Rac1 from the cytosol to the cell membrane. In other experiments in vascular smooth muscle, inhibition of geranylgeranylation reduced angiotensin II-mediated oxidative stress [172]. Statins also decreased oxidative stress in coronary smooth muscle via mechanisms involving suppression of phospholipase D (PLD) and protein kinase C-a (PKC-a) [173]. Overall, it is apparent that the net effect of inhibition of the mevalonate pathway is the reduction of oxidative stress.

In addition to the effects mediated by inhibition of the mevalonate pathway, statins have a pronounced intrinsic antioxidant activity. *In vitro* experiments have shown that statins antagonize oxidation by hydroxyl as well as peroxyl radicals [174]. Among several tested statins, simvastatin had the greatest scavenging capacity towards hydroxyl radicals, while fluvastatin was most effective in quenching peroxyl radicals. *In vivo*, statins have been shown to exert potent antioxidant effects including reduction of plasma levels of nitrotyrosine and chlorotyrosine [175].

It is likely that the above listed actions of statins may decrease inflammation and oxidative stress associated with endometriosis. Furthermore, in view of the autoimmune aspects of endometriosis, the immunomodulatory properties of statins may also have beneficial effects.

Statins and endometrium: increased expression of anti-inflammatory genes

While anti-inflammatory and antioxidant properties of statins are well established in many biological systems, little is known about how they affect endometrial/endometritotic tissues. To the best of our knowledge, only one report has addressed this issue in a study evaluating effects of atorvastatin on endometrial-endometriotic cells exposed to LPS in culture [91]. In that study, atorvastatin decreased mRNA and protein expression of COX-2, a rate-limiting enzyme in prostaglandin synthesis, and increased mRNA and protein expression of the anti-inflammatory and antioxidative genes: PPARγ and liver X receptor-α (LXR-α).

Other potential benefits of use of statins

In addition to the above discussed proven and proposed effects of statins on development of endometriosis, statins may also provide additional relevant benefits such as effects on pain, depression and bone density.

Pain is one of the most important symptoms of endometriosis and indirect evidence related to the actions of statins on NF-κB suggests that statins may reduce pain. One of the features of endometriosis is activation of NF-κB (e.g. by TNF-α) which in turn leads to expression of NF-κB-induced genes and release of cytokines [106,107,176,177]. NF-κB is also believed to underlie the complex regional pain syndrome (CRPS), including inflammation, ischemia and sensitization [178], interact with substance P [179] and modulate development of neuropathic pain [180]. Several studies have shown that statins decrease expression of NF-κB in various tissues [181–184]. Moreover, it was shown that atorvastatin inhibits nitroglycerin-induced activation of NF-κB in the trigeminal nucleus caudalis (TNC) and partly blocks transmission of experimentally induced migraine-related pain in the central nervous system [184]. These findings require verification, ideally in clinical trials on women with endometriosis.

An important aspect of endometriosis is its association with mood disorders including depression, anxiety and frustration due to typical symptoms of endometriosis such as dysmenorrhea, intermenstrual chronic pelvic pain, dyspareunia and infertility [185]. Mood disorders may also affect immune responses and even predispose to inflammatory diseases [186]. Interestingly, in an observational study of patients with coronary artery disease, long-term use of statins was shown to improve psychological well-being, as well as reducing risk of depression, anxiety and hostility [187]. The authors of the study postulated that statins directly affect the central nervous system. Wirleitner *et al* suggested a role of statins in the inhibition of an enzyme: indolamine (2,3)-dioxygenase (IDO) [188]. IDO degrades tryptophan, the precursor of the neurotransmitter serotonin (5-hydroxytryptamine), responsible for regulation of mood, appetite, sleep and some cognitive functions including memory and learning. Distorted serotonin production has a strong association with depression. Further studies evaluating the effect of statins on tryptophan metabolism in humans are needed.

Another possibly beneficial effect of statins in endometriosis treatment is related to their bone protective action which may be of particular benefit if statins were to be used in conjunction with GnRH analogs. Several studies have demonstrated that statins stimulate bone formation and inhibit bone resorption [189,190]. However, clinical studies evaluating the risk of bone fracture among users and non-users of statins have so far yielded conflicting results [191,192]. To date, there is no information regarding the effect of statins on bone density in users of GnRH analogs.

Statins: effects *in vivo* (rodent models of endometriosis)

At present, two studies have evaluated the effects of statins on animal models of endometriosis. The first study was published by Oktem *et al* [193] who evaluated effects of atorvastatin on experimentally induced endometriosis in the rat model. Wistar-Albino rats underwent laparotomy and endometrial tissue fragments were placed in the peritoneal cavity. Three weeks later the animals underwent a second laparotomy to evaluate the size of endometriotic implants. The rats were then randomly assigned into four groups: group I received 0.5 mg/kg/day oral atorvastatin (low-dose atorvastatin group), group II received 2.5 mg/kg/day oral atorvastatin (high-dose atorvastatin group), group III was given a single dose of 1 mg/kg SC leuprolide acetate (GnRH agonist group), and group IV received no medication (control group). After 21 days of treatment, the animals were euthanized and implant size, VEGF level in peritoneal fluid and histopathological scores evaluating the presence of epithelial cells in the implants were assessed. The mean areas of implants were smaller and VEGF levels in peritoneal fluid were lower in groups II and III than those in group I and the control group ($P < 0.05$). The mean areas of implants decreased from 41.2 ± 13.9 to $22.7 \pm 13.9 \, \text{mm}^2$ in group II ($P < 0.05$) and from 41.2 ± 18.1 to $13.1 \pm 13.8 \, \text{mm}^2$ in group III ($P < 0.05$). In group I, the mean area increased from 43.0 ± 12.7 to $50.5 \pm 13.9 \, \text{mm}^2$. In parallel, histopathological scores of implants also decreased following atorvastatin treatment. The authors concluded that high-dose atorvastatin caused a significant regression of endometriotic implants.

The second study evaluated the effects of simvastatin on a nude mouse model of endometriosis and the role of simvastatin in the modulation of MMP-3 [70,71]. Proliferative-phase human endometrial biopsies were obtained and established as organ cultures. To induce development of endometriosis in the nude mouse, endometrial tissues were first incubated in 1 nM estradiol (E_2) for 24 h and subsequently injected intraperitoneally into ovariectomized nude mice. All mice received E_2 (8 μg, silastic capsule implants). In addition, the animals received either placebo or simvastatin (5 and 25 mg/kg/day) by gavage for 10 days, beginning 1 day after injection of endometrial tissues. The animals were then euthanized and endometrial implants were evaluated. Simvastatin induced a significant dose-dependent inhibition of the number and the volume of endometrial implants (Plate 36.1). At the highest dose, simvastatin induced an 87%

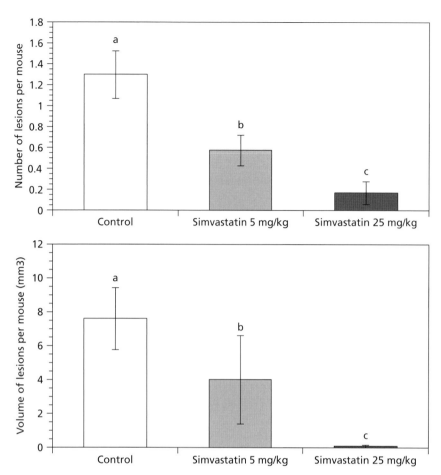

Figure 36.7 Effects of simvastatin on the number and volume of lesions per mouse; each *bar* represents mean ± SEM. Means with *no superscripts in common* are significantly different (*P* < 0.05). The figure summarizes three separate experiments on 37 mice: 13 in the control group, 12 treated with simvastatin at 5 mg/kg, and 12 treated with simvastatin at 25 mg/kg. Simvastatin protects against the development of endometriosis in a nude mouse model. Reproduced from Bruner-Tran *et al* [71] with permission from the Endocrine Society.

decrease in the number of lesions and 98% decrease in the volume of lesions per mouse (Fig. 36.7).

The above findings are encouraging and suggest that statins hold promise as a possible new treatment of endometriosis. However, in view of significant differences in the reproductive systems of humans and rodents, rat and mouse models of endometriosis are only distantly related to endometriosis in humans. Molecular cross-talk between xenograft and host tissue in animal model of endometriosis could be potentially distorted by species-different affinities of receptors to the ligands. Rodents do not undergo menstruation and do not develop spontaneous endometriosis. In addition, the above models involve the use of endometrial tissues in the absence of potentially important blood components present in retrograde menstruation in humans.

Future directions

Evaluation of statins as a potential novel treatment of endometriosis is still in its early stages. Promising findings of studies on rodent models of endometriosis and interesting results of *in vitro* experiments indicate that statins may provide a wide range of beneficial effects; however, the use of statins to treat endometriosis in clinical practice still cannot be recommended.

Ideally, further studies should include work on the primate model of endometriosis, such as the baboon. Subsequently, prospective randomized clinical trials in women with endometriosis will need to evaluate effectiveness of statins, optimal doses, appropriate duration of treatment and long-term safety.

Conclusion

Inhibition of the mevalonate pathway by statins, as well as their intrinsic antioxidant properties, may exert several beneficial effects on endometriosis, including decreased endometrial stromal cell adhesiveness, invasiveness, proliferation, angiogenesis, inflammation and oxidative stress. Available evidence suggests that statins alone or in combination with other therapeutic options may inhibit the initiation and progression of endometriosis.

References

1. Propst AM, Laufer MR. Endometriosis in adolescents. Incidence, diagnosis and treatment. J Reprod Med. 1999;44(9):751–758.

2. Panay N. Advances in the medical management of endometriosis. Br J Obstet Gynaecol 2008;115(7):814–817.

3. Mahmood TA, Templeton A. Prevalence and genesis of endometriosis. Hum Reprod 1991;6(4):544–549.

4. Giudice LC, Kao LC. Endometriosis. Lancet 2004;364(9447): 1789–1799.

5. Bulun SE, Cheng YH, Pavone ME et al. Estrogen receptor-beta, estrogen receptor-alpha, and progesterone resistance in endometriosis. Semin Reprod Med;28(1):36–43.

6. ACOG Committee Opinion No. 392, December 2007. Intrauterine device and adolescents. Obstet Gynecol 2007;110(6):1493–1495.

7. Romer T, Linsberger D. User satisfaction with a levonorgestrel-releasing intrauterine system (LNG-IUS): data from an international survey. Eur J Contracept Reprod Health Care 2009;14(6):391–398.

8. EHSRE Capri Workshop Group. Intrauterine devices and intrauterine systems. Hum Reprod Update 2008;14(3):197–208.

9. Ferrero S, Venturini PL, Ragni N, Camerini G, Remorgida V. Pharmacological treatment of endometriosis: experience with aromatase inhibitors. Drugs 2009;69(8):943–952.

10. Janni W, Hepp P. Adjuvant aromatase inhibitor therapy: outcomes and safety. Cancer Treat Rev 2010;36(3):249–261.

11. Mortimer JE. Managing the toxicities of the aromatase inhibitors. Curr Opin Obstet Gynecol;22(1):56–60.

12. Dorjgochoo T, Gu K, Kallianpur A et al. Menopausal symptoms among breast cancer patients 6 months after diagnosis: a report from the Shanghai Breast Cancer Survival Study. Menopause 2009;16(6): 1205–1212.

13. Pintiaux A, Chabbert-Buffet N, Foidart JM. Gynaecological uses of a new class of steroids: the selective progesterone receptor modulators. Gynecol Endocrinol 2009;25(2):67–73.

14. Mutter GL, Bergeron C, Deligdisch L et al. The spectrum of endometrial pathology induced by progesterone receptor modulators. Mod Pathol 2008;21(5):591–598.

15. Grady D, Sawaya GF, Johnson KC et al. MF101, a selective estrogen receptor beta modulator for the treatment of menopausal hot flushes: a phase II clinical trial. Menopause 2009;16(3):458–465.

16. Candiani GB, Fedele L, Vercellini P, Bianchi S, di Nola G. Repetitive conservative surgery for recurrence of endometriosis. Obstet Gynecol 1991;77(3):421–424.

17. Wheeler JM, Malinak LR. Recurrent endometriosis: incidence, management, and prognosis. Am J Obstet Gynecol 1983;146(3): 247–253.

18. Istvan ES, Deisenhofer J. Structural mechanism for statin inhibition of HMG-CoA reductase. Science 2001;292(5519):1160–1164.

19. Goldstein JL, Brown MS. Regulation of the mevalonate pathway. Nature 1990;343(6257):425–430.

20. Zhang FL, Casey PJ. Protein prenylation: molecular mechanisms and functional consequences. Annu Rev Biochem 1996;65:241–269.

21. Adam O, Laufs U. Antioxidative effects of statins. Arch Toxicol 2008;82(12):885–892.

22. Foyouzi N, Berkkanoglu M, Arici A, Kwintkiewicz J, Izquierdo D, Duleba AJ. Effects of oxidants and antioxidants on proliferation of endometrial stromal cells. Fertil Steril 2004;82 Suppl 3:1019–1022.

23. Santanam N, Murphy AA, Parthasarathy S. Macrophages, oxidation, and endometriosis. Ann N Y Acad Sci 2002;955:183–198; discussion 19–200, 396–406.

24. Danesh FR, Sadeghi MM, Amro N et al. 3-Hydroxy-3-methylglutaryl CoA reductase inhibitors prevent high glucose-induced proliferation of mesangial cells via modulation of Rho GTPase/ p21 signaling pathway: implications for diabetic nephropathy. Proc Natl Acad Sci USA 2002;99(12):8301–8305.

25. Mattingly RR, Gibbs RA, Menard RE, Reiners JJ Jr. Potent suppression of proliferation of a10 vascular smooth muscle cells by combined treatment with lovastatin and 3-allylfarnesol, an inhibitor of protein farnesyltransferase. J Pharmacol Exp Ther 2002;303(1):74–81.

26. Porter KE, Naik J, Turner NA, Dickinson T, Thompson MM, London NJ. Simvastatin inhibits human saphenous vein neointima formation via inhibition of smooth muscle cell proliferation and migration. J Vasc Surg 2002;36(1):150–157.

27. Levy HB, Kohlhaas HK. Considerations for supplementing with coenzyme Q10 during statin therapy. Ann Pharmacother 2006;40(2): 290–294.

28. Marcoff L, Thompson PD. The role of coenzyme Q10 in statin-associated myopathy: a systematic review. J Am Coll Cardiol 2007; 49(23):2231–2237.

29. Anfossi G, Massucco P, Bonomo K, Trovati M. Prescription of statins to dyslipidemic patients affected by liver diseases: a subtle balance between risks and benefits. Nutr Metab Cardiovasc Dis 2004; 14(4):215–224.

30. Edison RJ, Muenke M. Mechanistic and epidemiologic considerations in the evaluation of adverse birth outcomes following gestational exposure to statins. Am J Med Genet A 2004;131(3):287–298.

31. Kazmin A, Garcia-Bournissen F, Koren G. Risks of statin use during pregnancy: a systematic review. J Obstet Gynaecol Can 2007;29(11): 906–908.

32. Taguchi N, Rubin ET, Hosokawa A et al. Prenatal exposure to HMG-CoA reductase inhibitors: effects on fetal and neonatal outcomes. Reprod Toxicol 2008;26(2):175–177.

33. Witz CA, Thomas MR, Montoya-Rodriguez IA, Nair AS, Centonze VE, Schenken RS. Short-term culture of peritoneum explants confirms attachment of endometrium to intact peritoneal mesothelium. Fertil Steril 2001;75(2):385–390.

34. Lucidi RS, Witz CA, Chrisco M, Binkley PA, Shain SA, Schenken RS. A novel in vitro model of the early endometriotic lesion demonstrates that attachment of endometrial cells to mesothelial cells is dependent on the source of endometrial cells. Fertil Steril 2005;84(1):16–21.

35. Van der Linden PJ, de Goeij AF, Dunselman GA, Erkens HW, Evers JL. Amniotic membrane as an in vitro model for endometrium-extracellular matrix interactions. Gynecol Obstet Invest 1998;45(1): 7–11.

36. Koks CA, Groothuis PG, Dunselman GA, de Goeij AF, Evers JL. Adhesion of menstrual endometrium to extracellular matrix: the possible role of integrin alpha(6)beta(1) and laminin interaction. Mol Hum Reprod 2000;6(2):170–177.

37. Klentzeris LD. Adhesion molecules in reproduction. Br J Obstet Gynaecol 1997;104(4):401–409.

38. Schwartz MA, Denninghoff K. Alpha v integrins mediate the rise in intracellular calcium in endothelial cells on fibronectin even though they play a minor role in adhesion. J Biol Chem 1994;269(15): 11133–11137.

39. Chen Q, Kinch MS, Lin TH, Burridge K, Juliano RL. Integrin-mediated cell adhesion activates mitogen-activated protein kinases. J Biol Chem 1994;269(43):26602–26605.

40. Meredith JE Jr, Winitz S, Lewis JM et al. The regulation of growth and intracellular signaling by integrins. Endocr Rev 1996;17(3):207–220.

41. Klemmt PA, Carver JG, Koninckx P, McVeigh EJ, Mardon HJ. Endometrial cells from women with endometriosis have increased adhesion and proliferative capacity in response to extracellular matrix components: towards a mechanistic model for endometriosis progression. Hum Reprod 2007;22(12):3139–3147.

42. Kyama CM, Overbergh L, Mihalyi A et al. Endometrial and peritoneal expression of aromatase, cytokines, and adhesion factors in women with endometriosis. Fertil Steril 2008;89(2):301–310.

43. Hull ML, Escareno CR, Godsland JM et al. Endometrial-peritoneal interactions during endometriotic lesion establishment. Am J Pathol 2008;173(3):700–715.

44. Kim HO, Yang KM, Kang IS et al. Expression of CD44s, vascular endothelial growth factor, matrix metalloproteinase-2 and Ki-67 in peritoneal, rectovaginal and ovarian endometriosis. J Reprod Med 2007;52(3):207–213.

45. Goueffic Y, Guilluy C, Guerin P, Patra P, Pacaud P, Loirand G. Hyaluronan induces vascular smooth muscle cell migration through RHAMM-mediated PI3K-dependent Rac activation. Cardiovasc Res 2006;72(2):339–348.

46. Griffith JS, Liu YG, Tekmal RR, Binkley PA, Holden AE, Schenken RS. Menstrual endometrial cells from women with endometriosis demonstrate increased adherence to peritoneal cells and increased expression of CD44 splice variants. Fertil Steril 2010;93(6):1745–1749.

47. Heusinger-Ribeiro J, Fischer B, Goppelt-Struebe M. Differential effects of simvastatin on mesangial cells. Kidney Int 2004;66(1):187–195.

48. Fritz G, Kaina B. Rho GTPases: promising cellular targets for novel anticancer drugs. Curr Cancer Drug Targets 2006;6(1):1–14.

49. Raptis L, Arulanandam R, Vultur A, Geletu M, Chevalier S, Feracci H. Beyond structure, to survival: activation of Stat3 by cadherin engagement. Biochem Cell Biol 2009;87(6):835–843.

50. Bosco EE, Mulloy JC, Zheng Y. Rac1 GTPase: a "Rac" of all trades. Cell Mol Life Sci 2009;66(3):370–374.

51. Suzuki J, Jin ZG, Meoli DF, Matoba T, Berk BC. Cyclophilin A is secreted by a vesicular pathway in vascular smooth muscle cells. Circ Res 2006;98(6):811–817.

52. Pellegrin S, Mellor H. Actin stress fibres. J Cell Sci 2007;120 (Pt 20):3491–3499.

53. Nobes CD, Hall A. Rho, rac, and cdc42 GTPases regulate the assembly of multimolecular focal complexes associated with actin stress fibers, lamellipodia, and filopodia. Cell 1995;81(1):53–62.

54. Xu H, Zeng L, Peng H et al. HMG-CoA reductase inhibitor simvastatin mitigates VEGF-induced "inside-out" signaling to extracellular matrix by preventing RhoA activation. Am J Physiol Renal Physiol 2006;291(5):F995–1004.

55. Dobreanu M, Dobreanu D, Fodor A, Bacarea A. Integrin expression on monocytes and lymphocytes in unstable angina short term effects of atorvastatin. Rom J Intern Med 2007;45(2):193–199.

56. Nasu K, Yuge A, Tsuno A, Narahara H. Simvastatin inhibits the proliferation and the contractility of human endometriotic stromal cells: a promising agent for the treatment of endometriosis. Fertil Steril 2009;92(6):2097–2099.

57. Osteen KG, Yeaman GR, Bruner-Tran KL. Matrix metalloproteinases and endometriosis. Semin Reprod Med 2003;21(2):155–164.

58. Chung HW, Lee JY, Moon HS et al. Matrix metalloproteinase-2, membranous type 1 matrix metalloproteinase, and tissue inhibitor of metalloproteinase-2 expression in ectopic and eutopic endometrium. Fertil Steril 2002;78(4):787–795.

59. Kyama CM, Overbergh L, Debrock S et al. Increased peritoneal and endometrial gene expression of biologically relevant cytokines and growth factors during the menstrual phase in women with endometriosis. Fertil Steril 2006;85(6):1667–1675.

60. Bruner-Tran KL, Eisenberg E, Yeaman GR, Anderson TA, McBean J, Osteen KG. Steroid and cytokine regulation of matrix metalloproteinase expression in endometriosis and the establishment of experimental endometriosis in nude mice. J Clin Endocrinol Metab 2002;87(10):4782–4791.

61. Siristatidis C, Nissotakis C, Chrelias C, Iacovidou H, Salamalekis E. Immunological factors and their role in the genesis and development of endometriosis. J Obstet Gynaecol Res 2006;32(2):162–170.

62. Schweitzer M, Mitmaker B, Obrand D et al. Atorvastatin modulates matrix metalloproteinase expression, activity, and signaling in abdominal aortic aneurysms. Vasc Endovascular Surg;44(2):116–122.

63. Massaro M, Zampolli A, Scoditti E et al. Statins inhibit cyclooxygenase-2 and matrix metalloproteinase-9 in human endothelial cells: anti-angiogenic actions possibly contributing to plaque stability. Cardiovasc Res 2010;86(2):311–320.

64. Sluijter JP, de Kleijn DP, Pasterkamp G. Vascular remodeling and protease inhibition – bench to bedside. Cardiovasc Res 2006;69(3): 595–603.

65. Porter KE, Turner NA. Statins for the prevention of vein graft stenosis: a role for inhibition of matrix metalloproteinase-9. Biochem Soc Trans 2002;30(2):120–126.

66. Mastroianni CM, Liuzzi GM. Matrix metalloproteinase dysregulation in HIV infection: implications for therapeutic strategies. Trends Mol Med 2007;13(11):449–459.

67. Greenwood J, Steinman L, Zamvil SS. Statin therapy and autoimmune disease: from protein prenylation to immunomodulation. Nat Rev Immunol 2006;6(5):358–370.

68. Kamio K, Liu XD, Sugiura H et al. Statins inhibit MMP release from human lung fibroblasts. Eur Respir J 2010;35(3):637–646.

69. Grip O, Janciauskiene S, Lindgren S. Atorvastatin activates PPAR-gamma and attenuates the inflammatory response in human monocytes. Inflamm Res 2002;51(2):58–62.

70. Bruner-Tran KL, Osteen KG, Duleba AJ (eds). Simvastatin inhibits development of experimental endometriosis; role of inhibition of MMP-3. SGI 55th Annual Meeting, March 26–29 2008. San Diego: SAGE Publications.

71. Bruner-Tran KL, Osteen KG, Duleba AJ. Simvastatin protects against the development of endometriosis in a nude mouse model. J Clin Endocrinol Metab 2009;94(7):2489–2494.

72. Groothuis PG, Nap AW, Winterhager E, Grummer R. Vascular development in endometriosis. Angiogenesis 2005;8(2):147–156.

73. Eggermont J, Donnez J, Casanas-Roux F, Scholtes H, Van Langendonckt A. Time course of pelvic endometriotic lesion revascularization in a nude mouse model. Fertil Steril 2005;84(2):492–499.

74. Grummer R, Schwarzer F, Bainczyk K et al. Peritoneal endometriosis: validation of an in-vivo model. Hum Reprod 2001;16(8):1736–1743.

75. Ruegg C, Dormond O, Mariotti A. Endothelial cell integrins and COX-2: mediators and therapeutic targets of tumor angiogenesis. Biochim Biophys Acta 2004;1654(1):51–67.

76. Reddy KV, Mangale SS. Integrin receptors: the dynamic modulators of endometrial function. Tissue Cell 2003;35(4):260–273.

77. Machado DE, Berardo PT, Palmero CY, Nasciutti LE. Higher expression of vascular endothelial growth factor (VEGF) and its receptor VEGFR-2 (Flk-1) and metalloproteinase-9 (MMP-9) in a rat model of peritoneal endometriosis is similar to cancer diseases. J Exp Clin Cancer Res 2010;29(1):4.

78. Omwandho CO, Konrad L, Halis G, Oehmke F, Tinneberg HR. Role of TGF-betas in normal human endometrium and endometriosis. Hum Reprod;25(1):101–109.

79. Donnez J, Smoes P, Gillerot S, Casanas-Roux F, Nisolle M. Vascular endothelial growth factor (VEGF) in endometriosis. Hum Reprod 1998;13(6):1686–1690.

80. Walshe TE, Saint-Geniez M, Maharaj AS, Sekiyama E, Maldonado AE, d'Amore PA. TGF-beta is required for vascular barrier function, endothelial survival and homeostasis of the adult microvasculature. PLoS One 2009;4(4):e5149.

81. Chishima F, Hayakawa S, Sugita K et al. Increased expression of cyclooxygenase-2 in local lesions of endometriosis patients. Am J Reprod Immunol 2002;48(1):50–56.

82. Hindler K, Cleeland CS, Rivera E, Collard CD. The role of statins in cancer therapy. Oncologist 2006;11(3):306–315.

83. Weis M, Heeschen C, Glassford AJ, Cooke JP. Statins have biphasic effects on angiogenesis. Circulation 2002;105(6):739–745.

84. Skaletz-Rorowski A, Walsh K. Statin therapy and angiogenesis. Curr Opin Lipidol 2003;14(6):599–603.

85. Elewa HF, El-Remessy AB, Somanath PR, Fagan SC. Diverse effects of statins on angiogenesis: new therapeutic avenues. Pharmacotherapy 2010;30(2):169–176.

86. Endres M. Statins and stroke. J Cereb Blood Flow Metab 2005;25(9):1093–1110.

87. Bartoli M, Al-Shabrawey M, Labazi M et al. HMG-CoA reductase inhibitors (statin) prevents retinal neovascularization in a model of oxygen-induced retinopathy. Invest Ophthalmol Vis Sci 2009;50(10):4934–4940.

88. Park HJ, Zhang Y, Georgescu SP, Johnson KL, Kong D, Galper JB. Human umbilical vein endothelial cells and human dermal microvascular endothelial cells offer new insights into the relationship between lipid metabolism and angiogenesis. Stem Cell Rev 2006;2(2):93–102.

89. Zhang Y, Naggar JC, Welzig CM et al. Simvastatin inhibits angiotensin II-induced abdominal aortic aneurysm formation in apolipoprotein E-knockout mice: possible role of ERK. Arterioscler Thromb Vasc Biol 2009;29(11):1764–1771.

90. Esfandiari N, Khazaei M, Ai J, Bielecki R et al. Effect of a statin on an in vitro model of endometriosis. Fertil Steril 2007;87(2):257–262.

91. Sharma I, Dhawan V, Mahajan N, Chand Saha S, Dhaliwal LK. In vitro effects of atorvastatin on lipopolysaccharide-induced gene expression in endometriotic stromal cells. Fertil Steril 2010;94(5): 1639–1646.

92. Lee JW, Juliano R. Mitogenic signal transduction by integrin- and growth factor receptor-mediated pathways. Mol Cells 2004;17(2): 188–202.

93. Khan KN, Masuzaki H, Fujishita A et al. Regulation of hepatocyte growth factor by basal and stimulated macrophages in women with endometriosis. Hum Reprod 2005;20(1):49–60.

94. Arici A, Oral E, Attar E, Tazuke SI, Olive DL. Monocyte chemotactic protein-1 concentration in peritoneal fluid of women with endometriosis and its modulation of expression in mesothelial cells. Fertil Steril 1997;67(6):1065–1072.

95. Giudice LC, Dsupin BA, Jin IH, Vu TH, Hoffman AR. Differential expression of messenger ribonucleic acids encoding insulin-like growth factors and their receptors in human uterine endometrium and decidua. J Clin Endocrinol Metab 1993;76(5):1115–1122.

96. Kleinman D, Karas M, Roberts CT Jr et al. Modulation of insulin-like growth factor I (IGF-I) receptors and membrane-associated IGF-binding proteins in endometrial cancer cells by estradiol. Endocrinology 1995;136(6):2531–2537.

97. Giudice LC, Dsupin BA, Gargosky SE, Rosenfeld RG, Irwin JC. The insulin-like growth factor system in human peritoneal fluid: its effects on endometrial stromal cells and its potential relevance to endometriosis. J Clin Endocrinol Metab 1994;79(5):1284–1293.

98. Gebel HM, Braun DP, Tambur A, Frame D, Rana N, Dmowski WP. Spontaneous apoptosis of endometrial tissue is impaired in women with endometriosis. Fertil Steril 1998;69(6):1042–1047.

99. Dmowski WP, Ding J, Shen J, Rana N, Fernandez BB, Braun DP. Apoptosis in endometrial glandular and stromal cells in women with and without endometriosis. Hum Reprod 2001;16(9):1802–1808.

100. Garcia-Velasco JA, Mulayim N, Kayisli UA, Arici A. Elevated soluble Fas ligand levels may suggest a role for apoptosis in women with endometriosis. Fertil Steril 2002;78(4):855–859.

101. Lebovic DI, Mueller MD, Taylor RN. Immunobiology of endometriosis. Fertil Steril 2001;75(1):1–10.

102. Garcia-Velasco JA, Arici A, Zreik T, Naftolin F, Mor G. Macrophage derived growth factors modulate Fas ligand expression in cultured endometrial stromal cells: a role in endometriosis. Mol Hum Reprod 1999;5(7):642–650.

103. Selam B, Kayisli UA, Garcia-Velasco JA, Arici A. Extracellular matrix-dependent regulation of Fas ligand expression in human endometrial stromal cells. Biol Reprod 2002;66(1):1–5.

104. Meresman GF, Vighi S, Buquet RA, Contreras-Ortiz O, Tesone M, Rumi LS. Apoptosis and expression of Bcl-2 and Bax in eutopic endometrium from women with endometriosis. Fertil Steril 2000;74(4):760–766.

105. Jones RK, Searle RF, Bulmer JN. Apoptosis and bcl-2 expression in normal human endometrium, endometriosis and adenomyosis. Hum Reprod 1998;13(12):3496–3502.

106. Gonzalez-Ramos R, Donnez J, Defrere S et al. Nuclear factor-kappa B is constitutively activated in peritoneal endometriosis. Mol Hum Reprod 2007;13(7):503–509.

107. Gonzalez-Ramos R, van Langendonckt A, Defrere S et al. Agents blocking the nuclear factor-kappaB pathway are effective inhibitors of endometriosis in an in vivo experimental model. Gynecol Obstet Invest 2008;65(3):174–186.

108. Murk W, Atabekoglu CS, Cakmak H et al. Extracellularly signal-regulated kinase activity in the human endometrium: possible roles in the pathogenesis of endometriosis. J Clin Endocrinol Metab 2008;93(9):3532–3540.

109. Corsini A, Raiteri M, Soma MR, Bernini F, Fumagalli R, Paoletti R. Pathogenesis of atherosclerosis and the role of 3-hydroxy-3-methylglutaryl coenzyme A reductase inhibitors. Am J Cardiol 1995;76(2):21A–28A.

110. Rombouts K, Kisanga E, Hellemans K, Wielant A, Schuppan D, Geerts A. Effect of HMG-CoA reductase inhibitors on proliferation and protein synthesis by rat hepatic stellate cells. J Hepatol 2003;38(5):564–572.

111. Seeger H, Wallwiener D, Mueck AO. Statins can inhibit proliferation of human breast cancer cells in vitro. Exp Clin Endocrinol Diabetes 2003;111(1):47–48.

112. Izquierdo D, Foyouzi N, Kwintkiewicz J, Duleba AJ. Mevastatin inhibits ovarian theca-interstitial cell proliferation and steroidogenesis. Fertil Steril 2004;82(Suppl 3):1193–1197.

113. Gauthaman K, Fong CY, Bongso A. Statins, stem cells, and cancer. J Cell Biochem 2009;106(6):975–983.

114. Acquavella N, Quiroga MF, Wittig O, Cardier JE. Effect of simvastatin on endothelial cell apoptosis mediated by Fas and TNF-alpha. Cytokine 2010;49(1):45–50.

115. Lee SK, Kim YC, Song SB, Kim YS. Stabilization and translocation of p53 to mitochondria is linked to Bax translocation to mitochondria in simvastatin-induced apoptosis. Biochem Biophys Res Commun 2010;391(4):1592–1597.

116. Assmus B, Urbich C, Aicher A et al. HMG-CoA reductase inhibitors reduce senescence and increase proliferation of endothelial progenitor cells via regulation of cell cycle regulatory genes. Circ Res 2003;92(9):1049–1055.

117. Choi JA, Park MT, Kang CM et al. Opposite effects of Ha-Ras and Ki-Ras on radiation-induced apoptosis via differential activation of PI3K/Akt and Rac/p38 mitogen-activated protein kinase signaling pathways. Oncogene 2004 8;23(1):9–20.

118. Yoshino O, Osuga Y, Hirota Y et al. Possible pathophysiological roles of mitogen-activated protein kinases (MAPKs) in endometriosis. Am J Reprod Immunol 2004;52(5):306–311.

119. Piotrowski PC, Kwintkiewicz J, Rzepczynska IJ et al. Statins inhibit growth of human endometrial stromal cells independently of cholesterol availability. Biol Reprod 2006;75(1):107–111.

120. Noble LS, Takayama K, Zeitoun KM et al. Prostaglandin E2 stimulates aromatase expression in endometriosis-derived stromal cells. J Clin Endocrinol Metab 1997;82(2):600–606.

121. Bulun SE, Lin Z, Imir G et al. Regulation of aromatase expression in estrogen-responsive breast and uterine disease: from bench to treatment. Pharmacol Rev 2005;57(3):359–383.

122. Bukulmez O, Hardy DB, Carr BR et al. Androstenedione up-regulation of endometrial aromatase expression via local conversion to estrogen: potential relevance to the pathogenesis of endometriosis. J Clin Endocrinol Metab 2008;93(9):3471–3477.

123. Aghajanova L, Velarde MC, Giudice LC. Altered gene expression profiling in endometrium: evidence for progesterone resistance. Semin Reprod Med 2010;28(1):51–58.

124. Zeitoun K, Takayama K, Sasano H et al. Deficient 17beta-hydroxysteroid dehydrogenase type 2 expression in endometriosis: failure to metabolize 17beta-estradiol. J Clin Endocrinol Metab 1998;83(12):4474–4480.

125. Bulun SE, Cheng YH, Pavone ME et al. 17Beta-hydroxysteroid dehydrogenase-2 deficiency and progesterone resistance in endometriosis. Semin Reprod Med 2010;28(1):44–50.

126. Bulun SE, Imir G, Utsunomiya H et al. Aromatase in endometriosis and uterine leiomyomata. J Steroid Biochem Mol Biol 2005;95(1–5):57–62.

127. Wang W, Wong CW. Statins enhance peroxisome proliferator-activated receptor gamma coactivator-1alpha activity to regulate energy metabolism. J Mol Med 2010;88(3):309–317.

128. Ivashchenko CY, Bradley BT, Ao Z, Leiper J, Vallance P, Johns DG. Regulation of the ADMA-DDAH system in endothelial cells: a novel mechanism for the sterol response element binding proteins, SREBP1c and -2. Am J Physiol Heart Circ Physiol 2010;298(1):H251–258.

129. Song C, Wang J, Song Q et al. Simvastatin induces estrogen receptor-alpha (ER-alpha) in murine bone marrow stromal cells. J Bone Miner Metab 2008;26(3):213–217.

130. Kumar AS, Benz CC, Shim V, Minami CA, Moore DH, Esserman LJ. Estrogen receptor-negative breast cancer is less likely to arise among lipophilic statin users. Cancer Epidemiol Biomarkers Prev 2008;17(5):1028–1033.

131. Lin YC, Lin JH, Chou CW, Chang YF, Yeh SH, Chen CC. Statins increase p21 through inhibition of histone deacetylase activity and release of promoter-associated HDAC1/2. Cancer Res 2008;68(7):2375–2383.

132. Zhou Q, Atadja P, Davidson NE. Histone deacetylase inhibitor LBH589 reactivates silenced estrogen receptor alpha (ER) gene expression without loss of DNA hypermethylation. Cancer Biol Ther 2007;6(1):64–69.

133. Eaton M, Eklof J, Beal JR, Sahmoun AE. Statins and breast cancer in postmenopausal women without hormone therapy. Anticancer Res 2009;29(12):5143–5148.

134. Machado DE, Berardo PT, Landgraf RG et al. A selective cyclooxygenase-2 inhibitor suppresses the growth of endometriosis with an antiangiogenic effect in a rat model. Fertil Steril 2010;93(8):2674–2679.

135. Cipollone F, Fazia M, Iezzi A et al. Suppression of the functionally coupled cyclooxygenase-2/prostaglandin E synthase as a basis of simvastatin-dependent plaque stabilization in humans. Circulation 2003;107(11):1479–1485.

136. Cao X, Yang D, Song M, Murphy A, Parthasarathy S. The presence of endometrial cells in the peritoneal cavity enhances monocyte recruitment and induces inflammatory cytokines in mice: implications for endometriosis. Fertil Steril 2004;82 Suppl 3:999–1007.

137. Arici A. Local cytokines in endometrial tissue: the role of interleukin-8 in the pathogenesis of endometriosis. Ann N Y Acad Sci 2002;955:101–109; discussion 18, 396–406.

138. Fang CL, Han SP, Fu SL, Wang W, Kong N, Wang XL. Ectopic, autologous eutopic and normal endometrial stromal cells have altered expression and chemotactic activity of RANTES. Eur J Obstet Gynecol Reprod Biol 2009;143(1):55–60.

139. Pizzo A, Salmeri FM, Ardita FV, Sofo V, Tripepi M, Marsico S. Behaviour of cytokine levels in serum and peritoneal fluid of women with endometriosis. Gynecol Obstet Invest 2002;54(2):82–87.

140. Abrao MS, Podgaec S, Filho BM, Ramos LO, Pinotti JA, de Oliveira RM. The use of biochemical markers in the diagnosis of pelvic endometriosis. Hum Reprod 1997;12(11):2523–2527.

141. Chishima F, Hayakawa S, Hirata Y et al. Peritoneal and peripheral B-1-cell populations in patients with endometriosis. J Obstet Gynaecol Res 2000;26(2):141–149.

142. Gupta S, Goldberg JM, Aziz N, Goldberg E, Krajcir N, Agarwal A. Pathogenic mechanisms in endometriosis-associated infertility. Fertil Steril 2008;90(2):247–257.

143. Chuang PC, Wu MH, Shoji Y, Tsai SJ. Downregulation of CD36 results in reduced phagocytic ability of peritoneal macrophages of women with endometriosis. J Pathol 2009;219(2):232–241.

144. Bacci M, Capobianco A, Monno A et al. Macrophages are alternatively activated in patients with endometriosis and required for growth and vascularization of lesions in a mouse model of disease. Am J Pathol 2009;175(2):547–556.

145. Ngo C, Chereau C, Nicco C, Weill B, Chapron C, Batteux F. Reactive oxygen species controls endometriosis progression. Am J Pathol 2009;175(1):225–234.

146. Murphy AA, Santanam N, Morales AJ, Parthasarathy S. Lysophosphatidyl choline, a chemotactic factor for monocytes/T-lymphocytes is elevated in endometriosis. J Clin Endocrinol Metab 1998;83(6):2110–2113.

147. Ota H, Igarashi S, Hatazawa J, Tanaka T. Immunohistochemical assessment of superoxide dismutase expression in the endometrium in endometriosis and adenomyosis. Fertil Steril 1999; 72(1):129–134.

148. Ota H, Igarashi S, Kato N, Tanaka T. Aberrant expression of glutathione peroxidase in eutopic and ectopic endometrium in endometriosis and adenomyosis. Fertil Steril 2000;74(2):313–318.

149. Ota H, Igarashi S, Tanaka T. Xanthine oxidase in eutopic and ectopic endometrium in endometriosis and adenomyosis. Fertil Steril 2001;75(4):785–790.

150. Ota H, Igarashi S, Sato N, Tanaka H, Tanaka T. Involvement of catalase in the endometrium of patients with endometriosis and adenomyosis. Fertil Steril 2002;78(4):804–809.

151. Ando H, Takamura T, Ota T, Nagai Y, Kobayashi K. Cerivastatin improves survival of mice with lipopolysaccharide-induced sepsis. J Pharmacol Exp Ther 2000;294(3):1043–1046.

152. Dje N'Guessan P, Riediger F, Vardarova K et al. Statins control oxidized LDL-mediated histone modifications and gene expression in cultured human endothelial cells. Arterioscler Thromb Vasc Biol 2009;29(3):380–386.

153. Weber MS, Stuve O, Neuhaus O, Hartung HP, Zamvil SS. Spotlight on statins. Int MS J 2007;14(3):93–97.

154. Kwak B, Mulhaupt F, Myit S, Mach F. Statins as a newly recognized type of immunomodulator. Nat Med 2000;6(12):1399–1402.

155. Yilmaz A, Reiss C, Tantawi O et al. HMG-CoA reductase inhibitors suppress maturation of human dendritic cells: new implications for atherosclerosis. Atherosclerosis 2004;172(1):85–93.

156. Kuipers HF, van den Elsen PJ. Immunomodulation by statins: inhibition of cholesterol vs. isoprenoid biosynthesis. Biomed Pharmacother 2007;61(7):400–407.

157. Kuipers HF, Biesta PJ, Groothuis TA, Neefjes JJ, Mommaas AM, van den Elsen PJ. Statins affect cell-surface expression of major histocompatibility complex class II molecules by disrupting cholesterol-containing microdomains. Hum Immunol 2005;66(6):653–665.

158. Dunn SE, Youssef S, Goldstein MJ et al. Isoprenoids determine Th1/Th2 fate in pathogenic T cells, providing a mechanism of modulation of autoimmunity by atorvastatin. J Exp Med 2006;203(2):401–412.

159. Zapolska-Downar D, Siennicka A, Kaczmarczyk M, Kolodziej B, Naruszewicz M. Simvastatin modulates TNFalpha-induced adhesion molecules expression in human endothelial cells. Life Sci 2004;75(11):1287–1302.

160. Weitz-Schmidt G, Welzenbach K, Brinkmann V et al. Statins selectively inhibit leukocyte function antigen-1 by binding to a novel regulatory integrin site. Nat Med 2001;7(6):687–692.

161. Hillyard DZ, Jardine AG, McDonald KJ, Cameron AJ. Fluvastatin inhibits raft dependent Fcgamma receptor signalling in human monocytes. Atherosclerosis 2004;172(2):219–228.

162. Hillyard DZ, Nutt CD, Thomson J et al. Statins inhibit NK cell cytotoxicity by membrane raft depletion rather than inhibition of isoprenylation. Atherosclerosis 2007;191(2):319–325.

163. Bae YS, Kang SW, Seo MS et al. Epidermal growth factor (EGF)-induced generation of hydrogen peroxide. Role in EGF receptor-mediated tyrosine phosphorylation. J Biol Chem 1997;272(1):217–221.

164. Bae YS, Sung JY, Kim OS et al. Platelet-derived growth factor-induced H(2)O(2) production requires the activation of phosphatidylinositol 3-kinase. J Biol Chem 2000;275(14):10527–10531.

165. Wassmann S, Laufs U, Muller K et al. Cellular antioxidant effects of atorvastatin in vitro and in vivo. Arterioscler Thromb Vasc Biol 2002;22(2):300–305.

166. Turunen M, Olsson J, Dallner G. Metabolism and function of coenzyme Q. Biochim Biophys Acta 2004;1660(1–2):171–199.

167. Shibanuma M, Kuroki T, Nose K. Stimulation by hydrogen peroxide of DNA synthesis, competence family gene expression and phosphorylation of a specific protein in quiescent Balb/3T3 cells. Oncogene 1990;5(7):1025–1032.

168. Ernster L, Dallner G. Biochemical, physiological and medical aspects of ubiquinone function. Biochim Biophys Acta 1995; 1271(1):195–204.

169. Shi H, Noguchi N, Niki E. Comparative study on dynamics of antioxidative action of alpha-tocopheryl hydroquinone, ubiquinol, and alpha-tocopherol against lipid peroxidation. Free Radic Biol Med 1999;27(3–4):334–346.

170. Gregg D, Rauscher FM, Goldschmidt-Clermont PJ. Rac regulates cardiovascular superoxide through diverse molecular interactions: more than a binary GTP switch. Am J Physiol Cell Physiol 2003;285(4):C723–734.

171. Maack C, Kartes T, Kilter H et al. Oxygen free radical release in human failing myocardium is associated with increased activity of rac1-GTPase and represents a target for statin treatment. Circulation 2003;108(13):1567–1574.

172. Wassmann S, Laufs U, Baumer AT et al. Inhibition of geranylgeranylation reduces angiotensin II-mediated free radical production in vascular smooth muscle cells: involvement of angiotensin AT1 receptor expression and Rac1 GTPase. Mol Pharmacol 2001;59(3):646–654.

173. Yasunari K, Maeda K, Minami M, Yoshikawa J. HMG-CoA reductase inhibitors prevent migration of human coronary smooth muscle cells through suppression of increase in oxidative stress. Arterioscler Thromb Vasc Biol 2001;21(6):937–942.

174. Franzoni F, Quinones-Galvan A, Regoli F, Ferrannini E, Galetta F. A comparative study of the in vitro antioxidant activity of statins. Int J Cardiol 2003;90(2–3):317–321.

175. Shishehbor MH, Brennan ML, Aviles RJ et al. Statins promote potent systemic antioxidant effects through specific inflammatory pathways. Circulation 2003;108(4):426–431.

176. Huber AV, Saleh L, Prast J, Haslinger P, Knofler M. Human chorionic gonadotrophin attenuates NF-kappaB activation and cytokine expression of endometriotic stromal cells. Mol Hum Reprod 2007;13(8):595–604.

177. Taniguchi F, Harada T, Miyakoda H et al. TAK1 activation for cytokine synthesis and proliferation of endometriotic cells. Mol Cell Endocrinol 2009;307(1–2):196–204.

178. De Mos M, Laferriere A, Millecamps M et al. Role of NFkappaB in an animal model of complex regional pain syndrome-type I (CRPS-I). J Pain 2009;10(11):1161–1169.

179. Lieb K, Fiebich BL, Berger M, Bauer J, Schulze-Osthoff K. The neuropeptide substance P activates transcription factor NF-kappa B and kappa B-dependent gene expression in human astrocytoma cells. J Immunol 1997;159(10):4952–4958.

180. Tegeder I, Niederberger E, Schmidt R et al. Specific inhibition of IkappaB kinase reduces hyperalgesia in inflammatory and neuropathic pain models in rats. J Neurosci 2004;24(7):1637–1645.

181. Wang L, Zhang X, Liu L, Yang R, Cui L, Li M. Atorvastatin protects rat brains against permanent focal ischemia and downregulates HMGB1, HMGB1 receptors (RAGE and TLR4), NF-kappaB expression. Neurosci Lett 2010;471(3):152–156.

182. Li J, Li JJ, He JG, Nan JL, Guo YL, Xiong CM. Atorvastatin decreases C-reactive protein-induced inflammatory response in pulmonary artery smooth muscle cells by inhibiting nuclear factor-kappaB pathway. Cardiovasc Ther 2010;28(1):8–14.

183. Ozbek E, Cekmen M, Ilbey YO, Simsek A, Polat EC, Somay A. Atorvastatin prevents gentamicin-induced renal damage in rats through the inhibition of p38-MAPK and NF-kappaB pathways. Ren Fail 2009;31(5):382–392.

184. Yin Z, Fang Y, Ren L et al. Atorvastatin attenuates NF-kappaB activation in trigeminal nucleus caudalis in a rat model of migraine. Neurosci Lett 2009;465(1):61–65.

185. Sepulcri R de P, do Amaral VF. Depressive symptoms, anxiety, and quality of life in women with pelvic endometriosis. Eur J Obstet Gynecol Reprod Biol 2009;142(1):53–56.

186. Olff M. Stress, depression and immunity: the role of defense and coping styles. Psychiatry Res 1999;85(1):7–15.

187. Young-Xu Y, Chan KA, Liao JK, Ravid S, Blatt CM. Long-term statin use and psychological well-being. J Am Coll Cardiol 2003;42(4):690–697.

188. Wirleitner B, Sperner-Unterweger B, Fuchs D. Statins to reduce risk of depression. J Am Coll Cardiol 2004;43(6):1132; author reply 1133.

189. Mundy G, Garrett R, Harris S et al. Stimulation of bone formation in vitro and in rodents by statins. Science 1999;286(5446):1946–1949.

190. Staal A, Frith JC, French MH et al. The ability of statins to inhibit bone resorption is directly related to their inhibitory effect on HMG-CoA reductase activity. J Bone Miner Res 2003;18(1):88–96.

191. Pasco JA, Kotowicz MA, Henry MJ, Sanders KM, Nicholson GC. Statin use, bone mineral density, and fracture risk: Geelong Osteoporosis Study. Arch Intern Med 2002;162(5):537–540.

192. Van Staa TP, Wegman S, de Vries F, Leufkens B, Cooper C. Use of statins and risk of fractures. JAMA 2001;285(14):1850–1855.

193. Oktem M, Esinler I, Eroglu D, Haberal N, Bayraktar N, Zeyneloglu HB. High-dose atorvastatin causes regression of endometriotic implants: a rat model. Hum Reprod 2007;22(5):1474–1480.

8 Surgical Therapies for Pain

37 Surgical Therapies: Principles and Triage in Endometriosis

Alan Lam, Tommaso Bignardi and Su-Yen Khong

Department of Obstetrics and Gynaecology, Nepean Clinical School, University of Sydney, Sydney, Australia

Introduction

Despite tireless efforts in search of non-invasive diagnostic and medical cures, surgical therapies have continued to play an essential role for definitive confirmation or exclusion of endometriosis and for surgical destruction or removal of the disease.

By and large, the philosophy underlying surgical therapies for endometriosis is to remove all visible endometriotic lesions and associated adhesions, to repair damage or trauma to the affected organs/sites and to re-establish normal anatomy [1].

While surgical treatment has never claimed to eradicate or cure endometriosis, it has continued to play a crucial role in the diagnosis and management of this disease on the basis of proven benefits in relieving pain and improving fertility [2–7]. In cases of completed child bearing, intractable pain, severe or recurrent disease not responding to conservative measures, definitive surgical therapy in the form of hysterectomy and bilateral salpingo-oophorectomy may be indicated [8].

Laparoscopy should be the standard approach for diagnosis and for removal of most stages of endometriosis. With appropriate advanced training, laparoscopic surgery in the right settings can also deal with advanced-stage disease, reserving laparotomy for specific circumstances and indications only.

Beyond laparoscopic surgery for diagnostic purpose and removal of early-stage disease, it is increasingly recognized that complex endometriosis surgery is not for every gynecologist as this can be one of the most challenging and difficult types of pelvic surgery with potential for significant risks and complications [9]. Consequently, it has been suggested that complex endometriosis surgery should only be carried out after thorough preoperative counseling, ideally at dedicated centers with appropriately trained surgeons and multidisciplinary expertise and support [10,11].

Currently there are no clear guidelines regarding who should perform endometriosis surgery, where patients should be treated, what criteria should be used to determine which case to see-and-treat, which to see-and-discuss, or which to see-and-refer to a tertiary center. The objectives of this chapter are to discuss the rationale for a surgical triage system and to describe the principles of surgical therapies for endometriosis.

Triage

Why?

It is generally considered ideal practice to diagnose and remove endometriosis surgically at the same time [12], i.e. the "see-and-treat" policy. This approach offers several benefits: time-efficiency, cost-effectiveness, reduction of operative risks from multiple procedures, and optimal utilization of hospital resources. However, there is a valid argument why this *modus operandi* should be accompanied by a triage system when it comes to surgical therapies for endometriosis.

First, while endometriosis is a condition which can cause chronic, debilitating pain and infertility, and severely affect life quality, it is almost never life-threatening. As such, surgical treatment for endometriosis is almost always elective. Indeed, rarely does surgery have to be carried out for acute emergencies such as acute abdominal pain from rupture of endometrioma, for relief of loin pain from hydronephrosis or pyelonephritis secondary to ureteric obstruction, or for dealing with serious bowel complications in the course of treating endometriosis [12]. Accordingly, there should be ample time for comprehensive preoperative assessment, thorough counseling and careful case selection to ensure that surgical treatment can be performed under optimal circumstances [13].

Second, surgical treatment should be determined by the severity of disease found, the adequacy of preoperative counseling and consent, the suitability of the operating environment, the availability of surgical skills and expertise, and the level of postoperative care available [14].

Third, every surgeon treating endometriosis acknowledges the fact that the severity of disease found may not be apparent until the time of surgery [15]. In practice, this means that frequently the disease which appears superficial may on careful assessment be found to infiltrate deeply, causing intense fibrosis, obliteration of surgical spaces and/or involvement of blood vessels, bladder, ureter, bowels or even nerves [16].

Finally, as not all gynecologists are trained to deal with all stages of endometriosis adequately, it is therefore important to introduce a triage system with the objective of ensuring that women needing surgical therapies receive a level of care appropriate to the skills of the treating gynecologist. This fundamentally means that women with "high-risk" or advanced-stage disease should be cared for at centers with the necessary expertise [11].

How?

At present, there are no clear guidelines regarding whom should perform endometriosis surgery, where patients should be treated or when patients should be referred to a tertiary center. How, then, can the gynecologist exercise caution and judgment in deciding the extent of surgical therapy? And what criteria can he/she use to predict and triage women undergoing surgical therapies for endometriosis appropriately to ensure optimal outcomes?

History

While no correlation has been found between severity of dysmenorrhea, severity of symptoms and endometriosis stage, there is evidence showing correlation between different types of pelvic pain and specific locations of deep infiltrative endometriosis [17,18]. These researchers reported that deep dyspareunia is correlated with involvement of the uterosacral ligament, painful defecation with the vagina, non-cyclical pain with the bowel, lower urinary tract symptoms with the bladder, and gastrointestinal symptoms with the bowel and vagina. Vercellini *et al* reported a strong association between posterior cul-de-sac lesions and pain at intercourse [15], while dyschezia and, less commonly, cyclical rectal bleeding should raise clinical suspicion of deep infiltrative endometriosis involving the gastrointestinal tract, particularly rectum and sigmoid [19].

Examination

Regarding the value of physical examination, Ripps and Martin found correlation between localized tenderness and depth and volume of endometriosis affecting the cul-de-sac and the uterosacral ligaments [20]. Redwine and Wright found that 48% of 84 consecutive women undergoing laparoscopic treatment of endometriosis with complete cul-de-sac obliteration had nodularity on preoperative examination [21].

Imaging

Imaging techniques have been used for the diagnosis of superficial, ovarian and deep endometriosis. Transvaginal ultrasound is an accurate tool for the diagnosis of endometrioma [22] which in turn may be a marker of severe endometriosis, including an estimated one in five chance of complete cul-de-sac obliteration compared to one in 20 chances in women without ovarian endometriosis. In addition, when endometriomas are present, the relative risk of intestinal disease has been found to be increased by nearly three times compared to when ovaries are not involved [23].

To detect bowel lesions, several imaging techniques have been used, notably transrectal/transvaginal ultrasonography with or without bowel preparation, endoscopic transrectal sonography, magnetic resonance imaging (MRI) and barium enema [24–28]. At sonography, bowel nodules are visualized as elongated, solid, hypoechogenic lesions adherent to the wall of the intestinal loop. In most studies, ultrasound yielded a very high sensitivity for the detection of bowel nodules, varying between 95% and 100%. In some studies, ultrasound was also able to accurately predict the degree of submucosal infiltration, with great advantages for surgical planning [29]. However, we should note that these studies were conducted in tertiary centers for the treatment of endometriosis, by sonologists very experienced in the diagnosis of bowel involvement, and in selected women with a high clinical suspicion of bowel endometriosis [24–26]. It is likely that the performance of ultrasound in the detection of bowel involvement in low-risk women or by less experienced sonographers will be much lower. It is therefore important that high-risk women are evaluated in tertiary centers by sonologists who are specifically trained in the imaging of endometriosis.

Laparoscopy

At the time of diagnostic laparoscopy, the detection of stage 3–4 revised American Fertility Society (rAFS) endometriosis, typified by findings such as severe adhesions, ovarian endometrioma, obliteration of cul-de-sac, entrapped ovaries, pelvic sidewall, bowel, bladder, ureteric endometriosis, or suspicious lesions or masses, should give rise to caution and demand judgment by the treating gynecologist as to the extent of surgical therapies. A systematic assessment examination under anesthesia, combining vaginal and rectal examination, direct visualization of the cul-de-sac and the rectum with routine use of rectal probe, is essential for the diagnosis of rectovaginal endometriosis [30]. This should also include careful evaluation of appendix, ileum, cecum, rectosigmoid, liver and diaphragmatic surfaces.

In essence, a triage system could be based on information gained from *history taking*, *examination findings*, *imaging results* and *laparoscopic findings* to predict and determine the severity and stage of endometriosis. A suggested triage system found in Fig. 37.1 may be used to categorize cases needing surgical therapies into one of three groups: (1) *see-and-treat*, (2) *see-and-discuss*, or (3) *see-and-refer* (Fig. 37.1). The ultimate aim of this triage system is to help the gynecologist select the cases needing surgical

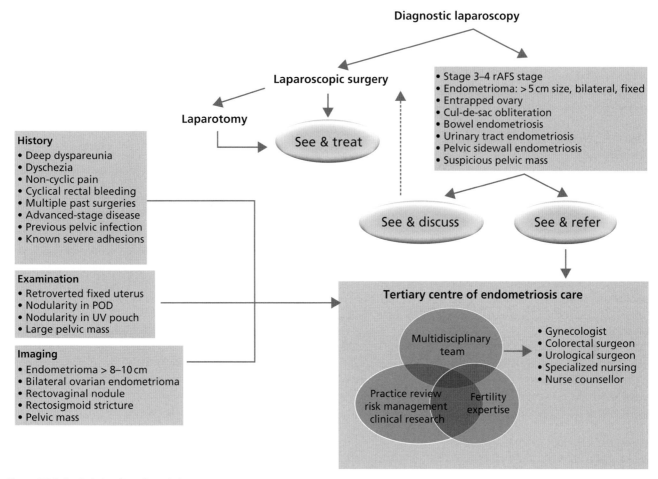

Figure 37.1 Surgical triage for endometriosis.

therapies based upon his/her training and experience, and refer others to an appropriate tertiary center of care.

Principles of surgical therapies

Despite the availability, sensitivity and specificity of imaging tests, the full extent and the depth of infiltration of endometriosis, more than any other pelvic pathology, are often not known until the time of surgery. Consequently, when contemplating surgical therapies for endometriosis, the following factors are considered essential for consistent, reproducible and optimal outcomes.

- Informed consent
- Teamwork
- Instrument selection
- Safe entry
- Knowledge of anatomy
- Energy selection

- Surgical techniques for removal of endometriosis
- Postoperative care

Informed consent

It is probably true to say that most women suffering from period or pelvic pain and/or infertility will have heard of the term "endometriosis" by the time they are referred to a specialist. Many may have undergone one or more surgeries or assisted reproductive technologies. Nevertheless, whether the patient is undergoing the first ever diagnostic laparoscopy or a repeat surgical therapy, it is essential that the patient considering surgical therapies for endometriosis should be given adequate time to understand:

- the diagnosis
- the purpose and nature of the recommended surgical therapy
- the benefits and risks of the procedure
- the expected outcomes of treatment and likelihood of success
- the alternative treatment options
- the prognosis if the treatment is refused [31].

As the amount of information can be overwhelming for the patient to understand, absorb or remember alone, it is often helpful for her to bring along a close family member or partner to the consultations [32]. In addition, it is also frequently advisable to incorporate diagrams, educational pamphlets and multimedia presentation in the process of informed consent.

Where resources allow, centers specializing in the management of endometriosis should employ nurse educators/counselors. In addition, any patient with complex disease or an unresolved management dilemma should be encouraged to seek more opinions from other experienced gynecological, urological or colorectal colleagues before proceeding with the surgical therapy [11].

Teamwork

With a see-and-treat *modus operandi* towards endometriosis, a gynecologist wishing to perform safe and adequate surgical therapies for endometriosis needs to have a supportive and experienced team. This includes an understanding anesthetist, experienced assistant (s), competent theater nurse and supportive theater and hospital managers.

Due to the unpredictability of endometriosis cases, a good working relationship with theater and hospital managers may well make the difference between being able to complete a case or having to defer or rearrange patient to a later time if ideal conditions for surgical therapies cannot be assured [33].

Instrument selection

Good surgical therapies for endometriosis do not necessarily require myriad complex instrumentation. The following list represents a selection of laparoscopic instruments which the author considers essential for a diagnostic and therapeutic procedure. For open surgery, the selection is similar.

* 0° 10 mm laparoscope
* Atraumatic ovum-grasping forceps
* Tooth-grasping forceps
* Merryland forceps
* Blunt-tip forceps
* Atraumatic bowel clamps
* Atraumatic vascular clamps
* Needle holder
* Irrigation and suction instrument
* Energy types: unipolar and bipolar diathermy, ultrasonic energy
* Uterine manipulator
* Scissors
* 5 mm ports × 3
* Sutures: 3–0 or 4–0 absorbable materials on a CT-2 or smaller needle size
* Optional: laser, 30° laparoscope

Safe entry

As laparoscopy is the main surgical technique used for diagnosis and treatment of endometriosis, and as more than 50% of all complications associated with laparoscopy occur during the abdominal entry phase, a safe entry technique is essential to avoid potential vascular, intestinal and urinary tract injuries and gas embolism [34].

The authors use a standardized open entry technique that involves:
* making a 1 cm vertical incision through the skin, the rectus sheath and the peritoneum at the umbilicus while elevating the abdominal wall with Littlewood clamps
* inserting a blunt or dilating tip trocar through the abdominal wall incision while elevating the abdominal wall
* insufflation of CO_2 gas only after confirmation of correct placement of the laparoscope.

Knowledge of anatomy

While superficial endometriosis is usually confined to pelvic peritoneum, deep endometriosis frequently infiltrates into pelvic ligamentous structures and surgical spaces. Endometriotic lesions may therefore firmly adhere to the ureter or uterine vessels, or cause partial or complete obliteration of the cul-de-sac or rectal adherence to the posterior uterine surface, the uterosacral junction and/or the posterior cervix. In more advanced cases, endometriosis may invade into the rectovaginal septum, through to the posterior vaginal fornix and rectal wall, and similarly into the uterovesical space, and at times through or into the bladder wall [35].

In order to achieve safe and complete excisional surgical therapy for endometriosis, it is essential that the gynecologist have a thorough knowledge of normal pelvic anatomy, including knowledge and ability to identify surgical spaces, anatomy of the pelvic sidewall, the ureter and the rectosigmoid.

Energy selection

While the scope of this chapter does not allow a detailed discussion of this topic, whatever energy sources the gynecologist chooses to use in the surgical treatment of endometriosis should be based upon a comprehensive understanding of biophysical properties and applied principles of the chosen energy. By combining scientific knowledge with surgical training and experience, the removal or destruction of endometriosis and associated adhesiolysis can be done efficiently and safely [36].

In the case of electrosurgery, the desired tissue effect depends on the power output setting, the chosen waveform (cutting, coagulating or blend), the size and shape of the electrode, and the duration of application. Acknowledging individual preferences, the author's usual electrosurgical setting is 50–60 W pure CUT, 30 W pure COAG current delivered through the tips of a disposable pair of scissors, and 30 W bipolar diathermy.

Using the pure CUT current in a non-contact mode via the tip of the scissors, endometriotic implants can be removed efficiently with little risk of lateral thermal spread to adjacent tissues. Deep endometriotic lesions infiltrating into dense ligamentous structures, surrounded by scar tissues and myriad small bleeding vessels, may be excised with pure CUT or blend CUT/COAG current. For larger blood vessels, the author's preference is bipolar diathermy before excision with ultrasonic energy.

Ultrasonic energy (harmonic scalpel) in the form of a laparoscopic coagulating shear (LCS) is an excellent energy and instrument choice for removal of moderate-to-severe endometriosis, particularly large implants or nodules on the pelvic sidewall, adjacent to large blood vessels, or infiltrating onto or into bladder, ureteric or bowel walls. The combination of an LCS for dissection and coagulation with a pair of bipolar grasping forceps has allowed the senior author to tackle many challenging, deep, vascular advanced cases of endometriosis.

CO_2 lasers have unique properties which can cut tissue with less risk of inadvertent tissue damage. Again, this should only be used after adequate training.

Finally, a point should be made with regard to the use of energy to remove endometriosis adjacent to ureter or from bowel walls, or to divide dense bowel adhesions, for example from the posterior uterine surface or cervix. In order to avoid or minimize the risk of delayed tissue damage, the authors prefer to cut these tissues using sharp scissors without electrosurgery. Hemostasis, if required, is achieved by coagulation using bipolar diathermy sparingly or with fine 3–0 or 4–0 absorbable sutures with a braided material.

Surgical techniques for removal of endometriosis

After achieving safe primary entry, the gynecologist should place one secondary port and proceed to systematically evaluate the extent and location of endometriosis, starting with the upper abdomen (diaphragm, liver, stomach, small and large bowels, appendix), then the pelvis (sigmoid, rectum, pouch of Douglas, uterovesical pouch, left and right pelvic sidewalls) and finally the uterus, fallopian tubes, and ovaries. Apart from confirming location and extent, the type (superficial or deep) of endometriosis, the degree of adhesions, the state of the cul-de-sac, and the rAFS stage should also be documented.

At this point, the treating gynecologist can decide whether the case is a see-and-treat, see-and-discuss, or see-and-refer.

If the decision is to see-and-treat, it is important that an adequate number of secondary ports (usually 2–3) is used. This is to ensure that there is adequate exposure of the operative field while at the same time protecting the bowels, ureter and blood vessels from harm. In addition, the location of the secondary ports should be planned so that the gynecologist can have maximal ease of access to the pathology for safe removal of the most significant disease. This usually means that the ports are sited in the upper half of the abdomen when dealing with pelvic sidewall or cul-de-sac disease.

Another important step is the mobilization of congenital sigmoid adhesions from the left pelvic brim to improve the view of and access to the left pelvic sidewall, the left ovary and the ureter. This step also reduces the risk of inadvertent electrosurgical bowel injury which may come into contact with the left iliac port outside the operative field.

Surgical principles for removal of peritoneal endometriosis

Peritoneal endometriotic lesions can either be ablated or excised with scissors, hook or spatula blade using a monopolar cutting current in non-contact mode, or CO_2 laser. In general, one should aim for 2–3 mm clear surgical margins from the endometriotic lesions to ensure complete removal of disease [37,38].

Superficial peritoneal endometriosis will easily lift away from underlying tissue with grasping forceps. Deep infiltrative lesions, on the other hand, are often anchored by variable depth of tissue penetration and surrounding fibrosis [39]. Gentle traction on these lesions with tooth-grasping forceps and excision using a monopolar CUT current, rather than ablation, will help to determine the lateral and vertical spread of the disease during removal.

Surgical principles for removal of endometriosis overlying ureter

Pelvic sidewall endometriosis may be found adjacent to the infundibulopelvic ligament, at the level of the pelvic brim, on the posterior leaf of the broad ligament, near the ureteric tunnel or at the uterosacral ligaments. As the subperitoneal fibrosis may distort the course of the ureter or cause it to be closely adhered to the endometriotic lesion, removal of endometriosis from these areas can put the ureter at risk of injury. Hence, this is another example where the surgeon must triage the case into see-and-treat, see-and-discuss, or see-and-refer. The over-riding principle is the ability to dissect and identify the ureter clearly before making any attempt to remove this type of endometriosis (Plate 37.1).

Where the ureter is clearly seen, the pelvic peritoneum containing the endometriotic lesion may be retracted and sharply incised above the ureter. The ureter can then be identified and bluntly dissected away to allow safe excision of the endometriotic lesion [40–42]. Minor bleeding can be controlled with bipolar diathermy.

If the ureter is not seen through the posterior leaf of the broad ligament, then it should be identified from the pelvic brim by making a peritoneal incision either medial or lateral to the infundibulopelvic ligament. Retroperitoneal dissection should lead to identification of the ureter. In turn, the ureter is then reflected away to allow excision of the attached endometriotic lesions.

Surgical principles for removal of ovarian endometriotic cyst

The approach to an endometriotic cyst should follow the same surgical principles as for any adnexal mass. This requires thorough intra-abdominal evaluation, followed by peritoneal washings and biopsies of any suspicious lesions at the start. Based on the appearance, size and mobility, extent of adhesions, degree of adherence or entrapment of the cyst to the pelvic sidewall, the gynecologist should determine the degree of difficulty and the likelihood of retroperitoneal dissection being required to identify the ureter in the course of dealing with ovarian endometriosis. Again, the surgeon needs to triage the case to see-and-treat, see-and-discuss, or see-and-refer, according to his/her surgical skills.

With strong evidence in favor of cystectomy over the cyst wall fenestration/drainage/ablation technique, every attempt should be made to remove endometriotic cysts completely [43]. This can be achieved by making a superficial longitudinal incision through the thinnest part of the ovarian cortex, using scissors with or without electrodiathermy or laser.

Using atraumatic ovum forceps to grasp the edges of the cortex and grasping forceps to retract the cyst wall, the cyst can usually be dissected out intact using a combination of blunt and hydro-dissection. If the cyst ruptures during dissection, the "chocolate" content should be confined to the pelvis for aspiration; the cyst cavity is then lavaged and inspected.

Removal of large, long-standing, thick-walled endometriomata can be difficult, with risk of profuse bleeding from the ovarian cortex, from the posterior leaf of the broad ligament or the pelvic sidewall to which the cyst is adherent. The surgeon will need to combine careful dissection with meticulous hemostasis using regular irrigation and bipolar diathermy, constantly checking anatomical landmarks to ensure that as much of the normal ovarian cortex as possible can be preserved along the way [44].

At times, when faced with very large and vascular endometrioma and the risk of oophorectomy, the surgeon may elect to perform a three-step therapy: (1) laparoscopic cyst drainage/cyst wall biopsy, (2) 2–3 months of hormonal suppression with a gonadotropin releasing hormone (GnRH) analog, (3) laparoscopic cystectomy [45]. The ovarian defect may close spontaneously after removal of endometrioma <5 cm diameter [46]. After removal of a large endometriotic cyst, the ovarian defect should be reconstructed to ensure hemostasis and to facilitate approximation of the cortex. This can be achieved by a vertical mattress closure, or alternatively by purse-string closure of the ovarian defect followed by superficial running closure of the ovarian cortex, with 3–0 or 4–0 absorbable sutures.

Small endometriotic cysts may be removed after being cut into small strips via the laparoscopic ports. Large endometrioma, and particularly cysts of a suspicious nature, should be placed and sealed securely inside a specimen bag for removal via the 10 mm umbilical port, under the guidance of a 5 mm laparoscope via the side port. If it is necessary to remove and reinsert ports during the procedure, one should rinse the ports and irrigate the port sites liberally with water. In addition, the surgeon should not remove tissue specimens directly through the abdominal wall to avoid the risk of incisional scar endometriosis [47].

Surgical principles for dealing with an entrapped endometriotic ovary

Endometriosis is one of the most common causes of ovarian entrapment in the pelvic sidewall. The peritoneum burying the ovary may contain endometriotic lesions and the embedded ovary itself may contain endometriomas. Frequently, the full extent of pathology will not be evident until adhesiolysis is performed to expose the pelvic sidewall.

Dealing with an entrapped endometriotic ovary is one of the most challenging gynecological operations, one which the gynecologist should triage to determine if it should be see-and-treat, see-and-discuss, or see-and-refer [33].

The surgical principles required are as follows.
- Mobilization of sigmoid adhesions to expose the pelvic brim in the case of left-sided pathology or, less commonly, appendix and cecum to expose the right pelvic brim in the case of right-sided pathology.
- Dissection, isolation of the infundibulopelvic ligament and the ureter at the level of the pelvic brim.
- Dissection and isolation of the pelvic ureter and, when required, dissection and isolation of the uterine vessel to which the ovary may attach.
- Hemostasis is controlled with bipolar diathermy during the dissection once vital structures such as the ureter are isolated.
- With the ureter protected, the entrapped ovary can then be dissected free from the pelvic sidewall and from rectosigmoid adhesions.
- Once endometriotic cystectomy and excision of surrounding peritoneal endometriosis are completed, the repaired ovary can be temporarily suspended to the abdominal wall at the end of the operation with non-absorbable 3–0 or 4–0 polypropylene sutures to prevent the ovary readhering to the pelvic sidewall. These sutures are removed 7 days later in the outpatient clinic. Where the entrapped ovary is to be removed, the steps involved are similar to those described above.

Surgical principles for dealing with obliteration of posterior cul-de-sac and removal of rectovaginal endometriosis

Faced with this kind of pathology, the gynecologist should triage the case into see-and-discuss, see-and-refer, or see-and treat. The see-and-treat option should only proceed if there has been adequate counseling, risk/benefit analysis and discussion with the patient. Beside assessing the surgeon's own skill level, this type of surgery requires adequate planning and availability of an appropriately trained surgical team, including colorectal and at times urological assistance [48].

The first step in this procedure involves mobilization of sigmoid from the left pelvic brim to improve the view of and access to the left pelvic sidewall, the left ovary and the ureter.

If endometriomas are present, attempts should be made to keep them intact as their ruptured contents may stain and obscure the surgical field. However, if endometriomas block or limit the view of and access to the posterior cul-de-sac, cystectomy should be performed, followed by suspension of the ovaries and tubes to the round ligaments or anterior abdominal wall using 2–0 polypropylene sutures during the procedure to keep them out of the surgical field.

Ureterolysis is often required to identify the route of the ureters from the pelvic brim, along the pelvic sidewalls to the ureteric tunnels. An incision may be required to release the ureter(s) from where endometriosis infiltrates into the broad ligaments and the uterosacral ligaments. Excision of these lesions can be performed using CUT monopolar current or harmonic scalpel, with bipolar diathermy for hemostasis of spot bleeding.

With the ureters and uterosacral ligaments identified and the pararectal spaces exposed, the rectal adhesion can be dissected off the posterior uterus using sharp scissors without energy source to reduce the risk of thermal injury to the bowel wall. During this critical dissection, regular irrigation and bipolar diathermy of spot bleeders are combined to keep the line of dissection clean and to check for air bubble which may indicate a breach of the bowel wall. Optimal visualization of the posterior cul-de-sac is facilitated by maintaining adequate anteversion of the uterus with a uterine manipulator. In addition, rectal and vaginal probes are helpful to delineate the rectum, the posterior vaginal fornix and the rectovaginal septum (Plate 37.2).

Once the disease is dissected off the posterior uterine surface, the uterosacral ligaments and the posterior vagina wall, it can then be reflected onto the anterior rectal wall. At this point, the decision to perform rectal shaving, disk or segmental bowel resection should be made with a colorectal surgeon depending on the site(s), size of the nodule(s), the length of bowel affected, and the degree of bowel stricture [49].

Finally, the integrity of the bowel wall after shaving, disk or segmental resection and anastomosis is tested by flooding the pelvic cavity with saline and insufflating air into the rectum using a bulb syringe while occluding the rectosigmoid proximal to the level of rectal surgery with atraumatic bowel clamps. Rectal wall defect leakage can be confirmed by the presence of bowel content spillage or air bubbles from the bowel loops submerged under irrigation fluid [50]. The rectal wall defect can be repaired laparoscopically or by exteriorizing the injured loop through a mini-laparotomy with one- or two-layered closure using 4–0 Vicryl or PDS sutures.

Postoperative management and follow-up

The majority of surgical therapies for endometriosis are suitable as day-case admissions. Women undergoing extensive and prolonged surgeries for advance-stage endometriosis may be kept for observations and analgesic for more days as indicated.

In general, the postoperative care protocol should include the following.
- Explanation of operative findings and procedure performed
- Advice regarding expected postoperative recovery and resumption of activities
- Instructions regarding analgesia
- Arrangement for follow-up appointment
- Advice to report abnormal recovery (fever, abdominal pain, nausea, vomiting, calf pain, shortness of breath) and contact point/phone number
- Close monitoring of the patient's condition, gastrointestinal rest, intravenous fluids, antibiotics and thromboprophylaxis where surgeries were performed for extensive endometriosis

Conclusion

Surgical therapies continue to play a crucial role in the diagnosis and treatment of endometriosis. Most cases of endometriosis can be managed by laparoscopic surgery, with laparotomy being reserved for the most challenging situations. To ensure that women needing surgical therapies receive a level of care appropriate to the skills of the treating gynecologist, a system based on history, examination findings, imaging results and laparoscopic findings may be used to triage each case into see-and-treat, see-and-discuss, or see-and-refer categories.

With sound surgical principles for dealing with the myriad presentations of this condition, it is possible to offer women suffering from endometriosis safe surgical care under optimal conditions.

References

1. Society of Obstetricians and Gynaecologists of Canada. Canadian consensus conference on endometriosis consensus statements. J SOGC 1999;21:471–473.
2. Jacobson TZ, Barlow DH, Garry R, Koninckx P. Laparoscopic surgery for pelvic pain associated with endometriosis (Cochrane Review). Cochrane Library, Issue 3. Chichester: John Wiley, 2004.
3. Jacobson TZ, Barlow DH, Koninckx PR, Olive D, Farquhar C. Laparoscopic surgery for subfertility associated with endometriosis (Cochrane Review). Cochrane Library, Issue 3. Chichester: John Wiley, 2004.
4. Abbott JA, Hawe J, Clayton RD, Garry R. The effects and effectiveness of laparoscopic excision of endometriosis: a prospective study with 2–5 year follow-up. Hum Reprod 2003;18:1922–1927.
5. Vercellini P, Somigliana E, Viganò P, Abbiati A, Barbara G, Crosignani PG. Surgery for endometriosis-associated infertility: a pragmatic approach. Hum Reprod 2009;24(2):254–269.
6. Vercellini P, Crosignani PG, Abbiati A, Somigliana E, Viganò P, Fedele L. The effect of surgery for symptomatic endometriosis: the other side of the story. Hum Reprod Update 2009;15(2):177–188.
7. Vercellini P, Fedele L, Aimi G, de Giorgi O, Consonni D, Crosignani PG. Reproductive performance, pain recurrence and disease relapse after conservative surgical treatment for endometriosis: the predictive value of the current classification system. Hum Reprod 2006;21(10):2679–2685.
8. Malinak LR. Surgical treatment and adjunctive therapy of endometriosis. Int J Gynaecol Obstet 1993;40:S43–47.
9. Lam A, Kaufman Y, Khong SY, Liew A, Ford S, Condous G. Dealing with complications in laparoscopy. Best Pract Res Clin Obstet Gynaecol 2009;23:631–646.
10. Kennedy S, Bergqvist A, Chapron C et al, ESHRE Special Interest Group for Endometriosis and Endometrium Guideline Development Group. ESHRE guideline for the diagnosis and treatment of endometriosis. Hum Reprod 2005;20(10):2698–2704.
11. D'Hooghe T, Hummelshoj L. Multi-disciplinary centres/networks of excellence for endometriosis management and research: a proposal. Hum Reprod 2006;21(11):2743–2748.

12. Mereu L, Gagliardi ML, Clarizia R, Mainardi P, Landi S, Minelli L. Laparoscopic management of ureteral endometriosis in case of moderate-severe hydroureteronephrosis. Fertil Steril 2010;93(1):46–51.

13. Catenacci M, Sastry S, Falcone T. Laparoscopic surgery for endometriosis. Clin Obstet Gynecol 2009;52(3):351–361.

14. Singh SS, Condous G, Lam A. Primer on risk management for the gynaecological laparoscopist. Best Pract Res Clin Obstet Gynaecol 2007;21(4):675–690.

15. Vercellini P, Fedele L, Aimi G, Pietropaolo G, Consonni D, Crosignani PG. Association between endometriosis stage, lesion type, patient characteristics and severity of pelvic pain symptoms: a multivariate analysis of over 1000 patients. Hum Reprod 2007;22(1):266–271.

16. Kwok A, Lam A, Ford R. Deeply infiltrating endometriosis: implications, diagnosis, and management. Obstet Gynecol Surv 2001;56(3):168–177.

17. Gruppo Italiano per lo Studio dell'Endometriosi. Relationship between stage, site and morphological characteristics of pelvic endometriosis and pain. Hum Reprod 2001;16(12):2668–2671.

18. Fauconnier A, Chapron C, Dubuisson JB, Vieira M, Dousset B, Bréart G. Relation between pain symptoms and the anatomic location of deep infiltrating endometriosis. Fertil Steril 2002;78(4):719–726.

19. Redwine DB. Laparoscopic en bloc resection for treatment of the obliterated cul-de-sac in endometriosis. J Reprod Med 1992;37(8):695–698.

20. Ripps BA, Martin DC. Correlation of focal pelvic tenderness with implant dimension and stage of endometriosis. J Reprod Med 1992;37:620–624.

21. Redwine DB, Wright JT. Laparoscopic treatment of complete obliteration of the cul-de-sac associated with endometriosis: long-term follow-up of en bloc resection. Fertil Steril 2001;76(2):358–365.

22. Moore J, Copley S, Morris J, Lindsell D, Golding S, Kennedy S. A systematic review of the accuracy of ultrasound in the diagnosis of endometriosis. Ultrasound Obstet Gynecol 2002;20(6):630–634.

23. Redwine DB. Ovarian endometriosis. A marker for more severe pelvic and intestinal disease. Fertil Steril 1999;73:310–315.

24. Chapron C, Dumontier I, Dousset B et al. Results and role of rectal endoscopic ultrasonography for patients with deep pelvic endometriosis. Hum Reprod 1998;13(8):2266–2270.

25. Bazot M, Detchev R, Cortez A, Amouyal P, Uzan S, Darai E. Transvaginal sonography and rectal endoscopic sonography for the assessment of pelvic endometriosis: a preliminary comparison. Hum Reprod 2003;18:1686–1692.

26. Abrao MS, Goncalves MO, Dias JA Jr, Podgaec S, Chamie LP, Blasbalg R. Comparison between clinical examination, transvaginal sonography and magnetic resonance imaging for the diagnosis of deep endometriosis. Hum Reprod 2007;22:3092–3097.

27. Goncalves MO, Dias JA Jr, Podgaec S, Averbach M, Abrao MS. Transvaginal ultrasound for diagnosis of deeply infiltrating endometriosis. Int J Gynaecol Obstet 2009;104:156–160.

28. Ribeiro HS, Ribeiro PA, Rossini L, Rodrigues FC, Donadio N, Aoki T. Double-contrast barium enema and transrectal endoscopic ultrasonography in the diagnosis of intestinal deeply infiltrating endometriosis. J Minim Invasive Gynecol 2008;15(3):315–320.

29. Goncalves MO, Podgaec S, Dias JA Jr, Gonzalez M, Abrao MS. Transvaginal ultrasonography with bowel preparation is able to predict the number of lesions and rectosigmoid layers affected in cases of deep endometriosis, defining surgical strategy. Hum Reprod 2010;25(3):665–671.

30. Griffiths AN, Koutsouridou RN, Penketh RJ. Rectovaginal endometriosis – a frequently missed diagnosis. J Obstet Gynaecol 2007;27(6):605–607.

31. Ward CJ. Professional liability and risk management for the gynecologic surgeon. In: Rock JA, Jones HW (eds) Te Linde's Operative Gynecology, 9th edn. Philadelphia: Lippincott Williams and Wilkins, 2003, pp. 43–66.

32. Markovic M, Manderson L, Warren N. Endurance and contest: women's narratives of endometriosis. Health (London) 2008;12(3):349–367.

33. Ball E, Koh C, Janik G, Davis C. Gynaecological laparoscopy: 'see and treat' should be the gold standard. Curr Opin Obstet Gynecol 2008;20(4):325–330.

34. Jansen FW, Kapiteyn K, Trimbos-Kemper T, Hermans J, Trimbos JB. Complications of laparoscopy: a prospective multicentre observational study. Br J Obstet Gynaecol 1997;104(5):595–600.

35. Chapron C, Bourret A, Chopin N et al. Surgery for bladder endometriosis: long-term results and concomitant management of associated posterior deep lesions. Hum Reprod 2010;25(4):884–889.

36. Soderstrom R. Principles of electrosurgery as applied to gynecology. In: Rock JA, Jones HW (eds) Te Linde's Operative Gynecology, 9th edn. Philadelphia: Lippincott Williams and Wilkins, 2003, pp. 291–308.

37. Redwine DB. Laparoscopic excision of endometriosis with 3-mm scissors: comparison of operating times between sharp excision and electro-excision. J Am Assoc Gynecol Laparosc 1993;1(1):24–30.

38. Wood C, Maher P. Peritoneal surgery in the treatment of endometriosis – excision or thermal ablation? Aust N Z J Obstet Gynaecol 1996;36(2):190–197.

39. Reich H, McGlynn F, Salvat J. Laparoscopic treatment of cul-de-sac obliteration secondary to retrocervical deep fibrotic endometriosis. J Reprod Med 1991;36(7):516–522.

40. Bosev D, Nicoll LM, Bhagan L, Lemyre M, Payne CK, Gill H, Nezhat C. Laparoscopic management of ureteral endometriosis: the Stanford University hospital experience with 96 consecutive cases. J Urol 2009;182(6):2748–2752.

41. Frenna V, Santos L, Ohana E, Bailey C, Wattiez A. Laparoscopic management of ureteral endometriosis: our experience. J Minim Invasive Gynecol 2007;14(2):169–171.

42. Scioscia M, Molon A, Grosso G, Minelli L. Laparoscopic management of ureteral endometriosis. Curr Opin Obstet Gynecol 2009;21(4):325–328.

43. Hart R, Hickey M, Maouris P, Buckett W, Garry R. Excisional surgery versus m ablative surgery for ovarian endometriomata: a Cochrane Review. Hum Reprod 2005;20(11):3000–3007.

44. Chapron C, Vercellini P, Barakat H, Vieira M, Dubuisson JB. Management of ovarian endometriomas. Hum Reprod Update 2002;8(6):591–597.

45. Donnez J, Lousse JC, Jadoul P, Donnez O, Squifflet J. Laparoscopic management of endometriomas using a combined technique of excisional (cystectomy) and ablative surgery. Fertil Steril 2010;94(1):28–32.

46. Dubuisson JB. Surgical treatment for endometriomas. J Gynecol Obstet Biol Reprod (Paris) 2003;32:S20–22.

47. Zhu Z, Al-Beiti MA, Tang L, Liu X, Lu X. Clinical characteristic analysis of 32 patients with abdominal incision endometriosis. J Obstet Gynaecol 2008;28(7):742–745.

48. Seracchioli R, Manuzzi L, Mabrouk M et al. A multidisciplinary, minimally invasive approach for complicated deep infiltrating endometriosis. Fertil Steril 2010;93(3):1007.

49. Remorgida V, Ferrero S, Fulcheri E, Ragni N, Martin DC. Bowel endometriosis: presentation, diagnosis, and treatment. Obstet Gynecol Surv 2007;62(7):461–470.

50. Beard JD, Nicholson ML, Sayers RD, Lloyd D, Everson NW. Intraoperative air testing of colorectal anastomoses: a prospective, randomized trial. Br J Surg 1990;77(10):1095–1097.

38 Surgical Therapies: Peritoneal Endometriosis Surgery

Michael P. Diamond and Valerie I. Shavell

Division of Reproductive Endocrinology and Infertility, Department of Obstetrics and Gynecology, Wayne State University School of Medicine, Detroit, MI, USA

Introduction

Since the introduction of laparoscopy, the diagnosis and treatment of endometriosis have been dramatically altered. Laparoscopy may be utilized to confirm the presence of endometriosis and to excise or ablate endometriotic lesions, often with reduced morbidity and comparable efficacy to laparotomy. Destruction of endometriotic lesions, restoration of normal anatomy, delay of disease progression, and symptomatic relief are the primary goals in the treatment of endometriosis [1].

Morphological appearance of endometriosis

Endometriosis is diagnosed in 15–80% of women undergoing laparoscopy for chronic pelvic pain, and in 21–65% of women undergoing evaluation for infertility [2]. During laparoscopic evaluation for endometriosis, endometriotic lesions may appear morphologically dissimilar. Red lesions, characterized by numerous proliferative glands, are highly active, vascularized lesions that are thought to be the first stage of peritoneal endometriosis [3,4]. In fact, it is often red lesions that are encountered in adolescents with endometriosis [5]. As the disease progresses, the implants become encased in a scarification process that renders them black from intraluminal debris [4]. Subsequent fibrosis and devascularization ensue, and white plaques and yellow-brown lesions form, often in association with adhesions to adjacent structures. These lesions are thought to represent quiescent or latent endometriosis. Compared with red lesions, white lesions have a lower mitotic index and a greater number of smaller vessels [6].

Aside from the color of the lesions, three different morphological types of peritoneal endometriosis have been described: polyp-type, plaque-type, and subperitoneal implant [7]. The polyp-type implant is a small mushroom-like lesion studded with endometriotic stroma while the plaque-type lesion is contiguous with the lining of the peritoneum. The subperitoneal implant is enclosed by normal peritoneum. These various types of lesions may reflect different etiologies, and may manifest varying likelihood of tissue invasiveness and symptomotology.

Diagnostic accuracy

While the diagnosis of peritoneal endometriosis may clinically often be based upon visual inspection at the time of laparoscopy, biopsy of suspected lesions provides definitive diagnosis of endometriosis. The proposed diagnostic accuracy of visualization in the diagnosis of endometriosis varies widely in the literature. Ueki *et al* [8] found that 73% of pigmented specimens obtained from the peritoneum were histologically confirmed endometriosis. Metller *et al* [9], however, reported that only 54% of suspected lesions were confirmed histologically: 100% of red lesions, 92% of black lesions, and 31% of white lesions. Contrary to these findings, Stratton *et al* [10] found that white or mixed-color lesions were more likely to be confirmed as endometriosis than black or red lesions, as were lesions greater than 5 mm, with an overall histological confirmation rate of 61%. Based on results from a prospective study, Walter *et al* [11] calculated a positive predictive value of 45%, sensitivity of 97%, negative predictive value of 99%, and specificity of 77% for the visual diagnosis of endometriosis. Much higher success has been reported by Martin *et al* [12], utilizing an approach in which only small tissue specimens thought to be the specific endometriotic lesions are provided to the pathologist for histological diagnosis.

Alternatively, atypical lesions not thought to be endometriosis may, in fact, represent true disease. In 24% of cases, atypical lesions that were not presumed to be endometriosis were histologically confirmed endometriotic lesions [13]. Furthermore, occult endometriosis has been discovered in biopsies of

Endometriosis: Science and Practice, First Edition. Edited by Linda C. Giudice, Johannes L.H. Evers and David L. Healy.
© 2012 Blackwell Publishing Ltd. Published 2012 by Blackwell Publishing Ltd.

normal-appearing peritoneum in 6% of patients [14]. Multiple biopsies of suspected lesions have been recommended to increase diagnostic accuracy during laparoscopy [15].

Excision of endometriosis

Laparoscopic excision of endometriotic lesions is the primary treatment for symptomatic endometriosis. Women who underwent laparoscopic excision of visually diagnosed endometriosis reported a 67% improvement in pain symptoms at 6–38 months of follow-up [16]. Furthermore, in a subgroup of patients found to have histologically confirmed endometriosis limited to the peritoneum, laparoscopic excision of endometriotic lesions has also been associated with a significant decrease in median pain scores at 3 months [17]. Redwine demonstrated that laparoscopic excision of endometriosis by sharp dissection resulted in a cumulative rate of recurrent or persistent disease in only 19% of women at 5 years of follow-up [18]. Compared with diagnostic laparoscopy alone, laparoscopic excision of endometriotic implants has been shown to result in an improvement in pain and quality of life at 6 months and up to 5 years after surgical intervention [19,20].

Laparoscopic excision of endometriotic implants may be performed using different techniques, including sharp dissection and electro-excision. In a retrospective study comparing sharp dissection with 3 mm scissors and monopolar electro-excision, operating time was reduced by 26–49% in the electro-excision group [21]. This may be due to the ability to cut and coagulate simultaneously with the use of electro-excision.

Disposable and reusable blunt-ended scissors with a monopolar electrode attachment are available for laparoscopic use. The peritoneum over the endometriotic lesion should be elevated in order to determine depth of involvement, and the lesion may then be excised with a 2–5 mm margin of normal-appearing peritoneum [14]. If multiple lesions are co-localized, a segment of peritoneum encompassing the lesions may be excised *en bloc*.

Ablation of endometriosis

In addition to excision of endometriotic implants, electrocautery may be utilized to vaporize or coagulate peritoneal endometriosis. Endometriotic lesions may be coagulated using a spoon, flat electrode, or bipolar electrocautery forceps. Bipolar forceps limit the spread of current between electrodes but may impede the total destruction of lesions that extend beyond visualizable portions. Endometriotic lesions may also be fulgurated with a cutting current of 50–70 W with an electrode held 1–2 mm from the tissue surface [14]. This technique limits the depth of tissue penetration but may result in deep penetration if the electrode accidentally touches the tissue surface. In a prospective randomized trial, laparoscopic fulguration of mild endometriosis was found to be associated with a significantly higher pregnancy rate compared with no intervention (60.8% versus 18.5%) [22].

The carbon dioxide laser has frequently been used in the treatment of endometriosis; however, fiber lasers such as the KTP-53, argon, and Nd:YAG laser may be utilized as well [1]. The laser has the advantage of precision coupled with the magnification afforded by the laparoscope [23]. The carbon dioxide laser may be used to coagulate lesions using a lower density of 2500–5000 W/cm^2 with single or repeat pulses, or a higher density superpulse may be used to vaporize endometriotic tissue [14]. Vaporization is recommended to attain deeper tissue penetration. The technique of hydrodissection, in which lactated Ringer's solution is injected subperitoneally, separating the peritoneum from underlying structures, has been described in the literature as a mechanism of safeguarding the penetration distance and increasing the safety of laser laparoscopy [24]. The carbon dioxide laser may also be used to excise endometriotic implants by tenting the peritoneum and undercutting the lesion [23].

In a study following 102 patients with infertility attributed to endometriosis, 60.7% conceived within 24 months after laser laparoscopy [25]. Compared with expectant management, medical treatment, and laparoscopic cautery of endometriotic implants, Paulson et al [26] found that there were significantly higher pregnancy rates in women with mild endometriosis who underwent laparoscopic laser treatment. Furthermore, Sutton et al [27] found that there was improvement or resolution of pain symptoms at 6 months in 63% of women who underwent laser treatment compared with 23% in the expectant management group, and 90% of those who initially responded were asymptomatic at 1 year [28]. The effect may be short-lived, however, as 61% of women with peritoneal endometriosis who were treated with the carbon dioxide laser were found to have recurrence of pelvic pain 18 months after surgery, compared with 39% at 6 months [29].

Of note, endometriosis may invade up to 3 cm beneath the peritoneal surface. Thus vaporization or coagulation of endometriotic implants may only address the superficial disease process [30]. Endometriosis has been found deep to areas that were previously vaporized on second-look laparoscopy [23]. Furthermore, thermal damage may obscure complete visualization of the lesions or adjacent vital structures [14]. Therefore, some surgeons think that careful sharp dissection and complete excision of peritoneal endometriosis may result in improved surgical outcomes.

Pathophysiology of endometriosis-associated pain

Destruction of endometriosis by either excision or ablation has been shown to decrease pelvic pain in numerous trials [2]. Although the pathophysiology of endometriosis-associated pain is not completely understood, endometriotic implants are theorized to incite pain due to factors related to neural innervation. Sensory, cholinergic, and adrenergic nerve fibers have been located in proximity to endometriotic glands, and the density of nerve fibers in peritoneal endometriotic lesions has been found to be greater than in normal peritoneum [31]. Furthermore, a greater number of nerve fibers appear to be present in the endometriotic lesions of women who are experiencing dysmenorrhea or pelvic pain [32].

Transforming growth factor (TGF)-β1 immunoreactive nerve fibers have been discovered in the endometriotic lesions of women with dysmenorrhea [33]. Via increased cyclo-oxygenase activity, TGF-β1 may augment prostaglandin production in sensory and sympathetic nerve fibers, which could result in the generation of endometriosis-associated pain. Peritoneal endometriotic lesions have also been shown to express several nerve growth factors such as neutrophin-3 (NT-3) and nerve growth factor (NGF), as well as pain-mediating substances such as histamine, kinins, and interleukins [32].

The mean density of macrophages in peritoneal endometriotic lesions has also been found to be greater than in normal peritoneum [34]. Macrophages may potentially facilitate the growth and repair of nerve fibers in endometriotic lesions by influencing the synthesis of substances such as NGF, brain-derived neurotropic factor (BDNF), and vascular endothelial growth factor (VEGF).

Endometriosis and peritoneal adhesions

Pelvic adhesions may result from mechanical damage to the peritoneum or peritoneal ischemia during surgery for endometriosis, or as a response to the inflammatory process of the disease itself [35]. Once formed, adhesions may contribute to pelvic pain, infertility, bowel obstruction, and difficulty in reoperation. Whether endometriotic lesions are excised or ablated, care must be taken to employ good surgical technique such as careful tissue handling, meticulous hemostasis, and copious irrigation in order to minimize postoperative adhesion formation.

Adhesions associated with endometriosis have a considerable presence of inflammatory, hemosiderin-laden, endometrial-like cells and fibrin deposits that may confer a propensity for adhesion re-formation after adhesiolysis [36]. After laser ablation of endometriotic lesions and lysis of adhesions, 43% of adhesions had re-formed at second-look laparoscopy [35]. Adhesion formation preferentially occurred at prior adhesion sites. The frequent re-formation of peritoneal adhesions after surgical treatment for endometriosis may play a role in the persistence of pelvic pain following surgical treatment of endometriosis.

Vaporization or coagulation of endometriotic lesions potentially complicates peritoneal healing. Laser vaporization of endometriotic lesions, for example, is associated with carbon deposition in ablated tissue [23]. Carbonization of the peritoneum potentially incites an inflammatory reaction that results in giant cell formation and delayed mesothelial repair [37]. Comparatively, sharp dissection incites less necrosis and foreign body reaction, but may cause bleeding which then requires interventions to achieve hemostasis that may incite adhesion development. Vaporization and coagulation, therefore, should be used judiciously.

Pneumoperitoneum during laparoscopic surgery for endometriosis may also contribute to adhesion formation. Adhesion formation in mice appears to be associated both with the duration of pneumoperitoneum and with insufflation pressure [38]. Mesothelial hypoxia is the proposed mechanism of pneumoperitoneum-associated adhesion formation.

Disease recurrence

Even after successful surgical treatment of endometriosis, symptoms may persist or recur. The rate of recurrent endometriosis following laparoscopic excision of endometriotic implants ranges from 33% to 44% in the literature [39]. One year after laser ablation for painful pelvic endometriosis, 29% of women who continued to be symptomatic were found to have progressive disease and 42% static disease at second-look laparoscopy [28].

Women may undergo additional surgical intervention as a result of persistent or worsening symptoms. The reoperation rate after laparoscopic treatment of endometriosis has been found to be 21% at 2 years and 58% at 7 years [40]. Similarly, Cheong et al [41] reported a 51% reoperation rate after 10 years of follow-up. The age of the patient at the time of surgery appears to be a major predictor of the need for reoperation – women 19–29 years had a 1.75 times higher rate of reoperation than women 30–39 years, and 4.76 times higher rate than women over 40 years of age [40].

Taylor and Williams [29] investigated patterns of disease recurrence at reoperation and found an overall probability of recurrence of 37%. Endometriosis was most likely to recur close to the original area of involvement, which may be a result of incomplete excision or ablation or a propensity for implantation at particular locations. Furthermore, there was no difference in the rate of recurrent endometriosis in areas that were initially excised versus ablated.

Reoperation may be warranted in symptomatic patients with endometriosis but should be undertaken with caution in patients desiring conception. Nineteen percent of patients were found to conceive after reoperation compared with 34% after initial intervention [42].

Incidental endometriosis

As there is no consensus on the management of asymptomatic minimal or mild endometriosis, the management of incidental endometriosis remains controversial. However, when endometriosis is incidentally discovered during surgery, destruction of endometriotic lesions may be warranted [43,44]. Excision of endometriotic implants has been especially advised in younger women, based upon the concept that the disease process could worsen and potentially incite adhesion formation [45]. In asymptomatic women who have endometriotic lesions identified during laparoscopy or laparotomy, postoperative medical treatment is not warranted as medical treatment has not been shown to alter the clinical course of minimal and mild endometriosis [44].

Adjuvant medical therapy

Adjuvant medical therapy prior to surgical treatment of endometriosis has been investigated with inconclusive results. Theoretically, medical pretreatment could reduce the inflammation and vascularization of endometriotic lesions, facilitating more efficient surgery [46]. On the other hand, preoperative medical therapy could result in regression of endometriotic lesions [47], resulting in incomplete excision or ablation at the time of surgery. Nonetheless, preoperative medical treatment does not appear to significantly affect reproductive outcome [46].

The use of postoperative adjuvant medical therapy has been proposed as a mechanism to decrease disease recurrence following surgical intervention. In a randomized placebo-controlled trial, the levonorgestrel-releasing intrauterine system (LNG-IUS) was shown to reduce the recurrence of moderate or severe dysmenorrhea in women who underwent laparoscopic treatment of endometriosis at 1 year of follow-up: dysmenorrhea recurred in 10% of women in the postoperative LNG-IUS group compared with 45% in the surgery-only group [48].

Postoperative administration of gonadotropin releasing hormone (GnRH) analogs has also been suggested to decrease the recurrence of endometriosis-associated pain. The effectiveness of a 6-month postoperative course of a GnRH analog was investigated by Vercellini *et al* [49]. Time to recurrence of symptoms was significantly delayed in the postoperative GnRH analog-treated group compared with those who underwent expectant management. This finding confirmed an earlier randomized controlled trial comparing postoperative GnRH analog treatment to placebo in which there was a significant decrease in physician-reported pain scores at 6 months in the GnRH analog-treated group [50]. A 3-month postoperative course of a GnRH analog, however, has not been shown to significantly reduce the recurrence of endometriosis-associated pain [51,52].

Postoperative administration of danazol appears to be clinically beneficial in the alleviation of endometriosis-associated pain as well. A 6-month postoperative course of danazol was found to significantly alleviate pelvic pain compared with placebo [53]. Furthermore, endometriotic lesions were found to be significantly smaller at second-look laparoscopy 6 months after initial intervention in the danazol-treated group. A 3-month postoperative course of danazol, however, was found to be ineffective in reducing the recurrence of endometriosis-associated pain compared with expectant management in women with stage III or IV endometriosis [54].

While postoperative adjuvant medical therapy may be beneficial in delaying symptomatic recurrence, it does not appear to affect the rate of conception in women with infertility associated with endometriosis [2]. However, the pretreatment of women with endometriosis with a GnRH agonist for 3–6 months prior to *in vitro* fertilization (IVF) has been shown to increase the odds of clinical pregnancy four-fold [55]. The improved pregnancy rate may be due to enhanced uterine receptivity or oocyte quality. Adjuvant medical therapy, therefore, should be considered in the proper setting.

Conclusion

Laparoscopy may be utilized to successfully diagnose and treat symptomatic endometriosis. Biopsy of suspected lesions is recommended to confirm the diagnosis. Excision and ablation of endometriotic lesions often result in symptomatic improvement but pain may recur, necessitating reoperation. Long-term postoperative adjuvant medical therapy may be considered to delay the recurrence of endometriosis-associated pain.

References

1. Valle RF, Sciarra JJ. Endometriosis: treatment strategies. Ann N Y Acad Sci 2003;997:229–239.
2. Yeung PP Jr, Shwayder J, Pasic RP. Laparoscopic management of endometriosis: comprehensive review of best evidence. J Minim Invasive Gynecol 2009;16:269–281.
3. Redwine DB. Age-related evolution in color appearance of endometriosis. Fertil Steril 1987;48:1062–1063.
4. Nisolle M, Donnez J. Peritoneal endometriosis, ovarian endometriosis, and adenomyotic nodules of the rectovaginal septum are three different entities. Fertil Steril 1997;68:585–596.
5. Goldstein MP, de Cholnoky C, Emans SJ et al. Laparoscopy in the diagnosis and management of pelvic pain in adolescents. J Reprod Med 1980;44:251–258.
6. Donnez J, Squifflet J, Casanas-Roux F. Typical and subtle atypical presentations of endometriosis. Obstet Gynecol Clin North Am 2003;30:83–93.
7. Brosens IA, Cornillie FJ. Peritoneal endometriosis. Morphological basis of the laparoscopic diagnosis. Contrib Gynecol Obstet 1987;16:125–137.
8. Ueki M, Saeki M, Tsurunaga T et al. Visual findings and histologic diagnosis of pelvic endometriosis under laparoscopy and laparotomy. Int J Fertil Menopausal Stud 1995;40:248–253.
9. Mettler L, Schollmeyer T, Lehmann-Willenbrock E et al. Accuracy of laparoscopic diagnosis of endometriosis. JSLS 2003;7:15–18.
10. Stratton P, Winkel CA, Sinaii N et al. Location, color, size, depth, and volume may predict endometriosis in lesions resected at surgery. Fertil Steril 2002;78:743–749.
11. Walter AJ, Hentz JG, Magtibay PM et al. Endometriosis: correlation between histologic and visual findings at laparoscopy. Am J Obstet Gynecol 2001;184:1407–1413.
12. Martin DC, Hubert GD, Vander Zwaag R, el-Zeky FA. Laparoscopic appearances of peritoneal endometriosis. Fertil Steril 1989;51:63–67.
13. Albee RB Jr, Sinervo K, Fisher DT. Laparoscopic excision of lesions suggestive of endometriosis or otherwise atypical in appearance: relationship between visual findings and final histologic diagnosis. J Minim Invasive Gynecol 2008;15:32–37.
14. Wood C. Endoscopy in the management of endometriosis. Baillière's Clin Obstet Gynaecol 1994;8:735–757.

15. Kazanegra R, Zaritsky E, Lathi RB et al. Diagnosis of stage I endometriosis: comparing visual inspection to histologic biopsy specimen. J Minim Invasive Gynecol 2008;15:176–180.

16. Wykes CB, Clark TJ, Chakravati S et al. Efficacy of laparoscopic excision of visually diagnosed peritoneal endometriosis in the treatment of chronic pelvic pain. Eur J Obstet Gynecol Reprod Biol 2006;125:129–133.

17. Kaiser A, Kopf A, Gericke C et al. The influence of peritoneal endometriotic lesions on the generation of endometriosis-related pain and pain reduction after surgical excision. Arch Gynecol Obstet 2009;280:369–373.

18. Redwine DB. Conservative laparoscopic excision of endometriosis by sharp dissection: life table analysis of reoperation and persistent or recurrent disease. Fertil Steril 1991;56:628–634.

19. Abbott JA, Hawe J, Clayton RD et al. The effects and effectiveness of laparoscopic excision of endometriosis: a prospective study with 2–5 year follow-up. Hum Reprod 2003;18:1922–1927.

20. Abbott J, Hawe H, Hunter D et al. Laparoscopic excision of endometriosis: a randomized, placebo-controlled trial. Fertil Steril 2004;82:878–884.

21. Redwine DB. Laparoscopic excision of endometriosis with 3-mm scissors: comparison of operating times between sharp excision and electro-excision. J Am Assoc Gynecol 1993;1:24–30.

22. Nowroozi K, Chase JS, Check JH et al. The importance of laparoscopic coagulation of mild endometriosis in infertile women. Int J Fertil 1987;32:442–444.

23. Davis GD, Brooks RA. Excision of pelvic endometriosis with the carbon dioxide laser laparoscope. Obstet Gynecol 1988;72:816–819.

24. Nezhat C, Nezhat FR. Safe laser endoscopic excision or vaporization of peritoneal endometriosis. Fertil Steril 1989;52:149–151.

25. Nezhat C, Crowgey SR, Garrison CP. Surgical treatment of endometriosis via laser laparoscopy. Fertil Steril 1986;45:778–783.

26. Paulson JD, Asmar P, Saffan DS. Mild and moderate endometriosis. Comparison of treatment modalities for infertile couples. J Reprod Med 1991;36:151–155.

27. Sutton CJ, Ewen SP, Whitelaw N et al. Prospective, randomized, double-blind, controlled trial of laser laparoscopy in the treatment of pelvic pain associated with minimal, mild, and moderate endometriosis. Fertil Steril 1994;62:696–700.

28. Sutton CJ, Pooley AS, Ewen SP et al. Follow-up report on a randomized controlled trial of laser laparoscopy in the treatment of pelvic pain associated with minimal to moderate endometriosis. Fertil Steril 1997;68:1070–1074.

29. Cibula D, Kuzel D, Fucíková Z et al. Long-term follow-up after complete treatment of peritoneal endometriosis with the CO2 laser [in Czech]. Ceska Gynekol 2003;68:63–68.

30. Broach AN, Mansuria SM, Sanfilippo JS. Pediatric and adolescent gynecologic laparoscopy. Clin Obstet Gynecol 2009;52:380–389.

31. Tokushige N, Markham R, Russell P et al. Nerve fibres in peritoneal endometriosis. Hum Reprod 2006;21:3001–3007.

32. Mechsner S, Kaiser A, Kopf A et al. A pilot study to evaluate the clinical relevance of endometriosis-associated nerve fibers in peritoneal endometriotic lesions. Fertil Steril 2009;92:1856–1861.

33. Tamburro S, Canis M, Albuisson E et al. Expression of transforming growth factor beta1 in nerve fibers is related to dysmenorrhea and laparoscopic appearance of endometriotic implants. Fertil Steril 2003;80:1131–1136.

34. Tran LV, Tokushige N, Berbic M et al. Macrophages and nerve fibres in peritoneal endometriosis. Hum Reprod 2009;24:835–841.

35. Parker JD, Sinaii N, Segars JH, Godoy H, Winkel C, Stratton P. Adhesion formation after laparoscopic excision of endometriosis and lysis of adhesions. Fertil Steril 2005;84:1457–1461.

36. Brosens IA, Campo R, Gordts S et al. An appraisal of the role of laparoscopy: past, present, and future. Int J Gynaecol Obstet 2001;74(Suppl 1):S9–14.

37. Di Zerega GS, Campeau JD. Peritoneal repair and post-surgical adhesion formation. Hum Reprod Update 2001;7:547–555.

38. Binda MM, Molinas CR, Koninckx PR. Reactive oxygen species and adhesion formation: clinical implications in adhesion prevention. Hum Reprod 2003;18:2503–2507.

39. Taylor E, Williams C. Surgical treatment of endometriosis: location and patterns of disease at reoperation. Fertil Steril 2010;93(1):57–61.

40. Shakiba K, Bena JF, McGill KM et al. Surgical treatment of endometriosis: a 7-year follow-up on the requirement for further surgery. Obstet Gynecol 2008;111:1285–1292.

41. Cheong Y, Tay P, Luk F, Gan HC, Li TC, Cooke I. Laparoscopic surgery for endometriosis: how often do we need to re-operate? J Obstet Gynaecol 2008;28:82–85.

42. Vercellini P, Somigliana E, Daguati R et al. The second time around: reproductive performance after repetitive versus primary surgery for endometriosis. Fertil Steril 2009;92:1253–1255.

43. Donnez J, Squifflet J, Pirard C et al. The efficacy of medical and surgical treatment of endometriosis-associated infertility and pelvic pain. Gynecol Obstet Invest 2002;54(Suppl 1):2–10.

44. Rossmanith WG. Minimal endometriosis: a therapeutic dilemma? Gynecol Endocrinol 2009;25:762–764.

45. Donnez J, Smets M, Jadoul P et al. Laparoscopic management of peritoneal endometriosis, endometriotic cysts, and rectovaginal adenomyosis. Ann N Y Acad Sci 2003;997:274–281.

46. Vercellini P, Somigliana E, Viganò P et al. Surgery for endometriosis-associated infertility: a pragmatic approach. Hum Reprod 2009;24:254–269.

47. Evers JL. The second-look laparoscopy for evaluation of the result of medical treatment of endometriosis should not be performed during ovarian suppression. Fertil Steril 1987;47:502–504.

48. Vercellini P, Frontino G, de Giorgi O et al. Comparison of a levonorgestrel-releasing intrauterine device versus expectant management after conservative surgery for symptomatic endometriosis: a pilot study. Fertil Steril 2003;80:305–309.

49. Vercellini P, Crosignani PG, Fadini R et al. A gonadotrophin-releasing hormone agonist compared with expectant management after conservative surgery for symptomatic endometriosis. Br J Obstet Gynaecol 1999;106:672–677.

50. Hornstein MD, Hemmings R, Yuzpe AA et al. Use of nafarelin versus placebo after reductive laparoscopic surgery for endometriosis. Fertil Steril 1997;68:860–864.

51. Parazzini F, Fedele L, Busacca M et al. Postsurgical medical treatment of advanced endometriosis: results of a randomized clinical trial. Am J Obstet Gynecol 1994;171:1205–1207.

52. Ozawa Y, Murakami T, Terada Y et al. Management of the pain associated with endometriosis: an update of the painful problems. Tohoku J Exp Med 2006;210:175–188.

53. Telimaa S, Rönnberg L, Kauppila A. Placebo-controlled comparison of danazol and high-dose medroxyprogesterone acetate in the treatment of endometriosis after conservative surgery. Gynecol Endocrinol 1987;1:363–371.

54. Bianchi S, Busacca M, Agnoli B et al. Effects of 3 month therapy with danazol after laparoscopic surgery for stage III/IV endometriosis: a randomized study. Hum Reprod 1999;14:1335–1337.

55. Sallam HN, Garcia-Velasco JA, Dias S, Arici A. Long-term pituitary down-regulation before in vitro fertilization (IVF) for women with endometriosis. Cochrane Database Syst Rev 2006;1:CD004635.

39 Surgical Therapies: Pouch of Douglas and Uterovaginal Pouch Resection for Endometriosis

Maurício S. Abrão, Sérgio Podgaec and Luiz Flávio Cordeiro Fernandes
Department of Obstetrics and Gynecology, University of São Paulo Medical School, São Paulo, Brazil

Introduction

One of the greatest challenges in the treatment of deep endometriosis is the surgical treatment of lesions located in the pouch of Douglas, including the retrocervical region, the vagina and the rectovaginal septum. In a continuous series of 426 patients with pelvic pain who were submitted to surgical treatment either by laparoscopy or laparotomy, Chapron et al studied the anatomical distribution of histologically confirmed deep endometriotic lesions and reported that they were found principally in the posterior pelvic compartment (uterosacral ligaments, vagina, ureter and bowel), more commonly on the left side [1]. In 52.7% of these patients, the lesions were on the uterosacral ligament, in 22.7% they were in the bowel, 16.2% in the vagina, 6.3% in the bladder and 2.1% in the ureter. Vaginal lesions were considered as those infiltrating the anterior rectovaginal pouch, the posterior vaginal fornix and the retroperitoneal area between the anterior rectovaginal pouch and the posterior vaginal fornix.

The difficulty involved in managing such cases is not only associated with complicated surgical access and the proximity of important structures such as the rectum, ureters and pelvic vessels and nerves, but also the need for a detailed presurgical diagnosis that will enable the surgeon to perform a thorough surgical procedure, which is crucial in improving pain and reducing the likelihood of a recurrence of the disease.

This chapter outlines the relevant anatomical considerations, the steps involved in selecting the optimal surgical technique to be performed, the details of the surgical procedure itself and the results obtained under these circumstances.

Anatomical points of reference

Before describing the anatomical features that need to be taken into consideration, it is important to define the regions that must be examined for lesions:
- the retrocervical region between the uterosacral ligaments, and the uterosacral ligaments themselves
- the posterior vaginal fornix, including the upper third of the vagina
- the rectovaginal septum, defined as the region between the rectum and the mid and lower thirds of the vagina, below the retrocervical region.

This chapter will discuss the areas affected by the lesions which, in order of frequency, are: the retrocervical region, the vaginal fornix and, less commonly, the rectovaginal septum. It should be mentioned that some authors refer to the retrocervical region as the uterine torus and to lesions in the vaginal fornix as rectovaginal lesions. Finally, there is some confusion in the literature, deep retrocervical and vaginal lesions sometimes being erroneously described as lesions of the rectovaginal septum.

First, from an anatomical point of view, the ureters represent important reference points in this region, their pelvic segment following the lateral wall of the pelvis in a posterior-inferior direction, where the posterior border of the ovarian fossa is located, reaching externally to the parietal peritoneum and anteriorly to the internal iliac arteries. They continue on this trajectory to around 1.5 cm above the ischiatic spines. At this point, each ureter curves anteromedially above the levator ani muscle where it is closely attached to the peritoneum. As it descends, the ureter passes medially to the point at which the uterine artery begins and continues as far as the ischiatic spine, where the uterine artery crosses above it. Next, it continues laterally to the posterior vaginal fornix and enters the posterior-superior angle of the bladder.

It is important to understand the system of arteries irrigating the pelvic portion of the ureter, since devascularization may result in fistulae. The blood supply to the pelvic segments of the ureters comes from the external and internal iliac arteries and the vesical arteries, the most constant vascular supply coming from branches of the uterine arteries [2]. The fact that the uterine artery crosses in front of and over the ureter, laterally to the vaginal fornix, is of extreme clinical importance, since the ureter may be inadvertently ligated or sectioned or may even suffer thermal lesions when this region is treated. In particular, the left ureter is more vulnerable, since it is located closer to the lateral surface of the cervix [2]. With this quirk of anatomy in mind, in 2008 Seracchioli *et al* re-evaluated data from 541 patients submitted to laparoscopic treatment for pelvic endometriosis and identified 30 patients with a histological diagnosis of ureteral endometriosis, 66.7% of whom (20/30) had no symptoms suggestive of involvement of the urinary tract [3]. Of these, four patients had ureterohydronephrosis as a silent complication. Nine patients were also found to have perimenstrual dysuria, all nine having associated bladder endometriosis. A presurgical diagnosis of ureteral involvement was suspected in only 40% of the patients (12/30). These investigators also showed that whenever there is ureteral involvement, the side most likely to be affected is the left, which is affected in 46.7% of cases, compared to the right side, which is involved in around 26.7% of cases, while in the remaining 26.7% of cases both sides are affected.

Another vitally important topic in the surgical management of the pelvis is the complex innervation of the pelvic region, since lesions to these structures may lead to prolonged and incapacitating postsurgical disorders. These include bladder, bowel and sexual disorders such as urinary retention and incontinence, atonic bladder, fecal incontinence and sexual dysfunction. This issue is made even more complex since these lesions may occur in young women as a result of the characteristics of the disease [4].

This innervation is principally provided by the superior and inferior hypogastric plexuses. Immediately below the promontory, the superior hypogastric plexus divides into two filaments referred to as the presacral or hypogastric nerves. This plexus extends towards the front of the sacrum, outside the anterior sacral foramina, and is located below and between the internal iliac vessels in the retroperitoneal fat. Medially, it is attached to the sigmoid and the rectum, then joins the inferior hypogastric plexus [5]. The inferior hypogastric plexus is triangular with its base in the posterior position and its vertex in the anterior-inferior position, its trajectory continuing at a distance of around 1 cm from the posterior margin of the inferior hypogastric artery. Below, it extends to the posterior leaf of the broad ligament, exactly at the point at which the ureter enters this structure [5].

The efferent branches of the inferior hypogastric plexus reach the vesicouterine pouch and the rectovaginal septum, the vaginal (or anterior) efferents extending in branches towards the bladder, vagina, uterus and rectum, with two trunks that originate immediately below the point at which the ureter crosses the uterine artery. The lateral trunk, which reaches the bladder, is situated laterally, beneath the ureter, following it until it reaches the trigone of

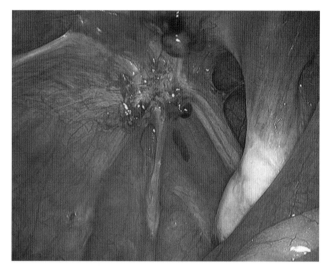

Figure 39.1 Cul-de-sac nodule involvement with endometriosis.

the bladder, whereas the medial trunk follows the lower margin of the uterine artery as far as the superior lateral wall of the vagina, where it subdivides into two groups: anterior and posterior. The anterior group is distributed along the vaginal wall, promoting innervation of the anterior two-thirds of this area. The posterior group is located immediately below the ureter and its branches perforate the posterior vaginal wall and are distributed along the rectovaginal septum. Branches emerging below the lower hypogastric plexus reach the rectum directly. Therefore, it is important to bear in mind the position of the lower hypogastric plexus, the ureter being used as a principal reference point. The point at which it crosses the uterine artery is where the bladder and vaginal branches are located, and this artery allows each one to be individualized, with the vaginal branches following the vessel and the vesicle branches following the terminal segment of the ureter [5,6].

Finally, the position at which it enters the rectum, which may be close to retrocervical lesions and to the posterior vaginal fornix, should always be examined, as well as the rectovaginal septum itself that divides the extraperitoneal portion of the rectum in relation to the vagina.

When is deep endometriosis suspected in the pouch of Douglas?

Concrete and decisive progress has been made in the diagnosis of lesions of deep endometriosis over the past 10 years, particularly as a result of interaction between the gynecologist and the radiologist and the evolution that has occurred in the ability to manipulate imaging methods, enabling data provided by imaging exams and data obtained during surgical procedures to be compared.

The clinical pillars of endometriosis are known to be pelvic pain and infertility; however, careful evaluation of the principal symptoms of the disease may guide the physician to the exact site of the lesions [7]. Patients with a complaint of deep dyspareunia may have deep lesions located in the cul-de-sac (Fig. 39.1). The clinical condition of the patient may include reports of dysmenorrhea, the most common complaint in women with endometriosis in addition to chronic (or acyclic) pelvic pain and changes in bowel habits, particularly during menstruation, that include pain on evacuation and an increase in the number of evacuations. It should be remembered that endometriosis may be present at other pelvic sites, possibly leading to a combination of these symptoms, including cases of infertility. In cases of endometriotic lesions affecting all the layers of the posterior vaginal fornix and exteriorized by the vaginal mucosa, the patients may report genital bleeding during or following sexual intercourse, which is sometimes confused with withdrawal bleeding related to the use of hormonal contraceptive methods [8].

In 2008, Abrão *et al* studied the association between vaginal lesions and bowel lesions affecting the rectosigmoid and found that the vagina was affected in 100% of cases in which the bowel lesions occupied more than 40% of the total circumference of the bowel lumen [9].

Seracchioli *et al* performed a retrospective analysis of 360 patients with a histological diagnosis of deep endometriosis of the posterior compartment [10]. In 240 of these cases, there was rectovaginal involvement (the posterior vaginal wall, the rectovaginal septum and the anterior wall of the rectum). The objective of the study was to establish a possible association between the intensity of perimenstrual dyschezia (pain during evacuation) and the anatomical location and diameter of the endometriotic lesions. The severity of dyschezia was found to be correlated with the presence of posterior deep endometriosis and there was also a positive association with the diameter of the rectovaginal lesion but not with involvement of the anterior wall of the rectum. These results are in agreement with the findings of Chapron *et al*, who performed a prospective study in 2005 and showed that dyschezia during menstruation is the strongest predictive factor for deep endometriosis of the posterior compartment [11]. In another retrospective analysis carried out in 2002 in which 225 patients with deep endometriosis were evaluated and a model of logistic regression was applied, it was found that perimenstrual dyschezia was more closely associated with involvement of the posterior vaginal wall and that the frequency of severe dysmenorrhea increased when adhesions were present in the pouch of Douglas. Also in that study, involvement of the uterosacral ligaments was associated with dyspareunia, whereas acyclic pelvic pain and functional bowel symptoms were found to be more closely linked to bowel endometriosis [12].

A crucial step in diagnosis concerns the physical examination, particularly speculum examination of lesions of the vaginal mucosa, and digital examination, which will detect any areas of thickening or nodules in the uterosacral ligaments, in the retrocervical region itself, the vaginal fornix or the rectovaginal septum [13,14]. In a study published by our group in 2007 that included cases of retrocervical and rectosigmoidal endometriosis, it was concluded that for every three cases of lesions at these sites, digital vaginal examination is capable of detecting this possibility in two, with an accuracy of a little over 60% [13]. This experience grows in a learning curve, with the greatest opportunity for learning being

during the surgical procedure when the patient is under anesthesia, at which time the pelvic cavity can be examined during videolaparoscopy in conjunction with carrying out digital vaginal examination. Of course, for lesions of the vaginal pouch itself, which consist of nodules in the posterior vaginal fornix and rectovaginal septum, digital examination may provide greater certainty of diagnosis. The principal limitation in this procedure lies in sexually inactive patients, obese patients and those who are reluctant to undergo the examination.

In the case of patients whose clinical status and physical examination are both suggestive of a diagnosis of endometriosis, an imaging method must then be used to map the pelvis. The information derived from this exam will serve to indicate the optimal form of management for each case. Transvaginal ultrasonography with simple bowel preparation prior to the exam is the method of choice for this purpose, since it permits adequate visualization of the internal genital organs and their interface with the urinary and intestinal tracts, hence being able to detect possible lesions of deep and ovarian endometriosis with a high degree of accuracy. Bowel preparation consists of the use of a mild oral laxative on the eve of the exam and a rectal enema consisting of 120 mL of dibasic sodium phosphate approximately 1 h prior to initiation of the exam. Bowel preparation is performed in order to eliminate any fecal residue and gases present in the rectosigmoid [9,15,16].

In 2009, Hudelist *et al* evaluated 200 patients referred to a tertiary referral center for endometriosis with symptoms suggestive of the disease and submitted them to physical examination of the pelvis associated with transvaginal ultrasonography [17,18]. These patients were then referred for laparoscopy. Comparing with subsequent histological diagnosis, the following sensitivity, specificity, positive and negative predictive values and accuracies were found with respect to the different sites of the disease: right uterosacral ligament (67%, 97%, 73%, 96% and 93%), left uterosacral ligament (84%, 86%, 62%, 95% and 86%), pouch of Douglas (87%, 98%, 90%, 98% and 97%), vagina (82%, 99%, 95%, 98% and 98%) and the rectovaginal septum (88%, 99%, 78%, 99% and 99%). These results highlight the extremely important association between physical examination and imaging exams in the diagnosis and presurgical preparation of the patient with endometriosis, allowing the surgeon to plan and decide on the optimal surgical therapy for each individual case [17,18].

Lesions of the posterior compartment that are not rectal lesions may be located anywhere from the rectovaginal septum through the vaginal fundus, uterosacral ligaments (that enter the cervix above the posterior vaginal fornix) and the uterine torus at the level of the isthmus. They may be medial or lateral and in the latter case there is a risk that the ureters will be affected, which, whenever possible, should be evaluated from the urinary meatus at least as far as their lateral passage to the cervix.

Donnez *et al* carried out a prospective evaluation of the prevalence of ureteral lesions in 405 patients treated for rectovaginal endometriotic nodules and identified ureteral involvement in 4.4% [19]. In none of these patients were the lesions confined to the ureter; in all cases, they were associated with rectovaginal endometriosis. They were not present at all in cases of rectovaginal nodules with a diameter of less than 2.0 cm; however, a prevalence of 0.6% was found for nodules ≥2.0 cm and <3.0 cm, this prevalence increasing to 11.2% when these nodules were ≥3.0 cm in diameter, highlighting the need for a thorough evaluation of the urinary tract in these cases.

In a case–control study of 609 patients submitted to laparoscopy with a histological diagnosis of endometriosis, Abrao *et al* identified 12 women with ureteral endometriosis and showed that this condition is not associated with bladder endometriosis but rather with a more advanced stage of the disease and with retrocervical and rectosigmoidal lesions [20]. When nodules are present in the topography of the vagina or adjacent areas and there is possible infiltration by contiguity, the procedure in this institute is to insert around 50–60 mL of ultrasound gel into the vagina to separate the cervix and distend the wall. This methodology allows us to assess whether the nodules are infiltrating the parietal layers of the vagina or whether they are simply fixed to the wall.

Magnetic resonance imaging (MRI) is also a good method for evaluating endometriosis; however, it has the limitation of not being as widely available as ultrasonography. Furthermore, it is more expensive and patients who are unable to tolerate the exam have to be sedated [21]. In a study comparing these imaging methods, our group reported sensitivity of 98.1% in cases of rectal endometriosis and 95.1% in retrocervical endometriosis with the use of transvaginal ultrasonography with prior bowel preparation, whereas sensitivity with MRI was 83.3% and 76% for rectal and retrocervical endometriosis, respectively [13].

Imaging methods, whether transvaginal ultrasonography, MRI or rectal echoendoscopy, may also be capable of defining the distance between the lowest portion of the lesion and the anal border [11,15,16,22]. This information may be very useful in defining the surgical technique and in enabling the surgeon to prevent any complications from occurring during the surgical treatment of low lesions a few centimeters from the anal border.

What is the best management of deep endometriosis in the pouch of Douglas?

In our institute, the initial treatment of the patient with pelvic pain and a suspicion of endometriosis is clinical, with the use of analgesics and hormones, except in cases of ovarian cysts and lesions of the appendix in which a differential diagnosis with malignant diseases is required, and in the case of obstructive lesions of the terminal ileum, cecum and rectosigmoid, all constituting situations for which the primary indication is for surgery. If no improvement is found with clinical treatment or if the lesions continue to grow, surgical intervention is also required. It must be emphasized that cases of infertility alone, when the patient has no complaints of pelvic pain, are not in principle treated surgically; however, each patient is evaluated individually.

Patients with pelvic pain, who are not interested in becoming pregnant and who have lesions in the vaginal pouch, are managed in accordance with this protocol and may be prescribed combined oral hormonal contraceptives, continuous progesterone therapy, either orally or by 3-monthly injection, or gonadotropin releasing hormone (GnRH) analogs. Alternatively, insertion of a levonorgestrel-releasing intrauterine system (LNG-IUS) may be recommended [23–25]. Response to treatment is followed up at 3-monthly outpatient visits, and imaging exams, preferably transvaginal ultrasonography with prior bowel preparation, are performed every 6 months to control the behavior and growth of lesions. In patients in whom response is positive, clinical treatment is maintained, although changes may be made in the type of hormonal treatment if the adverse side-effects that are characteristic to each class of hormones occur. If the patient fails to respond to the recommended treatment or if the endometriotic lesions continue to grow at the same speed and the infiltration rate remains unchanged, then surgical treatment is indicated.

Vercellini *et al* carried out a meta-analysis that included randomized observational, cohort and case–control studies in which the clinical treatment of rectovaginal endometriosis was evaluated [26]. The use of aromatase inhibitors, vaginal danazol, GnRH agonists, estrogen-progestin combinations (oral, transdermal and transvaginal), oral progestogens and the LNG-IUS were evaluated. Except for the use of aromatase inhibitors alone, the analgesic effect achieved with the other medications was high, ranging from 60% to 90%, and this effect persisted throughout the study period (6–12 months).

With the objective of evaluating the long-term results of the radical excision of rectovaginal endometriosis, Tarjanne *et al* followed up 60 patients for a mean period of 4 years and reported significant, prolonged relief from pain [27]. Furthermore, these investigators reported a recurrence rate, as established by clinical examination and ultrasonography, of 48%, although this recurrence was not associated with pain. Pharmaceutical treatments that induce amenorrhea (odds ratio (OR) 0.13; 95% confidence interval (CI) 0.02–0.65; $P = 0.01$) and bowel segmentary resection (OR 0.23; 95% CI 0.06–0.89; $P = 0.03$) reduce the risk of recurrence of rectovaginal endometriosis.

Angioni *et al* studied 31 patients with extensive, symptomatic endometriosis, which was unresponsive to pharmaceutical treatment and was affecting the pouch of Douglas, rectovaginal space and posterior vaginal fornix, with no bowel involvement [28]. It was reported that complete surgical removal, including excision of tissue from the adjacent posterior vaginal fornix, improves the quality of life and prolongs duration of the results (5 years). All the patients had severe pain that was exacerbated by clinical examination of the posterior vaginal fornix and uterosacral ligaments. The microscopic presence of endometriosis was identified in 10% of cases in which the vagina appeared to be unaffected. These investigators reported that complete remission from chronic pelvic pain was achieved in 38% of patients, while symptoms improved in another 22%; 38% of patients achieved total remission from dysmenorrhea, while in 22% the symptoms improved; and 45% of patients achieved full remission from dyspareunia, while in 25% this symptom improved partially. Indeed, 90% of the patients reported having avoided sexual intercourse prior to surgery, whereas more than 70% went on to have a satisfactory sexual life following surgery. This improvement in symptoms was statistically significant ($P < 0.001$) and persisted for 5 years with no recurrence of the disease.

It is appropriate here to mention a paper published in 2007 in which the highest rate of repeat operations in patients with endometriosis was related to having undergone previous surgeries that had been incompletely performed. Griffiths *et al* retrospectively analyzed 61 women with symptoms potentially indicative of rectovaginal endometriosis who had been submitted to laparoscopy previously and had received a negative diagnosis [29]. Of these, 16 were found to have rectovaginal endometriosis, 14 of whom had been previously submitted to videolaparoscopy without having been given a correct diagnosis, showing sensitivity and specificity for videolaparoscopy of 19% and 94%, respectively. This gives further strength to the hypothesis that when diagnostic surgery is performed by a general gynecologist, the correct diagnosis may not be reached in this type of disease, and raises the question that in many women rectovaginal endometriosis is not being diagnosed. In fact, many women are being told that their pelvic anatomy is normal when they actually have a severe form of deep endometriosis that is being ignored, leaving the patient to suffer unnecessarily, since this disease may cause debilitating symptoms, whereas surgical treatment is available and extremely effective [29].

Along the same lines, Carmona *et al* showed the importance of the surgeon's experience in the treatment of rectovaginal endometriosis [30]. These investigators analyzed 60 consecutive patients submitted to laparoscopy for symptomatic rectovaginal endometriosis and divided the patients into two groups, the first 30 being considered the early group and the next 30 the late group. They concluded that after the surgeon had gained experience in performing 30 cases, a reduction then occurred in the rate of conversion to laparotomy, in the time of surgery and in the amount of blood lost. Furthermore, they found a reduction in the cases of incomplete resection of the disease and in the recurrence rate as a function of the increased experience of the surgeon. They noted that recurrence of the disease was significantly associated with incomplete removal of the lesions, thereby suggesting persistence of the disease and highlighting the importance of the surgeon's experience in the treatment of this extremely challenging condition.

These studies stress the need for reflection on the part of the physician who wants to treat women with endometriosis. Much of what is currently defined as constituting a recurrence of endometriosis actually represents persistence of the disease, since different operations are performed in an attempt to remove all the ectopic lesions; however, for various reasons these foci remain untreated at their sites. The principal reason for lesions remaining untreated is inadequate presurgical evaluation, particularly as a consequence of not using specialized imaging methods to map the extent of the endometriotic lesions. If this critical step is not meticulously followed, the surgical team will be unprepared since, in certain cases, depending on the sites affected, the team should be multidisciplinary, particularly when the intestinal and urinary tracts are involved.

Therefore, when the option for treatment of endometriosis is surgical, the physician and his/her team should be trained to carry out complex procedures based on the information obtained from the specific imaging methods used for endometriosis that are available locally. In our own experience, we routinely use transvaginal ultrasonography with prior bowel preparation, which provides us with adequate mapping of the pelvis. Sometimes transvaginal ultrasonography is associated with ultrasonography of the urinary tracts and transabdominal pelvic ultrasonography to add further information on the urinary tracts, right colon and appendix. This operation should theoretically be the only one necessary, thereby avoiding repeat surgeries that generate vast technical difficulties, since manipulation, even by laparoscopy, may greatly increase the possibility of adherences. It is also important to remember that recurrent ovarian surgery may hamper the reproductive future of patients by reducing the number of follicles as a result of a thermal or even mechanical lesion.

Endometriosis in the pouch of Douglas affecting the rectum

Although a separate chapter deals specifically with bowel endometriosis, it is pertinent to include some considerations here on the specific situation in which the disease is present in the pouch of Douglas but is also infiltrating the rectum. Endometriosis of the bowel may be present in 3–37% of all cases of the disease [31] and the rectosigmoid is affected in 90% of these cases.

In such cases, we emphasize the importance of carrying out a careful, thorough preoperative critical analysis of the clinical data and all available imaging methods so as to avoid placing the surgical team in a situation that they are unable to resolve completely. The focus should be on the degree of complexity required to perform the ideal procedure for each situation. It is appropriate to include the participation of a multidisciplinary team composed of gynecologists, urologists and gastric surgeons, since only excision of all visible and palpable lesions of the disease will result in any real benefits to the patient.

Evaluating the symptoms of 70 patients with bowel endometriosis submitted to laparoscopic treatment, Abrão *et al* reported complaints of dysmenorrhea in all cases, and in 38.8% of patients the intensity of symptoms was sufficient to prevent them carrying out their routine activities [8]. Deep dyspareunia was present in 72.2% of cases, the probable cause of which was impact to the region affected by the lesion during coitus. Acyclic pelvic pain was present in 66.7% of patients. Cyclic bowel symptoms reported by 88.9% of patients represent significant clinical data and reflect a clear relationship with bowel endometriosis. In 50% of these patients (35 patients), this was their principal complaint, and included pelvic pain at evacuation and/or diarrhea during menstruation and, more characteristically, blood in the feces during menstrual periods. Physical examination was suggestive of deep endometriosis in 73.3% of evaluations. The value of the physical examination should not be underestimated, and this exam should be carried out methodically with this hypothesis in mind, since it may result in identification of areas of thickness and nodules in the anterior and posterior cul-de-sac and in the uterosacral ligaments, as well as in the rectovaginal septum.

For patients with severe pain, there is a certain consensus in the literature that treatment of endometriosis should be surgical whenever the patient has a complaint of pelvic pain. With respect to infertility, there are no randomized controlled studies or meta-analyses that support this conclusion. Access may be achieved by laparotomy or laparoscopy, depending on the surgeon's experience and the extent of the disease. However, in this institute we prefer laparoscopy, since this technique permits better visualization of the area affected by the disease and allows treatment to be sufficiently radical for each type of case.

As mentioned above, a preoperative analysis of the clinical and imaging data will define the indication for surgery and the procedure to be carried out. Imaging methods are able to provide information on the presence of deep retrocervical disease or endometriosis of the rectovaginal septum and whether or not the bowel is affected. In cases in which endometriosis has infiltrated the bowel wall and the deep submucous or mucous muscle layer has been affected, Abrão *et al* recommend resection of the affected segment [9]. On the other hand, when only the superficial or serous layer of the bowel wall is affected, these authors recommend resection only of the nodule without segmentary resection.

Since the disease being treated is benign and the principal concern is to extirpate all endometriotic lesions, bowel resection of varying proportions may be necessary.

Whenever deep endometriosis is clinically suspected, adequate presurgical bowel preparation is recommended. Usually we recommend preparation with an oral solution of polyethylene glycol (PEG) on the eve of surgery, associated with one or two rectal enemas or preparation with mannitol. Antibiotics should be given prophylactically during anesthesia induction, preferably using a second-generation cephalosporin at a dose of 2 g, administered intravenously.

Surgical tactics for managing the posterior cul-de-sac

Once the decision has been made to surgically treat the lesion on the posterior cul-de-sac, certain related factors should be taken into consideration. The patient should be aware of how the procedure will be performed and should be provided with information on issues ranging from presurgical preparation to the risk of complications. An informed consent form should be prepared containing all this information for the patient to read and sign, thus agreeing to and giving her consent for the surgery to take place.

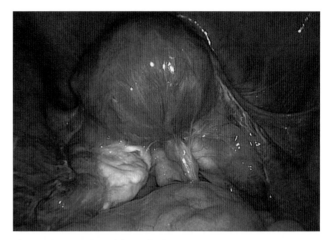

Figure 39.2 Complete cul-de-sac blockage.

Presurgical preparation includes clinical evaluation and laboratory and imaging exams in accordance with the individual requirement of each patient. The patient is generally admitted to hospital on the eve of surgery to undergo bowel cleansing with lactulose and enteroclysis. In the surgical theater, the patient is kept under general anesthesia, her arms extended alongside her body and her legs in comfortable stirrups, using elastic stockings to prevent thromboembolism, in a semi-gynecological position, with a long-term urinary catheter and uterine manipulator. This type of surgery is always performed by a team formed by the chief surgeon and two assistant surgeons, with particular importance being given to the assistant who manipulates the uterus, introduces a rectal probe when required and performs digital vaginal and rectal examination during surgery, which serves as a true guide to the location of the lesions in the pouch of Douglas and retrocervical lesions.

Pneumoperitoneum is achieved by introducing a Veress needle into the umbilical scar. The 11 mm trocar containing the 10 mm, 0° lens is introduced through an incision in the umbilical scar and the auxiliary tweezers are manipulated using 5 mm cannulae located in the right and left iliac fossa and right thigh. Initially, the overall appearance of the peritoneal cavity is evaluated, looking for signs of the presence of the endometriotic lesions suggested in the imaging exams, as well as any other lesions not previously identified, particularly any superficial lesions that may be present in the patient's pelvis.

The procedure of mapping the sites may also detect the presence of any adherences, which are common in advanced cases and in patients with a history of previous surgeries. The next step is to perform lysis of these adherences, which may involve loops of different bowel segments, the greater omentum and the internal genital organs. At this time, it is vital to identify and isolate the ureters. To do so, an incision is made to open the retroperitoneum and look for the point at which the ureter and the iliac artery cross, making it easier to follow the ureter along its trajectory up to the uterine artery, being careful in this dissection not to lose the internal vascularization of the ureters (Fig. 39.2).

Endometriosis is a disease that affects more than one site; however, this chapter deals specifically with lesions in the posterior cul-de-sac. As described above, these lesions may affect the retrocervical region, the posterior vaginal fornix and the rectovaginal septum. In these cases, in addition to dissecting the ureters, we must be absolutely sure about the location of the rectal wall, which may be adhered to the retrocervical region. This is achieved by making a lateral dissection in the rectal wall, taking advantage of the opening of the retroperitoneum to identify the ureters, and continuing close to the side of the rectal wall up to the anterior portion where it comes into contact with the retrocervical region. This dissection should only continue in the direction of the rectovaginal septum if the lesion has invaded deeply into the vaginal fornix or the rectovaginal septum itself. This procedure should be performed with extreme care in order to preserve the innervation described above and minimize the risk of complications. It should be emphasized once again that this step is facilitated by a conjunction of actions performed by the assistant surgeon, who manipulates the uterus forwards and the rectum backwards and carries out a digital vaginal examination to confirm the location of the lesion and of the normal tissue.

Once the rectum and the ureters have been isolated, the lesions should be completely excised. The retrocervical lesions that have not infiltrated into the vagina are removed without any need for local suturing; however, care must be taken not to go any deeper than necessary with the incision so as not to advance into the internal os of the cervix, keeping in mind that adenomyotic lesions may confuse a surgeon who is inexperienced in recognizing the characteristics of these tissues. Lesions of the vaginal fornix and rectovaginal septum are removed in a single block, together with part of the vaginal mucosa, since Matsuzaki *et al* analyzed the distance between the epithelium of the vaginal mucosa and the ectopic endometrial tissue and showed that in 98.4% of patients, this distance was less than 5 μm, thereby indicating that, in order to completely remove large rectovaginal nodules, the posterior vaginal fornix must be excised [32]. In this case, sutures are required to close the vagina. Separate sutures with 2–0 absorbable thread may be placed by laparoscopy or by the vaginal route, depending on the position of the opening and the ease with which the sutures can be made. If the option is made for laparoscopy, a gas-containing vaginal occlusion tampon must be introduced to maintain pneumoperitoneum and allow the needle holder to be manipulated.

Once the procedure is finalized, safety tests are performed on the rectum by introducing methylene blue and in general, drains are not retained. Antibiotic therapy is given prophylactically with second-generation cephalosporins and the urinary catheter is removed on the day after surgery, when the patient is also discharged from hospital if there are no complications.

Conclusion

Deep endometriosis is a common disease in which involvement of the pouch of Douglas demands specific attention. The specialist must pay particular attention to the patient's symptoms and perform a thorough gynecological examination to detect areas of pain and/or retrouterine nodules or even nodules of the rectovaginal septum. In our opinion, this information, in association with a good imaging exam, preferably transvaginal ultrasonography with prior bowel preparation, permits adequate presurgical identification of the foci of the disease and any bowel involvement. This information provides the physician with precise information, enabling him/her to decide whether surgery is indicated, which surgical procedure should be performed or, if the decision is for expectant management, how the patient should be followed up.

References

1. Chapron C, Chopin N, Borghese B et al. Deeply infiltrating endometriosis: pathogenetic implications of the anatomical distribution. Hum Reprod 2006;21(7):1839–1845.

2. Moore KL. Clinically Oriented Anatomy, 3rd edn. Philadelphia: Lippincott Williams and Wilkins, 1994.

3. Seracchioli R, Mabrouk M, Manuzzi L et al. Importance of retroperitoneal ureteric evaluation in cases of deep infiltrating endometriosis. J Minim Invasive Gynecol 2008;15(4):435–439.

4. Landi S, Ceccaroni M, Perutelli A et al. Laparoscopic nerve-sparing complete excision of deep endometriosis: is it feasible? Hum Reprod 2006;21(3):774–781.

5. Mauroy B, Demondion X, Bizet B, Claret A, Mestdagh P, Hurt C. The female inferior hypogastric (= pelvic) plexus: anatomical and radiological description of the plexus and its afferences – applications to pelvic surgery. Surg Radiol Anat 2007;29(1):55–66.

6. Mauroy B, Bizet B, Bonnal JL, Crombet T, Duburcq T, Hurt C. Systematization of the vesical and uterovaginal efferences of the female inferior hypogastric plexus (pelvic): applications to pelvic surgery on women patients. Surg Radiol Anat 2007;29(3):209–217.

7. Arruda MS, Petta CA, Abrao MS, Benetti-Pinto CL. Time elapsed from onset of symptoms to diagnosis of endometriosis in a cohort study of Brazilian women. Hum Reprod 2003;18(4):756–759.

8. Abrao MS, Neme RM, Averbach M. [Rectovaginal septum endometriosis: a disease with specific diagnosis and treatment]. Arq Gastroenterol 2003;40(3):192–197.

9. Abrao MS, Podgaec S, Dias JA Jr, Averbach M, Silva LF, Marino de Carvalho F. Endometriosis lesions that compromise the rectum deeper than the inner muscularis layer have more than 40% of the circumference of the rectum affected by the disease. J Minim Invasive Gynecol 2008;15(3):280–285.

10. Seracchioli R, Mabrouk M, Guerrini M et al. Dyschezia and posterior deep infiltrating endometriosis: analysis of 360 cases. J Minim Invasive Gynecol 2008;15(6):695–699.

11. Chapron C, Barakat H, Fritel X, Dubuisson JB, Breart G, Fauconnier A. Presurgical diagnosis of posterior deep infiltrating endometriosis based on a standardized questionnaire. Hum Reprod 2005;20(2):507–513.

12. Fauconnier A, Chapron C, Dubuisson JB, Vieira M, Dousset B, Breart G. Relation between pain symptoms and the anatomic location of deep infiltrating endometriosis. Fertil Steril 2002;78(4):719–726.

13. Abrao MS, Goncalves MO, Dias JA Jr, Podgaec S, Chamie LP, Blasbalg R. Comparison between clinical examination, transvaginal sonography and magnetic resonance imaging for the diagnosis of deep endometriosis. Hum Reprod 2007;22(12):3092–3097.

14. Bazot M, Lafont C, Rouzier R, Roseau G, Thomassin-Naggara I, Darai E. Diagnostic accuracy of physical examination, transvaginal sonography, rectal endoscopic sonography, and magnetic resonance imaging to diagnose deep infiltrating endometriosis. Fertil Steril 2009;92(6):1825–1833.

15. Goncalves MO, Dias JA Jr, Podgaec S, Averbach M, Abrao MS. Transvaginal ultrasound for diagnosis of deeply infiltrating endometriosis. Int J Gynaecol Obstet 2009;104(2):156–160.

16. Goncalves MO, Podgaec S, Dias JA Jr, Gonzalez M, Abrao MS. Transvaginal ultrasonography with bowel preparation is able to predict the number of lesions and rectosigmoid layers affected in cases of deep endometriosis, defining surgical strategy. Hum Reprod;25(3):665–671.

17. Hudelist G, Oberwinkler KH, Singer CF et al. Combination of transvaginal sonography and clinical examination for preoperative diagnosis of pelvic endometriosis. Hum Reprod 2009;24(5):1018–1024.

18. Hudelist G, Keckstein J. [The use of transvaginal sonography (TVS) for preoperative diagnosis of pelvic endometriosis]. Praxis (Bern 1994) 2009;98(11):603–607.

19. Donnez J, Nisolle M, Squifflet J. Ureteral endometriosis: a complication of rectovaginal endometriotic (adenomyotic) nodules. Fertil Steril 2002;77(1):32–37.

20. Abrao MS, Dias JA Jr, Bellelis P, Podgaec S, Bautzer CR, Gromatsky C. Endometriosis of the ureter and bladder are not associated diseases. Fertil Steril 2009;91(5):1662–1667.

21. Chamie LP, Blasbalg R, Goncalves MO, Carvalho FM, Abrao MS, de Oliveira IS. Accuracy of magnetic resonance imaging for diagnosis and preoperative assessment of deeply infiltrating endometriosis. Int J Gynaecol Obstet 2009;106(3):198–201.

22. Abrão MS, Neme RM, Averbach M, Petta CA, Aldrighi JM. Rectal endoscopic ultrasound with a radial probe in the assessment of rectovaginal endometriosis. J Am Assoc Gynecol Laparosc 2004;11(1):50–54.

23. Rosa e Silva AC, Rosa e Silva JC, Nogueira AA, Petta CA, Abrao MS, Ferriani RA. The levonorgestrel-releasing intrauterine device reduces CA-125 serum levels in patients with endometriosis. Fertil Steril 2006;86(3):742–744.

24. Petta CA, Ferriani RA, Abrao MS et al. Randomized clinical trial of a levonorgestrel-releasing intrauterine system and a depot GnRH analogue for the treatment of chronic pelvic pain in women with endometriosis. Hum Reprod 2005;20(7):1993–1998.

25. Petta CA, Ferriani RA, Abrao MS et al. A 3-year follow-up of women with endometriosis and pelvic pain users of the levonorgestrel-releasing intrauterine system. Eur J Obstet Gynecol Reprod Biol 2009;143(2):128–129.

26. Vercellini P, Crosignani PG, Somigliana E, Berlanda N, Barbara G, Fedele L. Medical treatment for rectovaginal endometriosis: what is the evidence? Hum Reprod 2009;24(10):2504–2514.

27. Tarjanne S, Sjoberg J, Heikinheimo O. Radical excision of rectovaginal endometriosis results in high rate of pain relief – results of a long-term follow-up study. Acta Obstet Gynecol Scand 2010;89(1):71–77.

28. Angioni S, Peiretti M, Zirone M et al. Laparoscopic excision of posterior vaginal fornix in the treatment of patients with deep endometriosis without rectum involvement: surgical treatment and long-term follow-up. Hum Reprod 2006;21(6):1629–1634.

29. Griffiths AN, Koutsouridou RN, Penketh RJ. Rectovaginal endometriosis – a frequently missed diagnosis. J Obstet Gynaecol. 2007;27(6):605–607.

30. Carmona F, Martinez-Zamora A, Gonzalez X, Gines A, Bunesch L, Balasch J. Does the learning curve of conservative laparoscopic surgery in women with rectovaginal endometriosis impair the recurrence rate? Fertil Steril 2009;92(3):868–875.

31. Jerby BL, Kessler H, Falcone T et al. Laparoscopic management of colorectal endometriosis. Surg Endosc 1999;13(11):1125–1128.

32. Matsuzaki S, Houlle C, Botchorishvili R, Pouly JL, Mage G, Canis M. Excision of the posterior vaginal fornix is necessary to ensure complete resection of rectovaginal endometriotic nodules of more than 2 cm in size. Fertil Steril 2009;91(4 Suppl):1314–1315.

40 Surgical Therapies: Randomized Controlled Trials in Endometriosis

Jason Abbott

Department of Obstetrics and Gynaecology, University of New South Wales, Sydney, Australia

Introduction

Given that the principal symptoms of endometriosis are infertility and pain [1], a significant number of surgical treatments are performed for one or both of these conditions. Laparoscopy is the gold standard in the diagnosis of endometriosis [2] and currently is the only way in which a histological diagnosis can be confirmed [3]. Women with endometriosis most commonly present with chronic pelvic pain, a symptom that accounts for 25% of all gynecological office visits [4]. Only one in four women will seek help for chronic pelvic pain [5] and of those, between 33% and 94% are diagnosed with endometriosis [4,6–9]. From a different perspective, 40% of women undergoing laparoscopy have at least one symptom of chronic pelvic pain [4].

Randomized controlled surgical trials

Unlike drug trials, which require a randomized clinical trial (RCT) before acceptance by regulating bodies such as the Food and Drug Administration (FDA) in the USA, surgery is not subject to such stringent regulation [10]. Surgical innovation is one of trial and error, and its use is at the discretion of the individual surgeon. If a surgical trial is performed, however, then it is viewed with more scrutiny than drug trials, owing to the ethical principal of non-maleficence, whereby the only expected benefit from "sham" surgery comes from the placebo effect, whilst the potential morbidity may be significantly greater than that arising from a sugar pill [11]. It is encouraging that there has been a marked increase in the number of randomized controlled trials in different areas of surgery in the last few years [12–16].

The success of surgery involves not just the surgical procedure but also a number of other factors including the patient's expectations and surroundings, the surgeon's personality, the anesthetic and the surgical incision [17]. Consequently, one of the reasons why surgery (new or existing) is not assessed by placebo-controlled trial is the difficulty in designing and conducting such studies where such factors can be taken into consideration [18]. Accordingly, many surgical trials do not control for either investigator bias or placebo effects. It is estimated that only 7% of surgeons use a randomized trial of any kind for assessing surgical techniques [19].

Randomized controlled studies examining surgery for endometriosis-related pain

There are three published randomized controlled studies of the effects of surgical treatment of endometriosis, comparing surgical treatment with expectant management by laparoscopy alone. Ethical limitations have been a factor in all three published studies, which possibly reflects the lack of equipoise in this condition, causing delays and restrictions that are not scientifically based. Additionally, the external validity of small RCTs with very strict entry criteria is generally low which may limit its applicability to a wider population.

Sutton's 1994 study examined the effect of laparoscopic laser surgery on endometriosis-related pain [20]. Table 40.1 summarizes the findings from this and the two subsequent studies. Prior medical or surgical treatments for this study are not stated, although women could not have received these for the 6 months prior to study inclusion. Women with stage IV disease were excluded, an ethics committee constraint. The primary outcome measure was overall pain improvement assessed by a visual analog scale (VAS). The study assessed dysmenorrhea, dyspareunia and pelvic pain individually, though these scores are not reported individually but rather as a median score from the combined VAS assessments.

The study duration was 6 months, with data collected blindly, patient group revealed and for women in the expectant surgery group, laser laparoscopy was offered as a treatment if pain symptoms persisted. Randomization appears adequate, and disease characteristics were similarly distributed across each of the arms of

Endometriosis: Science and Practice, First Edition. Edited by Linda C. Giudice, Johannes L.H. Evers and David L. Healy.
© 2012 Blackwell Publishing Ltd. Published 2012 by Blackwell Publishing Ltd.

Table 40.1 Methodological and outcome data from RCTs for excision of endometriosis and pain.

Author	(a) Recruited (b) Randomized (c) Lost to F/U	Power required (n)	rAFS distribution stage Treatment (n) Expectant (n)	Continued to 6 months n (%)	Pain reduction at study end	Possible pain reduction adjusting for loss to follow-up
Sutton 1994 [20]	(a) ?74 (b) 74 (c) *11 (15%)	Not stated	T: I 13; II 16; III 3; IV 0 E: I 16; II 12; III 3; IV 0	32 treatment 31 expectant	73% 20%	62–84% 17–23%
Abbott 2004 [23]	(a) 52 (b) 39 (c) *0 (0%)	40	T: I 0; II 8; III 2; IV 9 E: I 1; II 9; III 2; IV 8	20 treatment 19 expectant	80% 32%	80% 32%
Jarrell 2005 [24]	(a) 36 (b) 29 (c) **15 (52%)	84	T: I 3; II 10; III 0; IV 0 E: I 3; II 10; III 3; IV 0	7 treatment 9 expectant	45% 33%	22–68% 17–50%

* 6-month data; ** 12-month data; T, treatment group; E, expectant group; F/U, follow-up; rAFS, revised American Fertility Society.

the study. However, there were only six women who had stage III disease in the study sample (less than 10% of the entire sample).

At 3 months postoperatively, there was no statistically significant difference between the two groups with regard to pain. There was a statistically significant difference noted at 6 months with 62.5% of women reporting an improvement in pain symptoms in the surgery group compared to 22.6% in the placebo group ($P < 0.01$). The study reported an association between stage of disease and pain improvement, with the higher stages of disease accounting for a greater reduction in pain symptoms (of women with stage II or III disease at 6 months, 14/19 had pain relief with surgery compared to 3/20 who had placebo surgery). The very small numbers of women with moderate disease make this statement less robust.

Sixteen women in the expectant group had second surgery. Of these, 3/16 (19%) had progressed to a more advanced stage of disease, whilst none had spontaneously regressed. Five women who had laser laparoscopy and continued to have pain had a further laparoscopy. Three of these women had no visual endometriosis evident, and two had developed endometriosis in new sites, not previously treated.

The results at 1 year [21] indicate that there is good relief in those who respond initially, although recurrence of symptoms following surgical laser treatment was 44%. The longer term report [22] reiterates the recurrence of pain symptoms in 45%, and overall sustained improvement in symptoms is approximately one-third of the initial respondents, although recurrence of endometriosis is not always required for recurrence of pain symptoms.

In the second RCT from our own group, 52 women were recruited, with 39 having a histological diagnosis of endometriosis, since histological confirmation of disease was an inclusion criterion [23]. Randomization and blinding appear adequate and follow-up at 6 months with a cross-over design was a mandatory ethical requirement. Four different pain scores were assessed, and validated quality of life tools were analyzed for the two groups (see Table 40.1).

Thirteen women were excluded due to pregnancy (3), withdrawal prior to surgery (3) or no histological evidence of disease (7). Of those studied, 51% had previous medical treatment and

17% previous surgical treatment for endometriosis-related pain. A power calculation indicated that 40 women were required for a difference to be demonstrated and significantly more reported symptomatic improvement after excisional surgery compared with after placebo: 16/20 (80%) versus 6/19 (32%), $P = 0.002$. The addition of quality of life assessments to a VAS pain score indicated that there were also significant improvements in a number of areas for the excisional surgery group but not after expectant management.

At 6 months follow-up, 18/19 (94%) of the expectant group and 16/20 of the excisional group (80%) had a second surgery as per the protocol. Findings at cross-over surgery demonstrated that in the expectant management group, 8/18 (45%) had disease that was worse, six (33%) had disease that was unchanged, and four (22%) had disease that was improved from their original surgery. In the excisional group, 5/16 (31%) had no visual evidence of endometriosis, 4/16 (25%) had areas that were suspicious of disease but proved biopsy negative, and 7/16 (43%) had biopsy-proven disease. Overall, 14/16 (88%) had disease that was improved and one (6%) had worse disease than at her first surgery.

At follow-up 6 months from the second surgery (12 months from the original), 15/18 (83%) women in the expectant group reported pain improvement and 8/15 (53%) in the excisional surgical group reported further improvement in pain. The addition of a second surgical procedure to the first may give additional benefit, or alternatively, this may be placebo with an ongoing effect possible from the first surgical procedure.

The strengths of this study include histological confirmation of disease, the inclusion of all stages of disease (50% severe disease) and the inclusion of quality of life assessments rather than the single-dimension VAS pain score. The negatives of this study are its short follow-up time of 6 months, which is not reflective of the chronic nature of the disease, and power, which, although acceptable for primary difference, did not allow for differentiation of different pain parameters.

The most recent study by Jarrell reports on the longest blinded follow-up, with 29 patients having laparoscopy for severe pelvic pain asked to complete daily pain diaries monthly at baseline and then for three separate months during their 12-month follow-up period [24]. Randomization, concealment and blinding all appear adequate. Study entry included the assessment by a surgeon of possible safe excision of all disease. Of the 36 women recruited to the study, two had previous surgical treatments. Prior medical treatments are not stated. Seven women were excluded at surgery for diagnoses other than endometriosis.

Follow-up to 12 months was completed by eight women in the treatment group and seven in the expectant group, with nine (31%) completing all 4 months of pain diaries. No women with advanced disease were included in this study. All women who completed the study reported a significant reduction in pain scores from baseline ($P < 0.05$), with no differences between the groups, with pain reduction 45% in the treatment group and 33% in the expectant group.

One of the most unfortunate issues with this study was its premature closure due to external factors. This meant that less than one-third of the anticipated sample size were recruited and the 50% loss to follow-up of those recruited further decreases the generalizability of the study results.

The same authors reported a long-term follow-up of this cohort [25] indicating a repeat operation rate of 52% in the treatment group and 48% in the expectant group. The only factor that indicated likelihood of reoperation was preoperative pain experience.

A Cochrane review examining surgical treatment for endometriosis-associated pain concludes that laparoscopic surgical treatment is effective at reducing pain compared with diagnostic laparoscopy alone, but, not surprisingly, more research is required [26]. What we have to base this assessment on are data from 155 women recruited to published, randomized placebo-controlled studies, with 117 (75%) having follow-up data at 6–12 months following entry to their respective study in a blinded non-cross-over manner [23,24,27]. These numbers are small by any standards, yet the effort to produce these data is significant, with the paucity of such data in relation to the common performance of the procedure testimony to both the difficulties in performing such rigorous studies and the motivation of surgeons to act on the existing data for a treatment effect in their patient population without considering the need to seek additional information.

Several conclusions can be drawn from these studies. Surgical intervention in any form is likely to produce at least a 30% placebo response rate. This is not different from a placebo response rate in other surgical studies [20,28,30]. The placebo response reported in treatments for pain varies from 1% to 100% [31]. This wide range confirms the fact that pain is a subjective experience, reflecting interpretation by the individual and time, influenced by many factors. The authors of the three studies have tried to capture pain assessment using a VAS for total pain reduction, for individual pain parameters and as a comparison of improvement. The addition of quality of life assessment tools allows for comparative data with a non-disease-affected population and against other disease groups.

The additional response rate from the reported data above placebo is 12–48%. Extrapolated calculations give a possible range of 5–61% if the loss to follow-up is considered across all three studies. Given that the studies of Sutton and Abbott have good retention rates, these data would seem the most robust at this time, with additional responses of 40% and 48% respectively. Unfortunately, whilst the methodology of the study by Jarrell is likely to have been the best of the three RCTs, the loss to follow-up of 52% places the results in question and it has been estimated that a loss to follow-up of >30% renders results irrelevant to a wider population.

It is important to note that there were ethical constraints on all three studies. Sutton could not recruit patients with stage IV disease, Abbott had to have a cross-over design at 6 months and Jarrell's study had delays due to the "sham" surgical arm and was stopped prematurely when insurance reimbursement was obtained for the procedure. The best evidence indicated that the stage of disease is not relevant to the surgical response, and the only RCT to include stage IV disease (nearly 50% of the recruited population) supports this view [7,23,32–35].

From the perspective of recruitment and patient reaction to research, disclosure of the blinded, placebo nature of a surgical trial does not deter patients from enrolling in the study and does not eliminate the placebo effect [17]. The placebo response has been demonstrated in surgical trials, with some showing improvement in outcomes [13–15,23,27] whilst others have not [12,16,18,36]. From an ethical perspective, the use of a placebo in the clinical setting where patients are informed that this may be one of the therapeutic interventions does not include the same element of deception as when physicians in the truest sense of the word use a placebo, and the patient is not informed [37,38]. Therefore, patients who consent to participate in a randomized placebo-controlled trial are aware that they may not receive treatment, and accept this as a possibility. This is indeed good news for future placebo-controlled RCTs in this area and an increase in the evidence base would be most welcome.

Perhaps the other most significant factor arising from these studies is a non-response rate of at least 20% (but perhaps much higher). The studies of Jarrell and Sutton both had a majority of early-stage disease with a higher non-response rate, whilst the study of Abbott had the largest group of stage III/IV disease with the lowest non-response rate reported so far. Whilst it would be beneficial to determine which patients will or will not respond to surgical treatment, there is no evidence for predicting this outcome. Other non-randomized studies have determined that there is no link between stage of disease and likely response to surgical treatments.

In addition, there is no way of currently identifying in whom the disease will progress or present symptomatically [39]. There is evidence to suggest that the depth of penetration into the peritoneum may be responsible for some pain, due to mechanical compression of nociceptors and stretch placed on the peritoneal tissues [7,40], this perhaps being the basis for consideration of a greater response in the patient group with more advanced disease. However, for pain symptoms, the release of prostaglandin synthetase is not dependent on lesion size and may be higher in minimal or mild disease; therefore pain may be greater with this earlier disease, accounting for the discrepancy between size of lesion and perception of pain [41]. Similarly, there is no apparent correlation between the site of disease and the perception of pain [33,42].

Other data from non-randomized studies for surgical treatment of endometriosis

The lowest recurrence data for pain are reported by Redwine, who prospectively evaluated 359 women over a 10-year period [43]. These data from a single surgeon unit estimate the recurrence rate at 20% using life table analysis. There is no sensitivity analysis around patients lost to follow-up in this series. Outstanding surgical skill and technique could account for these impressive results and the skill of the surgeon is stated as a significant factor for the patient's outcome [44].

Our own group reported a prospective follow-up of 176 women with histologically confirmed endometriosis followed to 5 years post excisional surgery. Dysmenorrhea was reduced from VAS 9 to 3; non-menstrual pelvic pain 8 to 3; dyspareunia 7 to 0; and dyschezia 7 to 2. There were statistically significant improvements in the EuroQOL 5Dvas and 5Dindex scores and statistical improvement in pleasure and habit scores and reduction in pain assessed by a validated sexual activity questionnaire. The chance of requiring further surgical intervention was 36% at 5 years by Kaplan–Meier survival curve, with symptomatic recurrence being associated with biopsy-proven recurrent disease in 68% women [32,45]. This is equal to endometriosis being present in 22% of women with recurrent pain.

A large-scale prospective study by Vercellini *et al* reports on 425 women with first-line surgical outcomes following conservative laparoscopic surgery, with recurrence of dysmenorrhea at 3 years reported to be 24%, dyspareunia 15% and chronic pelvic pain 23% [46]. Stage of disease was not significantly associated with pain recurrence (33/117; 28% stage I versus 21/129; 16% stage IV). A multivariate regression analysis showed that only age was predictive of pain recurrence [46]. Pain recurrence was 12% at 3 years, with stage of disease again not associated with likelihood of recurrence.

Ferrero studied the quality of sex life in 170 women with endometriosis compared to a control group of 129 women [47]. Deep dyspareunia was more common in the endometriosis group (61% versus 35%; $P < 0.001$), and deep disease involving the uterosacrals was more likely to cause deep dyspareunia compared to endometriosis sufferers without uterosacral ligament involvement or controls [47].

Recent retrospective data reporting on 240 women indicate that the need for reoperation rate is estimated to be 56% at 7 years from conservative surgical treatment (120 women), compared with women who have hysterectomy at index surgery, with or without oophorectomy (120 women) where surgical reintervention was 23% [48].

Taken together, these data support the use of surgical treatment to improve endometriosis-related pain for the majority of women, although the need for reintervention in the longer term is high. Pain recurrence is not always associated with disease recurrence.

Mode of surgical treatment

Randomized studies

One study has compared excision and ablation in 24 women with minimal-to-mild disease (revised American Fertility Society (rAFS) score 1–2) [49]. Patients were assessed by questionnaire of symptoms at baseline and on physical signs, both of which were repeated at 6 months. A significant reduction in pain within the groups was found for symptoms but not signs and there was no difference in the outcomes between the groups. In this study, lack of power calculation, small sample size and no requirement for histological confirmation of endometriosis are negatives but it remains the only randomized study to examine the mode of surgery for pain relief in mild endometriosis. Another study has recently been published [74].

Non-randomized studies

Non-randomized studies of surgery by either laparoscopy or laparotomy have been reported to be effective for reducing pain associated with endometriosis [50–53]. These studies show no difference with regard to pain outcomes between the two surgical approaches, though costs and recovery time are shorter in the laparoscopy groups, even for women with advanced disease. Laparoscopic surgery seems to decrease the incidence of adhesion formation compared to laparotomy [54].

Ovarian endometriomas and pain

Randomized controlled studies

The first randomized trial in this area included 124 women with four different surgical techniques who had postoperative danazol and a repeat laparoscopy 8 weeks after treatment. The method of randomization was not adequate and follow-up time and symptom recurrence are not recorded [55]. The conclusions favor drainage of cysts, although these data have been superseded by more methodologically sound data.

The findings of two subsequent randomized trials are compared in Table 40.2 and include 164 patients, with treatments being cyst excision of drainage and coagulation [56,57]. From Beretta, excision compared with drainage and ablation of the cyst resulted in lower rates of dysmenorrhea (3/19; 15% versus 9/17; 53% $P < 0.05$); deep dyspareunia (3/15; 20% versus 9/12; 75% $P < 0.05$) and non-menstrual pelvic pain (2/20; 10% versus 9/17; 52% $P < 0.05$) respectively. From Alborzi, there were no differences in the excision compared to the drainage and ablation groups at 1 year, although by 2 years, recurrence of symptoms was greater (6/38; 15% versus 17/30; 56% $P < 0.001$) and reoperation rate lower (3/52; 6% versus 11/48; 23% $P < 0.003$) respectively. These studies favor surgical excision rather than drainage and coagulation to reduce pain symptoms and recurrence of endometrioma following treatment.

Table 40.2 Treatment of ovarian endometriomas and pain.

Author	(a) Recruited (b) Randomized (c) Lost to F/U	Power required (n)	Median time to follow-up	rAFS stage at time of surgery n (%)	Time to recurrence of moderate-to-severe pain (months)
Beretta 1998 [57]	(a) ?64 (b) 64 (c) ?0	Not stated	Ex: 20 months Dr: 20 months	Ex: III 25 (78%); IV 7 (22%) Dr: III 27 (85%); IV 5 (15%)	Ex: 19 months (range 13–24) Dr: 9 months (range 3–20) *P* < 0.05
Alborzi 2004 [56]	(a) ?100 (b) 100 (c) ?0	Not stated	24 months both groups	Ex: III 29 (56%); IV 23 (44%) Dr: III 33 (69%); IV 15 (31%) (no significant difference)	Not stated

Ex, excision group; Dr, drainage and ablation group; F/U, follow-up; rAFS, revised American Fertility Society.

Deeply invasive disease

Randomized studies

There are no randomized studies on the surgical treatment of deeply invasive endometriosis in the reduction of pain symptoms.

Non-randomized studies

There is one non-randomized, patient preference study examining laparotomy versus conservative treatment for severe, deeply invasive disease. In this study by Vercellini *et al* [58], 44/105 (42%) of women preferred surgery by laparotomy with excision of deep disease in all, anterior rectal resection in seven, ureteric resection of disease in six and partial urinary cystectomy in one for a full-thickness bladder nodule. Pain outcomes were in favor of the surgery group, with moderate-to-severe dysmenorrhea in 40% of the surgical group and 65% of the expectant group at 12 months and 61% and 75% at 24 months; dyspareunia in 14% and 43% at 12 months and 27% and 52% at 24 months; and dyschezia 14% and 35% at 12 months and 22% and 43% at 24 months in the surgical versus the conservative groups respectively.

Nerve ablation to treat endometriosis-related pain

Randomized trials

There are four RCTs for laparoscopic uterosacral nerve ablation (LUNA) with a combined total of 444 patients comparing this treatment with excision of endometriosis to surgical treatment without LUNA [59–62]. The outcomes for these studies are summarized in Table 40.3 and their results indicate that there is no advantage to this treatment in conjunction with surgical treatment of endometriosis compared with surgical treatment alone. The conclusion that can be made based on this good evidence is that this surgical therapy is not helpful for additional pain relief in women with endometriosis.

Three studies have compared excision of endometriosis with excision plus presacral neurectomy for endometriosis associated pain [63–65]. Two of these studies (total patients studied 227) show a decrease in pain for patients with central dysmenorrhea. Dyspareunia and non-menstrual pelvic pain are not improved. There was no relationship between pain reduction and the stage of endometriosis. Complications including intraoperative blood loss, constipation and bladder dysfunction can be problematic. These data suggest that presacral neurectomy should only be performed in selected cases with mainly central dysmenorrhea.

Hysterectomy to treat endometriosis-related pain

Randomized controlled studies

There are no RCTs on hysterectomy to reduce pain for women with endometriosis.

Non-randomized data

It has been suggested that hysterectomy is curative for women with endometriosis, with textbooks from more than a decade ago supporting this view [66,67] and recent reviews also stating this as fact [44]. What is apparent is that hysterectomy is not a definitive treatment, and that symptoms and disease may persist or recur. The term "definitive" should not be used when evidence indicates that even with this treatment, surgical intervention is likely in 8–23% of patients at 7 years following initial treatment [48]. Its judicious use for a woman who has completed her family may be of benefit for pain reduction. If hysterectomy is to be performed then it is important to remove all evidence of endometriosis, either by laparoscopy or laparotomy, with no difference between these modes [68].

Combined medical and surgical treatment

Randomized controlled trials

There are five RCTs that have evaluated the use of medical therapy after surgery for endometriosis [69–73]. In the first of these, 60 women were treated with either danazol or progesterone after surgery and their pain scores were significantly better than

Table 40.3 Randomized controlled studies examining surgical nerve ablation for endometriosis-associated pain.

Author	(a) Recruited (b) Randomized (c) Lost to F/U	Power required (n)	Endometriosis (nerve ablation/control)	Primary outcomes
Laparoscopic uterine nerve ablation (LUNA)				
Sutton 2001 [61]	(a) ?51 (b) 51 (c) 5	44	LUNA: I 12, II 12, III 3, IV 0 Con: I 12, II 12, III 3, IV 0 (control = excision endometriosis only)	Dysmenorrhea better in non-LUNA group at 3, 6 months ($P < 0.022$), no difference in non-menstrual pelvic pain
Vercellini 2003 [62]	(a) 273 (b) 180 (c) 24 (12 mths)	142	LUNA: I 35, II 20, III 18, IV 17 Con: I 29, II 17, III 23, IV 21 (control = excision endometriosis only)	23/78 (29%) recurrence dysmenorrhea 12 m 21/78 (27%) recurrence dysmenorrhea 12 m 36% versus 32% recurrence at 3 years (NS)
Johnson 2004 [60]	(a) 200 (b) 67* (c) 11	76	LUNA: I 10, II 13, III 6, IV 3 Con: I 12, II 13, III 5, IV 3 (control = treatment endometriosis only)	7/23 (33%) >50% reduction dysmenorrhea 12 m 11/24 (46%) >50% reduction dysmenorrhea 12 m (NS) NS for dyspareunia, dyschesia, non-menstrual pain
Daniels 2009 [59]	(a) 592 (b) 146* (c) ?	350	LUNA: I-II 41 not treated, 25 treated Cont: I-II 52 not treated, 28 treated	No difference in worst pain level, dysmenorrheal, non-cyclic pain or dyspareunia. No difference between the endometriosis groups treated or untreated.
Presacral neurectomy				
Tjaden 1990 [64]	(a) 26 (b) 8 (c) 0	Not stated	Eight women with stage III–IV disease randomized, all others chose group following early cessation by ethics committee	2/17 (randomized and self-chosen) had recurrent midline pain at 42 months follow-up 9/9 in the excision without PSN group had recurrence of pain Back and lateral pain and dyspareunia variable
Candiani 1992 [63]	(a)?78 (b) 78 (c) 7	80	T + PSN: III 23, IV 12 T only: III 26, IV 12	No statistical difference in recurrent moderate-to-severe dysmenorrhea survival curve between the two treatments. Pelvic pain absent in 86% versus 91% at 12 months
Zullo 2003 [65]	(a) 162 (b)141 (c) 15	116	T + PSN: I 16, II 22, III 17, IV 8 T only: I 18, II 21, III 17, IV 7	Cure rates at 12 months: stage I 61% versus 88%; II 57% versus 86%; III 58% versus 88%; IV 42% versus 75%. T versus T + PSN respectively ($P < 0.05$ for all stages, NS between stages)

* Only women in the endometriosis group are included in these data.
LUNA, laparoscopic uterosacral nerve ablation; NS, no significant difference; T, treatment by surgical resection; T + PSN, treatment + presacral neurectomy.

placebo [69]. In this study, pain scores had returned to preoperative levels 12 months after debulking of stage I–IV disease. In the second study, 109 women were given gonadotropin releasing hormone agonist (GnRHa) or placebo following surgery. The number of women requiring further treatment within 2 years was lower in the GnRHa group (31% versus 57%), but there was no difference in pain scores between these two groups [72]. In the third study, 75 women were given GnRHa or placebo following surgery and there was no difference in the pain scores at 1-year follow-up [70]. In the fourth study, 269 women having conservative surgery were randomized to receive GnRHa or expectant management for 6 months [71]. Women were followed up for 2 years after their surgery. There was no difference in pain relief following either of these treatments, though the study concluded that there was a significantly greater time to onset of symptoms in the group randomized to GnRHa following surgery. In the fifth study, 77 women were randomized to either danazol 600 mg per day for 3 months or expectant management following surgery for endometriosis.

There was no difference with regard to pain or fertility status in either group [73].

Overall, evidence suggest that postoperative medical treatment of any kind may delay the onset of recurrent symptoms, but there is no true realized pain reduction with time.

Conclusion

With currently available evidence, surgical treatment for endometriosis is successful for reducing pain compared with diagnostic surgical therapy in the short term. The duration of pain reduction is unknown and variable, with patient and physician factors likely to be involved. Recurrent pain symptoms seem at best 35% but up to 60% within 10 years of initial surgery. Pain recurrence is not always associated with disease recurrence.

The method of surgical treatment by ablation or excision is unlikely to be a significant factor, as long as all lesions are removed.

Laparoscopy offers no advantage over laparotomy with regard to pain reduction when all disease is removed, but the recovery time, cost and patient satisfaction are in favor of laparoscopy and this should be the preferred mode of treatment when the surgeon is sufficiently skilled.

When ovarian endometriomas are present, these should be treated by surgical excision rather than drainage and ablation. Uterosacral nerve ablation offers no improvement in addition to treatment of disease. Presacral neurectomy offers minimal benefit, with treatment of central dysmenorrhea being a possible indication for recurrent pain symptoms. The risk/benefit ratio must be considered with the patient.

Hysterectomy should not be considered the definitive treatment, since pain recurrence is reported. There may be pain reduction with hysterectomy, although its timing is clearly dependent on individual patient circumstances. There is no evidence that postoperative medical treatment confers any long-term advantage to surgery alone at this time.

There are no comparative trials of surgery versus medical treatments currently, although evidence in other chapters of this text indicates that simple, inexpensive medical treatments such as the oral contraceptive pill and progestins do offer symptomatic treatment with a reasonable side-effect profile. Because of the invasive nature of surgical treatments and until such studies become available, it would seem prudent to offer surgery for endometriosis-related pain only to those women in whom medical treatments were not effective or caused intolerable side-effects or who desire fertility where hormonal treatments are contraindicated.

It is apparent that surgery is not a panacea for endometriosis-related pain, but it is part of the approach to patient care. This complex and ever changing condition requires more study for the solution to become clear. I conclude with a quote from Proust, who sums up the issues that we face, not just as endometriosis surgeons but as the carers of women who suffer with this most frustrating of diseases.

> For, medicine being a compendium of the successive and contradictory mistakes of medical practitioners, when we summon the wisest of them to our aid the chances are that we may be relying on a scientific truth the error of which will be recognised in a few years' time. So that to believe in medicine would be the height of folly, if not to believe in it were not a greater folly still, for from this mass of errors a few truths have in the long run emerged. (Proust: *A La Recherche du Temps Perdu*, volume 3, The Guermantes Way)

References

1. Burns W, Schenken R. Pathophysiology of endometriosis-associated infertility. Clin Obstet Gynecol 1999;42(3):586–610.

2. Kennedy S, Gazvani M. The investigation and management of endometriosis. London: Royal College of Obstetricians and Gynaecologists, 2000.

3. Muse K. Clinical manifestations and classification of endometriosis. Clin Obstet Gynecol 1988;31:813–822.

4. Howard F. The role of laparoscopy in the evaluation of chronic pelvic pain: pitfalls with a negative laparoscopy. J Am Assoc Gynecol Laparosc 1996;4:85–94.

5. Winkel C. A cost-effective approach to the management of endometriosis. Curr Opin Obstet Gynecol 2000;12:317–320.

6. Carter J. Combined hysteroscopic and laparoscopic findings in patients with chronic pelvic pain. J Am Assoc Gynecol Laparosc 1994;2:43–47.

7. Koninckx P, Meuleman C, Demeyere S, Lesaffre E, Cornillie F. Suggestive evidence that pelvic endometriosis is a progessive disease, whereas deeply infiltrating endometriosis is associated with pelvic pain. Fertil Steril 1991;55(4):759–765.

8. Kresch A, Seifer D, Sachs L, Barrese I. Laparoscopy in 100 women with chronic pelvic pain. Obstet Gynecol 1984;64:672–674.

9. National Center for Health Statistics. National health interview series (CD-ROM), series 10 number 5. Maryland: Public Health Service, 1993.

10. Spodick D. Numerators without denominators: there is no FDA for the surgeon. JAMA 1975;232:35–36.

11. Macklin R. The ethical problems with sham surgery in clinical research. N Engl J Med 1999;341(13):992–996.

12. Moseley J, O'Malley K, Petersen N et al. A controlled trial of arthroscopic surgery for osteoarthritis of the knee. N Engl J Med 2002;347(2):81–88.

13. Guyuron B, Reed D, Kreigler J, Davis J, Pashmini N, Amini S. A placebo controlled surgical trial of the treatment of migraine headaches. Plast Reconstr Surg 2009;124(2):461–468.

14. Rodriguez L, Reyes E, Fagalde P et al. Pilot clinical study of an endoscopic removable duodenal-jejunal bypass liner for the treatment of type 2 diabetes. Diabetes Technol Therapeut 2009;11(11):725–732.

15. Shaheen N, Sharma P, Overholt B et al. Radiofrequency ablation in Barrett's esophagus with dysplasia. N Engl J Med 2009;360(22):2277–2288.

16. Burchbinder R, Osborne R, Ebeling P et al. A randomized trial of vertebroplasty for painful osteoporotic vertebral fractures. N Engl J Med 2009;361(6):557–568.

17. Johnson A. Surgery as a placebo. Lancet 1994;344(8930):1140–1142.

18. Freeman T, Vawter D, Leaverton P et al. Use of placebo surgery in controlled trials of a cellular-based therapy for Parkinson's disease. N Engl J Med 1999;341(13):988–992.

19. Reeves B. Health-technology assessment in surgery. Lancet 1999;353(Suppl 1):S13–S15.

20. Sutton C, Ewen S, Whitelaw N, Haines P. Prospective, randomized, double-blind trial of laser laparoscopy in the treatment of pelvic pain associated with minimal, mild and moderate endometriosis. Fertil Steril 1994;62(4):696–700.

21. Sutton C, Pooley A, Ewen S, Haines P. Follow-up report on a randomized controlled trial of laser laparoscopy in the treatment of pelvic pain ssociated with minimal to moderate endometriosis. Fertil Steril 1997;68(6):1070–1074.

22. Jones K, Haines P, Sutton C. Long-term follow-up of a controlled trial of laser laparoscopy for pelvic pain. J Soc Laparoendosc Surg 2001;5:111–115.

23. Abbott J, Hawe J, Hunter D, Holmes M, Finn P, Garry R. Laparoscopic excision of endometriosis: a randomized, placebo-controlled trial. Fertil Steril 2004;82(4):878–884.

24. Jarrell J, Mohindra R, Ross S, Taenzer P, Brant R. Laparoscopy and reported pain among patients with endometriosis. J Obstet Gynaecol Can 2005;27(5):477–485.

25. Jarrell J, Brant R, Leung W, Taenzer P. Women's pain experience predicts future surgery for pain associated with endometriosis. J Obstet Gynaecol Can 2007;29:988–991.

26. Jacobson T, Duffy J, Barlow D, Koninckx P, Garry R. Laparoscopic surgery for pelvic pain associated with endometriosis. Cochrane Database Syst Rev 2009;4:CD001300.

27. Sutton C, Ewen S, Whitelaw N. Prospective, randomized, double-blind, controlled trial of laser laparoscopy in the treatment of pelvic pain associated with minimal, mild, and moderate endometriosis. Fertil Steril 1994;62(4)):696–700.

28. Spiller R. Problems and challenges in the design of irritable bowel syndrome clinical trials: Experience from published trials. Am J Med 1999;107(5A):91S–97S.

29. Diener H-C, Dowson A, Ferrari M, Nappi G, Tfelt-Hansen P. Unbalanced randomization influences the placebo response: scientific versus ethical issues around the use of placebo in migraine trials. Cephalagia 1999;19:699–700.

30. Freeman E, Rickels K. Characteristics of placebo responses in medical treatment of premenstrual syndrome. Am J Psychiatry 1999;156(9):1403–1408.

31. Wall P. The placebo effect: an unpopular topic. Pain 1992;51:1–3.

32. Garry R, Clayton R, Hawe J. The effect of endometriosis and its radical laparoscopic excision on quality of life indicators. Br J Obstet Gynaecol 2000;107(1):44–54.

33. Fedele L, Parazzini F, Bianchi S. Stage and localization of pelvic endometriosis and pain. Fertil Steril 1990;53:155–158.

34. Muzii L, Murana R, Pedulla S, Catalano G, Mancuso S. Correlation between endometriosis associated dysmenorrhea and the presence of typical or atypical lesions. Fertil Steril 1997;68:19–22.

35. Nezhat C, Seidman D, Nezhat F, Nezhat C. Long-term outcome of laparoscopic presacral neurectomy for the treatment of central pelvic pain attributed to endometriosis. Obstet Gynecol 1998;91(5):701–704.

36. Cobb L, Thomas G, Dillard D, Merendino K, Bruce R. An evaluation of internal mammary artery ligation by a double-blind technic. N Engl J Med 1959;260(22):1115–1118.

37. Levine J. Ethics, Regulation Of Clinical Trials, 2nd edn. New Haven: Yale University Press, 1986.

38. Horng S, Miller F. Is placebo surgery unethical? N Engl J Med 2002;347(2):137–139.

39. Martin D. Letter to the editor. Fertil Steril 1991;56:792.

40. Cornillie F, Oosterlynck D, Lauweryns J, Koninckx P. Deeply infiltrating pelvic endometriosis: histology and clinical significance. Fertil Steril 1990;53(6):978–983.

41. Vernon M, Beard J, Graves K. Classification of endometriotic implants by morphologic appearance and capacity to synthesize prostaglandin. Fertil Steril 1985;46:801–806.

42. Ripp B, Martin D. Focal pelvic tenderness, pelvic pain and dysmenorrhea in endometriosis. J Reprod Med 1991;36:470–472.

43. Redwine D. Conservative laparoscopic excision of endometriosis by sharp dissection: life table analysis of reoperation and persistent or recurrent disease. Fertil Steril 1991;56(4):628–634.

44. Vercellini P, Crosignani P, Abbiati A, Somigliana E, Vigano P, Fedele L. The effect of surgery for symptomatic endometriosis: the other side of the story. Hum Reprod Update 2009;15(2):177–188.

45. Abbott J, Hawe J, Clayton R, Garry R. The effects and effectivness of laparoscopic excision of endometriosis: a prospective study with 2–5 years follow-up. Hum Reprod 2003;18(9):1922–1927.

46. Vercellini P, Fedele L, Aimi G, de Giorgi O, Consonni D, Crosignani P. Reproductive performance, pain recurrence and disease relapse after conservative surgical treatment for endometriosis: the predictive value of the current classification system. Hum Reprod 2006;21:2679–2685.

47. Ferrero S, Esposito F, Abbamonte LH, Anserini P, Remorgida V, Ragni N. Quality of sex life in women with endometriosis and deep dyspareunia. Fertil Steril 2005;83(3):573–579.

48. Shakiba K, Bena J, McGill K, Minger J, Falcone T. Surgical treatment of endometriosis: a 7 year follow-up on the requirement for further surgery. Obstet Gynecol 2008;111(6):1285–1292.

49. Wright J, Lotfallah H, Jones K, Lovell D. A randomized trial of excision versus ablation for mild endometriosis. Fertil Steril 2005;83(6):1830–1836.

50. Bateman B, Kolp L, Mills S. Endosopic versus laparotomy management of endometriomas. Fertil Steril 1994;62:690–695.

51. Catalano G, Marana R, Caruana P, Muzii, L, Mancuso S. Laparoscopy versus microsurgery by laparotomy for excision of ovarian cysts in patients with moderate or severe endometriosis. J Am Assoc Gynecol Laparosc 1996;3:267–270.

52. Crosignani P, Vercellini P, Biffignandi F, Constantini W, Cortesi I, Imparato E. Laparoscopy versus laparoscopy in conservative surgical treatment for severe endometriosis. Fertil Steril 1996;66(5):706–711.

53. Busacca M, Fedele L, Bianchi S et al. Surgical treatment of recurrent endometriosis: laparotomy versus laparoscopy. Hum Reprod 1998;13(8):2271–2274.

54. Diamond M. Post-operative adhesion development after operative laparoscopy: evaluation at early second look procedures. Fertil Steril 1991;55:700–704.

55. Fayez J, Vogel M. Comparison of different treatment methods of endometriomas by laparoscopy. Obstet Gynecol 1991;78:660–665.

56. Alborzi S, Momtahan M, Parsanezhad M, Dehbashi S, Zolchadri J, Alborzi S. A prospective randomized study comparing ovarian cystectomy versus fenestration and coagulation in patients with endometriomas. Fertil Steril 2004;82:1633–1637.

57. Beretta P, Franchi M, Ghezzi F. Randomised clinical trial of two laparoscopic treatments of endometriomas: cystectomy versus drainage and coagulation. Fertil Steril 1998;70:1176–1180.

58. Vercellini P, Fedele L, Aimi G et al. Reproductive performance in infertile women with rectovaginal endometriosis: is surgery worthwhile? Am J Obstet Gynecol 2006;195:1303–1310.

59. Daniels, Gray R, Hills R et al. Laparoscopic uterosacral nerve ablation for alleviating chronic pelvic pain. JAMA 2009;302(9):955–961.

60. Johnson N, Farquar C, Crossley S et al. A double-blind randomised controlled trial of laparoscopic uterosacral nerve ablatio for women with chronic pelvic pain. Br J Obstet Gynaecol 2004;111(9):950–959.

61. Sutton C, Pooley A, Jones K, Dover R, Haines P. A prospective, randomized, double-blind controlled trial of laparoscopic uterine nerve

ablation in the treatment of pelvic pain associated with endometriosis. Gynaecol Endosc 2001;10(4):217–222.

62. Vercellini P, Aimi G, Busacca M, Apolone G, Uglietti A, Crosignani P. Laparocopic uterosacral ligament resection for dysmenorrhea associated with endometriosis: results of a randomised controlled trial. Fertil Steril 2003;80(2):310–319.

63. Candiani G, Fedele L, Vercellini P, Bianchi S, di Nola G. Presacral neurectomy for the treatment of pelvic pain associated with endometriosis: a controlled study. Am J Obstet Gynecol 1992;167:100–103.

64. Tjaden B, Schlaff W, Kimball A. The efficacy of presacral neurectomy for the relief of midline dysmenorrhea. Obstet Gynecol 1990;76:89–91.

65. Zullo F, Palomba F, Zupi E et al. Effectiveness of presacral neurectomy in women with sever dysmenorrhea caused by endometriosis who were treated with laparoscopic conservative surgery: a 1-year prospective randomized double-blind controlled trial. Am J Obstet Gynecol 2003;189(1):5–10.

66. Reddy S, Rock J. Treatment of endometriosis. Clin Obstet Gynecol 1998;41(2):387–392.

67. Metzger D. Treating endometriosis pain: a multidisciplinary approach. Semin Reprod Endocrinol 1997;15(3):245–250.

68. Soysal M, Soysal S, Vicdan K. Laparoscopically assisted definative treatment of severe endometriosis. Int J Obste Gynecol 2001; 72:191–192.

69. Telimaa S, Ronnberg L, Kauppila A. A placebo-controlled comparison of danazol and high dose medroxyprogesterone acetate in the treatment of endometriosis after conservative surgery. Gynecol Endocrinol 1987;1:363–371.

70. Parazzini F, Fedele L, Bussaca M et al. Postsurgical medical treatment of advanced endometriosis: results of a randomized clinical trial. Am J Obstet Gynecol 1994;171(5):1205–1207.

71. Vercellini P, Crosignani P, Fadini R, Radici E, Belloni C, Sismondi P. A gonadotropin-releasing hormone agonist compared with expectant management after conservative surgery for symptomatic endometriosis. Br J Obstet Gynaecol 1999;106:672–677.

72. Hornstein M, Hemmings R, Yuzpe A, Heinrichs W. Use of nafarelin versus placebo after reductive laparoscopic surgery for endometriosis. Fertil Steril 1997;68:860–864.

73. Bianchi S, Busacca M, Agnoli B, Candiani M, Calia C, Vignali M. Effects of three month therapy with danazol after laparoscopic surgery for stage III/IV endometriosis: a randomised study. Hum Reprod 1999;15(5):1335–1337.

74. Healey M, Ang WC, Cheng C. Surgical treatment of endometriosis: a prospective randomized double-blinded trial comparing excision and ablation. Fertil Steril 2010;94(7):2536–2540.

41 Surgical Therapies: Rectal/Bowel Endometriosis

Jim Tsaltas

Gynaecological Endoscopy, Monash Medical Centre and Southern Health Care Network; Department of Obstetrics and Gynaecology, Monash University, Melbourne, Australia

Introduction

Endometriosis is one of the most significant benign gynecological disorders. It is a chronic disease found most commonly in women of reproductive age. It has a suspected prevalence of 8–15% [1]. This chapter will outline surgical therapies in the management of rectal and bowel endometriosis, symptoms relating to this disease, techniques for the diagnosis of the disease, surgical techniques, indications for surgery and, importantly, preoperative consent. The chapter focuses on endometriosis of the rectum/bowel, its impact and the relevant surgical therapies.

Symptoms of rectal/bowel endometriosis

Symptoms of endometriosis include dysmenorrhea, ovulation pain, chronic pelvic pain, infertility and deep dyspareunia. Endometriosis of the bowel is estimated to affect 5.3–12% of all women affected by endometriosis [2–4]. The most common sites of bowel endometriosis are the rectum, the rectosigmoid junction and the sigmoid. These areas alone account for 70–93% of all bowel lesions [2,5]. The appendix, cecum and distal ileum may also be affected, with incidences of 3–18%, 2–3% and 2–16% reported respectively when the bowel is involved [6,7]. It is very rare to have histologically proven bowel endometriosis without any other site of endometriosis in the pelvis [8]. Bowel disease is multifocal and lesions are seen in more than one intestinal area. This is observed in 15–35% of cases [9,10].

The symptoms of rectal endometriosis can be very severe. In some cases the symptoms can be debilitating, particularly in the days leading up to and during menstruation. One of the most significant symptoms correlating with the extent of disease by rectal wall invasion is rectal pain on defecation (dyschezia) [11]. The classic symptoms of rectal/sigmoid endometriosis (which make up the majority of all intestinal endometriosis) are:

- rectal bleeding during menstruation, which is not a very common presenting symptom. It is, however, the one symptom that is often quoted in textbooks. Even in patients who have infiltrative disease right through from the serosa to the mucosa, the chance of rectal bleeding at the time of menses is actually very small [11]. This has certainly been the author's experience
- deep rectal pain during the time of menstruation
- dyschezia, which is severe rectal pain during defecation at the time of menstruation. This symptom is the one that should alert all gynecologists to the potential of a patient having infiltrating rectal/sigmoid endometriosis.

As well as painful defecation, some patients describe difficulty in passing stools, describing their bowels as feeling "blocked." Some women may describe the rectal pain as extremely sharp and knife-like. These symptoms should suggest to the gynecologist that the patient may have severe rectovaginal endometriosis. These symptoms are in the author's view the most significant indicators of and most definitive of infiltrative disease [12,13]. It is important to note that some patients have infiltrative disease but remain asymptomatic. There will also be many patients whose primary symptom will be infertility alone.

Definition of bowel endometriosis

The term "bowel endometriosis" should be used when endometrial-like glands and stroma infiltrate the bowel wall, reaching at least the subserous fat tissues or adjacent to the neurovascular branches (subserous plexus) [13,14]. It has been suggested that endometriosis foci located on the bowel serosa should be considered as peritoneal endometriosis and not bowel endometriosis. Peritoneal endometriosis should not be considered as deep

Endometriosis: Science and Practice, First Edition. Edited by Linda C. Giudice, Johannes L.H. Evers and David L. Healy.
© 2012 Blackwell Publishing Ltd. Published 2012 by Blackwell Publishing Ltd.

infiltrative endometriosis (DIE). (Serosal superficial lesions can often be easily excised without impact on the outer longitudinal fibers of the bowel wall. If during surgery these fibers are compromised then simple interrupted sutures using 2.0 Vicryl will deal with this issue.)

Investigations

The starting point in the investigation of bowel endometriosis is the taking of a thorough history. The symptoms should be recorded and then a thorough examination undertaken, including an abdominal examination At this point, masses may be felt which could be a sign of large endometriomas. A speculum examination should follow wherein the examiner should look for infiltrative nodules of endometriosis in the posterior fornix. Finally a bimanual examination should then be performed. The palpation of a nodule in the pouch of Douglas should alert the gynecologist to potential infiltrative bowel disease [15]. The patient may have tenderness but no lesions palpable in the posterior fornix.

Once an examination has been performed, the next step should be transvaginal ultrasound. This is often the easiest and most readily available imaging modality in gynecology. There are other modalities that can be employed if bowel disease is suspected, including magnetic resonance imaging (MRI) and transrectal ultrasound [16,17]. In Australia, MRI is not funded for the assessment of gynecological disorders. Transrectal ultrasound is not readily available to gynecologists, outside specialized colorectal practices. These modalities will be covered in Chapter 29. Colonoscopy does not have a place in the diagnosis of sigmoid and rectal endometriosis. It is of little assistance in the diagnosis of bowel endometriosis because lesions are typically submucosal and usually are not visible during examination [18,19]. If a lesion is seen through the bowel mucosa and a colonoscopy is performed, then biopsy may be positive. Colonoscopy does, however, have a role in excluding other pathology, particularly if the patient has bowel symptoms such as change in bowel habit and bleeding that is not cyclical [19].

Sometimes the diagnosis of infiltrative bowel disease is difficult. Often patients have lesions in multiple pelvic locations and it is not easy to locate the precise source of the patient's complaint. However, in the event of a clear-cut diagnosis or where the gynecologist suspects DIE in the bowel, preoperative assessment is important. A diagnosis in the preoperative work-up gives the opportunity to plan surgical strategy.

If bowel disease is suspected the author's practice now includes a transvaginal ultrasound with preoperative bowel preparation. This is a mild bowel preparation involving Dulcolax SP (fluid solution) 10 drops the night before or Dulcolax one tablet of 5 mg. A Fleet enema is used 1 h before the scan. This technique has been well described in the published literature [15,20,21] and is helpful in predicting the extent of bowel involvement and planning surgical management of these patients [22]. Transvaginal ultrasound also allows identification of other pelvic pathology relevant to these patients of reproductive age. Ultrasound can image the uterus and diagnose any anomalies including fibroids, adenomyosis and polyps. Significant hydrosalpinges may also be seen. Ultrasound can detect endometriomas which can be a significant marker of progressive and severe DIE [23,24].

Although imaging techniques are helpful in the diagnosis of bowel endometriosis, they are not widely available widespread. Diagnostic laparoscopy is still one of the most common methods used to diagnose infiltrative bowel endometriosis [19]. Obviously patients who have symptoms of DIE of the bowel should have imaging to try and delineate the position, size and extent of the lesion. Unfortunately, advanced imaging will not be available for all patients, depending on local expertise and access to imaging centers and in particular the expertise of the person performing and interpreting the imaging modality used. Such experts will most likely be attached to a center of excellence with expertise in dealing with advanced DIE of the bowel.

For many patients laparoscopy will still be a first-line investigation. As part of this investigation standard transvaginal ultrasound can precede the laparoscopy and focus on the pathology of the uterus and ovaries. An indication for diagnostic laparoscopy may also be infertility, and DIE of the bowel may be diagnosed incidentally at this time.

Laparoscopy

Often a laparoscopy is performed to investigate symptoms of both pain and infertility. This may be the first time a significant bowel lesion is diagnosed. At the time of this initial laparoscopy, it is important to document the extent of the disease, the degree of anatomical distortion and the presence of DIE lesions in the pelvis. In nearly all cases patients will not have been counseled or prepared for advanced endometriosis surgery. Often the diagnostic laparoscopy will have been performed by a general gynecologist. The severity of the disease is unexpected by both the patient and the gynecologist. Certainly, it is possible to deal with pelvic side wall and adnexal disease at this time. This will depend on the laparoscopic surgical skills of the operating gynecologist. The deep infiltrative disease in the pouch of Douglas should be left to a multidisciplinary team [19].

At this early stage it is important to stop, bring the patient back into the practice and discuss the findings in detail, the implications of the findings and further management, be it medical, *in vitro* fertilization (IVF) or surgical. This will depend on the reasons for the patient's presentation and her symptoms. When advanced surgery is appropriate, patients should be referred to an appropriate center of excellence with a multidisciplinary team equipped to deal with the problem [19,25,26].

Indications for bowel surgery

The most common indication for fertility-sparing bowel surgery is debilitating chronic pain affecting the patient's quality of life [5,19,27–29]. These patients are suffering and they want and need help with their pain. This will often be the most common indication for surgery. It is now well documented that bowel resection for DIE will significantly improve the quality of life of these patients [27,28,30]. The symptoms of potential infiltrative bowel disease were mentioned above.

There are some patients who complain of almost complete obstruction of the colon from the disease. This is rare but has been reported [13]. There are also patients who have mild symptoms or who are relatively asymptomatic and are not trying to conceive. These patients can be offered expected management with careful observation. Monitoring for these patients could be a yearly speculum examination, vaginal examination and ultrasound. Patients who may fall into this category are those women who at routine gynecological review are found to have a rectovaginal nodule; they may have a "blue" nodule seen infiltrating through the posterior fornix or a nodule felt at digital examination [13,31]. The exact number of patients with severe disease which is asymptomatic is unknown.

Infertility and bowel endometriosis

Another group who will require surgery are those patients who present with infertility and infertile patients with endometriosis who are already undergoing IVF. Patients in this group who have been diagnosed with severe infiltrative endometriosis will need advice on the management of their problem. In the infertile couple (not already on IVF), the overall clinical picture of the couple should be considered. Endometriosis and its impact on infertility and IVF will be addressed in Chapters 44–47. This chapter addresses the impact of bowel endometriosis and its implications for infertility from a surgeon's perspective. There is constant debate about surgery versus IVF in this patient group but the following discussion is confined to infertile patients with severe bowel disease.

In couples with infertility and severe bowel endometriosis, the overall infertility picture of the couple should be considered and not just the endometriosis. In the circumstance of severe male-factor infertility then IVF should be considered as first-line treatment. Where there is no male factor then the age of the female partner will act as a guide for treatment. In this scenario, the gynaecologist should be able to formulate a reproductive prognosis which should estimate the expected benefit (if any) of intervention over the spontaneous probability of conception. This is particularly important with radical fertility-sparing bowel surgery. This surgery may be challenging and the risks of intraoperative and postoperative morbidity are not negligible. A publication by Vercellini *et al* provides an excellent guide to the parameters of the prognosis [32].

It is reasonable that if the female partner is under 35 then surgery can be offered as first-line therapy. The aim of surgery is to normalize the anatomy and improve the chance of spontaneous pregnancy [33–36]. Following surgery, a very strict time line needs to be implemented that the couple can follow. If no pregnancy has occurred after 6 months then IVF should be offered. Obviously at this point, it is the couple's choice whether they would like to proceed with advanced reproductive technologies. They should, however, be given the choice. There will be patients under the age of 35 who do not want to have

surgery because of the risks of major endometriosis bowel surgery [13,19,37]. These patients will elect to either continue to try for spontaneous conception or move on to IVF.

Patients over 35 may consider IVF as first-line treatment prior to surgery. This is certainly now more feasible given the improved success rates of IVF that have been seen over the past decade. Factors that will influence the decision will be length of infertility, the degree of associated pain and the perception of the patient about her chances of conceiving on IVF and the potential risk/benefit of the surgery. Other factors that will influence this decision include the degree of pain and the presence and size of associated endometriomas [38], the age of the patient, the extent of disease and previous failed IVF attempts [39]. As mentioned earlier, an improved IVF success rate will have an influence on this decision [39]. The patient's concerns about surgical complications or the extent of the surgery required will be another key factor in the decision-making process.

The availability of an appropriate multidisciplinary team will also influence the decision for surgical intervention. Waiting times for surgery can be up to 6 months, during which IVF is a feasible alternative. Many couples will opt for this, hoping to conceive prior to scheduled surgery. Surgery is, however, planned in case patients have not conceived in this period. Patients undergoing IVF in this time will have had potentially 3–5 embryos transferred. It is vital that patients are not subjected to multiple unsuccessful cycles of IVF without the issue of endometriosis being reassessed. In such patients, strong consideration should be given to surgical excision of the endometriosis. A recent publication has indeed tried to address this issue. In the study from Bianchi *et al*, extensive laparoscopic treatment of DIE significantly improved IVF pregnancy rates of women with infertility associated with this DIE [40]. Surgery in this situation not only seems to improve IVF pregnancy rates but will normalize anatomy, and spontaneous pregnancy rates will also improve.

Preoperative surgical consent

Patient understanding and consent prior to this surgery are of paramount importance. Most patients are young women of reproductive age who are undergoing major surgery to improve their quality of life and/or their fertility. They need to understand the potential complications of the surgery. The most common and significant complications from this surgery are as follows.

Conversion to laparotomy
It is arguable whether conversion to laparotomy is a complication of laparoscopic bowel surgery. In some cases it is a prudent necessity performed at the time of the surgery [4]. Conversion rates vary from 0% to 13% [19].

Urinary tract infection and urinary retention
Urinary retention due to autonomic nerve damage is not a common problem following this surgery. Transient neurogenic

bladder effects can occur, presenting as urinary retention or dysuria [25,30,31,41]. Urinary tract infection will occur but is not a difficult problem to treat.

Stoma and rectovaginal fistula

These two complications are of most concern to patients and are discussed at greatest length. A stoma may be required electively or as a result of a postoperative leak. The requirement for an elective stoma because of an ultra-low anastomosis is not common. In our series, there was one elective stoma in 177 cases followed [36]. The stoma rates following anastomotic leaks vary from 0% to 10% [5,19,42–44]. This can be devastating to a patient and as such they need to understand that this is a risk of this surgery. The incidence of rectovaginal fistula is low and appears to be more common when the vagina is also opened [19]. The incidence varies from 0.3% to 2% [30]. It will usually present 5–10 days postoperatively.

Alteration of bowel habit

Alteration in bowel function is common after bowel surgery. Patients can have urgency, diarrhea and constipation, which may last for 6–12 months following the surgery. Rectal stenosis after anastomosis is not common, affecting only 1% of patients [19,45].

General laparoscopic risks

The general risks of laparoscopy, such as vascular injury, entry complications and gas embolism, also need to be clearly outlined.

General surgical complications

Rare complications such as blood transfusion, pelvic hematoma, pelvic infection, postoperative chest infection, venous thrombosis and pulmonary embolus should be outlined to patients. These complications fortunately are very rare; an incidence of less than 1% has been reported [19,36,45].

Surgical procedure

Preparation

For this type of surgery it is imperative that a multidisciplinary approach is adhered to. Once an assessment has been made of the potential extent of the disease then a surgical date is planned. In our unit, the gynecologist and the colorectal surgeon perform the surgery together. For this procedure, we put aside a whole operating list which is usually 4.5 h.

Preoperatively, the patient is seen by both the gynecologist and the colorectal surgeon. Assessment by both surgeons ensures the patient has full and informed consent for whatever is necessary to completely excise the deep pelvic endometriosis at operation. Patients are aware that the extent of rectal surgery may range from shave excision of the exterior rectal wall to a segmental excision of the rectum and rarely a diverting stoma. In this type of operation, there are three categories of surgery that need to be considered.

- Shave (dissection of the endometriosis off the rectal wall)
- Full-thickness excision of the anterior rectal wall (usually with a transanal stapler)
- Segmental resection of the bowel

Preoperatively all patients will have bowel preparation with PicoPrep (sodium picosulfate oral powder, Pharmatel Fresenius Kabi, Australia).

At the time of surgery patients are given a general anesthetic and intubated. They are then placed in a low dorso/lithotomy position. An indwelling catheter is inserted into the bladder.

Insufflation

A Veress needle is inserted into the umbilicus or at Palmer's point. Once it is established that the Veress needle is in the intra-abdominal cavity, insufflation pressure is increased to 25 mmHg for entry. This is then followed by a visual entry using the Visiport™ plus RPF 5–12 mm single-use optical trochar with fixation (Covidien). If Palmer's point is used due to potential lower abdominal adhesions then a 5 mm trocar is inserted at this point; we use a 5 mm Endopath® xcel™ (Ethicon Endo-Surgery). Three lower 5 mm ports are then inserted: one suprapubically and two lateral to the inferior epigastric arteries.

Instruments that will potentially be used

- 5 mm tooth laparoscopic graspers × 2
- 5 mm bowel grasper – ATRAC Direct Drive® reusable grasper 5 mm × 32 cm (Applied Medical USA)
- One other 5 mm non-tooth reusable grasper
- Preferred scissors are the 5 mm Endo mini shears™ (Covidien)
- Suction irrigation system
- Bipolar forceps
- Rectal and vaginal probes

Basic technique

The abdomen and pelvis are carefully inspected. The extent of the endometriotic lesions is defined. The cecum, appendix and small bowel are inspected, looking for other sites of possible bowel endometriosis. Once the extent of the endometriosis is determined, the surgery commences.

A critical component of the surgery is normalization of the anatomy. Obviously, the principles of traction and countertraction should be employed to facilitate surgical dissection. The ATRAC is an excellent bowel grasper allowing safe steady traction on the bowel. Endometriomas which are found should be dealt with first to allow visualization of the pouch of Douglas, particularly if they are extremely large. As part of this procedure, the ovary/ovaries will be mobilized. As part of the mobilization, the ureters and their course will need to be identified. Once the endometriomas have been removed by stripping and dissection of the ovary wall, it is our practice to suture the ovary closed. There is some evidence that this reduces postoperative adhesions around the ovary [46]. One of the concerns when a large endometrioma has been dealt with and there is significant side wall dissection is that the ovary can be embedded/buried in a pelvic side wall or peritoneum, making any future procedures difficult. The ovary/ies are closed with 4.0 Prolene. In the past, many laparoscopists would have left the ovary unsutured, knowing that it would heal well after cystectomy. It will certainly heal well but evidence shows that suturing may reduce adhesions. Suturing is a vital part of advanced laparoscopic surgical skills. It is important to encourage gynecologists and trainees in advanced endoscopic surgery to suture as often as they can. This will allow them to suture quickly and efficiently in all endoscopic procedures.

Endometriomas

Often the indication for endometriosis surgery may simply be the presence of a large unilateral endometrioma or bilateral endometriomas. Once the endometrioma/s have been dealt with surgically, the infiltrating lesion of the rectum/sigmoid can be discovered. As this may be the first time that the bowel lesion has been recognized, it is our current practice to deal with the endometriomas, suture the ovaries closed, identify the lesion and then *stop*. The reason for this is to allow time to discuss with the patient the implications of bowel surgery and obtain formal consent before proceeding with bowel surgery with the multidisciplinary team. Bowel surgery in the uninformed and unprepared patient is totally inappropriate. It is also preferable to try and dissect the ureters and the rectovaginal septum only once, at the time of the definitive surgery [19].

An integral part of the surgery is normalization of the anatomy, adhesiolysis and ureteric dissection. It is paramount that the ureters are well clear of the dissection margin to allow complete excision. Also if the ureters are safely dissected free then if there is any bleeding from the pelvic side and the pouch of Douglas, this prior identification of the ureter will allow safe and efficient control of any bleeding vessels.

In bowel disease the rectum/sigmoid will often be densely adherent to the vagina, cervix or uterine body. The planes need to be identified. The rectum is mobilized from the back of the vagina/cervix/uterine body and the aim is to identify the rectovaginal septum. To facilitate dissection of the rectum from the vagina/cervix, a rectal probe and a vaginal probe are used. Our preferred method is to completely separate the rectum from the vagina and identify the rectovaginal septum and then mobilize the rectum to below the level of the lesion. Once the extent of the rectal lesion is identified then, depending on this lesion, the rectal lesion can be shaved, removed with an anterior disk excision or a formal bowel segmental resection is performed. In principle, a rectal nodule greater than 2 cm in size or occupying more than one-third of the rectal circumference is not suitable for anterior wall disk excision.

Once a decision has been made for segmental dissection of the rectum, the sigmoid is mobilized on the left-hand side to the level of the descending colon. This is to increase the length of mobile sigmoid for the anastomosis. As mentioned earlier, the rectum is dissected below the level of the disease. The pararectal spaces are opened and this facilitates further rectal mobilization. To allow better mobilization of the bowel, the inferior mesenteric artery is electrocoagulated using bipolar or sealed using the Ligasure™ laparoscopic instrument (Covidien). Once the mesenteric artery is divided, the posterior rectum/sigmoid is mobilized from the presacral space. The mesorectum is cleaned from the rectal tube and then the rectum is stapled below the lesion. The Covidien Endo GIA™ universal stapler is used to staple and divide the rectum. The staple reload used is the Endo GIA™ Universal Roticulator™ 60 3.5 single-use loading unit (Covidien). The rectal mobilization is an integral part of the procedure, as is the pelvic side wall dissection. Prior to the rectum being stapled below the level of the lesion, all other visible pelvic endometriosis needs to be excised.

The next component of the procedure is to staple and divide the rectum. Once the rectum has been transected, the proximal bowel is then exteriorized by extending the suprapubic incision. Usually 2.5–3 cm in total length is adequate. To widen the entire incision at this point, an Alexis drape is used to expand the incision without increasing its cut length (Alexis® Wound Retractor 5–9 cm, medium, Applied Medical, USA). Once the wound is prepared, the proximal bowel is then exteriorized. A decision is then made as to the length of bowel to be resected. The bowel is then cut proximal to the lesion. The head of the rectal circular stapler is then inserted and placed in the lumen of the bowel and a purse-string suture is placed to close the bowel lumen around the stapler head in a watertight fashion. The suture used is 0 Prolene. The circular stapler is a DST™ Series EEA™ either 28 or 31 mm in diameter.

The bowel with the head of the stapler attached is then placed back into the abdomen. The suprapubic incision is then occluded to allow reinsufflation. The Alexis drape then simply needs to be rotated and twisted and this then occludes the lumen of the drape and establishes the pneumoperitoneum, allowing continuation with further surgery. In the past we would close the suprapubic incision but we have found it more efficient to close the incision at the end when all the port sites are being closed.

Once the pneumoperitoneum is established, a rectal stapler is passed transanally and the spike pushed through the rectal stump. It is important to make sure the rectum is aligned correctly at this stage. Once the spike is through, the head of the stapler is engaged over the spike. The two ends of the rectal stapler are brought together, tightened and the circular rectal stapler is then fired. The stapler is removed transanally and the two donuts of tissue within the cutting blade are inspected for complete circular cutting. It is important that there is complete resection of all endometriosis before the rectal excision is performed. It is inappropriate to use a rectal probe once the stapling has occurred so as not to traumatize the staple line.

Once the resection is complete, the integrity of the rectum/sigmoid is checked with the insufflation of per rectum betadine under pressure transanally. Any areas of leakage (which are very rare) are reinforced by intracorporeal laparoscopic suture using 2/0 Vicryl.

The last component of the procedure is a final inspection phase. The pelvis is inspected, irrigated and checked for completeness of hemostasis. A drain tube is placed in the pelvis under suction. The ports are then removed and skin incisions sutured. The suprapubic port is closed. As part of the closure of the suprapubic incision, the sheath and peritoneum are also sutured. The skin is closed with 3/0 Prolene.

It is rare that a defunctioning colostomy/ileostomy will be required. This would be considered in an ultra-low anastomosis, repeat rectal resection, incomplete donuts and/or a betadine leak. The decision is up to the surgical team on the day of the surgery. The patient should have been informed about the potential for this.

Non-segmental bowel surgery

When a lesion does not require a segmental resection then it is either shaved off the rectum or stapled transrectally. These techniques will be briefly described below.

Transrectal stapling of an endometriotic lesion

Transanal removal of a rectal endometriotic lesion using the circular stapler is used if the lesion is infiltrating the bowel wall, it is small enough (less than 2 cm) and occupying less than a third of the anterior circumference of the rectum. Again, the decision is made once all the pelvic endometriosis is removed as well as the bulk of the endometriosis being shaved off the rectum.

Once the decision is made, a 2/0 Vicryl suture is placed into the lesion. The ends are left long, to allow manipulation of the lesion by being able to simply pull on the ends of the suture. This allows correct alignment of the lesion into the rectal stapler which is most valuable if the lesion is slightly off center. Also, it allows the surgeons to push the rectal lesion into the head of the transanal stapler. The circular stapler is then placed transanally. In this situation the head of the stapler has remained attached to the circular stapler. The stapler is opened enough to allow the anterior wall to be put into the head of the stapler. The handle of the stapler is pushed down so that the head of the stapler is anteverted which reduces the risk of capturing some of the posterior rectal mucosa when the stapler is closed and fired (maintaining the anteverted position of the stapler). The stapler is then opened. The head of the stapler tilts 45° and allows easy removal. It is then removed and again it is important to ensure that only a portion of the anterior wall of the stapler has been removed without capturing any of the posterior wall. The rectal wall integrity is then checked with PR betadine.

Rectal shaving

Once the lesion is isolated, it may be that shaving is all that is required. This can be achieved with scissors and diathermy for any bleeding points. The lesion is cut away from the rectum. If there is any breach of the outer longitudinal fibers of the rectal wall, it should be sutured with interrupted 2/0 Vicryl sutures.

Conclusion

Severe infiltrative bowel endometriosis must be managed by an appropriate multidisciplinary team. It is a complex problem requiring careful assessment of the patient, her symptoms and future fertility being paramount considerations. Prior to surgery, a full explanation of the surgical procedure recommended and all potential complications should be discussed with the patient. Infiltrative endometriosis bowel disease causes a significant reduction in women's quality of life and fertility. Diagnostic and surgical advances with appropriate management on a case-by-case basis will ensure effective medical and social rewards.

Acknowledgments

I would like to acknowledge the contribution of Mr Rod Woods, colorectal surgeon, who kindly reviewed this manuscript prior to submission.

References

1. Eskenazis B, Warner MC. Epidemiology of endometriosis. Obstet Gynecol Clin North Am 1997;24:235–258.
2. Thomassin I, Bazot M, Detcher R et al. Symptoms before and after surgical removal of colorectal endometriosis that are assessed by magnetic resonance imaging and rectal endoscopic sonography. Am J Obstet Gynecol 2004;190:1264–1271.
3. Darai E, Marpeau O, Thomassin I et al. Fertility after laparoscopic colorectal resection for endometriosis: preliminary results. Fertil Steril 2005;84:945–950.
4. Darai E, Ackerman G, Bazot M et al. Laparoscopic segmental colorectal resection for endometriosis: limits and complications. Surg Endosc 2007;21:1572–1577.
5. Dubernaud G, Pikethy M, Rouzier R et al. Quality of life after laparoscopic colorectal resection for endometriosis. Hum Reprod 2006;21:1243–1247.
6. Campagnacci R, Perretta S, Guerriers M et al. Laparoscopic colorectal resection for endometriosis. Surg Endosc 2005;19:662–664.
7. Bailey H, Ott M, Hartendorp P. Aggressive surgical management for advanced colorectal endometriosis. Dis Colon Rectum 1994;10: 182–189.
8. Redwine DB. Intestinal endometriosis. In: Redwine DB (ed) Surgical Management of Endometriosis. London: Taylor and Francis, 2004, pp.157–173.
9. Redwine DB. Ovarian endometriosis: a marker for more extensive pelvic and intestinal disease. Fertil Steril 1999;72:310–315.
10. Keckstein J, Wiesinger H. The laparoscopic treatment of intestinal endometriosis. In: Sutton C, Jones K, Adamson GD (eds) Modern Management of Endometriosis. London: Taylor and Francis, 2005.
11. Jaron AK, Solomon MJ, Young J et al. Laparoscopic management of rectal endometriosis. Dis Colon Rectum 2005;49:169–174.
12. Seracchioli R, Mabrouk M, Guerrini M et al. Dyschezia and posterior deep infiltrating endometriosis: analysis of 300 cases. J Minim Invasive Gynecol 2008;16:695–699.
13. Remorgida V, Ferreno S, Fulcheri E et al. Bowel endometriosis: presentation, diagnosis and treatment. Obst Gynecol Surv 2007;7:461–470.
14. Chapron C, Fauconnier A, Viera M et al. Anatomical distribution of deeply infiltrating endometriosis: surgical implications and proposition for a classification. Hum Reprod 2003;18:157–161.

15. Hudelist G, Oberwinkler KH, Singer CF et al. Combinations of transvaginal sonography and clinical examination for preoperative diagnosis of pelvic endometriosis. Hum Reprod 2009;5:1018–1024.

16. Dumontier I, Roseau G, Vincent B et al. Comparison of endoscopic ultrasound and magnetic resonance imaging in pelvic endometriosis. Gastroenterol Clin Biol 2000;24:1197–1204.

17. Kinkel K, Chapron C, Balleyguier C et al. Magnetic resonance imaging characteristics of deep endometriosis. Hum Reprod 1999;14:1080–1086.

18. Redwine DB, Sharpe DR. Laparoscopic surgery for intestinal and urinary endometriosis. Baillière's Clin Obst Gynaecol 1995;9:775–794.

19. Brouwer R, Woods RJ. Rectal endometriosis: results of radical excision and review of published work. Aust NZ J Surg 2007;77:562–571.

20. Goncalves MO, Dias JA, Podgaec S et al. Transvaginal ultrasound for diagnosis of deeply infiltrating endometriosis. Int J Gynaecol Obstet 2009;2:156–160.

21. Pereira RM, Zanatha A, de Mello Bianchi PH et al. Transvaginal ultrasound after bowel preparation to assist surgical planning for bowel endometriosis resection. Int J Gynaecol Obstet 2009;2:161.

22. Abrao MS, Podgaec S, Dias JA et al. Endometriosis lesions that compromise the rectum deeper than the inner muscular layer have more than 40% of the circumference of the rectum affected by the disease. J Minim Invasive Gynecol 2007;3:280–285.

23. Chapron C, Pietri-Vialle C, Borghese B et al. Associated ovarian endometriosis is a marker for greater severity of deeply infiltrating endometriosis. Fertil Steril 2009;2:453–457.

24. Banerjee SK, Ballard KD, Wright JK. Endometriosis as a marker of disease severity. J Minim Invasive Gynecol 2008;5:536–540.

25. Slack A, Child T, Lindsey I et al. Urological and colorectal complications following surgery for rectovaginal endometriosis. Br J Obstet Gynaecol 2007;114:1278–1282.

26. Darai E, Bazet M, Rouzier R et al. Outcome of laparoscopic colorectal resection for endometriosis. Curr Opin Obstet Gynecol 2007;4:308–313.

27. Abbott JA, Haive J, Clayton RO et al. The effects and effectiveness of laparoscopic excision of endometriosis: a prospective study with 2–5 year follow up. Hum Reprod 2003;18:1922–1927.

28. Lyons SD, Chew SS, Chorenor AJ et al. Clinical and quality-of-life outcomes after fertility-sparing laparoscopic surgery with bowel resection for severe endometriosis. J Minim Invasive Gynecol 2006;13:436–441.

29. Wills HJ, Reid GD, Cooper MJ et al. Fertility and pain outcomes following laparoscopic segmental bowel resection for colorectal endometriosis: a review. Aust NZ J Obstet Gynaecol 2008;48:292–295.

30. Darai E, Thomassin I, Barranger E et al. Feasibility and clinical outcome of laparoscopic colorectal resection for endometriosis. Am J Obstet Gynecol 2005;192:394–400.

31. Fedele L, Bianchi S, Zancanto G et al. Is rectovaginal endometriosis a progressive disease? Am J Obstet Gynecol 2004;191:1539–1542.

32. Vercellini P, Pietropaolo G, de Giorgi O et al. Reproductive performance in infertile women with rectovaginal endometriosis: is surgery worthwhile? Am J Obstet Gynecol 2005;195:1303–1310.

33. Adamson GD, Pasta DJ. Surgical treatment of endometriosis-associated infertility: meta-analysis compared with survival analysis. Am J Obstet Gynecol 1994;171:1488–1504.

34. Adamson GD, Hurd SJ, Pasta DJ et al. Laparoscopic endometriosis treatment: is it better? Fentil Steril 1993;59:35–44.

35. Maroux S, Maheux R, Berube S. Laparoscopic surgery in infertile women with minimal or mild endometriosis. N Engl J Med 1997;337:217–222.

36. Wills HJ, Reid GD, Cooper MJ et al. Bowel resection for severe endometriosis. An Australian series of 177 cases. Aust NZ J Obstet Gynaecol 2009;49:415–418.

37. Donnes J, Squifflet J. Laparoscopic excision of deep endometriosis. Obstet Gynecol Clin North Am 2004;31:567–580.

38. Kennedy S, Bergquist A, Chapron C et al. ESHRE guidelines for the diagnosis and treatment of endometriosis. Hum Reprod 2005;20:2698–2704.

39. Littman ED, Giudice LC, Berker B et al. Role of laparoscopic treatment of endometriosis in patients with failed in vitro fertilization cycles. Fertil Steril 2005;84:1574–1578.

40. Bianchi PH, Pereira RM, Zanatha A et al. Extensive excision of deep infiltrative endometriosis before in vitro fertilization significantly improves pregnancy rates. J Minim Invasive Gynecol 2009;16:174–180.

41. Fedele L, Bianchi S, Zancanato G et al. Long-term follow up after conservative surgery for rectovaginal endometriosis. Am J Obstet Gynecol 2004;190:1020–1024.

42. Campagnacci R, Perretta S, Guernier M et al. Laparoscopic colorectal resection for endometriosis. Surg Endosc 2005;19:662–664.

43. Duepree H, Senagore A, Delaney C et al. Laparoscopic resection of deep pelvic endometriosis with rectosigmoid involvement. J Am Coll Surg 2002;195:754–758.

44. Fleisch M, Xafis D, DeBruyne F et al. Radical resection of invasive endometriosis with bowel and bladder involvement – long term results. Eur J Obstet Reprod Biol 2005;123:224–229.

45. Seracchioli R, Poggioli G, Pierangel F et al. Surgical outcome and longterm follow up after laparoscopic rectosigmoid resection in women with deep infiltrating endometriosis. Br J Obstet Gynaecol 2007;114:889–895.

46. Pellicano M, Bromante S, Guida M et al. Ovarian endometrioma: postoperative adhesions following bipolar coagulation and suture. Fertil Steril 2008;89:796–799.

42 Surgical Therapies: Ureteric Dissection and Urological Endometriosis

Anna Rosamilia[1] and Caroline Dowling[2]
[1]Department of Obstetrics and Gynaecology and
[2]Department of Surgery, Monash University, Melbourne, Australia

Incidence

Involvement of the urinary tract by endometriosis is rare; 1–2% of cases of endometriosis will include the bladder, kidney, ureter or urethra [1]. In the majority, the bladder is involved, and this accounts for 85% of urological endometriosis. The kidney is involved in 4% of cases, though this is often a pathological finding after removal and not one that is readily recognized at surgery or on preoperative imaging. The urethra is involved in 2% of cases [1,2].

As with other presentations of the condition, urological endometriosis affects women most commonly in the 25–40-year-old age group. When it presents in the postmenopausal age group, there is often a history of estrogen replacement or obesity accounting for high serum levels of estrogen [1].

Ureteric endometriosis only accounts for 0.1–0.4% of all cases. The management is complex and so cases of ureteric endometriosis seem over-represented in the literature surrounding the management of urological disease [3]. The majority of ureteric endometriosis involves the lower third of the ureter and there is a propensity for left-sided disease.

Left-sided involvement is reported in 41% by Weingertner [4] but larger series show less bias to the left side with more equal rates; left 38/80 and right 34/80 [5]. Left-to-right asymmetry provides support for the theory of retrograde menstruation and implantation of endometrial cells as the basis of the genesis of endometriotic deposits. Nezhat et al [6] have also observed that where ureteric involvement occurred, it did so most frequently at or below the level of the uterosacral ligaments, suggesting retrograde flow and implantation.

Bilateral ureteric involvement occurs with varying frequency, though with lower numbers in the larger series by Camanni (10%) [5] and Ghezzi (12%) [7].

Ureteric and bladder involvement with endometriosis, as would be expected, is associated with a more advanced stage of endometriosis. Of 80 patients with ureteric disease, 70% had stage III or IV disease according to the revised American Fertility Society (rAFS) classification [5]. Nearly all patients with ureteric endometrosis will subsequently be found to have extraurinary pelvic endometriosis. Ureteric disease is more likely to be associated with multifocal disease in the pelvis and in sites other than the bladder [8]; in particular, there is an association between retrocervical lesions and ureteric disease.

Pathogenesis

Urological endometriosis, whether involving bladder or ureter, can be considered pathologically to exist as an intrinsic or extrinsic disease entity. Extrinsic vesical lesions involve the serosal or peritoneal surface. Intrinsic vesical disease involves the detrusor muscle. Some series do not include cases with only the peritoneal serosal surface involved in vesical disease, because this has few complications compared with the intrinsic detrusor disease [9] and is more likely to be asymptomatic.

Intrinsic bladder lesions are more likely to have resulted from iatrogenic implantation and as many as 50% will have a history of pelvic surgery when sought [10,11]. There is an association between bladder endometriosis and cystitis cystica, a benign inflammatory condition of the bladder caused by hyperplasia in the submucosa in response to inflammatory disorder resulting from chronic irritation. Intrinsic disease is also more likely to be symptomatic. Intrinsic vesical involvement occurs only in 12% of cases of vesical disease overall [12].

Ureteric disease has been suggested to be a complication of severe ovarian endometriosis [13,14]. It is also highly correlated with uterosacral ligament involvement, with 65% in one series [7] and up to 100% found by other authors [15]. As with bladder involvement, ureteric endometriosis can be considered histologically to be

Endometriosis: Science and Practice, First Edition. Edited by Linda C. Giudice, Johannes L.H. Evers and David L. Healy.
© 2012 Blackwell Publishing Ltd. Published 2012 by Blackwell Publishing Ltd.

extrinsic or intrinsic. Extrinsic endometriosis of the ureter is four times more common than intrinsic disease [16]. Intrinsic endometriosis is that which involves the muscular layer or muscularis mucosae of the ureter. Extrinsic endometriosis involves only the adventitia or periureteral tissues. Intrinsic endometriosis is more commonly associated with ureteric stenosis and hydronephrosis.

Whether or not bladder and ureteric endometriosis have distinctly different origins is controversial. Bladder and ureteric endometriosis co-exist in approximately 10% [5]. There are series describing cases where the bladder is not affected in any patient with ureteric endometriosis. Abrao *et al* [8] looked at a series of 690 cases of laparoscopically and histologically confirmed pelvic endometriosis and found that 12/690 had ureteric and 26/690 bladder involvement. Therefore there may be a different pathogenesis for the two urinary tract sites. The theory of retrograde menstruation and extrinsic involvement is perhaps etiological for ureteric pathology. Bladder endometriosis has long centered around the theory of implantation at previous surgery, but the Abrao series did not show a positive correlation with previous pelvic surgery [8].

Pathological findings in urinary tract endometrosis

The pathological definition of ureteral endometriosis is described as: "usually unilateral, confined to the lower one third of the ureter and associated with endometriosis elsewhere in the pelvis. Involvement of the overlying peritoneum, uterosacral ligament, or ovary may result in compression of the ureteric wall. Less commonly, the endometriosis is intrinsic, resulting in a thickened ureteric wall with fibrosis and proliferation of the ureteric muscularis, rarely the mucosa may also be involved with a polypoid tumour-like mass projecting into the lumen" [17].

In cases where the diagnosis is difficult, it is suggested that specific histological stains such as progesterone and estrogen receptor status along with CD10, CD7 and occasionally CA125 (67% positive) may assist [18].

Bladder endometriosis is most usually non-polypoid but can be of the polypoid type [19]. In the polypoid type, a lack of periglandular stromal hypercellularity, stromal atypia and intraglandular stromal papillae help distinguish it from adenosarcoma.

Controversy about the diagnosis of ureteric endometriosis

It is suggested by some authors that the term "ureteric endometriosis" should be confined only to those cases where there is histological evidence of intrinsic disease. Donnez does not consider that extrinsic disease, especially in the absence of histological confirmation or ureteric stenosis causing upper tract changes, should be classified as ureteric disease [20].

Clinical presentation

The presentation of urinary tract endometriosis is similar to other urological conditions with symptoms that could be confused with urinary tract infection, such as storage lower urinary

---

Box 42.1 Symptoms associated with vesical endometriosis

• Frequency	41–71%
• Urgency	41–78%
• Dysuria	14–21%
• Suprapubic pain	38–78%
• Nocturia	50–75%
• Urge incontinence	21%
• Hematuria	19–30%
• Pelvic mass	50%

Source: Comiter [1].

---

tract symptoms (LUTS) including frequency, urgency, suprapubic pressure or pain relieved by voiding (up to 80%) or less frequently with upper tract involvement with loin pain. The link to the presence of endometriosis is the cyclical nature of symptoms as related to menses, particularly where there is bladder pathology. One-third of patients will present with the classic symptom of cyclical hematuria with bladder involvement [11,21].

Examination findings in endometriosis of the bladder may include tenderness of the anterior vaginal wall and in 50% of cases there is a palpable pelvic mass [1].

Cyclical connection to symptoms with ureteric disease is far less absolute [8]. Indeed, the hallmark of ureteric involvement seems to be its vague and insidious presentation, mandating that it is remembered in the context of the condition where other pelvic involvement is recognized as severe. Otherwise it is likely to be missed until the time of surgical exploration. The Abrao study showed that 50% of cases with ureteric involvement did have symptoms and these were often severe or incapacitating dysmenorrhea (75%) when this group was compared with the bladder and control groups [8].

Box 42.1 shows the symptoms associated with vesical endometriosis [1].

Diagnostics and investigation

Bladder: role of cystoscopy

In the assessment for potential bladder involvement, cystocopy can be performed as a rigid procedure with general anesthesia or, less preferably but more conveniently, as a flexible local anesthetic procedure to ascertain the presence, size and location of lesions. Rigid cystoscopy allows biopsy by resection to confirm the diagnosis. Cold cup biopsy may be insufficient owing to the transmural nature of the vesical endometrial pathology.

Ninety percent with vesical involvement will have an abnormal cystoscopic examination [1]. A laparoscopy and hysteroscopy should be performed concomitantly. The laparoscopic view is shown in Plate 42.1 A. Vesical lesions are typically located close to the dome as they involve the peritoneal surface of the bladder and show a bluish irregular submucosal hue as seen in Plate 42.1 B. Cystoscopy should be considered in all who present with any lower urinary tract symptoms or hematuria in the context of pelvic pain or other symptoms of endometriosis. Vesical disease may mimic carcinoma of the bladder on ultrasound examination and hence a cystoscopy and biopsy or resection to confirm pathology may be required. Endoscopic biopsy may, however, be reserved for those cases where there is some diagnostic doubt, such as in a patient with additional risk factors for malignancy such as heavy smoking. The endoscopic appearance of endometriosis in concert with other positive pelvic sites at laparoscopy is often enough for diagnosis and biopsy has been associated with torrential bleeding requiring blood transfusion and open exploration (personal communication, A Clarke). Therefore it should be undertaken with caution.

Assessment of the upper tracts

As most patients with bladder or ureteric involvement usually have stage III or IV disease, it is prudent in these cases to undertake thorough assessment of the urinary tract prior to definitive surgery to document the extent of urinary tract involvement. Most patients as a part of their diagnostic work-up will have had an ultrasound study of the pelvis but adequate views of the kidneys are required to ensure their presence and size. If there is any degree of hydronephrosis further functional studies are recommended.

Computed tomography (CT) with intravenous contrast and delayed studies that give an accurate pyelogram (CT/IVP) and ureteric images to the level of obstructive pathology should be the first choice of study in those with upper tract changes on ultrasound scan. Prior to imaging with contrast, serum creatinine, urea and electrolytes are required to ensure there is adequate renal function for contrast administration.

More than one-third of cases involving the ureter will have some impairment of renal excretion and identifiable pathology on CT scanning [9]. Changes ranging from delayed excretion of contrast to complete loss of function may be present. In cases of very poor function, drainage with a percutaneous nephrostomy tube or stenting may be required to reassess function in the absence of obstruction.

Further studies depend on the initial findings but may include nuclear medicine scans for differential renal function and assessment for presence of obstruction.

In recent series, up to 11% of renal units [9] are found to have irreversible renal atrophy. This may lead to the decision for renal removal, usually now via laparoscopic nephrectomy. This is an important decision to make preoperatively as realistically, where a renal unit has less than 10% function despite drainage and there is a normal contralateral renal unit, the patient is best served by nephrectomy and not complex reconstruction. Rates of irreversible atrophy vary amongst authors and older series quote higher rates in the order of 30% [22]. However, more recent series such as Nezhat [6] and Antonelli [9] show rates of irreversible renal loss in the order of 4–11%.

At the time of cystoscopy, if there is suspicion regarding the presence of ureteral involvement, retrograde ureteropyelography as shown in Plate 42.2 and possible ureteroscopic assessment can be performed. As previously stated, endoscopic bladder biopsy should be undertaken with caution. Where there is a diagnostic dilemma, biopsy can be achieved via a 22 Fr sheath with rigid biopsy forceps and then coagulation undertaken using a diathermy electrode (e.g. 6 Fr Bugbee). It is possible to biopsy using a resectoscope and diathermy loop but this will create a much larger defect and potentially increase the risk of hemorrhage. If the cold cup biopsy sites cannot be controlled with a diathermy electrode, the next step will be to use the resectoscope loop or a roller ball to coagulate. Great care needs to be exercised in the dome area, where these lesions most frequently occur, as there is a high risk of full-thickness perforation of the bladder wall with deeper biopsy and attempted cogaulation and this places intraperitoneal structures, in particular bowel, at risk of injury.

If there is need to investigate the ureter in a retrograde fashion, the first step is to cannulate the affected side with a ureteric catheter and inject radiographic contrast with the aid of an image intensifier and perform retrograde pyelography. The ureteric catheter is advanced only into the lower ureter and this is studied first, prior to attempted gentle advancement of the catheter to inject contrast into the upper ureter. In cases of severe scarring, this may not be possible and the classic appearance of extrinsic ureteric compression with a "rat tail" like tapering of the pelvic ureter may be seen.

If further investigation of the lumen is sought, a guidewire is passed under image intensification via the ureteric catheter and then a ureteroscope; either a fine-gauge rigid 7 Fr or flexible scope can be passed. If there is a luminal lesion, which is less often the case and would usually be associated with intrinsic disease, a biopsy via the ureteroscope can be performed. However, as in the case of the bladder, this would be in circumstances where there was doubt about the presence of another pathology, the specimens gained are usually tiny and difficult to interpret histologically and there is a distinct risk of causing bleeding. Where there is functional obstruction, there will be need for further laparoscopic exploration with possible excision and the need for biopsy prior to this is not mandatory in cases where the clinical picture is consistent with endometriosis.

As most patients will undergo a diagnostic laparoscopy as part of their overall work-up, it is pertinent to organize multidisciplinary involvement where urological endometriosis is suspected, such that concomitant cystoscopy and/or ureteric studies with imaging or ureteroscopy can occur. It should also be noted that at laparoscopy, the diagnosis of ureteral endometriosis may be missed as the overlying peritoneum may remain unaffected even in the presence of significant retroperitoneal disease[7].

Role of magnetic resonance imaging

A review by Kinkel *et al* [23] suggests that magnetic resonance imaging (MRI) offers the best overall assessment of not only the whole urinary tract but all pelvic sites of endometriosis.

Endometriotic lesions demonstrate high signal intensity on T1-weighted spin echo and low signal on T2-weighted spin echo. Bladder endometriosis may be identified on MRI as submucosal masses with characteristic MRI features of hemorrhagic foci and reactive fibrosis [24]. In current clinical practice where access may be limited, MRI is reserved for those cases which are particularly complex or there is need for imaging without the administration of intravenous contrast.

Planning of management and general issues

Management of urinary tract endometriosis is complex and relies on a team with a multidisciplinary approach and expertise in this specific area [6]. It is notable that isolated urological endometriosis is rare and if present, the bladder is most frequently involved [9]. Many patients will have extraurinary pelvic sites of endometriosis and therefore the urinary tract will be but one consideration in the care of multiple organ systems that may be involved.

The management of bladder endometriosis is aimed at relief of symptoms, restoration of function, preservation of fertility and avoidance of recurrence. Consideration of age, fertility, extent of vesical disease, severity of urinary symptoms, impact on menstrual function and presence of other pelvic disease must be undertaken. The aims for management of ureteric endometriosis are similar, with a particular emphasis on recovery of any impaired renal function where possible and the maintenance of drainage of the upper tracts for the long term.

Medical management

Medical management of vesical and ureteral endometriosis is suboptimal. There are only small numbers of cases managed this way reported in the literature and there is a high associated failure rate.

Intrinsic disease of the bladder treated medically is often unresponsive owing to the desmoplastic reaction within the bladder wall caused by repeated intramural cyclical bleeding. Medical management is feasible but long-term follow-up is required as there is a high rate of recurrence after cessation of therapy [11]. There is also morbidity associated with long-term medical therapy [25].

Endoscopic management: transurethral resection and ureteric stenting

Management of vesical lesions with transurethral resection of endometriosis (TURE) is often unsuccessful. By their very transmural nature, it is virtually impossible to safely and completely resect the endometriotic nodules without causing perforation and potential damage to intraperitoneal structures. Transurethral resection is therefore associated with a high rate of recurrence [9] and up to a 35% relapse rate is quoted [26]. Successful series such as that of Schneider *et al* [21] demonstrate that one-third of cases (five of 15) could be managed with TURE with a mean of 20 months follow-up. The remaining 10 patients in the series had a laparoscopic partial cystectomy.

Equally, management of ureteric lesions by endoscopic means, with passage of double J stents, with or without prior attempts at dilation, is unlikely to be successful as the lesion remains, is often encasing and periureteric and recurrence is therefore high.

Role of ureteroscopy in ureteric endometriosis

A single case report of ureteroscopic ablation with holmium laser and then hormonal therapy with leuprolide [16] may be worthy of comment as a "conservative" option where the patient was unfit for surgery, the lesion was high or there was an issue about renal preservation, etc.

A further paper discussed the use of medical therapy for ureteric endometrosis with gonadotropin releasing hormone agonist (GnRHa) in three patients, two of whom responded; the one who failed had intrinsic disease [25].

Definitive surgical management of bladder and ureteric endometriosis

Initial management in many patients is with endoscopy and transurethral resection of the endometriotic nodule in order to confirm the histological diagnosis. However, as discussed, the nodules are by definition full thickness, as they begin on the peritoneal surface and are difficult to completely resect endoscopically. Even with addition of hormonal therapy, there is a high recurrence rate. Therefore, optimal definitive management in most cases is partial cystectomy, which can now be achieved laparoscopically.

Most lesions are simple dome lesions and are readily identifiable by transperitoneal access and hence amenable to this technique. Excision of simple dome lesions laparoscopically can be achieved with low morbidity and good long-term results [9].

Where lesions are lower and more intimately involved with surrounding structures and the trigone, laparotomy has traditionally been the preferred approach. However, improved laparoscopic techniques continue to push the boundaries of what can be achieved in this more difficult area, with case reports of successful laparoscopic clearance of lesions close to the trigone and right ureteric orifice described recently [27].

Laparoscopic partial cystectomy: surgical technique
Preparation
Patients should undergo bowel preparation prior to laparoscopy for bladder or ureteric endometriosis. Prophylactic antibiotics with both gram-positive and -negative cover are given. They are not required postoperatively unless there is concomitant bowel resection. Thromboprophylaxis should be considered.

Equipment
Laparoscopic surgery for endometriosis is very complex and requires optimal equipment and usually takes place in a tertiary referral setting. An experienced subspecialist team of surgical nursing, technical and anesthetic staff is needed to bring the patient through these types of complex reconstructive laparoscopy.

A team allowing for a combined laparoscopic and cystoscopic surgical approach is ideal.

A combined approach allows initial endoscopic incision of the bladder by resection with Collings knife around the lesion until perivesical fat is reached. The removal and suturing is then done laparoscopically. This protects the ureters but also gives a clean margin which is easier to suture (personal communication, A Clarke).

High-quality laparoscopes, good light sources and adjustable LED screens, including one for the assistant, provide the correct environment for surgery to take place. Disposable trocars are preferable and with the best possible safety features to avoid injury. Two 5 mm and one adjustable, such as a 5–10 mm Versaport™, are required along with the main 10 mm laparoscope port.

Entry is per the surgeon's preference with either Verres needle or Hassan technique and insufflation with high- and low-flow capabilities is required with flow rate around 14 mmHg usually maintained.

A variety of subspecialized instruments is available and these have increasing capabilities in terms of articulation and energy sources (monopolar, bipolar and laser) that may be applied for dissection and hemostasis. At least two high-quality needle holders are required for the intracorporeal suturing. A combined suction irrigation device is used.

Anesthesia

Laparoscopic surgery for endometriosis is performed under general anesthesia and precautions for pressure areas, thromboembolic and antibiotic prophylaxis need to be taken in accordance with the long length of the surgery.

Operation

Position

The patient is placed in the lithotomy position with the legs flat at the hip joints and bent at the knees; ideally, multijoint supported stirrups such as the Allen® Yellofin® Elite Stirrups are used and pneumatic sequential calf compression applied. The patient is shaved as per the surgeon's preference and then preparation of the abdomen, perineum and vagina is performed.

Cystoscopy

The cystoscopy is performed using a 30° telescope with 22 Fr sheath which delineates the site and extent of the endometriotic nodule. Ureteric stenting is performed at this point if necessary using a 4 or 5 Fr ureteric catheter. The bladder is emptied prior to the laparoscopic entry.

Uterine manipulation

With the aid of a Sims speculum, the anterior lip of the cervix is grasped, the cervix is dilated and a medium curette or uterine manipulator introduced to allow for uterine movement during the case.

Pneumoperitoneum and port placement

Umbilical Verres, Hassan or Palmer's point entry is achieved, depending on the surgeon's preference or the presence of abdominal scars, and a 10 mm laparoscope introduced. Two 5 mm ports are placed lateral to the superficial epigastric vessels and one suprapubic port to facilitate suturing is sited, such as a 5–10 mm Versaport™.

Opening the peritoneum

The most difficult part of the procedure is the dissection of the bladder from the uterus, cervix and vagina with care to identify the ureters and uterine arteries; the latter is shown in Plate 42.3A. A McCartney tube is a useful instrument that helps put upward traction on the vaginal fornices and aids with bladder dissection. The retropubic space is also entered using a transverse incison with, for example, monopolar scissors or spade with the obliterated umbilical artery as a lateral landmark and the urachus in the midline. The bladder needs to be completely mobilized above, below and lateral to the lesion and the retropubic dissection helps with mobilization so the bladder can be closed without tension after excision of the nodule.

Cystotomy and resection of endometriotic nodule

Simultaneous cystoscopic delineation with monopolar diathermy around the perimeter of the endometriotic nodule with clear margins is then followed by perforating the full thickness of the bladder to the peritoneal cavity to commence the partial cystotomy. This can then be completed laparoscopically.

Cystotomy must be planned if there is concomitant ureteric disease and a possible bladder flap is required. In that instance, a curvilinear incision for a flap with its base at the corresponding apical corner of the bladder to the side of the ureteric deficit is needed. Occasionally, the lesion is not full thickness and the mucosa can be spared, but this is an uncommon scenario and most require a full-thickness excision.

Bladder closure

The bladder is closed with 2/0 polyglactin (e.g. Vicryl) or Monocryl suture material using intra- or extracorporeal knot tying. This can be performed as a double-layer closure; however, in large lesions a double layer can further compromise final bladder capacity and therefore techniques such as using a continuous monolayer suture with clips applied at intervals to maintain tension can be utilized.

Completion of the procedure

Cystoscopy to a volume of 150–200 ml is performed at the end after administration of intravenous indigo carmine (if no stents) 5 ml to ensure ureteric integrity and (cystoscopic instillation) water-tight bladder closure. A drain tube is left *in situ*.

Postoperative management

A urethral catheter is left *in situ*, ideally a larger bore such as 16 or 18 Fr for 7–14 days. A cystogram is performed prior to catheter removal.

Complications and outcome of laparoscopic partial cystectomy

Initial postoperative complications include an anastomotic leak or hematuria which may require a careful bladder wash-out.

Long-term complications may include urinary urgency and a decreased bladder capacity.

Management of the ureter and ureteric dissection

The requirement for complete excision of endometriotic nodules, for recurrence-free recovery, makes ureteric involvement and management some of the most challenging surgery in endometriosis care. Initial attempts to manage ureters with drainage, either by stenting retrograde or percutaneous nephrostomy placement and antegrade stenting, are only ever temporary, to relieve obstruction and assess subsequent renal function in what may be a permanently compromised renal unit.

It is useful to consider the classification of ureteric involvement according to Frenna [28] as shown in Box 42.2.

Patients in Frenna's categories B and C are often amenable to "conservative" laparoscopic management by "simple" laparoscopic ureterolysis as shown in Plate 42.3 B. There are six published case series [5,6,13,15,28,32], including one with 96 patients with no recurrence over a 2–50-month follow-up using the laparoscopic ureterolysis technique in all but two patients [5].

Antonelli [9] states that simple ureterolysis is only recommended in the case of a non-obstructing, extrinisic, isolated ureteric lesion, i.e. a Frenna type C lesion. Ureteroneocystostomy (UNC), according to Antonelli, is preferable if there is more extensive disease.

Some patients will have disease that is suitable for ureteric resection and a spatulated end-to-end anastomosis but, as will be explored, this procedure has several caveats and is often inferior to UNC for the pelvic or lower third of the ureter. There are increasing reports of laparoscopic UNC and reconstruction, with laparoscopic bladder hitch and Boari or bladder flap described laparoscopically, even in the presence of a duplex ureter [29]. The feasibility and description of these complex reconstructive surgeries will be reviewed in the next section.

Anatomy of the ureter

To understand how endometriosis may affect the ureter and then how it may be optimally managed surgically, it is worth reviewing the anatomy, particularly the layers of the ureter and its blood supply.

The ureter receives its blood supply from the medial side more proximally taking branches from the renal, aortic and ovarian arteries. As it descends, this supply becomes more laterally based

from superior and inferior vesical arteries and ureteral vessels arising from the internal iliac arteries. Hence there is a potential watershed area around the middle portion of the ureter from the lower pole of the kidney and brim of the pelvis, where the ureter is the most poorly vascularized and the risk of ischemia is higher.

A rich anastomosis forms in the adventitia itself, also piercing the adventitial layer and running the entire length of the ureter. The ureter can then be divided along its length at many sites without risk of ischemia but it does affect the viability of the end of the ureter, especially in the instance where it has been previously mobilized and the adventitia disrupted. This may be relevant when a failed ureterolysis requires subsequent excision and UNC. Maintenance of overlying peritoneal branches is also important for viability, especially in the lower ureter.

The ureteral sheath is a loose layer derived from the retroperitoneal connective tissue lying just under the peritoneum to which it is adherent. As with the adventitial layer, it begins at the renal pelvis and continues to Waldeyer's sheath of the trigone. Close association with the uterovaginal and vesicovaginal plexuses of veins within the parametrium makes the ureter more difficult to free during surgery on the uterus.

The sheath provides a barrier between inflammatory and neoplastic processes and the underlying adventitia. The ureter may remain mobile within the attenuated sheath when the process results in its thickening, and this may be the case with extrinsic endometriosis. However, when the process is more infiltrative, such as in the case of intrinsic disease, there is greater threat to function.

The adventitia is loose over the muscular layer, composed of three bundles of inner, middle and outer "interlacing helices." There are independent nexuses between each smooth muscle cell allowing for intrinsic electrical activity transfer with little extraneuronal supply. Within the muscularis is a transitional epithelium-lined inner epithelium on a lamina propria with no submucosa.

General principles of ureteric repair and reimplantation

When approaching ureteric repair, whether open or laparoscopically, it is useful to observe the following principles.

- Sufficient mobilization for reimplantation or repair without tension
- Excision of any non-viable ureter
- Avoiding skeletonization of the ureter and preservation of its blood supply
- Spatulated or oblique ureteral margins
- A water-tight anastomosis with absorbable sutures
- Support of the anastomosis with a double J stent

Direct ureteroureterostomy is ideally applied where repair of the upper or middle thirds of the ureter is required. The distribution of most endometriotic lesions means that this will not usually be the best choice of management as most will be found in the lower third or pelvic ureter.

When ureteroureteostomy is performed, the initial steps are as for laparoscopic ureterolysis. The ends of the ureter are then spatulated for 5 mm or cut cleanly at an oblique angle. Double J stent insertion at this point facilitates realignment of the ureter for anastomosis with interrupted 4/0 polyglactin (e.g. Vicryl™) or poliglecaprone 25 (e.g. Monocryl™) sutures.

A surgeon's preference for a direct anastomosis, and not bypassing the distal diseased segment and opting for a UNC, may be influenced by the requirement for lengthening steps, such as a hitch or flap, in order to achieve tension-free anastomosis in the more proximal pelvic ureter. This may be particularly the case in the laparoscopic approach to ureteric resection.

Ureteroneocystostomy is a straightforward open procedure when the very distal ureter is involved and hence a direct anastomosis without any lengthening procedures is achieved.

Simple open UNC is achieved by the extravesical tunnel or Lich–Gregoir technique. The ureter is isolated and the diseased section excised, bearing in mind all the principles of the direction of the blood supply and preservation of the adventitia but dividing the obliterated umbilical artery, the perforating vessels behind the ureter and the uterine artery where necessary. A suitable site on the upper lateral aspect of the dome of the bladder for reanastomosis is chosen. This is facilitated by having the bladder filled retrograde with saline, via the Foley catheter, which is prepped into the operative field at the commencement of the case.

Stay sutures may be placed in the detrusor at the proximal and distal ends of the incision, which is a 2–3 cm groove in an almost vertical direction with the bladder elevated and rotated medially. The end result will be that the site runs in the direction of the course of the ureter once the bladder is allowed to fall back into its natural position.

The detrusor is undermined against the subepithelium to create muscular flaps for later closure. A mucosa-to-mucosa anastomosis is then created over a double J stent with 4/0 polyglactin (e.g. Vicryl™) or poliglecaprone 25 (e.g. Monocryl™) sutures. 2/0 sutures can then be used in an interrupted fashion to close the muscle over the anastomosis. The steps are almost identical, whether open or laparoscopic. Where there is a duplex ureter, the mobilization is the same and the two are left within their common sheath and reimplanted as a single unit, with care taken on mucosa-to-mucosa anastomosis with the bladder not to compromise the narrow lumen; two double J stents are required.

Reimplantation does not need to be achieved in an antireflux fashion. There are disadvantages to fashioning an antirefluxing anastomosis: a greater length of ureter is required and the risk of subsequent stenosis is higher. Antirefluxing technique is not required for reimplantation in the setting of injury or excision for tumor, as is the case in ureteric endometriosis.

Ureteroneocystostomy was first performed laparoscopically by Nezhat in 1992 [30]. As with laparoscopic ureterolysis, laparoscopic UNC has advantages including less blood loss, less postoperative pain, shorter hospital stay and quicker return to normal activities.

Since the Nezhat case report, there have been several other reports of small numbers of laparoscopic UNC. Seracchioli [15] describes creation of a non-refluxing anastomosis in three patients.

Laparoscopic ureterolysis for endometriosis

The operative technique for laparoscopic ureteric dissection begins very similarly to laparoscopic partial cystectomy and, as discussed, the two conditions frequently co-exist and are managed at the same operative sitting.

Preparation, equipment, anesthesia, patient positioning and establishment of pneumoperitoneum and initial dissection to open the peritoneum proceed as per the description in the preceding section on laparoscopic partial cystectomy. The principal difference in the two procedures initially relates to the cystoscopy and possible placement of a double J stent or ureteric catheter electively at the start of the case where ureteric surgery is planned, prior to entry into the abdomen. The advantages and disadvantages of double J stent placement are explored in the following section.

Opening the peritoneum and commencement of ureterolysis

After incision of the peritoneum along the pelvic side wall, the ureter is mobilized commencing with blunt dissection of the unaffected ureter above the level of the lesion down to the uterosacral ligaments. Start the dissection where the ureter is clearly visible, usually through the peritoneum, high on the pelvic side wall, healthy and free of adhesions, and progress it in the direction of the uterosacral ligaments until the ureterovesical junction is reached. The use of multiple techniques with irrigation and laser (CO_2) is described to facilitate the mobilization.

Care is taken where possible, and especially with the unaffected ureter, to minimize handling, maintain the adventitia and avoid excessive skeletonization with the resultant risk of postoperative stricture.

The ureteric blood supply becomes more laterally based as the ureter crosses the pelvic brim and it is at its most vulnerable at the middle third where there is a transition of supply picked up medially above and laterally below.

Ureterolysis: resection of endometriotic nodules

Begin ureterolysis prior to attempting to resect the adenomyotic lesion and complete the ureterolysis as far as is practicable. This may require resection of the adventitial layer, leaving the muscularis intact in areas where there is endometriotic tissue. Small breaches of the wall can be left [6,7]. Where there is uncertainty about the degree of breach, IV indigo carmine can be used to assess the laceration.

In some instances, resection of adenomyotic lesions may require resection of the uterine vessels.

A preoperative double J stent or ureteric catheter may help with identification of the ureter and will also rapidly demonstrate any breach in the ureteric wall. For those cases where after mobilization it is evident that resection of a segment of the ureter is required in order to completely resect the endometriosis, a double J stent should be placed at that point in a retrograde fashion via cystoscopy. Where there is entry to the lumen, it is repaired with 4/0 polyglactin (e.g. Vicryl™) or poliglecaprone 25 (e.g. Monocryl™) sutures.

If the lumen is completely occluded then the next step is to assess for suitability for an excision and end-to-end anastomosis over a double J stent. An end-to-end repair can be achieved where there is a short, less than 2 cm segment of ureter involved and there is sufficient mobility to achieve a tension-free anastomosis. The ureter is spatulated and then closed with interrupted 4/0 polyglactin (e.g. Vicryl™) or poliglecaprone 25 (e.g. Monocryl™) sutures, about four in number to achieve adequate opposition of the two ends. Where there is a longer defect or the defect is close to the bladder or below the level of the pelvic brim and there is sufficient mobility, ureteric reimplantation is required and this is dealt with in the next section.

Where there has been a ureteric repair and double J stent insertion, the stents should be left for 6 weeks and then removed with a flexible cystoscope. Six weeks after this removal, a contrast study such as a CT/IVP is performed to ensure there is no narrowing of the repair. This should then be repeated at 6 months and 1 year and annually to 3 years postoperative or in the instance of recurrence of any symptoms suggestive of obstruction.

The use of double J stents

The use of double J stenting, electively in all cases for potential ureterolysis, where the stent is inserted at the commencement of the procedure, is controversial, with critics arguing that it adds unnecessary time and cost for unproven benefit. Camanni [5] does not routinely stent, claiming the low risk of subsequent fistula (3.7%) in his series, along with the possibility that fistula would not be avoided by stenting.

In the Weingertner study [4], which looked specifically at the need for double J stents in a series of 145 patients requiring laparoscopy for deep pelvic endometriosis, only 17 or 11% needed stenting at some point. Preoperatively, seveh cases were electively stented for hydronephrosis, gross ureteral distortion on imaging or previous ureteral lesion at previous operation. Per-operative stenting was required in seven cases for aggressive dissection with injury, resection or doubt about integrity or dilated ureter not previously identified and in a single case of vesical endometriosis requiring resection of the trigone. Postoperative stenting was required in three cases: one ureterovaginal fistula, one obstruction and one case of doubt about ureteric integrity. Overall, five major complications (two vesicovaginal fistulae, three ureteric complications) occurred despite stenting.

Conversely, placement of a double J stent is a relatively quick and simple procedure and if it avoids an unnecessary, potentially open operation, its disadvantages are justifiable. It is not necessary to leave the patient on antibiotic prophylaxis, as many papers suggest, and removal of the stent is a simple and very quick procedure under local anesthetic.

Some 70% of ureteric injuries are diagnosed postoperatively [31] but if a stent was present and the injury identified, these would largely be obviated by elective double J stent insertion. Between 61% and 100% of these injuries require subsequent open management at present [4]. If stenting facilitates a laparoscopic approach, where otherwise a laparotomy would be required, the insertion of the stent is easily justified.

Outcomes and complications of ureterolysis for endometriosis

When considering the outcome of ureterolysis, several factors require consideration, not all of which are uniformly presented in the literature. First, the utility of "simple" ureterolysis as a single technique without the need to resort to excision and reanastomosis should be examined as an endpoint. The immediate and long-term surgical complications of the technique should be assessed and then the recurrence of the endometriosis requiring reintervention should be ascertained.

On this basis, ureterolysis was adequate definitive management for 75 of 80 patients, if those who required UNC at the outset (four, for deeply infiltrating intrinsic endometriosis of the ureter) and those who required reoperation for complications that included the need for repeat reconstruction (one) are excluded [5].

Reported complication rates vary in the literature. A large series of 80 patients undergoing ureterolysis had a 3.7% rate of long-term complications. All three patients developed fistulae and all three had more than a 4 cm length of ureter involved at the initial surgery [5].

If reoperation is taken as the endpoint, the Camanni series shows a low need for reintervention with 96% intervention free at 12 months and 87% intervention free at 24 months [5]. Smaller series show higher reoperation rates of the order of 15% [7] or as high as 30%. These series had more cases of intrinsic and higher volume disease. Reoperation takes both the laparoscopic and open form depending on the original pathology found. Early complications, such as urinomas and fistulae, and late complications, such as strictures, are equally managed with open and laparoscopic approaches. Minimally invasive techniques, such as double J stenting or percutaneous drainage, may suffice in some instances.

Further study of the Frenna series [28] reveals that of the 54 patients, only three actually had stenosis of the ureter involved. Complications of the ureterolysis in that series included ureteric injury requiring repair intraoperatively and stenting (1/54), two of 54 patients stented per-operatively, to prevent obstruction where there had been "significant " dissection required, one ureterovaginal fistula and two cases of transient urinary retention. Pain scores postoperatively showed high levels of satisfaction (76%), four patients required recurrent resection of disease with complete resolution and the total follow-up period reported on was 1 year. It is not clear if those patients who had ureteric obstruction at the time of diagnosis were in this latter group.

The ureteric injury rate is overall 0.2–2% in laparoscopic gynecological surgery but occurs in 38% of cases where surgery is for endometriosis [4].

The Antonelli series [9] reports no urological complications for 25 of the 31 patients who had initial non-endoscopic management, and this is with a minimum follow-up period of 1 year. Two patients with simple ureterolysis had disease recurrence detected and one patient who had an end-to-end ureteroureterostomy had recurrence which required reoperation.

Patients who require repeat surgery for recurrent disease after ureterolysis are few in number. Ghezzi et al [7] strongly contend that most cases will be amenable to "conservative" management, i.e. laparoscopic ureterolysis. Their study supports the findings of Nehzat and Donnez, who present some of the earliest work in this area. Nezhat reports no recurrences from the series in 1996 in which 10 patients in total underwent laparoscopic ureterolysis.

The role of laparoscopy versus laparotomy for ureteric management is unanswered in the literature in proper well-constructed prospective randomized trials. It is only possible to infer from the larger series of experience that despite long operative times of the order of 3–4 h (Camanni mean 167 mins, up to 750 mins [5]), laparoscopy offers a potential benefit in terms of lowered morbidity and more rapid recovery with less postoperative pain. Patients treated in the Nezhat series [6] had a mean length of stay of 1.8 days (range 1–6). Laparoscopy also has intraoperative benefits such as magnification and visualization and superior access to the deep pelvis despite body habitus.

Long-term follow-up is required not only to assess for late ureteric stricture as a result of the reconstructive surgery alone, but because, particularly with cessation of any hormonal treatment, there is a high rate of recurrence of symptomatic disease [9].

The largest series of ureterolysis describes 96 patients and in all but one, the primary complaint was pain and only a third had urinary symptoms. The left ureter was affected in 64% of cases and disease was bilateral in 10%. Four patients had hydroureter and two had hydronephrosis. All patients underwent ureterolysis with endometriotic excision or ablation. Two patients underwent resection and UNC with a psoas hitch because of extensive involvement and obstruction of the distal part of the ureter and six patients required a double J stent intraoperatively after extensive ureterolysis. During the 2–50-month follow-up no patient had recurrent urinary tract disease. This series summarized that laparoscopic ureterolysis represents an effective treatment option in most cases that can be safely accomplished even in cases of moderate or severe hydroureteronephrosis [32].

Indications for resection and when ureterolysis is not enough

Most centers recommend avoiding ureteric resection owing to the added complexity of reconstruction and therefore the risk of urinary leakage, ureteric stricture, compromise in bladder function where large flaps are required to bridge the deficit and overall increased morbidity when compared with ureterolysis. However, there are instances where ureterolysis is insufficient and indeed, most series report some failures in their ureterolysis groups that subsequently required UNC for definitive repair [9,28,33].

Situations that may require consideration for resection of the affected ureter include those where there is an intrinsic lesion of the ureter, lesions greater than 3 cm in size and where viability is in question [4,32].

As the definition of intrinsic endometriosis is a pathological distinction and it may not always be possible to determine this pre- or even intraoperatively, opting for a more conservative approach and accepting the possibility that further intervention may be required for a small number is not an unreasonable strategy. However, where intrinsic or very large lesions are recognized, there is benefit in resection and definitive treatment as opposed to a more conservative laparoscopic approach and subsequent hormonal therapy, as this group of patients is at risk of silent renal loss due to fibrosis and stenosis [6]. There is always the risk that the reconstruction will fail if there is downstream disease or tension on the anastomosis, so the preferred option is excision and reimplantation of the ureter (UNC) where possible as opposed to an end-to-end repair.

Ultimately, Camanni is correct to write "The choice between conservative and aggressive surgical approach depends more on the surgeon's personal opinion than scientific evidence" but the presence of adverse factors such as length of ureteric involvement and the possibility for intrinsic disease should suggest a more aggressive approach [5].

Resection of disease and reimplantation, usually with direct bladder neocystostomy, is the preferred treatment for more extensive disease. This is traditionally performed via an open approach. This is due to the complexity of the reconstruction, the need for possible lengthening maneuvers such as a psoas hitch or Boari flap creation and the likelihood of management of other organs such as the gastrointestinal tract at the same operation, given that many of these patients have high grades of endometriotic disease.

However, laparoscopy and the use of robotics are facilitating a move towards a more minimally invasive approach to the problem of extensive ureteric disease, though only in large volume centers, in which owing to the rarity of the disorder only a few cases are seen.

Advanced laparoscopic and open reconstruction for ureteric reimplantation

As discussed, the length and location of endometrial involvement will determine the reconstructive approach to the ureter. Most disease involves the distal third of the ureter and hence excision and reimplantation can be achieved usually with direct reimplantation, especially where the ureter is within a few centimeters of the intramural course. Where the excised segment is longer or the diseased area higher and towards the pelvic brim, lengthening to allow reanastomosis without tension is achieved by hitching the bladder on the ipsilateral side to the psoas minor tendon, or by creation of a bladder flap.

A psoas hitch is the first lengthening maneuver to bridge a gap which will not allow direct reimplantation without tension. A cystotomy is required and it is best to fashion this as if a subsequent flap is required as the ultimate length to be achieved is not always apparent.

The bladder is filled retrograde via a Foley catheter and then an abbreviated U-shaped incision, slightly tilted with the inferior point of the U towards the opposite lower corner of the bladder, is marked out with diathermy. It is not necessary to immediately extend the lateral and medial limbs of the U fully to the lateral

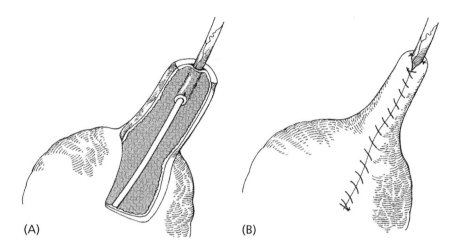

Figure 42.1 Diagram of Boari flap.(A) Developing the flap from the bladder wall. (B) Suturing the flap to form a tube over the antireflux anastomosis.

(A)　　　　　　(B)

bladder wall and dome respectively. After incision, using two fingers or a laparoscopic instrument within the bladder, the ipsilateral corner is pushed towards the defect and mobilized ureter to assess if a psoas hitch alone will bridge the gap. If the ureter reaches the top of the bladder once it is helped up toward the psoas minor tendon, the bladder can be fixed to the tendon with three absorbable sutures (e.g. 3/0 polyglactin) placed in a vertical direction through the tendon in shallow bites so as not to catch or compromise the branches of the lumbar plexus that pass through the underlying psoas musculature. Additional length can also be obtained prior to hitching by division of the contralateral superior vesical pedicle.

The ureter is then reimplanted as described for a direct UNC with a refluxing anastomosis over a double J stent. It is useful for all instances to have a 4/0 absorbable stay suture in the ureter to facilitate manipulation at the time of anastomosis. Place this at the apex of the spatulation.

Creation of a bladder flap will allow a section of up to 7 cm to be bridged. Bladder flap creation was originally described by Boari [34] as shown in Figure 42.1. Prior to cystotomy, bladder mobilization with optional division of the contralateral superior vesical pedicle is performed. The bladder is filled retrograde via a Foley catheter and then a U-shaped incision, slightly tilted with the inferior point of the U towards the opposite lower corner of the bladder, is marked out with diathermy. It is then useful to place stay sutures in the bladder at the proximal ends of the U and the tip with 2/0 polyglactin (e.g. Vicryl™) for later manipulation. The flap needs to be made wide enough and despite a wide-based U, shrinkage after fashioning can be deceptive.

The flap is then reflected cranially and it is optional to place lengthening incisions halfway up the medial side of the flap and at the junction of the upper one-third and lower two-thirds of the flap, allowing closure in the style of a Z-plasty [35]. In practice this is usually not required.

The flap is then secured to the psoas minor tendon as previously described. There are then two options for reanastomosing the ureter. The first method is by direct spatulation and anastomosis to the tip of the flap, creating a wide tunnel. The anastomosis is done with interrupted absorbable suture material such as 4/0 polyglactin (e.g. Vicryl™) or poliglecaprone 25 (e.g. Monocryl™) sutures. The second method is to make a cystotomy with a small right angle towards the tip of the flap and bring the spatulated ureter through the cystotomy and suture mucosa to mucosa with interrupted absorbable sutures. In both instances a double J stent is inserted.

The flap is then closed with a running, locked watertight 2/0 absorbable suture, preferably a 2/0 polyglactin (e.g. Vicryl™). An indwelling catheter (IDC) of at least 18 Fr is left *in situ* and drainage recorded hourly for the first 24 h to ensure that there is no blockage that may place strain on the cystotomy and increase the leak rate. If there is concern about the repair, placement of an additional suprapubic catheter is an option. A low suction drain is left in the pelvis and removed between day 2 and 4, depending on drainage.

After a cystogram at day 10 the IDC may be removed and a trial of voiding performed. The double J stent is removed with a flexible cystoscope at 6 weeks and then a follow-up contrast study, such as an IVP, is performed 2 weeks after stent removal to ensure anastomotic patency. This should then be rechecked at 6 months and 1 year and then yearly thereafter to 3 years.

Beyond creation of a bladder flap, ileal ureteral substitution or even autotransplantation are the final options where there is an absolute requirement for renal preservation. These are complex procedures with additional complications that make their risks outweigh their benefits in the presence of a functioning contralateral renal unit. The reader is referred to urological reconstructive texts for further information on these procedures.

Laparoscopy and advanced reconstruction

Nezhat first described laparoscopic UNC with accompanying psoas hitch in 1999 [36]. Since then there has been increasing enthusiasm for more complex laparoscopic reconstruction.

In the literature looking at ureteral reimplantation for other benign conditions, Teber *et al* [37] report a recent series of 24 laparoscopic reimplantations where five cases had a simple Lich–Gregoir extravesical ureteric reimplantation, 10 cases had a psoas hitch and the remaining nine both a psoas hitch and Boari flap. Twenty-three patients had good drainage at follow-up imaging with a mean follow-up interval of 35 months.

The use of robotics in ureteric endometriosis

Robotic surgical systems, such as the DaVinci® surgical system (Intuitive Surgical, Sunnyvale, CA), have provided a quantum leap forward in minimally invasive management of benign and malignant pelvic disease.

The advantages of robotics include operating with a three-dimensional view, magnification, motion scaling and seven degrees of movement, compared with four degrees with conventional laparoscopy, and elimination of hand tremor.

While they offer these advantages, they are at present expensive and not always accessible and with the good results from conventional laparoscopic approaches for ureterolysis, the robotic approach is currently better reserved for more complex reconstructive surgery. The surgeon must also overcome the lack of tactile feedback with the robotic approach, instead relying entirely on visual cues.

The robotic procedure for ureteral surgery is described by Williams and Leveillee [38]. Their series included one patient with ureteric endometriosis from a total of seven patients with benign stricture disease of the distal ureter. They utilized a three-arm technique with port placement in a triangulated fashion similar to most laparoscopic techniques; a 12 mm port was placed in the umbilical position and two further 8 mm robotic trocars in each of the lower quadrants.

The dissection then proceeds similarly to laparoscopic ureterolysis and the ureter is then transected just above the level of the obstruction and spatulated using robotic Potts scissors. A double J stent is placed retrograde to the renal pelvis.

The bladder is filled retrograde via the Foley catheter as with the open procedure and then mobilized. Williams notes that they did not have to divide the contralateral superior vesical pedicle for additional mobility. The procedure then described is for a UNC with a refluxing, interrupted, watertight anomosis with 4/0 poliglecaprone 25 over the double J stent. The anastomosis is sited above and lateral to the native ureteric orifice and the mobile bladder dome is avoided to reduce the risk of ureteral kinking. 3/0 polyglactin is used to secure the ureter to the detrusor muscle for stability prior to anastomosis. A leak test with bladder filling is conducted at the end.

This description of the robotic technique did not include any cases requiring a psoas hitch. The operative times were comparable to the laparoscopic technique.

The utility of the robotic technique is further demonstrated in a series of 11 patients with an admixture of benign and malignant ureteric disease which were successfully managed with robotic-assisted laparoscopic distal ureteric surgery by Schimpf and Wagner [39].

The role of nephrectomy in ureteric endometriosis

Historical series demonstrate very high rates (up to 47%) of nephrectomy for obstruction secondary to endometriosis [40]. Nephrectomy is uncommon in most of the contemporary series presented. It should be noted that functional renal loss may be a result of injudicious use of diathermy on the pelvic side wall for previous attempts at endometriotic excision and management with resultant ureteric structuring rather than from involvement by endometriosis itself, which as stated previously is an uncommon presentation.

The need for nephrectomy is assessed preoperatively with assessment of the function of the obstructed unit once decompression with double J stent or percutaneous nephrostomy is performed. Occasionally, if the process has been very chronic and the parenchyma of the affected renal unit is severely thinned as seen on imaging, usually a CT or MRI, a decision for extirpation without assessment of function will be undertaken.

Where there is less than 15–20% of total function on the affected side, a decision for nephrectomy may be made. However, there are several important caveats, including the patient's other co-morbidities, the possibility for future function on the unaffected side and the potential feasibility of reanastomosis or reimplantation of the ureter, depending on the severity and level of the endometriosis.

Almost all nephrectomies in this setting will now be achieved via a transperitoneal laparoscopic approach and as these cases, whilst rare, often have complicated pelvic disease, there will often be a multidisciplinary approach with other pelvic surgery taking place concomitantly [41].

Acknowledgments
The authors are grateful to Dr Anita Clarke, urologist, and Dr Jim Tsaltas, gynecologist, for their communications and advice.

References

1. Comiter C. Endometriosis of the urinary tract. Urol Clin North Am 2002;29(3):625–635.
2. Abeshouse B, Abeshouse G. Endometriosis of the urinary tract: a review of the literature and a report of four cases of vesical endometriosis. J Int Coll Surg 1960;34:43–63.
3. Antonelli A et al. Surgical treatment of ureteral obstruction from endometriosis: our experience with thirteen cases. Int Urogynecol J Pelvic Floor Dysfunct 2004;15(6):407–412; discussion 412.
4. Weingertner AS et al. The use of JJ stent in the management of deep endometriosis lesion, affecting or potentially affecting the ureter: a review of our practice. Br J Obstet Gynaecol 2008;115(9):1159–1164.
5. Camanni M et al. Laparoscopic conservative management of ureteral endometriosis: a survey of eighty patients submitted to ureterolysis. Reprod Biol Endocrinol 2009;7:109.
6. Nezhat C et al. Urinary tract endometriosis treated by laparoscopy. Fertil Steril 1996;66(6):920–924.
7. Ghezzi F et al. Outcome of laparoscopic ureterolysis for ureteral endometriosis. Fertil Steril 2006;86(2):418–422.
8. Abrao MS et al. Endometriosis of the ureter and bladder are not associated diseases. Fertil Steril 2009;91(5):1662–1667.

9. Antonelli A et al. Clinical aspects and surgical treatment of urinary tract endometriosis: our experience with 31 cases. Eur Urol 2006;49(6):1093–1097; discussion 1097–1098.

10. Chatterjee S. Scar endometriosis: a clinicopathologic study of 17 cases. Obstet Gynecol 1980;56(1):81–84.

11. Westney O, Amundsen C, McGuire E. Bladder endometriosis: conservative management. J Urol 2000;163(6):1814–1817.

12. Sircus S, Sant G, Ucci A Jr. Bladder detrusor endometriosis mimicking interstitial cystitis. Urology 1988;32(4):339–342.

13. Donnez J, Nisolle M, Squifflet J. Ureteral endometriosis: a complication of rectovaginal endometriotic (adenomyotic) nodules. Fertil Steril 2002;77(1):32–37.

14. Vercellini P et al. The pathogenesis of bladder detrusor endometriosis. Am J Obstet Gynecol 2002;187(3):538–542.

15. Seracchioli R et al. Importance of retroperitoneal ureteric evaluation in cases of deep infiltrating endometriosis. J Minim Invasive Gynecol 2008;15(4):435–439.

16. Generao S, Keene K, Das S. Endoscopic diagnosis and management of ureteral endometriosis. J EndoUrol 2005;19(10):1177–1179.

17. Clement PB. Endometriosis, lesions of the secondary mullerian system, and pelvic mesothelial proliferations. In: Kurman R (ed) Blaustein's Pathology of the Female Genital Tract, 3rd edn. New York: Springer-Verlag, 1987, pp. 516–559.

18. Al-Khawaja M et al. Ureteral endometriosis: clinicopathological and immunohistochemical study of 7 cases. Hum Pathol 2008;39(6):954–959.

19. Parker RL et al. Polypoid endometriosis: a clinicopathologic analysis of 24 cases and a review of the literature. Am J Surg Pathol 2004;28(3):285–297.

20. Donnez J, Brosens I. Definition of ureteral endometriosis? Fertil Steril 1997;68(1):178–180.

21. Schneider A et al. Endometriosis of the urinary tract in women of reproductive age. Int J Urol 2006;13(7):902–904.

22. Stillwell T, Kramer S, Lee R. Endometriosis of ureter. Urology 1986;28(2):81–85.

23. Kinkel K et al. Diagnosis of endometriosis with imaging: a review. Eur Radiol 2006;16(2):285–298.

24. Wong-You-Cheong JJ et al. From the archives of the AFIP: inflammatory and nonneoplastic bladder masses: radiologic-pathologic correlation. Radiographics 2006;26(6):1847–1868.

25. Rivlin ME et al. Leuprolide acetate in the management of ureteral obstruction caused by endometriosis. Obstet Gynecol 1990;75 (3 Pt 2):532–536.

26. Perez-Utrilla Perez M et al. Urinary tract endometriosis: clinical, diagnostic, and therapeutic aspects. Urology 2009;73(1):47–51.

27. Walid M, Heaton R. Laparoscopic partial cystectomy for bladder endometriosis. Arch Gynecol Obstet 2009;280(1):131–135.

28. Frenna V et al. Laparoscopic management of ureteral endometriosis: our experience. J Minim Invasive Gynecol 2007;14(2):169–171.

29. Nezhat C, Rottenberg H. Laparoscopic ureteroneocystostomy and vesicopsoas hitch with double ureter for infiltrative endometriosis: a case report. J Reprod Med 2009;54(6):407–410.

30. Nezhat C, Nezhat F. Laparoscopic repair of ureter resected during operative laparoscopy. Obstet Gynecol 1992;80(3 Pt 2):543–544.

31. Ostrzenski A, Radolinski B, Ostrzenska K. A review of laparoscopic ureteral injury in pelvic surgery. Obstet Gynecol Surv 2003; 58(12):794–799.

32. Bosev D, Nicoll LM, Bhagan L et al. Laparoscopic management of ureteral endometriosis: the Stanford University Hospital experience with 96 consecutive cases. J Urol 2009;182:2748–2752.

33. Chen HY et al. Failure of laparoscopy to relieve ureteral obstruction secondary to endometriosis. Taiwan J Obstet Gynecol 2006;45(2): 142–145.

34. Boari A. Contributo sperimentale alla plastica dell'uretere. Atti Accad Sci Med E Nat In Ferrara 1894;68:149.

35. Passerini-Glazel G et al. Technical options in complex ureteral lesions: 'ureter-sparing' surgery. Eur Urol 1994;25(4):273–280.

36. Nezhat CH et al. Laparoscopic vesicopsoas hitch for infiltrative ureteral endometriosis. Fertil Steril 1999;71(2):376–379.

37. Teber D et al. Prevention and management of ureteral injuries occurring during laparoscopic radical prostatectomy: the Heilbronn experience and a review of the literature. World J Urol 2009; 27(5):613–618.

38. Williams S, Leveillee R. Expanding the horizons: robot-assisted reconstructive surgery of the distal ureter. J EndoUrol 2009;23(3): 457–461.

39. Schimpf M, Wagner J. Robot-assisted laparoscopic distal ureteral surgery. JSLS 2009;13(1):44–49.

40. Klein R, Cattolica E. Ureteral endometriosis. Urology 1979;13(5): 477–482.

41. Seracchioli R et al. A multidisciplinary, minimally invasive approach for complicated deep infiltrating endometriosis. Fertil Steril 2010; 93(3):1007.

43 Surgical Therapies: Robotics and Endometriosis

Camran Nezhat, Arathi Veeraswamy and Chandhana Paka

Center for Special Minimally Invasive and Robotic Surgery and Stanford University Medical Center, Palo Alto, CA, USA

Introduction

Since the late 1990s, the use of computer-assisted or robotic technology in minimally invasive gynecological surgery has increased. Advocates of robotic-assisted gynecological surgery revere the system's wristed instrumentation, ergonomic positioning, and three-dimensional high-definition vision system as significant improvements over laparoscopic equipment's four degrees of freedom (DOF) and the two-dimensional laparoscope which means the surgeon has to stand throughout a procedure. With improvements in operative times, decreased blood loss, and decrease in length of stay after surgery, the computer-enhanced technology (robot) has enabled surgeons to perform procedures laparoscopically which were formerly performed by laparotomy, while giving patients the benefits of minimally invasive surgery. However, the cost, lack of haptic feedback, and the bulky size of the equipment make robotics less attractive to others. Robotic assistance has also been applied to multiple procedures for infertility, myomectomies [1], urogynecology problems and gynecological oncology [2] with good success and relatively low morbidity.

The current debate regarding robotic-assisted laparoscopy is being met with the same skepticism that advanced operative laparoscopy met in the 1980s and 1990s [3,4]. However, without a doubt, Nezhat's introduction of video laparoscopy has revolutionalized minimally invasive surgery, making it a feasible and appropriate option for many surgical procedures [5]. Now, no one would argue that open would be a better route when a procedure can be done laparoscopically.

Surgeons who have adopted minimally invasive techniques are embracing the clinical benefits of laparoscopy, including shorter postoperative hospital stays and improved cosmesis. Moreover, these surgeons are responding to the market pressure of what patients want. It is just a matter of time until technology allows surgeons to perform all elective procedures through smaller incisions or no incisions at all. Robotics is a major example of the technology that will contribute to the advancement of minimally invasive surgery (MIS).

Slow adoption into minimally invasive surgery

Since Nezhat's collaborative work with robotic pioneers Ajit Shah and Phil Green from the Stanford Research Institute, who developed the Da Vinci robot in the 1990s, others have successfully applied this technology to various fields [6]. We have reported a variety of gynecological surgeries, such as myomectomies, treatment of endometriosis, total and supracervical hysterectomy, ovarian cystectomy, sacral colpopexy and the Moskowitz procedure [6]. In 2001, the da Vinci™ robotics platform by Intuitive was approved for use by the Food and Drug Administration. This platform is a master-slave system where the surgeon sits at a console and directs either 8 mm or 5 mm instruments inside the patient through endoscopic trocars. The robot eliminates the counterintuitive motion of standard laparoscopy and aligns the eyes and hands over the area of interest with improved ergonomics. It allows an increased freedom of instrument movement by allowing wristed and finger movements that standard laparoscopic instruments do not have. This increases the DOF from four movements to seven, allowing more precision in the surgical field which more closely mimics open surgery. The robot minimizes instrument tremor from the console to the patient. It has three-dimensional stereoscopic vision with its dual-camera technology. This allows depth perception not seen on a standard laparoscopic monitor. However, the greatest weakness of the current platform is decreased tactile feedback on the tissue, requiring the surgeon to utilize visual

Endometriosis: Science and Practice, First Edition. Edited by Linda C. Giudice, Johannes L.H. Evers and David L. Healy.
© 2012 Blackwell Publishing Ltd. Published 2012 by Blackwell Publishing Ltd.

cues over tactile cues. Despite this limitation, the platform is a reliable and durable way to be very precise in surgical dissection and reconstruction.

The three basic factors for adoption of technology such as the surgical robot into MIS are the surgeon's endoscopic skill level, equipment limitations and procedure complexity high enough to justify the need for robotic precision. If these three factors balance, there will be greater adoption of robotics in gynecological surgery.

The robot currently has limited instrumentation for surgical stapling or a sealing and cutting instrument. Many general laparoscopic procedures require movement in many quadrants around the abdomen, which is also difficult for the robot. During surgery for endometriosis, after initial evaluation of the abdomen and pelvis with the laparoscope, the more complex procedures may lend themselves to robotic maneuvering.

Factors to consider when choosing a robotic surgical approach include disease type, extent of disease, preoperative imaging, stage, patient age, Body Mass Index, parity, size of lesion(s), and equipment availability. There are currently no published guidelines on patient selection as it relates to robotic surgery in gynecology. We recommend that the robot be used to convert laparotomy to laparoscopies. The size and weight of the patient often play a limited role in the decision to proceed with robotic surgery. The main factor is the ability of the patient to tolerate steep Trendelenburg, which is necessary to complete the surgery. Patients with multiple (non-pulmonary) co-morbidities need not be excluded from a robotic surgical approach if anesthesia clears them.

Diagnostic laparoscopy

Initially, the surgeon explores the pelvic cavity to assess the extent of disease and identify abnormalities or distortions of the pelvic organs. The location and boundaries of the bladder, ureter, colon, rectum, pelvic gutters, uterosacral ligaments, and major blood vessels are noted. The upper abdominal organs, abdominal walls, liver, and diaphragm should be evaluated for endometriosis or any other condition that may contribute to the patient's symptoms. The omentum and the small bowel are evaluated for disease and to ensure that they were not injured during insertion of the Veress needle or trocar. A rectovaginal examination is accomplished to evaluate deep and retroperitoneal endometriosis found in the lower pelvis in the rectovaginal septum, uterosacral ligament, lower colon, and pararectal area. Deep retroperitoneal endometriosis is rare without a connection to the surface peritoneum. In 15% of patients with endometriosis, the appendix is involved and should be examined [7]. An implant that has penetrated several centimeters retroperitoneally is called an "iceberg" lesion. It can be detected laparoscopically by palpating areas of the pelvis and bowel with the suction-irrigator probe. With the forceps or probe, endometriotic implants are examined to gauge size, depth, and proximity to normal pelvic structures.

Surgical management of endometriosis

The optimum management of endometriosis remains as problematic as ever. Endometriosis may be either symptomatic or associated with minor symptoms and lesions that are sometimes self-limiting. It may also be associated with very severe symptoms and major pathological lesions involving the vital structures of the pelvis. Different levels of symptomatology and pathology require different levels of therapeutic intervention [8]. The extent of surgery is thus dependent on the preoperative symptoms and the severity of disease. Most clinicians use the revised American Society for Reproductive Medicine (ASRM) scoring system for endometriosis, which comprises four groups:
- minimal (stage I)
- mild (stage II)
- moderate (stage III)
- severe (stage IV)

according to the operative findings [9].

With the appropriate facilities, the experienced surgeon can perform complex endometriosis operations. These include extensive peritoneal dissection, cul-de-sac and rectovaginal dissection, resection of invasive bowel endometriosis, appendectomy, treatment of invasive ovarian endometriosis or endometriomas, removal of tubal endometriosis, resection of bladder endometriosis, resection of ureteral endometriosis, removal of uterine endometriosis, uterosacral nerve ablation, presacral neurectomy, endometriosis of diaphragm, lungs and liver [10–13].

Many surgeons early on are best advised to dock only three arms of the system until the potential trocar and arm interference issues are understood and managed. After the procedure has been tried and analyzed, adding the fourth arm to the operation makes great sense. Again, robotic general surgeons need to evolve their procedures because a standard robotic approach does not usually exist [6]. Various treatment modalities are available for use in robotic surgery [14]. These include cautery hook, scissors with monopolar electrocautery, and bipolar coagulation, all of which allow resection, cauterization and vaporization of endometriosis. In a prospective study, laparoscopic excision of endometriosis significantly reduced pain and improved quality of life for up to 5 years [15]. The above results could be extrapolated to robotic surgery as we gain more experience and more studies are done. Promising results have been obtained with more radical surgery, including extensive excision of deep disease and also removal of portions of bowel and bladder containing significant endometriosis [14].

There may be a continuing role for hysterectomy in the management of endometriosis, but the evidence for concomitant oophorectomy is less convincing. Farquhar and Steiner [16] reported that only 10% of hysterectomies were performed minimally invasively with the assistance of laparoscopy. Robotics has been looked upon as an enabling device to facilitate the trend towards laparoscopy [17]. Robotic surgery may bridge the gap between laparotomy and laparoscopy for trachelectomy in complicated cases [18]. Although robots may not alter the outcomes of endoscopic surgery, they will enable more laparotomies to be converted to minimally invasive surgery.

Gastrointestinal involvement

The gastrointestinal tract is believed to be involved in 3–37% of women with endometriosis [19]. Severe endometriosis commonly involves the uterosacral ligaments, rectovaginal septum, and rectosigmoid colon with partial or complete posterior cul-de-sac obliteration. Patients may present with lower abdominal pain, back pain, dysmenorrhea, dyspareunia, diarrhea, constipation, tenesmus, and occasionally rectal bleeding. Symptoms usually occur cyclically or are temporarily related to the time of menstruation.

We have reported the frequency and spectrum of histologically proven diseases of the appendix in patients undergoing laparoscopic surgery for chronic pelvic pain in conjunction with endometriosis [20]. Incidental robotic appendectomy can be performed safely without the need for switching to conventional laparoscopy. It should be considered in patients undergoing robotic pelvic surgery for pelvic pain and ovarian malignancy [7,21].

Though slower to gain acceptance, laparoscopic colorectal surgery has gained in popularity, and in experienced hands is now regarded as a safe and feasible alternative to open surgery. Robotic approaches to the rectum appear attractive for the same reasons that robotic prostatectomy has been accepted. The pelvis is a small area with limited visibility and room for dissection. The robotic precision and visualization should allow for excellent rectal dissection in the pelvis.

Robotics in colorectal surgery have demonstrated several advantages over traditional laparoscopic surgery [22]. First, the operating surgeon has a unique three-dimensional stereoscopic view of the operative field, with adjustable magnification (×10) and a stable camera platform, directly controlled (using a foot-pedal) and thus not reliant on an assistant. Second, the surgeon also gains three extra degrees of motion that are lost with conventional laparoscopy by using articulated instruments which more closely simulate the movements of the human wrist. In addition, robotic surgeons benefit from tremor filtering and motion scaling (up- or downscaling). In short, the robotic surgeon can achieve an unparalleled level of precision and control during operative dissection.

It has been postulated that these characteristics of robotic surgery can facilitate certain steps in colorectal procedures and thereby reduce conversion rates. These include dissection of the inferior mesenteric vessels [22], autonomic nerve preservation, rectal mobilization, ureter and gonadal vessel identification, dissection in the narrow pelvis, and suturing [22].

A recently published paper by Nezhat *et al* discusses the various procedures performed via laparoscopy and robotically [23]. While intracorporeal anastomosis is not routinely required in colorectal surgery, the ability to suture accurately is advantageous in certain instances, including rectopexy and salvage of a disrupted staple line in the pelvis. A total of 31 complications of robotic colorectal surgery have been reported from all studies reviewed, representing an 11% morbidity rate. Only two of these were specific to use of the robot. The aforementioned injuries to the bowel by robotic graspers

are proposed to result from a lack of force feedback in the current generation of robots. The absence of tensile feedback necessitates the use of visual clues to sense undue pull on the bowel or mesentery to reduce tissue damage [22]. Wexner *et al* recently suggested that this drawback may be so significant as to offset benefits such as tremor filtering [24].

In patients who have severe disease of the bowel wall, resection may be necessary [25,26]. Nezhat *et al* reported the first series of laparoscopic partial proctectomies performed without a separate surgical incision for rectovaginal endometriosis [26–28]. Sixteen women were treated for extensive endometriosis invading the rectal wall [26]. Laparoscopically assisted anterior rectal wall resection and anastomosis were described in 1991 to treat symptomatic, infiltrative rectosigmoid endometriosis [28,29]. A hybrid technique of laparoscopic and robotic assistance in the resection of mid- to low-rectal cancer (total mesorectal excision) has been published [30]. Laparoscopic approach was used to isolate the inferior mesenteric artery and for mobilization of the left colon. The da Vinci robot was used in the dissection of the rectum down to the pelvic floor. A similar technique with modifications could be applied with deep infiltrating endometriosis.

Suturing is one of the main tasks in advanced laparoscopic surgery, but limited degrees of freedom, two-dimensional vision, fulcrum and pivoting effect make it difficult to perform. Performance studies have shown that the needle can be grabbed and handled more easily with the robot due to motion scaling, tremor filtration and three-dimensional view. The additional DOF allows intuitive motion and manipulation of the needle. These benefits increase the dexterity and accuracy of grabbing the needle at the right position. The robotic system allows easy tying, as in hand-sewn anastomoses, due to the endowrist instrument tip. Especially inexperienced users profit from the easy and intuitive loading of the thread in a loop on the instrument and from being able to precisely catch the end of it [31,32]. However, the lack of haptic feedback may result in an increased risk of damaging threads, especially when performed by inexperienced users [33]. It has to be emphasized that for experienced robotic surgeons, this does not represent a problem because they develop a "visual feeling" for the tension of the suture. The magnified view gives the surgeon a relatively small view of the operation area. Therefore the largest part of the thread is usually out of sight, especially when the view is blocked by an instrument. As a consequence, it can easily happen that the thread is pulled out and out when drawing the thread through. Moreover, grasping and handling the suture material with the power of robotic instruments in combination with the lack of haptic feedback may easily lead to thread breakage or damage, resulting in weaker sutures or additional working time [34]. However, after a short learning curve, most users are able to handle the instruments safely [35].

During robotic procedures a short, preliminary part of the operation, consisting of proper positioning of the loops of small bowel and lysis of major adhesions between the loops of bowel and the abdominal wall, is performed laparoscopically. The rest of the procedure, including the lysis of adhesions between the loops of bowel, complete dissection, and transection of the colon, is then completely performed with the robot. After exteriorization of the specimen, transanal anastomosis is done laparoscopically. If the anastomosis is hand sewn, it can be done intracorporeally with the robot or extracorporeally.

In left colon and sigmoid disease, the patient is placed supine with the legs apart in a 25–30° Trendelenburg position with a 10–15° right lateral rotation and shoulder supports. The assistant surgeon stands on the patient's left side. An intraumbilical port is inserted after achieving pneumoperitoneum and a 30° standard 12 mm robotic laparoscope is inserted through the port. The da Vinci trocars are placed under direct vision: one 8 mm instrument port in the right hypochondrium between the umbilicus and the costal margin for a grasping forceps and the other in the right suprapubic area, 3 or 4 cm to the right of the mini-laparotomy line, for the ultrasound dissector, shears, and other tools. An additional 12 mm port is created in the right McBurney area for the assistant surgeon to insert the stapler and mechanical suture instruments. The da Vinci system is positioned beside the patient's left shoulder.

For resections of the lower rectum, there are two steps involved in the robotic system's placement. The first is the same as for left colon and sigmoid colon resections, to mobilize the spleen flexure. The second consists of moving the da Vinci system down to the coxa area and introducing another trocar (the fifth) in the left McBurney area on the lateral margin of the abdominis rectus muscle for the grasping forceps. In the right McBurney area, the right robot arm is replaced with the ultrasound dissector. Then the assistant surgeon uses the 12 mm port in the right hypochondrium. A Pfannenstiel mini-laparotomy is performed to extract the resected colon in both procedures. In the Miles procedure, the steps are the same as for rectum resection but the resected colon is removed from the abdomen through the left McBurney laparotomy used to perform the colostomy.

Robotic suturing tends to be superior to laparoscopic suturing in terms of time, safety and patency. D'Annibale *et al* demonstrated that robotic and laparoscopic techniques can achieve the same operative and postoperative results. The dexterity and flexibility of the da Vinci system may be useful in certain stages of the surgical procedure (dissection of the inferior mesenteric artery with identification of the nervous plexus, and dissection of a narrow pelvis). As experience is gained with this device, it will likely be recommended for use in selected patients and institutions [36].

Genitourinary endometriosis

Endometriosis may spread to the urinary system in 1–2% of women with symptomatic endometriosis. Endometriosis of the urinary tract tends to be superficial but may be invasive and cause complete ureteral obstruction [37–39], decreased bladder capacity and stability unresponsive to conventional therapy. Clinicians should consider endometriosis in cases of refractory and unexplained urinary complaints. If urinary tract endometriosis is suspected, an intravenous pyelogram (IVP), ultrasound of the kidneys, and routine blood and urine work-up are indicated. In selected cases of recurrent hematuria, cystoscopy is suggested.

Vesical endometriosis

Although the bladder wall is one of the sites least frequently involved with endometriosis, the bladder is the most commonly affected site in the urinary system, followed by the ureter and the kidney in a ratio of 40:5:1 [40,41]. Patient presentation is quite variable, and symptoms may consist of suprapubic discomfort, pelvic pain, dysmenorrhea, dysuria, urinary frequency, urgency, microscopic hematuria, and even cyclical gross hematuria.

Endometriomas are typically solitary and most frequently involve the dome and posterior wall of the bladder because of the relative location of the uterus to the bladder. However, involvement of other locations of the bladder may occur. The lesions tend to invade the detrusor musculature in an extrinsic fashion and often remain submucosal. If the lesions are superficial, hydrodissection and vaporization or excision may be adequate for removal. Using hydrodissection, the areolar tissue between the serosa and muscularis beneath the implants is dissected. The lesion is circumcised, and fluid is injected into the resulting defect. The lesion is grasped with forceps and dissected. Treatment of a patient with severe pelvic and infiltrative bladder endometriosis with mucosal involvement using robotic-assisted laparoscopic excision and partial bladder resection was first reported in 2008 [42,43].

Ureteral involvement by endometriosis is rare and occurs in 0.1–0.4% of cases. It most commonly affects the distal ureter, less commonly the mid-ureter, and rarely the proximal ureter [44,45]. Lesions are typically extrinsic, with a smaller fraction of cases involving the lumen of the ureter (i.e. intrinsic). The extrinsic-to-intrinsic ratio has been reported at 3:1 to 4:1, and the left ureter appears to be more frequently involved [46,47]. In cases of ureteral involvement, the patient typically has concomitant pelvic endometriosis that causes external compression, inflammation, and fibrosis of the involved ureter. The patient may present with symptoms of renal colic, hematuria, or silent urinary obstruction with loss of renal function.

In cases in which extrinsic ureteral involvement is minimal, ureterolysis alone may be all that is needed. The principles of success include atraumatic handling of the ureter and, when feasible, interposition of normal tissue, such as omentum. Superficial implants over the ureter are treated with hydrodissection, vaporization or excision of lesions with a circumference of 1–2 cm. When the lesions are large or excision is preferred, a circular line with a 1–2 cm margin is made around the lesion. The peritoneum is held with grasping forceps and peeled away with the help of a robotic cautery hook. As a result, depending on the extent of ureteral involvement, ureterolysis with or without ureteral resection can be performed safely and effectively with the robot.

In the majority of cases, only the distal third of the ureter is involved, and when the length of the involved ureter is short (≤2 cm), resection followed by an end-to-end ureteroureterostomy may be performed. The ultimate goal is to avoid ureteral obstruction and loss of renal function. Success is dependent on careful preoperative evaluation, surgical planning, and careful postoperative follow-up. Radiological imaging, laparoscopy, and ureteroscopy are useful techniques for disease staging that the laparoscopic surgeon should be familiar with. Complete resection remains the mainstay of therapy in cases refractory to conservative medical management. Urinary symptoms generally resolve, and recurrence generally does not occur provided that the lesion is completely resected.

Laparoscopic reconstructive surgery may be performed for the management of distal and mid-ureteric strictures, but difficulty with intracorporeal suturing and prolonged operative times remain distinct disadvantages. The robotic surgical system is particularly well suited for the management of complex reconstructive procedures like ureteroneocystostomy.

Ureteral reimplantation

The first laparoscopic ureteroneocystostomy was reported by Nezhat *et al* in 1992 [48]. As the world-wide experience with laparoscopic procedures has increased, surgeons are including robotic surgery in their armamentarium. Reusable instruments for the robotic system include forceps, needle drivers and curved scissors.

The procedures begin by incising the retroperitoneum along the line of Toldt and medializing the colon (cecum on the right and sigmoid colon on the left). The ureter can then be visualized at this level in the groove between the psoas muscle and the common iliac artery.

The ureter once identified is carefully dissected down to the level of the obstruction. Isolation of the obstructed segment may occasionally be challenging because of previous inflammation, infection or scarring. It is essential that during ureteric dissection, care is taken to preserve the ureteric blood supply to prevent excessive devascularization. The ureter is transected just superior to the level of the obstruction and spatulated using robotic Pott's or curved scissors. A suitably sized double J ureteral stent is passed with the aid of a guidewire through the assistance trocars in a retrograde manner into the proximal ureter and kidney.

The bladder is then filled with approximately 500 ml of normal saline via an indwelling Foley catheter. This aids dissection and mobilization of the bladder from surrounding peritoneal attachments and in the development of the space of Retzius. The division of the contralateral superior vesicle pedicle may achieve additional bladder mobilization, although this step can be skipped for mid-ureteral strictures.

A detrusor incision is made on the bladder dome posteriorly for a distance of 2–3 cm, a 2 cm ellipse of bulging mucosa is then excised and tagged with an absorbable stitch to prevent mucosal retraction. The ureter is placed in the bed thus made and the muscle closed loosely over the ureter. The distal end of the J stent is threaded into the bladder , after the posterior wall of the anastomosis is completed, a watertight drain is placed near the anastomosis and brought out through the most lateral abdominal skin incision.

The robot provides distinct advantages over standard laparoscopy for reconstruction. It allows for precision in movement by the elimination of hand tremor, which is essential for the meticulous dissection of the ureter. This precision in movement is important for adequate preservation of the tenuous ureteral

blood supply and surrounding vital structures, particularly when the ureter is embedded in dense fibrous tissue. Robotic instruments have seven degrees of freedom of motion which allows for bidirectional articulation and grasp that mimics the hand movements of the surgeon and makes intracorporeal suturing within the pelvis more precise. Adequate dissection of the bladder and ureter and precise suturing are essential to create a tension-free, well-vascularized anastomosis [49].

If additional ureter length is needed, a vesicopsoas hitch with or without a vesical flap may be performed [47]. The detrusor fiber of the bladder is tacked down to the psoas with either an absorbable or non-absorbable suture to minimize tension on the reimplanted ureter [50]. The surgeon should be aware of the location of the genitofemoral nerve as it crosses the surface of the psoas. The stitch is usually placed parallel to the nerve, either lateral or medial to it to avoid nerve entrapment. Should additional length be required, the contralateral superior vesical pedicles can be divided to give upward mobility to the bladder. Rarely, a vesical flap or an ileal ureter may also be used for replacement of the entire ureter [47–51].

Except for simple cases of ureterolysis in which ureter manipulation is minimal, a double J ureteral stent is placed and left indwelling for 3–6 weeks. In clinic follow-up, the stent is removed and an IVP is typically obtained in 3–4 weeks to assess ureter anatomy and rule out strictures. A renal bladder ultrasound may also be useful in assessment of hydronephrosis.

Restoration of tubo-ovarian anatomy

Once all lesions are resected or ablated and the adnexa are freed of adhesions, the anatomical relationship between the ovary and ipsilateral tube is evaluated and any distortion caused by adhesions is corrected. The mesosalpinx often adheres to the ovarian cortex along the ampullary segment of the tube. These adhesions cover a significant part of the surface of the ovarian cortex and may interfere with the ovulatory process at oocyte release. Moreover, the fimbriae frequently are agglutinated, inhibiting their ability to capture the oocyte. Adhesiolysis along the ovarian surface and mesosalpinx can be accomplished; the ovary and tube are grasped with atraumatic forceps and pulled apart, and the plane between them is dissected with electrode or scissors.

Relief of pain

A randomized, blinded, cross-over study was done to examine the effect on pain and quality of life for women with all stages of endometriosis undergoing minimally invasive surgery compared with placebo surgery [52]. Thirty-nine women were randomized to receive initially either a diagnostic procedure or full excisional surgery. After 6 months, repeat laparoscopy was performed, with removal of any pathology present. More women in the group who were operated on according to protocol reported symptomatic improvement after excisional surgery than in the placebo group: 16/20 (80%) versus 6/19 (32%). Other aspects of quality of life were also significantly improved 6 months after excisional surgery but not after placebo. Progression of disease at second surgery was demonstrated for women having only an initial diagnostic procedure in 45% of cases, with disease remaining static in 33% and improving in 22% of cases. Non-responsiveness to surgery was reported in 20% of cases.

As a conclusion, laparoscopic excision of endometriosis was more effective than placebo at reducing pain and improving quality of life. Our recent paper discusses use of robots for complex endometriosis [23].

Fertility outcomes after minimally invasive surgery for endometriosis

A 50% pregnancy rate was obtained after laparoscopic management in a series of 814 women with endometriomas [53]. It could be that the removal or destruction of endometriomas provides further benefit than simply restoring the normal anatomy and ovarian structure. However, because of the progressive nature of the disease in many patients, combined with the largest prospective, randomized trial demonstrating improved fecundity with therapy at the time of surgery, it appears prudent to ablate endometriotic lesions at the time of endoscopic surgery in patients with minimal and mild endometriosis [54–56].

The question of whether the presence of endometriosis affects the outcome of women undergoing IVF has not been resolved, with some authors noting negative associations and others noting no association. In a meta-analysis, Barnhart *et al* [57] investigated the IVF outcome for patients with endometriosis and found that patients with endometriosis have a more than 50% reduction in pregnancy rate after IVF compared with women with tubal factor infertility. In May 2004, the Practice Committee of the ASRM recommended that when laparoscopy is performed, the surgeon should consider safely ablating or excising visible lesions of endometriosis [58]. In younger women with stage I/II endometriosis-associated infertility, expectant management or superovulation/intrauterine insemination (IUI) after laparoscopy may be considered. Women 35 years of age or older should be treated with superovulation/IUI or IVF embryo transfer. In women with stage III/IV endometriosis-associated infertility, conservative surgical therapy with laparoscopy and possible laparotomy is indicated.

Conclusion

At the current time we do not have adequate controlled studies with the robot. Nonetheless, the next few years are likely to show an explosion in minimally invasive robotic surgery as more operations are being described and published showing clinical benefits. Areas of improvement presently being developed include systems with improved tactile feedback, multifunctioning instruments and robotic miniaturization. New instrumentation such as robotically controlled stapling devices will push the adoption even further. It is likely that robotic surgery will replace standard laparoscopy for complex procedures, as well as simple cases which will be performed through single incision or natural orifice approaches. Digital platforms have the power to interact with other informational systems such as computed tomography to allow augmented reality of the surgical field. Promising innovations in scaling down the footprint of robotic platforms, the early experience with mobile miniaturized *in vivo* robots, advances in endoscopic navigation systems using augmented reality technologies and tracking devices, the emergence of technologies for robotic natural orifice transluminal endoscopic surgery and single-port surgery, advances in flexible robotics and haptics, the development of new virtual reality simulator training platforms compatible with the existing da Vinci system, and recent experiences with remote robotic surgery and telestration all suggest that robotic surgery may become the standard minimally invasive surgical technique and that standard mechanical laparoscopy is a passing phase [59].

References

1. Nezhat C, Lavie O, Hsu S, Watson J, Barnett O, Lemyre M. Robotic-assisted laparoscopic myomectomy compared with standard laparoscopic myomectomy – a retrospective matched control study. Fertil Steril 2009;91(2):556–559.

2. Nezhat FR, Datta MS, Liu C, Chuang L, Zakashansky K. Robotic radical hysterectomy versus total laparoscopic radical hysterectomy with pelvic lymphadenectomy for treatment of early cervical cancer. JSLS 2008;12(3):227–237.

3. Nezhat C, Garrison CP. Surgical treatment of endometriosis via laser laparoscopy. Fertil Steril 1986;45:778–83.

4. Kelley WE. The evolution of laparoscopy and the revolution in surgery decade of the 1990s. JSLS. 2008;12(4):351–7.

5. Page B. Camran Nezhat & the advent of advanced operative video-laparoscopy. In: Nezhat C, editor. Nezhat's History of Endoscopy. Tuttlingen, Germany: Endo Press; 2011:159–87.

6. Nezhat C, Saberi NS, Shahmohamady B, Nezhat F. Robotic-assisted laparoscopy in gynecological surgery. JSLS 2006;10(3):317–320.

7. Nezhat C, Nezhat F. Incidental appendectomy during videolaseroscopy. Am J Obstet Gynecol 1991;165(3):559–564.

8. Garry R. The effectiveness of laparoscopic excision of endometriosis. Curr Opin Obstet Gynecol 2004;16(4):299–303.

9. Revised American Fertility Society classification of endometriosis: 1985. Fertil Steril 1985;43(3):351–352.

10. Nezhat C, Seidman DS, Nezhat F. Laparoscopic surgical management of diaphragmatic endometriosis. Fertil Steril 1998;69(6): 1048–1055.

11. Nezhat C, Nicoll LM, Bhagan L et al. Endometriosis of the diaphragm: four cases treated with a combination of laparoscopy and thoracoscopy. J Minim Invasive Gynecol 2009;16(5):573–580.

12. Nezhat C, Nezhat F. Surgery for endometriosis of the bowel, bladder, ureter, and diaphragm. Ann N Y Acad Sci 1997;828:332–340.

13. Nezhat C, Kazerooni T, Berker B, Lashay N, Fernandez S, Marziali M. Laparoscopic management of hepatic endometriosis: report of two cases and review of the literature. J Minim Invasive Gynecol 2005;12(3):196–200.

14. Nezhat C, Lavie O, Lemyre M, Unal E, Nezhat CH, Nezhat F. Robot-assisted laparoscopic surgery in gynecology: scientific dream or reality? Fertil Steril 2009;91(6):2620–2622.

15. Davis CJ, McMillan L. Pain in endometriosis: effectiveness of medical and surgical management. Curr Opin Obstet Gynecol 2003;15(6):507–512.

16. Farquhar CM, Steiner CA. Hysterectomy rates in the United States 1990–1997. Obstet Gynecol 2002;99(2):229–234.

17. Nezhat C, Lavie O, Lemyre M, Gemer O, Bhagan L. Laparoscopic hysterectomy with and without a robot: Stanford experience. JSLS 2009;13(2):125–128.

18. Nezhat CH, Rogers JD. Robot-assisted laparoscopic trachelectomy after supracervical hysterectomy. Fertil Steril 2008;90(3):850.

19. Samper ER, Slagle GW, Hand AM. Colonic endometriosis: its clinical spectrum. South Med J 1984;77(7):912–914.

20. Berker B, Lashay N, Davarpanah R, Marziali M, Nezhat CH, Nezhat C. Laparoscopic appendectomy in patients with endometriosis. J Minim Invasive Gynecol 2005;12(3):206–209.

21. Akl MN, Magrina JF, Kho RM, Magtibay PM. Robotic appendectomy in gynaecological surgery: technique and pathological findings. Int J Med Robot 2008;4(3):210–213.

22. Mirnezami AH, Mirnezami R, Venkatasubramaniam AK, Chandrakumaran K, Cecil TD, Moran BJ. Robotic colorectal surgery: hype or new hope? A systematic review of robotics in colorectal surgery. Colorectal Dis 2010;12(11):1084–1093.

23. Nezhat C, Lewis M, Kotikela S et al. Robotic versus standard laparoscopy for the treatment of endometriosis. Fertil Steril 2010;94(7):2758–2760.

24. Wexner SD, Bergamaschi R, Lacy A et al. The current status of robotic pelvic surgery: results of a multinational interdisciplinary consensus conference. Surg Endosc 2009;23(2):438–43.

25. Nezhat C, Hood J, Winer W, Nexhat F, Crowgey SR, Garrison CP. Videolaseroscopy and laser laparoscopy in gynaecology. Br J Hosp Med 1987;38(3):219–224.

26. Nezhat F, Nezhat C, Pennington E, Ambroze W Jr. Laparoscopic segmental resection for infiltrating endometriosis of the rectosigmoid colon: a preliminary report. Surg Laparosc Endosc 1992;2(3):212–216.

27. Nezhat C, Nezhat FR. Safe laser endoscopic excision or vaporization of peritoneal endometriosis. Fertil Steril 1989;52(1):149–151.

28. Nezhat C, Pennington E, Nezhat F, Silfen SL. Laparoscopically assisted anterior rectal wall resection and reanastomosis for deeply infiltrating endometriosis. Surg Laparosc Endosc 1991;1(2):106–108.

29. Nezhat F, Nezhat C, Pennington E. Laparoscopic proctectomy for infiltrating endometriosis of the rectum. Fertil Steril 1992;57(5):1129–1132.

30. Prasad LM, de Souza AL, Marecik SJ, Park JJ, Abcarian H. Robotic pursestring technique in low anterior resection. Dis Colon Rectum 2010;53(2):230–234.

31. Hanly EJ, Talamini MA. Robotic abdominal surgery. Am J Surg 2004;188(4A Suppl):19S–26S.

32. Gutt CN, Oniu T, Mehrabi A, Kashfi A, Schemmer P, Buchler MW. Robot-assisted abdominal surgery. Br J Surg 2004;91(11):1390–1397.

33. Kuang W, Shin PR, Matin S, Thomas AJ Jr. Initial evaluation of robotic technology for microsurgical vasovasostomy. J Urol 2004;171(1):300–303.

34. Schoor RA, Ross LS, Niederberger CS. Re: initial evaluation of robotic technology for microsurgical vasovasostomy. J Urol 2004;172(2):780; author reply 781.

35. Begin E, Gagner M, Hurteau R, de Santis S, Pomp A. A robotic camera for laparoscopic surgery: conception and experimental results. Surg Laparosc Endosc 1995;5(1):6–11.

36. D'Annibale A, Morpurgo E, Fiscon V et al. Robotic and laparoscopic surgery for treatment of colorectal diseases. Dis Colon Rectum 2004;47(12):2162–2168.

37. Nezhat CH, Nezhat F, Seidman D, Nezhat C. Laparoscopic uretero-ureterostomy: a prospective follow-up of 9 patients. Prim Care Update Obstet Gynecol 1998 1;5(4):200.

38. Nezhat C, Nezhat F, Nezhat CH, Nasserbakht F, Rosati M, Seidman DS. Urinary tract endometriosis treated by laparoscopy. Fertil Steril 1996;66(6):920–924.

39. Nezhat CR, Nezhat F, Admon D, Seidman D, Nezhat CH. Laparoscopic management of genitourinary endometriosis. J Am Assoc Gynecol Laparosc 1994;1(4, Part 2):S25.

40. Abeshouse BS, Abeshouse G. Endometriosis of the urinary tract: a review of the literature and a report of four cases of vesical endometriosis. J Int Coll Surg 1960;34:43–63.

41. Nezhat C, Nezhat F. Laparoscopic repair of ureter resected during operative laparoscopy. Obstet Gynecol 1992;80(3 Pt 2):543–544.

42. Liu C, Perisic D, Samadi D, Nezhat F. Robotic-assisted laparoscopic partial bladder resection for the treatment of infiltrating endometriosis. J Minim Invasive Gynecol 2008;15(6):745–748.

43. Bosev D, Nicoll LM, Bhagan L et al. Laparoscopic management of ureteral endometriosis: the Stanford University hospital experience with 96 consecutive cases. J Urol 2009;182(6):2748–2752.

44. Antonelli A, Simeone C, Canossi E et al. Surgical approach to urinary endometriosis: experience on 28 cases. Arch Ital Urol Androl 2006; 78(1):35–38.

45. Gagnon RF, Arsenault D, Pichette V, Tanguay S. Acute renal failure in a young woman with endometriosis. Nephrol Dial Transplant 2001;16(7):1499–1502.

46. Bornstein A, Gaasch WH, Harrington J. Assessment of the cardiac effects of hemodialysis with systolic time intervals and echocardiography. Am J Cardiol 1983;51(2):332–335.

47. Antonelli A, Simeone C, Frego E, Minini G, Bianchi U, Cunico SC. Surgical treatment of ureteral obstruction from endometriosis: our experience with thirteen cases. Int Urogynecol J Pelvic Floor Dysfunct 2004;15(6):407–412; discussion 412.

48. Nezhat C, Nezhat F, Green B. Laparoscopic treatment of obstructed ureter due to endometriosis by resection and ureteroureterostomy: a case report. J Urol 1992;148(3):865–868.

49. Williams SK, Leveillee RJ. Expanding the horizons: robot-assisted reconstructive surgery of the distal ureter. J Endourol 2009;23(3):457–461.

50. Nezhat CH, Malik S, Nezhat F, Nezhat C. Laparoscopic ureteroneo-cystostomy and vesicopsoas hitch for infiltrative endometriosis. JSLS 2004;8(1):3–7.

51. Vercellini P, Pisacreta A, Pesole A, Vicentini S, Stellato G, Crosignani PG. Is ureteral endometriosis an asymmetric disease? Br J Obstet Gynecol 2000;107(4):559–561.

52. Abbott J, Hawe J, Hunter D, Holmes M, Finn P, Garry R. Laparoscopic excision of endometriosis: a randomized, placebo-controlled trial. Fertil Steril 2004;82(4):878–884.

53. Donnez J, Nisolle M, Gillet N, Smets M, Bassil S, Casanas-Roux F. Large ovarian endometriomas. Hum Reprod 1996;11(3): 641–646.

54. Winkel CA. Evaluation and management of women with endometriosis. Obstet Gynecol 2003;102(2):397–408.

55. Buyalos RP, Agarwal SK. Endometriosis-associated infertility. Curr Opin Obstet Gynecol 2000;12(5):377–381.

56. Nezhat C, Winer WK, Cooper JD, Nezhat F. Endoscopic infertility surgery. J Reprod Med 1989;34(2):127–134.

57. Barnhart K, Dunsmoor-Su R, Coutifaris C. Effect of endometriosis on in vitro fertilization. Fertil Steril 2002;77(6):1148–155.

58. Practice Committee of the ASRM. Endometriosis and infertility. Fertil Steril 2004;81(5):1441–1446.

59. Wilson EB. The evolution of robotic general surgery. Scand J Surg 2009;98(2):125–129.

9   Infertility and Endometriosis

44 Medical Therapy of Endometriosis: Subfertility

Johannes L. H. Evers

Centre for Reproductive Medicine and Biology, GROW, School of Oncology and Developmental Biology, Maastricht University Medical Centre, Maastricht, The Netherlands

Introduction

The fact that we live in the age of evidence-based medicine will not have escaped anyone. Clinical quality assurance and health technology assessment programs have moved into the focus of both political as well as medical attention. Whereas authority-driven medicine has served an important role for many years, patients nowadays request and deserve that we do not impose unfounded diagnostic tests and treatments on them, but provide evidence of their proven efficacy, their potential harm, and their eventual shortcomings.

Unfortunately, hard evidence is rare in reproductive medicine. Many of the diagnostic procedures we perform are not based on sound scientific evidence and many treatments lack robust objective evaluation. In endometriosis, numerous uncertainties come together, we do not understand the disease, we fail to appreciate its relationship – if any – with impaired fertility, we disagree on the means to make a firm diagnosis, and the disease so far escapes rational treatment. Endometriosis-associated impairment of fertility has been a heavily disputed issue among clinicians. The advent of clinical epidemiology, and later of evidence-based medicine, has introduced many question marks in our discourse of the causes and consequences of the disease.

Clinical epidemiology has long relied on Robert Koch's famous postulates for establishing causality. Wheeler and Malinak [1] have looked at these postulates in relation to endometriosis-associated subfertility. They concluded that no sound evidence exists from experiments in humans for the putative relationship between endometriosis and subfertility, that there is no strong statistical correlation – if any – of endometriosis with subfertility except for the severe cases with adhesions and endometriomas, that their association is not consistent from study to study, that the temporal relationship between the two is not correct

(endometriosis preceding subfertility complaints in some patients and vice versa in others), that there does not exist a dose–response relationship, that the association is not specific and that the situation in subfertile endometriosis patients does not show a clear analogy to proven causal relations in other fields of medicine. They concluded that they only could confirm that the association between clinically recognized endometriosis and decreased fertility may make some epidemiological and perhaps some biological sense [1]. From applying Koch's postulates to the endometriosis literature, they inferred that, in a clinical and epidemiological sense, there is insufficient scientific evidence for endometriosis and impaired fertility to be causally related.

When considering fertility in endometriosis patients, two clinical questions prevail: Do endometriosis patients suffer from impairment of fertility, and, if so, does treatment improve their pregnancy chances? In other words, does endometriosis affect fertility, and does its elimination restore fertility?

Does endometriosis affect fertility?

Whether endometriosis *per se* decreases fertility is an intriguing question but one that is difficult to answer. It can best be studied in a prospective observational cohort study of two groups of patients without any fertility-impairing factors, one group with and one without documented endometriosis (and endometriosis only), with all other factors (age, sexual activity, socio-economic class) being equal. This means comparing, from the very moment they wish to start a family, the spontaneous pregnancy rate in proven normal young couples with that in proven normal young couples of whom the female partner has endometriosis as the only abnormal finding. Since it would require a laparoscopy to be performed in perfectly healthy young women even before they started attempting to achieve a pregnancy, a study like this will

Endometriosis: Science and Practice, First Edition. Edited by Linda C. Giudice, Johannes L.H. Evers and David L. Healy.
© 2012 Blackwell Publishing Ltd. Published 2012 by Blackwell Publishing Ltd.

Study	Cases	Cases pregnant	Controls	Controls pregnant	OR	95% CI
Thomas & Cooke [2]	20	5	17	4	1.1	0.2–4.9
Bayer et al [3]	37	13	36	17	0.6	0.2–1.5
Telimaa et al [4]*	18	6	14	6	0.7	0.2–2.8
Telimaa [5]	17	7	(14)	(6)	0.9	0.2–3.9
Fedele 6]	35	10	36	11	0.9	0.3–2.5
Parrazzini et al [7]	36	7	39	7	1.1	0.3–3.5
Bianchi et al [10]	15	5	15	6	0.8	0.2–3.3
Harrison et al [11]	50	0	50	3	0.3	0.03–3.1
Shawki et al [12]	34	16	34	5	5.2	1.6–16.5
Loverro et al [13]	14	5	13	6	0.8	0.2–3.5
Combined	*276*	*74*	*254*	*65*	*1.1*	*0.7–1.6*

Table 44.1 Odds ratios of 10 randomized controlled studies of medical treatment of minimal and mild endometriosis.

CI, confidence interval; OR, odds ratio.

*Telimaa's was a three-arm trial, controls only counted once.

Table 44.2 Odds ratios in two randomized controlled studies of surgical treatment of minimal and mild endometriosis.

Study	Cases	Cases pregnant	Controls	Controls pregnant	OR	95% CI
Marcoux et al [8]	172	63	169	37	2.1	1.3–3.3
GISE [9]	54	12	47	13	0.7	0.3–1.8
Combined	*226*	*75*	*216*	*50*	*1.6*	*1.1–2.5*

CI, confidence interval; OR, odds ratio.

From Marcoux et al [8] and GISE [9], as adapted by Crosignani and Vercellini [28].

obviously never be performed. For obvious reasons also, the most powerful clinical study design, a randomized controlled trial (RCT), implanting endometrial fragments in the pelvis of one group of patients and not in the other, and studying their subsequent fertility, will never be done.

These potent clinical study designs being an illusion, several less robust trial designs remain. One is to compare spontaneous pregnancy rates in patients with unexplained subfertility after a complete fertility work-up to those in patients with endometriosis but otherwise also unexplained subfertility, the ages and durations of subfertility being equal in both groups (more than a few published studies suffer from the fact that endometriosis patients on average are several years older than patients with unexplained subfertility, thus confounding the issue by introducing an age effect in a very critical period of decreasing female fertility, i.e. the mid and late 30s). One way to assess spontaneous pregnancy rates in endometriosis patients is to study non-treated control patients participating in randomized controlled trials. Twelve studies have been reported from which figures like these can be derived [2–13]. Together, they involved 470 control patients, who achieved a crude spontaneous pregnancy rate of 25% (Tables 44.1 and 44.2). This approaches the combined spontaneous pregnancy rate of 33% from 20 studies (involving 2026 unexplained subfertility patients) as reported by Taylor and Collins [14] in their literature review of unexplained subfertility.

Studying the results of artificial insemination in women with azoospermic husbands offers an alternative way of addressing the issue. Three studies may offer some insight in this respect [15–17]. The crude pregnancy rates during 12 months of inseminating donor sperm ranged from a low figure of 29% in the few patients in one study (2/7 [16]) to a "normal" conception rate of 81% in another, not much bigger study (17/21 [17]) in women with endometriosis, as compared to 51% in women without endometriosis [16]. Overall, pregnancies occurred in 38/59 cases (64%) and 46/91 controls (51%), i.e. if anything a more favorable outcome in endometriosis patients than in controls.

Also, international registry studies have shown comparable success rates of assisted reproductive technologies (ART) in patients with endometriosis (33.1%) and unexplained subfertility (31.7%) [18]. The issue of surgical treatment will be dealt with in Chapter 45. For the sake of this discussion of minimal and mild endometriosis affecting fertility in otherwise unexplained subfertility patients, however, we need to have a quick look at studies removing lesions and reporting the effect on fertility. No RCT has been published so far reporting spontaneous pregnancy rates following surgical treatment of endometriosis (and endometriosis only) in patients with otherwise unexplained subfertility. Two medium-sized studies, one from Canada involving 341 patients and one from Italy involving 101 patients, have been published reporting surgical removal of endometriosis *and adhesions* [8,9] in subfertility patients with mild or minimal endometriosis and no other fertility-decreasing factors (see Table 44.2).

Both studies have been criticized, not only because they also removed adhesions along with the lesions, but also because after surgery, the patients were informed about the ablation of lesions having been or not having been performed in their specific case. It cannot be excluded that this might have affected the outcome.

The Canadian study is by far the largest published RCT on any treatment of endometriosis in subfertility patients so far. It offers evidence that surgical treatment of minimal and mild endometriosis improves the pregnancy chances in a subfertility patient, although it does not restore it to the level one would expect in patients like these, and most definitely not to normal. During the 36 weeks of follow-up, 50 patients (29%) of the 172 randomized to have surgery conceived and 29 (17%) of those randomized to no treatment. The (36 weeks) pregnancy rate of 17% in the untreated patients from this surgical RCT compares unfavorably to the combined (6 months) pregnancy rate of 27% in the untreated patients from the 10 medical RCTs mentioned above. Since there is no reason to presume that being an untreated control patient in a medical RCT provides for better pregnancy chances than being an untreated control patient in a surgical RCT, it is not yet possible to draw firm conclusions from the findings of the Canadian study [8].

The Italian study [9] included 101 patients. During the 12 months of follow-up, 12 patients (22%) of the 54 randomized to have surgery conceived and 13 (28%) of those (n = 47) randomized to no treatment. The (1 year) pregnancy rate of 28% in the untreated patients from this surgical RCT is similar to the combined pregnancy rate of 27% in the untreated patients from the 10 medical RCTs mentioned before, although the latter was obtained after only 6 months of follow-up. Calculating the pregnancy rate in patients after surgical removal of endometriosis lesions only (i.e. in those patients who did not have or did not need lysis of adhesions) would give the only clear answer to the question whether removal of lesions as such will improve a patient's subsequent pregnancy chances.

The authors of the two studies were kind enough to provide these data (Table 44.3). A pooled estimate of the odds ratio (OR) for the occurrence of an ongoing pregnancy, as derived from these two studies, allowed the conclusion that resection or ablation of minimal and mild endometriosis appears to modestly enhance fecundity in women with otherwise unexplained subfertility, but that the 95% confidence interval (CI) of the combined OR still includes unity.

From these findings, it seems safe to conclude that endometriotic implants as such may have a negative effect on fertility and that

their removal may cause a (probably temporary) improvement of the patient's pregnancy chances. How long it will take before residual occult lesions develop into manifest ones, only to decrease fertility again, remains to be elucidated.

Does medical treatment restore fertility?

Based on the (erroneous) assumption that endometriosis regresses during anovulation, medical therapies used to treat endometriosis-associated pain have also been tried in subfertility patients. The theory behind all medical therapies is to block the hormonal support of the endometrial tissue by ovarian steroid hormones, thus stopping retrograde menstruation and creating a suboptimal environment for escaped menstrual fragments to implant on the peritoneal surface, invade, proliferate and reseed from secondary lesions. Involution, atrophy and regression are supposed to take place instead. Among the drugs that have been used to 'treat' endometriosis-associated subfertility are the following.

• Progestogens, both derivatives from progesterone as well as derivatives of 19-nortesterone, have been used to counteract the estrogen effect on the endometrium and (presumably) endometriosis.

• Danazol and gestrinone, synthetic steroid derivatives of 17α-ethinyltestosterone, that block cyclic changes in ovarian estrogen production and increase serum free testosterone by suppressing circulating sex hormone binding globulin (SHBG) concentrations.

• Combined oral contraceptives, often used in a continuous way (continuous combined oral contraceptives (CCOC), the contraceptive patch, the contraceptive vaginal ring), for their atrophic effect on endometrial development.

• Gonadotropin releasing hormone (GnRH) agonists and antagonists, for depleting or blocking the pituitary GnRH receptors, inducing a profound hypoestrogenic state. Due to often severe estrogen deprivation symptoms, their use has been combined with low-dose estrogen add-back.

• Aromatase P450 inhibitors, blocking the conversion of androstenedione and testosterone to estrone and estradiol respectively. Their use in (premenopausal) subfertility patients will lead to ovarian hyperstimulation (cyst formation) due to their abolishing the negative estrogen feedback on the hypothalamus and pituitary, causing hypergonadotropism. If it is confirmed in larger studies that aromatase activity is not detectable in the endometrium of healthy women but occurs exclusively in eutopic endometrium and implants of patients with endometriosis [19], inhibiting aromatase activity may become a selective way of suppressing endometriosis in patients without the desire for children.

• Chinese herbal medicines and different kinds of alleged immunomodulators, e.g. pentoxifylline, have been used, as have (in experimental set-ups) progesterone receptor modulators, TNF-α inhibitors, angiogenesis blockers, matrix metalloproteinase inhibitors and estrogen receptor β agonists.

Table 44.3 Achievement of a pregnancy continuing beyond 20 weeks, following removal of lesions in a subgroup of women with unexplained subfertility and minimal or mild endometriosis only, without pelvic adhesions (cases) compared to women in whom removal of lesions was not performed (controls).

Study	Cases	Cases pregnant	Controls	Controls pregnant	OR	95% CI
Marcoux *et al* [8]	145	41	139	25	1.8	1.0–3.2
GISE [9]	36	9	32	10	0.7	0.3–2.1
Combined	*181*	*50*	*171*	*35*	*1.5*	*0.9–2.4*

CI, confidence interval; OR, odds ratio.
From Marcoux *et al* [8], GISE [9] and R Maheux, S Berube, PG Crosignani, F Parazzini, 2001, personal communication.

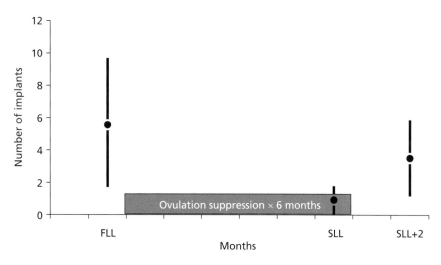

Figure 44.1 Activity of endometriosis, classified according to the number of implants visible at first-look laparoscopy (FLL) compared to second-look laparoscopy (SLL) in endometriosis patients who had their SLL performed during ovarian suppression in the final week of treatment by danazol (n = 10) and those patients (n = 11) who were randomized to have their SLL performed after return of ovarian activity, in the follicular phase of the second spontaneous menstrual cycle after the end of treatment (SLL+2) [23].

No specific drug has been proven superior to any other or, more importantly, to placebo with regard to restoring fertility in endometriosis patients. Ten RCTs have shown that medical treatment does not improve pregnancy chances in subfertile endometriosis patients [2–7,10–13] (see Table 44.1). Hughes and co-workers [20], who did a Cochrane review on ovulation suppression for endometriosis in women with subfertility, concluded, based on the combined data of trials comparing danazol, gestrinone or medroxyprogesterone acetate (MPA) with placebo or no treatment, that there is no evidence of benefit in the use of ovulation suppression in subfertile women with endometriosis who wish to conceive. They established that to reach this conclusion, a reasonably strong body of clinical evidence existed with little inconsistency and minimal heterogeneity: the available evidence (providing 80% power to detect a benefit of 20%, two-tailed α 0.05) consistently failed to do so. In the opinion of these authors more, larger trials comparing ovulation suppression in subfertile endometriosis patients do not appear warranted. They anticipate no new data for this topic and consider the review closed. As of 2010 it will no longer be updated [20].

Estimating the effect of medical treatment: a fallacy

The American Fertility Society (AFS) classification for staging the severity of disease in endometriosis was designed originally to study the subsequent pregnancy rates in patients after conservative surgery [21]. The classification was never intended to evaluate the resolution of disease during medical therapy. Brosens and co-workers [22] have warned against such misuse of the revised AFS classification in comparing the pelvic scores before and upon termination of medical suppression of endometriosis. The pelvic organs and the endometriosis lesions should be studied under identical conditions, with the same,

physiological hormonal stimulation. Comparing active, hemorrhagic, productive implants in a moist, inflammatory or even hyperemic pelvis during spontaneous ovarian activity with subdued, suppressed or even concealed, unproductive lesions in a dry, inactive pelvis during ovarian suppression will confound objective ascertainment of the effect of medical therapy. The size of the implants may be overestimated before therapy as a result of the endometriotic secretions and the surrounding peritoneal inflammatory response; the number of implants may be underestimated during ovarian suppression, because of the difficulty in discerning the smaller implants when secretory products are lacking and the hyperemic inflammatory surroundings have faded.

We studied the change in appearance of endometriotic lesions during medical treatment from first-look laparoscopy (FLL) to second-look laparoscopy (SLL) when the SLL was performed during the last week of ovarian suppression and compared it to the situation when the SLL was performed in the follicular phase of the second spontaneous menstrual cycle after the end of treatment [23]. Both the number of implants and their cumulative diameter appeared to have decreased significantly when the SLL was performed during ovarian suppression (5.9 to 0.8 implants; 16.9 to 2.7 mm cumulative diameter), whereas the difference was no longer statistically significant when the SLL was performed after return of ovarian activity (5.7 to 3.5 and 12.5 to 8.3 respectively). From these findings we concluded that at least part of the "cure rate" of medical endometriosis therapy can be attributed to the difference in pelvic environment at the time of SLL. For comparative classification of the activity of disease, but above all of its resolution during medical therapy, SLL, if performed during ovarian suppression, is a misleading procedure (Fig. 44.1).

The problem is further compounded by the fact that there exists a small but definite tendency for spontaneous regression of endometriosis lesions. Mahmood and Templeton [24] documented progression in 64% of untreated endometriosis patients between FLL and SLL; in 9% the extent of endometriosis was unchanged, and in 27% spontaneous regression had occurred. The comparative figures from those studies that included a SLL in the non-treated control patients [2–5] were roughly one-third progression, one-third regression, and no change in the remaining one-third of patients [25].

Other medical treatments

There was no evidence of an increase in clinical pregnancy in subfertile endometriosis patients treated with pentoxifylline compared to placebo (three RCTs, OR 1.54, 95% CI 0.89–266) [26]. With respect to restoring fertility in endometriosis patients, no RCTs comparing the effect of Chinese herbal medicine with placebo have been published [27], and neither have other medical treatments been subjected to robust objective clinical evaluation. Medical ovarian suppression in preparation for the application of assisted reproductive technologies will be discussed in Chapter 46.

Conclusion

From the study reports available today, it seems reasonable to conclude that there exists no or only very limited evidence to support the contention that the simple endometriosis lesion *per se* causes subfertility. Fertility figures in non-treated endometriosis patients who serve as controls in clinical trials approach those of patients with unexplained subfertility. This is corroborated by findings from international ART registries, which show that in assisted reproduction, patients with endometriosis perform as well as patients with unexplained subfertility, showing similar pregnancy rates. However, there is statistical evidence for a slight beneficial effect of surgical removal of the lesions. The clinical relevance of this seems only limited and the effect may be short-lived. There is no support for the contention that medical treatment of minimal and mild endometriosis improves pregnancy chances in subfertile couples. On the contrary, it will prevent them from conceiving as long as ovulations are suppressed. Medical treatment will render minimal and mild disease only temporarily invisible, allowing the lesions to re-emerge with time. There exists no rationale for treating occult endometriosis, and available treatments for minimal and mild endometriosis are necessarily (theoretically and in practice) ineffective in patients with occult disease since, if anything, they will leave numerous occult lesions behind. Finally, if, for research purposes, a second-look laparoscopy is to be performed in endometriosis patients to establish the effect of medical (or for that matter surgical) treatment, this procedure should not be performed during ovarian suppression but after resumption of ovarian activity, in the same phase of the menstrual cycle as the original first-look laparoscopy.

References

1. Wheeler JM, Malinak LR. Does mild endometriosis cause infertility? Semin Reprod Endocrinol 1988;6:239–251.
2. Thomas EJ, Cooke ID. Successful treatment of asymptomatic endometriosis: does it benefit infertile women? BMJ 1987;294:1117–1119.
3. Bayer SR, Seibel MM, Saffan DS et al. Efficacy of danazol treatment for minimal endometriosis in infertile women. A prospective, randomised study. J Reprod Med 1988;33:179–183.
4. Telimaa S, Ronnberg L, Kauppila A. Placebo-controlled comparison of danazol and high-dose medroxyprogesterone acetate in the treatment of endometriosis after conservative surgery. Gynecol Endocrinol 1987;1:363–371.
5. Telimaa S. Danazol and medroxyprogesterone acetate inefficacious in the treatment of infertility in endometriosis. Fertil Steril 1988;50:872–875.
6. Fedele L, Parazzini F, Radici E et al. Buserelin acetate versus expectant management in the treatment of infertility associated with minimal or mild endometriosis: a randomized clinical trial. Am J Obstet Gynecol 1992;166:1345–1350.
7. Parrazzini F, Fedele L, Busaca M et al. Postsurgical medical treatment of advanced endometriosis: results of a randomized clinical trial. Am J Obstet Gynecol 1994;171:1205–1207.
8. Marcoux S, Maheux R, Berube S, and the Canadian Collaborative Group on Endometriosis. Laparoscopic surgery in infertile women with minimal or mild endometriosis. N Engl J Med 1997;337:217–222.
9. Gruppo Italiano per lo Studio dell'Endometriosi. Ablation of lesions or no treatment in minimal-mild endometriosis in infertile women: a randomised trial. Hum Reprod 1999;14:1332–1334.
10. Bianchi S, Busaca M, Agnoli B et al. Effects of 3 months therapy with danazol after laparoscopic surgery for stage III/IV endometriosis: a randomized study. Hum Reprod 1999;14:1335–1337.
11. Harrison RF, Barry-Kinsela C. Efficacy of medroxyprogesterone treatment in infertile women with endometriosis: a prospective, randomized, placebo controlled study. Fertil Steril 2000;74:24–30.
12. Shawki O, Hamza H, Sattar M. Mild endometriosis, to treat or not to treat: randomized controlled trial comparing diagnostic laparoscopy with no further treatment versus post-operative Zoladex in cases with infertility associated with stage I-II endometriosis. Fertil Steril 2002;13(Suppl):O-36.
13. Loverro G, Carriero C, Rossi A et al. A randomized study comparing triptorelin or expectant management following conservative laparoscopic surgery for symptomatic stage III-IV endometriosis. Eur J Obstet Gynaecol Reprod Biol 2008;136:194–198.
14. Taylor PJ, Collins JA. Unexplained Infertility. Oxford: Oxford Medical Publications, 1992.
15. Portuondo JA, Echanojauregui AD, Herran C, Alijarte I. Early conception in patients with untreated mild endometriosis. Fertil Steril 1983;39:22–25.
16. Jansen RPS. Minimal endometriosis and reduced fecundability: prospective evidence from an artificial insemination by donor program. Fertil Steril 1986;46:141–143.

17. Rodriguez-Escudero FJ, Neyro JL, Corcostegui B, Benito JA. Does minimal endometriosis reduce fecundity? Fertil Steril 1988;50:522–524.

18. Centers for Disease Control. 2006 Assisted Reproductive Technology Report: Section 2 – ART cycles using fresh, nondonor eggs or embryos. www.cdc.gov/ART/ART2006.

19. Noble LS, Simpson ER, Johns A, Bulun SE. Aromatase expression in endometriosis. J Clin Endocrinol Metabol 1996;81:174–179.

20. Hughes E, Brown J, Collins JJ et al. Ovulation suppression for endometriosis for women with subfertility. Cochrane Database Syst Rev 2010;1:CD000155.

21. American Fertility Society. Revised classification of endometriosis. Fertil Steril 1985;43:351–352.

22. Brosens IA, Cornillie F, Koninckx P, Vasques G. Evolution of the revised American Fertility Society classification of endometriosis (letter). Fertil Steril 1985;44:714.

23. Evers JL. The second-look laparoscopy for evaluation of the result of medical treatment of endometriosis should not be performed during ovarian suppression. Fertil Steril 1987;47:502–504.

24. Mahmood TA, Templeton A. The impact of treatment on the natural history of endometriosis. Hum Reprod 1990;5:965–970.

25. Evers JL. The pregnancy rate of the no-treatment group in randomized clinical trials of endometriosis therapy. Fertil Steril 1989;52:906–907.

26. Lv D, Song H, Li Y, Clarke J, Shi G. Pentoxifylline versus medical therapies for subfertile women with endometriosis. Cochrane Database Syst Rev 2009;3:CD007677.

27. Flower A, Liu JP, Chen S et al. Chinese herbal medicine for endometriosis. Cochrane Database Syst Rev 2009;3:CD006568.

28. Crosignani PG, Vercellini P. Evidence may change with more trials: concepts to be kept in mind (letter). Hum Reprod 2000;15:2448.

45 Infertility Therapies: The Role of Surgery

Oswald Petrucco[1] and David L. Healy[2]

[1]The Robinson Institute, University of Adelaide, Adelaide, Australia
[2]Department of Obstetrics and Gynaecology, Monash University, Melbourne, Australia

Introduction

In the new millennium, gynecologists are witnessing less division between minimal access and conventional surgery. As predicted [1], endoscopic surgery is expanding in parallel with advances in fiberoptics, ceramics and computer technology. High-definition endocameras, monitors and robotic systems, incorporating three-dimensional and stereoscopic imaging, are facilitating and obviating difficulties with hand–eye co-ordination and depth perception.

Ancillary systems to ensure optical clarity and maintenance of clear vision include pressure-controlled carbon dioxide insufflation, variable electrocautery, suction, temperature-controlled irrigation and electronically controlled light sourcing. On-demand video for proximal and telemedicine transmission allows simulation and training to be achieved at remote distances from the surgical site. Virtual-reality display technology has also facilitated training and development of new methods and procedures. Telemedicine, teleassistance and telemanipulation have enabled guidance of telescopes and surgical instruments by experts teaching new procedures intercontinentally, the only limitation being image transmission over longer distances.

Globally gynecologists are capitalizing on these advances and incorporating and integrating new endoscopic techniques to treat women with endometriosis-related infertility.

Endometriosis surgery has benefited from these new endoscopic advances and the most important aspects are discussed in other chapters of this book.

The aims of this chapter include the substantiation that endometriosis surgery plays an important role in the management of endometriosis-related infertility. We explore how it can best be taught at trainee and postgraduate levels, how to evaluate the most appropriate setting for efficient assessment, team-related surgery and postoperative support for endometriosis patients.

It is not our intention to debate whether artificial reproductive technology (ART) should be considered instead of surgery to achieve fertility as fertility is often not the only problem affecting endometriosis patients.

The most significant factors determining a need for surgical intervention in women with proven endometriosis include:
- age
- previous therapies
- nature and severity of symptoms
- location and severity of disease process.

For many women the presence or absence of pelvic pain, as well as infertility, will influence their decision to undergo surgery. For obvious reasons, the regular occurrence of dysmenorrhea, pelvic pain, dyschezia, dysuria and dyspareunia significantly influences the ability to enjoy and be involved in coitus at the appropriate time of the menstrual cycle. We believe that deeply infiltrating endometriosis is often incompletely excised because not all treating gynecologists have sufficient skills to carry out definitive treatment.

When fertility is not an issue, definitive surgery is usually performed because of failed medical or conservative surgery, or the presence of deeply invading disease process in the pelvis or ovaries when pelvic clearance may be required.

Equally significant decisions have to be made when fertility is the principal concern. The implications of surgery and skills required to perform that surgery are of paramount importance. Maintenance of ovarian function, particularly when the ovaries are primarily involved by endometriosis, must be the primary objective. We suggest that endometriosis lesions are often overtreated surgically without a strong evidence base.

Because endometriosis may involve the bladder, ureters and the gastrointestinal tract in often close proximity to pelvic vasculature, definitive surgery often requires either advanced endoscopy training or a team approach involving urologists and colorectal surgeons. The practice of superficial cautery to visible pelvic

Endometriosis: Science and Practice, First Edition. Edited by Linda C. Giudice, Johannes L.H. Evers and David L. Healy.
© 2012 Blackwell Publishing Ltd. Published 2012 by Blackwell Publishing Ltd.

deposits of endometriosis or simple drainage of endometriomas has rightfully been replaced by complete excision of the disease process no matter where sited in the abdomen or pelvis.

Not all gynecologists have the opportunity or indeed the innate potential to learn, develop and perform the advanced surgical procedures required for endometriosis surgery. The opportunity for learning has been influenced by the introduction of medical treatment for many gynecological conditions previously treated by surgery which means less surgical exposure for trainees. Teachers also may not be able to maintain or indeed want to pursue surgical skills to the detriment of their trainees. Training programs need to allow for the separate development of medical/fetomaternal or surgical gynecology specialists in the future.

Subspecialization in tertiary referral centers has also influenced the debate about separating obstetrics from gynecology despite parent bodies maintaining the status quo.

Competence to perform surgical procedures has become a major factor in medicolegal litigation. Particularly in endoscopic surgery, gynecologists must be able to confirm having received adequate training under supervision before embarking on complex endoscopic surgical procedures. Hospital credentialing should be mandatory.

Effective gynecological day surgery

It is important to define different terms used in assessing new technology and surgical operations for endometriosis.
- *Efficacy* refers to an ideal situation when a new technique is practiced by experts and results have been substantiated by controlled clinical trials.
- An *effective* operation is one that achieves satisfactory results by the majority of surgeons and one which fulfils most patients' expectations.
- When a new technique has been proven to be cost-effective with least complications, it is labeled *efficient*. This status is usually only achieved after adequate comparison with other conservative nonsurgical approaches or previously available surgical practices [2]. Effective gynecological day surgery is not as easy as it sounds. The speed at which a large number of new operations for endometriosis have been introduced since the mid-1980s is bewildering. Which of these operations is effective is not clear. This rapid change in technique makes the assessment of endometriosis surgery much more difficult than the assessment of procedures in obstetrics.

Gynecological day surgery operations have only been available for a relatively short time, even in the most expert of hands. Many gynecologists are still learning to perform these new operations for endometriosis. It is clear that many sound and experienced gynecologists will never be able to become confident with these new operations. Some will not even wish to try. This is quite different from operative obstetrics, where the same range of operations has been available and taught to all specialists for many years. Standard obstetric operations, capable of being performed by any specialist obstetrician and gynecologist in all areas of any country, have been

taught to trainee specialists over many years. This represents a much more stable surgical base from which to assess whether an obstetric operation is effective or not. The contrast with modern endometriosis surgery could hardly be more stark.

The quality of current medical evidence from examination of the effectiveness of gynecological day surgery operations is generally poor. As emphasized above, this is not for want of trying but because most gynecological day surgery operations are still relatively new. Medical articles often include what is conventionally believed to be the lowest quality of medical evidence, i.e. individual case reports.

Nevertheless, the impact of individual surgical case reports, in contrast to their epidemiological impact, can be significant. For example, the case report of the first laparoscopic hysterectomy or the case report of the first baby born after *in vitro* fertilization (IVF) had major impacts upon specialists in obstetrics and gynecology and their patients, if not upon epidemiologists and public health experts.

A series of such individual patient operations placed together provides a case series or observational series. Many surgeons report their favorite operation in this way. This is not necessarily a bad thing provided it does not end there. Case series of endometriosis surgical operations can be difficult to interpret. Are these the surgeon's best results, best patients or typical subjects? After these case reports and series, there should be participation in surgical trials, which provide experimental evidence that one similar operation is better than another. Endometriosis surgeons have ethical and social responsibilities to participate in such studies.

Case–control and cohort epidemiological trials are examples of the next stage of medical evidence. Such studies reduce bias and delusion on the part of surgeons that one operation for endometriosis is best because they believe it to be so. Increasingly, epidemiologists in hospitals, insurance companies and governments are demanding at least this quality of evidence as proof of an effective new operation.

Case–control studies are typically retrospective. In a case–control study, a group of patients will undergo an endoscopic operation or gynecological day surgery operation and the results are compared with those from a similar group of patients who underwent a conventional operation or an operation in a conventional operating theater. In the case–control method, the frequency with which the point of interest occurs is then compared between the cases and the controls. For example, the complication rate or patient satisfaction could be analyzed in this way (Box 45.1).

Typically, the selection of control patients is the most controversial part of a case–control study and usually its weakest link. It is vital that the controls are as similar to the cases as possible. The introduction of bias in making this selection of surgical controls and cases is the major weakness of the case–control method. Bias may be seen in many ways in such a surgical case–control study. There may be referral bias in which the hardest or easiest cases are referred unfairly to one or other group. There may be selection bias in which the easier or more difficult cases are allocated one or other group. Classification bias, especially, is commonly seen in

Box 45.1 Clinical indicators for gynecological day surgery

- Blood transfusion for gynecological day surgery
- Injury, unplanned repair or unplanned removal of an organ or structure during a gynecological day surgery procedure
- Unplanned return to operating room during the same day
- Patient having evidence of a wound or infection after the fifth postoperative day
- Unplanned hospital readmission

studies of endometriosis. Recall bias is prevalent when patients with cancer are asked to recall earlier medications or health treatments. Nevertheless, there are significant advantages in the case–control approach. The above issues can be accounted for and bias minimized. Case–control studies are usually easy to understand and not technically difficult to undertake.

Cohort epidemiological trials are usually prospective studies. In this approach, a group of patients who have undergone endoscopic surgery, say, are compared over time with a group of similar patients who have not had the same treatment. Both of these subsets of patients could be followed until their rates of pregnancy, if this was the endpoint to be studied, were clear. This would be an example of a cohort study. Cohort studies are less prone to bias than are case–control studies.

Randomized controlled trials sit near the top of the pyramid of medical evidence as the best medical data (Fig. 45.1). Effective gynecological day surgery operations can be proven in a randomized controlled trial by randomly assigning patients between the new operation and the conventional procedure. The Cochrane Pregnancy and Childbirth Database was able to be assembled after a series of randomized controlled trials in perinatal medicine.

Such randomized controlled trials of the high-priority questions in gynecological day surgery are now required. This would establish whether several surgery operations for endometriosis are effective or not. There seems no reason to us why an international Cochrane collaboration could not be commenced on endometriosis surgery. Alternatively, the various national or international endoscopy societies could undertake quality studies of the high-priority questions in gynecological day surgery.

After several randomized controlled trials have been reported on a key question in gynecological day surgery, meta-analysis of these trials is then an option (see Fig. 45.1). Meta-analysis of several controlled trials should give added strength to any conclusions of their effectiveness. Meta-analysis of satisfactory randomized controlled trials is commonplace in many branches of medicine but still in its infancy in gynecology.

Evidence-based surgery is one of the motherhood statements of modern hospital practice. Most gynecologists would hope that they are practicing evidence-based medicine and surgery. They are typically bewildered with much of the modern hospital with its economic and epidemiological medical approach. This

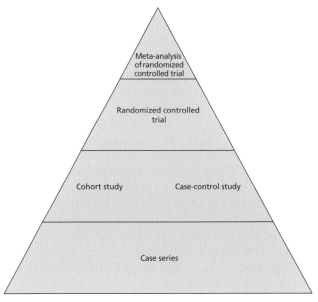

Figure 45.1 An evidence pyramid, showing many case reports but few meta-analyses, in endometriosis surgery. Reproduced from Healy and Petrucco [2] with permission from Springer.

Table 45.1 Levels of medical research design quality.

Evidence	Level	Study
Best	Level 1	Meta-analysis of randomized controlled trial (RCT)
	Level 2	Randomized controlled trial (RCT)
	Level 3	Non-randomized controlled trials – cohort studies and case–control studies
Worst	Level 4	Case series/expert consensus

bewilderment stems from the many years which they have invested in training and surgical knowledge to acquire a good working knowledge of the consensus of "experts."

This consensus of "experts" is developed from the surgical practices of the leading surgeons and teachers of trainee gynecologists and obstetricians in every community. It has been the educational path for most specialists in most centers in the world. Discovering that the expert consensus is the lowest and least regarded of four levels of medical evidence is a major shock to many skilled and competent surgeons (Table 45.1; see also Fig. 45.1).

Cost-effectiveness

Health administrators and insurance companies are typically concerned with reducing costs for any operation. For a cost-effectiveness analysis to be undertaken, it first needs to be demonstrated that a new operation is indeed medically effective. Such studies need to be supported by health economists. It should be possible to include economic assessments in randomized controlled trials. This would establish if the new endometriosis operation is indeed cheaper than the existing operation.

In a cost-effectiveness analysis, the individual cost per endometriosis patient can be determined by regarding each patient and her operation as a unique final output of the hospital production process. Managers can capture from each computerized system throughout the hospital the actual resources consumed by each patient during her stay in hospital and related outpatient or general practitioner treatment. These resources include the hours of nursing and doctoring care in a day surgery or conventional hospital setting, theater time, laboratory tests, radiology, pharmaceutical products and any allied health services.

The direct costs of administration and infrastructure services can be included in any cost presented and typically are one-third of the total cost per patient. For endometriosis surgery, operating theater cost must include the relevant instrument costs and can be allocated to patients according to the minutes of surgical table-top time recorded for each patient.

In many healthcare systems, a cost-effectiveness analysis as above is probably all that will be realistic. Achieving the same operation or output at a cheaper cost is typically all that many governments and medical insurance companies are concerned about. Other medical economic analyses are possible, however, and can include cost-benefit analysis and cost-utility analysis. The result of these studies may not count exclusively the financial cost but other endpoints including quality-adjusted life-years (QALYs).

Current status of endoscopic endometriosis surgery

The last 20 years have seen the formation of endoscopy societies by groups of enthusiasts. These promote and teach endoscopic surgery. Their provision of forums for meetings and education has lead to the establishment of guidelines for credentialing and accreditation of individuals wanting to practice advanced endoscopic surgery.

In 1992 the Australian Gynaecological Endoscopy Society (AGES) proposed and had accepted by the Royal Australian College of Obstetricians and Gynaecologists (RACOG) its *Guidelines for Training in Advanced Operative Laparoscopy in the Speciality of Obstetrics and Gynaecology*. These guidelines were last reviewed in March 2009 and have resulted in a "consensus statement" formulated by the now amalgamated Royal Australian and New Zealand College of Obstetricians and Gynaecologists (RANZCOG) and the AGES.

General considerations include:
- acceptance o f minimal access surgery
- maintenance of satisfactory standard of training, expertise in case selection and performance of appropriate safe surgery
- acceptance that not all individuals will be competent to perform all procedures, e.g. excision of level IV/V endometriosis requires further training and supervision prior to unsupervised surgery

- acceptance that the award of hospital operating privileges is the responsibility of relevant hospitals
- promotion of ethical research and evaluation of any new procedures
- adherence to principles of informed consent and explanation of potential risks and benefits and indicating if procedures are experimental or unproven
- familiarization with guidelines for performing advanced operative laparoscopy.

Such guidelines emphasize the fact that minimal access procedures are still major surgical procedures with risks and hazards requiring minimal standards related to training, practice, skills and familiarization with appropriate equipment.

The guidelines should suggest levels of skill ranging from skill level I, encompassing diagnostic laparoscopic procedures, to skill level V, total laparoscopic hysterectomy, Burch colposuspension and myomectomy. Skill level VI includes laparoscopic pelvic floor repair and excisional American Fertility Society (AFS) level 4 endometriosis surgery. Laparoscopic removal of residual ovaries, oncological procedures involving pelvic and para-aortic lymph node dissection and radical hysterectomy are also in this group.

Training in advanced techniques commences with assisting followed by supervision by experienced and credentialed colleagues. Regular attendance at endoscopic workshops and educational courses is strongly encouraged. Performance of level V, level VI surgery and laparoscopy suturing "requires formal preceptorships under the supervision of appropriately skilled laparoscopic surgeons" [3,4].

The use of lasers in obstetrics and gynecology, including laparoscopic surgery, also has requirements for training and accreditation [5].

The Royal College of Obstetricians and Gynaecologists (RCOG)'s publication *The Investigation and Management of Endometriosis* (Green-top Guideline No. 24, October 2006) includes the following.

For a definitive diagnosis of endometriosis usual inspection of the pelvis at laparoscopy is the gold standard investigation, unless disease is visible in the posterior vaginal fornix or elsewhere. Positive histology confirms the diagnosis of endometriosis; negative histology does not exclude it. Whether histology should be obtained if peritoneal disease alone is present is controversial.

Depending upon the severity of disease found, ideal practice is to diagnose and remove endometriosis surgically.

Endometriosis-associated pain can be reduced by removing the entire lesions in severe and deeply infiltrating disease.

Ablation of endometriosis lesions plus adhesiolysis to improve fertility in minimal-to-mild endometriosis is effective compared with diagnostic laparoscopy alone (A).

The rate of surgery in improving pregnancy rates for moderate-to-severe disease is uncertain (B).

Laparoscopic cystectomy for ovarian endometriosis is better than drainage and coagulation (A).

The French College of Obstetricians and Gynaecologists (CNGOF)'s *Guidelines for the Management of Endometriosis* (2006) similarly highlight the following.

When laparoscopy is carried out, surgical treatment of the lesions, if feasible, is recommended in order to improve fertility (Grade B). However, there is still insufficient data to make the same conclusions in cases of deeply infiltrating endometriosis.

Endometriosis has no impact on the final result of IVF. For endometriomas less than 6 cm, neither repeat surgery nor drainage of the endometriomas is recommended prior to IVF (Grade B).

Simple laparoscopic drainage of endometriomas is not recommended because it results in immediate recurrence (Grade B). Laparoscopic cystectomy is superior to drainage followed by destruction of the cyst wall by bipolar coagulation for endometriomas measuring at least 3 cm in diameter regardless of the indication (infertility, pain or adnexal mass) (NP1). Cystectomy should be performed wherever technically feasible (Grade A).

It is recommended that surgery for the most severe lesions of endometriosis be treated by teams experienced in the management of endometriosis.

The rate of major complications of surgery for endometriosis is between 0.1% to 15% depending on the extent of the lesions (NP3). These complications can have an adverse effect on spontaneous fertility.

The European Society of Human Reproduction and Embryology *Guidelines for the Diagnosis and Treatment of Endometriosis* (2005) also suggest the following.

Surgical ablation of endometriosis lesions plus adhesiolysis to improve fertility in minimal-mild endometriosis is effective compared to diagnostic laparoscopy alone [6]. This recommendation was based upon a systematic review and a meta-analysis of two similar but contradictory RCTs comparing laparoscopic surgery (I adhesiolysis) with laparoscopy alone (Evidence Level Ia).

No RCTs or meta-analysis are available to answer the question whether surgical excision of moderate-to-severe endometriosis enhances pregnancy rate. Based upon three studies [7–9], there seems to be a negative correlation between the stage of endometriosis and the spontaneous cumulative pregnancy rate after surgical removal of endometriosis but statistical significance was only reached in one study [9].

Laparoscopic cystectomy for ovarian endometriomas >4 cm diameter improves fertility compared to drainage and coagulation [10,11].

Resident training in obstetrics and gynecology in the United States

In the United States, all resident trainees in the speciality of obstetrics and gynecology must keep a log book of mentor surgical cases as the surgeon or first assistant. This book must be signed by the chairman of the residency program or other authorized person to confirm that the cases were actually performed. This is important for hospitals when the recently graduated resident is requesting surgical privileges.

The development and use of standards in the ongoing evaluation and certification of specialists in obstetrics and gynecology in the United States is conducted through the American Board of Medical Specialities (ABMS) [12]. The American Board of Obstetrics and Gynecology is an approved ABMS member. ABMS member boards certify obstetricians and gynecologists in the general specialty as well as in the subspecialty of reproductive endocrinology/infertility. The subspecialty group for all aspects of reproductive endocrinology/infertility, including surgical infertility, is the American Society for Reproductive Medicine (ASRM).

The ASRM *Guidelines for Practice – Endometriosis and Infertility Relating to Surgery and Endometriosis* (2006) state the following.

In stage I/II endometriosis laparoscopic ablation of endometrial implants has been associated with a small but significant improvement in live birth rates.

Compared to no treatment, for every 12 patients having stage I/II endometriosis diagnosed at laparoscopy there will be one additional successful pregnancy if ablation/resection of visible endometriosis is performed.

A non-randomized study and other observational studies that are not free from bias suggest that in women with stage III/IV endometriosis without other identifiable infertility factors, conservative surgical treatment with laparoscopy and possible laparotomy may increase fertility [13,14]. It thus seems that there is general consensus among these groups apart from issues relating to management of endometrioma.

On current available evidence, therefore, the following conclusions and recommendations for surgical treatment of endometriosis can be given.

- There is a lack of evidence from RCTs to make strong recommendations for treatment of pelvic endometriosis.
- Patients' age, duration of infertility, pelvic pain and stage of endometriosis are of paramount importance when considering surgical intervention.
- In suitable circumstances (preoperative counseling), a finding of visible endometriosis at laparoscopy should be followed by ablation/resection of the lesions.
- Treatment of stage I/II endometriosis in infertile patients leads to improved livebirth rate.
- For infertile patients with stage III/IV endometriosis, conservative laparoscopic surgery is indicated, particularly when other significant symptoms are present, i.e. pelvic pain and dyspareunia.
- Combined conservative surgical and ART therapies must be considered particularly for patients in the post-35 year age group.

Controversies

Controversies abound with any new medical procedure, especially a new method of surgery in which the operations are not proven to be of benefit.

Hospital administrators, health department administrators and insurance companies can see immediate cost savings in gynecological day surgery. For this reason, these groups welcome day surgery with the promise of rapid discharge of patients home. From their perspective, surgeons should undertake day surgery more and more frequently and if not, why not?

Surgeons who have not learnt a range of operative laparoscopic procedures may be jealous of gynecological day surgery. Jealousy is a common emotion in surgery and can be part of a rationale not to learn endoscopic operations. If I can do conventional endometriosis surgery by laparotomy upon anybody in 45 min, why take weeks learning to fiddle around with a 3 h laparoscopic operation for endometriosis and then do it half as well?

Complications inevitably occur in any surgical or medical procedure. The penalties of complications in gynecological day surgery are sometimes tragic. Opponents of day surgery will nudge each other and "I told you so!" Of course, similar complications have occurred during the learning phase of any traditional gynecological operation.

Patients requiring gynecological surgery are strong advocates for day surgery procedures. The avoidance of large abdominal scars and the more rapid return home promised by day surgery are powerful reasons in their choice. Patient satisfaction should be high with this positive view of "keyhole" surgery.

A further controversy of surgery for endometriosis is medical research. Randomized controlled trials of the high-priority questions in any branch of medicine are accepted as vital to the advancement of that discipline. Nevertheless, some endometriosis surgeons believe that controlled trials of day surgery operations are impractical, inappropriate, impossible or, perhaps, even unethical.

Our view is the opposite of this. We believe that properly designed medical research trials are vital for gynecological day surgery for endometriosis. These studies should be funded by medical research councils or national institutes of health and are just as important for nation health as studies in basic science and molecular biology. They should be given equal priority and funding. It is the role of national and international day surgery societies to develop high-quality protocols of important surgical questions about endometriosis which can be realistically answered. The President of the World Endometriosis Society has recently highlighted these controversies [15].

Audit

Effectiveness of surgery for endometriosis can be monitored by audit. Evaluation may occur by various criteria (Box 45.2; see also Box 45.1). Gynecological day surgery can be audited by monitoring the complications of day surgery operations. The return of patients to hospital within 1 day or 1 week can be compared with other day surgery centers. This helps determine best practice for one surgeon, in one hospital, one state or one nation.

Box 45.2 Advanced endoscopic surgery at a local hospital level

Hospital administrators should be made aware that:

- delineation of hospital privileges is the responsibility of hospital accreditation committees

- hospital accreditation committees should consist only of medical practitioners and preferably include a Fellow who is not a member of hospital staff

- hospital accreditation committees should be provided with evidence that competence has been achieved by a Fellow in performing a new advanced technique before granting privileges to perform the surgery

- before privileges can be granted to perform a new surgical procedure, the hospital will ensure that adequate facilities to perform that procedure safely are in place

- following the introduction of a new technique, in-house quality assurance studies and surgical audits are carried out to assess the safety and effectiveness of the new technique

- the relevant group will facilitate the appointment where necessary of a Preceptor who will decide whether a Fellow has reached a level of competence at different levels of training to have accreditation. The number of procedures to be performed before accreditation is given will vary between individuals and an agreement would have to be reached between the Preceptor and Fellow that a satisfactory level of training and competence has been reached

Source: Adapted from Guidelines of the Royal Australian College of Obstetricians and Gynaecologists.

Computerized patient records can monitor the total time of a patient's care from entry to exit through the gynecological day surgery hospital. The preoperative time, time in the operating theater, time in recovery and exit from the hospital can all be recorded. This can be compared between surgeons at the same hospitals, between different operations at the same hospital and between different gynecological day surgery hospitals. The financial cost of each section of the day surgery hospital experience can be determined. This cost will be the sum of the direct as well as the indirect costs.

Audit of patient satisfaction with a surgery experience for endometriosis is another measure of assessment of gynecological day surgery. Involving patients, and developing a patients' support group, may provide new ideas to improve the experience of endometriosis surgery within the hospital.

Five clinical indicators are shown in Box 45.1.

Future directions: endometriosis surgical centers

Laparoscopic endometriosis surgery for stage I/II endometriosis can be adequately performed by credentialed gynecologists with adequate training. More advanced laparoscopic surgery requires further training and possibly the involvement of urological and colorectal colleagues.

Pioneering centers in Europe have recently been established to achieve quality improvement in the overall management of patients with endometriosis [16]. The aims of these centers are to bring together medical and paramedical staff and scientists to carry out investigations, treatment and research on endometriosis, and to provide relevant information not only to patients but also to the public, healthcare providers, politicians and industry.

The German Endometriosis Center in Berlin, established in 2006 by the German Endometriosis Research Foundation, has recently presented results involving over 1400 patients, with 300 having advanced surgery, 110 of these for deep infiltrating endometriosis involving bowel, vagina, appendix, diaphragm and/ or bladder and ureters. Core medical partners (gynecology, visceral surgery, general surgery, urology, radiology, and pathology) are supported by co-operative partner groups providing patient interest/support, nutritional counseling, physiotherapy, pain therapy, ART and rehabilitation. Interdisciplinary co-operation is achieved by case discussion, documentation of decision-making process and control of finances. Co-operation with general and private practice physicians ensures that patient well-being is maintained once primary treatment is completed. Information for patients is provided at symposia as well as by written brochures.

Such a center can best provide advanced surgical training because of the larger throughput of cases. Documentation on diagnosis, therapy and aftercare compiled in annual reports and disseminated to all groups can form the basis for future developments. The assessment of data on medical and surgical therapies, relapses, infertility, pain and supplementary therapy of larger groups of patients should hopefully provide much needed answers for future management of this difficult condition.

Similar centers of excellence in other countries are currently being planned, the limiting factor being federal or community funding for such proposals. Two epidemiological studies undertaken by the World Endometriosis Research Foundation, the Global Study of Women's Health and the Women's Health Symptoms Study, are addressing the global impact of endometriosis involving 19 centers in 15 countries.

These measures auger well for a better understanding and management of endometriosis and may resolve controversies such as the endometriosis-ovarian cancer connection [17].

Acknowledgments

We would like to thank Dr David Adamson for his assistance in the preparation of this chapter.

References

1. Petrucco OM. Endoscopy in the new millennium. In: O'Brien P (ed) Yearbook of Obstetrics and Gynaecology, vol 8. London: RCOG Press, 2000, pp.325–343.

2. Healy DL, Petrucco O. Effective Gynecological Day Surgery. London: Chapman and Hall Medical, 1998.

3. www.ranzcog.edu.au/publications/statements/C-trg1.pdf

4. www.ranzcog.edu.au/publications/statements/C-trg2.pdf

5. www.ranzcog.edu.au/publications/statements/C-trg4.pdf

6. Jacobson TZ, Duffy JMN, Barlow D, Farquhar C, Koninckx PR, Olive D. Laparoscopic surgery for subfertility associated with endometriosis. Cochrane Database Syst Rev 2010;1:CD001398.

7. Adamson GD, Hurd SJ, Pasta DJ, Rodriguez BD. Laparoscopic endometriosis treatment: is it better? Fertil Steril 1993;59(1): 35–44.

8. Guzick DS, Silliman NP, Adamson GD et al. Prediction of pregnancy in infertile women based on the American Society for Reproductive Medicine's revised classification of endometriosis. Fertil Steril 1997;67(5):822–829.

9. Osuga Y, Koga K, Tsutsumi O et al. Role of laparoscopy in the treatment of endometriosis-associated infertility. Gynecol Obstet Invest 2002;53(Suppl 1):33–39.

10. Beretta P, Franchi M, Ghezzi F, Busacca M, Zupi E, Bolis P. Randomized clinical trial of two laparoscopic treatments of endometriomas: cystectomy versus drainage and coagulation. Fertil Steril 1998;70(6):1176–1180.

11. Chapron C, Vercellini P, Barakat H, Vieira M, Dubuisson JB. Management of ovarian endometriomas. Hum Reprod Update 2002;8(6):591.

12. www.abms.org/Maintenance_of_Certification/ABMS_MOC.aspx

13. Al-Inany HG, Crosignani PG, Vercellini P. Evidence may change with more trials: concepts to be kept in mind (letters). Hum Reprod 2000;15:2447–2811.

14. Shenken RS. Modern concepts of endometriosis. Classification and its consequences for therapy. J Reprod Med 1998;43:269–275.

15. www.endometriosis.ca/WES%20e-Journal%20March-April%20 2010.pdf

16. Ebert AD, Rosenow G, Kruger K et al. Development of centres of excellence for endometriosis – the Berlin experiences. Hum Reprod 2009;24(Suppl 1):Abstract 0–134.

17. www.endometriosis.ca/WES%20e-Journal%20March-April%20 2010.pdf

46 Infertility Therapies: The Role of Assisted Reproductive Technologies

Kimberly Moon, Jeris Cox and Alan DeCherney

Program in Reproductive and Adult Endocrinology, Eunice Kennedy Shriver National Institute of Child Health and Human Development, National Institutes of Health, Bethesda, MD, USA

Introduction

Endometriosis is found in 25–50% of women with infertility compared to 2–5% in the general population [1]. This suggests, but does not confirm, a causal role of endometriosis in infertility. Proposed treatment options for endometriosis-associated infertility include expectant management, ovarian suppression, surgical treatment, and ovarian stimulation with intrauterine insemination or assisted reproductive technologies (ART). With expectant management, infertile women with endometriosis can expect monthly fecundity of 0.02–0.10 compared to 0.15–0.20 in normal fertile couples [1]. Evidence to date indicates that medical therapy alone does not promote spontaneous conception for patients with endometriosis and infertility [2]. Data are insufficient regarding efficacy of surgical treatment alone in stage III/IV disease. The value of surgical treatment alone in stage I/II disease is also controversial. Based on a meta-analysis of two studies, ablation of endometriotic lesions plus adhesiolysis is effective in improving fertility compared to diagnostic laparoscopy alone [3]. The strength of evidence is highly questioned, however. There has been some success with increasing fecundity in endometriosis-associated infertility with ovulation induction and intrauterine insemination [4]. There are no large randomized controlled trials definitively demonstrating that *in vitro* fertilization (IVF) is more effective than expectant management in the treatment of stage-specific infertility associated with endometriosis. It is, however, routinely offered as an effective treatment that likely bypasses some of the impairments of endometriosis and is especially appropriate with co-existing infertility factors such as tubal or male factor or when other treatments have failed.

An attempt has been made to develop a classification system with a dose–response relationship to pregnancy following treatment. The current classification devised by the American Society of Reproductive Medicine (ASRM) in 1996 is based on a 20-point system dividing the disease into four stages. Stage I (minimal) and stage II (mild) disease are characterized by scattered superficial implants and filmy adhesions. Stage III (moderate) disease is characterized by multiple superficial and deep implants, small endometriomas (≤2 cm), and partial obliteration of the cul-de-sac. Stage IV (severe) disease is characterized by superficial and deep implants, dense ovarian and tubal adhesions, complete obliteration of the cul-de-sac and large endometriomas [5]. This system provides a standardized form for recording location and extent of disease, allowing clinicians and researchers to communicate effectively; however, it suffers from its subjectivity. It unfortunately has not been found to be a sensitive predictor of pregnancy following treatment [1].

A number of theories have been suggested for the discrepancy between the classification system and fertility outcomes. Although infertility and endometriosis are clearly associated, a cause-and-effect relationship has yet to be definitively established. While medical and surgical management of endometriosis have been shown to reduce pain symptoms, attempted medical or surgical eradication of clinical manifestations of disease has not resulted in increases in fertility. Further, pelvic adhesions and distorted pelvic anatomy could theoretically cause mechanical disruption of ovulation or efficient gamete transport. However, this does not explain infertility in cases where there is no mechanical alteration in the reproductive tract as in stage I/II endometriosis. It is fair to conclude that there may be important anatomical or biochemical factors beyond the visible lesions that are responsible for the reduced fecundity seen in women with endometriosis.

In vitro fertilization outcomes in patients with endometriosis

Analysis of IVF outcomes in patients with endometriosis is not only important for patient counseling and management

Endometriosis: Science and Practice, First Edition. Edited by Linda C. Giudice, Johannes L.H. Evers and David L. Healy.
© 2012 Blackwell Publishing Ltd. Published 2012 by Blackwell Publishing Ltd.

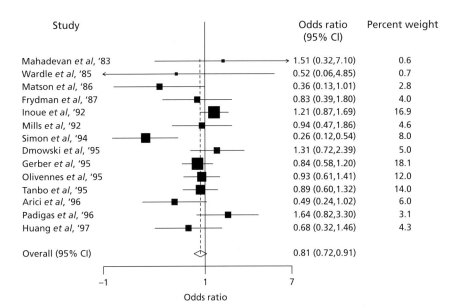

Study		Odds ratio (95% CI)	Percent weight
Mahadevan *et al*, '83		1.51 (0.32,7.10)	0.6
Wardle *et al*, '85		0.52 (0.06,4.85)	0.7
Matson *et al*, '86		0.36 (0.13,1.01)	2.8
Frydman *et al*, '87		0.83 (0.39,1.80)	4.0
Inoue *et al*, '92		1.21 (0.87,1.69)	16.9
Mills *et al*, '92		0.94 (0.47,1.86)	4.6
Simon *et al*, '94		0.26 (0.12,0.54)	8.0
Dmowski *et al*, '95		1.31 (0.72,2.39)	5.0
Gerber *et al*, '95		0.84 (0.58,1.20)	18.1
Olivennes *et al*, '95		0.93 (0.61,1.41)	12.0
Tanbo *et al*, '95		0.89 (0.60,1.32)	14.0
Arici *et al*, '96		0.49 (0.24,1.02)	6.0
Padigas *et al*, '96		1.64 (0.82,3.30)	3.1
Huang *et al*, '97		0.68 (0.32,1.46)	4.3
Overall (95% CI)		0.81 (0.72,0.91)	

Odds ratio (−1, 1, 7)

Figure 46.1 Odds ratio of pregnancy after IVF in patients with endometriosis compared to tubal factor controls. Reproduced from Barnhart *et al* [22] with permission from Elsevier.

but these studies also may facilitate our understanding of the pathophysiology of the disease.

Implantation and pregnancy rates compared to other infertility diagnoses

Some studies report lower implantation and pregnancy rates in women with endometriosis-associated infertility treated with IVF compared to those with tubal factor or unexplained infertility or both [6–9]. Other studies show no statistically significant differences in the implantation and pregnancy rates between these two groups of women [10–21].

A meta-analysis of 22 non-randomized trials reported that women with endometriosis have lower pregnancy rates after IVF (odds ratio (OR) 0.81, 95% confidence interval (CI) 0.72–0.91) when compared to women with tubal factor infertility (Fig. 46.1). Also demonstrated were lower peak E2 concentrations, reduced fertilization and implantation rates, and a significant decrease in the number of oocytes retrieved with endometriosis [22].

This finding is inconsistent with the data demonstrated in two large databases, SART and HFEA, where endometriosis has not been shown to adversely affect pregnancy rates. Templeton *et al* examined 52,507 IVF cycles reported to the Human Fertilization and Embryology Authority in the UK and found that after adjustment for age and duration of infertility, there was no significant effect of etiology of infertility on livebirth rate per treatment cycle [23]. Results from the Society for Assisted Reproductive Technology (SART) 2008 database demonstrated similar results, with livebirth rates similar among women with endometriosis, unexplained infertility or tubal factor infertility [24].

Outcomes by severity of disease

When looking at outcomes by severity of disease, some studies suggest that stage of disease is an important predictor of pregnancy outcome with IVF while others do not. A few authors have reported no difference in terms of severity [10,12,17,25]. In a larger number of studies, pregnancy rates in women with stage I/II endometriosis do not differ from those with tubal factor infertility but patients with stage III/IV disease have reduced pregnancy rates [8,26–31].

Kuivasaari *et al* compared 98 surgically confirmed endometriosis patients divided into stage I/II and stage III/IV with infertility with 87 patients with tubal factor infertility undergoing IVF/intracytoplasmic sperm injection (ICSI). There were no differences in the mean number of oocytes retrieved, the fertilization rate or the quality of embryos between the groups. There was no difference in pregnancy rates between the stage I/II and tubal factor groups but the pregnancy rates were significantly lower in the stage III/IV group when compared to the tubal factor group (22.6% versus 36.6%, *P* = 0.009) [28]. Similarly, the Barnhart meta-analysis demonstrated poorer success with IVF with stage III/IV disease when compared with stage I/II disease (OR 0.60, 95% CI 0.42–0.87) [22].

While IVF outcome studies may provide important information for counseling patients as well as insights about the pathophysiological mechanisms of endometriosis in infertility, it is important to note that results may be altered by the IVF process itself. For example, defects in folliculogenesis or the endometrium might be overcome by the administration of gonadotropin releasing hormone (GnRH) analogs and hormone therapies. Mild-to-severe disease may be very different entities. Overall, while success with IVF for endometriosis may or may not be lower than other infertility diagnoses, the current data suggest that success with IVF for endometriosis is worsened in stage III/IV disease compared to stage I/II disease. Nonetheless, the overall success rate in all stages of disease is good and higher than with expectant management.

Medical treatment prior to *in vitro* fertilization

In an attempt to increase pregnancy and implantation rates in women with endometriosis undergoing IVF, a number of medical pretreatments have been proposed with various claims of success.

Since endometriosis is predominantly found during the reproductive years and regression occurs in menopause and other hypoestrogenic states, a hormonal dependence has been suggested and is the basis for its medical management.

Danazol and gestrinone

Danazol and gestrinone are two medical treatments for endometriosis that received much more attention in the past; however, due to their shared hyperandrogenic adverse side-effects, including weight gain, acne, hirsuitism, and unfavorable lipid profile changes, they have largely been replaced by available medical treatments that are equally effective and better tolerated. Danazol, an isoxazol derivative of 17α-ethinyl testosterone, suppresses the hypothalamic-pituitary-ovarian axis, increases serum androgen levels, and decreases serum estrogen levels. It was the first medication approved by the US FDA for the treatment of endometriosis and was once the gold standard for treatment of endometriosis-associated pain symptoms [32].

Gestrinone, a 19-norsteroid derivative, blocks follicular development and estradiol production. It binds androgen receptors and has agonist and antagonist effects on progesterone receptors. It has been shown to provide pain symptom relief in patients with endometriosis similar to danazol [32].

Two studies have demonstrated favorable outcomes with the use of danazol and gestrinone prior to IVF in endometriosis patients. Infertility patients with mild endometriosis pretreated for 6–9 months with danazol or gestrinone demonstrated a comparable number of embryos to patients with tubal factor infertility (1.9 in treated group versus 2.1 in tubal factor patients, not significant (NS)) and a greater number than the untreated endometriosis patients (1.7) [33]. A prospective trial with 82 women randomized to pretreatment with danazol or no treatment before ART after prior failed cycles demonstrated increased pregnancy rates compared to control subjects (40% versus 19.5%, $P < 0.05$) although the number of embryos with optimal morphology was decreased in the treatment group (1.07 versus 2.04, $P < 0.05$) [34].

Gonadotropin releasing hormone agonists

Gonadotropin releasing hormone is a decapeptide released in a pulsatile fashion into the hypophyseal-portal circulation binding to anterior pituitary gonadotropic cells and thus activating intracellular signaling pathways involved in the production and release of follicle-stimulating hormone (FSH) and luteinizing hormone (LH). A large number of structural analogs have been developed. Analogs have a greater affinity for the receptor than endogenous GnRH and therefore have an immediate "flare" effect or increase in secretion of FSH and LH followed by an inhibition of secretion of these hormones or a downregulation. The ultimate effect is to produce a hypoestrogenic state so not surprisingly, GnRH agonists have demonstrated success in reducing endometriosis-associated pain. They are not, however, capable of eradicating the disease [32].

If endometriosis interferes with fertilization or implantation or causes a reduction in embryo quality, as many suspect, effective treatment strategies that diminish size or activity of endometriotic implants might be expected to restore normal fecundity [35]. However, while GnRH analogs have a firm place in the treatment of fertility disorders in preventing premature LH surges, for providing the flare effect during hyperstimulation and for synchronization of donor/recipient cycles, there is no indication for ovarian suppression alone to improve spontaneous pregnancy rates in minimal-to-mild disease and the evidence is lacking for more severe endometriosis [3]. The pathological processes associated with the disease may be suppressed during treatment but may resume by the time ovarian function returns even if patients remain asymptomatic [36].

Gonadotropin releasing hormone agonists do not improve results when given to a general IVF population prior to undergoing ART. In a prospective study, women matched for age, diagnosis (tubal, unexplained, and mild endometriosis) and number of prior IVF attempts were randomized to GnRH agonist suppression for 4 months or a standard long protocol. The two groups had a similar ovarian response and similar clinical pregnancy rates (23.35 versus 16.6%, NS). Interestingly, the GnRH agonist group was found to have lower peak E2 levels at human chorionic gonadotropin (hCG) administration (1393 pg/mL versus 2376 pg/mL, $P < 0.001$) and required an almost statistically significant higher amount of ampoules of gonadotropins (31.1 versus 27.8, $P = 0.06$) [37].

A number of non-randomized studies have asserted that prolonged treatment with GnRH agonists in patients with endometriosis prior to ART improves outcomes (Table 46.1). In a retrospective analysis, 53 infertile women with staged endometriosis pretreated with 6 weeks of GnRH agonist were compared to 153 patients with tubal factor infertility given 3 weeks of GnRH agonist downregulation prior to IVF. The fertilization rate per oocyte was lower in the moderate/severe endometriosis group compared to the tubal factor infertility group (2.6 versus 3.7, $P < 0.05$); however, the number of mature eggs per cycle, fertilization rate per cycle and pregnancy rates per embryo transfer were similar between the groups [38]. This supported the hypothesis that GnRH agonist pretreatment in endometriosis patients would allow comparable performance in IVF cycles to tubal factor infertility patients. This study was limited by a lack of control without endometriosis and no GnRH agonist treatment group with tubal infertility for comparison.

Dicker et al retrospectively analyzed 31 infertile women with surgically confirmed moderate and severe endometriosis who underwent a repeat IVF cycle after 6 months of pretreatment with GnRH agonist [39]. The number of oocytes recovered (4.3 versus 2.2, $P < 0.0006$) and pregnancy rates per cycle (30% versus 0%, $P < 0.0001$) were significantly increased after GnRH agonist treatment when compared to their own prior unsuccessful cycles as a control [39]. There was no control group receiving no pretreatment in the second IVF cycle for comparison. In another non-randomized trial, Nakamura et al examined 32 infertile patients with surgically confirmed endometriosis failing to conceive in prior IVF cycles and divided them into two groups: (1) 21 women (four minimal, one mild,

Table 46.1 Trials of GnRH agonists as pretreatment prior to IVF.

	Study design	Interventions	Results
Curtis 1993 [38]	Retrospective (n = 331) Tubal infertility versus stage I/II versus stage III/IV endometriosis	Tx: endometriosis, GnRH agonist × 6 weeks Control: tubal infertility, no pretreatment	Decreased fertilization rates per oocyte between treated mod/severe endometriosis group and tubal infertility patients (51% versus 63%, $P < 0.001$) Fertilization and pregnancy rates per transfer were not different
Dicker 1990 [39]	Retrospective (n = 31) Moderate and severe endometriosis failing prior IVF	Tx: GnRH agonist × 6 months Control: same patient in prior failed cycle of IVF	Greater # of oocytes retrieved (170 versus 106, $P < 0.0006$) and higher pregnancy rates/cycle (30% versus 0%, $P < 0.0001$) after GnRH agonist
Nakamura 1992 [40]	Retrospective (n = 32) All stages endometriosis failing prior IVF	Tx: GnRH agonist × 60 days Control: no pretreatment	Higher # of embryos implanted (1.2 versus 0.4, $P < 0.05$) and clinical pregnancy rates (67% versus 27%, $P < 0.05$) in long-term GnRH group versus standard protocol
Marcus 1994 [41]	Prospective controlled trial (n = 84) Stage III/IV endometriosis previously treated with danazol, laser, surgery or progestins	Tx: GnRH agonist × 2–7 months Control: no pretreatment	Pregnancy rate higher per embryo transfer in patients undergoing IVF after at least 4 months of downregulation (18/42, 42.8%) compared to controls (17/134, 12.7%), $P < 0.001$

GnRH, gonadotropin releasing hormone; IVF, *in vitro* fertilization.

seven moderate, nine severe endometriosis) treated with a GnRH agonist for 60 or more days and (2) 11 women (four minimal, two moderate, five severe endometriosis) treated with a GnRH agonist in the midluteal phase prior to IVF. There was a significant difference found in the number of embryos implanted (1.2 versus 0.4, $P < 0.05$) and clinical pregnancy rates (67% versus 27%, $P < 0.05$) [40].

Finally, Marcus *et al* prospectively followed 84 patients with stage III/IV endometriosis previously treated with danazol, laser, surgery and progestins. Patients received a GnRH agonist for 2–7 months prior to IVF or they underwent an ultrashort or short GnRH agonist protocol. Pregnancy rates per embryo transfer were higher in patients undergoing IVF after 3 or more months of downregulation (18/42, 42.8%) compared to controls (17/134, 12.7%), $P < 0.001$ [41].

There have also been three prospective randomized controlled trials that have investigated the same topic (Table 46.2). The first trial analyzed 67 women with severe endometriosis undergoing 6 months of GnRH agonist treatment or no treatment prior to IVF. The findings included a higher number of oocytes retrieved and higher clinical pregnancy rate per cycle and per transfer in the GnRH agonist group versus control (25.0 versus 3.9, $P < 0.0001$; 33.3 versus 5.3, $P < 0.0001$). There were more preclinical pregnancies in the control group (1 versus 8, $P < 0.0001$) [42]. Surrey *et al* performed a trial of 51 infertile women with surgically confirmed stage I to IV endometriosis. Twenty-five women received GnRH agonist for 3 months before starting a standard luteal GnRH agonist down-regulation protocol. The second group of 26 women received no pretreatment. Again, higher pregnancy rates were found in the long-acting GnRH regimen group when compared to the control group (80 versus 53.9%, $P < 0.05$) [36]. The third randomized trial by Rickes *et al* included 110 infertile women with surgically confirmed II to IV endometriosis with prior surgical treatment for the disease.

These patients were assessed for cumulative pregnancy rates after three cycles of IVF/intrauterine insemination (IUI). The treatment group (n = 55) received 6 months of GnRH agonist therapy before ART (28 had IVF/ICSI with controlled ovarian hyperstimulation (COH) starting 2 weeks after last depot injection, 27 had gonadotropin/IUI). The control group (n = 55) received surgical treatment only before ART (19 had IVF with GnRH downregulation starting CD18 prior to COH with rFSH (recombinant follicle stimulating hormone), 36 had gonadotropin/IUI). Pregnancy rates were higher in patients with stage III/IV endometriosis who received GnRH agonist pretreatment before IVF compared to the group undergoing surgery alone (82% versus 40%, $P = 0.037$) but not in the stage II endometriosis group [43]. None of these three studies used blinding or a placebo for the control groups. Further, none reported livebirth rates, number of embryos obtained and number frozen, ectopic rates, multigestation rates, fetal abnormality rates or incidence of adverse events.

A Cochrane meta-analysis was performed based on the prior three randomized controlled trials with 165 women. The number of oocytes retrieved was found to be significantly higher in women who received the GnRH agonist compared with the control group. No difference was found in the ampoules of gonadotropins required or in the spontaneous abortion rates. Clinical pregnancy rates in women receiving GnRH agonist compared to no pretreatment were 53/88 and 25/77, respectively. This review suggested that in women with endometriosis, pretreatment with a GnRH agonist for a period of 3–6 months prior to IVF or ICSI increases the odds of clinical pregnancy by approximately fourfold (OR 4.28, 95% CI 2.00–9.15) [44]. The authors concluded that based on the current available evidence, women with endometriosis-associated infertility should receive GnRH agonist pretreatment for a minimum of 3 months.

Table 46.2 Trials of GnRH agonists as pretreatment prior to IVF.

	Study design	Interventions	Results
Randomized trials			
Dicker 1992 [42]	RCT (n = 67) Severe endometriosis	Tx: GnRH agonist × 6 months Control: no pretreatment	GnRH agonist group had more oocytes retrieved ($P < 0.0006$) and higher clinical pregnancy rates per cycle (25% versus 3.9%, $P < 0.0001$)
Rickes 2002 [43]	RCT (n = 110) Stage II to IV endometriosis with prior surgical treatment	Tx: GnRH agonist × 6 months Control: no pretreatment	Pregnancy rates higher in stage III to IV endometriosis receiving GnRH agonist pretreatment before IVF compared to surgery alone (82% versus 40%, $P = 0.037$)
Surrey 2002 [36]	RCT (n = 51) Stage I to IV endometriosis	Tx: GnRH agonist × 3 months Control: no pretreatment	Pregnancy rates higher in long-acting GnRH regimen group compared to control (80 versus 53.9%, $P < 0.05$)
Non-randomized trials			
Dicker 1990 [39]	Retrospective (n = 31), moderate and severe endometriosis failing prior IVF	Tx: GnRH agonist × 6 months Control: same patient in prior failed cycle of IVF	Greater number of oocytes retrieved (170 versus 106, $P < 0.0006$) and higher pregnancy rates per cycle (30% versus 0%, $P < 0.0001$) after GnRH agonist
Nakamura 1992 [40]	Retrospective (n = 32), endometriosis failing prior IVF	Tx: GnRH agonist × 60 days Control: no pretreatment	Greater number of embryos implanted (1.2 versus 0.4, $P < 0.05$) and clinical pregnancy rates (67% versus 27%, $P < 0.05$) in long-term GnRH group versus standard protocol
Curtis 1993 [38]	Retrospective (n = 331) *Group 1*: Tubal infertility *Group 2*: Minimal/mild endometriosis *Group 3*: Moderate/severe endometriosis	Tx: endometriosis, GnRH agonist × 6 weeks Control: tubal infertility, no pretreatment	Decreased fertilization rates per oocyte between treated mod/severe endometriosis group and tubal infertility patients (51% versus 63%, $P < 0.001$) Fertilization and pregnancy rates per transfer were not different
Marcus 1994 [41]	Prospective controlled trial (n = 84) Stage III/IV endometriosis previously treated with danazol, laser, surgery and progestins	Tx: GnRH agonist × 2–7 months Control: no pretreatment	Pregnancy rate higher per embryo transfer in patients undergoing IVF after at least 4 months of downregulation (18/42, 42.8%) compared to controls (17/134, 12.7%), $P < 0.001$

GnRH, gonadotropin releasing hormone; IVF, *in vitro* fertilization; RCT, randomized controlled trial.

The above studies suggest an improvement in IVF outcomes with a GnRH agonist for a period of 3–6 months. Caruso *et al* examined whether patients might benefit from more than 3 months of treatment and found that pregnancy rates after ART were similar in patients with endometriosis who were pretreated with a GnRH agonist for 10–90 days before COH when compared to a group treated for >90 days [45]. While limited by its retrospective nature, this study suggests that treatment within the 10–90-day range is sufficient for an effect.

While outcomes were assessed in the above studies, they did not address the etiology of the effect. It is not known whether the improvement is a result of a change in uterine receptivity or in the quality of oocytes or whether it is a result of the direct effects of GnRH agonists or the consequence of the hypoestrogenic state.

Based on studies in hypogonadal women given hormone replacement therapy and donor oocytes, it is thought that the endometrium may be more responsive to implantation after long-term amenorrhea when compared to cycling women of a similar age. Steroid-sensitive structures such as pinopods may recover cell function [43,46]. However, Surrey and Halme found

that GnRH agonists do not appear to have a direct effect on endometrial tissue [47].

Several other studies have postulated at the beneficial effects of GnRH agonist on fertility in endometriosis. Seli and Arici argue that a heightened immune response in endometriosis facilitates rather than inhibits the development of endometriosis. Secretory products such as cytokines and prostaglandins contribute to the pelvic inflammation and development of pain although it is unclear if these immunological alterations are a consequence of endometriosis or induce its presence. This inflammatory environment may lead to adhesion formation and scarring as well as impaired folliculogenesis, fertilization, and embryo implantation. GnRH agonists downregulate the cellular and humoral immune responses which are associated with endometriosis, including an elevation in natural killer cell activity, a suppression of autoantibodies, and a reduction of elevated interleukin (IL)-1 and tumor necrosis factor (TNF) in peritoneal fluid [48].

Other theories include attenuation of production of tissue inhibitors of metalloproteinases (TIMPs), a regulator of extracellular matrix modeling. TIMPs are altered in patients with endometriosis but restored after GnRH agonist administration

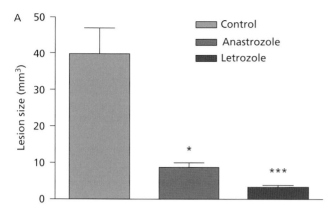

Figure 46.2 Effect of aromatase inhibitors on endometriotic lesion size. Reproduced from Bilotas *et al* [54] with permission from Elsevier.

[49]. Alternatively, spontaneous apoptosis is significantly lower in endometriotic tissue than in control subjects. Exposure of this endometriotic tissue to a GnRH agonist resulted in an increased apoptotic rate of endometrial cells while the control endometrium was not affected [50].

Lessey hypothesized that aberrant expression of integrin subtype αvβ3, a purported marker of uterine receptivity, has been described in endometriosis patients with return of function reported with GnRH agonist administration [35]. This theory was tested in a prospective randomized controlled trial examining expression of integrin αvβ3 vitronectin as a predictor of patients with endometriosis that may benefit from pretreatment with prolonged GnRH agonist therapy, however, no significant differences were found in the integrin expression strata [51].

Aromatase inhibitors

High levels of aromatase are present in endometriotic tissue [52]. Aromatase catalyzes the rate-limiting step in the biosynthesis of estrogen. Since endometriosis is an estrogen-dependent disease, aromatase inhibitors are obvious candidates for treatment of endometriosis and have been shown to have promising results in the treatment of endometriosis-related pain [53]. The effect of anastrozole and letrozole on ectopic endometrial growth was evaluated by Bilotas *et al* in a mouse model. Neither aromatase inhibitor prevented the establishment of lesions, but they did cause a significant decrease in their size [54] (Fig. 46.2).

A prospective observational study of 20 infertile women aged 20–39 with endometriomas (largest diameter 20–70 mm) with an indication for IVF were given anastrozole 1 mg daily for 69 days and goserelin on days 1, 28, and 56 followed by controlled ovarian hyperstimulation with rFSH. Inactivation of endometriosis during treatment was measured by a change in endometriomal volume (median change was 29%) and change in CA-125 (median change was 61%). When compared to 15 patients who served as their own controls, no difference in number of stimulation days, total FSH dose, oocytes retrieved, fertilization rate or number of embryos was found. The numbers were too small to analyze

for pregnancy rates [55]. Further studies are needed to clearly establish whether there is a role for these compounds prior to IVF.

Summary

In conclusion, there is some evidence to support medical pretreatment with GnRH agonists prior to IVF in patients with endometriosis but this is far from unanimous. An emerging therapy for endometriosis is the use of aromatase inhibitors but more studies are needed. Time to pregnancy is an important consideration in older IVF patients due to concern for diminished ovarian reserve with aging and it is important to remember that courses of medical therapies before IVF postpone treatment.

Surgical treatment prior to *in vitro* fertilization

Whether surgical treatment prior to IVF affects outcomes is also a controversial topic. For supporters of surgical treatment, the benefits include reduction of disease burden, excision of endometriomas that may affect oocyte retrieval either by location or size, potential improvement in IVF outcomes and improvement of pain symptoms. Opponents, however, argue that surgery may be detrimental to ovarian reserve as normal ovarian tissue may be compromised during removal of diseased tissue. Further, surgical treatment has the potential to worsen pelvic anatomical distortion, introduce scar tissue, and worsen pain symptoms.

Postsurgical *in vitro* fertilization outcomes

While it appears that surgical intervention does not necessarily improve pregnancy rates, the literature also does not definitely establish that treatment is detrimental. A number of studies have analyzed the effect of surgical intervention on subsequent ovarian responsiveness to controlled ovarian hyperstimulation and on IVF outcomes including fertilization and pregnancy rates, specifically in patients with endometriomas.

A number of non-randomized studies have demonstrated a difference in ovarian response to stimulation including number of developing follicles and oocytes retrieved in patients undergoing endometrioma resection when compared to tubal factor infertility controls but failed to demonstrate a difference in IVF outcomes, including pregnancy rates [56–60].

Tsoumpou *et al* performed a meta-analysis of five non-randomized studies [61–65] (Table 46.3) to evaluate the effect of surgical treatment for endometriomas on IVF outcomes including both ovarian stimulation response and pregnancy rates. The treatment group was women undergoing endometrioma resection and the control group was no treatment for an endometrioma prior to IVF. The authors did not report significant differences in number of oocytes retrieved, number of ampoules of gonadotropin required, or peak E2 levels. They also failed to detect a difference in pregnancy rates per cycle between the resection group when compared to the controls (OR 0.92, 95% CI 0.61–1.38) [66].

In the only RCT on this topic, Demirol *et al* reported a significantly longer stimulation (14 versus 10.8), higher dose of

Table 46.3 Studies comparing IVF outcomes in patients with treated and untreated endometriomas.

	Groups	Total ampoules	Peak E2	# Oocytes	Fertilization rate	Pregnancy rate
Garcia-Velasco 2004 [61]	133 treated 56 untreated	52 versus 45, $P = 0.035$	1910 versus 2472, $P = 0.018$	NS	NS	NS
Pabuccu 2004 [62]	44 treated 40 untreated	NS	NS	NS	NS	NS
Suganuma 2002 [63]	36 treated 20 untreated	–	–	7.2 versus 9.7, $P < 0.05$	NS	NS
Tinkanen 2000 [64]	55 treated 45 untreated	NS	–	NS	NS	NS
Wong 2004 [65]	36 treated 38 untreated	NS	NS	NS	87 versus 81, $P < 0.05$	NS

NS, non-significant.

gonadotropins (4575 versus 3675 IU), and lower mean number of mature oocytes (7.8 versus 8.6) in the surgically treated versus untreated groups with endometriomas. But again, there was no difference in fertilization, implantation, or pregnancy rates [67].

Ragni *et al* described the diminished response to stimulation as a quantitative rather than a qualitative damage to ovarian reserve. In a retrospective study of 38 subjects comparing operated to contralateral intact ovaries of the same patient, there was a marked reduction in the number of dominant follicles, oocytes retrieved, total embryos, and high-quality embryos. However, the rate of fertilization and the rate of high-quality embryos did not differ between oocytes retrieved from the operated and contralateral ovary [68] (Fig. 46.3).

Collectively, insights from these studies have shown a trend that oocytes may be affected quantitatively, whether as a result of the endometrioma itself or as a result of surgical removal, which may result in decreased ovarian responsiveness. Oocyte quality, as reflected in IVF outcomes including fertilization, implantation, and pregnancy rates, does not appear to be affected by surgery.

International guidelines on surgery prior to *in vitro* fertilization

The ASRM, the European Society of Human Reproduction and Embryology (ESHRE), and the Royal College of Obstetricians and Gynaecologists (RCOG) have all published guidelines for the management of endometriosis, summarized by Vercellini *et al* [69] (Table 46.4). The Practice Committee of the ASRM [1] reports that conclusions are difficult regarding surgical treatment prior to IVF due to limited data but with advanced age, longer duration of fertility, concomitant pelvic pain, and prior infertility operations, a therapeutic plan moving directly to IVF is often a better option. Both the RCOG [70] and the ESHRE [3] guidelines state that, based on expert opinion, laparoscopic ovarian cystectomy for endometriomas $\geq 4\,\mathrm{cm}$ is recommended in order to confirm histology, reduce the risk of infection, improve access to follicles, possibly improve ovarian response, and prevent endometriosis progression.

Other considerations for surgical intervention

The fertility treatment outcomes and the effect on ovarian responsiveness are not the only issues that need to be addressed with

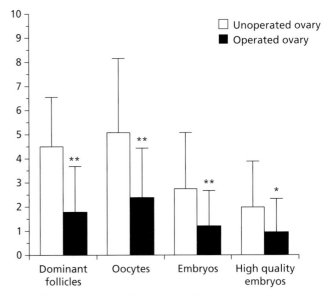

Figure 46.3 Response to ovarian hyperstimulation in an ovary status post endometrioma excision compared to the unoperated contralateral ovary. *$P = 0.005$, **$p < 0.001$. Reproduced from Ragni *et al* [68] with permission from Elsevier.

regard to a patient with endometriosis considering surgery prior to ART. Many patients have moderate-to-severe burden of disease, and thus surgery itself does not come without complications. In a meta-analysis by Chapron *et al*, the rates of major and minor surgical complications associated with laparoscopy are 1.4% and 7.5%. With patients who have severe disease, the likelihood of adhesions affecting successful surgery and an increase in bowel and bladder complications is real and must be considered when choosing surgery, reoperation, or movement directly towards IVF [71].

While endometriomas are generally accurately diagnosed by ultrasonography, a level of suspicion must remain for any complex adnexal mass, especially if enlarging over time. Surgical removal and pathological examination are required for accurate diagnosis of concerning adnexal masses in order to definitively rule out malignancy. Reported incidence of occult malignancy in endometriotic samples ranges from 0.8% to 0.9% [72,73]. While this risk is quite low, careful sonographic evaluation and

Table 46.4 International guidelines on surgical treatment of endometriosis-associated infertility in asymptomatic women.

	Recommendation		
Clinical condition	ESHRE 2005	ASRM2006	RCOG 2006
Minimal-mild endometriosis (stage I to II disease)	Limited benefit: surgery recommended	Small benefit: surgery recommended	Demonstrated benefit: surgery recommended
Moderate-severe endometriosis (stage III to IV disease)	Possible but unproven benefit: surgery recommended	Possible benefit: surgery recommended	Possible benefit: recommendation uncertain
Post-operative adjuvant treatment	No benefit: not recommended	No benefit: not recommended	No benefit: not recommended
Surgery before IVF	Recommended if endometrioma ≥ 4 cm	Doubtful benefit: no recommendation	Recommended if endometioma ≥ 4 cm
Recurrent endometriosis	No recommendation	Second-line surgery not recommended	No recommendation

Source: Vercellini P *et al* [69] with permission from Wiley-Blackwell.

consideration for surgical intervention should be a priority in any concerning masses.

Proceeding directly to IVF may reduce the time to pregnancy, avoid potential surgical complications, and limit costs. Surgery should be considered when patients have concomitant pain symptoms refractory to medical management, when malignancy cannot be ruled out, or in the presence of large cysts in symptomatic patients. Based on lack of improvement in pregnancy outcomes and the potential for damage to normal ovarian tissue, multiple factors must be considered when deciding whether to operate or to proceed directly to ART.

In vitro fertilization complications associated with endometriosis

Pelvic abscess following oocyte retrievals in patients with endometriomas has been reported in several case reports in the literature [74,75]. While the above studies have supported the view that surgical intervention does not improve fertility rates significantly and may affect ovarian responsiveness, other concerns are that patients with larger endometriomas may be at risk for infection after oocyte retrieval. It has been reported that the bloody content of an endometrioma may serve as an excellent culture medium and may facilitate the spread of infection [76]. Benaglia *et al* attempted to identify the frequency of pelvic abscess in women with endometriomas who underwent ultrasound-guided oocyte retrieval. In the 214 retrievals they evaluated, six cases had known punctures of endometriomas and in none of these six cases did patients acquire an infection, suggesting that the incidence of this complication is very rare. While a rare complication, it is reasonable to consider surgical removal if oocyte removal is hindered due to size or location of the cyst so as to prevent possible infection, but also to prevent pain to the patient [77].

Endometriosis has been considered an estrogen-dependent disease and it is well known that this disease has the potential for recurrence even after medical or surgical therapy. Due to the high levels of hormones a patient is exposed to when undergoing ovarian stimulation, a question that has been proposed is: Could it be possible that ovarian stimulation actually increases the burden of disease or recurrence? D'Hooghe *et al* published a retrospective cohort study in 2006 examining the recurrence rate of endometriosis in patients after ovarian stimulation for IUI or IVF with prior surgical treatment of endometriosis [78]. Their results suggested that temporary exposure to high estrogen levels is not a risk factor for endometriosis recurrence [78]. Furthermore, a prospective study by Benaglia *et al* in 2008 evaluated 48 women with endometriomas undergoing IVF and measured the size of the endometriomas before and at 2- and 6-month follow-ups. They also failed to document any increase in size of the endometriomas [77]. Further studies are needed to evaluate this question, but to date no supporting evidence for further progression of endometriosis with ovarian stimulation exists.

Obstetrical complications in patients with endometriosis have also been reported. It is believed that abnormal endometrium, its decidualized stroma, and impaired placentation may lead to preterm birth, intrauterine growth restriction, and babies small for gestational age (SGA). Fernando *et al* retrospectively examined women with and without endometriosis who underwent ART in order to conceive [79]. Rates of preterm birth and SGA babies doubled in infertility patients with ovarian endometriomata who required ART. This study suggests that some pathological changes occur in patients with endometriomas that may further increase the risk of preterm birth and intrauterine growth retardation. However, it is important to note that the majority of patients who deliver after ART with the previous diagnosis of endometriosis have healthy babies. Further studies are needed to elucidate the frequency of preterm births and SGA babies in this population.

Stimulation protocols

It has been theorized that if there are differences in response to IVF with varying stages of endometriosis then it is possible that individualized IVF protocols may improve clinical outcomes.

Pabuccu *et al* examined the outcomes in a GnRH agonist versus antagonist protocol for stage I/II endometriosis and endometrioma. Considering implantation and clinical pregnancy rates, COH with either analog demonstrated similar outcomes in all groups [80].

Conclusion

Endometriosis is common in women with infertility. A number of factors need to be taken into account when formulating a management plan for infertile patients with endometriosis, including age, duration of infertility, family history, pelvic pain, co-existing infertility diagnoses, number of prior fertility treatment cycles, stage of endometriosis, and cost. In general, early aggressive treatment with IVF is recommended as an effective means to treat endometriosis-associated infertility. There is some evidence to support medical pretreatment with GnRH agonists as well as emerging evidence for aromatase inhibitors prior to IVF, but medical treatment may unnecessarily delay time to pregnancy. Surgical treatment prior to IVF may result in a reduced ovarian response to hyperstimulation but this does not translate into poorer IVF outcomes. In general, surgery is not necessary and may even be detrimental prior to IVF unless there is concern for malignancy or a need to improve access for oocyte aspiration.

References

1. Practice Committee of the American Society for Reproductive Medicine. Endometriosis and infertility. Fertil Steril 2006;86: S156–160.

2. Hughes E, Brown J, Collins J et al. Ovulation suppression for endometriosis. Cochrane Database Syst Rev 2007;3:CD000155.

3. Kennedy S, Bergqvist A, Chapron C et al. ESHRE guidelines for the diagnosis and treatment of endometriosis. Hum Reprod 2005;20: 2698–2704.

4. Guzick D, Silliman N, Adamson G et al. Prediction of pregnancy in infertile women based on the American Society for Reproductive Medicine's revised classification of endometriosis. Fertil Steril 1997;67:822–829.

5. American Society for Reproductive Medicine. Revised American Society for Reproductive Medicine classification of endometriosis: 1996. Fertil Steril 1997;67:817–821.

6. Arici A, Oral E, Bukulmez O, Duleba A, Olive D, Jones E. The effect of endometriosis on implantation: results from the Yale University in vitro fertilization and embryo transfer program. Fertil Steril 1996;65:603–607.

7. Cahill D, Wardle P, Maile L, Harlow C, Hull M. Pituitary-ovarian dysfuction as a cause for endometriosis-associated and unexplained infertility. Hum Reprod 1995;10:3142–3146.

8. Matson PL, Yovich JL. The treatment of infertility associated with endometriosis with in vitro fertilization. Fertil Steril 1986;46:432–434.

9. Trinder J, Cahill D. Endometriosis and infertility: the debate continues. Hum Fertil 2002;5(Suppl):S21–27.

10. Dmowski WP, Rana N, Michalowska J, Friberg J, Papierniak C, El-Roeiy A. The effect of endometriosis, its stage and activity, and of autoantibodies on in vitro fertilization and embryo transfer success rates. Fertil Steril 1995;63:555–562.

11. Frydman R, Belaisch-Allart JC. Results of in vitro fertilization for endometriosis. Contr Gynecol Obstet 1987;16:328–331.

12. Geber S, Paraschos T, Atkinson G, Margara R, Winston R. Results of IVF in patients with endometriosis: the severity of the disease dose not affect outcome or the incidence of miscarriage. Hum Reprod 1995;10:1507–1511.

13. Huang HY, Lee CL, Lai YM, Chang MY, Chang SY, Soong YK. The outcome of in vitro fertilization and embryo transfer therapy in women with endometriosis failing to conceive after laparoscopic conservative surgery. J Am Assoc Gynecol Laparosc 1997;4:299–303.

14. Inoue M, Kobayashi Y, Honda I, Awaji H, Fujii A. The impact of endometriosis on the reproductive outcome of infertile patients. Am J Obstet Gynecol 1992;167:278–282.

15. Mahadevan M, Trounson A, Leeton J. The relationship of tubal blockage, infertility of unknown cause, suspected male infertility, and endometriosis to success of in vitro fertilizaiton and embryo transfer. Fertil Steril 1983;40:755–762.

16. Mills MS, Eddowes HA, Cahill DJ et al. A prospective controlled study of in-vitro fertilzation, gamete intra-Fallopian transfer and intrauterine insemination combined with superovulation. Hum Reprod 1992;7:490–494.

17. Olivennes F, Feldberg D, Liu HC, Cohen J, Moy F, Rosenwaks Z. Endometriosis: a stage by stage analysis – the role of in vitro fertilization. Fertil Steril 1995;64:392–398.

18. Pagidas K, Falcone T, Hemmings R, Miron P. Comparison of reoperation for moderate (stage III) and severe (stage IV) endometriosis-related infertility with in vitro fertilization-embryo transfer. Fertil Steril 1996;65:791–795.

19. Suzuki T, Izumi S, Matsubayashi H, Awaji H, Yoshikata K, Makino T. Impact of ovarian endometrioma on oocytes and pregnancy outcome in invitro fertilization. Fertil Steril 2005;83:908–913.

20. Tanbo T, Omland A, Dale PO, Abyholm T. In vitro fertilization/ embryo transfer in unexplained infertility and minimal peritoneal endometriosis. Acta Obstet Gynecol Scand 1995;74:539–543.

21. Wardle PG, Mitchell JD, McLaughlin EA, Ray BD, McDermott A, Hull MG. Endometriosis and ovulatory disorder: reduced fertilization in vitro compared with tubal and unexplained infertility. Lancet 1985;2:236–239.

22. Barnhart K, Dunsmoor-Su R, Coutifaris C. Effect of endometriosis on in vitro fertilization. Fertil Steril 2002;77:1148–1155.

23. Templeton A, Morris J, Parslow W. Factors that affect outcome of in-vitro fertilization treatment. Lancet 1996;348:1402–1406.

24. Sunderam S, Chang J, Flowers L et al. Assisted reproductive technology surveillance – United States, 2006. MMWR Survill Summ 2009;12:1–25.

25. Diaz I, Navarro J, Blasco L, Simon C, Pellicer A, Remohi J. Impact of stage III-IV endometriosis on recipients of sibling oocytes: matched case-control study. Fertil Steril 2000;74:31–34.

26. Azem F, Lessing J, Geva E et al. Patients with stages III and IV endometriosis have a poorer outcome of in vitro fertilization-embryo transfer than patients with tubal infertility. Fertil Steril 1999;72:1107–1109.

27. Chilik C, Acosta A, Garcia J et al. The role of in vitro fertilization in infertile patients with endometriosis. Fertil Steril 1985;44:56–61.

28. Kuivasaari P, Hippelainen M, Anttila M, Heinonen. Effect of endometriosis on IVF/ICSI outcome: stage III/IV endometriosis worsens cumulative pregnancy and live-born rates. Hum Reprod 2005;20:3130–3135.

29. Oehninger S, Acosta A, Kreiner D, Muasher S, Jones H, Rosenwaks Z. In vitro fertilization and embryo transfer (IVF/ET): an established and successful therapy for endometriosis. J In Vitro Fertil Embryo Transf 1988;5:249–256.

30. O'Shea RT, Chen C, Weiss T, Jones WR. Endometriosis and in vitro fertilization. Lancet 1985;2:723.

31. Pellicer A, Oliveira N, Ruiz A, Remohi J, Simon C. Exploring the mechanism(s) of endometriosis-related infertility: an analysis of embryo development and implantation in assisted reproduction. Hum Reprod 1995;10:91–97.

32. Vercellini P, Somigliana E, Vigano P, Abbiati A, Barbara G, Crosignani P. Endometriosis: current therapies and new pharmacological developments. Drugs 2009;69:649–675.

33. Wardle P, Foster P, Mitchell J, McLaughlin E, Sykes J, Corrigan E. Endometriosis and IVF: effect of prior therapy. Lancet 1986;327:276–277.

34. Tei C, Miyazaki T, Kuji N, Tanaka M, Sueoka K, Yoshimura Y. Effects of Danazol on the pregnancy rate in patients with unsuccessful in vitro fertilization-embryo transfer. J Reprod Med 1998;43:541–546.

35. Lessey B. Medical management of endometriosis and infertility. Fertil Steril 2000;73:1089–1096.

36. Surrey E, Silverberg K, Surrey M, Schoolcraft W. Effect of prolonged gonadotropin-releasing hormone agonist therapy on the outcome of in vitro fertilization – embryo transfer in patients with endometriosis. Fertil Steril 2002;78:699–704.

37. Fabregues F, Balasch J, Creus M et al. Long-term down-regulation does not improve pregnancy rates in an in vitro fertilization program. Fertil Steril 1998;70:46–51.

38. Curtis P, Jackson A, Bernard A, Shaw R. Pretreatment with gonadotropin releasing hormone (GnRH) analogue prior to in vitro fertilisation for patients with endometriosis. Eur J Obstet Gynecol 1993;52:211–216.

39. Dicker D, Goldman G, Ashkenazi J, Feldberg D, Voliovitz I, Goldman J. The value of pre-treatment with gonadotropin releasing hormone (GnRH) analogue in IVF-ET therapy of severe endometriosis. Hum Reprod 1990;5:418–420.

40. Nakamura K, Oosawa M, Kondou I et al. Menotropin stimulation after prolonged gonadotropin releasing hormone agonist pretreatment for in vitro fertilization in patients with endometriosis. J Assist Reprod Genet 1992;9:113–117.

41. Marcus S, Edwards R. High rates of pregnancy after long-term down-regulation of women with severe endometriosis. Am J Obstet Gynecol 1994;171:812–817.

42. Dicker D, Feldberg D, Goldman J, Ashkenazi J, Levy T. The impact of long-term gonadotropin-releasing hormone analogue treatment in preclinical abortions in patients with severe endometriosis undergoing in vitro fertilization-embryo transfer. Fertil Steril 1992;57:597–600.

43. Rickes D, Nickel I, Kropf S, Kleinstein J. Increased pregnancy rates after ultralong postoperative therapy with gonadotropin-releasing hormone analogs in patients with endometriosis. Fertil Steril 2002;78:757–762.

44. Sallam H, Garcia-Velasco J, Dias S, Arici A. Long-term pituitary down-regulation before in vitro fertilization (IVF) for women with endometriosis. Cochrane Database Syst Rev 1996;1:CD004635.

45. Caruso A, Rawlings RG, Radmeuslla E. The effect of GnRH agonist suppression in infertility treatment outcome in patients with endometriosis. In: 53rd Annual Meeting of the American Society for Reproductive Medicine, October 18–27, 1997, Cincinnati, OH. Abstract P-166.

46. Edwards RG, Morcos S, MacNamee M, Balmaceda JP, Walters DE, Asch R. High fecundity of amenorrhoeic women in embryo-transfer programmes. Lancet 1991;338:292–294.

47. Surrey E, Halme J. Direct effects of medroxyprogesterone acetate, danazol, and leuprolide acetate on endometrial stromal cell proliferation in vitro. Fertil Steril 1992;58:273–278.

48. Seli E, Arici A. Endometriosis: interaction of immune and endocrine systems. Semin Reprod Med 2003;21:135–144.

49. Sharpe-Timms K. Keisler L, McIntush E, Keisler D. Tissue inhibitor of metalloproteinase-1 concentrations are attenuated in peritoneal fluid and sera of women with endometriosis and restored in sera by gonadotropin-releasing hormone agonist therapy. Fertil Steril 1998;69:1128–1134.

50. Imai A, Takagi A, Tamaya T. Gonadotropin-releasing hormone analog repairs reduced endometrial cell apoptosis in endometriosis in vitro. Am J Obstet Gynecol 2000;182:1142–1146.

51. Surrey E, Lietz A, Gustofson R, Minjarez D, Schoolcraft W. Does endometrial integrin expression in endometriosis parients predict enhanced in vitro fertilization cycle outcomes after prolonged GnRH agonist therapy? Fertil Steril 2010;93:646–651.

52. Bulun S, Imir G, Utsunomiya H et al. Aromatase in endometriosis and uterine leiomyomata. J Steroid Biochem Mol Biol 2005;95:57–62.

53. Ailawadi R, Jobanputra S, Kataria M. Treatment of endometriosis and chronic pelvic pain with letrozole and norethindrone acetate: a pilot study. Fertil Steril 2004;81:290–296.

54. Bilotas M, Meresman G, Stelia I, Sueldo C, Baranao RI. Effect of aromatase inhibitors on ectopic endometrial growth and peritoneal environment in a mouse model of endometriosis. Fertil Steril 2010;93:2513–2518.

55. Lossl K, Loft A, Freiesleben N et al. Combined down-regulation by aromatase inhibitor and GnRH-agonist in IVF patients with endometriomas – a pilot study. Eur J Obstet Gynecol Reprod Biol 2009;144:48–53.

56. Esinler I, Bozdag G, Aybar F, Bayar U, Yarali H. Outcome of in vitro fertilization/intracytoplasmic sperm injection after laparoscopic cystectomy for endometriomas. Fertil Steril 2006;85:1730–1735.

57. Geber S, Ferreira DP, Prates LF, Sales L, Sampaio M. Effects of previous ovarian surgery for endometriosis on the outcome of assisted reproduction treatment. Reprod Biomed Online 2002;5:162–166.

58. Loo TC, Lin M, Chen SH et al. Endometrioma undergoing laparoscopic ovarian cystectomy: its influence on the outcome of in vitro fertilization and embryo transfer (IVF-ET). J Assist Reprod Genet 2005;22:329–333.

59. Marconi G, Vilela M, Qunitana R, Sueldo C. Laparoscopic ovarian cystectomy of endometriomas does not affect the ovarian response to gonadotrophin stimulation. Fertil Steril 2002;78:876–878.

60. Matalliotakis IM, Cakmak H, Mahutte N, Fragouli Y, Arici A, Sakkas D. Women with advanced-stage endometriosis and previous surgery respond less well to gonadotropin stimulation, but have similar IVF implantation and delivery rates compared with women with tubal factor infertility. Fertil Steril 2007;88:1568–1572.

61. Garcia-Velasco JA, Mahutte NG, Corona J et al. Removal of endometriomas before in vitro fertilization does not improve fertility outcomes: a matched, case-control study. Fertil Steril 2004;81: 1194–1197.

62. Pabuccu R, Onalan G, Goktolga U, Kucuk T, Orhon E, Ceyhan T. Aspiration of ovarian endometriomas before intracytoplasmic sperm injection. Fertil Steril 2004;82:705–711.

63. Suganuma N, Wakahara Y, Ishida D et al. Pretreatment for ovarian endometrial cyst before in vitro fertilization. Gynecol Obstet Invest 2002;54(Suppl):36–42.

64. Tinkanen H, Kujansuu E. In vitro fertilization in patients with ovarian endometriomas. Acta Obstet Gynecol Scand 2000;79:119–122.

65. Wong BC, Gillman NC, Oehninger S, Gibbons WE, Stadtmauer LA. Results of in vitro fertilization in patients with endometriomas: is surgical removal beneficial? Am J Obstet Gynecol 2004;191:597–606.

66. Tsoumpou I, Kyrgiou M, Gelbaya T, Nardo L. The effect of surgical treatment for endometrioma on in vitro fertilization outcomes: a systematic review and meta-analysis. Fertil Steril 2009;92:75–87.

67. Demirol A, Guven S, Baykal C, Gurgan T. Effect of endometrioma cystectomy on IVF outcome: a prospective randomized study. Reprod Biomed Online 2006;12:639–643.

68. Ragni G, Somigliana E, Benedetti F, Paffoni A, Vegetti W, Restelli L. Damage to ovarian reserve associated with laparoscopic excision of endometriomas: a quantitative rather than a qualitative injury. Am J Obstet Gynecol 2005;193:1908–1914.

69. Vercellini P, Somigliana E, Vigano P, Abbiati A, Barbara G, Crosignani PG. Surgery for endometriosis-associated infertility: a pragmatic approach. Hum Reprod 2009;24:254–269.

70. Royal College of Obstetricians and Gynaecologists. The Investigation and Management of Endometriosis. Guideline No. 24. London: RCOG Press, 2006.

71. Chapron C, Fauconnier A, Goffinet F, Breart G, Dubuisson JB. Laparoscopic surgery is not inherently dangerous for patients presenting with benign gynaecologic pathology: results of a meta-analysis. Hum Reprod 2002;17:1334–1342.

72. Mostoufizadeh M, Scully RE. Malignant tumors arising in endometriosis. Clin Obstet Gynecol 1980;23:951–963.

73. Stern RC, Dash R, Bentley RC, Snyder MJ, Haney AF, Robboy SJ. Malignancy in endometriosis: frequency and comparison of ovarian and extraovarian types. Int J Gynecol Pathol 2001;20:133–139.

74. Padilla SL. Ovarian abscess following puncture of an endometrioma during ultrasound-guided oocyte retrieval. Hum Reprod 1993;8: 1282–1283.

75. Younis JS, Ezra Y, Laufer N, Ohel G. Late manifestation of pelvic abscess following oocyte retrieval, for in vitro fertilization, in patients with severe endometriosis and ovarian endometriomata. J Assist Reprod Genet 1997;14:343–346.

76. Chen MJ, Yang JH, Yang YS, Ho HN. Increased occurrence of tubo-ovarian abscesses in women with stage III and IV endometriosis. Fertil Steril 2004;82:498–499.

77. Benaglia L, Somigliana E, Iemmello R, Colpi E, Nicolosi AE, Ragni G. Endometrioma and oocyte retrieval-induced pelvic abscess: a clinical concern or an exceptional complication? Fertil Steril 2008;89: 1263–1266.

78. D'Hooghe TM, Denys B, Spiessens C, Meuleman C, Debrock S. Is the endometriosis recurrence rate increased after ovarian hyperstimulation? Fertil Steril 2006;86:283–290.

79. Fernando S, Breheny S, Jaques AM, Halliday JL, Baker G, Healy D. Preterm birth, ovarian endometriomata, and assisted reproduction technologies. Fertil Steril 2009;91:325–330.

80. Pabuccu R, Onalan G, Kaya C. GnRH agonist and antagonist protocols for stage I-II endometriosis and endometrioma in in vitro fertilization/intracytoplasmic sperm injection cycles. Fertil Steril 2007;88:832–839.

47 Ovarian Endometrioma: Surgery and Fertility Preservation

Luk J.F. Rombauts

Department of Obstetrics and Gynaecology, Monash University, Melbourne, Australia

Ontogenesis

There are three main theories of endometrioma formation:
- invagination secondary to bleeding of a superficial implant
- invagination secondary to metaplasia of coelomic epithelium in cortical inclusion cysts
- endometriotic transformation of functional cysts.

They were postulated as separate theories by different research groups, but there is no reason to believe that they are mutually exclusive.

Brosens *et al* performed a number of studies involving ovarioscopy to argue that endometriotic cysts in the ovary are pseudocysts [1]. They described how active endometrial implants in the ovarian fossa cause the lateral aspect of the ovary to become adherent to it. With subsequent menstruations, blood and debris become trapped between the adhesions, eventually invaginating the ovarian cortex to form a pseudocyst. The important implication is that the thickened wall of the pseudocyst consists of ovarian cortex and excision of the endometrioma therefore means loss of ovarian cortex.

Nisolle and Donnez have presented evidence supporting the alternative view that endometriomas are the consequence of metaplasia of epithelial inclusions in the ovary [2].

Nehzat *et al* have postulated that there is another class of endometriomas in addition to those that originate through invagination. Type I endometriomas usually are <5 cm in size, contain a dark fluid, and have capsules that are difficult to remove because they are associated with dense fibrosis and adhesions. Type II endometriomas, on the other hand, are thought to develop following endometriotic overgrowth of functional ovarian cysts [3].

Histopathology

Classically, endometriomas are described as ovarian cysts, sometimes loculated, and at least partially lined by an endometrium-like epithelium, stroma and hemosiderin-laden macrophages.

A histological evaluation of the whole endometrioma wall reveals that the cyst wall has at least some endometriosis in 100% of cases, covering the inner aspect of the cyst for approximately 60% of its surface [4]. Knowing the depth of "invasion" may also be important for deciding on the best surgical approach. Unfortunately, studies vary widely in their reporting of this. One study reported an average penetration into the cyst wall for a mean depth of 0.6 mm, and only rarely up to 1.5 mm [4]. Nehzat *et al* noted that the capsule of endometriomas could be up to 4–5 mm in thickness [5]. There is also growing evidence that the surrounding ovarian tissue undergoes morphological changes [6]. In particular, the follicular densities in the ovarian cortex surrounding endometriomas appear to be much lower than in other benign cysts such as dermoid cysts [7]. These changes may be caused by oxidative stress [8].

Diagnosis and classification

Blood tests have so far not been reliable for diagnosing endometriosis, let alone endometriomas. The tumor marker CA-125 can be elevated in the presence of an endometrioma, but it has been shown to be wanting as a useful serological test for the diagnosis of endometriomas [9]. However, a new marker, follistatin, is showing more promise [10].

One distinct advantage of endometriomas is that they can be reliably diagnosed with transvaginal ultrasound. Sensitivity and specificity of transvaginal ultrasound for the diagnosis of endometriomas have been reported to range between 84–100% and 90–100%, respectively [11–14]. Endometriomas can have a range of appearances on ultrasound, varying from anechoic cysts to solid-appearing masses but typically, in over 80% of cases, an endometrioma is a thick-walled ovarian cyst with a homogenous "ground-glass" content. The differential diagnosis includes primarily hemorrhagic cysts and dermoids. Endometriomas can be uni- or multilocular and often have hyperechogenic wall foci or nodularities. There is no internal vascularity and typically the low-level echoes that fill the cyst do not display acoustic streaming. Commonly, multiple lesions are seen, in one or both ovaries. There is a general trend for endometriosis to be more common on the left side of the pelvis. Endometriomas also appear to follow this tendency, but the discrepancy appears to weaken with age [15].

The diagnosis of an ovarian endometrioma on ultrasound is significant. Redwine [16] found that 99% of women with ovarian endometriosis had endometriosis in other locations as well. Ovarian endometriomas are also associated with a higher number of deeply infiltrating endometriotic lesions elsewhere, compared to women without an endometrioma [17]. These lesions were also found to be more severe with an increased rate of vaginal, intestinal, and ureteral lesions.

An ultrasound diagnosis of an ovarian endometrioma is also important given that it needs to be differentiated from an ovarian malignancy, particularly when confronted with larger endometriomas in older women. For this reason, the European Society of Human Reproduction and Embryology (ESHRE) guidelines [18] refer back to locally developed guidelines for the investigation and management of suspected ovarian malignancies. Essentially, they recommend biopsy and preferably removal of the cyst for histological confirmation if the cyst is >3 cm diameter.

The most widely accepted classification system for endometriosis is the revised American Fertility Society (rAFS) system [19]. It is based on the appearance, size, and depth of peritoneal and ovarian implants, the presence, extent, and type of adnexal adhesions and also the degree of cul-de-sac obliteration. The classification was developed primarily to assess fertility and adnexal adhesions were thus given a disproportionate weight in the scoring system. Despite the revisions, the current rAFS system does not reliably predict the outcome of treatment [18]. Nevertheless, high rAFS scores are usually obtained in the presence of endometriomas and/or cul-de-sac obliteration. The impact of deep ovarian endometriosis on fertility was also recognized by Adamson and Pasta in the Endometriosis Fertility Index [20].

Impact on fertility

When deciding how to best treat an ovarian endometrioma, it is important to assess how much of an impact the cyst may have on a woman's fertility. It would appear logical to assume that a very small endometrioma will have less impact than large bilateral endometriomas ("kissing ovaries").

It is well documented that endometriosis causes infertility. A meta-analysis of 22 non-randomized studies by Barnhart et al [21] found that the pregnancy rate was significantly lower for women with endometriosis compared to women with tubal infertility. This effect seems at least partly mediated through an effect on oocyte quality [22]. Unfortunately, there is little information on the specific adverse effects of ovarian endometriomas. The issue is also not helped by the lack of appropriate animal models for deep ovarian endometriosis.

In a retrospective study by Suzuki et al fewer oocytes were retrieved during in vitro fertilization (IVF) from women with endometriosis compared with women without endometriosis. Interestingly, the egg yield was not more affected in women with ovarian endometriomas [23].

Other evidence comes from a series of experiments carried out in the late 1990s by the group from the Instituto Valenciano de Infertilidad. They reported on the outcomes of oocyte donor cycles involving oocyte donors and recipients with and without endometriosis [24]. Although their results have not been confirmed by others, they support the view that endometriosis has a direct effect on oocyte quality. Oocyte recipients with endometriosis had normal implantation rates as long as they received eggs from women without the disease. However, oocyte recipients without endometriosis had lower implantation rates when they received eggs from women with the disease. These findings suggest that pelvic endometriosis may affect oocyte quality, perhaps through an altered intrafollicular milieu [22] and increased granulosa cell apoptosis [25].

However, new evidence is also emerging that deep ovarian endometriosis alters the local environment through intraovarian oxidative damage [8,26]. Other studies have shown that the spontaneous ovulation rate in the affected ovary is significantly lower than expected [27,28]. Moreover, in the study from Benaglia et al [28], a dose–response effect was observed. When only one endometrioma was present the ovulation rate in the affected ovary was 35%. When an ovary contained two or more cysts, the ovulation rate was only 19%.

The direct effects of endometriomas on ovarian function require further elucidation, in particular whether the damage, if any, is permanent or transient. This particular question is echoed in the ongoing debate regarding the impact of endometrioma surgery. It remains unclear to what extent the postoperative reduction in ovarian function is caused by the surgery itself or by a pre-existing direct effect of the endometrioma.

Although it is difficult at this stage to ascertain the impact of an isolated endometrioma on fertility, there are a number of other points to raise. Firstly, in the rAFS classification deep ovarian endometriosis receives high scores, up to a maximum of 40 points, not taking into account the presence of adhesions [19]. The Endometriosis Fertility Index similarly assigns a high score to the presence of ovarian endometriomas in recognition of their impact on a woman's fertility [20].

Secondly, an ovarian endometrioma tends to be a sentinel marker of more disseminated endometriosis. In a study with 1785 cases with endometriomas, only 1% of the patients had ovarian disease exclusively [16]. Often the additional endometriosis is widespread, severe and in locations which would easily escape diagnosis with routine imaging techniques [29].

In light of this, it is somewhat academic to try and single out the impact of ovarian endometriosis. The reality is that ovarian endometriosis is usually accompanied by other pelvic lesions and adhesions. The combined effect is that of more severe disease, which is associated with lower fertility rates. Indeed, Barnhart *et al* concluded in their meta-analysis of 22 non-randomized studies that IVF pregnancy rates for women with severe disease were significantly lower than for women with mild endometriosis (odds ratio (OR) 0.60, 95% confidence interval (CI) 0.42–0.87) [21].

Treatment

The treatment of ovarian endometriomas in the context of infertility remains a difficult and hotly debated topic. It has been customary to treat endometriomas surgically to improve a patient's fertility, but that dogmatic approach is now being questioned, in particular since the arrival of IVF. There are growing concerns that surgery may be causing more harm than good.

This section will be divided into three main parts. First, the non-surgical options will be explored (*First: do no harm*). The second part will deal with a variety of surgical approaches. Different techniques will be discussed with special emphasis on their relative impact on ovarian reserve (*Second: minimize further harm*). Finally, the third part will briefly cover options to preserve fertility, when conservative surgery is not an option (*Third: when harm is inevitable, preserve fertility*).

First, do no harm

Is it always appropriate to intervene surgically when ovarian endometriomas are diagnosed with ultrasound? The answer to this question depends on a variety of factors. In the context of fertility treatment, factors such as age, parity, duration of infertility, associated pain, previous surgery and affordability of treatment need to be taken into account when making a decision. Where considered appropriate, a number of non-surgical treatment options are available, including expectant management, medical treatment and assisted reproductive technologies. These have been discussed in more detail in previous chapters in this book and will only be touched upon where relevant for the treatment of ovarian endometriomas.

Expectant management

There may be a number of situations where delaying intervention is appropriate. Although transvaginal ultrasound is good at diagnosing endometriomas, it is worth repeating the scan in 2–3 months to exclude the possibility of a functional cyst, in particular a hemorrhagic corpus luteum cyst, which will resolve with time. In contrast, endometriomas have an average growth rate of approximately 0.5 cm per 6 months [30].

Also, expectant management may be appropriate when counseling patients about their fertility treatment options.

Consider the following example: a small likely endometrioma is an incidental finding during an ultrasound in a young woman presenting with heavy periods. She has also been trying to conceive for the last 6 months. Even though there may be more widespread disease, one of the treatment options for discussion should include further expectant management for 6 months.

Medical management

There is specific evidence showing that medical pretreatment with either gonadotropin releasing hormone (GnRH) agonists or danazol is effective in shrinking the size of endometriomas by approximately 50% [31]. Whether this is clinically relevant is a different matter. A meta-analysis by Sallam *et al* [32] argued in favor of medical suppression with GnRH agonists prior to IVF for women with any endometriosis. The meta-analysis of three randomized controlled trials (RCTs) concluded that the administration of GnRH agonists for a period of 3–6 months prior to IVF in women with endometriosis increases the odds of clinical pregnancy fourfold. The benefits were most obvious for women with stage III/IV endometriosis, and by extension this is relevant for women with endometriomas larger than 3 cm. However, two of the included studies were characterized by flaws that called the validity of those conclusions into question [33].

Controlled ovarian hyperstimulation and intrauterine insemination

There are a growing number of arguments against the use of controlled ovarian hyperstimulation and intrauterine insemination (COH-IUI) in women with endometriosis. In an analysis of nearly 15,000 COH-IUI cycles, endometriosis was found to be one of the unfavorable predictors for an ongoing pregnancy [34]. In another study in women with endometriosis, one cycle of IVF was more effective than six cycles of COH-IUI and this was even more obvious for women with more severe disease [35]. This would be particularly relevant in women with endometriomas where it can be expected that the tubo-ovarian anatomy is more significantly altered.

The implication that IVF may be a better choice gains further support from the observation by D'Hooghe *et al* that the endometriosis recurrence rate after surgery for endometriosis stage III or IV is higher following COH-IUI compared to IVF, suggesting that temporary exposure to high estradiol levels during IVF is not a significant risk factor for endometriosis recurrence [36].

In vitro fertilization

Endometriomas can present technical issues during the oocyte retrieval procedure. It is generally not recommended to puncture an endometrioma because of the associated risk of abscess formation (see below). Depending on the size and position of the endometrioma, this may make the retrieval of oocytes from the ipsilateral side more hazardous or even impossible. In addition, ovaries with endometriomas are often adherent to the posterior serosal surface of the uterus where they may be out of reach. In addition, without surgical classification of the endometriosis, it will be difficult to ascertain whether bowel loops may be fixed in the path of the aspiration needle.

Endometriomas may also have relevant pathophysiological effects on the ovary. They have been linked with higher cumulative doses of follicle-stimulating hormone and the production of fewer follicles following stimulation [37]. Although this suggests that the ovarian function is compromised in the presence of an endometrioma, some studies have failed to demonstrate an adverse effect of endometriomas on key IVF outcomes, such as clinical pregnancy rates [38].

More recent reports on the effects of an endometrioma during IVF have not resolved the uncertainty. In a study by Fernando *et al*, 95 patients with ovarian endometriomas, 535 patients with endometriosis but without ovarian endometriomas and 1201 without endometriosis were compared [39]. The authors reported a higher risk of preterm birth in the women with endometriomas, but the fertilization rates and embryological endpoints were otherwise similar in all IVF groups.

In another study comparing similar groups (80 cycles in women with ovarian endometriomas, 248 cycles in women with endometriosis but without ovarian endometriomas and 283 cycles in women without endometriosis), endometriosis was found to affect oocyte number but not embryo quality or pregnancy outcome, irrespective of the presence of an ovarian endometrioma [23].

Kumbak *et al* investigated whether the space-occupying effect of an endometrioma, rather than the endometriosis within the cyst itself, affects IVF results [40]. In their study, 85 normoresponder patients with untreated endometriomas of 10–50 mm were compared with 83 normoresponder patients with untreated simple ovarian cysts of 10–35 mm. The presence of an endometriotic cyst during the IVF cycle was demonstrated to be associated with a lower embryo quality and implantation rate, although pregnancy success was unaffected.

Risks of non-surgical treatment
Spontaneous rupture
Without surgical intervention, the spontaneous evolution of an ovarian endometrioma is progressive growth and eventually leakage or spontaneous rupture, leading to acute abdominal pain and often emergency surgery. The intra-abdominal spill of chocolate fluid leads not only to severe pain but also to inflammatory reactions which promote dissemination of the disease and further adhesion formation [41].

Pelvic abscess
There have been several case reports of pelvic abscesses following the inadvertent puncture of endometriomas during oocyte collection for IVF. The accidental inoculation of the cyst filled with chocolate fluid, a perfect natural culture medium, can lead to the rapid development of an ovarian abscess. It is hard to estimate the incidence but in a series of 214 IVF cycles in women with endometriomas, the complication was never recorded, indicating that the risk is very low (95% CI 0.0–1.7%) [42].

The concern is that the diagnosis of an abscess is often delayed, because IVF patients generally show the same early clinical signs

following oocyte retrieval: lower abdominal pain, subfebrility and raised inflammatory markers. In addition, the diagnosis on ultrasound is more difficult in the presence of multiple resolving follicle cysts. It is therefore generally recommended to prescribe prophylactic antibiotics before oocyte retrieval and to carefully monitor the patient's progress following oocyte retrieval.

Cancer
Another concern is the missed diagnosis of a co-existing ovarian malignancy. It has long been known that women with certain epithelial ovarian cancers have a higher prevalence of endometriosis. Indeed, the prevalence rates of endometriosis in epithelial ovarian cancer have been calculated to be 4.5%, 1.4%, 35.9%, and 19.0% for serous, mucinous, clear cell and endometrioid ovarian carcinoma, respectively [43].

So, is it possible to estimate the risk of endometrioma-related ovarian cancer? There are a number of ways to look at this. There are two large studies that are worth highlighting. The first one is a case–control study by Brinton *et al* [44] which included 20,686 women with a mean 11.4-year follow-up period. Compared to women who had never been diagnosed with endometriosis, their relative risk (RR) for developing a malignancy of the ovary was significantly increased to 1.92 (95% CI 1.3–2.8). The RR was increased to 4.20 (95% CI 2.0–7.7) when the endometriosis was confined to the ovary.

To work out how many women this roughly represents, we need to do a few calculations. The incidence rate (new cases per year) of ovarian cancer is about 1 per 10,000 women (or 100/1,000,000 women). These 100 new ovarian cancers per year arise in a population of 1,000,000 women with and without endometriosis. Let's assume that the population prevalence of endometriosis is 10%. This means that 100,000 of these 1,000,000 women will have endometriosis. If we accept Brinton's findings that the RR in women with endometriosis is approximately twofold increased, then 18 of the 100 ovarian malignancies will have arisen in women with endometriosis; 18/100,000 is twice as high as 82/900,000. Given that the RR is approximately two, half of those 18 malignancies would have arisen anyway, the other nine because of the association with endometriosis; this equates to an excess risk of about one ovarian cancer in every 10,000 women with endometriosis.

When contemplating this excess risk of 1/10,000, it is important to remember that when Brinton stratified the risk for length of follow-up, a statistically significant increase in the RR was only observed in the subgroup of women with >10 years follow-up (RR 2.51, 95% CI 1.4–4.1). So the risk of 1/10,000 is a lot lower again in the age group where we may consider delaying excision until after fertility treatment.

The second report is a recent study by Kobayashi *et al* [45], prospective and longitudinal in design. The study estimates the standardized incidence ratio (SIR: ratio of the observed number of cancer cases to the expected number of cases) to be almost 9 (95% CI 4.1–15.3). However, the vast majority of these cancers originated in menopausal women with endometriomas >9 cm in diameter.

Although the risk of a malignancy should always be taken seriously, it would appear that the risk is very low in women within the normal reproductive window. In the next section, the risks of surgery will be discussed and these may well be greater and more relevant for women in this age group.

Pregnancy complications

Women with endometriosis have a higher risk of preterm birth, antepartum bleeding/placental complications, preeclampsia and cesarean section [46], although the increased risk of preeclampsia was not confirmed in a smaller population-based study [47]. Interestingly, in an IVF population, Fernando et al [39] found that the increased risk of preterm birth appeared to be confined to women with endometriomas.

Second, minimize further harm

In many situations, conservative surgery may be the best treatment option. Surgeons have a number of interventions at their disposal, ranging from cyst aspiration to cyst excision. The choice will again depend on patient-specific factors but even though more RCTs are needed in this area, some universal truths are emerging to offer us a guide to the best treatment options.

Aspiration

Some investigators have hypothesized that the endometriotic lining of an endometrioma may undergo pressure atrophy and that spontaneous resolution of the endometrioma can be achieved by simple aspiration of its content. The advantage of aspiration of endometriotic cysts in the ovary is that it is a relatively simple and minimally invasive procedure. It can be carried out transabdominally, but the more common route is transvaginal.

In one prospective non-randomized study [48], aspiration of endometriotic cysts was carried out transvaginally in nine and transabdominally in 13 patients, followed by intranasal buserelin in eight and danazol in 14 patients. Reaspiration was performed when recurrence was observed. A total of 47 aspirations were done, with reaspiration required in six patients and a surgical intervention in one. No procedure-related complications were reported. The effect of cyst aspiration on subsequent IVF pregnancy rates is controversial given that both better [49] and worse [50] outcomes have been reported.

Other reports have also cast doubt on the long-term effectiveness of endometrioma aspiration. In a prospective study, eight endometriomas (range 18–46 mm) were aspirated in six patients. Although there were no major complications, within 3 months six ovarian cysts recurred in five women (83.3%) [51]. In addition, the procedure may not be without risk. Similar to accidental puncture of an endometrioma during an IVF oocyte retrieval, pelvic abscesses have been reported following intentional aspiration of ovarian endometriomas [52].

Chemoablation

The chemoablation technique was developed as a further extension of the aspiration technique, the rationale being that

sclerotherapy of the cyst with a solution of tetracycline, methotrexate, interleukin-2 or ethanol may more effectively destroy the epithelial lining and hereby reduce the recurrence rate. Hsieh et al report various studies with a recurrence rate for sclerotherapy varying between 9.1% and 66.7% [53]. In their own study, the observed overall 12-month recurrence rate was 26.9% for ethanol sclerotherapy, but they managed to decrease the recurrence rate to 13.3.% by leaving the 95% ethanol in situ.

The available studies are too small to allow for any meaningful conclusions regarding the impact of sclerotherapy on further fertility. Furthermore, this procedure has also been associated with postoperative pelvic abscesses [54].

Laparoscopy

A strong argument can be made in favor of laparoscopic treatment of ovarian endometriomas. According to Redwine [16], 99% of patients with an ovarian endometrioma will have other lesions, mostly in pelvic and/or intestinal locations. The probability of peritubal/periovarian adhesions in these patients is high and a proper laparoscopic staging should therefore be considered. Thus if one accepts the value of a diagnostic laparoscopy, it seems almost irrational not to convert the procedure to a surgical intervention if the anatomy can be adequately and safely restored. Not everyone agrees, however, and there is now growing support to move straight to IVF following the ultrasound diagnosis of an endometrioma. This section will discuss both the benefits and drawbacks of cyst ablation/enucleation to put this new debate in perspective.

On one hand, drainage and ablation of the endometriotic implants on the cyst wall interior can be performed with electrical or laser energy. This delivery of energy is a potential risk to healthy follicles which may be contained within the cyst wall (invaginated cortex).

On the other hand, excision of the cyst wall ("stripping") is achieved following drainage of the cyst. The cleavage plane between the cortex and the cyst wall is carefully developed and the cyst wall is dissected free from the healthy cortex and underlying stroma. This obviously leads to the surgical removal of any healthy follicles within the cyst wall and it also often leads to bleeding of the vascular bed in the hilus, which requires meticulous hemostatic control.

A recently updated Cochrane review gives us some guidance regarding the relative benefits of both procedures [55]. The review included two randomized studies [56,57] comparing laparoscopic ablation and excision for ovarian endometriomas greater than 3 cm in size for the primary symptom of pain. Laparoscopic excision of the cyst wall was more successful in reducing all types of endometriosis-related pain. The recurrence rate was also lower (OR 0.41, 95% CI 0.18–0.93) with a reduced requirement for further surgery (OR 0.21, 95% CI 0.05–0.79) and, more importantly for this chapter, the subsequent spontaneous pregnancy rate in women with prior subfertility was fivefold higher (OR 5.21, 95% CI 2.04–13.29). The benefits of excisional surgery could not be demonstrated in another randomized controlled study in which patients received COH-IUI following surgery. The ovary in which an endometrioma was ablated or excised responded equally well and comparably to the unaffected contralateral ovary [58].

Although the evidence appears to favor excision over ablation, it remains unclear whether excision is actually better than no intervention at all. A meta-analysis of five non-randomized studies on this topic concluded that surgical management of endometriomas has no significant effect on ovarian response to stimulation and IVF pregnancy rates compared with no treatment [59]. Unfortunately, the authors of the review excluded the only RCT to date on the basis that the endometriomas in the control group were drained at the time of oocyte retrieval. The findings of this RCT [60] indicate that excision leads to a poorer ovarian response but similar pregnancy and implantation rates.

How important the observed loss of ovarian responsiveness is for the cumulative livebirth rate remains to be established. It is possible that ovarian surgery, in particular repeat surgery, can lead to reduced ovarian reserve in the longer term. Clearly, more RCTs are required and this was named as one of the endometriosis research priorities in a recent position paper [61]. Until then, it is best to keep in mind that excision of endometriomas can occasionally lead to iatrogenic ovarian failure [62,63].

It is worth looking at a number of relevant studies that have been published since the two systematic reviews. Some have looked at measures to prevent or minimize the reduction in ovarian reserve following laparoscopic excision. In a non-randomized study, Li *et al* [64] followed up the ovarian reserve for 12 months after surgical treatment of unilateral or bilateral benign ovarian cysts using three different modalities: bipolar electrocoagulation, harmonic scalpel or suturing. Compared to the other modalities, electrocoagulation was associated with a reduction in ovarian reserve, which was at least partly ascribed to a worse impact on the ovarian vasculature. Another study showed that suturing may also reduce the postoperative formation of ovarian adhesions compared with bipolar surgery [65]. The theme of achieving proper hemostasis without compromising the ovarian vasculature is carried forward with the development of a new gelatine-thrombin matrix. Clinical studies have shown this to be a clinically effective, topical hemostatic agent for the control of minor bleeding of the ovarian wall at the end of laparoscopic stripping [66,67].

Another theme has been the prevention of recurrences following surgery. Recently, three RCTs investigated the benefits of postoperative hormonal suppression. The first of these studies [68] randomized 70 patients to either 6 months of cyclic low-dose combined oral contraceptives (COC) or no treatment following laparoscopic excision of ovarian endometriomas. At 12 months the cumulative recurrence rate was lower for patients receiving COC versus control subjects, but this difference disappeared by 24 months. The second study [69] compared the recurrence rate following continuous COC, GnRH agonist, dietary therapy or placebo in 259 randomized patients. This study found no differences in the recurrence

rates between the groups after 6 months. Finally, the most recent study [70] measured endometrioma recurrence following cyclic COC, continuous COC or no treatment in 239 patients. The crude recurrence rate within 2 years was significantly lower in cyclic (14.7%) and continuous users (8.2%) compared with non-users (29%). There was no obvious benefit of continuous COC over cyclic COC. Taken together, two of the three RCTs indicate that recurrences can be delayed by the simple postoperative use of COC.

Third, preserve fertility

Fertility preservation is generally used in the context of gonadotoxic cancer treatment and not of endometriosis. Nevertheless, situations may very exceptionally arise where infertile patients have to consider radical surgery for the treatment of very severe endometriosis. In these cases removal of all remaining ovarian tissue may be necessary and it may not be possible to delay the procedure to allow for a number of IVF cycles. For these women the treatment principles of fertility preservation are essentially the same.

Currently the preferred option for cancer patients is cryopreservation of embryos or, in the absence of a male partner, oocytes. These fertility preservation techniques are currently associated with the highest delivery rates [71]. However, these techniques may not be suitable for patients with endometriosis in whom radical surgery cannot be further delayed. The best option here would be to recover and freeze the remaining healthy ovarian cortex during the oophorectomy procedure, which is straightforward. The ideal conditions for cryopreservation of ovarian tissue are relatively well understood, but they do require the scientific expertise of an IVF laboratory. The thawing and transplantation techniques, on the other hand, are only in their infancy and will require further research before they can be considered effective. Only nine livebirths have been reported to date following transplantation of cryopreserved ovarian tissue [72]. Nevertheless, these unfortunate, often young women often consider this to be their only option to preserve some of their own gametes in the hope that later scientific advances may bring better livebirth rates. The limited success of fertility preservation at the present time puts clinicians under great pressure to try and avoid radical surgery in women who have not completed their family.

References

1. Brosens IA, Puttemans PJ, Deprest J, The endoscopic localization of endometrial implants in the ovarian chocolate cyst. Fertil Steril 1994;61:1034–1038.
2. Nisolle M, Donnez J. Peritoneal endometriosis, ovarian endometriosis, and adenomyotic nodules of the rectovaginal septum are three different entities. Fertil Steril 1997;68:585–596.
3. Nezhat F, Nezhat C, Allan CJ, Metzger DA, Sears DL. A clinical and histological classification of endometriomas: implications for a mechanism of pathogenesis. J Reprod Med 1992;37:771–776.

4. Muzii L, Bianchi A, Bellati F et al. Histologic analysis of endometriomas: what the surgeon needs to know. Fertil Steril 2007;87:362–366.

5. Nezhat C, Nezhat C, Seidman D, Berker B, Nezhat F. An expert forum for the histology of endometriomas. Fertil Steril 2007;8(4):1017–1018.

6. Muzii L, Bianchi A, Croce C, Manci N, Panici PB. Laparoscopic excision of ovarian cysts: is the stripping technique a tissue-sparing procedure? Fertil Steril 2002;77:609–614.

7. Schubert B, Canis M, Darcha C et al. Human ovarian tissue from cortex surrounding benign cysts: a model to study ovarian tissue cryopreservation. Hum Reprod 2005;20:1786–1792.

8. Matsuzaki S, Schubert B. Oxidative stress status in normal ovarian cortex surrounding ovarian endometriosis. Fertil Steril 2010;93(7):2431–2432.

9. Bedaiwy MA, Falcone T. Laboratory testing for endometriosis. Clin Chim Acta 2004;340:41–56.

10. Florio P, Reis FM, Torres PB et al. High serum follistatin levels in women with ovarian endometriosis. Hum Reprod 2009;24:2600–2606.

11. Mais V, Guerriero S, Ajossa S, Angiolucci M, Paoletti AM, Melis GB. The efficiency of transvaginal ultrasonography in the diagnosis of endometrioma. Fertil Steril 1993;60:776–780.

12. Kurjak A, Kupesic S. Scoring system for prediction of ovarian endometriosis based on transvaginal color and pulsed Doppler sonography. Fertil Steril 1994;62:81–88.

13. Alcázar JL, Laparte C, Jurado M, López-García G. The role of transvaginal ultrasonography combined with color velocity imaging and pulsed Doppler in the diagnosis of endometrioma. Fertil Steril 1997;67:487–491.

14. Eskenazi B, Warner M, Bonsignore L, Olive D, Samuels S, Vercellini P. Validation study of nonsurgical diagnosis of endometriosis. Fertil Steril 2001;76:929–935.

15. Bazi T, Nader KA, Seoud MA, Charafeddine M, Rechdan JB, Zreik TG. Lateral distribution of endometriomas as a function of age. Fertil Steril 2007;87:419–421.

16. Redwine DB. Ovarian endometriosis: a marker for more extensive pelvic and intestinal disease. Fertil Steril 1999;72:310–315.

17. Chapron C, Pietin-Vialle C, Borghese B, Davy C, Foulot H, Chopin N. Associated ovarian endometrioma is a marker for greater severity of deeply infiltrating endometriosis. Fertil Steril 2009;92:453–457.

18. Kennedy, S. Bergqvist, A, Charpon, C et al. ESHRE guideline for the diagnosis and treatment of endometriosis. Hum Reprod 2005;20:2698–2704.

19. American Society for Reproductive Medicine. Revised American Society for Reproductive Medicine classification of endometriosis: 1996. Fertil Steril 1997;67:817–821.

20. Adamson GD, Pasta DJ. Endometriosis fertility index: the new, validated endometriosis staging system. Fertil Steril 2010;94(5):1609–1615.

21. Barnhart K, Dunsmoor-Su R, Coutifaris C. Effect of endometriosis on in vitro fertilization. Fertil Steril 2002;77:1148–1155.

22. Garrido N, Navarro J, Remohi J, Simón C, Pellicer A. Follicular hormonal environment and embryo quality in women with endometriosis. Hum Reprod Update 2000;6:67–74.

23. Suzuki T, Izumi SI, Matsubayashi H, Awaji H, Yoshikata K, Makino T. Impact of ovarian endometrioma on oocytes and pregnancy outcome in in vitro fertilization. Fertil Steril 2005;83:908–913.

24. Garrido N, Navarro J, García-Velasco J, Remohi J, Pellicer A, Simón C. The endometrium versus embryonic quality in endometriosis-related infertility. Hum Reprod Update 2002;8:95–103.

25. Nakahara K, Saito H, Saito T et al. Ovarian fecundity in patients with endometriosis can be estimated by the incidence of apoptotic bodies. Fertil Steril 1998;69:931–935.

26. Schubert B, Canis M, Darcha C et al. Human ovarian tissue from cortex surrounding benign cysts: a model to study ovarian tissue cryopreservation. Hum Reprod 2005;20:1786–1792.

27. Horikawa T, Nakagawa K, Ohgi S. The frequency of ovulation from the affected ovary decreases following laparoscopic cystectomy in infertile women with unilateral endometrioma during a natural cycle. J Assist Reprod Genet 2008;25:239–244.

28. Benaglia L, Somigliana E, Vercellini P, Abbiati A, Ragni G, Fedele L. Endometriotic ovarian cysts negatively affect the rate of spontaneous ovulation. Hum Reprod 2009;24:2183–2186.

29. Chapron C, Pietin-Vialle C, Borghese B, Davy C, Foulot H, Chopin N. Associated ovarian endometrioma is a marker for greater severity of deeply infiltrating endometriosis. Fertil Steril 2009;92:453–457.

30. Seracchioli R, Mabrouk M, Frascà C et al. Long-term cyclic and continuous oral contraceptive therapy and endometrioma recurrence: a randomized controlled trial. Fertil Steril 2010;93:52–56.

31. Rana N, Thomas S, Rotman C, Dmowski WP. Decrease in the size of ovarian endometriomas during ovarian suppression in stage IV endometriosis. Role of preoperative medical treatment. J Reprod Med 1996;41:384–392.

32. Sallam HN, Garcia-Velasco JA, Dias S, Arici A. Long-term pituitary down-regulation before in vitro fertilization (IVF) for women with endometriosis. Cochrane Database Syst Rev 2006;1:CD004635.

33. Rombauts L. GnRH agonist therapy after surgical treatment of endometriosis improved the results of fertility treatment, Evidence-Based Obstet Gynecol 2003;5:81–83.

34. Steures P, van der Steeg JW, Mol BW et al, CECERM (Collaborative Effort in Clinical Evaluation in Reproductive Medicine). Prediction of an ongoing pregnancy after intrauterine insemination. Fertil Steril 2004;82:45–51.

35. Kissler S, Hamscho N, Zangos S et al. Diminished pregnancy rates in endometriosis due to impaired uterotubal transport assessed by hysterosalpingoscintigraphy. Br J Obstet Gynaecol 2005;112:1391–1396.

36. D'Hooghe TM, Denys B, Spiessens C, Meuleman C, Debrock S. Is the endometriosis recurrence rate increased after ovarian hyperstimulation? Fertil Steril 2006;86:283–290.

37. Al-Azemi M, Bernal AL, Steele J, Gramsbergen I, Barlow D, Kennedy S. Ovarian response to repeated controlled stimulation in in-vitro fertilization cycles in patients with ovarian endometriosis. Hum Reprod 2000;15:72–75.

38. Garcia-Velasco JA, Mahutte NG, Corona J et al. Removal of endometriomas before in vitro fertilization does not improve fertility outcomes: a matched, case-control study. Fertil Steril 2004;81:1194–1197.

39. Fernando S, Breheny S, Jaques AM, Halliday JL, Baker G, Healy D. Preterm birth, ovarian endometriomata, and assisted reproduction technologies. Fertil Steril 2009;91:325–330.

40. Kumbak B, Kahraman S, Karlikaya G, Lacin S, Guney A. In vitro fertilization in normoresponder patients with endometriomas: comparison with basal simple ovarian cysts. Gynecol Obstet Invest 2008;65:212–216.

41. Pratt JH, Shamblin WR. Spontaneous rupture of endometrial cysts of the ovary presenting as an acute abdominal emergency. Am J Obstet Gynecol 1970;108:56–62.

42. Benaglia L, Somigliana E, Iemmello R, Colpi E, Nicolosi AE, Ragni G. Endometrioma and oocyte retrieval-induced pelvic abscess: a clinical concern or an exceptional complication? Fertil Steril 2008;89:1263–1266.

43. Van Gorp T, Amant F, Neven P, Vergote I, Moerman P. Endometriosis and the development of malignant tumours of the pelvis. A review of literature. Best Pract Res Clin Obstet Gynaecol 2004;18:349–371.

44. Brinton LA, Gridley G, Persson I et al. Cancer risk after a hospital discharge diagnosis of endometriosis. Am J Obstet Gynecol 1997;176:572–579.

45. Kobayashi H, Sumimoto K, Kitanaka T et al. Ovarian endometrioma – risk factors of ovarian cancer development. Eur J Obstet Gynecol Reprod Biol 2008;138:187–193.

46. Stephansson O, Kieler H, Granath F, Falconer H. Endometriosis, assisted reproduction technology, and risk of adverse pregnancy outcome. Hum Reprod 2009;24:2341–2347.

47. Hadfield RM, Lain SJ, Raynes-Greenow CH, Morris JM, Roberts CL. Is there an association between endometriosis and the risk of preeclampsia? A population based study. Hum Reprod 2009;24:2348–2352.

48. Mittal S, Kumar S, Kumar A, Verma A. Ultrasound guided aspiration of endometrioma – a new therapeutic modality to improve reproductive outcome. Int J Gynaecol Obstet 1999;65:17–23.

49. Dicker D, Goldman JA, Feldberg D, Ashkenazi J, Levy T. Transvaginal ultrasonic needle-guided aspiration of endometriotic cysts before ovulation induction for in vitro fertilization. J In Vitro Fert Embryo Transf 1991;8:286–289.

50. Suganuma N, Wakahara Y, Ishida D et al. Pretreatment for ovarian endometrial cyst before in vitro fertilization. Gynecol Obstet Invest 2002;54(Suppl 1):36–40.

51. Chan LY, So WW, Lao TT. Rapid recurrence of endometrioma after transvaginal ultrasound-guided aspiration. Eur J Obstet Gynecol Reprod Biol 2003;109:196–198.

52. Younis JS, Ezra Y, Laufer N, Ohel G. Late manifestation of pelvic abscess following oocyte retrieval, for in vitro fertilization, in patients with severe endometriosis and ovarian endometriomata. J Assist Reprod Genet 1997;14:343–346.

53. Hsieh CL, Shiau CS, Lo LM, Hsieh TT, Chang MY. Effectiveness of ultrasound-guided aspiration and sclerotherapy with 95% ethanol for treatment of recurrent ovarian endometriomas. Fertil Steril 2009;91:2709–2713.

54. Mikamo H, Kawazoe K, Sato Y, Itoh M, Tamaya T. Ovarian abscess caused by Peptostreptococcus magnus following transvaginal ultrasound-guided aspiration of ovarian endometrioma and fixation with pure ethanol. Infect Dis Obstet Gynecol 1998;6:66–68.

55. Hart RJ, Hickey M, Maouris P, Buckett W. Excisional surgery versus ablative surgery for ovarian endometriomata. Cochrane Database Syst Rev 2008;2:CD004992.

56. Alborzi S, Momtahan M, Parsanezhad ME, Dehbashi S, Zolghadri J, Alborzi S. A prospective, randomized study comparing laparoscopic ovarian cystectomy versus fenestration and coagulation in patients with endometriomas. Fertil Steril 2004;82:1633–1637.

57. Beretta P, Franchi M, Ghezzi F, Busacca M, Zupi E, Bolis P. Randomized clinical trial of two laparoscopic treatments of endometriomas: cystectomy versus drainage and coagulation. Fertil Steril 1998;70:1176–1180.

58. Alborzi S, Ravanbakhsh R, Parsanezhad ME, Alborzi M, Alborzi S, Dehbashi S. A comparison of follicular response of ovaries to ovulation induction after laparoscopic ovarian cystectomy or fenestration and coagulation versus normal ovaries in patients with endometrioma. Fertil Steril 2007;88:507–509.

59. Tsoumpou I, Kyrgiou M, Gelbaya TA, Nardo LG. The effect of surgical treatment for endometrioma on in vitro fertilization outcomes: a systematic review and meta-analysis. Fertil Steril 2009;92:75–87.

60. Demirol A, Guven S, Baykal C, Gurgan T. Effect of endometrioma cystectomy on IVF outcome: a prospective randomized study. Reprod Biomed Online 2006;12:639–643.

61. Rogers PA, D'Hooghe TM, Fazleabas A et al. Priorities for endometriosis research: recommendations from an international consensus workshop. Reprod Sci 2009;16:335–346.

62. Reich H, Abrao MS. Post-surgical ovarian failure after laparoscopic excision of bilateral endometriomas: is this rare problem preventable? Am J Obstet Gynecol 2006;195:339.

63. Benaglia L, Somigliana E, Vighi V, Ragni G, Vercellini P, Fedele L. Rate of severe ovarian damage following surgery for endometriomas. Hum Reprod 2010;25:678–682.

64. Li CZ, Liu B, Wen ZQ, Sun Q. The impact of electrocoagulation on ovarian reserve after laparoscopic excision of ovarian cysts: a prospective clinical study of 191 patients. Fertil Steril 2009;92:1428–1435.

65. Pellicano M, Bramante S, Guida M et al. Ovarian endometrioma: postoperative adhesions following bipolar coagulation and suture. Fertil Steril 2008;89:796–799.

66. Ebert AD, Hollauer A, Fuhr N, Langolf O, Papadopoulos T. Laparoscopic ovarian cystectomy without bipolar coagulation or sutures using a gelantine-thrombin matrix sealant (FloSeal): first support of a promising technique. Arch Gynecol Obstet 2009;280:161–165.

67. Angioli R, Muzii L, Montera R et al. Feasibility of the use of novel matrix hemostatic sealant (FloSeal) to achieve hemostasis during laparoscopic excision of endometrioma. J Minim Invasive Gynecol 2009;16:153–156.

68. Muzii L, Marana R, Caruana P, Catalano GF, Margutti F, Panici PB. Postoperative administration of monophasic combined oral contraceptives after laparoscopic treatment of ovarian endometriomas: a prospective, randomized trial. Am J Obstet Gynecol 2000;183:588–592.

69. Sesti F, Capozzolo T, Pietropolli A, Marziali M, Bollea MR, Piccione E. Recurrence rate of endometrioma after laparoscopic cystectomy: a

comparative randomized trial between post-operative hormonal suppression treatment or dietary therapy vs. placebo. Eur J Obstet Gynecol Reprod Biol 2009;147:72–77.

70. Seracchioli R, Mabrouk M, Frascà C et al. Long-term cyclic and continuous oral contraceptive therapy and endometrioma recurrence: a randomized controlled trial. Fertil Steril 2010;93:52–56.

71. Schmidt KT, Larsen EC, Andersen CY, Andersen AN. Risk of ovarian failure and fertility preserving methods in girls and adolescents with a malignant disease. Br J Obstet Gynecol 2010;117:163–174.

72. Ernst E, Bergholdt S, Jørgensen JS, Andersen CY. The first woman to give birth to two children following transplantation of frozen/thawed ovarian tissue. Hum Reprod 2010;25(5):1280–1281.

10 Associated Disorders

48 Endometriosis and Autoimmunity

Srinu Pathivada and Thomas D'Hooghe

Department of Obstetrics and Gynaecology, University Hospitals Leuven, Leuven, Belgium

Introduction

Endometriosis is an important gynecological disease, defined as the presence of endometrial glands and stroma in sites outside the uterine cavity, primarily on the pelvic peritoneum and ovaries [1]. The disease is clinically associated with dysmenorrhea, pelvic pain and infertility. While much progress has been made in recent years towards diagnosing endometriosis, the pathogenesis, spontaneous evolution and endometriosis-associated infertility are not well understood. Several theories have been proposed to explain the mechanism of endometriosis. The most widely accepted theory is Sampson's retrograde menstruation theory which states that, during a woman's menstrual flow, some of the endometrial fragments are displaced into the peritoneal cavity through the fallopian tube and develop into endometriotic lesions [2]. Although retrograde menstruation occurs in 76–90% of women, only 8–10% are known to develop endometriosis, suggesting the involvement of other factors in the development of endometriosis [3]. In contrast, the coelomic metaplasia theory proposes that the differentiation of mesothelial cells into endometrium-like tissue results in the formation of endometriotic lesions within the peritoneal cavity [4]. The induction theory, an extension of the metaplasia theory, proposes that endometriosis results from differentiation of mesenchymal cells, activated by substances released by degenerating endometrium that ends up in the abdominal cavity [5,6]. However, no single theory can explain all cases of endometriosis. In addition to the classic theories, altered cellular and humoral immune function has been proposed as a key factor in the pathogenesis of endometriosis.

A systemic or specific immune deficiency resulting in incomplete rejection of autologous endometrial tissue has been proposed by several investigators to be involved in the pathogenesis of endometriosis [7–10]. It is proposed that endometrial cells arriving in the peritoneal cavity escape from immunosurveillance by increased expression of specific proteins such as human leukocyte antigen (HLA)-G [11], soluble intercellular adhesion molecule (sICAM)-1 [12] and FasL [13] which may provide immune tolerance and in turn support survival of the ectopic graft. These results have contributed to the hypothesis [3,14,15] that endometriosis is an autoimmune disease. According to this theory, endometrial cells in the peritoneal cavity are processed by activated macrophages and presented to T-cells. Under the influence of macrophage-released cytokines, T-cells proliferate and differentiate into functional subsets with helper, suppressor-inducer and cytotoxic properties. A host of T-cell-derived factors then play a critical role in the activation of B-cells from the resting state, which facilitates further differentiation and antibody secretion. Autoantibodies may then be produced against endometrial cells or against endometrial cell-derived phospholipids, histones or nucleotides. Autoantibodies may in turn reduce fertility by interfering with ovum capture or implantation, or by increasing the frequency of miscarriages [16]. These antiendometrial autoantibodies have also been suggested as possible peripheral blood markers for the presence of endometriosis [17–19]. In addition, the immune and inflammatory alterations observed in women with endometriosis share many similarities with those reported in other autoimmune diseases such as rheumatoid arthritis (RA), Crohn's disease, and psoriasis [20]. Furthermore, a high incidence of occurrence of autoimmune disorders such as hypothyroidism, fibromyalgia, chronic fatigue syndrome, multiple sclerosis, allergies and asthma is significantly more common in women affected by endometriosis [21].

In this chapter we will discuss the role of immune tolerance and autoimmunity in the context of endometriosis, focusing on defective immunosurveillance, the role of altered immune cells, immunomodulation via the HLA system, autoimmunity, inflammation and anti-inflammatory agents in endometriosis.

Endometriosis: Science and Practice, First Edition. Edited by Linda C. Giudice, Johannes L.H. Evers and David L. Healy.
© 2012 Blackwell Publishing Ltd. Published 2012 by Blackwell Publishing Ltd.

Endometriosis: role of defective immunosurveillance

The lack of adequate immune surveillance in the peritoneal cavity is considered to be a causative factor in endometriosis. Evasion of immunosurveillance might be accomplished via the secretion of proteins that interfere with immunocyte-endometrial implant recognition [22]. It has been speculated that lymphocytes can adhere to endometrial cells through the lymphocyte function antigen (LFA)-1 via the intercellular adhesion molecule (ICAM)-1-dependent pathway and present them as a target to natural killer (NK) cells [12]. Soluble forms of ICAM (sICAM)-1 secreted by peritoneal fluid (PF) endometrial cells/endometriotic lesions can also bind to LFA-1-presenting lymphocytes and could prevent the recognition of endometrial cells by these lymphocytes and prevent subsequent NK cell-mediated cytotoxicity [12]. Furthermore, interleukin (IL)-6 secreted by endometriotic cells in concert with interferon-γ may upregulate sICAM-1 production by macrophages of patients with endometriosis [23]. As a result, increased secretion of sICAM-1 may allow endometrial fragments to evade immunosurveillance, to survive and to implant.

Another major abnormal mechanism involves apoptosis or programmed cell death via the Fas/Fas ligand (FasL) expression system in women with endometriosis when compared to controls [10]. The Fas/FasL system is implicated in several aspects of immune regulation and development including modulation of T-cell selection and clonal deletion of activated T-cells by the thymus. New evidence points to expression of FasL in women with endometriosis as a possible mediator to escape immune surveillance [24]. Indeed, during their attachment to the peritoneum during retrograde menstruation, endometrial stromal cells show increased FasL expression, together with increased expression of laminin, fibronectin and collagen IV [25]. These data suggest that increased FasL expression of endometrial stromal cells after adhesion to the extracellular matrix may provide immune tolerance by inducing apoptosis of Fas-bearing cytotoxic T-lymphocytes, which would allow further development of ectopic implants [25].

Levels of soluble FasL (sFasL) have also been reported to be elevated in serum and PF from women with moderate-to-severe endometriosis compared to women with minimal or mild endometriosis and women without endometriosis [13]. The elevated levels of sFasL may result in increased apoptosis of Fas-bearing immune cells, thereby decreasing immune cell scavenger activity, which ultimately leads to increase of the survival of endometrial cells in the peritoneal cavity [24].

Role of defective immune system

Reduced natural killer cell activity

Natural killer cells are important cytotoxic lymphocytes of the immune system, which are also known to decrease in number and cytotoxicity in patients with autoimmune disease, such as systemic lupus erythematosus (SLE) [26]. A deficiency in cellular immunity, particularly in peritoneal NK cell or cytotoxic T-cell function, has also been proposed to underlie the initiation, maintenance and progression of endometriotic lesions [8]. Peritoneal NK cells and activated T-lymphocytes display reduced cytotoxicity against autologous endometrium from women with endometriosis when compared to controls, which correlated negatively with the stage of the disease [7,27–29]. However, D'Hooghe and colleagues documented no difference in lymphocyte-mediated cytotoxicity and NK cell activity between baboons with and without endometriosis [30].

A dysfunction of two subclasses of NK cells may nurture autoimmunity associated with endometriosis [3]. One subset, NK T-cells, is characterized by the capacity to kill cell targets and secrete cytokines, such as IL-4 and IL-10, which are important in the regulation of autoimmunity [31]. Another subset of NK cells, CD16/CD56 NK cells, kill autologous dentritic cells (DCs) presenting self-antigens to autoreactive T-cells. The inability of NK cells to eliminate autologous DCs expressing endometrial self-antigens may allow the presentation of these self-antigens by DCs to autoreactive T-cells and lead to the production of autoantibodies [3]. The failure of NK cells to scavenge autologous endometrial cells may allow the development and progression of ectopic endometrium [3].

Decreased T-lymphocyte cytotoxicity

CD4 cells are important lymphocytes of the immune system. CD4 T-cells are divided into type 1 helper (Th1) cells and type 2 helper (Th2) cells. Th1 cells secrete interleukin (IL)-2, IL-12 and interferon (IFN-γ) and trigger an immune cell process that involves the participation of NK cells, macrophages, CD8 T-lymphocytes. Th2 cells, which secrete IL-4, IL-5, IL-6, IL-10, and IL-13, and their response are characterized by activation of B-lymphocytes, eosinophils, basophils and tissue mastocytes [32]. It is well known that cell-mediated immunity, including T-cell-mediated cytotoxicity, is activated or suppressed by cytokines produced by Th1 and Th2 cells. Under normal conditions, there is a tightly regulatory control mechanism between Th1 and Th2 cells. For instance, Th1 cells secrete IL-12, which activates cytotoxic NK cell activity, whereas Th2 cells may reduce NK cell activity by producing IL-10.

In women with endometriosis, Th2 cells from PF are reported to aberrantly suppress cell-mediated immunity by upregulating IL-4 and IL-10 secretions in PF from women with endometriosis [33]. Many study groups [32,34–36] have reported significantly elevated levels of IL-2, IL-4, IL-6, IL-10 and IFN-γ in the serum, PF and endometriotic tissue of women with advanced stages (stages III–IV) of endometriosis when compared to those with early stages (stages I, II) [37]. The presence of these elevated proinflammatory cytokines suggests that endometriosis is a disease with a complex inflammatory behavior with a clear Th1 component and also with a shift towards Th2 cytokine production [32,34]. The Th2 differentiation at the systemic and local levels is associated with a humoral-type immune response and may also play a role in enhancement of autoantibody production [35].

Activation of humoral immunity

In addition to alterations in cell-mediated immunity, alterations in humoral immunity such as increased B-cell activity and increased incidence of autoantibodies have also been described in women with endometriosis [20]. Importantly, B-cell responses have been subdivided into thymus-independent, B-1-like and related subsets, which may not require T-cell help to make antibodies, and thymus-dependent B-2 responses. B-1 cells are known to exist in the human body and typically recognize antigens that induce multivalent cross-linking of the B-cell receptor. The B-cell repertoire is likely selected by self-antigens, which make them potentially autoreactive and allow the production of autoreactive antibodies against self-antigens like DNA, involved in SLE and RA [38]. The percentage of B-1 cells in the peripheral blood (PB) has been reported to be higher in women with endometriosis and antinuclear antibodies (ANAs) than in those without ANAs or in controls with a normal pelvis [39]. In endometriosis, higher levels of B-1 cells may play an important role in the development of endometriosis through autoantibody production.

The presence of endometriotic lesions has been proposed to trigger a specific B-cell response, leading to production of antibodies directed against specific endometrial antigens [40]. Endometriotic lesions are characterized by the presence of abundant plasma cells, many of which produce immunoglobulin (Ig) M, and macrophages that produce B-lymphocyte stimulator (BlyS), a member of the tumor necrosis factor (TNF) superfamily implicated in other autoimmune diseases including RA, SLE and Sjögren syndrome (SS) [41]. Recently, BlyS levels were found to be upregulated in serum and endometriotic lesions from women with endometriosis when compared to controls with a normal pelvis but not in women with adenomyosis and uterine fibroids [42]. In the light of evidence from research in other autoimmune diseases, these high levels of BlyS can stimulate B-cell responses and thus lead to the initiation of autoimmune responses also in women with endometriosis [42].

Endometriosis: immune tolerance

Tolerance to self-antigens is a fundamental property of the immune system and its loss leads to autoimmune diseases.

Role of human leukocyte antigen system in autoimmune disease

The major histocompatibility complex (MHC) or HLA system in humans is involved in the pathogenesis of many autoimmune diseases. HLA molecules play a key role in T-cell clonal selection during fetal development, presentation of processed peptide antigens to T-cells, regulation of immune response and maintenance of immune tolerance [43]. Based on their functional diversity,

HLA genes are divided into two classes: the class I region that contains the classic HLA-A, HLA-B and HLA-C and non-classic HLA-G, HLA-E and HLA-F genes, and the class II region that contains the HLA-DR gene family (DRB1–DRB9) and HLA-DR antigen specificities (i.e. DR1–DR18). HLA class I molecules are expressed on the surface of all nucleated cells but HLA class II molecules are expressed only on B-lymphocytes, antigen-presenting cells (monocytes, macrophages, and dendritic cells) and activated T-lymphocytes [43]. The available information suggests that the HLA molecules also play a major role in autoimmune disease by presenting self-antigens to autoreactive T-cells in disease conditions, for example, type II collagen in RA, myelin basic protein and proteoline protein in multiple sclerosis, acetylcholine receptors in myasthenia gravis, and thyrotropin receptors in Graves disease [44]. However, the nature of the association of self-proteins with HLA molecules has not been fully elucidated in any of these autoimmune diseases.

Increased expression of human leukocyte class I inhibitory receptors in natural killer cells from women with endometriosis

Endometrial cells that express specific HLA class molecules interact with particular killer-activating and killer-inhibiting receptors on NK cells [45]. These receptors together with HLA class molecules are thought to be of fundamental importance in mediating immune tolerance to endometrial cells. In humans, NK cells are known to express two distinct types of HLA class I specific inhibitory receptors: killer immunoglobulin-like receptors (KIR), that recognize both classic HLA-I and non-classic HLA-G antigen [46], and C-type lectin protein CD94/NKG2A that binds to the non-classic HLA-I antigen HLA-E [47].

Natural killer cells from PB and PF have been reported to have a higher number of subclass KIR receptors such as KIR2DL1$^+$, CD158a(+) in women with endometriosis compared to controls [48–50]. Furthermore, the proportion of peritoneal NK cells positive for CD94/NKG2A and its ligand HLA-E is higher in women with endometriosis than in controls [51]. The increased expression of these HLA class I inhibitory receptors in peritoneal NK cells from women with endometriosis may mediate the resistance of endometriotic tissue to NK cell-mediated lysis [51]. Taken together, these data suggest the existence of a local and systemic decrease in NK cell activity against ectopic endometrium in women with endometriosis [52].

Increased expression of human leukocyte antigen class molecules in endometrial cells from women with endometriosis

It has been suggested that a higher expression of surface HLA class I molecules in endometrial cells may contribute to the resistance against immune cell attack in women with endometriosis. Conversely, downregulation of HLA class I molecules enhances susceptibility to NK cell and lymphokine-mediated cell lysis [53]. *In vitro,* endometrial cells derived from endometriosis lesions have been shown to have an increased expression of HLA class I molecules when compared to those originating from eutopic endometrium in women with endometriosis [53,54], and that this increased expression can be normalized after treatment with IFN-γ [54]. A higher expression of HLA class I molecules has also been reported in endometrial stromal cells in eutopic endometrium from women with endometriosis when compared to controls [55]. The endometrial membrane expression of HLA class I molecules may be regulated by both local cytokine-mediated IFN-γ and hormone-controlled mechanisms [53].

Endometrial expression of immune modulator human leukocyte antigen-G in endometriosis

Human leukocyte antigen G, a non-classic MHC class I molecule, is important for immune tolerance during pregnancy [56]. HLA-G is a non-classic molecule, which differs from classic HLA class I molecules in its genetic diversity, expression, structure and function [57]. Ectopic expression of HLA-G can be induced in pathological conditions such as transplantation, cancer and autoimmune diseases like multiple sclerosis (MS) [58]. The expression of HLA-G in damaged cells and tissues is upregulated by cytokines such as IL-10, interferons, TNF-α, and transforming growth factor (TGF)-β, and by hypoxia [59]. These altered immune mechanisms can induce a Th2 cytokine profile which may contribute to the long-term efficient immune escape or tolerance and lead to the development of autoimmunity [60].

Human leukocyte antigen G interacts with inhibitory receptors such as immunoglobulin-like transcript (ILT)-2 (NK cells, T-cells, antigen-presenting cells), ILT-4 (myeloid cells) and KIR2DL4 (NK cells and T-cells). This interaction of HLA-G at the surface of T- or NK cells not only inhibits their immune function but also renders them immunosuppressive as it could inhibit T-cell alloproliferation as well as NK cell cytolytic function [61].

The expression of HLA-G has been reported only in the glandular epithelium of 93.3% peritoneal endometriotic lesions, but not in stromal cells and eutopic endometrium of women with and without endometriosis [11]. This observation has led to the suggestion that inflammation or cellular stress may upregulate HLA-G expression by promoting ectopic endometrial survival [11]. However, in women with adenomyosis, HLA-G expression was lower in ectopic endometrium than in glandular and stromal cells of eutopic endometrium [62]. In PF, epithelial cells expressing HLA-G were only detectable during the menstrual stage, and no difference was observed between women with and without endometriosis [63].

Based on these results, it has been hypothesized that endometrial cells bearing HLA-G may enter the peritoneal cavity during retrograde menstruation, allowing the antigen to react locally with specific receptors on immune cells which might in turn suppress the NK cell activity [63]. The reasons for the differential HLA-G expression pattern between endometriosis and adenomyosis are unclear. In contrast to the above results, one group failed to detect HLA-G protein in the peritoneal fluid, normal and ectopic endometrium and stromal cells of endometriosis patients and age-matched normal controls [64]. Therefore, it can be concluded that the role of HLA-G expression on endometrial cells in the pathogenesis of endometriosis needs further investigation.

Interaction between human leukocyte antigen G and dendritic cells in women with endometriosis

Dendritic cells are professional antigen-presenting cells which have also been implicated in the development of autoimmune diseases such as SLE [65]. HLA-G can inhibit the development of immature dendritic cells into mature and stimulatory dendritic cells through the induction of anergic and immunosuppressive CD4+ and CD8+ effector T-cells [66]. An increased number of immature dendritic cells has been associated with the development of endometriotic lesions in women with endometriosis and in the nude mouse model for endometriosis [67,68]. Depending on the maturation or activation state, all DCs have the capacity for initiating tolerance or immunity [69]. In women with endometriosis, an interaction between endometrial HLA-G and ILT on dendritic cells may play an important role in immature dendritic cell generation and their functional regulation which in turn may play a role in the generation of autoantibodies through the altered presentation of self-antigens to T-cells [67].

Downregulation of human leukocyte antigen DR in macrophages from women with endometriosis

The presence of class II HLA-DR, which is involved in efficiently transmitting antigen-related information to T-cells via an immunological synapse, could be considered as an index of activation in macrophages [70]. HLA-DR is also involved in several autoimmune conditions, disease susceptibility and disease resistance [71].

Increased expression of HLA-DR antigen was reported in glandular cells of both eutopic and ectopic endometrium from patients with endometriosis compared to controls with a normal pelvis [72,73]. The surface of PF macrophages also contains HLA-DR localization and a homogenous distribution of HLA-ABCs [70]. The percentage of HLA-DR-positive macrophages as well as intensity of HLA-ABC has been found to be lower in the PF of women with advanced-stage endometriosis compared to controls [70,74,75]. This decreased HLA-DR expression of PF macrophages suggests a limitation of their antigen presentation capability in women with endometriosis compared to controls [70]. Low levels of IFN-γ, normally produced by lymphocytes and mainly NK cells through their cytotoxic action, can downregulate HLA-DR expression in PF macrophages from women with endometriosis [76], limiting the immune response to the peritoneal cavity antigens such as implanted or metaplastic endometrial tissue [75].

Association of specific human leukocyte haplotypes with endometriosis

Genetic studies have shown that people who have certain HLA alleles have a higher risk of specific autoimmune diseases than those without these alleles [77]. In addition, HLA typing has led to some improvement and acceleration in the diagnosis of some autoimmune diseases such as celiac disease and type 1 diabetes [78]. The strongest association is between HLA-B27 and autoimmune ankylosing spondylitis (AS) [79]. It is now possible to estimate the relative risk of developing a disease with every known HLA allele [80]. Similarly, HLA allele associations have also been found between class II MHC genes and autoimmune diseases like insulin-dependent diabetes and rheumatoid arthritis [81].

A significant positive association of the HLA-B7 allele with endometriosis has been reported in Japanese women [82], but was not correlated with the stage of endometriosis or the presence of adenomyosis and/or leiomyomas. However, the distribution of HLA-A and -B alleles was similar in patients with endometriosis and a general control group in the Korean population [83]. A higher prevalence of the HLA class II alleles HLA-DRB1, HLA-DQA1, HLA-DQB1 and HLA-DPB1 has been found in patients with endometriosis when compared to the general female population in Japan [84–86]. In Caucasian women, a positive association was observed between endometriosis and HLA-DR(2) 15 and HLA-DR(3) 17 alleles, that are also associated with an increased risk of multiple sclerosis and autoimmune thyroiditis [87].

However, other investigators [88–90] failed to find statistically significant HLA associations with endometriosis, probably because different HLA frequency patterns exist in different ethnic populations and different serological methods have been used for HLA-A, -B, -C, and -DR antigen typing. Furthermore, it should be added that disease-associated HLA sequences are also found in the normal population and conversely, alleles commonly present in normal individuals are also found in some patients with autoimmune diseases. Therefore, the expression of a particular HLA gene is not itself the cause of an autoimmune disease [80]. In conclusion, the association of endometriosis with particular HLA haplotypes requires further investigation.

Antigen presentation by endometrial cells

Apart from professional antigen-presenting cells, it has also been demonstrated that the epithelial and stromal cells from eutopic endometrium are able to constitutively express MHC class II molecules and present antigen directly to CD4+ T-cells [91]. *In vitro* upregulation of MHC class II antigen has been observed in endometrial epithelial cells after treatment with IFN-γ [91,92]. These data suggest that the local inflammatory response of endometriosis, consisting in part of IFN-γ production by lymphoid and other stromal cells, may regulate antigen presentation by endometrial epithelial cells.

Autoimmunity

Autoimmunity results from a breakdown or failure of the mechanisms that are normally responsible for maintaining self-tolerance. Immune responses against self (autologous) antigens, called autoimmunity, are usually abnormal. In normal individuals, potentially self-reactive lymphocytes that encounter self-antigens prior to attaining a stage of functional maturity are either deleted or inactivated (clonal deletion and clonal anergy).

Endometriosis and autoantibodies

Autoantibodies do exist in normal individuals and are stimulated in low levels during an immune response to foreign antigens. These autoantibodies are low-affinity IgM antibodies and are neither generated with T-cell help nor produce tissue injury. Thus, the potential for autoreactivity normally occurs. Pathological autoimmunity with tissue damage may develop if larger amounts of high-affinity autoantibodies are produced, presumably with assistance provided by autoreactive T-cells. This concept emphasizes the importance of T-cell tolerance in maintaining unresponsiveness to self-antigens [80]. In order to prove that a particular disease is caused by antibodies, demonstration of disease must be confirmed in a normal animal following the adoptive transfer of Ig purified from the blood or affected tissues of individuals with the disease. A natural experiment is often seen in neonates of mothers suffering from antibody-mediated diseases. These infants may be born with transient expression of the disease because of transplacental passage of IgG antibodies. However, in clinical situations it is not possible to experimentally transfer diseases with antibodies. Therefore, the diagnosis of antibody-mediated disease is usually based on the following criteria [80,93].

- Demonstration of antibodies, complement and/or immune complexes deposited in the tissues.
- Presence of anti-tissue antibodies or immune complexes in the circulation; increased complement activation products in the circulation.
- Clinicopathological similarities with experimental diseases that are proved to be antibody mediated by adoptive transfer.

Presence of antibodies in endometrium

Some studies [94–97] using immunofluorescence, immunoperoxidase and Western blot techniques, have demonstrated a higher prevalence of endogenous IgG in the endometrium of women with endometriosis than in those without the disease. In another report [98], moderate-to-intense staining with anti-IgG (immunoperoxidase) was noted in the endometrium of patients with endometriosis (75%), adenomyosis (50%), and leiomyomata (70%) compared to only 6% in the endometrium of women with a normal pelvis. These studies suggest that there is a high prevalence of endogenous IgG in the endometrium of women with benign gynecological diseases, but not specifically related to endometriosis. In conclusion, the presence of endogenous IgG in endometrium has not been proven to be specifically associated with endometriosis or to be related to infertility.

In one study, little endogenous IgA or IgM was detected by Western blot in endometrium from either endometriosis patients or controls [97]. In an earlier study, these same investigators, using immunofluorescence, reported IgA to be equally present in endometriosis patients and in controls [95].

In conclusion, evidence for the presence and specificity of endogenous IgA or IgM in endometrium from endometriosis patients is, at present, equivocal.

Presence of antibodies in endometriosis lesions

Using Western blot techniques, it was reported that endogenous IgG from endometriotic tissue was directed against antigens with a molecular weight (MW) of 27, 34, 50/52, 54, 80 and 110 kDa [97] and endogenous antigens of 27, 50/52 or 54 kDa present in both eutopic and ectopic endometrium from 78% of endometriosis patients and 22% of fertile controls [97]. However, other studies have been unable to confirm these results [99–102]. Positive staining of ovarian endometriotic foci for IgA revealed a higher tendency in infertile women with endometriosis (60%) than in fertile women with endometriosis (25%) [96]. Similar results were reported for IgM, but statistical analysis was not reported for either IgA or IgM [96].

In conclusion, endogenous IgG seems to be present in endometriotic implants, but it has not yet been established if there are differences between ovarian and peritoneal implants and if there is a relationship with infertility.

Presence of antibodies in serum and peritoneal fluid

Several studies have reported that antiendometrial antibodies (AEAB) against the 26, 34, 52, 58, 82, 94, 100, 120 kDa antigens were found in serum of endometriosis patients [97,99,101,102]. Increased levels of serum AEAB have been reported in 45% of patients with endometriosis stage III compared to 7.4% of patients with stage I endometriosis and healthy fertile women [103]. The presence of IgG and IgM type AEAB response to multiple endometrial antigens of 30, 45, 75, 105 and 160 kDa has been reported in sera from 60% of endometriosis patients who had dysmenorrhea or infertility [104]. A good relationship has been observed between serum AEAB and the laparoscopic verification of endometriosis [105]. Both IgA and IgG AEAB to endometrial antigens ranging from 10 to 200 kDa have been found in serum from patients with endometriosis but also in serum from women with tubal factor infertility (TFI), and AEAB to a 47 kDa protein-enolase was found to be more prevalent in TFI patients [106].

Immunoglobulin G AEAB against antigens of 26 and 34 kDa [99,97] were present in PF from women with endometriosis, but not in PF from controls. Furthermore, in women with endometriosis but not in controls, both serum and PF contained IgG AEAB against antigens with MW of 34, 46/48, 64, 84, 94 and 120 kDa [107]. Increased autoantibody reactivity to endometrial

antigens has been reported to be associated with the stage of endometriosis, with maximum reactivity observed against the plasma membrane fraction and reduced reactivity observed against nucleus and cytosol fractions derived from endometrial and ovarian cells of patients with endometriosis [108]. However, other authors reported that the reactivity to endometrial antigens of a specific molecular weight could not be related to stage or severity of endometriosis [104,105,109]. The lack of a clear correlation between the severity of the endometriosis and the titer of AEAB suggests that the production of autoantibodies is a secondary event [27] and may be regulated differently when compared to autoimmune disorders where the increase of antibody titer is correlated with increasing severity of the disease.

Complement deposition in endometrium/endometriosis lesions

At present there is no proof that complement activation specifically occurs in the endometrium of women with endometriosis. Earlier studies using endometrium in culture support this conclusion [110–112]. However, when different AFS stages were analyzed, endometrial C3 was produced in significantly greater amounts in patients with minimal endometriosis than in patients without endometriosis or in patients with severe endometriosis [110].

Few data are available regarding the presence of complement in endometriosis lesions. *In vitro* incubation of endometriotic tissue from ovarian or peritoneal origin has revealed the secretion of a 180 kDa protein very similar to human C3 which was only produced and secreted by epithelial cells [111]. The clinical significance of this finding is unclear, since two other studies have reported the presence of complement in both eutopic and ectopic endometrium [113,114]. The incidence of moderate-to-intense staining of endometriotic tissue from patients with histologically proven adenomyosis was 80% for C3 (endometrium: 80%) and 71% for C4 (endometrium: 83%) [113]. In another study [114], specific staining for C3d and for the presence of the terminal membrane attack complex (MAC, C5b-9) was not observed on the glandular epithelium of ectopic endometrium, while in the stromal compartment, complement deposition was colonized with terminal complement inhibitors/cell–cell attachment factors, clusterin and vitronectin on elastic fibers. The results of this study suggested that, like eutopic endometrium, ectopic endometrial lesions may "benefit" from intrinsic mechanisms (inhibition of complement activation) protecting glandular cells from autologous complement attack *in vivo* [114].

Presence of autoantibodies against specific endometrial antigens

Autoimmunity can also be caused by mechanisms other than polyclonal activation [80], such as antigen mimicry (immunological cross-reactions of foreign and self-antigens). An immune response is induced by a foreign antigen or a altered self-antigen but the disease develops because the response is also directed against the homologous self-antigen. Because autoimmune responses induced by immunological cross-reactions are likely to generate autoantibodies specific for one or a few related antigens, it is likely that the lesions that develop are organ or tissue specific [80]. It is important to note that antibodies against self tissues are not always pathogenic. For instance, tissue injury due to ischemia or infection may lead to autoantibody production because of alterations in self-antigens or exposure of antigens that are normally sequestered from the immune system. In such situations, the autoantibodies may be the result and not the cause of tissue necrosis. For example, some patients who suffer myocardial infarctions develop antibodies against their own cardiac cells. Many tissue- or organ-specific immunological diseases are associated with the production of, and are thought to be caused by, autoantibodies: Goodpasture syndrome, autoimmune hemolytic anemia and thrombocytopenia, bullous pemphigoid, myasthenia gravis, Graves disease, and insulin-resistant diabetes mellitus. Autoantibodies against cell surface receptors may lead to functional abnormalities without the involvement of any other effector mechanisms. Examples include Graves disease (autoantibodies against thyroid stimulating hormone receptor on thyroid epithelial cells) and myasthenia gravis (autoantibodies against acetylcholine receptors in the motor endplates of neuromuscular junctions).

Carbonic anhydrase

Autoantibodies to carbonic anhydrase (CA) isoenzymes have been demonstrated in many autoimmune diseases such as SLE and RA [115]. It has been reported that 70% and 66% of women with endometriosis and endometriosis-associated infertility respectively had serum antibodies directed against carbonic anhydrase [116,117]. A positive correlation has been reported between the stage of endometriosis and the prevalence of autoantibodies against CA (55% of stage I, 50% of stage II, 73% of stage III, and 85% of stage IV endometriosis); these autoantibodies were also found in 38% of infertile women without endometriosis, but not in fertile controls [118].

α2-Heremans Schmidt glycoprotein and transferrin

Using two-dimensional gel electrophoresis of endometrial extracts, elevated antibody levels to two proteins, α2-Heremans Schmidt (α2-HS) glycoprotein and transferrin with MW of 64 kDa and 72 kDa were found in all patients with endometriosis but not in controls [119]. The concentration of α2-HS glycoprotein (serum and PF) and transferrin (PF only) was significantly elevated in patients with endometriosis compared to those without [120], allowing the non-invasive diagnosis of endometriosis with a sensitivity and specificity of at least 90% [121]. As HS glycoprotein and transferrin are detrimental to egg quality and sperm motility, increased levels of autoantibodies to both of these proteins may be relevant to infertility associated with endometriosis [122].

Laminin-1

Laminin-1 is a base membrane protein involved in embryogenesis, implantation and placentation. There is evidence that autoantibodies to laminin-1 may be important in the development of autoimmune-mediated reproductive failures [123]. Antibodies

against anti-laminin-1 have been observed in 17/42 infertile patients with endometriosis but not in women with infertility related to tubal factor, hormonal abnormalities or uterine anomalies [124]. However, increased levels of antibodies against laminin-1 have also been found in serum and PF from subfertile patients with stage II/III endometriosis, and in women with polycystic ovaries [125]. It has been suggested that anti-laminin-1 antibodies in infertile patients with endometriosis may play a role in endometriosis-associated infertility [123].

Thomsen–Friedenreich-like carbohydrate antigen

Women with endometriosis have antibody responses to a number of serum and tissue antigens such as α2-HS glycoprotein, transferrin, CA, human chorionic gonadotropin, hemopexin and α-chain of IgA1 [126]. A common carbohydrate epitope, the Thomsen–Friedenreich-like (T) antigen, which is present on all these diverse proteins, elicits this autoantibody response [127]. All of the above mentioned antigens bind to the lectin jacalin, which in turn specifically binds the T antigen [127].

Potential involvement of anti-Thomsen–Friedenreich-like antigen autoantibodies in endometriosis progression

In vitro culture of T antigen-specific lectin jacalin with cultured PB mononuclear cells can enhance the secretion of high levels of IL-1, IL-6, and TNF-α [128]. This observation suggests that autoantibodies recognizing the T antigen could directly trigger the synthesis of several cytokines such as IL-1, TNF-α, and IL-6 in women with endometriosis. These cytokines can favor in turn the expression of aromatase and 17β-hydroxysteroid dehydrogenase enzymes [129] and immunological mediators, such as prostaglandin E$_2$ (PGE$_2$) in endometriotic lesions [130]. Overall, these data suggest a possible link between T-like autoantibody response and expression of aromatase and 17β-hydroxysteroid dehydrogenase enzymes in endometriosis lesions.

A hemopexin domain with high sequence homology to plasma hemopexin is expressed by matrix metalloproteinases, except MMP-7, and can be recognized by T-like autoantibodies in women with endometriosis [126]. It has been postulated that the hemopexin domain expressed by most MMPs is involved in the process of MMP upregulation. The binding of T-like autoantibodies to the hemopexin domain may lead to dysregulation of the expression of MMPs and tissue inhibitors of metalloproteinases (TIMPs) in ectopic lesions, leading to increased invasiveness of these lesions in women with endometriosis [131].

Presence of autoantibodies against phospholipid antigens, histones and nucleotides in peripheral blood and peritoneal fluid

As previously discussed, autoimmunity can result from antigen-independent stimulation of self-reactive clones that are not deleted during development. Polyclonal activators stimulate a large number of T- and B-lymphocytes irrespective of antigen specificity and often without interacting with antigen receptors (e.g. lipopolysaccharid injection in mice). This form of autoimmunity, being a component of a polyclonal response, is usually associated with the production of multiple autoantibodies.

Immune complexes composed of a soluble (foreign or self) antigen and specific antibody (IgG or IgM) produce immunological disease by formation in the circulation and deposition in vessel walls virtually anywhere in the body [80]. Immune complex (IC) diseases tend to be systemic with little or no specificity for a particular antigen located in a particular tissue or organ. Clinical examples include SLE, serum sickness, polyarteritis nodosa and post-streptococcal glomerulonephritis.

In endometriosis patients, an increased prevalence of autoantibodies against phospholipid antigens (cardiolipin, phosphatidylserine, phosphatidylglycerol, phosphatidylethanolamine, phosphatidylinositol, phosphatidic acid), histone proteins (H1, H2A, H2B, H3, H4) and polynucleotides (ssDNA, dsDNA, Poly (I), Poly (dT)) has been reported in various studies using enzyme-linked immunosorbent assay (ELISA) techniques [132–134] or immunofluorescence, counter immunoelectrophoresis, double immunodiffusion and Western blots [135]. Higher levels of antiphospholipid antibodies, detected by passive hemagglutination, have been found in serum and PF from women with endometriosis stage I/II compared to those with endometriosis stage III/IV [19]. Higher levels of antiphospholipid antibodies (aPLs) IgG, IgM, sIgA and antinuclear antibodies have also been documented in PF than in serum from women with primary infertility [136,137].

Two studies have assessed serum levels of anticardiolipin (aCL) in endometriosis patients versus healthy controls who had not undergone a laparoscopy to exclude endometriosis [138,139]. Comparable values were found in one study [139], but higher levels in endometriosis patients were reported in the other [138]. In yet another report, the concentration of aCL in PF and lymphocyte culture fluid was found to be significantly higher in women with endometriosis compared to healthy women with a normal pelvis [140].

Antinuclear antibodies are serological findings in autoimmune diseases and are well known for tissue damage and correlation with disease activity of several autoimmune syndromes (e.g. SLE and SS) [141]. The ANAs are found in the serum of 29–47% patients with endometriosis, but are not related to pain, infertility or stage of endometriosis [142]. Therefore, the presence of ANA in patients with pelvic endometriosis appears to be an immunological secondary effect and does not represent an aggravating factor in patients with pelvic endometriosis. The lack of clear evidence that autoantibodies are important in endometriosis is not surprising. Endometriosis is defined as the ectopic presence of endometrium on several organs in and/or outside the pelvis, but cannot really be considered as a multiorgan disease.

Presence of immunoglobulin and complement in the circulation
Immunoglobulin
Most studies have reported comparable IgG levels in PB of endometriosis patients and fertile controls [127,143,145], and infertile women without endometriosis [8,144]. One study [146] reported normal levels during the luteal phase, but lower IgG values during the follicular phase in infertile endometriosis patients versus fertile controls. Similarly, most studies have reported comparable PB levels of IgA, IgE and IgM between endometriosis patients and controls [8,135,143,145–147]. In conclusion, at present there is no evidence that PB or PF IgG, IgA or IgM levels are significantly and specifically increased in patients with endometriosis when compared to women without the disease.

Complement
Most studies have reported comparable levels of C3, C4, factor B and properdin in the PB from patients with endometriosis or adenomyosis and controls [8,135,146,148]. In PF, increased C3, C3c and C4 levels, but normal factor B and properdin concentrations were reported in infertile patients with endometriosis versus infertile controls by one group of investigators [145]. Elevated levels of C3c (the final product of C3), C4, and SC5b-9 and a decreased concentration of iC3b have been reported in PF and serum from infertile women with endometriosis compared with healthy women [149]. However, plasma levels of proteolytic fragment C3a (anaphylatoxin) were similar in women with and without endometriosis [150].

In conclusion, currently there is no evidence of complement activation or consumption in either PB or PF from patients with endometriosis. However, previous studies were compromised by several methodological factors. Measurement of the split products of C3 (C3b, C3c, C3d), C4 and the C5b-9 complex (MAC) has been shown to be particularly useful as an index of complement activation [151] and should be used to further explore the role of complement activation in endometriosis, but should be verified with more specific state-of-the-art techniques.

Genetic polymorphisms associated with autoimmune diseases and endometriosis

Single nucleotide polymorphisms (SNPs) often provide correlative evidence for the involvement of specific genes in human diseases. It has been demonstrated that the function of crucial components of the T-cell antigen receptor (TCR) signaling pathways of the immune system and autoimmune diseases is usually affected by SNPs [152]. Protein tyrosine phosphatases (PTPs), currently one of the few known shared-autoimmune genes, are particularly good candidates for carrying disease-related SNPs [153] which may play a major role in preventing spontaneous T-cell activation and restrict the response to antigen.

Autoimmunity-predisposing allelic variation in the lymphoid tyrosine phosphatase (LYP) protein of the PTPN22 gene has been associated with the development of autoimmune diseases such as type 1 diabetes, SLE, RA and Graves disease [154]. PTPN22 polymorphism studies in endometriosis have been carried out in Italian, Polish and Brazilian populations [155–157] with and without a history of endometriosis and/or autoimmune diseases. In advanced-stage disease conditions, an allelic variation of the PTPN22 gene with endometriosis has been reported in Italian and Brazilian women [155,157] but not in Polish women [156].

Cytotoxic T-lymphocyte antigen (CTLA) 4 gene is recognized as a primary determinant for autoimmunity since specific polymorphisms of this gene have been associated with several autoimmune disorders [158], but not with endometriosis [159]. However, a positive association has been found in Japanese and Korean populations between severe endometriosis and five common polymorphisms of the gene for TNF-α, a multifunctional inflammatory cytokine known to be associated with various inflammatory and autoimmune diseases [160,161].

Many association studies are limited by the low number of patients included, and by the inclusion of controls without laparoscopic exclusion of endometriosis. In future association studies, efforts should be made to control for other risk factors in endometriosis and to select a proper control group, with laparoscopic confirmation of a normal pelvis and without other pelvic causes of pain or subfertility (i.e. women undergoing tubal ligation) [162].

Hormonal influences

Endometriosis affects only females, probably because only women menstruate and are thus at risk for development of this disease. This female preponderance has been used as an argument to propose an autoimmune etiology for endometriosis [163], in analogy with other autoimmune diseases such as SLE which affects females 10 times more frequently than males. It is not known whether this is due to the influence of sex hormones or other factors.

Common features in endometriosis and autoimmune diseases

If there is an increase in the frequency of organ-specific and organ-non-specific autoantibodies, one might suspect that endometriosis may be an autoimmune disease. This theory was first introduced by Gleicher and colleagues, and strong evidence would indicate that endometriosis fulfills most of the classification criteria of an autoimmune disease [132]. Endometriosis, like other classic autoimmune diseases, is associated with increased B-cell activation, polyclonal B-cell activation, immunological abnormalities in T- and B-cell functions, increased apoptosis, tissue damage, multiorgan involvement, familial occurrence, possible genetic basis (HLA typing), involvement of environmental co-factors (dioxins) and association with other autoimmune diseases [20].

In addition to the above similarities, some of the common recurring pathophysiologies such as increased inflammation, elevated levels of tissue remodeling components, and altered apoptosis exist both in women with endometriosis and in patients with autoimmune diseases such as RA, Crohn's disease, and psoriasis [20].

Inflammation

Endometriosis is a chronic inflammatory condition with abnormal local production of proinflammatory cytokines such as IL-1, IL-6, IL-8, TNF-α, IFN-γ and elevated concentration of nitric oxide (NO) [164]. The increased cytokines can modulate chemotactic factors, which in turn may recruit macrophages and T-lymphocytes to the peritoneum that could promote tissue damage and induce antibody secretion [20]. In addition, endometriotic implants surviving in the context of chronic inflammation may stimulate weakly self-reactive lymphocytes and thereby lead to the development of autoimmunity in response to local inflammatory processes. Altered cytokines like TNF-α and IL-1 can stimulate endometrial cell adhesion to the peritoneal mesothelial cell monolayers *in vitro* in endometriosis patients compared to those without endometriosis [165,166]. Eutopic and ectopic endometrium of patients with endometriosis secrete MMPs, which may enhance the adhesion process to the peritoneum [167].

Dysregulated apoptosis

Another important similarity that exists between endometriosis and autoimmune diseases is the deregulation of the apoptotic process [20]. In endometriosis, several studies have demonstrated the decreased susceptibility of eutopic and ectopic endometrial cells to apoptosis from women with endometriosis compared to fertile controls [168]. However, it remains unclear if these alterations in apoptosis in women with endometriosis are the cause or result of the process.

Environment

It is well established that chronic exposure to dioxin is immunosuppressive to murine SLE [169]. Some studies have shown an association between endometriosis and exposure to dioxins [170–172] that are known to suppress cell-mediated immunity [173] and promote inflammation [174]. However, serious concerns have been published regarding the quality of the studies "proving" the link between endometriosis and dioxins [171,172,175–177], and more studies are needed to address this issue, especially in view of the fact that in many countries the exposure to dioxins has diminished during the last 10 years.

High frequency of autoimmune and endocrine disorders among women with endometriosis

To test the hypothesis that women with endometriosis are more susceptible to autoimmune and endocrinological disorders, the US Endometriosis Association and the US National Institutes of Health conducted a cross-sectional survey in women with endometriosis in 1998 [21]. Women with endometriosis had higher rates of hypothyroidism, fibromyalgia, chronic fatigue syndrome, RA, SLE, SS and MS but no increased prevalence of hyperthyroidism or diabetes compared to the general female population [21]. In Caucasian women, endometriosis has been associated with the triad of alopecia universalis, autoimmune thyroiditis and

MS [178]. However, other studies have reported that prevalence and severity of SLE or SS, asthma, thyroid dysfunction and autoimmune thyroid disease were similar in women with and without endometriosis [179–181]. More well-designed epidemiological research in various ethnic groups is needed to investigate the hypothesis that women with endometriosis have an increased prevalence of other autoimmune diseases.

Peritoneal and systemic inflammation in endometriosis

Activated immune response and abnormal local production of proinflammatory cytokines have been proposed to play a major role in the pathogenesis of endometriosis. In women with endometriosis, PF volume is found to be increased with increased inflammation, including increased concentration of white blood cells and macrophages, and increased activation status of macrophages [131]. In addition, aberrant expression of several cytokines by activated macrophages, such as IL-1, IL-6, IL-8 and TNF-α, in the PF of women with endometriosis may contribute to a peritoneal microenvironment which favors the implantation of endometrial cells and the establishment of endometriosis [131]. It remains unclear whether inflammation is a cause or consequence in the pathophysiology of endometriosis. Obviously, these cause–effect relationships cannot be studied in women for ethical reasons.

Baboon model for the study of endometriosis-associated inflammation and immunomodulatory treatment of endometriosis

It has been well demonstrated that baboons with spontaneous endometriosis [182] or induced endometriosis after intrapelvic injection of menstrual endometrium [183] are a validated relevant preclinical model in which to study the pathophysiology and development of new drugs for endometriosis [184]. One month after induction of endometriosis, PF volume, PF white blood cell (WBC) concentration, macrophages, cytotoxic T-cells and inflammatory cytokines like TNF-α and ICAM-1 are significantly increased [184]. The increased percentage of CD4+ and IL-2R+ cells found in the peripheral blood of baboons with stage II/IV spontaneous endometriosis, when compared to those with stage I endometriosis or a normal pelvis, suggests that alterations in PB WBC populations may be an effect rather than the cause of endometriosis. Taken together, the above-mentioned baboon data support the notion that peritoneal inflammation is a consequence, not a cause of endometriosis [185]. Even if this is true, then the co-existence of endometriosis and peritoneal inflammation may offer new anti-inflammatory therapeutic options in the treatment of endometriosis.

Baboon model to test new drugs for treatment or prevention of endometriosis

The management of endometriosis today is almost exclusively accomplished through the use of gonadotropin releasing hormone analog and steroidogenic compounds, which are also known to be associated with side-effects including suppression of the menstrual cycle and hypoestrogenic state [186]. The use of immunomodulatory agents to treat endometriosis-associated infertility and suppress endometriotic implant growth has been well recommended [187,188]. In baboons, it has been shown that both TNF-α inhibitors and peroxisome proliferator-activated receptor-γ agonists can either prevent or treat peritoneal endometriosis, especially red lesions that represent angiogenic inflammatory active disease, as effectively as luteinizing hormone-releasing hormone antagonists without affecting the menstrual cycle or ovulation [182,189–192]. If these drugs are acceptable in terms of side-effects, they may represent a new medical treatment for women with peritoneal endometriosis.

Conclusion

There is increasing evidence that immune cells such as macrophages, NK cells, and dendritic cells and immune mediators such as IL-2, IL-10, and TNF-α cytokines are involved in the development and progression of endometriosis. In addition, the presence of both organ-specific and organ-non-specific endometrial antibodies and high serum concentrations of antiphospholipid and antinuclear antibodies may play a role in the onset and development of endometriosis and endometriosis-related infertility. The novel expression of immune modulator molecules such as HLA-G, sICAM-1 and FasL by endometrium and endometriotic lesions may offer another protective mechanism in the maintenance of immune tolerance of endometrial cells in the peritoneal environment. The link between autoimmunity and endometriosis may result from a common etiological origin (genetic, hormonal or environmental factors). Furthermore, endometriosis and autoimmune diseases like Crohn's disease, RA and psoriasis share important features including elevated levels of inflammatory cytokines, MMPs and altered apoptosis. In addition, patients with endometriosis appear to be more susceptible to other autoimmune and endocrinological disorders.

In order to better understand the complex relationship between endometriosis, autoimmunity and autoantibodies, more research is needed in well-defined patient populations (endometriosis, normal pelvis, other pelvic pathology) with or without pain and/or infertility, applying robust and reproducible assays in peripheral blood, peritoneal fluid and both eutopic and ectopic endometrium.

References

1. Bulun SE. Endometriosis. N Engl J Med 2009;360(3):268–279.

2. Sampson JA. Peritoneal endometriosis due to menstrual dissemination of endometrial tissue into the pelvic cavity. Am J Obstet Gynecol 1927;14:422–469.

3. Matarese G, de Placido G, Nikas Y et al. Pathogenesis of endometriosis: natural immunity dysfunction or autoimmune disease? Trends Mol Med 2003;9(5):223–228.

4. Ferguson BR, Bennington JL, Haber SL. Histochemistry of mucus substances and histology of mixed müllerian pelvic lymph node glandular inclusions. Evidence for histogenesis by müllerian metaplasia of coelomic epithelium. Obstet Gynecol 1969;33(5):617–625.

5. Levander G, Normann P. The pathogenesis of endometriosis: an experimental study. Acta Obstet Gynecol Scand 1955; l34(4):366–398.

6. Merrill JA. Endometrial induction of endometriosis across Millipore filters. Am J Obstet Gynecol 1966;94(6):780–790.

7. Dmowski WP, Steele RW, Baker GF. Deficient cellular immunity in endometriosis. Am J Obstet Gynecol 1981;141(4):377–383.

8. Steele RW, Dmowski WP, Marmer DJ. Immunologic aspects of endometriosis. Am J Reprod Immunol 1984;6:33–36.

9. Oosterlynck D, Cornillie FJ, Waer M et al. Women with endometriosis show a defect in natural killer cell activity resulting in a decreased cytotoxicity to autologous endometrium. Fertil Steril 1991; 56:45–51.

10. Lebovic DI, Mueller MD, Taylor RN. Immunobiology of endometriosis. Fertil Steril 2001;75(1):1–10.

11. Barrier BF, Kendall BS, Ryan CE et al. HLA-G is expressed by the glandular epithelium of peritoneal endometriosis but not in eutopic endometrium. Hum Reprod 2006;21(4):864–869.

12. Viganò P, Gaffuri B, Somigliana E et al. Expression of intercellular adhesion molecule (ICAM)-1 mRNA and protein is enhanced in endometriosis versus endometrial stromal cells in culture. Mol Hum Reprod 1998;4(12):1150–1156.

13. Garcia-Velasco JA, Mulayim N, Kayisli UA et al. Elevated soluble Fas ligand levels may suggest a role for apoptosis in women with endometriosis. Fertil Steril 2002;78(4):855–859.

14. Dmowski WP. Etiology and histogenesis of endometriosis. Ann N Y Acad Sci 1991;622:236–241.

15. Mathur SP. Autoimmunity in endometriosis: relevance to infertility. Am J Reprod Immunol 2000;44(2):89–95.

16. Zegers-Hochschild F, Adamson GD, de Mouzon J et al. The International Committee for Monitoring Assisted Reproductive Technology (ICMART) and the World Health Organization (WHO) Revised glossary on ART terminology. Hum Reprod 2009;24(11):2683–2687.

17. Wild RA, Hirisave V, Bianco A et al. Endometrial antibodies versus CA-125 for the detection of endometriosis. Fertil Steril 1991;55:90–94.

18. Wild RA, Hirisave V, Podczaski ES et al. Autoantibodies associated with endometriosis: can their detection predict presence of the disease? Obstet Gynecol 1991;77(6):927–931.

19. Ulcová-Gallová Z, Bouse V, Svábek L et al. Endometriosis in reproductive immunology. Am J Reprod Immunol 2002;47(5):269–274.

20. Nothnick WB. Treating endometriosis as an autoimmune disease. Fertil Steril 2001;76(2):223–231.

21. Sinaii N, Cleary SD, Ballweg ML et al. High rates of autoimmune and endocrine disorders, fibromyalgia, chronic fatigue syndrome and atopic diseases among women with endometriosis: a survey analysis. Hum Reprod 2002;10:2715–2724.

22. Ulukus M, Arici A. Immunology of endometriosis. Minerva Ginecol 2005;57(3):237–248.

23. Fukaya T, Sugawara J, Yoshida H et al. Intercellular adhesion molecule-1 and hepatocyte growth factor in human endometriosis: original investigation and a review of literature. Gynecol Obstet Invest 1999;47(1):11–16.

24. Agic A, Djalali S, Diedrich K et al. Apoptosis in endometriosis. Gynecol Obstet Invest 2009;68(4):217–223.

25. Selam B, Kayisli UA, Garcia-Velasco JA et al. Extracellular matrix-dependent regulation of Fas ligand expression in human endometrial stromal cells. Biol Reprod 2002;66(1):1–5.

26. Perricone R, Perricone C, de Carolis C et al. NK cells in autoimmunity: a two-edged weapon of the immune system. Autoimmun Rev 2008;7(5):384–390.

27. Oosterlynck DJ, Lacquet FA, Waer M et al. Lymphokine-activated killer activity in women with endometriosis. Gynecol Obstet Invest 1994;37(3):185–190.

28. Ho HN, Chao KH, Chen HF et al. Peritoneal natural killer cytotoxicity and CD25+ CD3+ lymphocyte subpopulation are decreased in women with stage III-IV endometriosis. Hum Reprod 1995;10(10):2671–2675.

29. Ho HN, Wu MY, Yang YS. Peritoneal cellular immunity and endometriosis. Am J Reprod Immunol 1997;38(6):400–412.

30. D'Hooghe TM, Bambra CS, Raeymaekers BM et al. The effects of immunosuppression on development and progression of endometriosis in baboons (Papio anubis). Fertil Steril 1995;64(1):172–178.

31. Wilson MT, Van Kaer L. Natural killer T cells as targets for therapeutic intervention in autoimmune diseases. Curr Pharm Des 2003;9(3):201–220.

32. Podgaec S, Abrao MS, Dias JA Jr et al. Endometriosis: an inflammatory disease with a Th2 immune response component. Hum Reprod 2007;22(5):1373–1379.

33. Hsu CC, Yang BC, Wu MH et al. Enhanced interleukin-4 expression in patients with endometriosis. Fertil Steril 1997;67(6):1059–1064.

34. Li JX, Dai SZ, Liu H et al. Study on the changes of T-lymphocyte subsets in the patients with endometriosis. Zhonghua Fu Chan Ke Za Zhi 2005;40(1):17–20.

35. Antsiferova YS, Sotnikova NY, Posiseeva LV et al. Changes in the T-helper cytokine profile and in lymphocyte activation at the systemic and local levels in women with endometriosis. Fertil Steril 2005;84(6):1705–1711.

36. OuYang Z, Hirota Y, Osuga Y et al. Interleukin-4 stimulates proliferation of endometriotic stromal cells. Am J Pathol 2008;173(2):463–469.

37. American Society for Reproductive Medicine. Revised classification of endometriosis. Fertil Steril 1997;67:817–821.

38. Casali P, Burastero SE, Nakamura M et al. Human lymphocytes making rheumatoid factor and antibody to ssDNA belong to Leu-1+ B-cell subset. Science 1987;236(4797):77–81.

39. Chishima F, Hayakawa S, Hirata Y et al. Peritoneal and peripheral B-1-cell populations in patients with endometriosis. J Obstet Gynaecol Res 2000;26(2):141–146.

40. Weed JC, Arquembourg PC. Endometriosis: can it produce an autoimmune response resulting in infertility? Clin Obstet Gynecol 1980;23:885–893.

41. Gross JA, Dillon SR, Mudri S et al. TACI-Ig neutralizes molecules critical for B cell development and autoimmune disease: impaired B cell maturation in mice lacking BLyS. Immunity 2001;15(2):289–302.

42. Hever A, Roth RB, Hevezi P et al. Human endometriosis is associated with plasma cells and overexpression of B lymphocyte stimulator. Proc Natl Acad Sci USA 2007;104(30):12451–12456.

43. Choo SY. The HLA system: genetics, immunology, clinical testing, and clinical implications. Yonsei Med J 2007;48(1):11–23.

44. Flavell RA, Hafler DA. Autoimmunity. Curr Opin Immunol 1999;11:635–707.

45. Somigliana E, Viganò P, Vignali M. Endometriosis and unexplained recurrent spontaneous abortion: pathological states resulting from aberrant modulation of natural killer cell function? Hum Reprod Update 1999;5(1):40–51.

46. Moretta L, Moretta A. Killer immunoglobulin-like receptors. Curr Opin Immunol 2004;16(5):626–633.

47. Borrego F, Masilamani M, Kabat J et al. The cell biology of the human natural killer cell CD94/NKG2A inhibitory receptor. Mol Immunol 2005;42(4):485–488.

48. Maeda N, Izumiya C, Yamamoto Y et al. Increased killer inhibitory receptor KIR2DL1 expression among natural killer cells in women with pelvic endometriosis. Fertil Steril 2002;77(2):297–302.

49. Matsuoka S, Maeda N, Izumiya C et al. Expression of inhibitory-motif killer immunoglobulin-like receptor, KIR2DL1, is increased in natural killer cells from women with pelvic endometriosis. Am J Reprod Immunol 2005;53(5):249–254.

50. Zhang C, Maeda N, Izumiya C et al. Killer immunoglobulin-like receptor and human leukocyte antigen expression as immunodiagnostic parameters for pelvic endometriosis. Am J Reprod Immunol 2006;55(2):106–114.

51. Galandrini R, Porpora MG, Stoppacciaro A et al. Increased frequency of human leukocyte antigen-E inhibitory receptor CD94/NKG2A-expressing peritoneal natural killer cells in patients with endometriosis. Fertil Steril 2008;89(5):1490–1496.

52. Berkkanoglu M, Arici A. Immunology and endometriosis. Am J Reprod Immunol 2003;50(1):48–59.

53. Semino C, Semino A, Pietra G et al. Role of major histocompatibility complex class I expression and natural killer-like T cells in the genetic control of endometriosis. Fertil Steril 1995;64(5):909–916.

54. Xin Y, Xu X, Ling H. Expression of major histocompatibility complex-class I antigen on endometrial stroma cells in patients with Endometriosis. Zhonghua Fu Chan Ke Za Zhi 2000;35(9):530–532.

55. Vernet-Tomás Mdel M, Pérez-Ares CT, Verdú N et al. The endometria of patients with endometriosis show higher expression of class I human leukocyte antigen than the endometria of healthy women. Fertil Steril 2006;85(1):78–83.

56. Aldrich CL, Stephenson MD, Karrison T et al. HLA-G genotypes and pregnancy outcome in couples with unexplained recurrent miscarriage. Mol Hum Reprod 2001;7(12):1167–1172.

57. Carosella ED, Favier B, Rouas-Freiss N et al. Beyond the increasing complexity of the immunomodulatory HLA-G molecule. Blood 2008;111(10):4862–4870.

58. Wiendl H, Feger U, Mittelbronn M et al. Expression of the immune-tolerogenic major histocompatibility molecule HLA-G in multiple sclerosis: implications for CNS immunity. Brain 2005; 128(11):2689–2704.

59. Mouillot G, Marcou C, Zidi I et al. Hypoxia modulates HLA-G gene expression in tumor cells. Hum Immunol 2007;68(4):277–285.

60. Le Maoult J, Rouas-Freiss N, Le Discorde M et al. HLA-G in organ transplantation. Pathol Biol (Paris) 2004;52(2):97–103.

61. Favier B, LeMaoult J, Carosella ED. Functions of HLA-G in the immune system. Tissue Antigens 2007;69(1):150–152.

62. Wang F, Wen Z, Li H et al. Human leukocyte antigen-G is expressed by the eutopic and ectopic endometrium of adenomyosis. Fertil Steril 2008;90(5):1599–1604.

63. Kawashima M, Maeda N, Adachi Y et al. Human leukocyte antigen-G, a ligand for the natural killer receptor KIR2DL4, is expressed by eutopic endometrium only in the menstrual phase. Fertil Steril 2009;91(2):343–349.

64. Hornung D, Fujii E, Lim KH et al. Histocompatibility leukocyte antigen-G is not expressed by endometriosis or endometrial tissue. Fertil Steril 2001;75(4):814–817.

65. Crispin JC, Alcocer-Varela J. The role myeloid dendritic cells play in the pathogenesis of systemic lupus erythematosus. Autoimmun Rev 2007;6(7):450–456.

66. Chui CS, Li D. Role of immunolglobulin-like transcript family receptors and their ligands in suppressor T-cell-induced dendritic cell tolerization. Hum Immunol 2009;70(9):686–691.

67. Schulke L, Berbic M, Manconi F et al. Dendritic cell populations in the eutopic and ectopic endometrium of women with endometriosis. Hum Reprod 2009;24(7):1695–1703.

68. Fainaru O, Adini A, Benny O et al. Dendritic cells support angiogenesis and promote lesion growth in a murine model of endometriosis. FASEB J 2008;22(2):522–529.

69. Wu J, Horuzsko A. Expression and function of ILTs on tolerogenic dendritic cells. Hum Immunol 2009;70(5):353–356.

70. Kusume T, Maeda N, Izumiya C et al. Human leukocyte antigen expression by peritoneal macrophages from women with pelvic endometriosis is depressed but coordinated with costimulatory molecule expression. Fertil Steril 2005;83(1):1232–1240.

71. Muixí L, Alvarez I, Jaraquemada D et al. Peptides presented in vivo by HLA-DR in thyroid autoimmunity. Adv Immunol 2008;99:165–209.

72. Ota H, Igarashi S. Expression of major histocompatibility complex class II antigen in endometriotic tissue in patients with endometriosis and adenomyosis. Fertil Steril 1993;60(5):834–838.

73. Liu Y, Luo L, Zhao H. Immunohistochemical study of HLA-DR antigen in endometrial tissue of patients with endometriosis. J Huazhong Univ Sci Technolog Med Sci 2002;22(1):60–61.

74. Izumiya C, Maeda N, Kusume T et al. Coordinated but depressed expression of human leukocyte antigen-DR, intercellular adhesion molecule-1, and CD14 on peritoneal macrophages in women with pelvic endometriosis. Fertil Steril 2003;80(2):768–775.

75. Yamamoto Y, Maeda N, Izumiya C et al. Decreased human leukocyte antigen-DR expression in the lipid raft by peritoneal macrophages from women with endometriosis. Fertil Steril 2008;89(1):52–59.

76. Watson CA, Petzelbauer P, Zhou J et al. Contact-dependent endothelial class II HLA gene activation induced by NK cells is mediated by IFN-gamma-dependent and -independent mechanisms. J Immunol 1995;154(7):3222–3233.

77. Thorsby E. Invited anniversary review: HLA associated diseases. Hum Immunol 1997;53:1–11.

78. Lavant EH, Carlson JA. A new automated human leukocyte antigen genotyping strategy to identify DR-DQ risk alleles for celiac disease and type 1 diabetes mellitus. Clin Chem Lab Med 2009;47(12):1489–1495.

79. Benjamin R, Parham P. Guilt by association: HLA-B27 and ankylosing spondylitis. Immunol Today 1990;11:137–142.

80. Abbas AK, Lichtman AH, Pober JS. Cellular and Molecular Immunology. Philadelphia: W.B. Saunders, 1991.

81. Balsa A, Cabezon A, Orozco G et al. Influence of HLA DRB1 alleles in the susceptibility of rheumatoid arthritis and the regulation of antibodies against citrullinated proteins and rheumatoid factor. Arthritis Res Ther 2010;12(2):R62.

82. Kitawaki J, Obayashi H, Kado N et al. Association of HLA class I and class II alleles with susceptibility to endometriosis. Hum Immunol 2002;63(11):1033–1038.

83. Whang DH, Kim SH, Park MH et al. Association of HLA-A, B antigens with susceptibility to advanced endometriosis in Koreans. Korean J Lab Med 2008;28(2):118–123.

84. Ishii K, Takakuwa K, Adachi H et al. Studies on the human leukocyte antigen class I antigens in Japanese patients with macroscopically diagnosed endometriosis. Gynecol Obstet Invest 2002; 54(3):150–153.

85. Ishii K, Takakuwa K, Kashima K et al. Associations between patients with endometriosis and HLA class II: the analysis of HLA-DQB1 and HLA-DPB1 genotypes. Hum Reprod 2003;18(5):985–989.

86. Zong L, Pan D, Chen W et al. Comparative study of HLA-DQA1 and HLA-DRB1 allele in patients with endometriosis and adenomyosis. Zhonghua Yi Xue Yi Chuan Xue Za Zhi 2002;19(1):49–51.

87. Alviggi C, Carrieri PB, Pivonello R et al. Association of pelvic endometriosis with alopecia universalis, autoimmune thyroiditis and multiple sclerosis. J Endocrinol Invest 2006;29(2):182–189.

88. Simpson JL, Malinak LR, Elias S. HLA associations in endometriosis. Am J Obstet Gynecol 1984;148(4):395–397.

89. Moen M, Bratlie A, Moen T. Distribution of HLA-antigens among patients with endometriosis. Acta Obstet Gynecol Scand 1984;123(Suppl):25–27.

90. Maxwell C, Kilpatrick DC, Haining R et al. No HLA-DR specificity is associated with endometriosis. Tissue Antigens 1989; 34:145–147.

91. Wallace PK, Yeaman GR, Johnson K et al. MHC class II expression and antigen presentation by human endometrial cells. J Steroid Biochem Mol Biol 2001;76(1–5):203–211.

92. Hershberg RM, Framson PE, Cho DH et al. Intestinal epithelial cells use two distinct pathways for HLA class II antigen processing. J Clin Invest 1997;100(1):204–215.

93. Cooper NR. The complement system. In: Lange-Fundenberg H, Stites D, Caldwell J et al (eds) Basic and Clinical Immunology, 3rd edn. Los Altos, CA: Lange Medical Publications, 1980, p.83.

94. Startseva NV. Clinico-immunological aspects of endometriosis. Akush Ginekol 1980;3:23–26.

95. Mathur S, Peress MR, Williamson HO et al. Autoimmunity to endometrium and ovary in endometriosis. Clin Exp Immunol 1982;50:259–266.

96. Saifuddin A, Buckley CH, Fox H. Immunoglobulin content of the endometrium in women with endometriosis. Int J Gynecol Pathol 1983;2:255–263.

97. Mathur S, Garza DE, Smith LF. Endometrial autoantigens eliciting immunoglobulin (Ig) G, Ig A and Ig M responses in endometriosis. Fertil Steril 1990;54:56–63.

98. Ota H, Maki M. Content of immunoglobulin G and complement components C3 and C4 in endometriotic tissue or endometrium in women with adenomyosis or endometriosis. Med Sci Res 1990;18:727–728.

99. Mathur S, Chihal HJ, Homm RJ et al. Endometrial antigens involved in the autoimmunity of endometriosis. Fertil Steril 1988; 50:860–863.

100. Switchenko AC, Kauffman RS, Becker M. Are there antiendometrial antibodies in sera of women with endometriosis? Fertil Steril 1991;56:235–241.

101. Rajkumar K, Malliah V, Simpson CW. Identifying the presence of antibodies against endometrial antigens. A preliminary study. J Reprod Med 1992;37:552–556.

102. Gorai I, Ishikawa M, Onose R et al. Antiendometrial auto antibodies are generated in patients with endometriosis. Am J Reprod Immunol 1993;29:116–123.

103. Iborra A, Palacio JR, Ulcova-Gallova Z et al. Autoimmune response in women with endometriosis. Am J Reprod Immunol 2000;44(4):236–241.

104. Gajbhiye R, Suryawanshi A, Khan S et al. Multiple endometrial antigens are targeted in autoimmune endometriosis. Reprod Biomed 2008;16:817–824.

105. Randall GW, Gantt PA, Poe-Zeigler RL. Serum antiendometrial antibodies and diagnosis of endometriosis. Am J Reprod Immunol 2007;58(4):374–382.

106. Sarapik A, Haller-Kikkatalo K, Utt M et al. Serum anti-endometrial antibodies in infertile women – potential risk factor for implantation failure. Am J Reprod Immunol 2010;63(5):349–357.

107. Mathur S, Butler WJ, Chihal HJ et al. Target antigen(s) in endometrial autoimmunity of endometriosis. Autoimmunity 1995; 20(4):211–222.

108. Bohler HC, Gercel-Taylor C, Lessey BA et al. Endometriosis markers: immunologic alterations as diagnostic indicators for endometriosis. Reprod Sci 2007;14(6):595–604.

109. Chihal HJ, Mathur S, Holtz GL. An endometrial antibody assay in the clinical diagnosis and management of endometriosis. Fertil Steril 1986;46:408–411.

110. Isaacson KB, Coutifaris C, Garcia CR et al. Production and secretion of complement component C3 by endometriotic tissue. J Clin Endocrinol Metab 1989;69:1003–1009.

111. Isaacson KB, Galman M, Coutifaris C et al. Endometrial synthesis and secretion of complement-component-3 by patients with and without endometriosis. Fertil Steril 1990;53:836–841.

112. Bischof P, Planas D, Campana A. The third factor of the complement cascade (C3) is produced by human endometrial cells cultured in vitro. Abstract 159, presented at the 39th Annual Meeting of the Society for Gynecological Investigation, San Antonio, 1992, p.188.

113. Ota H, Maki M. Content of immunoglobulin G and complement components C3 and C4 in endometriotic tissue or endometrium in women with adenomyosis or endometriosis. Med Sci Res 1990;18:727–728.

114. D'Cruz OJ, Wild RA. Evaluation of endometrial tissue specific complement activation in women with endometriosis. Fertil Steril 1992;57:787–795.

115. Itoh Y, Reichlin M. Antibodies to carbonic anhydrase in systemic lupus erythematosus and other rheumatic diseases. Arthritis Rheum 1992;35(1):73–82.

116. Kiechle FL, Quattrociocchi-Longe TM, Brinton DA. Carbonic anhydrase antibody in sera from patients with endometriosis. Am J Clin Pathol 1994;101(5):611–615.

117. D'Cruz OJ, Wild RA, Haas GG Jr et al. Antibodies to carbonic anhydrase in endometriosis: prevalence, specificity, and relationship to clinical and laboratory parameters. Fertil Steril 1996;66(4):547–556.

118. Brinton DA, Quattrociocchi-Longe TM, Kiechle FL et al. Endometriosis: identification by carbonic anhydrase auto antibodies and clinical features. Ann Clin Lab Sci 1996;26(5):409–420.

119. Pillai S, Zhou GX, Arnaud P et al. Antibodies to endometrial transferrin and alpha 2-Heremans Schmidt (HS) glycoprotein in patients with endometriosis. Am J Reprod Immunol 1996;35(5):483–494.

120. Mathur SP, Lee JH, Jiang H et al. Levels of transferrin and alpha 2-HS glycoprotein in women with and without endometriosis. Autoimmunity 1999;29(2):121–127.

121. Mathur SP, Holt VL, Lee JH et al. Levels of antibodies to transferrin and alpha 2-HS glycoprotein in women with and without endometriosis. Am J Reprod Immunol 1998;40(2):69–73.

122. Pillai S, Zhou GX, Arnaud P et al. Antibodies to endometrial transferrin and alpha 2-Heremans Schmidt (HS) glycoprotein in patients with endometriosis. Am J Reprod Immunol 1998;35(5):483–494.

123. Inagaki J, Kondo A, Lopez LR et al. Anti-laminin-1 auto antibodies, pregnancy loss and endometriosis. Clin Dev Immunol 2004;11(3–4):261–266.

124. Inagaki J, Sugiura-Ogasawara M, Nomizu M et al. An association of IgG anti-laminin-1 auto antibodies with endometriosis in infertile patients. Hum Reprod 2003;18(3):544–549.

125. Cervená R, Bibková K, Micanová Z et al. IgG antibodies against laminin-1 in serum and in peritoneal fluid in patients with decreased fertility. Ceska Gynekol 2009;74(3):188–192.

126. Yeaman GR, Collins JE, Lang GA. Autoantibody responses to carbohydrate epitopes in endometriosis. Ann N Y Acad Sci 2002;955:174–182.

127. Lang GA, Yeamen GR. Auto antibodies in endometriosis sera recognize a Thomsen-Friedenreich-like carbohydrate antigen. J Autoimmun 2001;16(2):151–161.

128. Taimi M, Dornand J, Nicolas M et al. Involvement of CD4 in interleukin-6 secretion by U937 monocytic cells stimulated with the lectin jacalin. J. Leukocyte Biol 1994;55:214–220.

129. Bulun SE, Zeitoun KM, Takayama K et al. Estrogen biosynthesis in endometriosis: molecular basis and clinical relevance. J Mol Endocrinol 2000;25(1):35–42.

130. Zeitoun KM, Bulun SE. Aromatase: a key molecule in the pathophysiology of endometriosis and a therapeutic target. Fertil Steril 1999;72(6):961–969.

131. Kyama CM, Debrock S, Mwenda JM et al. Potential involvement of the immune system in the development of endometriosis. Reprod Biol Endocrinol 2003;2:1–123.

132. Gleicher N, El-Roeiy A, Confino E et al. Is endometriosis an autoimmune disease? Obstet Gynecol 1987;70:115–122.

133. El-Roeiy A, Gleicher N. Definition of normal autoantibody levels in an apparently healthy population. Obstet Gynecol 1988;72:596–602.

134. Confino E, Harlow L, Gleicher N. Peritoneal fluid and serum autoantibody levels in patients with endometriosis. Fertil Steril 1990;53:242–245.

135. Taylor PV, Maloney MD, Campbell JM et al. Autoreactivity in women with endometriosis. Br J Obstet Gynaecol 1991;98(7):680–684.

136. Ulcová-Gallová Z, Krauz V, Bouse V et al. Correlation between peritoneal fluid and serum antiphospholipid antibodies in women with primary infertility. Int J Fertil Womens Med 1998;43(5):267–272.

137. Lucena E, Cubillos J. Immune abnormalities in endometriosis compromising fertility in IVF-ET patients. J Reprod Med 1999;44(5):458–464.

138. Kennedy SH, Nunn B, Cederholm-Williams SA et al. Cardiolipin antibody levels in endometriosis and systemic lupus erythematosus. Fertil Steril 1989;52:1061–1062.

139. Kilpatrick DC, Haining REB, Smith SSK. Are cardiolipin antibody levels elevated in endometriosis? Fertil Steril 1991;55:436–437.

140. Sikora J, Mielczarek-Palacz A, Kondera-Anasz Z et al. Concentration of anticardiolipin antibodies in peritoneal fluid and in fluid from lymphocyte culture in women with endometriosis. Ginekol Pol 2009;80(6):419–423.

141. Pradhan VD, Patwardhan MM, Ghosh K et al. Anti-nucleosome antibodies as a disease marker in systemic lupus erythematosus and its correlation with disease activity and other auto antibodies. Indian J Dermatol Venereol Leprol 2010;76(2):145–149.

142. Dias JA Jr, de Oliveira RM, Abrao MS. Antinuclear antibodies and endometriosis. Int J Gynaecol Obstet 2006;93(3):262–263.

143. El-Roeiy A, Dmowski WP, Gleicher N et al. Danazol but not gonadotropin-releasing hormone agonists suppresses auto antibodies in endometriosis. Fertil Steril 1988;50:864–871.

144. El-Roeiy A, Gleicher N. Definition of normal autoantibody levels in an apparently healthy population. Obstet Gynecol 1988;72:596–602.

145. Badawy SZ, Cuenca V, Stitzel A et al. Autoimmune phenomena in infertile patients with endometriosis. Obstet Gynecol 1984;63:271–275.

146. Meek SC, Hodge DD, Musich JR. Autoimmunity in infertile patients with endometriosis. Am J Obstet Gynecol 1988;158:1365–1373.

147. Eidukaite A, Tamosiunas V. Activity of eosinophils and immunoglobulin E concentration in the peritoneal fluid of women with endometriosis. Clin Chem Lab Med 2004;242(6):590–594.

148. Ota H, Maki M, Shidara Y et al. Effects of danazol at the immunologic level in patients with adenomyosis, with special reference to auto antibodies: a multi-center cooperative study. Am J Obstet Gynecol 1992;167:481–486.

149. Kabut J, Kondera-Anasz Z, Sikora J et al. Levels of complement components iC3b, C3c, C4, and SC5b-9 in peritoneal fluid and serum of infertile women with endometriosis. Fertil Steril 2007;88(5):1298–1303.

150. Fassbender A, D'Hooghe T, Mihalyi A et al. Plasma C3a-des-Arg levels in women with and without endometriosis. Am J Reprod Immunol 2009;62(3):187–195.

151. Morgan BP. Assays of complement and complement activation. In: Morgan PB (ed) Complement. San Diego: Academic Press, 1990, pp.195–203.

152. Bottini N, Vang T, Cucca F et al. Role of PTPN22 in type 1 diabetes and other autoimmune diseases. Semin Immunol 2006; 18(4):207–213.

153. Wu J, Katrekar A, Honigberg LA et al. Identification of substrates of human protein-tyrosine phosphatase PTPN22. J Biol Chem 2006;281:11002–11010.

154. Vang T, Miletic AV, Bottini N et al. Protein tyrosine phosphatase PTPN22 in human autoimmunity. Autoimmunity 2007; 40(6):453–461.

155. Ammendola M, Bottini N, Pietropolli A et al. Association between PTPN22 and endometriosis. Fertil Steril 2008;89:993–994.

156. Płoski R, Dziunycz P, Kostrzewa G et al. PTPN22/LYP 1858C>T gene polymorphism and susceptibility to endometriosis in a Polish population. J Reprod Immunol 2009;79(2):196–200.

157. Gomes FM, Bianco B, Teles JS et al. PTPN22 C1858T polymorphism in women with endometriosis. Am J Reprod Immunol 2010;63(3):227–232.

158. Pociot F. CTLA4 gene and autoimmune endocrinopathies: a new marker? J Endocrinol Invest 2002;25(11):1001–1005.

159. Viganò P, Lattuada D, Somigliana E et al. Variants of the CTLA4 gene that segregate with autoimmune diseases are not associated with endometriosis. Mol Hum Reprod 2005;11(10):745–749.

160. Asghar T, Yoshida S, Kennedy S et al. The tumor necrosis factor-alpha promoter -1031C polymorphism is associated with decreased risk of endometriosis in a Japanese population. Hum Reprod 2004;19(11):2509–2514.

161. Lee GH, Choi YM, Kim SH et al. Association of tumor necrosis factor-{alpha} gene polymorphisms with advanced stage endometriosis. Hum Reprod 2008;23(4):977–981.

162. Falconer H, D'Hooghe T, Fried G. Endometriosis and genetic polymorphisms. Obstet Gynecol Surv 2007;62(9):616–628.

163. Dmowski WP, Braun D, Gebel H. Endometriosis: genetics and immunologic aspects. In: Chadha DR, Buttran VC (eds) Current Concepts in Endometriosis. New York: Alan R Liss, 1990, pp.99–122.

164. Ota H, Igarashi S, Hatazawa J et al. Endothelial nitric oxide synthase in the endometrium during the menstrual cycle in patients with endometriosis and adenomyosis. Fertil Steril 1998;69(2):303–308.

165. Zhang RJ, Wild RA, Ojago JM et al. Effect of tumor necrosis factor-alpha on adhesion of human endometrial stromal cells to peritoneal mesothelial cells: an in vitro system. Fertil Steril 1993; 59(6):1196–1201.

166. Sillem M, Prifti S, Monga B et al. Integrin-mediated adhesion of uterine endometrial cells from endometriosis patients to extracellular matrix proteins is enhanced by tumor necrosis factor alpha (TNF alpha) and interleukin-1 (IL-1). Eur J Obstet Gynecol Reprod Biol 1999;87(2):123–127.

167. Collette T, Maheux R, Mailloux J, Akoum A. Increased expression of matrix metalloproteinase-9 in the eutopic endometrial tissue of women with endometriosis. Hum Reprod 2006;21(12):3059–3067.

168. Gebel HM, Braun DP, Tambur A et al. Spontaneous apoptosis of endometrial tissue is impaired in women with endometriosis. Fertil Steril 1998;69(6):1042–1047.

169. Li J, McMurray RW. Effects of chronic exposure to DDT and TCDD on disease activity in murine systemic lupus erythematosus. Lupus 2009;18(11):941–949.

170. Bruner-Tran KL, Osteen KG. Dioxin-like PCBs and endometriosis. Syst Biol Reprod Med 2010;56(2):132–146.

171. Guo SW. The link between exposure to dioxin and endometriosis: a critical reappraisal of primate data. Gynecol Obstet Invest 2004;57(3):157–173.

172. Guo SW, Simsa P, Kyama CM et al. Reassessing the evidence for the link between dioxin and endometriosis: from molecular biology to clinical epidemiology. Mol Hum Reprod 2009;15(10):609–624.

173. Smith SK. The aetiology of endometriosis. Hum Reprod 1995;10(5):1274.

174. Bruner-Tran KL, Yeaman GR, Crispens MA et al. Dioxin may promote inflammation-related development of endometriosis. Fertil Steril 2008;89(5):1287–1298.

175. Zhao D, Pritts EA, Chao VA et al. Dioxin stimulates RANTES expression in an in-vitro model of endometriosis. Mol Hum Reprod 2002;8(9):849–854.

176. Anger DL, Foster WG. The link between environmental toxicant exposure and endometriosis. Front Biosci 2008;13:1578–1593.

177. Foster WG. Endocrine toxicants including 2,3,7,8-terachlorodibenzo-p-dioxin (TCDD) and dioxin-like chemicals and endometriosis: is there a link? Toxicol Environ Health B Crit Rev 2008;11(3–4):177–187.

178. Alviggi C, Carrieri PB, Pivonello R. Association of pelvic endometriosis with alopecia universalis, autoimmune thyroiditis and multiple sclerosis. J Endocrinol Invest 2006;29(2):182–189.

179. Ferrero S, Petrera P, Colombo BM et al. Asthma in women with endometriosis. Hum Reprod 2005;20(12):3514–3517.

180. Matorras R, Ocerin I, Unamuno M et al. Prevalence of endometriosis in women with systemic lupus erythematosus and Sjogren's syndrome. Lupus 2007;16(9):736–740.

181. Petta CA, Arruda MS, Zantut-Wittmann DE et al. Thyroid autoimmunity and thyroid dysfunction in women with endometriosis. Hum Reprod 2007;22(10):2693–2697.

182. Barrier BF, Bates GW, Leland MM et al. Efficacy of anti-tumor necrosis factor therapy in the treatment of spontaneous endometriosis in baboons. Fertil Steril 2004;81(1):775–779.

183. D'Hooghe TM, Bambra CS, Raeymaekers BM et al. Intrapelvic injection of menstrual endometrium causes endometriosis in baboons (Papio cynocephalus and Papio anubis). Am J Obstet Gynecol 1995;173(1):125–134.

184. D'Hooghe TM, Kyama CM, Chai D et al. Nonhuman primate models for translational research in endometriosis. Reprod Sci 2009;16(2):152–161.

185. D'Hooghe TM, Bambra CS, Xiao L et al. Effect of menstruation and intrapelvic injection of endometrium on inflammatory parameters of peritoneal fluid in the baboon (Papio anubis and Papio cynocephalus). Am J Obstet Gynecol 2001;184(5):917–925.

186. Nothnick WB, D'Hooghe TM. Medical management of endometriosis: novel targets and approaches towards the development of future treatment regimes. Gynecol Obstet Invest 2003;55(4):189–198.

187. Balasch J, Creus M, Fábregues F et al. Pentoxifylline versus placebo in the treatment of infertility associated with minimal or mild endometriosis: a pilot randomized clinical trial. Hum Reprod 1997;12(9):2046–2050.

188. Nothnick WB, Curry TE, Vernon MW. Immunomodulation of rat endometriotic implant growth and protein production. Am J Reprod Immunol 1994;31(2–3):151–162.

189. D'Hooghe TM, Nugent NP, Cuneo S et al. Recombinant human TNFRSF1A (r-hTBP1) inhibits the development of endometriosis in baboons: a prospective, randomized, placebo- and drug-controlled study. Biol Reprod 2006;74(1):131–136.

190. Falconer H, Mwenda JM, Chai DC et al. Treatment with anti-TNF monoclonal antibody (c5N) reduces the extent of induced endometriosis in the baboon. Hum Reprod 2006;21(7):1856–1862.

191. Lebovic DI, Mwenda JM, Chai DC et al. PPAR-gamma receptor ligand induces regression of endometrial explants in baboons: a prospective, randomized, placebo- and drug-controlled study. Fertil Steril 2007;88(4):1108–1119.

192. Lebovic DI, Mwenda JM, Chai DC et al. Peroxisome proliferator-activated receptor-(gamma) receptor ligand partially prevents the development of endometrial explants in baboons: a prospective, randomized, placebo-controlled study. Endocrinology 2010; 151(4):1846–1852.

49 Endometriosis and Cancer: Epidemiology

Paola Viganò[1], Edgardo Somigliana[2], Fabio Parazzini[3] and Paolo Vercellini[3]

[1] Scientific Institute San Raffaele and Center for Research in Obstetrics and Gynecology, Milan, Italy
[2] Department of Obstetrics, Gynecology and Neonatology, Fondazione Cà Granda, Ospedale Maggiore Policlinico, Milan, Italy
[3] Prima Clinica Ostetrico Ginecologica, Università di Milano, Milan, Italy

Introduction

Endometriosis is generally regarded as a benign condition although it exhibits some characteristics reminiscent of malignancy, such as development of local and distant foci and attachment to and invasion of other tissues with subsequent damage to the target organs [1].

The relationship between endometriosis and cancer is still an intriguing and poorly investigated issue. This overview will cover the certainties and doubts of this problem. Specifically: (1) observational, case–control and cohort studies aiming to assess a possible association between endometriosis and various types of cancer will be critically analyzed; (2) the magnitude of this potential association will be examined and discussed; (3) evidence will be presented in favor of or against a possible causative link between the two entities versus the sharing of similar risk factors, employing the nine criteria proposed by Austin Bradford Hill, which still stand as foundation milestones for causal inference [2]. Establishing an argument of causation between endometriosis and ovarian cancer, where causation is intended in terms of precursor lesions, would imply a reappraisal of the current long-term management of patients with endometriosis.

Endometriosis and ovarian cancer

Observational clinical studies

Based on Sampson's [3] and Scott's [4] criteria for identifying malignant tumors raised from endometriosis, few groups have evaluated the prevalence of ovarian malignancy in large series of patients operated for endometriosis. Mostoufizadeh and Scully [5] and Stern et al [6] reported similar (0.8% and 0.9%, respectively) prevalence of cancer in about 1000 cases of ovarian endometriosis.

Stern et al have pointed out that this prevalence rose to 3.8% if "arising in" was defined according to Sampson's criteria only [3]. Unfortunately, all currently available series are retrospective, and thus probably unable to properly address this point. In support of this idea, the same prevalence proposed by Stern et al differed significantly according to the pathologists who performed the analysis [6]. This rate was as high as 8.9% (27 out of 305) if pathologists with specific gynecological experience were involved. The percentage dropped to 1.3% (nine out of 695) if reports from other pathologists were considered. A prospective, sufficiently large and unbiased series on the frequency of the concomitant presence of endometriosis and cancer is currently unavailable.

More interesting insights have been provided by studies addressing the frequency of endometriosis among patients with ovarian malignancies [7–17]. A 4–29% frequency of endometriosis was found in cases operated for ovarian tumors (Table 49.1). These percentages do not appear to be very different from the 10% supposed prevalence of the disease in the reproductive age group. On the other hand, it is important to note that a consistent body of evidence has documented a clear association between endometriosis and some specific histological subtypes of ovarian epithelial cancers, namely endometrioid and clear cell carcinoma. Studies that have estimated the presence of endometriosis in relation to cancer histological histotypes are shown in Table 49.1. This epidemiological observation currently represents one of the most relevant aspects supporting a relationship between endometriosis and ovarian cancer.

With regard to the clinical behavior and prognostic factors in ovarian cancer patients with or without concomitant endometriosis, patients affected tended to be younger and to be diagnosed in earlier stages and with lower grade lesions [18–20]. A better prognosis could be demonstrated in these patients. It remains to be clarified whether the less frequent dissemination outside the ovaries in cancers arising from endometriosis may be due to different

Table 49.1 Studies on the frequency of endometriosis in patients with ovarian cancers according to the malignant histotype.

Authors	Ovarian cancer histotype					Total
	Serous	Mucinous	Endometrioid	Clear cell	Other	
Aure et al, 1971	0%(0/357)	1%(1/203)	9%(20/212)	24%(14/59)	–	4%(35/831)
Kurman et al, 1972	6%(7/118)	4%(2/47)	11%(4/37)	8%(2/28)	–	7%(15/230)
Russel, 1979	3%(7/233)	4%(3/69)	28%(20/72)	48%(16/33)	–	11%(46/407)
Vercellini et al, 1993	4%(8/220)	6%(6/94)	26%(30/114)	21%(8/38)	12%(11/88)	11%(63/556)
De La Cuesta et al, 1996[a]	0%(0/10)	6%(1/18)	39%(9/23)	41%(7/17)	45%(5/11)	28%(22/79)
Toki et al, 1996	10%(9/88)	9%(3/33)	30%(16/54)	50%(22/44)	0%(0/16)	21%(50/235)
Jimbo et al, 1997	9%(8/92)	3%(1/35)	23%(3/13)	41%(13/32)	–	15%(25/172)
Fukunaga et al, 1997	10%(6/63)	6%(2/35)	42%(13/31)	54%(27/50)	67%(2/3)	27%(50/182)
Ogawa et al, 2000	7%(4/60)	0%(0/17)	43%(3/7)	70%(30/43)	–	29%(37/127)
Vercellini et al, 2000	3%(2/61)	3%(1/30)	20%(13/66)	14%(5/35)	6%(1/17)	10%(22/209)
Oral et al, 2003	4%(3/70)	6%(2/35)	22%(4/18)	9%(1/11)	8%(4/49)	8%(14/183)

Those studies evaluating association with at least endometrioid, clear cell and seromucinous histotypes have been included.

[a] Only stage I cancers were included.

Reproduced from Somigliana et al. Association between endometriosis and cancer: a comprehensive review and a critical analysis of clinical and epidemiological evidence. Gynecol Oncol 2006;101:331–341, with permission from Elsevier.

pathological behavior of the malignancy *per se* or whether it may be related to the destruction of endometriotic lesions in more advanced cancers. Furthermore, a diagnostic bias could also explain, at least in part, the increased diagnosis in initial stages. The typical symptoms of endometriosis might facilitate earlier diagnosis.

Population-based studies

Data from the majority of the available cohort and case–control studies tend to suggest an association between endometriosis and ovarian cancer, although it is difficult to precisely estimate the effect size as the observed increase in risk is quite variable (Table 49.2).

Some limitations of the available studies have to be considered.
• Confounders have not always been controlled adequately. It is well known that parity and oral contraceptive use represent strong preventive factors [21]. Measures of association should at least be controlled for these two factors. Adjustments for these two confounders have not been performed in all epidemiological studies. Of note, it cannot be ruled out that some medical treatment options of endometriosis may also influence the hazard of ovarian cancer. A recent study has suggested that danazol, an antiandrogenic medication that was commonly used in the treatment of endometriosis in the past, may increase the risk of ovarian cancer [22]
• Studies assume that the identification of endometriotic lesions during a surgical intervention corresponds to the presence of the disease in that particular patient. However, surgery is aimed at

eradicating the disease. Since recurrence of endometriosis is not a systematic occurrence, the assumption that all operated patients remain affected may lead to an underestimation of the risk.
• The generalization of the results to all women with endometriosis might be incorrect, as most of the observations refer to women affected by advanced forms necessitating hospitalization and surgery.
• Insights from clinical series indicate that endometriosis is linked only to endometrioid and clear cell ovarian carcinomas and not to other malignant histotypes (see Table 49.1). None of the largest cohort epidemiological studies has analyzed results according to the different tumor histotypes while the smallest studies that have evaluated this aspect consistently found a much higher risk. Hence, some limitations may have biased results towards the null hypothesis whereas others may have led to overestimation of the association.

Cohort studies

The Swedish National Board of Health and Welfare started collecting data on individual hospital discharges in an inpatient register in 1964. Since each record contains precise medical data including diagnosis of endometriosis, this tool has been used to investigate the potential association between endometriosis and cancer. The frequency of cancer in the general population adjusted for age was used as a referral group. A cohort study [23] and the following expansions [24,25] and two cohort nested case–control studies [26,27] have so far been derived from this register.

Table 49.2 Relationship between endometriosis and ovarian cancer.

Studies	Study design	Entity of the association	
		OR, SIR or RR	95% CI
Brinton et al, 1997	Cohort	1.9	1.3–2.8
Ness et al, 2000	Case–control	1.7	1.2–2.4
Ness et al, 2002	Case–control	1.7	1.1–2.7
Brinton et al, 2004	Cohort	1.3	0.6–2.6
Borgfeldt and Andolf, 2004	Case–control	1.3	1.0–1.7
Modugno et al, 2004	Case–control	1.3	1.1–1.6
Melin et al, 2006	Cohort	1.4	1.2–1.7
Melin et al, 2007	Cohort	1.3	1.1–1.6
Rossing et al, 2008	Case–control	1.3	1.0–1.8
Nagle et al, 2008[a]	Case–control	2.2	1.2–3.9
Nagle et al, 2008[b]	Case–control	3.0	1.5–5.9

CI, confidence interval; OR, odds ratio; RR, relative risk; SIR, standardized incidence ratio.

[a] Endometrioid subtype.

[b] Clear cell subtype.

Modified from Somigliana et al. Association between endometriosis and cancer: a comprehensive review and a critical analysis of clinical and epidemiological evidence. Gynecol Oncol 2006;101:331–341, with permission from Elsevier.

In the first study, the records of 20,686 women who were hospitalized for endometriosis from 1969 to 1983 were linked with the National Swedish Cancer Registry through 1989 to detect all subsequent diagnoses of cancer [23]. The mean follow-up was 11.4 years and the cohort contributed 216,851 woman-years. Standardized incidence ratios (SIR) and relative 95% confidence interval (95% CI) were computed using age- and period-specific incidence rates derived from the Swedish population. A total of 738 malignancies was detected among the study subjects, resulting in an overall SIR of 1.2 (95% CI 1.1–1.3). Significant risk increases were observed for cancer of the breast (SIR 1.3, 95% CI 1.1–1.4), of the ovary (SIR 1.9, 95% CI 1.3–2.8), and for all hematopoietic malignancies (SIR 1.4, 95% CI 1.0–1.8). This latter increase was largely determined by an excess risk of non-Hodgkin lymphoma (SIR 1.8, 95% CI 1.2–2.6), which was limited to patients admitted after age 40. The risk of ovarian cancer was particularly elevated among subjects with a long-standing history (≥10 years) of ovarian endometriosis (SIR 4.2, 95% CI 2.0–7.7).

The first expansion of this study [24] enrolled a total of 64,492 women after a hospital discharge diagnosis of endometriosis from 1969 to 2000 but the previously reported increased overall cancer risk was not confirmed (SIR 1.0, 95% CI 0.9–1.0). Conversely, this study still documented an increase in risk for ovarian cancer (SIR 1.4, 95% CI 1.2–1.7), non-Hodgkin lymphoma (SIR 1.2, 95% CI 1.0–1.5), endocrine tumors (SIR 1.3, 95% CI 1.1–1.6) and brain tumors (SIR 1.2, 95% CI 1.0–1.4). Supporting a trend found in the original study, the risk of cervical cancer decreased (SIR 0.6, 95% CI 0.5–0.8).

In the second expansion [25], data were also linked to the Swedish Multi-Generation Register to calculate parity and age at first birth and enrolled 63,630 women from 1969 to 2002. Again, the overall cancer risk was not confirmed (SIR 1.0, 95% CI 0.9–1.0) and an increase in risk of ovarian cancer (SIR 1.3, 95% CI 1.1–1.9), renal cancer (SIR 1.3, 95% CI 1.1–1.6), thyroid cancer (SIR 1.3, 95% CI 1.0–1.7), endocrine tumors (SIR 1.3, 95% CI 1.1–1.6), melanoma (SIR 1.2, 95% CI 1.0–1.4), breast cancer (SIR 1.08, 95% CI 1.0–1.1) and brain tumors (SIR 1.2, 95% CI 1.0–1.4) was demonstrated. There was no significant difference between nulliparous and parous women with endometriosis regarding risk of any of the cancer types.

Using the same Swedish register, Borgfeldt and Andolf [27] evaluated whether women born before 1970 and discharged from hospital during the period 1969–1996 with a diagnosis of ovarian cyst (n = 42,217), functional ovarian cyst (n = 17,998) or endometriosis (n = 28,163) had an increased risk of developing gynecological cancers. For each case, three controls were matched. Women with endometriosis had an overall increased risk for gynecological malignancy (odds ratio (OR) 1.1, 95% CI 1.0–1.3), and specifically for ovarian cancer (OR 1.3, 95% CI 1.0–1.7). The risk was even more pronounced after more than 10 years from the diagnosis of endometriosis (OR 1.5, 95% CI 1.0–2.1) and was inversely related to parity, being almost twofold in nulliparous subjects (OR 1.9, 95% CI 1.2–3.0). Finally, women with endometriosis had a decreased risk of both cervical (OR 0.6, 95% CI 0.4–0.9) and endometrial cancer (OR 0.6, 95% CI 0.4–0.8), whereas no change in breast cancer risk was found (OR 1.1, 95% CI 1.0–1.2).

The Iowa Women's Health Study is a prospective study designed to use the Iowa Cancer Registry to identify risk factors for cancer and other chronic diseases in postmenopausal women [28]. Self-reported history of endometriosis diagnosis was recorded on a baseline questionnaire and its association with cancer evaluated. Of the 37,434 women at risk, 1392 (3.8%) reported at baseline that they had ever been diagnosed with endometriosis. Endometriosis was not associated with risk of all cancers combined (relative risk (RR) 0.9, 95% CI 0.8–1.0). Unfortunately, the power of this study was insufficient to draw conclusions on the risk of ovarian cancer. The only specific cancer type found to be associated was non-Hodgkin lymphoma with a 1.8 RR (95% CI 1.0–3.0) even after adjustment for transfusion history, marital status and alcohol intake (RR 1.7, 95% CI 1.0–2.9), known risk factors for this type of tumor.

In 2007, another cohort study was published by a Japanese group, a prospective study involving women in the Shizuoka Ovarian Cancer Program who had a clinical diagnosis of ovarian endometrioma during the period 1985–1995 with follow-up through 2002 [29]. The study aimed to assess the long-term risk of ovarian cancer following ovarian endometrioma. Forty-six ovarian cancers were identified in the ovarian endometrioma cohort of 6398 women compared to 5.14 expected, yielding an overall SIR of 8.9 (95% CI 4.1–15.3). The excess risk for ovarian cancer increased markedly with increasing age at ovarian endometrioma diagnosis. Endometrioma diameter of 9 cm or more and postmenopausal status were independent predictive factors for the development of ovarian cancer.

Since endometriosis is associated with infertility, association between the disease and cancer should be interpreted with caution since an increased risk may be due to nulliparity rather than to endometriosis *per se*. This bias may be particularly relevant for ovarian and breast cancer. In this context, interesting findings were derived from cohort studies specifically enrolling infertile women. Venn *et al* evaluated the incidence of gynecological malignancies in a cohort of 29,700 infertile women using data from 10 Australian infertile clinics. The authors failed to observe an increased risk of breast cancer (SIR 1.0, 95% CI 0.7–1.5). The recruited sample size did not allow reliable analysis for uterine and ovarian cancers [30].

More recently, a large US study has assessed the risk of ovarian cancer according to the different causes of infertility (endometriosis, ovulation disorders, tubal disease and pelvic adhesions, male factors or uterine/cervical disorders, and unexplained causes/incomplete work-ups) among 12,193 women recruited between 1965 and 1988 in five different centers [31]. Infertile patients were found to have a significantly higher risk of ovarian cancer (SIR 2.0, 95% CI 1.4–2.6); the risk was higher for patients with primary (SIR 2.7, 95% CI 1.8–4.0) rather than secondary infertility (SIR 1.4, 95% CI 0.9–2.3). Among infertile women, patients with endometriosis had the highest risk with a SIR of 2.5 (95% CI 1.3–4.2) compared to the general population, with a SIR of 4.2 (95% CI 2.0–7.7) for the group with primary infertility. When comparisons by cause of infertility were performed within the infertile population, the SIR for ovarian cancer was 1.3 (95% CI 0.6–2.6) in women with endometriosis. When restricting the analysis only to women with endometriosis and primary infertility, the SIR rose to 2.7 (95% CI 1.1–6.7). This group of patients might represent those with more advanced stages of the disease. Data from the same series of patients have been successively analyzed with the specific aim of assessing the risk of cancers in extraovarian sites [32]. A statistically significant association between endometriosis and melanoma (RR 2.1, 95% CI 1.0–4.4) has emerged. The risk for non-Hodgkin lymphoma was not increased (data not reported) although the small number of events did not allow definitive conclusions.

Case–control studies

The association between endometriosis and ovarian cancer has also been investigated using a case–control study design.

In a large population-based case–control study, 767 cases 20–69 years of age with a recent diagnosis of epithelial ovarian cancer were compared with 1367 community controls. After adjustment for reproductive and contraceptive factors that reduce the risk, such as age, number of pregnancies, family history of ovarian cancer, race, oral contraceptive use, tubal ligation, hysterectomy, and breast feeding, women with ovarian cancer were 1.7-fold more likely (95% CI 1.2–2.4) to report a history of endometriosis [33].

Ness *et al* pooled data on infertility and fertility drug use from eight case–control studies conducted between 1989 and 1999 in the United States, Denmark, Canada, and Australia to examine the relationship between infertility and relative treatments and ovarian cancer. Included in the analysis were 5207 cases and 7705 controls. Endometriosis and unknown cause of infertility were independently associated with elevation in ovarian cancer risk after adjustment for standard confounding factors (OR 1.7, 95% CI 1.1–2.7 and OR 1.2, 95% CI 1.0–1.4 respectively) [34].

Modugno *et al* pooled data on the history of endometriosis from four population-based, ovarian cancer case–control studies that recruited women from four regions of the United States from 1993 through 2001. Of the 2098 cases and 2953 control subjects included in the combined analysis, 177 cases (8.5%) and 184 control subjects (6.3%) reported a history of endometriosis. After adjustments for study site, duration of oral contraceptive use, parity, age, tubal ligation, and family history of ovarian cancer, women with endometriosis were more likely to develop ovarian cancer than women without a history of the disease (adjusted OR 1.3, 95% CI 1.1–1.6). As expected, cases were less likely to have borne children, to have had a tubal ligation and have used oral contraceptives. Compared with never-users of oral contraceptives, use for >10 years was associated with a substantial reduction in risk among women with endometriosis (adjusted ORs for <10 years and >10 years of use were 0.58 and 0.21, respectively). Among women without endometriosis, the adjusted ORs were 0.70 and 0.47, respectively [35].

In a population-based case–control study of epithelial ovarian cancer conducted in Washington State, Rossing and co-workers assessed the risk of ovarian cancer associated with a prior diagnosis of ovarian cysts or endometriosis and with ovarian surgery [36]. Information was collected during in-person interviews with 812 women affected by ovarian cancer and 1313 population-based controls. Women with a history of endometriosis had an OR of 1.3 (95% CI 1.0–1.8) to develop an ovarian cancer in general and an OR of 2.8 (95% CI 1.7–4.7) for endometrioid and clear cell carcinomas, with a lesser risk increase among women who underwent subsequent ovarian surgery.

Finally, an Australian case–control study specifically addressed risks factors for endometrioid and clear cell ovarian cancers in a population of 142 women with endometrioid ovarian tumors, 90 with clear cell tumors and 1508 population controls [37]. Women with a self-reported history of endometriosis had an increased risk for both subtypes (OR 2.2, 95% CI 1.2–3.9 for endometrioid and OR 3.0, 95% CI 1.5–5.9 for clear cell).

Risk factors for endometriosis and ovarian cancer

The association between endometriosis and some forms of ovarian cancer might be explained by the sharing of similar risk factors. Therefore, an indirect way to analyze the relation between endometriosis and cancer is to compare the epidemiological characteristics of women affected by the two conditions.

Risk factors for endometriosis

Age is the main determinant of risk for endometriosis: the condition is rare before the menarche, probably increases with age until menopause and decreases after menopause [38–40]. The role of menstrual factors as determinants of endometriosis risk has been suggested, women with early menarche (2–3 years before the mean age), and with short and heavy menstrual cycles being at a higher risk [41–44]. These determinants are explained in light of the menstrual reflux hypothesis according to which endometriosis development would depend on implantation of endometrial fragments regurgitated in peritoneum with retrograde menses.

Parity is inversely associated with the risk of endometriosis [40,42,45,46]. However, it is still unclear whether nulliparity is a cause or consequence of endometriosis. In some studies, the risk of the disease was lower among current oral contraceptive users [47] but higher in ex-users [47–54]. Oral contraceptives may temporarily suppress endometriosis, but previous use could increase the risk of the disease, being a cause of regular menstrual cycles. Probably, treatment with oral contraceptives does not cure endometriosis, and ectopic endometrial implants survive, although in an atrophic form, ready for reactivation when treatment is stopped. Dysmenorrhea is a frequent symptom of endometriosis and also an important indication for oral contraceptive use; thus, the higher risk for ever and past users of oral contraceptives may be due to selective mechanisms and indication biases.

Other reported risk factors for endometriosis are:
- family history of the condition [55–59]
- smoking (heavy smokers are at decreased risk of endometriosis) [38,41,48]
- alcohol and coffee drinking and a diet rich in saturated fats [38,60]
- exposure to dioxin [61,62] and personal history of immune disorders: rheumatoid arthritis, systemic lupus erythematosus, hypo- or hyperthyroidism, multiple sclerosis or non-Hodgkin lymphomas [23,28,63].

Available data on these factors are, however, scanty and further studies are needed.

Risk factors for ovarian cancer

Menstrual and reproductive factors, as well as female hormones, have long been related to ovarian carcinogenesis [64,65]. Most studies found a moderately increased risk in women with early menarche. The relative risks were approximately 1.2–1.3 in women reporting earlier menarche [66,67].

Likewise, several studies showed a direct relation between late age at menopause (2–3 years after the mean age) and the risk of ovarian cancer [64]. Nulliparity and low parity have been consistently related to ovarian cancer risk. Oral contraceptive use lowers the subsequent ovarian cancer risk. The favorable effect of oral contraceptives against ovarian cancer risk seems to persist for at least 10–15 years after stopping use [67].

With reference to hormone replacement therapy (HRT) in menopause, some studies reported moderately elevated risks and others no consistent association [68]. Garg et al [69], in a meta-analysis, reported an OR of 1.15 for ever-users. Coughlin et al [70], in a subgroup analysis of four case–control studies from the US, found a borderline association between HRT and ovarian cancer (OR 1.3). Negri et al, in a meta-analysis of four European studies, found an OR of 1.7 for ever-HRT users [71].

Among other main risk factors for ovarian cancer, an increased risk has been reported in women with a family history of ovarian and breast cancer [64–72]. Some interest has been recently focused on the effect of a diet rich in fats.

The incessant ovulation and the stimulation by gonadotropin hypotheses have been proposed to explain the role of hormonal and reproductive factors in the etiology of epithelial ovarian cancer. The protective effect conferred by parity and oral contraceptives would suggest an unfavorable role of ovulation, but the limited effect of age at menarche and at menopause does not fully support this vision [73]. The lack of protection from HRT (which suppresses pituitary hormones) does not support the existence of a favorable role of gonadotropin stimulation on ovarian carcinogenesis [68]. A more complex mechanism of carcinogenesis is consequently likely to be involved in the etiology of epithelial ovarian cancer.

The potential different impact of risk factors on the different histological types of the disease has not been widely investigated. Of note, some reports have suggested that non-contraceptive estrogen use may increase the risk of endometrioid ovarian cancer, but not of other subtypes, although this observation has not been confirmed in other studies [74–80].

A protective role of oral contraceptive use for serous and endometrioid tumors, but not for mucinous ones, has been reported in studies conducted in the USA, Canada, Norway and in the WHO Collaborative Study of Neoplasia and Steroid Contraceptives [76,81–83].

Therefore, nulliparity and menstrual characteristics (early age at menarche, regular menstrual cycles) are determinants of the risk for both endometriosis and ovarian cancer, but the biological interpretations generally reported to explain the associations differ, being related to retrograde menses for endometriosis and to incessant ovulation for ovarian cancer. Other risk factors common to both conditions are a diet rich in saturated fats and alcohol and coffee consumption. Unclear is the relation between oral contraceptive use (a well-recognized protective factor for ovarian cancer) and risk of endometriosis.

In conclusion, endometriosis does share some risk factors with ovarian cancer. It is currently difficult to clarify whether the similarity of these risk factors may totally explain the association between two completely unrelated conditions or whether this observation should be interpreted as evidence supporting a continuum between the two conditions.

Endometriosis and other cancers

Breast cancer

Data from previously mentioned cohort studies on the association of endometriosis and breast cancer are inconclusive, since an increase in risk was initially found in the Swedish studies [23,26] but not in studies from other countries [28,30]. Using the Swedish register, data involving 15,844 women who underwent gynecological operations between 1965 and 1983 were analyzed to assess the risk of breast cancer in relation to indication for surgery. Endometriosis as the sole indication for surgery was associated with a more than threefold increase in risk [23,26] (Table 49.3). One of the expansions of the original cohort study demonstrated a limited but significantly increased in the risk (SIR 1.08, 95% CI 1.0–1.1) [25]. Two case–control studies have specifically focused on this possible association [84,85]. One of these studies has reported an elevated OR of borderline significance in premenopausal women (OR 4.3, 95% CI 0.9–20.4) but an OR <1 in postmenopausal women [84]. The second study did not find significant variation in breast cancer risk in association with a history of surgery for endometriosis (OR 1.1, 95% CI 0.7–1.8) [85].

Therefore, the potential association between endometriosis and breast cancer remains unclear although the issue is of particular importance given the relatively high incidence of both conditions; even a minor increase in breast cancer risk would have a major clinical impact. Epidemiological findings are summarized in Table 49.3. Three possible explanations for the slight, if any, increase in breast cancer risk among women with endometriosis, especially premenopausal ones, can be hypothesized:
- the two diseases may share a common pathogenetic insult. Of note, both conditions have a hormonal-dependent etiology
- endometriosis, a possible cause of infertility, is particularly evident in nulliparous women or in women who have delayed childbearing, both risk factors for breast cancer
- treatment of endometriosis with medications such as danazol, progestational agents and oral contraceptives could have an adverse effect on the breast.

Melanoma

A single research group has repeatedly reported an association between melanoma and endometriosis [86–89] (see Table 49.3). In general, these studies collected a limited number of subjects, were concerned with dysplastic nevi, a well-known precursor of melanoma, rather than the cancer itself and were characterized by too many subanalyses in relation to the casistics evaluated. Based on one of these studies, among 7559 female college and university alumni, a higher number of subjects with melanoma reported procedures related to the reproductive system, including surgery for endometriosis (OR 3.2, 95% CI 1.0–10.1 versus the non-melanoma skin cancer group, and OR 3.9, 95% CI 1.2–12.4 versus women with neither malignancy). However, when the reproductive history of a group of women attending the Pigmented Lesion Unit of the Massachusetts General Hospital was investigated, the risk of endometriosis was not increased in the group of women with melanoma with and without dysplastic nevi (OR 1.1, 95% CI 0.5–2.3) [87].

Results from large independent observational studies are controversial in this regard (see Table 49.3). Holly *et al* [90] investigated oral contraceptive use and reproductive factors in a

Table 49.3 Relationship between endometriosis and non-ovarian gynecological cancers.

Studies	Study design	Entity of the association	
		OR, SIR or RR	95% CI
Breast cancer			
Moseson *et al*, 1993	Case–control	4.3	0.9–20.4
Schairer *et al*, 1997 (A)	Cohort	3.2	1.2–8.0
Schairer *et al*, 1997 (B)	Cohort	3.0	0.7–4.1
Brinton *et al*, 1997	Cohort	1.3	1.1–1.4
Weiss *et al*, 1999	Case–control	1.1	0.7–1.8
Venn *et al*, 1999	Cohort	1.0	0.7–1.5
Olson *et al*, 2002	Cohort	1.0	0.8–1.2
Borgfeldt and Andolf, 2004	Case–control	1.1	1.0–1.2
Brinton *et al*, 2005	Cohort	0.8	0.6–1.1
Melin *et al*, 2006	Cohort	1.4	1.2–1.7
Melin *et al*, 2007	Cohort	1.1	1.0–1.1
Cervical cancer			
Brinton *et al*, 1997	Cohort	0.7	0.4–1.3
Borgfeldt and Andolf, 2004	Case–control	0.6	0.4–0.9
Melin *et al*, 2006	Cohort	0.6	0.4–0.8
Melin *et al*, 2007	Cohort	0.7	0.5–0.9
Endometrial cancer			
Brinton *et al*, 1997	Cohort	1.1	0.6–1.9
Olson *et al*, 2002	Cohort	1.2	0.6–2.5
Borgfeldt and Andolf, 2004	Case–control	0.6	0.4–0.8
Brinton *et al*, 2005	Cohort	0.8	0.3–1.9
Melin *et al*, 2006	Cohort	1.2	0.9–1.4
Melin *et al*, 2007	Cohort	1.1	0.9–1.4
Melanoma			
Wyshak *et al*, 1989	Case–control	3.9	1.2–12.4
Frish and Wyshak, 1992	Case–control	1.1	0.5–2.3
Holly *et al*, 1995	Case–control	0.9	0.5–1.4
Brinton *et al*, 1997	Cohort	1.0	0.7–1.5
Olson *et al*, 2002	Cohort	0.7	0.2–1.8
Brinton *et al*, 2005	Cohort	2.1	1.0–4.4
Melin *et al*, 2006	Cohort	1.1	1.0–1.3
Melin *et al*, 2007	Cohort	1.2	1.1–1.4
Kvaskoff *et al*, 2007	Cohort	1.6	1.1–2.2
Non-Hodgkin lymphoma			
Brinton *et al*, 1997	Cohort	1.8	1.2–2.6
Olson *et al*, 2002	Cohort	1.7	1.0–2.9
Melin *et al*, 2006	Cohort	1.2	1.0–1.5
Melin *et al*, 2007	Cohort	1.1	0.9–1.3

CI, confidence interval; OR, odds ratio; RR, relative risk; SIR, standardized incidence ratio.
The study from Scharer *et al* focused on two different cohorts: patients who underwent hysterectomy (A) and those who underwent oophorectomy (B). Modified from Somigliana *et al*. Association between endometriosis and cancer: a comprehensive review and a critical analysis of clinical and epidemiological evidence. Gynecol Oncol 2006;101:331–341, with permission from Elsevier.

population-based case–control study of 452 women aged 25–59 years with a cutaneous malignant melanoma and 930 controls. No consistent association was observed between melanoma risk and oral contraceptive use as well as any considered reproductive factors, including endometriosis (OR 0.9, 95% CI 0.5–1.4). These findings were subsequently confirmed in the first study by Brinton *et al* (SIR 1.0, 95% CI 0.7–1.5) [23] and in the Iowa Women's Health Study (RR 0.7, 95% CI 0.2–1.8) [28], but in the latter report, the number of expected cases was very low. However, the most recent study by Melin *et al* has again proposed this possible association (SIR 1.2, 95% CI 1.0–1.4) [25].

The US study that assessed the risk of cancers according to the different causes of infertility in five different centers found a statistically significant association between endometriosis and melanoma (RR 2.1, 95% CI 1.0–4.4) [32].

Importantly, in a large prospective cohort study involving 98,995 French women aged 40–65 years insured by a national health system, 363 melanoma cases were ascertained during 12 years of follow-up and a history of endometriosis was significantly associated with a higher risk of melanoma (RR 1.3, 95% CI 1.0–6) [91].

However, independently of the melanoma risk, in recent years a positive dose–effect relationship between endometriosis and skin sensitivity to sun exposure and number of nevi and freckles has been emphasized [92,93].

Non-Hodgkin lymphoma

The largest population-based cohort studies have independently documented an association with non-Hodgkin lymphoma [23,24,28] albeit not consistently [25] (see Table 49.3). However, the statistically significant results from these studies are based on a small number of observed cases and need further confirmation. Case–control studies aiming to verify this association are lacking.

Potential explanations for an increase in risk of non-Hodgkin lymphoma in women with endometriosis are currently speculative. Three different explanations for this association have been suggested:
• humoral immunity abnormalities have been documented in women with endometriosis. More specifically, there may be a link between B-cell activation in endometriosis and development of B-cell lymphoma
• the association may be consequent upon medications prescribed to treat endometriosis
• the link between the two conditions may be due to a common etiological agent.

Cervical cancer

Supporting a trend found in the first Swedish cohort study, the expansions of this study documented a decreased risk of cervical cancer (SIR 0.6, 95% CI 0.5–0.8) [23–25] (see Table 49.3). If confirmed, this unexpected association could be interpreted in terms of increased number of referrals to a gynecologist of patients with endometriosis, and the consequent more regular performance of cervical smears.

Endometrial cancer

The relationship between endometriosis and endometrial carcinoma is potentially interesting because it could suggest a "baseline" genetic predisposition of the endometrium of some women to undergo malignant transformation. In other words, the eutopic endometrium, and not endometriosis *per se*, would be the origin of eutopic and ectopic adenocarcinomas. However, no association has been found between endometriosis and endometrial carcinoma in population-based studies [23–25,28] (see Table 49.3).

Discussion

Population-based and observational studies do not unequivocally support an overall increased risk of malignancies in women with endometriosis [23–25,28]. Nevertheless, these patients may be at increased risk of specific forms of cancer. Thus far, evidence supporting an association, whether causative or not, with breast cancer, melanoma and non-Hodgkin lymphoma is generally scanty (see Table 49.3). Conversely, a consistent body of literature is in favor of an increased risk of ovarian cancer in women with endometriosis. Cohort studies have reported a significant increased risk, with a SIR that varied between 1.3 and 1.9 [23–25,28]. However, given the limitations of these studies, this risk remains to be better clarified. A crucial point is to establish whether this increased association is or is not based on a causative effect.

Two possible hypotheses may explain the link between endometriosis and ovarian cancer: endometriosis may directly undergo malignant transformation or endometriosis and cancer may simply share common antecedent mechanisms and/or predisposing factors. In order to disentangle this debated issue, we have decided to apply specific guidelines for causation. These guidelines, commonly referred to as the Bradford Hill criteria for causal association, have been used by epidemiologists and others when addressing causation of disease in a broad range of situations [2].

A first and major aspect to be considered is the *strength* of the association. In epidemiology, a relative risk of less than 2 is considered to indicate a weak association and weak associations are more likely to be explained by unrelated biases [94]. The reported strength of association between endometriosis and ovarian cancer is within this range, varying between 1.3 and 1.9. However, it should be noted that most population-based studies did not generally control for cancer histotype. A threefold risk emerged when association between endometriosis and endometrioid/clear cell carcinoma was specifically investigated [36,37]. Indeed, in case series of ovarian cancer, endometriosis was repeatedly found to be strongly associated only with these two histological histotypes (see Table 49.1).

Temporal evolution of risk following exposure favors a causal relation between the two entities. For most epithelial tumors, one expects a latent period of at least 15 years. Typically, when exposure is continuous there is little risk of cancer development until some 10–15 years after exposure starts; the relative risk then increases to reach a plateau after 30 years or more [94].

Epidemiological data concerning age at diagnosis for the two entities fulfill this model. Ovarian cancer is typically a disease of peri- and postmenopausal women whereas endometriosis is a reproductive age condition.

Demonstration of a *risk reduction after exposure has terminated* is further persuasive evidence, although the absence of a reduction is no indication of lack of causality. No data are available regarding endometriosis and ovarian cancer since no study has controlled for this factor.

There is evidence supporting the *biological plausibility* of a causative relation between endometriosis and cancer. Clonality analyses confirm that a single endometriotic cell can grow into a focus of ectopic tissue [1]. If ovarian carcinomas do arise from endometriosis, one would expect to find genetic alterations common to both endometriosis and malignant tumors. Conversely, if endometriosis represents a distinct entity then one would expect to find alterations unique to the pathway that leads to this pathology. From results of the various techniques, it is evident that poor consistency exists in relation to the DNA abnormalities present in endometriotic samples [1]. According to some studies, a significant proportion (from about one-third to one-half for allelotyping and more than two-thirds for comparative genomic hybridization) of endometriosis lesions harbors somatic genetic changes in chromosomal regions supposed to contain genes involved in tumorigenesis, especially for endometrioid carcinoma [1]. Since the frequency of loss of heterozygosity (LOH) events in ovarian endometrioid cancers is estimated at 60–90%, these results would be consistent with the progression model for carcinogenesis where some ovarian tumors are expected to harbor a greater number of genetic alterations than their benign precursors. Moreover, the frequency of genetic aberrations is shown to increase for cases of endometriosis adjacent or contiguous to ovarian cancer and, more importantly, these cases tend to share the same genetic changes, which supports the idea of a common developmental pathway through the inactivation of the same tumor suppressor genes [1]. Data on the tumor suppressor gene PTEN are particularly suggestive in this context since loss of PTEN function is an early event in endometrial rather than ovarian tumorigenesis. Somatic mutations in the PTEN gene and modifications of the protein level in endometriosis would indicate that ectopic endometrium is likely to undergo specific genetic alterations similarly to the eutopic tissue [1]. On the other hand, other studies cannot replicate these findings and fail to detect evidence supporting the concept that endometriosis may be a preneoplastic condition [1].

The observation that an association is confined to *specific subcategories of disease* can be persuasive evidence of causality. True associations are specific. The documentation that cigarette smoking was associated with a specific lung cancer histotype, the squamous carcinoma, was used to support causality. In the field of endometriosis, a clear association between endometriosis and ovarian endometrioid or clear cell carcinomas has emerged (see Table 49.1). As previously mentioned, according to some authorities, clear cell carcinoma should be properly classified as a subtype of the endometrioid malignancy of the ovary [95]. Moreover, an overall SIR of 8.9 (95% CI 4.1–15.3) was found when the risk evaluation was limited to the cohort of women with ovarian endometrioma [29].

Consistency of findings provides additional support for causal associations. A single study seldom furnishes conclusive evidence. Accessible population-based studies tend to support an increased risk of ovarian cancer in women suffering from endometriosis (see Table 49.2). Moreover, present evidence derives from different populations and different methodological study designs.

In pharmacovigilance, a causal association is supported when an adverse event occurs in a *dose-dependent manner* or from cumulative exposure over a prolonged period of time. Unfortunately, data on ovarian cancer risk in relation to severity of endometriosis are lacking. Conversely, it has been shown that the cancer risk markedly increases in women with a long-standing history of endometriosis [23,24,27].

Cause-and-effect interpretation does not seriously conflict with known facts concerning the natural history and biology of the two diseases. Some aspects are, however, not *coherent* with contemporary knowledge. If the neoplastic transformation of endometriosis would simply replicate the mechanisms recognized for endometrial cancer in an ectopic location, localization of tumors should be much more diffuse in the peritoneal cavity consistent with the wide dissemination of endometriosis rather than concentrated in the ovary. Indeed, in 80% of cases, the site involved in the carcinogenic process is the ovary [96]. However, a similar dogma is currently widely accepted in explaining the origin of epithelial ovarian cancer from the superficial ovarian coelomic epithelium even if this type of epithelium covers the entire peritoneal cavity.

Experimental evidence as a supportal causal inference is another criterion. A single study did succeed in establishing a model of endometriosis transformation into cancer in genetically engineered mice [97]. In mice harboring an oncogenic allele of K-ras resulting in the development of benign lesions reminiscent of endometriosis, a conditional deletion of PTEN caused progression toward the ovarian endometrioid tumor. Although this model is probably not perfect as a genocopy of endometriosis, it supports the potential existence of a mechanism of tumorigenesis conforming to a progression model from the benign lesion to the malignant ovarian disease based on the combination of two mutations in tumor-related genes.

Analogy supports causation if similar causal relationships can be found in other areas of medicine. A consistent body of literature supports the vision that, in some cancers, the inflammatory process is a co-factor in carcinogenesis. Increased risk of malignancy is associated with the chronic inflammation caused by chemical and physical agents and autoimmune and inflammatory reactions of uncertain etiology [98]. Classic examples of this pathogenetic process are ulcerative colitis and colorectal cancer, asbestos fibers and mesothelioma, hepatitis B and C and liver cancer. Endometriosis is a condition well known to be associated with an inflammatory process [99].

The application of Bradford Hill criteria represents a helpful but not conclusive tool to investigate causative relationships between exposure and cancer development. One should not simply follow rules of thumb when considering all the guidelines together. There are no simple algorithms to be applied from a checklist. Epidemiological and clinical judgment become important when one has considered each criterion in turn. In the context of the association between endometriosis and ovarian cancer, it has to be underlined that specific answers to some of these criteria are lacking. Three of the most important criteria, namely strength, biological plausibility and experimental model of carcinogenesis in animals, tend to support a causal relationship but require definitive confirmations. Five of the Bradford Hill criteria are fulfilled. Although there is some support for causality, on the basis of this still uncertain pattern, a cautious approach has to be adopted.

References

1. Vigano P, Somigliana E, Chiodo I, Abbiati A, Vercellini P. Molecular mechanisms and biological plausibility underlying the malignant transformation of endometriosis: a critical analysis. Hum Reprod Update 2006;12:77–89.

2. Bradford-Hill A. The environment and disease: association or causation. Proc R Soc Med 1965;58:295–330.

3. Sampson JA. Endometrial carcinoma of the ovary arising in endometrial tissue in that organ. Arch Surg 1925;10:1–72.

4. Scott RB. Malignant changes in endometriosis. Obstet Gynecol 1953;2:283–289.

5. Mostoufizadeh H, Scully RE. Malignant tumours arising in endometriosis. Clin Obstet Gynecol 1980;23:951–963.

6. Stern RC, Dash R, Bentley RC, Snyder MJ, Haney AF, Robboy SJ. Malignancy in endometriosis: frequency and comparison of ovarian and extraovarian types. Int J Gynecol Pathol 2001;20:133–139.

7. Aure JC, Hoeg K, Kolstad P. Carcinoma of the ovary and endometriosis. Acta Obstet Gynecol Scand 1971;50:63–67.

8. Kurman RJ, Craig JM. Endometrioid and clear cell carcinoma of the ovary. Cancer 1972;29:1653–1664.

9. Russel P. The pathological assessment of of ovarian neoplasms: I. Introduction to the common "epithelial" tumors and analysis of benign "epithelial" tumors. Pathology 1979;11:5–26.

10. Vercellini P, Parazzini F, Bolis G et al. Endometriosis and ovarian cancer. Am J Obstet Gynecol 1993;169:181–182.

11. De La Cuesta RS, Eichhorn JH, Rice LW, Fuller AF, Nikrui N, Goff BA. Histologic transformation of benign endometriosis to early epithelial ovarian cancer. Gynecol Oncol 1996;60:238–244.

12. Toki T, Nakayama K. Proliferative activity and genetic alterations in TP53 in endometriosis. Gynecol Obstet Invest 2000;50:33–38.

13. Jimbo H, Yoshikawa H, Onda T, Yasugi T, Sakamoto A, Taketani Y. Prevalence of ovarian endometriosis in epithelial ovarian cancer. Int J Gynaecol Obstet 1997;59:245–250.

14. Fukunaga M, Nomura K, Ishikawa E, Ushigome S. Ovarian atypical endometriosis: its close association with malignant epithelial tumours. Histopathology 1997;30:249–255.

15. Ogawa S, Kaku T, Amada S et al. Ovarian endometriosis associated with ovarian carcinoma: a clinicopathological and immunohistochemical study. Gynecol Oncol 2000;77:298–304.

16. Vercellini P, Scarfone G, Bolis G, Stellato G, Carinelli S, Crosignani PG. Site of origin of epithelial ovarian cancer: the endometriosis connection. Br J Obstet Gynaecol 2000;107:1155–1157.

17. Oral E, Ilvan S, Tustas E et al. Prevalence of endometriosis in malignant epithelial ovary tumours. Eur J Obstet Gynecol Reprod Biol 2003;109:97–101.

18. McMeekin DS, Burger RA, Manetta A, DiSaia P, Berman ML. Endometrioid adenocarcinoma of the ovary and its relationship to endometriosis. Gynecol Oncol 1995;59:81–86.

19. Komiyama S, Aoki D, Tominaga E, Susumu N, Udagawa Y, Nozawa S. Prognosis of Japanese patients with ovarian clear cell carcinoma associated with pelvic endometriosis: clinicopathologic evaluation. Gynecol Oncol 1999;72:342–346.

20. Erzen M, Rakar S, Klancnik B, Syrjanen K, Klancar B. Endometriosis-associated ovarian carcinoma (EAOC): an entity distinct from other ovarian carcinomas as suggested by a nested case-control study. Gynecol Oncol 2001;83:100–108.

21. Parazzini F, Braga C, La Vecchia C, Negri E, Acerboni S, Franceschi S. Hysterectomy, oophorectomy in premenopause, and risk of breast cancer. Obstet Gynecol 1997;90:453–456.

22. Cottreau C, Ness RB, Modugno F, Allen GO, Goodman MT. Endometriosis and its treatment with danazol or lupron in relation to ovarian cancer. Clin Cancer Res 2003;9:5142–5144.

23. Brinton LA, Gridley G, Persson I, Baron J, Bergqvist A. Cancer risk after a hospital discharge diagnosis of endometriosis. Am J Obstet Gynecol 1997;176:572–579.

24. Melin A, Sparen P, Persson I, Bergqvist A. Endometriosis and the risk of cancer with special emphasis on ovarian cancer. Hum Reprod 2006;21:1237–1242.

25. Melin A, Sparen P, Bergqvist A. The risk of cancer and the role of parity among women with endometriosis. Hum Reprod 2007;22:3021–3026.

26. Schairer C, Persson I, Falkeborn M, Naessen T, Troisi R, Brinton LA. Breast cancer risk associated with gynecologic surgery and indications for such surgery. Int J Cancer 1997;70:150–154.

27. Borgfeldt C, Andolf E. Cancer risk after hospital discharge diagnosis of benign ovarian cysts and endometriosis. Acta Obstet Gynecol Scand 2004;83:395–400.

28. Olson JE, Cerhan JR, Janney CA, Anderson KE, Vachon CM, Sellers T. Postmenopausal cancer risk after self-reported endometriosis diagnosis in the Iowa Women's Health Study. Cancer 2002;94:1612–1618.

29. Kobayashi H, Sumimoto K, Moniwa N et al. Risk of developing ovarian cancer among women with ovarian endometrioma: a cohort study in Shizuoka, Japan. Int J Gynecol Cancer 2007;17:37–43.

30. Venn A, Watson L, Bruinsma F, Giles G, Healy D. Risk of cancer after use of fertility drugs with in-vitro-fertilization. Lancet 1999;354:1586–1590.

31. Brinton LA, Lamb EJ, Moghissi KS et al. Ovarian cancer risk associated with varying causes of infertility. Fertil Steril 2004;82:405–414.

32. Brinton LA, Westhoff CL, Scoccia B et al. Causes of infertility as predictors of subsequent cancer risk. Epidemiology 2005;16:500–507.

33. Ness RB, Grisso JA, Cottreau C et al. Factors related to inflammation of the ovarian epithelium and risk of ovarian cancer. Epidemiology 2000;11:111–117.

34. Ness RB, Cramer DW, Goodman MT et al. Infertility, fertility drugs, and ovarian cancer: a pooled analysis of case-control studies. Am J Epidemiol 2002;155:217–224.

35. Modugno F, Ness RB, Allen GO, Schildkraut JM, Davis FG, Goodman MT. Oral contraceptive use, reproductive history, and risk of epithelial ovarian cancer in women with and without endometriosis. Am J Obstet Gynecol 2004;191:733–740.

36. Rossing MA, Cushing-Haugen KL, Wicklund KG, Doherty JA, Weiss NS. Risk of epithelial ovarian cancer in relation to benign ovarian conditions and ovarian surgery. Cancer Causes Control 2008;19:1357–1364.

37. Nagle CM, Olsen CM, Webb PM, Jordan SJ, Whiteman DC, Green AC. Endometrioid and clear cell ovarian cancers – a comparative analysis of risk factors. Eur J Cancer 2008;44:2477–2484.

38. Missmer SA, Cramer DW. The epidemiology of endometriosis. Obstet Gynecol Clin North Am 2003;30:1–19.

39. Houston DE, Noller KL, Melton LJ, Selwyn BJ. The epidemiology of pelvic endometriosis. Clin Obstet Gynecol 1988;31:787–800.

40. Gruppo Italiano per lo Studio dell'Endometriosi. Prevalence and anatomical distribution of endometriosis in women with selected gynaecological conditions: results from a multicentric Italian study. Hum Reprod 1994;9:1158–1162.

41. Cramer DW, Wilson E, Stillman RJ et al. The relation of endometriosis to menstrual characteristics, smoking, and exercise. JAMA 1986;255:1904–1908.

42. Signorello LB, Harlow BL, Cramer DW, Spiegelman D, Hill JA. Epidemiologic determinants of endometriosis: a hospital-based case-control study. Ann Epidemiol 1997;7:267–741.

43. Darrow SL, Vena JE, Batt RE, Zielezny MA, Michalek AM, Selman S. Menstrual cycle characteristics and the risk of endometriosis. Epidemiology 1993;4:135–142.

44. Meiling H, Lingya PL, Baozhen W. A case-control epidemiologic study of endometriosis. Clin Med Sci 1994;9:114–118.

45. Candiani GB, Danesino V, Gastaldi A, Parazzini F, Ferraroni M. Reproductive and menstrual factors and risk of peritoneal and ovarian endometriosis. Fertil Steril 1991;56:230–234.

46. Smith SK. The aetiology of endometriosis. Hum Reprod 1995;10:1274.

47. Sangi-Haghpeykar H, Poindexter AN. Epidemiology of endometriosis among parous women. Obstet Gynecol 1995;85:983–992.

48. Vessey MP, Villard-Mackintosh L, Painter R. Epidemiology of endometriosis in women attending family planning clinics. BMJ 1993;306:182–184.

49. Moen MH. Endometriosis in women at interval sterilization. Acta Obstet Gynecol Scand 1987;66:451–454.

50. Kirshon B, Poindexter AN. Contraception: a risk factor for endometriosis. Obstet Gynecol 1988;7:829–831.

51. Moen MH. Is a long period without childbirth a risk factor for developing endometriosis? Hum Reprod 1991;6:1404–1407.

52. Parazzini F, Ferraroni M, Bocciolone L, Tozzi L, Rubessa S, La Vecchia C. Contraceptive methods and risk of pelvic endometriosis. Contraception 1994;49:47–55.

53. Royal College of General Practitioners. Oral Contraceptives and Health. An interim report from the Oral Contraceptive Study of the Royal College of General Practitioners. London: Pitman Medical Publishing, 1974.

54. Walnut Creek Contraceptive Drug Study. A Prospective Study on the Side Effects of Oral Contraceptives. Bethesda, MD: National Institutes of Health, 1981, p. 3.

55. Simpson JL, Elias S, Malinak LR, Buttram VC Jr. Heritable aspects of endometriosis. Am J Obstet Gynecol 1980;137:327–331.

56. Lamb K, Hoffmann RG, Nichols TR. Family trait analysis: a case-control study of 43 women with endometriosis and their best friends. Am J Obstet Gynecol 1986;154:596–601.

57. Moen MH, Magnus P. The familial risk of endometriosis. Acta Obstet Gynecol Scand 1993;72:560–564.

58. Moen MH. Endometriosis in monozygotic twins. Acta Obstet Gynecol Scand 1994;73:59–62.

59. Treloar S, Hadfield R, Montgomery G et al. The International Endogene Study: a collection of families for genetic research in endometriosis. Fertil Steril 2002;78:679–685.

60. Parazzini F, Chiaffarino F, Surace M. Selected food intake and risk of endometriosis. Hum Reprod 2004;19:1755–1759.

61. Koninckx PR, Braet P, Kennedy SH, Barlow DH. Dioxin pollution and endometriosis in Belgium. Hum Reprod 1994; 9:1001–1002.

62. Eskenazi B, Mocarelli P, Warner M et al. Serum dioxin concentrations and endometriosis: a cohort study in Seveso, Italy. Environ Health Perspect 2002;110:629–634.

63. Sinaii N, Cleary SD, Ballweg ML, Nieman LK, Stratton P. High rates of autoimmune and endocrine disorders, fibromyalgia, chronic fatigue syndrome and atopic diseases among women with endometriosis: a survey analysis. Hum Reprod 2002;17:2715–2724.

64. Parazzini F, Franceschi S, La Vecchia C, Fasoli M. The epidemiology of ovarian cancer. Gynecol Oncol 1991;43:9–23.

65. Risch HA. Hormonal etiology of epithelial ovarian cancer, with a hypothesis concerning the role of androgens and progesterone. J Natl Cancer Inst 1998;90:1774–1786.

66. Parazzini F, La Vecchia C, Negri E, Gentile A. Menstrual factors and the risk of epithelial ovarian cancer. J Clin Epidemiol 1989;42:443–448.

67. Franceschi S, La Vecchia C, Booth M. Pooled analysis of 3 European case-control studies of ovarian cancer: II. Age at menarche and at menopause. Int J Cancer 1991;49:57–60.

68. IARC. Hormonal contraception and post-menopausal hormonal therapy. In: IARC (ed) Monographs on the Evaluation of Carcinogenic Risks of Humans. Lyon: IARC, 1999, p. 72.

69. Garg PP, Kerlikowske K, Subak L, Grady D. Hormone replacement therapy and the risk of epithelial ovarian carcinoma: a meta-analysis. Obstet Gynecol 1998;92:472–479.

70. Coughlin SS, Giustozzi A, Smith SJ, Lee NC. A meta-analysis of estrogen replacement therapy and risk of epithelial ovarian cancer. J Clin Epidemiol 2000;53:367–375.

71. Negri E, Tzonou A, Beral V, Lagiou P, Trichopoulos D. Hormonal therapy for menopause and ovarian cancer in a collaborative re-analysis of European studies. Int J Cancer 1999;80:848–851.

72. Parazzini F, Negri E, La Vecchia C. Family history of reproductive cancers and ovarian cancer risk: an Italian case-control study. Am J Epidemiol 1992;135:35–40.

73. Whiteman DC, Murphy MF, Cook LS et al. Multiple births and risk of epithelial ovarian cancer. J Natl Cancer Inst 2000;68:1172–1177.

74. Weiss NS, Lyon JL, Krishnamurthy S, Dieteri SE, Liff JM, Dailing JR. Non contraceptive estrogen use and the occurrence of ovarian cancer. J Natl Cancer Inst 1982;68:95–98.

75. La Vecchia C, Liberati A, Franceschi S. Noncontraceptive estrogen use and the occurrence of ovarian cancer. J Natl Cancer Inst 1982;69:1207.

76. Risch H, Marrett LD, Jain M, Howe GR. Difference in risk factors for epithelial ovarian cancer by histologic type. Results of a case-control study. Am J Epidemiol 1996;136:1184–1203.

77. Kaufman DW, Kelly JP, Welch WR, Rosemberg L, Stolley PD, Warshauer ME. Noncontraceptive estrogen use and ephitelial ovarian cancer. Am J Epidemiol 1989;130:1184–1203.

78. Whittemore AS, Harris R, Itnyre J, Collaborative Ovarian Cancer Group. Characteristics relating to ovarian cancer risk: collaborative analysis of 12 US case-control studies. Invasive epithelial ovarian cancers in white women. Am J Epidemiol 1992;136:1184–1203.

79. Kvale G, Heuch I, Nilssen S, Beral V. Reproductive factors and risk of ovarian cancer: a prospective study. Int J Cancer 1988;42:246–251.

80. Tung KH, Goodman MT, Wu AH et al. Reproductive factors and epithelial ovarian cancer risk by histologic type: a multiethnic case-control study. Am J Epidemiol 2003;158:629–638.

81. Wittenberg J, Cook LS, Rossing MA, Weiss NS, Wittenberg L. Reproductive risk factors for mucinous and non-mucinous epithelial ovarian cancer. Epidemiology 1999;10:761–763.

82. Cramer DW, Hutchison GB, Welch WR, Cully RE, Knapp RC. Factors affecting the association of oral contraceptives and ovarian cancer. N Engl J Med 1982;307:1047–1051.

83. WHO Collaborative Study of Neoplasia and Steroid Contraceptive. Epithelial ovarian cancer and combined oral contraceptives. Int J Cancer 1989;18:538–545.

84. Moseson M, Koenig KL, Shore RE, Pasternack BS. The influence of medical conditions associated with hormones on the risk of breast cancer. Int J Epidemiol 1993;22:1000–1009.

85. Weiss HA, Brinton LA, Potischman NA et al. Breast cancer risk in young women and history of selected medical conditions. Int J Epidemiol 1999;28:816–823.

86. Wyshak G, Frisch RE, Albright NL, Albright TE, Schiff I. Reproductive factors and melanoma of the skin among women. Int J Dermatol 1989;28:527–530.

87. Frisch RE, Wyshak G, Albert LS, Sober AJ. Dysplastic nevi, cutaneous melanoma, and gynecologic disorders. Int J Dermatol 1992;31:331–335.

88. Hornstein MD, Thomas PP, Sober AJ, Wyshak G, Albright NL, Frisch RE. Association between endometriosis, dysplasic naevi and hystory of melanoma in women of reproductive age. Hum Reprod 1997;12:143–144.

89. Wyshak G, Frisch RE. Red hair color, melanoma and endometriosis: suggestive associations. Int J Dermatol 2000;39:795–800.

90. Holly EA, Cress RD, Ahn DK. Cutaneous melanoma in women: III. Reproductive factors and oral contraceptive use. Am J Epidemiol 1995;141:943–950.

91. Kvaskoff M, Mesrine S, Fournier A, Boutron-Ruault MC, Clavel-Chapelon F. Personal history of endometriosis and risk of cutaneous melanoma in a large prospective cohort of French women. Arch Intern Med 2007;167:2061–2065.

92. Kvaskoff M, Mesrine S, Clavel-Chapelon F, Boutron-Ruault MC. Endometriosis risk in relation to naevi, freckles and skin sensitivity to sun exposure: the French E3N cohort. Int J Epidemiol 2009;38:1143–1153.

93. Somigliana E, Viganò P, Abbiati A et al. 'Here comes the sun': pigmentary traits and sun habits in women with endometriosis. Hum Reprod 2010;25:728–733.

94. Shakir SAW, Layton D. Causal association in pharmacovigilance and pharmacoepidemiology. Drug Safety 2002;25:467–470.

95. Morrow CP, Cutin JP. Tumors of the ovary: neoplasms derived from celomic epithelium. In: Morrow CP, Cutin JP (eds) Synopsis of Gynecologic Oncology. New York: Churchill Livingstone, 1998, pp. 223–280.

96. Heaps JM, Nieberg RK, Berek JS. Malignant neoplasms arising in endometriosis. Obstet Gynecol 1990;75:1023–1028.

97. Dinulescu DM, Ince TA, Quade BJ, Shafer SA, Crowley D, Jacks T. Role of K.ras and Pten in the development of mouse models of endometriosis and endometrioid ovarian cancer. Nat Med 2005;11:63–70.

98. Balkwill F, Mantovani A. Inflammation and cancer: back to Virchow? Lancet 2001;357:539–545.

99. Vignali M, Infantino M, Matrone R et al. Endometriosis: novel etiopathogenetic concepts and clinical perspectives. Fertil Steril 2002;78:665–678.

50 Molecular Mechanisms Underlying Endometriosis and Endometriosis-Related Cancers

Daniela Dinulescu

Division of Women's and Perinatal Pathology, Harvard Medical School, Boston, MA, USA

Epidemiology

Geographic distribution, incidence, mortality

Endometriosis is very common in the general population, affecting up to 10–15% of women in the reproductive age group [1,2], While it is known that endometriosis is a wide-ranging disease that affects at least 5.5 million women in North America at any one time, it is difficult to provide exact statistics for its prevalence because of complications that arise with diagnosis [1–3].

Endometriosis, a benign disease defined as the presence of functional uterine-like tissue outside the uterus, is frequently associated with endometrioid and clear cell ovarian adenocarcinomas [1–3]. The presence of stroma around the benign-appearing endometrioid glands is a histological hallmark of endometriosis and diagnostically distinguishes it from neoplastic endometrioid carcinoma implants that are never associated with such a stromal component. The clinical definition for endometriosis is the presence of ectopic endometrial glands and stroma. However, some protocols have allowed a diagnosis simply with a complaint of pelvic pain or infertility. With such a broad diagnosis, creating control groups becomes problematic. Applying epidemiological principles to the study of endometriosis is also difficult because diagnostic tools are not always available to all women. For example, surgical biopsies to investigate a genetic predisposition to the disease are not only invasive surgical procedures but are also associated with relatively high medical costs; consequently the procedure is not feasible for all patients [1–3].

Studies indicate that 5.5 million women in the US and Canada are affected and the healthcare costs associated with this disease are substantial since approximately 4 in 1000 patients are hospitalized with endometriosis each year [3]. Endometriotic implants are commonly associated with the surface of pelvic/peritoneal organs, including ovaries, uterus, fallopian tubes, stomach, pancreas, liver, bladder, intestine, and kidney; the presence of such implants results in fibrous adhesions between organs [1–3]. However, despite being extremely debilitating due to dysmenorrhea, dyspareunia, and chronic abdominal, pelvic, and back pain and a major cause of infertility, endometriosis is rarely fatal [1–13].

Age and genetic factors

Endometriosis affects women of child-bearing age but it is also found in adolescents and postmenopausal women who are receiving hormone replacement therapy [4]. Interestingly, endometriosis is common to all ethnic and social groups [4]. It is important to mention that endometriosis has a strong genetic component and it is not an autoimmune disease, as was previously thought. In support of this assertion, it was noted that women with endometriosis were significantly more likely to report a family history of cancer compared to women in control groups [5]. Endometriosis is known to share numerous characteristics with neoplastic processes, such as cell proliferation, angiogenesis, and tissue invasion. It is possible, therefore, that some of the genetic factors that predispose a woman to the development of neoplasia could also predispose her to the development of endometriosis [5].

In addition, related women with endometriosis are known to have a 4–8 times greater risk of developing endometriosis than women from an unaffected family [3]. Furthermore, the risk of developing the disease drastically increases dramatically up to 10-fold in women with an affected first-degree relative [6,7]. It is likely that some families carry genes that allow abnormal cells to survive and grow ectopically in the pelvic cavity. Interestingly, a study of cousin pairs provided further genetic evidence that endometriosis was found in both maternally and paternally connected women [6]. Moreover, a genome-wide association study (GWAS) has recently identified a locus at 7p15.2 that is associated with the development of endometriosis [8]. Interestingly, this locus shows the strongest association with moderate-to-severe disease and is located in an intergenic region upstream of two candidate

Endometriosis: Science and Practice, First Edition. Edited by Linda C. Giudice, Johannes L.H. Evers and David L. Healy.
© 2012 Blackwell Publishing Ltd. Published 2012 by Blackwell Publishing Ltd.

genes: NFE2L3 and HOXA10 [8]. HOXA10, a homeobox allotype gene of the HOXA family, in particular is believed to play an important role in ovarian endometrioid and clear cell cancer development by promoting the proliferation, migration, and invasion of tumor cells [9]. For example, HOXA10 is overexpressed in ovarian clear cell cancer and is correlated with poor survival [9]. In addition, HOXA10 promotes tumor lineage specificity by inducing the morphogenesis of endometrioid ovarian tumors [10].

Reproductive factors: risk factors and productive factors

Numerous studies, including a 6-year retrospective review at the Yale University School of Medicine, have indicated that the factors associated with an increased risk for endometriosis include lower body weight, alcohol use, early menarche, shorter cycle length, and heavier menstrual cycles [5]. For this study, 535 diagnosed cases of endometriosis were compared with 200 control patients who had all been treated at the hospital between the years of 1996 and 2002 and patient information was compiled from various sources [5].

In general, exposure to estrogen is one of the primary risk factors for endometriosis, whereas progesterone appears to be protective against the disease. For this reason, greater parity in women indicates a lower incidence of the disease, due to the influence of progesterone during pregnancy. However, it is difficult to calculate the exact risk for a particular patient due to a large number of contributing risk factors, some of which have confounding influences and may in fact be the result rather than the cause of disease development [5].

Etiology and pathogenesis

It is believed that endometriosis is inherited as a complex genetic trait, as many factors seem to interact during the progression of the disease; thus, beyond genetic factors, multiple environmental cues and a malfunction in the immune system can also affect the development of endometriosis [1,7]. There are two prevailing theories that explain the pathogenesis of this disease. First, the "implantation theory" postulates that endometriosis arises through seeding of the peritoneum or ovary with uterine endometrial cells derived from retrograde menstruation. The alternative view, known as the "metaplastic theory," is that endometriosis arises directly from the surface of the involved organs. While there is clinical evidence for both mechanisms, molecular studies from patient material have been inconclusive to date.

Implantation theory (retrograde menstruation)

The implantation theory proposes that viable endometrial cells travel backwards through the fallopian tubes via retrograde menstruation. These cells are then deposited on pelvic and peritoneal organs, where they acquire an enhanced capability to seed and grow. Due to their stem cell-like properties, it is possible that the cells initiating the disease are capable of surviving in ectopic environments [1].

Metaplastic theory (*de novo* metaplasia for pelvic and ovarian endometriosis)

The second theory is supported by the fact that induction of endometriosis is possible in animal models and *in vitro* human cultures. For example, ovarian endometriotic lesions can arise directly from the ovarian surface epithelium through a metaplastic differentiation process induced by genetic and/or immune events [4]. In addition, it is speculated that endogenous biochemical factors present in menstrual fluid are capable of inducing the metaplastic differentiation of undifferentiated peritoneal cells, allowing the development and propagation of endometriotic tissue [4].

Key genes and pathways associated with the development and propagation of endometriosis

Oncogenes and growth factor receptors

Multiple studies have found higher levels for multiple proto-oncogenes, such as c-myc, c-fms, c-erbB-1/2, and RAS, in endometriosis patients compared to levels found in the normal endometrium of healthy controls. These data suggest that alterations in proto-oncogene expression may be responsible for the aberrant growth and differentiation of endometriotic cells. Monoclonal cell expansion in endometriosis has also been observed. In addition, another study indicated overexpression of c-myc and erbB-1/2 in an established endometriosis cell line [11]. Comparative genomic hybridization reports identified alteration of DNA copy numbers on several chromosomes in endometriosis patients: 1p, 22q, X, 6p, and 17q. Fluorescent *in situ* hybridization studies further confirmed that the gain of 17q resulted in amplification of the HER-2/neu proto-oncogene in endometriosis cases [12].

Tumor suppressor genes

The disruption of the PTEN tumor suppressor function has been proven to facilitate the development of endometriosis [12,13]. The loss of function of a single PTEN allele is sufficient to provide a growth advantage to cells due to a gene inactivation event. Reduced expression of this tumor suppressor gene is commonly seen in women with late-stage disease [13]. Furthermore, a comprehensive study using a cDNA microarray made up of 23,040 genes, which investigated genes that were downregulated in endometriotic cysts versus normal endometrium, identified multiple key tumor suppressor genes, such as PTEN and TP53, in addition to genes involved in cellular apoptosis [7]. In addition, loss of heterozygosity at 5q, 6q, 9p, 11q, 22q, p16, and others has been identified in endometriotic tissue [12]. Such relatively frequent loss of heterozygosity (LOH) events indicate a loss of multiple tumor suppressor genes in endometriosis cases [12].

Abnormal regulation of signaling pathways

Abnormal regulation of multiple key signaling pathways, PTEN/PI3K, MAPK, WNT, and others, has been implicated in the etiology of this disease. For example, when WNT signaling is abrogated, the cytoplasmic enzyme glycogen synthase kinase-3β is able to phosphorylate and activate downstream effectors with proliferation-promoting properties, which in turn allow endometriotic cells to rapidly divide without any inhibition. Cells begin to acquire neoplastic properties, eventually developing transformative capability that encourages the progression from endometriosis to cancer [14]. Interestingly, one study confirmed abnormal activation and increased expression of Wnt7a, Wnt2, and F2D1 in endometriotic tissue, further indicating that the WNT pathway was disrupted in endometriosis [15].

Apoptosis

Overexpression of the bcl-2 gene is known to decrease the rate of cell death. Normally, the gene functions in the endometrium tissue to maintain cellular homeostasis. Overexpression of bcl-2 in ectopic endometrial tissue has been reported, indicating that endometriotic cells fail to undergo apoptosis. Apoptosis was also found to be significantly decreased in eutopic endometrial tissue of women with endometriosis, compared with fertile women who did not have the disease, further indicating that it plays a key role in the etiology of this disease [11].

Epigenetic changes

Aberrant methylation and deregulation of microRNA expression have been found in endometriotic tissue. For example, a close association was reported between the development of endometriosis and epigenetic changes that involve genes coding for DNA methylation (DNMTs). Thus, DNMT1, DNMT3A, and DNMT3B were found to be overexpressed in endometriotic tissue compared to normal endometrium of healthy women [16].

Telomerase

Recent studies have demonstrated that abnormal telomerase expression in the endometrium helps to enhance cellular proliferation and contributes to the pathogenesis of endometriosis [17].

Steroid hormones and receptors

It was also noted that aromatase, which catalyzes the rate-limiting step in the synthesis of estrogen, is abnormally expressed in endometriotic tissue [1]. In addition, prostaglandin E_2 (PGE_2) is known to stimulate aromatase activity in endometriotic tissues. Both PGE_2 and cyclo-oxygenase (COX)-2, the key enzyme in the biosynthesis of prostaglandins, are produced in excess in endometrial and endometriotic tissues of endometriosis patients [1]. Consequently, increases in COX-2 and PGE_2 signaling upregulate estrogen production in endometriosis via a positive feedback loop. As a result, aromatase and prostaglandin inhibitors have been proposed as possible therapies, especially since they are known to reduce pelvic pain and disease[1]. In addition to these important players in the progression of endometriosis, levels of the steroidogenic factor (SF)1 were significantly higher in ectopic endometria compared to normal endometrium, and further correlated with the severity of disease [1]. This suggests a potential role for these genes in locally induced steroidogenesis in

endometriotic cells, which is important for both the initiation and propagation of the disease.

Modeling endometriosis: animal models of disease

Genetic models

The chicken chorio-allantoic membrane (CAM) model has been used extensively to study the human disease. CAM contains extracellular matrix that is very similar to human peritoneal extracellular matrix, therefore making it an important model to study the attachment and invasion of ectopic endometrial cells, which is the hallmark of endometriosis [18]. A further development was provided by Dinulescu *et al* who generated the first *de novo* mouse models for endometriosis and endometrioid adenocarcinoma of the ovary, and in the process provided evidence for a genetic link between endometriosis and certain subtypes of ovarian cancer [19]. These models are significant because they share the histopathology and biological behavior of the human disease (Plates 50.1, 50.2) [19].

The possibility that ovarian cancer arises through the malignant transformation of endometriosis has long been suggested; a clear genetic link between endometriosis and ovarian cancer was first identified in *de novo* mouse models [19] and further validated in more recent clinical studies [20–24]. The results of the animal model study suggest that common molecular genetic pathways, such as the K-RAS/MAPK and PTEN/PI3K pathways, are involved in the pathogenesis of both endometriosis and endometrioid ovarian carcinoma (Plate 50.3) [19]. Further molecular genetic evidence that endometriosis is a precursor of endometrioid and clear cell ovarian cancer had recently been shown in a key patient study [20]. A total of 63 LOH events were reported in human carcinoma samples; interestingly, 22 of these were also detected in the corresponding endometriosis samples. In each case, the same allele was lost in both endometriosis and cancer [20].

Furthermore, a separate microarray analysis study has identified upregulation of multiple genes within the RAS/RAF/MAPK and PI3K pathways in endometriosis patients compared to controls [21]. Moreover, a key study establishes a functional role for the constitutive activation of the MAPK pathway in endometriosis by suggesting that it is responsible for the maintenance of proliferative changes, which are normally associated only with the secretory-phase endometrium. The maintenance of these permanent proliferative events further explains the abnormal propagation of endometriotic lesions [22]. Of note, PTEN and K-RAS mutations were found to play a role in the development of low-grade ovarian endometrioid carcinomas, a histological tumor subtype that is frequently associated with the presence of endometriosis in patients [23]. In addition, synchronous PTEN and K-RAS mutations were identified in uterine and ovarian endometrioid tumors associated with endometriosis [24].

Disease xenografts

Rodent and rabbit models are commonly used to study the development of endometriosis. However, these animals are estrous, which means that their endometrial tissue is reabsorbed rather than released and, therefore, spontaneous endometriosis cannot occur. Transplants derived from either homologous or heterologous sources are used to implant the disease tissue into these models [18]. For example, syngeneic or autologous uterine tissue surgically transplanted to ectopic sites on the peritoneum in mice has been used successfully as an animal model to study endometriosis [18].

Link between endometriosis and cancer

Association of endometriosis with endometrioid cancer: genes and pathways

Endometriosis has long been associated with an increased risk for certain malignant tumors, notably ovarian (endometrioid and clear cell) cancer and non-Hodgkin lymphoma. Thus, 15–40% of endometrioid ovarian carcinoma cases are associated with endometriosis [19]. Based on this frequent association, numerous reports have even implicated endometriosis as a precursor lesion in endometrioid ovarian cancer [19,25]. The possibility that ovarian cancer arises through the malignant transformation of endometriosis has long been suggested. The first documentation of the association between endometriosis and endometrioid ovarian cancer was noted by Sampson in 1925 [25]. He suggested that the association between the two diseases had to fulfill certain criteria in order to indicate the malignant transformation of endometriosis. First, there had to be a clear example of endometriosis in the area directly surrounding the tumor. Second, the histology of the cancer needed to be consistent with an endometriotic origin. Third, there could be no other primary site for the tumor [25].

The risk of ovarian cancer among women with endometriosis is higher, by 30–40%, than among women without endometriosis [26]. The majority of ovarian cancers associated with endometriosis are either clear cell or endometrioid carcinomas [26]. Bell and Kurman's analysis of benign ovarian endometrioid tumors and well-differentiated endometrioid carcinomas found frequent co-existence of endometriosis and endometrioid neoplasms, further supporting a genetic link between the two [27,28]. It has been suggested that carcinoma arises from endometriosis through a multi-step process where typical endometriosis acquires severe atypia with or without hyperplasia and then transforms into carcinoma [27,28]. In about 60% of endometriosis-associated ovarian cancer (EAOC), the cancer is adjacent to or arises directly from endometriosis tissue, clearly indicating that malignant transformation can occur [27,28].

It is thought that endometriosis can give rise to endometrioid carcinomas through accumulation of abnormal mutations in multiple signaling pathways, such as the WNT and PI3K/PTEN pathways [27]. Multiple studies have shown frequent LOH events where identical alleles are lost in both endometriosis and ovarian

cancer, which statistically would be very unlikely to occur as independent events; this provides further evidence that endometriosis is a clonal precursor to EAOC [27,28]. LOH studies have implicated the involvement of numerous chromosomal regions, including 1q, 5q, 9p, 10q, 11q, 17q, and 22q, in this process. These genetic loci contain candidate oncogenes and tumor suppressor genes that are involved in the initiation, promotion, and progression of endometriosis to EAOC [27,28]. For example, loss of the PTEN tumor suppressor gene has been implicated in progression from endometriosis to endometrioid ovarian carcinoma [12,27,28]. Specifically, three out of five cases of endometrioid ovarian carcinomas associated with endometriosis displayed LOH events at the PTEN 10q23.3 locus in both the ovarian carcinoma and endometriosis lesions [12,19,27,28]. In addition, somatic mutations in the PTEN gene have been identified in 20% of endometrioid ovarian carcinoma cases as well as 20% of ovarian endometriotic cysts, suggesting that PTEN inactivation occurs early on in the malignant process of endometriosis [12,19,27,28].

Interestingly, although considered benign, endometriosis shares certain characteristics with cancer, such as tissue invasion, unrestrained growth, and angiogenesis; in addition, some cases are monoclonal in origin. Similarities between endometriosis and endometriosis-associated ovarian cancer are mentioned in numerous studies and summarized in Table 50.1 [11,12,21,22,27–32].

Currently, the screening in use for the detection of endometriosis is the measurement of CA-125 levels, a cancer antigen marker, in blood samples. An elevated level of this protein in a patient sample could indicate endometriosis, but it could also indicate ovarian cancer, pregnancy or pancreatitis. Therefore, a significantly elevated CA-125 level cannot be used to accurately diagnose endometriosis. There have been documented cases involving patients with high CA-125 levels and ovarian cysts, but upon laparoscopic evaluation, there was no evidence of malignancy but only endometriosis, which later went on to develop into ovarian cancer. While CA-125 is not an ideal biomarker to detect endometriosis, it can be used to determine a further course of action for women until a more exact marker is discovered [29,30]. In the future, more sensitive diagnostic blood tests need be developed in order to specifically diagnose endometriosis [29,30].

Association of endometriosis with ovarian clear cell cancer: genes and pathways

Ovarian clear cell carcinoma comprises 10% of epithelial ovarian cancers and is one of the most aggressive types because it is refractory to standard platinum-based chemotherapy [31]. Like endometrioid carcinoma, morphological and molecular studies suggest that clear cell carcinomas can develop from a common progenitor disease, such as endometriosis, and then proceed to malignancy [31].

Recently, Jones *et al* and Wiegand *et al* have found that the ARID1A tumor suppressor gene is frequently disrupted in ovarian clear cell and endometrioid carcinomas [31,32]. ARID1A encodes BAF250a, a key component of the SWI-SNF chromatin remodeling complex [31,32]. It is hypothesized that somatic inactivating mutations in the ARID1A gene induce changes in chromatin

Table 50.1 Common factors and pathogenetic mechanisms link endometriosis and endometriosis-associated ovarian cancer.

Protective factors	Risk factors	Pathogenetic mechanisms of disease
Pregnancy	Nulliparity	Abnormal expression of PTEN/PI3K and DNA mismatch repair gene hMLH1
Oral contraceptive pill	Early onset of menstruation	Hyperactivation of the WNT pathway
Surgery (hysterectomy, tubal ligation)	Family history	Overexpression of the bcl-2 gene
	Exposure to estrogen	ARID1A inactivation
	Late onset of menopause	Hyperactivation of the MAPK pathway
	Elevated gonadotropins	Overamplification of the HER-2/neu gene
	Chronic inflammation	Mutation or loss of p53
		Abnormal expression of the hepatic nuclear factor (HNF-1b)
		Abnormal expression of CA-125 tumor and serum biomarker

remodeling and thereby influence the epigenetic regulation of multiple genes playing a role in malignant transformation [31]. Thus, ARID1A genetic mutations were present in 46% of ovarian clear cell carcinomas and 30% of endometrioid carcinomas, but were not identified in any of the high-grade serous ovarian carcinomas screened [31,32]. Interestingly, in two of the cases, endometriotic lesions next to the malignant tumor had the same ARID1A mutations; this was not true for lesions distant from the tumor [32]. Molecular analysis of the adjacent lesions also shows loss of TP53 and PTEN, as well as similar LOH patterns [32]. Consequently, data presented by Weigand et al strongly suggest that ARID1A and PTEN inactivation occurs early in the development of these tumors, during transformation of endometriosis [32].

Risk for malignant transformation of endometriosis

There are several questions of great interest for patients: is there a subtype of endometriosis patients who carry the highest risk of malignant transformation? How to detect those at high risk? What is the risk of malignant transformation for ovarian versus pelvic/peritoneal (non-ovarian) endometriosis?

In answer to these questions, one report describes a large-scale study run in Japan with 6398 participants in order to determine the risk factors for developing ovarian cancer after having been diagnosed with ovarian endometriomas [28]. The study suggests that the severity of endometriosis lesions may predispose a woman to clear cell and endometrioid ovarian cancers. In addition, advancing age and the size of endometriomas were independent predictors of the development of ovarian cancer in women with endometriosis. Thus, ovarian endometriomas greater than 9 cm in diameter found in postmenopausal women of 45 years or older were found to be strong predictors of malignant transformation. Of note, this study is important because of the large number of patients enrolled and followed up after the initial ultrasound scan confirming the presence of endometriosis. Weaknesses of the study include the lack of a comprehensive study of some patients after a diagnosis of endo-

metriosis is given, and the use of prevention therapies (hormone treatments, surgery), which make it difficult to establish a specific age and lesion size which correspond to the development of cancer [28].

Additional evidence suggests that atypical epithelia in endometriosis may be a precursor for malignancy [33]. Atypical endometriosis has genetic events that support the intermediate nature of this lesion between benign endometriosis and ovarian cancer. Furthermore, atypical endometriosis is more frequently found in endometriosis accompanied by ovarian malignant tumors than in benign endometriotic cysts [33]. Moreover, atypical endometriotic foci were observed in 61% of endometriosis cases associated with ovarian malignant tumors compared to only 1.7% of endometriosis patients with no cancer [33].

Current surgical and medical therapeutic strategies for endometriosis

Current therapeutic strategies for endometriosis focus on treating the symptoms rather than curing the cause or preventing the disease. Endometriosis can be effectively cured with up to 85% pain relief by non-conservative surgery (i.e. hysterectomy and bilateral oophorectomy), but most young patients are wary of this option as it affects future fertility. Conservative surgery typically only provides temporary relief, and symptoms usually recur [34]. While many clinical trials involving different treatments for endometriosis have taken place, the results of very few have been published. This implies that the data collected in these studies did not prove the efficacy of various treatments. Consequently, currently there is no successful drug on the market for the eradication of endometriosis [29]. As ectopic and eutopic tissue are extremely similar, a treatment would have to be created that could differentiate between the healthy and diseased tissues in order to protect the normal endometrium [34]. Different trials have been conducted in which treatments interfere with various events that characterize endometriosis, including implantation of endometriotic cells, neo-angiogenesis, proliferation, atypical metabolism, abnormal immunological reactions, inflammation, and apoptotic activity. None of these treatments has been shown to efficiently block the development of the disease without causing serious risk to an otherwise healthy patient [34].

Future options
Treatment of endometriosis using key pathway inhibitors

Recent studies have produced data showing that protein kinase inhibitors can control endometriotic cell proliferation *in vitro* and *in vivo*. Extracellular signal-regulated kinases (ERK 1 and 2) are members of a MAPK subfamily and are important in cellular proliferation, survival, differentiation, and adhesion. In endometriotic tissue, the MAPK (ERK1/2) pathway was found to be hyperactivated compared with the endometrial tissue from control patients [21,22,35]. When endometriotic tissue samples were treated with protein kinase inhibitors, such as A771726, PD98059, and U0126, cell proliferation was dramatically decreased. A future treatment could involve the use of protein kinase inhibitors in patients, as the *in vitro* and *in vivo* experiments have so far proven to be successful [35].

Chemopreventive treatment for endometriosis patients carrying the highest risk for malignant transformation

Endometriosis presents a serious risk factor, which can accelerate the development of ovarian cancer by 5.5 years [36]. The mean age at diagnosis of ovarian cancer is 54 years compared to the diagnosis of ovarian cancer in endometriosis patients, which averages 48 years [36].

Endometriosis-associated ovarian cancer has specific features; it usually gives rise to endometrioid and clear cell subtypes and tends to be found in earlier stages and have a favorable prognosis [33]. As outlined above, the allotyping of endometriosis along with adjacent ovarian carcinoma lesions identified common genetic alterations in most cases, providing molecular evidence that endometriosis, which appears benign, has genetic defects that may give rise to ovarian cancer [33]. Advances in mass spectrometry and medical imaging (optical and positron emission tomography) technologies are improving our ability to detect malignant disease in its earliest stages.

Ultimately, optimal early detection of malignancy will need to rely on detecting early preneoplastic lesions (i.e. endometriosis, precursor lesions in fimbriae) before they have a chance to develop into ovarian cancer. Cancer prevention research is an imperative for the better management of the disease. Thus, it is critical that we identify women at increased risk for the development of ovarian cancer, not only those carrying BRCA1, BRCA2 familial mutations but also women with severe/atypical ovarian endometriosis carrying mutations in the PTEN/PI3K and/or K-RAS/MAPK pathways or "p53 signatures" in the fallopian tube. Such patients who have the highest risk for developing ovarian

cancer may benefit from the use of chemopreventive agents or surgical treatment.

References

1. Bulun SE. Endometriosis. N Engl J Med 2009;360(3):268–279.
2. Giudice LC. Clinical practice. Endometriosis. N Engl J Med 2010; 362(25):2389–2398.
3. McLeod BS, Retzloff MG. Epidemiology of endometriosis: an assessment of risk factors. Clin Obstet Gynecol 2010;53:389–396.
4. Carrell DT, Peterson CM. Reproductive Endocrinology and Infertility: Integrating Modern Clinical and Laboratory Practice. New York: Springer, 2010.
5. Matalliotakis IM, Cakmak H, Fragouli YG et al. Epidemiological characteristics in women with and without endometriosis in the Yale series. Arch Gynecol Obstet 2008;277:389–393.
6. Stefansson H, Geirsson RT, Steinthorsdottir V et al. Genetic factors contribute to the risk of developing endometriosis. Hum Reprod 2002;17:555–559.
7. Barlow DH, Kennedy S. Endometriosis: new genetic approaches and therapy. Annu Rev Med 2005;56:345–356.
8. Painter JN, Anderson CA, Nyholt DR et al. Genome wide association study identifies a locus at 7p15.2 associated with endometriosis. Nat Genet Dec 2011;43(1):51–54.
9. Li B, Jin H, Yu Y et al. HOXA10 is overexpressed in human ovarian clear cell adenocarcinoma and correlates with poor survival. Int J Gynecol Cancer 2009;19(8):1347–1352.
10. Cheng W, Liu J, Yoshida H, Rosen D, Naora H. Lineage infidelity of epithelial ovarian cancers is controlled by HOX genes that specify regional identity in the reproductive tract. Nat Med 2005; 11(5):531–537.
11. Simpson JL, Bischoff FZ. Heritability and molecular genetic studies of endometriosis. Ann N Y Acad Sci 2002;955:239–239; discussion 293–293, 396–406.
12. Nezhat F, Datt, MS, Hanson V, Pejovic T, Nezhat C, Nezhat C. The relationship of endometriosis and ovarian malignancy: a review. Fertil Steril 2008;90:1559–1570.
13. Vigano P, Somigliana E, Chiodo I, Abbiati A, Vercellini P. Molecular mechanisms and biological plausability underlying the malignant transformation of endometriosis: a critical analysis. Hum Reprod Update 2008;12:77–89.
14. Weinberg RA. The Biology of Cancer. New York: Garland Science, 2007.
15. Sonderegger S, Pollheimer J, Knofler M. Wnt signaling in implantation, decidualisation and placental differentiation – review. Placenta 2010;31:839–847.
16. Guo SW. Epigenetics of endometriosis. Mol Hum Reprod 2009;15:587–607.
17. Hapangama DK, Turner MA, Drury JA et al. Endometriosis is associated with aberrant endometrial expression of telomerase and increased telomere length. Hum Reprod 2008;23:1511–1519.
18. Jensen JR, Coddington CC 3rd. Evolving spectrum: the pathogenesis of endometriosis. Clin Obstet Gynecol 2010;53:379–388.

19. Dinulescu DM, Ince TA, Quade BJ et al. Role of K-RAS and Pten in the development of mouse models of endometriosis and endometrioid ovarian cancer. Nat Med 2005;11:63–70.

20. Prowse AH, Manek S, Varma R et al. Molecular genetic evidence that endometriosis is a precursor of ovarian cancer. Int J Cancer 2006; 119(3):556–562.

21. Matsuzaki S, Canis M, Pouly J et al. Differential expression of genes in eutopic and ectopic endometrium from patients with ovarian endometriosis. Fertil Steril 2006;86(3):548–553.

22. Velarde MC, Aghajanova L, Nezhat CR, Giudice LC. Increased mitogen-activated protein kinase kinase/extracellularly regulated kinase activity in human endometrial stromal fibroblasts of women with endometriosis reduces 3′,5′-cyclic adenosine 5′-monophosphate inhibition of cyclin D1. Endocrinology 2009;150(10):4701–4712.

23. Kolasa IK, Rembiszewska A, Janiec-Jankowska A et al. PTEN mutation, expression and LOH at its locus in ovarian carcinomas. Relation to TP53, K-RAS and BRCA1 mutations. Gynecol Oncol 2006; 103(2):692–697.

24. Irving JA, Catasús L, Gallardo A et al. Synchronous endometrioid carcinomas of the uterine corpus and ovary: alterations in the beta-catenin (CTNNB1) pathway are associated with independent primary tumors and favorable prognosis. Hum. Pathol 2005; 36(6):605–619.

25. Valenzuela P, Ramos P, Redondo S, Cabrera Y, Alvarez I, Ruiz A. Endometrioid adenocarcinoma of the ovary and endometriosis. Eur J Obstet Gynecol Reprod Biol 2007;134:83–86.

26. Birrer MJ. The origin of ovarian cancer – is it getting clearer? N Engl J Med 2010;363:1574–1575.

27. Cho KR, Shih IM. Ovarian cancer. Annu Rev Pathol 2009;4:287–313.

28. Kobayashi H, Kajiwara H, Kanayama S et al. Molecular pathogenesis of endometriosis-associated clear cell carcinoma of the ovary (review). Oncol Rep 2009;22:233–240.

29. Kitawaki J, Ishihara H, Koshiba H et al. Usefulness and limits of CA-125 in diagnosis of endometriosis with associated endometriomas. Hum Reprod 2005;20:1999–2003.

30. Check JH. CA-125 as a biomarker for malignant transformation of endometriosis. Fertil Steril 2009;91:e35; author reply e36.

31. Jones S, Wang TL, Shih IeM et al. Frequent mutations of chromatin remodeling gene ARID1A in ovarian clear cell carcinoma. Science 2010;330:228–231.

32. Wiegand KC, Shah SP, Al-Agha OM et al. ARID1A mutations in endometriosis-associated ovarian carcinomas. N Engl J Med 2010; 363:1532–1543.

33. Mandai M, Yamaguchi K, Matsumura N, Baba T, Konishi I. Ovarian cancer in endometriosis: molecular biology, pathology, and clinical management. Int J Clin Oncol 2009;14:383–391.

34. Vercellini P, Crosignani P, Somigliana E, Vigano P, Frattaruolo M, Fedele L. 'Waiting for Godot': a commonsense approach to the medical treatment of endometriosis. Hum Reprod 2011;26(1):3–13.

35. Ngo C, Nicco C, Leconte M et al. Protein kinase inhibitors can control the progression of endometriosis in vitro and in vivo. J Pathol 2010;222:148–157.

36. Aris A. Endometriosis-associated ovarian cancer: a ten-year cohort study of women living in the Estrie Region of Quebec, Canada. J Ovarian Res 2010;3:2.

51 Pregnancy and Obstetric Outcomes in Women with Endometriosis

Henrik Falconer

Department of Women's and Children's Health, Karolinska Institute, Stockholm, Sweden

Introduction

The association between endometriosis and decreased fecundity is well known and has been the subject of intense research the last decades [1]. Advances in assisted reproductive technologies (ART) have increased the chances for women with endometriosis to become pregnant. However, little is known about the effect of pregnancy on the disease and vice versa. This particular area of endometriosis is difficult to study and it could be assumed that both doctors and patients have been quite satisfied in the event of a pregnancy (spontaneous or assisted). The potential risks or benefits have simply not been a major concern. A widespread idea is that pregnancy relieves endometriosis-associated pain and other related symptoms. The support for this belief is weak with a minimal scientific foundation. With the massive rise in estradiol associated with early pregnancy, a deterioration of symptoms could be expected. However, the endocrine changes during pregnancy are complex and the alterations in progesterone metabolism in combination with amenorrhea may have a healing effect.

Until very recently, barely anything was known about the effects of endometriosis on pregnancy outcome. Many other chronic inflammatory diseases, including rheumatoid arthritis and Crohn's disease, are associated with preterm birth and other risks during pregnancy. Identifying risk factors for preterm birth, stillbirth and preeclampsia is important as it may be possible to intervene during pregnancy and thus reduce the risks.

This chapter will focus on two entities: the effects of pregnancy on endometriosis and the effects of endometriosis on pregnancy.

Effects of pregnancy on endometriosis

A widespread myth, especially on patient-orientated websites, is that pregnancy improves or even cures endometriosis. Women with endometriosis are often encouraged to consider family formation early in life and many patients are left with the impression that a pregnancy is the ultimate solution for their symptoms. Endometriosis is associated with a reduced fecundity rate and many women are concerned about their fertility. A pregnancy will most likely have a positive effect on the general well-being which in turn may affect the perceived symptoms. Whether this relief is purely psychological or the result of decreased disease activity is uncertain.

Early observations by Meigs and Sampson suggested beneficial effects, at least histological, of pregnancy exerted on endometriosis [2,3]. In 1952, Gainey reported that a minority of women examined post partum revealed objective improvement [4]. Subjectively, however, a majority (80%) of women reported improvement of complaints related to endometriosis. These observations lead to the development of "pseudo-pregnancy" as a treatment option for endometriosis. Kistner proposed a combined regimen of high doses of estrogens and progestagens for periods up to 7 months [5]. However, it was quickly discovered that this regimen was not curative and it was later modified [6,7].

The findings by Meigs and Sampson were not questioned until the early 1960s, when McArthur and Ulfelder examined 24 cases of endometriosis during pregnancy [8]. The authors found that the effects of pregnancy on endometriosis were very variable. They observed a few cases with regression of endometriotic lesions, but in most cases the disease progressed. These observations were supported by a few case reports published in the 1960s [9] but apart from that, quality studies in humans are limited.

Observing the natural course of events would require serial biopsies or laparoscopies in pregnant women, which for ethical

Endometriosis: Science and Practice, First Edition. Edited by Linda C. Giudice, Johannes L.H. Evers and David L. Healy.
© 2012 Blackwell Publishing Ltd. Published 2012 by Blackwell Publishing Ltd.

Table 51.1 Studies of endometriosis and adverse pregnancy outcome. Figures refer to odds ratio (OR) and 95% confidence interval (CI) except for the study by Brosens *et al.*

	Cases	Controls	Subtype	Preterm	SGA	Preeclampsia	Antepartum hemorrhage	Cesarean section
Kortelahti *et al* 2003 [23]	137	137	All	NS	NA	NS	NS	NS
Brosens *et al* 2007 [19]	245	274	All	NA	NA	0.8% vs 5.8% P = 0.002	NA	NA
Juang *et al* 2007 [25]	104*	208	Adenomyosis	1.96 (1.23–4.47)	NA	NA	NA	NA
Fernando *et al* 2009 [27]	95+535**	3757	Endometrioma	1.98 (1.09–3.62)	1.95 (1.06–3.60)	NA	NA	NA
Stephansson *et al* 2009 [28]	13,090	1429 585	All	1.33 (1.23–1.44)	NS	1.13 (1.02–1.26)	1.76 (1.56–1.99)	1.47 (1.40–1.54)
Hadfield *et al* 2009 [24]	3239	205,640	All	NA	NA	NS	NA	NA

* Number of cases and controls refers to preterm v term deliveries. The total number of women with adenomyosis was 35.
** 95 women with endometriomata and 535 women with non-ovarian endometriosis.
NA, not analyzed; NS, not statistically significant; SGA, small for gestational weight.

reasons would be very difficult to carry out. However, the findings by McArthur and Ulfelder have some support in an animal study performed in pregnant baboons. The baboon model has been used successfully in the study of various aspects of endometriosis and the reproductive behavior of this non-human primate is very similar to humans. D'Hooghe and co-workers performed serial laparoscopies in non-pregnant and pregnant animals during the first and second trimesters of gestation [10]. The results suggested no effect of pregnancy on the extent of peritoneal endometriosis. Previous experiments in cynomolgus monkeys and rats had shown regression of endometriotic implants in pregnant animals, although the effect may be attributed to the anestrus postpartum period [11,12].

Unfortunately, interest in the effects of pregnancy upon endometriosis has been very limited in the scientific community. In the past 10–15 years, virtually nothing has been published in this area at all. As summarized in this section, current knowledge rests on a weak foundation and further studies are necessary.

Effects of endometriosis on pregnancy

In contrast to the previous section, all studies regarding potential effects on pregnancy have been conducted within the last 10 years. This is most likely the result of better and more efficient epidemiological methods, which is the foundation of risk analysis studies. In order to study the effects of a certain factor on a condition or disease (in this case endometriosis on pregnancy), a large number of exposed cases is normally required. If an outcome is rare (e.g. stillbirth), an even larger sample size (cohort) is necessary. This can only be obtained through epidemiological methods which in turn require well-organized registers, spanning a substantial period of time [13].

Epidemiology has the advantage of not requiring a specific hypothesis prior to analysis. The method is rather hypothesis generating and may constitute the basis of experimental studies. Its strength, however, is that it may give an idea whether an effect (any effect) is potentially existing or not. Moreover, epidemiology will tell very little of the underlying mechanisms of an observed effect.

In endometriosis, there are no more than a handful of well-designed studies of the effect of the disease on pregnancy. A PubMed search using the search terms endometriosis, preterm birth, adverse pregnancy outcome, and preeclampsia results in only six publications (Table 51.1). Out of these, only four meet the standards for good case–control studies [14]. In addition to these studies, a few publications in adjacent areas contribute to current knowledge. A recent publication indicates that subfertile women are at risk for several obstetric complications, including preeclampsia and placental abruption [15]. These results may be true for women with endometriosis but well-designed, specific studies are imperative. The lack of research is quite remarkable, especially considering the association between endometriosis and assisted reproductive technologies. However, these studies require large and well-organized registers.

In other areas, the association between intercurrent diseases and poor pregnancy outcome has gained substantial interest in the past 10–20 years. It is now well known that inflammatory diseases such as rheumatoid arthritis and Crohn disease are associated with adverse pregnancy outcome [16,17]. The most commonly studied outcome variable is preterm birth. This is mainly due to the fact that preterm birth is increasing in Western countries and constitutes a large economic factor in modern healthcare. Furthermore, the strong association between neonatal death, morbidity, and preterm birth has strongly influenced the study of adverse pregnancy outcome [18]. Whether the

Table 51.2 Crude and adjusted odds ratios for adverse pregnancy outcome in women with and without endometriosis among singleton births in Sweden between 1992 and 2006 (Stephansson et al, 2009 [28]).

	Endometriosis n (%) 13 090	No endometriosis n (%) 1 429 585	Crude (95% CI)	Adjusted (95% CI)*
Preterm birth	883 (6.78)	70 806 (4.98)	1.39 (1.30–1.49)	1.33 (1.23–1.44)
SGA birth	361 (2.77)	33 795 (2.38)	1.17 (1.05–1.30)	1.04 (0.92–1.17)
Stillbirth	53 (0.40)	4725 (0.33)	1.23 (0.94–1.61)	1.02 (0.74–1.40)
Preeclampsia	441 (3.37)	41 377 (2.89)	1.17 (1.06–1.29)	1.13 (1.02–1.26)
Antepartum hemorrhage	344 (2.63)	19 482 (1.36)	1.95 (1.75–2.18)	1.76 (1.56–1.99)
Cesarean section	2815 (21.50)	193 082 (13.51)	1.76 (1.69–1.84)	1.47 (1.40–1.54)

* Odds ratios have been adjusted for maternal age, smoking, Body Mass Index, parity, years of formal education and year of birth of the child.
CI, confidence interval; SGA, small for gestational age.

identification of adverse pregnancy outcome allows for intervention (and subsequent reduction of risks) is unknown.

Two of the existing publications have tried to answer more specific questions and thus only four have looked at adverse obstetric outcome in general (see Table 51.1). In the former category, an attempt was made to clarify the potential association between endometriosis and preeclampsia in a case–control study from Belgium. It has been proposed that preeclampsia arises from a defective remodelling of junctional zone myometrial spiral arteries in the placental bed [19] and studies by Leyendecker and co-workers suggest a relationship between endometriosis and dysregulation of the junctional zone [20]. This finding implies an association between endometriosis and preeclampsia. Furthermore, studies by Lockwood and co-workers of soluble fms-like tyrosine kinase-1 (sFlt-1) suggest a link between endometriosis and preeclampsia which involves inhibition of the proangiogenetic factor, vascular endothelial growth factor [21,22]. However, in the study by Brosens and co-workers, the risk of preeclampsia was in fact decreased. The authors suggested that the lower incidence may reflect the increased local expression of angiogenetic factors and enhanced endometrial perfusion in women with endometriosis. These results are to some extent in agreement with a previous report from Finland, although the lower risk of preeclampsia in this case–control study was non-significant [23]. However, these two studies suffer from methodological shortcomings, where the limited number of cases is the most apparent.

The latest and by far the largest study of endometriosis and subsequent risk of preeclampsia was published in 2009 [24]. In this longitudinal study, a total of 3239 women with endometriosis were identified among 208,879 women with a singleton birth. In contrast to the findings by Brosens et al, no association was found between endometriosis and the development of preeclampsia during pregnancy. This result remained unchanged after adjusting for maternal age and gestation.

The first quality study with a more general approach was published by Juang and co-workers in 2007 [25]. In this 1:2 nested case–control study, the potential effects of adenomyosis on pregnancy outcome were studied in a Taiwanese population. The investigators noticed an

increased risk of preterm birth and premature preterm rupture of membranes (PPROM). These results were based on the observation of 35 women with adenomyosis and the authors concluded that there may be a common pathway in the development of preterm birth and PPROM. Apart from the apparent limitation with only a certain subgroup of the disease, the results may be affected by misclassification of exposure variable (adenomyosis). Adenomyosis was diagnosed either by magnetic resonance imaging (MRI) or ultrasonography and neither method has a sensitivity above 80% [26].

The observation of preterm birth in the Taiwanese population was supported by results from an Australian retrospective cohort study, where pregnancy outcome was reported among women with ovarian endometriosis undergoing ART [27]. In this study, 95 singleton births from women with endometriomata and 535 babies born to women with non-ovarian endometriosis were compared with non-endometriosis controls. The main result suggests that women with endometriomata have an increased risk of both preterm birth and small for gestational age (SGA) babies. Interestingly, none of these associations was observed among women with non-ovarian endometriosis. The authors speculated that abnormal endometrium, with subsequent disturbances in implantation, may be the cause of preterm birth among these women.

The largest study to date was conducted by our group in Sweden 2009 [28]. This retrospective cohort study was based on more than 1,400,000 births during 1992–2006 from the Swedish Medical Birth Register (MBR) and the Patient Register (PAR). The population-based MBR includes prospectively collected information including demographic data, reproductive history and complications during pregnancy, delivery and the neonatal period among more than 98% of all births in Sweden [29]. The PAR started in 1964 and since 1987 the register has covered all public, inpatient care in Sweden. Since 2001, it has also included diagnoses from specialized outpatient clinics. As mentioned previously, high-quality registers with a high coverage are essential for this type of cohort study. Our results showed that endometriosis is associated with preterm birth (Table 51.2). Moreover, women with endometriosis seem to be at risk for developing preeclampsia and antepartum hemorrhage during pregnancy. Also, an almost twofold increase in cesarean section (CS) was observed among women with endometriosis. This association was most evident for prelabor CS and suggests that women with endometriosis more often are scheduled for elective CS, possibly due to antepartum hemorrhage.

There are several well-known risk factors for preterm birth, including the use of ART [30]. This is obviously a potential effect modifier and we found that women with endometriosis required ART 10 times more often than control subjects. However, the relative risk of preterm birth remained relatively unchanged when stratified for the use of ART. A limitation of the study is that we did not know to what extent the diagnosis of endometriosis was based on histological verification after surgery. In a previous study of endometriosis and cancer risk based on the Swedish PAR, the diagnosis of endometriosis was histologically confirmed in 81% of the patients [31]. Furthermore we only had information on diagnosis of endometriosis for hospitalized women between 1964 and 2006 or those who attended outpatient clinics at hospitals between 2001 and 2006. It is therefore likely that such data are limited to the more severe stages of endometriosis. However, if some women were misclassified according to diagnosis of endometriosis, this would dilute the effect of endometriosis since there is no reason to assume that diagnosis misclassification is related to the outcome under study. On the other hand, it may not be possible to generalize the findings of an increased risk of adverse pregnancy outcomes to women with mild endometriosis. Another limitation of this study was the inability to assess the influence of treatment of endometriosis on the risk of adverse pregnancy outcome.

The underlying causes of the observed risks during pregnancy are largely unknown. The Taiwanese group speculated about altered prostaglandin (PG) metabolism as a common pathway for preterm birth, PPROM, and adenomyosis. There are several studies in support of PG changes in peritoneal and menstrual fluid from women with endometriosis [32,33]. Fernando and co-workers suggested that endometrial abnormalities may impair placentation. This is to some extent supported by the findings of aberrant expression of integrins and HOX genes which could affect endometrial receptivity and subsequent placentation [34,35]. However, it should be noted that none of the existing epidemiological studies have been able to confirm or deny these potential physiological explanations.

Conclusion

In contrast to many other areas of endometriosis, the field of pregnancy and endometriosis is largely unexplored. The effects of pregnancy on the disease are more or less unknown since many of the available publications are either obsolete or anecdotal. Moreover, questionnaire studies regarding pain experience and quality of life before and after pregnancy are completely absent. Animal models, especially non-human primates, may be one solution to this problem. These models allow for repeated laparoscopies before, during and after pregnancy, a crucial aspect in studies of disease progression/regression.

Until recently, obstetricians and gynecologists were unaware of the potential risks of endometriosis during pregnancy. Taking into consideration the changes in immunity and angiogenesis associated with endometriosis, the lack of risk analysis is remarkable. However, recent epidemiological studies have shed light on the association between endometriosis and adverse pregnancy outcome. The results from these studies strongly indicate an association between endometriosis and preterm birth. Due to conflicting results, an association with preeclampsia is less certain, although the largest study did show a positive correlation. There is also evidence suggesting that women with endometriosis are at risk for antepartum haemorrhage and subsequent cesarean section. Many of these findings are in agreement with observations of other chronic inflammatory diseases during pregnancy.

Endometriosis is a complex trait with multiple pathophysiological mechanisms. Some of these, including increased levels of PGs and endometrial abnormalities, may be related to obstetric events such as preterm birth, antepartum haemorrhage due to placental complication and preeclampsia. Endometriosis is common among women of child-bearing age and recent data provide important information in the search for etiological factors in preterm birth. From a clinical perspective, women with endometriosis may need extra attention during pregnancy.

References

1. Barnhart K, Dunsmoor-Su R, Coutifaris C. Effect of endometriosis on in vitro fertilization. Fertil Steril 2002;77:1148–1155.
2. Meigs JV. Endometrial hematomas of the ovary. Boston Med Surg J 1922;187:1–13.
3. Sampson JA. The life history of ovarian hematomas (hemorrhagic cysts) of endometrial (Mullerian) type. Am J Obstet Gynecol 1922;4:451.
4. Gainey HL, Keeler JE, Nicolay KS. Endometriosis in pregnancy, clinical observations. Am J Obstet Gynecol 1952;63:511–523.
5. Kistner RW. The treatment of endometriosis by inducing pseudopregnancy with ovarian hormones. Fertil Steril 1959;10: 539–555.
6. Andrews MC, Andrews WC, Strauss AF. Effects of progestin-induced pseudopregnancy on endometriosis: clinical and microscopic studies. Am J Obstet Gynecol 1959;78:776–785.
7. Scott RB, Wharton LR Jr. Effects of progesterone and norethindrone on experimental endometriosis in monkeys. Am J Obstet Gynecol 1962;84:867–875.
8. McArthur JW, Ulfelder H. The effect of pregnancy upon endometriosis. Obstet Gynecol Surv 1965;20:709–733.
9. Hanton EM, Malkasian GD, Dockerty MB, Pratt JH. Endometriosis: symptomatic during pregnancy. Am J Obstet Gynecol 1966;95: 1165–1166.
10. D'Hooghe TM, Bambra CS, de Jonge I, Lauweryns JM, Raeymaekers BM, Koninckx PR. The effect of pregnancy on endometriosis in

baboons (Papio anubis, Papio cynocephalus). Arch Gynecol Obstet 1997;261:15–19.

11. Schenken RS, Williams RF, Hodgen GD. Effect of pregnancy on surgically induced endometriosis in cynomolgus monkeys. Am J Obstet Gynecol 1987;157:1392–1396.

12. Barragan JC, Brotons J, Ruiz JA, Acien P. Experimentally induced endometriosis in rats: effect on fertility and the effects of pregnancy and lactation on the ectopic endometrial tissue. Fertil Steril 1992;58:1215–1219.

13. Adami HO, Trichopoulos D. Epidemiology, medicine and public health. Int J Epidemiol 1999;28:S1005–1008.

14. Zondervan KT, Cardon LR, Kennedy SH. What makes a good case-control study? Design issues for complex traits such as endometriosis. Hum Reprod 2002;17:1415–1423.

15. Thomson F, Shanbhag S, Templeton A, Bhattacharya S. Obstetric outcome in women with subfertility. Br J Obstet Gynaecol 2005;112: 632–637.

16. Skomsvoll JF, Ostensen M, Irgens LM, Baste V. Obstetrical and neonatal outcome in pregnant patients with rheumatic disease. Scand J Rheumatol 1998; 107(Suppl):109–112.

17. Cornish J, Tan E, Teare J et al. A meta-analysis on the influence of inflammatory bowel disease on pregnancy. Gut 2007;56:830–837.

18. Goldenberg RL, Culhane JF, Iams JD, Romero R. Epidemiology and causes of preterm birth. Lancet 2008;371:75–84.

19. Brosens IA, Robertson WB, Dixon HG. The role of the spiral arteries in the pathogenesis of preeclampsia. Obstet Gynecol Annu 1972;1:177–191.

20. Leyendecker G, Kunz G, Herbertz M et al. Uterine peristaltic activity and the development of endometriosis. Ann N Y Acad Sci 2004;1034: 338–355.

21. Cho SH, Oh YJ, Nam A et al. Evaluation of serum and urinary angiogenic factors in patients with endometriosis. Am J Reprod Immunol 2007;58:497–504.

22. Lockwood CJ, Krikun G, Caze R, Rahman M, Buchwalder LF, Schatz F. Decidual cell-expressed tissue factor in human pregnancy and its involvement in hemostasis and preeclampsia-related angiogenesis. Ann N Y Acad Sci 2008;1127:67–72.

23. Kortelahti M, Anttila MA, Hippelainen MI, Heinonen ST. Obstetric outcome in women with endometriosis – a matched case-control study. Gynecol Obstet Invest 2003;56:207–212.

24. Hadfield RM, Lain SJ, Raynes-Greenow CH, Morris JM, Roberts CL. Is there an association between endometriosis and the risk of pre-eclampsia? A population based study. Hum Reprod 2009;24: 2348–2352.

25. Juang CM, Chou P, Yen MS, Twu NF, Horng HC, Hsu WL. Adenomyosis and risk of preterm delivery. Br J Obstet Gynaecol 2007;114:165–169.

26. Bazot M, Cortez A, Darai E et al. Ultrasonography compared with magnetic resonance imaging for the diagnosis of adenomyosis: correlation with histopathology. Hum Reprod 2001;16: 2427–2433.

27. Fernando S, Breheny S, Jaques AM, Halliday JL, Baker G, Healy D. Preterm birth, ovarian endometriomata, and assisted reproduction technologies. Fertil Steril 2009;91:325–330.

28. Stephansson O, Kieler H, Granath F, Falconer H. Endometriosis, assisted reproduction technology, and risk of adverse pregnancy outcome. Hum Reprod 2009;24:2341–2347.

29. Cnattingius S, Ericson A, Gunnarskog J, Kallen B. A quality study of a medical birth registry. Scand J Soc Med 1990;18:143–148.

30. Helmerhorst FM, Perquin DA, Donker D, Keirse MJ. Perinatal outcome of singletons and twins after assisted conception: a systematic review of controlled studies. BMJ 2004;328:261.

31. Melin A, Sparen P, Persson I, Bergqvist A. Endometriosis and the risk of cancer with special emphasis on ovarian cancer. Hum Reprod 2006;21:1237–1242.

32. Bieglmayer C, Hofer G, Kainz C, Reinthaller A, Kopp B, Janisch H. Concentrations of various arachidonic acid metabolites in menstrual fluid are associated with menstrual pain and are influenced by hormonal contraceptives. Gynecol Endocrinol 1995;9: 307–312.

33. Karck U, Reister F, Schafer W, Zahradnik HP, Breckwoldt M. PGE2 and PGF2 alpha release by human peritoneal macrophages in endometriosis. Prostaglandins 1996;51:49–60.

34. Lessey BA, Castelbaum AJ. Integrins in the endometrium of women with endometriosis. Br J Obstet Gynaecol 1995;102:347–348.

35. Taylor HS, Bagot C, Kardana A, Olive D, Arici A. HOX gene expression is altered in the endometrium of women with endometriosis. Hum Reprod 1999;14:1328–1331.

52 Sexuality in Endometriosis

Brigitte Leeners

Clinic for Reproductive Endocrinology, University Hospital Zürich, Zürich, Switzerland

Introduction

Sexual quality of life is a multifactorial construct including desire, arousal, physical functioning, beliefs and values, comfort with sexual and emotional intimacy, sexual satisfaction, body image, self-esteem, etc. Endometriosis-associated symptoms may interfere with sexual function on all of these levels [1]. Consequently, adequate medical support includes addressing questions of sexual health. Unfortunately, in most countries, gynecologists are not trained in sexual issues and sexologists are lay persons with respect to endometriosis.

In addition, physicians as well as patients may still consider sexuality either a taboo or a non-medical style luxury issue. Therefore, sexual counseling and therapy have, until now, played no part in the routine care of women with endometriosis.

Factors involved in sexual disorders

Individual patient sexual functioning is determined by person-related pre-existing factors and disease-specific implications as well as the patient's and partner's general response to disease [2,3].

Person-related pre-existing factors

Person-related pre-existing factors include age, body image, general well-being, individual sexual needs, and fantasies [4]. An individual's personality and general attitude towards sexuality define the framework of their sexual life. One of the most stable predictors for sexual dysfunction after a distressing event is subjective satisfaction with previous sexual activity [5,6]. Although there is great interindividual variation of the development of sexuality throughout the lifespan, increasing age is associated with a higher risk for impaired sexual function. Body image has

an impact on sexual motivation, withdrawal, contact, behavior, and satisfaction [7–9]. Also cognitive, emotional and behavioral coping elements determine sexual function. Women who give up, lose hope, withdraw, catastrophize, focus on negative thoughts, and are depressed and anxious will have a greater risk of suffering from sexual difficulties or will avoid sexuality completely [10,11].

Last but not least, media messages, literature, art, and even scientific research transmit a model of human sexuality which is very much oriented towards male sexuality. Predominance of visual stimulation, focus on intercourse, and a linear model of sexual reaction reflect male sexual needs and experiences. Women's needs and experiences are socially much less represented and may therefore contribute to women's sexual insecurity and finally dissatisfaction [12].

Disease-specific implications

Endometriosis and its treatment side-effects may lead to reduced mobility, chronic pain, dyspareunia, and fatigue. Each of these symptoms is associated with impaired sexual function [12–16].

Removal of hormone-producing organs and medically induced hormonal changes, e.g. estrogen deficiency, may lead to vaginal dryness, hot flushes, palpitations, and sleep disturbances which may interfere with a fulfilling sexual life [17]. Clinical symptoms of endometriosis and side-effects from surgical and medical treatment may cause a loss of physical attractiveness, female identity, self-acceptance, and self-esteem which may in turn lead to sexual disorders.

For many couples, sexuality is at least during a certain phase of life combined with the wish for a child. When couples experience infertility, sexual activity may start to lack emotional involvement and spontaneity, be limited to fertile periods and be perceived to be of reduced value. In addition, the discovery that endometriosis interferes with reproduction may distort a patient's positive evaluation of her own body.

Endometriosis: Science and Practice, First Edition. Edited by Linda C. Giudice, Johannes L.H. Evers and David L. Healy.
© 2012 Blackwell Publishing Ltd. Published 2012 by Blackwell Publishing Ltd.

Anxiety and depression, which are at the same time well-known consequences of endometriosis and pathogenic factors in sexual function, may enhance avoidant behavior. Patients may develop subclinical disturbances that manifest primarily in the domain of sexuality [17–19]. At the same time, sexual problems may aggravate affective disorders [20].

Finally, endometriosis-associated symptoms may disturb affectionate relationships. Consequently, an important cause for lack of sexual activity in women with severe endometriosis is having no partner [21].

Patient's and partner's general response to disease

With the onset of disease symptoms, sexual possibilities as well as sexual needs may change considerably. Partners have to modify their sexual relationship as otherwise such changes may create chronic incongruence, conflict, and avoidance behavior [22,23]. An indispensable precondition to creating a new balance is adequate communication about sexual needs and limitations. A study investigating the effect of dyspareunia on sexuality of women suffering from endometriosis showed that 33% were unable to discuss this symptom with their partners [24]. Difficulties in communicating can cause loss of intimacy and emotional closeness, which then may result in sexual withdrawal.

Affective response, coping style, and changes in relationship dynamics will further determine sexual response to endometriosis of both partners [4]. Patients may sometimes express an increased need for tenderness and non-genital physical closeness, and need to feel that they are desired and that the partner is taking an active, positively aggressive role in sexuality. Also, the partner may experience difficulties in moving from the caretaker role to that of sexual partner. He might assume that the unwell woman does not want to be sexually active or even feel inadequate.

Endometriosis-related sexual disorders

According to the *International Classification of Diseases* (ICD) 10 and the *Diagnostic and Statistical Manual* (DSM) IV, a sexual dysfunction is present when the sexual symptom leads to personal distress and/or interpersonal difficulties. The leading symptom is endometriosis-related sexual pain and disturbances may occur on each level of the sexual response cycle: desire, arousal, orgasm, and resolution phase. However, there seems to be no correlation with endometriosis stage [25–29].

Dyspareunia

Deep dyspareunia is a frequent component of endometriosis-associated pain [30]. It is defined as painful intercourse with deep vaginal penetration. In contrast, pain with initial penetration of the vaginal introitus, called superficial, introital or entry dyspareunia, more likely has to be attributed to causes other than endometriosis [31]. Depending on onset of the symptoms, deep dyspareunia may be classified as primary or secondary, and both forms may be associated with endometriosis.

Epidemiology

Studies on endometriosis patients show prevalence rates of dyspareunia between 32.6% and 68.2% [16,24,26,32–35] which is higher than the prevalence of 8–41.2% found in women with chronic pelvic pain [36,37]. Also, the prevalence of primary deep dyspareunia, i.e. pain at first intercourse, is significantly higher among women with endometriosis than in controls [16]. Deep dyspareunia affects between 60% and 79% of women with endometriosis undergoing surgery [16,38–40] and between 53% and 90% of those using medical therapies [41,42]. More than 50% of women with endometriosis report having suffered from dyspareunia throughout their entire sex lives [16]. Luckily, a relatively high percentage of women diagnosed with endometriosis-related dyspareunia experience minimal to light forms of this symptom [24] but reliable data on this correlation are still insufficient.

Pathophysiology

In women with endometriosis, deep dyspareunia is most severe before menstruation and usually decreases with changing positions [43].

An association between dyspareunia and endometriosis on the uterosacral ligaments as well as the extent of pelvic adhesions has been described by several authors [27,30,38]. This correlation can be explained by the fact that the uterosacral ligaments contain a considerable amount of nerve tissue, including major nerve trunks, ganglia, and free nerve fibers with an important sensory and sensorimotor content [44,45]. Women with lesions on the uterosacral ligaments also show higher pain scores than women without this type of lesion. However, the presence of mono- or bilateral endometriotic lesions on the uterosacral ligament seems not to affect the intensity of dyspareunia.

Among subjects with dyspareunia, those with deep infiltrating endometriosis of the uterosacral ligament have the most severe impairment of sexual function, i.e. a reduced number of intercourses per week, less satisfying orgasm, and feeling less relaxed and fulfilled after sex. Women diagnosed with endometriosis who show no lesion of the uterosacral ligaments show the same frequency of intercourse as healthy controls; nevertheless they report a worse perception of their sexuality [16].

Moreover, rectovaginal endometriosis seems to be associated with dyspareunia [26]. The intraneural and perineural invasion in the rectovaginal endometriotic nodules is associated with pain severity [46]. Also dyspareunia is more frequently reported in women with only atypical endometriosis (that is, clear vesicles, clear or red papules, red polypoid lesions compared to typical lesions such as black nodules or stellate scars) [26]. However, there are also opposite results [47].

Besides an eventual neural and perineural invasion, dyspareunia seems to be the result of stretching of scarred and inelastic tissue, mechanical pressure on enlarged ovaries, endometriotic lesions, or adhesions, release of chemical mediators of pain or increased pelvic perfusion [26,38]. In addition, the immobilization of pelvic organs during coital activity may contribute to pathogenesis [43]. It remains speculative whether changes in the

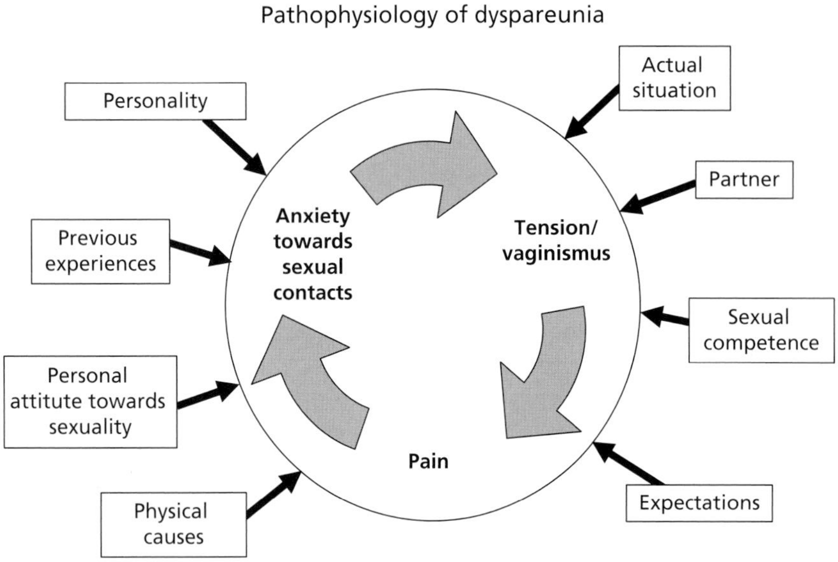

Pathophysiology of dyspareunia

Figure 52.1 Pathophysiological model of dyspareunia in endometriosis.

secretion of immune and neurological modulators, as well as the modified pain perception in women with endometriosis, are also involved in dyspareunia.

There is also increasing evidence for the role of neuropathic pain mechanisms in the pathophysiology of sexual pain disorders [48].

Differential diagnosis

Deep dyspareunia is a heterogeneous disorder, and other conditions may overlap with endometriosis, contributing to the pathogenesis of pain during intercourse. Pelvic adhesions, pelvic congestion, pelvic inflammatory disease, and interstitial cystitis may also cause deep dyspareunia [49–52].

Secondary sexual disorders

Dyspareunia has been associated with anxiety and a negative attitude toward sexuality [53,54]. When the cycle of pain, fear and more pain continues, women suffering from dyspareunia may avoid sexual intercourse altogether [53–57]. With regard to the pathophysiological role of the pelvic floor in sexual pain disorders, it is important to investigate vaginismus, which may be a secondary sexual disorder when dyspareunia is present as well as a co-morbidity (Fig. 52.1). Careful investigation of muscle tone/strength differences may help in differentiation [48]. The anticipation of pain is as destructive as the pain itself, inhibiting sexual desire and sexual arousal which prevents lubrication, hence making any subsequent pain worse [57]. When sexual arousal is impaired, women will also have more difficulty achieving orgasm. As a whole, sexual contact becomes less satisfying. Instead, it represents a source of pain and frustration.

Lack of sexual desire

The diagnosis "sexual desire/interest disorder" is described as a lack of interest in sexual activity and a lack of responsive sexual desire. Notably, the lack of spontaneous sexual desire before a sexual encounter has begun is not considered to be a sexual dysfunction.

Poor physical health is consistently found to be associated with decreased desire [57,58]. Sexual desire is also profoundly influenced by emotion. Repetitive experiences of failure increase personal vulnerability, performance anxiety, anger and distress, which can in a self-enforcing way maintain the sexual problem [57,59]. Disorders of the desire phase occur when anxiety occurs early in the cycle. Also, depressed mood is a leading cause of decreased desire [60].

Decline of sex steroid hormones due to medical and/or surgical treatment of endometriosis may be accompanied by a diminution of the biologically determined part of the sexual drive [61–63].

A low level of sexual desire, difficulty in arousal, and orgasm as well as sexual dissatisfaction are often associated with dyspareunia [58].

Sexual arousal disorder

Female sexual arousal has been conceptualized as a complex interaction between physiological and psychological components, which can be expressed as either a lack of subjective excitement or a lack of genital lubrication or swelling that results in distress. The presence or anticipation of pain may result in lower sexual arousal [57]. Also, consequences of surgery or side-effects of medical treatments, for example gonadotropin releasing hormone analogs, may lead to a reduced vascular supply, which may diminish lubrication and lead to changes in genital mucosa, resulting in discomfort and pain [61–63].

Vaginismus

Vaginismus is defined as persistent or recurrent difficulty of a woman to allow vaginal entry of penis, a finger or any object, despite the women's expressed wish to do so [64]. Affected women experience involuntary pelvic muscle contraction and fear or actually experience pain in sexual contact, resulting in avoidance of intercourse. In endometriosis, vaginismus most often occurs as a secondary disorder of dyspareunia.

Resistance to penetration resulting from fear of pain may provoke pelvic floor hypertonus, restricting vaginal entry and causing both dyspareunia and mechanical trauma of the vestibular mucosa and urethra. Pelvic floor muscles are indirectly innervated by the limbic system and are thus potentially reactive to emotional states; central nervous system changes have been confirmed in women with vaginismus [48,65].

Orgasm disorder

Women diagnosed with endometriosis believe significantly more often than healthy controls that pain affects their intensity of orgasm [16]. Also, women with dyspareunia may experience fewer orgasms [57]. To determine the relevance of such orgasm problems for sexual well-being, it is important to know that for women, orgasm is not always the most important factor in sexual satisfaction. Therefore, it has to be investigated in each individual woman whether quality and frequency of orgasm have indeed to be changed to achieve sexual fulfillment.

Secondary effects of impaired sexual activity

When sexuality becomes a domain associated with conflicts, often affectionate contacts and the closeness of partners are also perturbed. Women may not dare to initiate any affectionate contact because they are afraid that they will find themselves in a situation where they feel obliged to have intercourse. Most people perceive petting contact as less valuable than intercourse. If an attempt at a fulfilling sexual contact fails, both partners may remain frustrated so that each attempt at sexual activity is associated with a high risk for sexual dissatisfaction and resulting non-sexual strain on the partnership. Consequently, women with endometriosis and their partners need a higher motivation to start sexual contact compared to couples without any sexual disorders. As a result, sexual disorders resulting from endometriosis may create marital difficulties at a time when a woman needs support, affection, and intimacy from her partner. Sexual difficulties may lead to increased feelings of inadequacy and guilt [54]. While women with sexual disorders due to endometriosis worry that they are inadequate sexual partners and therefore sometimes force themselves to have intercourse despite intense pain, male partners also report not daring to initiate sexual contact because they fear hurting their partners. The strain sexual difficulties put on matrimonial relationships is an important factor in separation or marriage breakdown [66,67].

Diagnosis of sexual disorders

Even today, taking a sexual history is hampered by shame, the fact that sexuality is still a taboo subject and the lack of adequate education of gynecologists on how to diagnose and treat sexual disorders [4,12]. Women with endometriosis report that they feel embarrassed to discuss personal issues such as sexual function and/or dyspareunia with anyone [66,68]. Women may also estimate that sexual problems in the context of endometriosis are not important enough to be mentioned to their physicians. Consequently, they often experience particularly limited medical support in this domain [67]. However, an increasing knowledge about sexual aids has made patients aware of therapeutic possibilities and has increased their demand.

History taking

The diagnostic process for sexual dysfunction in endometriosis has to be multidimensional, including biological, psychological, and sociocultural factors [12]. It should carefully investigate person-related pre-existing factors and disease-specific implications as well as the patient's and partner's general response to endometriosis and the sexual problem. In order to adapt medical support to the couple's needs, physicians need to discuss how important sexual activity is for each single partner as well as both partners together and how much energy they want to spend to improve their sexual life.

As sexual problems are a frequent consequence of chronic endometriosis and as patients cannot be expected to take the initiative to discuss sexuality, physicians should actively offer to discuss sexual problems. Such an offer can be promoted either by a direct question on sexual activity when taking a history or by information brochures on sexuality, for example in waiting rooms. The latter approach shows a patient very discreetly that her doctor is willing to talk about her sexual health.

Gynecological examination

The exact location of pain spots should be identified by gynecological examination and assigned to anatomical structures. It has to be differentiated carefully whether pain might be due to endometriotic lesions, for example on the sacrouterine ligaments, or due to other causes of chronic pelvic pain. In cases of tightness of the levator ani, vaginismus should be suspected.

Clinical assessments lead to better results when the patient is informed about the aims of assessment and the pathophysiological background. It is imperative that the woman has control over the examination, i.e. that the gynecologist stops immediately if the patient wishes. Each step should be explained and before it is started, permission should be sought.

Therapeutic options

Surgery

If chronic pelvic pain can be reduced by surgery, this will also ameliorate sexual function. Many studies have proven the efficacy of radical excision of endometriotic lesions for the intensity of deep dyspareunia and the quality of sexual activity [21,39,69–74]. Different studies report improvement rates between 77.8% and 88.2% [70,71,75,76]. About 23–81% of women investigated report that dyspareunia disappeared completely after surgery [7,75]; however, data are scarce and differences in study groups with regard to the location of endometriotic lesions and/or the time of investigation in relation to surgery hamper a final conclusion with regard to effect size. Amelioration after surgical excision of endometriotic lesions seems to be better when lesions of the uterosacral ligaments are present [76]. In cases of dyspareunia due to deep rectovaginal endometriosis with rectal involvement, nodule excision has resulted in better outcomes than segmental resection [75].

Radical laparoscopic excision of endometriotic lesions has a positive effect on a variety of factors related to sexual function. Improvements have been demonstrated for sex life in general, desire, pleasure, reduction of dyspareunia/discomfort, habit, frequency, satisfaction level with orgasm, relaxation during and fulfillment after sexual activity [21,30,69–71,75,77]. Although long-term studies are lacking, currently available data show that such enhancement can be confirmed up to 2 years following surgery [70,71,78]. About 88% of women with deep dyspareunia prior to laparoscopy report satisfactory improvement when investigated 20 months after surgery [70].

Even though surgery may lead to significant improvement, sexual functions often remain impaired when endometriosis patients are compared to healthy control women [71]. After surgery, about 20% of women experience no change and a few patients even deteriorate [71]. Postoperative fibrosis resulting from dissection of the rectovaginal pouch of Douglas, shortening and narrowing of the upper vagina caused by closure and/or resection may contribute at least in part to some residual postoperative pain [60,79]. Also, surgery may induce new adhesions which result in additional pain. Horizontal closure of the vagina might help avoid narrowing of the upper part of the vagina and subsequent dyspareunia.

The importance of a uterus for female sexual satisfaction varies greatly. Consequently, the impact of hysterectomy is different in each individual case. Chronic pelvic pain is the main indication for hysterectomy in women with endometriosis. When hysterectomy succeeds in resolving pain, about 80–90% of women show an improvement of sexual function [60]. A subgroup of 10–20% of women report negative outcomes such as reduced sexual interest, arousal, and orgasm, as well as depressive symptoms and impaired body image [60]. There is little evidence to suggest that the removal of the uterus alone causes lowered sexual desire. However, hysterectomy with concurrent oophorectomy can result in low libido [60].

Several mechanisms have been suggested for the reduction in sexual arousal after hysterectomy. First, the reduced quantity of tissue resulting from removal of the uterus, cervix and/or vagina reduces pelvic vasocongestion [80]. Second, the disruption in the blood circulation may impair an adequate lubrication response [81]. Third, the formation of scar tissue may prevent the full ballooning of the vagina [60]. However, the empirical evidence with regard to changes in sexual arousal due to the removal of the uterus is weak. While hysterectomy seems to have no systematic negative effect on orgasmic potential in most women, again a subgroup of 15–25% appears to experience adverse changes in the frequency of orgasm [60]. In this context, the lack of uterine contractions and of a possibility for cervical stimulation after hysterectomy are potential underlying factors. Further, hysterectomy is theorized to cause depression because of the perceived loss of feminine self-image, strength, vitality and self-esteem, as well as feelings of deformation, mutilation, and the mourning of the loss of child-bearing capacity [60]. The wish for future children is correlated with posthysterectomy depression, independent of whether the woman has already borne children. Scarring following abdominal hysterectomy can be interpreted as a form of mutilation and may result in impaired body image.

Hormonal treatment

Continuous treatment with combined oral contraceptive pills, desogestrel-only contraceptive pill, cyproterone acetate, norethindrone acetate, or levonorgestrel-releasing intrauterine device may reduce the intensity of deep dyspareunia with limited side-effects [41,42,82]. Gonadotropin releasing hormone analogs may improve dyspareunia; however, the hypoestrogenic stage within the vagina leading to reduced lubrication as well as an increased risk for vaginal infections may require add-back therapy with local or systemic estrogens or drugs with estrogenic activity [31]. More recently, aromatase inhibitors have been proposed for the treatment of endometriosis. While a combination of letrozole and norethisterone acetate significantly reduced the severity of deep dyspareunia, pain recurred after the interruption of treatment [83]. These findings were confirmed in another study combining letrozole with the desogestrel-only contraceptive pill [84]. Recurrence of symptoms after interruption of treatment is a problem in any hormonal treatment of endometriosis-associated symptoms, which has not satisfactory been resolved yet. Although several drugs are currently under investigation for the treatment of endometriosis, it seems unlikely that they may effectively treat deep dyspareunia and other pain symptoms in all women with endometriotic lesions.

Sexual counseling

Sexual counseling may provide important support to enable women with endometriosis to establish a fulfilling sexual relationship. Gynecologists should actively offer to integrate sexual counseling into their healthcare. Basic sexual counseling includes the following.

• *Information:* many couples are not aware of the physiology and psychology of sexual function in general or of the potential endometriosis-specific consequences on sexuality. Explaining the sexual disorder(s) diagnosed and how endometriosis may influence sexuality is an important step in empowering the couple to better understand the limiting factors of their sexuality. A model of general predisposing, maintaining and disease-specific factors adapted to their individual situation should be discussed with the couple.

• *Communication:* communication difficulties represent a main factor leading to sexual problems in any couple as well as in couples where the woman is diagnosed with endometriosis. Therefore, it is important to help partners to communicate with regard to their sexual needs. Physicians may support the couple to become more aware of their often only semi-conscious concepts of sexuality which are not only partially unknown to themselves but are frequently completely unknown to the partner [12]. These concepts should be carefully adapted to the actual situation, i.e. basic conditions determined by endometriosis symptoms should be taken into account. Patients consider such help in communication as very important [12].

• *Range of sexual activities:* partners should be encouraged to broaden their sexual knowledge by experimenting with petting techniques in order to enrich their pain-free pleasurable sexual possibilities.

• *Positions:* in cases of dyspareunia, positions where the woman has control over movements and penetration depth are preferable [13,67]. A position where the woman is on top of her partner may facilitate intercourse as it allows ready control over angle and depth of vaginal penetration [85].

• *Referral to sexual therapist:* whenever deep dyspareunia or any other sexual problem persists despite adequate sexual counseling and a couple wants to improve sexual function, a referral to a sexual therapist, ideally a specialist who is familiar with endometriosis-associated symptoms, should be considered [30].

Sexual therapy

While sexual counseling can and should be offered by any physician with basic knowledge of sexual medicine, sexual therapy should only be performed by adequately trained sexual therapists. To give any interested physician an idea of the procedure and possibilities of sexual therapy, some of the established methods will be briefly described.

As both partners are involved in the development and persistence of a sexual problem, it is helpful to integrate both partners into sexual therapy. First, both partners' background of current sexuality should be investigated in detail. This includes the parents' attitude towards sexuality and nudeness, whether and from whom the patient received any sexual education, masturbation experiences as well as former partner sexual experiences from the first love to the current relationship. With the background of this history, a differentiated look at the actual sexual life helps to identify predisposing, precipitating and maintaining factors of the sexual problem(s).

The first important step in dealing with sexual dysfunction is to discuss the status quo and the aims of eventual sexual therapy with both partners, taking into account the limitations imposed by the disease. The explicit discussion of the objectives of therapy is a prerequisite to clarify the individual woman's and man's changes and whether these wishes coincide or not [12]. Communication about these issues helps couples to understand the advantages of the actual situation and to balance these advantages against the potential risk of any changes.

The spectrum of psychotherapeutic interventions reaches from individual body and fantasy-centered approaches such as body awareness and masturbation exercises to couple-oriented interventions which combine the classic sensate focus technique by Masters and Johnson with different psychotherapeutic approaches (psychodynamic, cognitive-behavioral and systemic) [12,86,87]. One of the basic elements of the psychotherapeutic interventions is to help the couple to create awareness of the blockages and destructive interventions which hinder desired change and to replace these patterns by either more effective repair mechanisms or new patterns of communication. A second common element is

the importance given to activating the resources and experiences both partners have. It is not so much the disclosure of defects, deficits and weaknesses, but much more the support of the individual strengths and shared experiences and history [12]. Finally, these approaches encourage the couples to learn about their own and their partner's often hidden sexual wishes and dreams, to express them, and to integrate them into a newly created sexual script [88]. Relaxation techniques, for example progressive relaxation, may be used to manage anxiety after unpleasant or painful sexual experiences [89].

Sensate focus programs are very effective in treating sexual disorders. A sensate focus program is a series of structured touching activities designed to help couples overcome anxiety and increase comfort with physical intimacy. Intercourse is initially banned and couples use homework exercises to gradually move through stages of intimacy to penetration [89]. The aims of this program are to improve communication between partners, to increase body awareness, to become able to influence body tension, especially in the pelvis, and to identify positive sexual stimuli. Also, partners learn creatively to increase their range of sexual techniques and to integrate their own needs and wishes into partner sexuality.

Treatment of vaginismus consist of education, counseling, and behavioral exercises [89]. The aim of treatment is to enable the woman to become more comfortable with her genitals, by teaching relaxation techniques to be used in conjunction with self-exploration of the genitals and insertion of "vaginal trainers." These are rods graduated in size and length which may help women to increase body awareness, i.e. tension of the vaginal wall. Such trainers can be integrated into a sensate focus program. It has to be emphasized that integrating rods into sexual therapy aims in no way to dilate the introitus. Indeed, any attempt at dilation is counterproductive in the therapy of vaginismus.

Prognosis

The prognosis of sexual disorders in endometriosis is strongly linked to pelvic pain and dyspareunia. Despite adequate application of currently available therapies, pain cannot be resolved in all women, so remaining pain will influence sexual function. In contrast, the prognosis of vaginismus is excellent when adequate sex therapy is performed [90,91]. In most couples, sexual counseling combined with sexual therapy allows them to realize a fulfilling and affectionate sexual life despite endometriosis-associated sexual symptoms.

Conclusion

Endometriosis disturbs sexual function and may lead to any of the known sexual disorders, i.e. dyspareunia, desire, arousal, orgasm disorder and vaginismus, with all the resulting secondary effects. Improvement based on pain reduction is limited, but adequate sexual counseling combined with sexual therapy when needed may enable couples to improve sexual satisfaction.

References

1. Hatzichristou D, Rosen RC, Broderick G et al. Clinical evaluation and management strategy for sexual dysfunction in men and women. J Sex Med 2004;1(1):49–57.

2. Segraves R, Woodard T. Female hypoactive sexual desire disorder: history and current status. J Sex Med 2006;3(3):408–418.

3. Nappi R, Salonia A, Traish AM et al. Clinical biologic pathophysiologies of women's sexual dysfunction. J Sex Med 2005;2(1):4–25.

4. Bitzer J, Platano G, Tschudin S, Alder J. Sexual counseling for women in the context of physical diseases: a teaching model for physicians. J Sex Med 2007;4(1):29–37.

5. Dennerstein L, Lehert P. Modeling mid-aged women's sexual functioning: a prospective, population-based study. J Sex Marital Ther 2004;30(3):173–183.

6. Moreira ED Jr, Kim SC, Glasser D, Gingell C. Sexual activity, prevalence of sexual problems, and associated help-seeking patterns in men and women aged 40–80 years in Korea: data from the Global Study of Sexual Attitudes and Behaviors (GSSAB). J Sex Med 2006;3(2):201–211.

7. Schover LR, Yetman RJ, Tuason LJ et al. Partial mastectomy and breast reconstruction. A comparison of their effects on psychosocial adjustment, body image, and sexuality. Cancer 1995;75(1):54–64.

8. Sheppard C, Whiteley R. Psychosexual problems after gynaecological cancer. J Br Menopause Soc 2006;12(1):24–27.

9. Basson R, Brotto LA, Laan E, Redmond G, Utian WH. Assessment and management of women's sexual dysfunctions: problematic desire and arousal. J Sex Med 2005;2(3):291–300 .

10. Devine D, Parker PA, Fouladi RT, Cohen L. The association between social support, intrusive thoughts, avoidance, and adjustment following an experimental cancer treatment. Psychooncology 2003;12(5):453–462.

11. Graziottin A, Basson R. Sexual dysfunction in women with premature menopause. Menopause 2004;11(6 Pt 2):766–777.

12. Bitzer J, Platano G, Tschudin S, Alder J. Sexual counseling in elderly couples. J Sex Med 2008;5(9):2027–2043.

13. Weinstein K. The emotional aspects of endometriosis: what the patient expects from her doctor. Clin Obstet Gynecol 1988;31(4):866–873.

14. Bodden-Heidrich R, Hilberink M, Frommer J et al. Qualitative research on psychosomatic aspects of endometriosis. Zsch Psychosom Med 1999;45:372–389.

15. Strauß B, Didzus A, Speidel H. A study concerning the psychosomatics of endometriosis. Psychother Psychosom Med Psychol 1992; 42:242–252.

16. Ferrero S, Esposito F, Abbamonte LH, Anserini P, Remorgida V, Ragni N. Quality of sex life in women with endometriosis and deep dyspareunia. Fertil Steril 2005;83(3):573–579.

17. Hawton K, Gath D, Day A. Sexual function in a community sample of middle-aged women with partners: effects of age, marital, socioeconomic, psychiatric, gynecological, and menopausal factors. Arch Sex Behav 1994;23(4):375–395.

18. Dunn KM, Croft PR, Hackett GI. Association of sexual problems with social, psychological, and physical problems in men and women: a cross sectional population survey. J Epidemiol Commun Health 1999;53(3):144–148.

19. Amsterdam A, Carter J, Krychman M. Prevalence of psychiatric illness in women in an oncology sexual health population: a retrospective pilot study. J Sex Med 2006;3(2):292–295.

20. Lindau ST, Schumm LP, Laumann EO, Levinson W, O'Muircheartaigh CA, Waite LJ. A study of sexuality and health among older adults in the United States. N Engl J Med 2007;357(8):762–774.

21. Garry R, Clayton R, Hawe J. The effect of endometriosis and its radical laparoscopic excision on quality of life indicators. Br J Obstet Gynaecol 2000;107(1):44–54.

22. Basson R, Leiblum S, Brotto L et al. Definitions of women's sexual dysfunction reconsidered: advocating expansion and revision. J Psychosom Obstet Gynaecol 2003;24(4):221–229.

23. Walker BL. Adjustment of husbands and wives to breast cancer. Cancer Pract 1997;5(2):92–98.

24. Oehmke F, Weyand J, Hackethal A, Konrad L, Omwandho C, Tinneberg HR. Impact of endometriosis on quality of life: a pilot study. Gynecol Endocrinol 2009;25(11):722–725.

25. Sinaii N, Plumb K, Cotton L et al. Differences in characteristics among 1,000 women with endometriosis based on extent of disease. Fertil Steril 2008;89(3):538–545.

26. Gruppo Italiano per lo Studio dell'Endometriosi. Relationship between stage, site and morphological characteristics of pelvic endometriosis and pain. Hum Reprod 2001;16(12):2668–2671.

27. Porpora MG, Koninckx PR, Piazze J, Natili M, Colagrande S, Cosmi EV. Correlation between endometriosis and pelvic pain. J Am Assoc Gynecol Laparosc 1999;6(4):429–434.

28. Vercellini P, Trespidi L, de Giorgi O, Cortesi I, Parazzini F, Crosignani PG. Endometriosis and pelvic pain: relation to disease stage and localization. Fertil Steril 1996;65(2):299–304.

29. Parazzini F, Ferraroni M, Fedele L, Bocciolone L, Rubessa S, Riccardi A. Pelvic endometriosis: reproductive and menstrual risk factors at different stages in Lombardy, northern Italy. J Epidemiol Commun Health 1995;49(1):61–64.

30. Ferrero S, Abbamonte LH, Giordano M, Ragni N, Remorgida V. Deep dyspareunia and sex life after laparoscopic excision of endometriosis. Hum Reprod 2007;22(4):1142–1148.

31. Ferrero S, Ragni N, Remorgida V. Deep dyspareunia: causes, treatments, and results. Curr Opin Obstet Gynecol 2008; 20(4):394–399.

32. Fagervold B, Jenssen M, Hummelshoj L, Moen MH. Life after a diagnosis with endometriosis – a 15 years follow-up study. Acta Obstet Gynecol Scand 2009;88(8):914–919.

33. Matalliotakis IM, Cakmak H, Fragouli YG, Goumenou AG, Mahutte NG, Arici A. Epidemiological characteristics in women with and without endometriosis in the Yale series. Arch Gynecol Obstet 2008;277(5):389–393.

34. Flores I, Abreu S, Abac S, Fourquet J, Laboy J, Rios-Bedoya C. Self-reported prevalence of endometriosis and its symptoms among Puerto Rican women. Int J Gynaecol Obstet 2008;100(3):257–261.

35. Carlton D. Awareness of endometriosis. Practice Nurse 1996;12:514–515.

36. Latthe P, Latthe M, Say L, Gulmezoglu M, Khan KS. WHO systematic review of prevalence of chronic pelvic pain: a neglected reproductive health morbidity. BMC Public Health 2006;6:177.

37. Zondervan KT, Yudkin PL, Vessey MP et al. Chronic pelvic pain in the community – symptoms, investigations, and diagnoses. Am J Obstet Gynecol 2001;184(6):1149–1155.

38. Fauconnier A, Chapron C, Dubuisson JB, Vieira M, Dousset B, Breart G. Relation between pain symptoms and the anatomic location of deep infiltrating endometriosis. Fertil Steril 2002;78(4):719–726.

39. Chopin N, Vieira M, Borghese B et al. Operative management of deeply infiltrating endometriosis: results on pelvic pain symptoms according to a surgical classification. J Minim Invasive Gynecol 2005;12(2):106–112.

40. Nardo LG, Moustafa M, Gareth Beynon DW. Laparoscopic treatment of pelvic pain associated with minimal and mild endometriosis with use of the Helica Thermal Coagulator. Fertil Steril 2005;83(3):735–738.

41. Fedele L, Bianchi S, Zanconato G, Portuese A, Raffaelli R. Use of a levonorgestrel-releasing intrauterine device in the treatment of rectovaginal endometriosis. Fertil Steril 2001;75(3):485–488.

42. Vercellini P, de Giorgi O, Mosconi P, Stellato G, Vicentini S, Crosignani PG. Cyproterone acetate versus a continuous monophasic oral contraceptive in the treatment of recurrent pelvic pain after conservative surgery for symptomatic endometriosis. Fertil Steril 2002; 77(1):52–61.

43. Olive DL, Blackwell RE, Copperman AB. Endometriosis and pelvic pain. In: Blackwell RE, Olive DL, editors. Chronic Pelvic Pain. New York: Springer-Verlag, 1998. pp. 61–83.

44. Butler-Manuel SA, Buttery LD, A'Hern RP, Polak JM, Barton DP. Pelvic nerve plexus trauma at radical and simple hysterectomy: a quantitative study of nerve types in the uterine supporting ligaments. J Soc Gynecol Invest 2002;9(1):47–56.

45. Butler-Manuel SA, Buttery LD, A'Hern RP, Polak JM, Barton DP. Pelvic nerve plexus trauma at radical hysterectomy and simple hysterectomy: the nerve content of the uterine supporting ligaments. Cancer 2000;89(4):834–841.

46. Anaf V, Simon P, El Nakadi I et al. Relationship between endometriotic foci and nerves in rectovaginal endometriotic nodules. Hum Reprod 2000;15(8):1744–1750.

47. Vercellini P, Bocciolone L, Vendola N, Colombo A, Rognoni MT, Fedele L. Peritoneal endometriosis. Morphologic appearance in women with chronic pelvic pain. J Reprod Med 1991;36(7):533–536.

48. Weijmar Schultz W, Basson R, Binik Y, Eschenbach D, Wesselmann U, van Lankveld J. Women's sexual pain and its management. J Sex Med 2005;2(3):301–316.

49. Beard RW, Reginald PW, Wadsworth J. Clinical features of women with chronic lower abdominal pain and pelvic congestion. Br J Obstet Gynaecol 1988;95(2):153–161.

50. Steege JF, Ling FW. Dyspareunia. A special type of chronic pelvic pain. Obstet Gynecol Clin North Am 1993;20(4):779–793.

51. Koziol JA, Clark DC, Gittes RF, Tan EM. The natural history of interstitial cystitis: a survey of 374 patients. J Urol 1993;149(3):465–469.

52. Parsons CL, Dell J, Stanford EJ et al. Increased prevalence of interstitial cystitis: previously unrecognized urologic and gynecologic cases identified using a new symptom questionnaire and intravesical potassium sensitivity. Urology 2002;60(4):573–578.

53. Meana M, Binik YM, Khalife S, Cohen DR. Biopsychosocial profile of women with dyspareunia. Obstet Gynecol 1997;90(4 Pt 1):583–589.

54. Jones G, Jenkinson C, Kennedy S. The impact of endometriosis upon quality of life: a qualitative analysis. J Psychosom Obstet Gynaecol 2004;25(2):123–133.

55. Walker E, Katon W, Jones LM, Russo J. Relationship between endometriosis and affective disorder. Am J Psychiatry 1989; 146(3):380–381.

56. Low WY, Edelmann RY. Psychosocial aspects of endometriosis: a review. J Psychosom Obset Gynaecol 1991;12:3–12.

57. Laumann EO, Paik A, Rosen RC. Sexual dysfunction in the United States: prevalence and predictors. JAMA 1999;281(6):537–544.

58. Carey JC. Disorders of sexual desire and arousal. Obstet Gynecol Clin North Am 2006;33(4):549–564.

59. Althof SE, Leiblum SR, Chevret-Measson M et al. Psychological and interpersonal dimensions of sexual function and dysfunction. J Sex Med 2005;2(6):793–800.

60. Flory N, Bissonnette F, Binik YM. Psychosocial effects of hysterectomy: literature review. J Psychosom Res 2005;59(3):117–129.

61. Bachmann GA, Leiblum SR. The impact of hormones on menopausal sexuality: a literature review. Menopause 2004; 11(1):120–130.

62. Myers LS, Dixen J, Morrissette D, Carmichael M, Davidson JM. Effects of estrogen, androgen, and progestin on sexual psychophysiology and behavior in postmenopausal women. J Clin Endocrinol Metab 1990; 70(4):1124–1131.

63. Dennerstein L, Dudley EC, Hopper JL, Burger H. Sexuality, hormones and the menopausal transition. Maturitas 1997;26(2):83–93.

64. Basson R, Althof S, Davis S et al. Summary of the recommendations on sexual dysfunctions in women. J Sex Med 2004;1(1):24–34.

65. Frasson E, Graziottin A, Priori A et al. Central nervous system abnormalities in vaginismus. Clin Neurophysiol 2009;120(1):117–122.

66. Cox H, Henderson L, Andersen N, Cagliarini G, Ski C. Focus group study of endometriosis: struggle, loss and the medical merry-go-round. Int J Nurs Pract 2003;9(1):2–9.

67. Denny E. Women's experience of endometriosis. J Adv Nurs 2004;46(6):641–648.

68. Denny E. "You are one of the unlucky ones": delay in the diagnosis of endometriosis. Div Health Soc Care 2004;1:39–44.

69. Chapron C, Dubuisson JB. Laparoscopic treatment of deep endometriosis located on the uterosacral ligaments. Hum Reprod 1996; 11(4):868–873.

70. Chapron C, Dubuisson JB, Fritel X et al. Operative management of deep endometriosis infiltrating the uterosacral ligaments. J Am Assoc Gynecol Laparosc 1999;6(1):31–37.

71. Anaf V, Simon P, El Nakadi I, Simonart T, Noel J, Buxant F. Impact of surgical resection of rectovaginal pouch of Douglas endometriotic nodules on pelvic pain and some elements of patients' sex life. J Am Assoc Gynecol Laparosc 2001;8(1):55–60.

72. Abbott JA, Hawe J, Clayton RD, Garry R. The effects and effectiveness of laparoscopic excision of endometriosis: a prospective study with 2–5 year follow-up. Hum Reprod 2003;18(9):1922–1927.

73. Seracchioli R, Poggioli G, Pierangeli F et al. Surgical outcome and long-term follow up after laparoscopic rectosigmoid resection in women with deep infiltrating endometriosis. Br J Obstet Gynaecol 2007;114(7):889–895.

74. Abbott J, Hawe J, Hunter D, Holmes M, Finn P, Garry R. Laparoscopic excision of endometriosis: a randomized, placebo-controlled trial. Fertil Steril 2004;82(4):878–884.

75. Roman H, Loisel C, Resch B et al. Delayed functional outcomes associated with surgical management of deep rectovaginal endometriosis with rectal involvement: giving patients an informed choice. Hum Reprod 2010;25(4):890–899.

76. Ferrero S, Abbamonte LH, Parisi M, Ragni N, Remorgida V. Dyspareunia and quality of sex life after laparoscopic excision of endometriosis and postoperative administration of triptorelin. Fertil Steril 2007;87(1):227–229.

77. Kristensen J, Kjer JJ. Laparoscopic laser resection of rectovaginal pouch and rectovaginal septum endometriosis: the impact on pelvic pain and quality of life. Acta Obstet Gynecol Scand 2007; 86(12):1467–1471.

78. Dubernard G, Piketty M, Rouzier R, Houry S, Bazot M, Darai E. Quality of life after laparoscopic colorectal resection for endometriosis. Hum Reprod 2006;21(5):1243–1247.

79. Aumeerally Z, Lilford RJ, Johnson NJ. The disappearing vagina syndrome. Eur J Obstet Gynecol Reprod Biol 1996;69(2):141–142.

80. Meston CM. The effects of hysterectomy on sexual arousal in women with a history of benign uterine fibroids. Arch Sex Behav 2004; 33(1):31–42.

81. Thakar R, Manyonda I, Stanton SL, Clarkson P, Robinson G. Bladder, bowel and sexual function after hysterectomy for benign conditions. Br J Obstet Gynaecol 1997;104(9):983–987.

82. Vercellini P, Pietropaolo G, de Giorgi O, Pasin R, Chiodini A, Crosignani PG. Treatment of symptomatic rectovaginal endometriosis with an estrogen-progestogen combination versus low-dose norethindrone acetate. Fertil Steril 2005;84(5):1375–1387.

83. Remorgida V, Abbamonte HL, Ragni N, Fulcheri E, Ferrero S. Letrozole and norethisterone acetate in rectovaginal endometriosis. Fertil Steril 2007;88(3):724–726.

84. Remorgida V, Abbamonte LH, Ragni N, Fulcheri E, Ferrero S. Letrozole and desogestrel-only contraceptive pill for the treatment of stage IV endometriosis. Aust N Z J Obstet Gynaecol 2007;47(3):222–225.

85. Steege JF, Lamvu GM, Zolnoun D. Treatment of pain associated with endometriosis. In: Sutton C, Jones K, Adamson GD, editors. Modern Management of Endometriosis. London: Taylor and Francis, 2005, pp. 273–287.

86. Masters WH, Johnson VE. Human Sexual Inadequacy. Boston, MA: Little, Brown, 1970.

87. Levine SB, Risen CB, Althof SE. Handbook of Clinical Sexology for Mental Health Professionals. New York: Houve Brunner Routledge, 2003.

88. Althof SE, Banner L. Difficult cases: psychologic treatment of desire, arousal and orgasm disorders. In: Goldstein I, Meston CM, Davis SR, Traish AM, editors. Women's Sexual Function and Dysfunction: Study, Diagnosis and Treatment. London: Taylor and Francis, 2006, pp. 462–467.

89. Crowley T, Goldmeier D, Hiller J. Diagnosing and managing vaginismus. BMJ 2009;338:b2284.

90. Jeng CJ, Wang LR, Chou CS, Shen J, Tzeng CR. Management and outcome of primary vaginismus. J Sex Marital Ther 2006;32(5):379–387.

91. McGuire H, Hawton K. Interventions for vaginismus. Cochrane Database Syst Rev 2001;2:CD001760.

53   Psychosomatic Aspects

Brigitte Leeners

Clinic for Reproductive Endocrinology, University Hospital Zürich, Zürich, Switzerland

Introduction

With a prevalence of 7–10%, endometriosis is one of the most common gynecological diseases in women during their reproductive period [1,2]. Symptoms of endometriosis include a broad spectrum, from accidental diagnosis without clinical significance to a chronic disabling disease [3]. About 20% of women show recurrent disease symptoms, especially pelvic pain, within 12 months after treatment and another 50% within 5 years, independent of the treatment implemented [4,5]. Endometriosis seems to be one of the chronic gynecological conditions with the most negative effect on women's lives [6].

Surprisingly, there has been little research which explores the reality of living with endometriosis. Although it is evident that a chronic painful disease such as endometriosis will have an important impact on health-related quality of life, the research on psychosomatic aspects of the disease is only in its infancy. Medical support tends to concentrate on somatic therapies and offers little help to integrate a chronic disease into daily life. Accordingly, current models for medical support lack adequate strategies regarding psychosomatic aspects of the disease.

The interface between gynecology and mental health has only recently become a subject of research. In particular, the investigation of psychosomatic aspects in specific gynecological disorders is a very young field. The prevailing method of managing disease and conducting research is based on a biomedical model that targets organic causes of disease, but there is increasing recognition of the benefits of adapting a biopsychosocial model to clinical practice and research. In applying a biopsychosocial approach, the psychological and social determinants of disease are considered simultaneously with the biological ones as factors which act by predisposing, precipitating, and maintaining the progression of the disease condition [7]. If medical investigators overlook the psychosocial aspect when making a differential diagnosis for a condition with a biopsychosocial etiology, efficient evaluation as well as treatment are hampered [7]. A psychosomatic approach to management can also increase patient compliance, and prevent the overutilization of healthcare resources [8].

As a whole, the methodological quality of the currently available literature on psychosomatic aspects of endometriosis is poor. Most publications are based on clinical experiences, while the few systematic investigations present results from small study groups, show methodological deficits, and do not differentiate between stages of disease. Many reports lack accurate differentiation between causes and effects. Consequently, the results of many studies should be treated with considerable caution. Studies reporting psychosocial interventions in the management of chronic pelvic pain in endometriosis are missing. Despite these limitations, results from existing studies give us an idea where to put the focus of future research projects.

This chapter will summarize current knowledge on psychosomatic aspects of endometriosis based on clinical experiences and qualitative research as well as the few systematic investigations available.

Psychosomatic and psychosocial factors in the genesis of endometriosis

Few authors consider psychosomatic factors as being causally involved in the development of endometriosis.

Gender role conflicts

Collins [9] assumed that chronic emotional disturbances based on a gender role conflict might first provoke dysfunctions of the pelvic organs, which would later lead to morphologically verifiable disease. A comparison of women with endometriosis to healthy controls more often showed conflicts with parents during childhood, a lower

Endometriosis: Science and Practice, First Edition. Edited by Linda C. Giudice, Johannes L.H. Evers and David L. Healy.
© 2012 Blackwell Publishing Ltd. Published 2012 by Blackwell Publishing Ltd.

interest of fathers in their daughters and a problematic attitude towards sexuality in the family [10]. The authors take these findings as a cause for an increased uncertainty of gender identity, which is associated with an augmented risk for endometriosis. However, as this investigation was retrospective, it should be interpreted with caution. Strauss *et al* [11] found specific gender role conflicts in women diagnosed with endometriosis, which present predominantly as a negative perception of menarche and puberty with early manifestation of gynecological disorders and negative sexual experiences. According to their results, part of this perception has to be attributed to increased fearfulness and oversensitivity towards physical changes in women with endometriosis.

Perception of menstruation

A rejection of menstruation stimulated by family convictions, a culturally fixed judgment of menstruation as something dirty/malodorous as well as menstruation as a cause for mood swings and reduced resilience in women are also discussed as potential causes of endometriosis [12]. The underlying hypothesis is based on the idea that (unconscious) rejection of menstruation might lead to dysmenorrhea, which could facilitate retrograde menstruation by unphysiological uterine contractions and consequently enable transfer of basal cells into the abdominal cavity.

Sexual abuse

An increasing number of research results confirm that chronic pelvic pain is associated with sexual abuse experiences [13,14]. Also several studies have shown a correlation between physical abuse during childhood as well as lifetime sexual abuse and endometriosis [15,16]. In 2006, Belaisch and Allart formulated the hypothesis that traumatic events during childhood could have an unfavorable effect on the immune system and psychoneuroendocrinological regulation processes which facilitate the development of endometriosis [17]. According to the clinical experiences of the authors, women with endometriosis more frequently report sexual abuse experiences than women without endometriosis, which was confirmed by quantitative research results [18]. Furthermore, sexual abuse experiences may be associated with increased pain perception [19]. However, underlying pathophysiological mechanisms explaining how sexual abuse experiences can contribute to the development of endometriosis remain unclear.

Psychosomatic strain/stress

Psychosomatic strain may represent a further factor in the etiopathology of endometriosis. Harrison *et al* presented a woman with endometriosis who showed an increased number of familial psychosomatic strain situations which led to a higher stress level with the resulting psychoneuroendocrinological changes when compared to a healthy control woman [20]. Differences between both women and both families were present in at least three generations. Differences were demonstrated in modifications of the electroencephalogram (EEG), digital skin temperature, dermal reaction to electrical impulses, and electromyography. The authors assume that such differences could also be confirmed

in a larger study group and interpret these changes as being involved in the etiopathology of endometriosis.

The following arguments have been used in the discussion of whether endometriosis might to some extent be a consequence of stress

• Stress is known to be associated with abnormalities of the immune system [21] and a variety of basic research results confirm that immunological reactions are involved in the genesis of endometriosis [22].
• Stress may lead to modifications of the endocrine system and different endocrinological changes have been described in endometriosis.
• An increased release of catecholamines and prostaglandin E_2 which modifies uterine and tubal motility may represent a pathophysiological link between the psyche and endometriosis [17].

However, women with endometriosis have been demonstrated to show a pathological reaction to stress. The secretion of cortisol under stressful conditions provides a protection for the organism, including mobilization of energy supplies and suppression of immune/inflammatory responses [23]. Although endometriosis patients show higher levels of perceived stress than controls, they present hypocortisolism which seems to be independent of pain and mental health [23]. Recent evidence has shown that insufficient glucocorticoid signaling (hypocortisolism) may play a role in the development and expression of pathology in stress-related disorders [24]. When accompanied by hypocortisolemia, these disorders can share a syndrome characterized by a triad of enhanced stress sensitivity, pain, and fatigue [23,25]. Hypocortisolemia may promote increased vulnerability to autoimmune disorders, inflammation, and chronic pain [23]. Whether hypocortisolism is an adaptive response to the aversive symptoms of the disorder or a feature related to the etiology of endometriosis remains to be elucidated [23].

Although there is a correlation between stress and immunological as well as endocrinological changes, there are currently no data confirming a pathophysiological mechanism between stress and the development of endometriosis on an immunological or endocrine basis. Before stress can be investigated as an underlying pathophysiological factor acting on immune and endocrinological factors in the development of endometriosis, the role of these factors in the development of the disease has to be clarified.

Depression

Few reports raise the question of whether depression represents a predisposing factor for endometriosis. However, currently it seems more likely that depression is a consequence and not a cause of the disease [26–28].

Personality

The correlation between specific features of personality and endometriosis is controversial [9,13,29].

Psychosocial factors

Because of its association with a delay in child bearing and a diminished number of pregnancies, endometriosis has been described as a disease of career women, which is more likely a result than a cause of the disease [27,30]. Women diagnosed with endometriosis tend to be from a higher social class [31]. However, such class-dependent prevalence rates might also be due to diagnostic failure in lower social classes [32]. Single investigations report a higher prevalence in women with a lower socio-economic background [13]. Conversely, specific risk factors in these women may not be identified yet. Hence, endometriosis is a disease which has to be diagnosed in any social class.

Indirect effect through modification of risk factors

Theoretically psychological factors can have an indirect effect through their influence on different health risk behaviors. Data on the relationship between alcohol, coffee, smoking, and endometriosis risk are limited and controversial [33–35]. Consequently, the psychological influence of such factors does not seem to play a major role in the development of endometriosis.

Summary

Currently, the question of whether psychological factors are a cause or a consequence of endometriosis cannot fully be answered [36]. No systematic methodologically well-designed studies on these correlations are available. Especially, longitudinal studies allowing differentiation between causes and symptoms of endometriosis are lacking. As today we know that retrograde menstruation is physiological but only about 10% of women develop endometriosis [37], any psychosomatic factor postulated to augment retrograde menstruation loses its significance. Future investigations will have to prove which interactions between psyche, endocrine, and immune system wll increase the risk for endometriosis.

Diagnostic delay

The average time between first symptoms and diagnosis is more than 6 years in Australia and Norway, 7 years in Brazil, nearly 8 years in England, and between 6 and more than 11 years in the USA [38–42]. Variations in reported delays were large in all studies, with a range from 0 to 44 years [38,39]. This diagnostic delay in endometriosis can be attributed to a variety of reasons.

• *Subjectivity of disease symptoms:* besides infertility, the effects of endometriosis are subjective and difficult to quantify [43]. It is also difficult to decide whether symptoms represent minor inconveniences or demand immediate effective therapies [44].

• *Unspecificity of symptoms:* the symptoms and complications of endometriosis are not specific and overlap with symptoms of other gynecological or non-gynecological conditions such as pelvic inflammatory disease or irritable bowel syndrome [45,46]. In fact, many women with endometriosis and pain also have other painful pelvic conditions. Consequently, correct diagnosis may be hampered by co-morbidity.

• *Diversity of symptoms:* the few investigations designed to determine the influence of clinical symptoms, i.e. pelvic pain and infertility, on diagnostic delay report controversial results [40,41].

• *Interpretation of symptoms:* if women have had painful menstrual periods from menarche and/or their mothers have experienced similar symptoms, they tend to consider such menstruation as normal [47]. As it may be difficult to make clear distinctions between normal and abnormal menstrual experiences [47], some women are misguidedly taught to view disease symptoms as normal [40,48]. Consequently, no medical investigation is started and women do not think of/dare to seek more adequate medical care [42,48].

• *Confidence in patients' reports:* attitudes among gynecologists and general practitioners of not taking women's description of symptoms such as period pain seriously lead to a delayed diagnosis [48]. If doctors do not listen attentively and try to understand their patient's complaints, they fail to comprehend the full picture of her situation. Such an attitude is one more reason why no medical support is provided; women doubt their symptoms and hesitate to seek medical support.

• *Psychologizing of disease symptoms:* often physicians falsely label symptoms as psychogenic [49,50]. Symptoms of clinical disease in women are more likely than in men to be labeled neurotic or their complaints as psychogenic [51]. Transvaginal ultrasound may lead to an incorrect exclusion of endometriosis. A false psychogenic interpretation will lead to referral to a psychiatrist or psychologist, i.e. specialists who are even less well educated about endometriosis than the referring physician [48,49].

• *Embarrassment:* embarrassment as well as the fear of appearing weak and unable to cope with disease symptoms may inhibit women from disclosing endometriosis-associated symptoms [47].

• *Socio-economic factors:* no correlation has been found between the patient's years of formal school education and the time interval for a diagnosis of endometriosis [40]. Data investigating the influence of socio-economic level on diagnostic delay are controversial [13,27,30,31,52].

• *Age at onset of disease symptoms:* the diagnostic delay in women whose pain symptoms begin during adolescence is particularly long, i.e. about 9 years longer than in adults [40,53]. In addition to the factors mentioned above, adolescents might be less convincing and persuasive than older women when reporting symptoms, and may feel even more uncomfortable when reporting dysmennorhea or dyspareunia [40].

• *Limited value of clinical examination:* clinical examination may be helpful, and abnormal clinical findings correlate with laparoscopic finding in 70–90% [54]. However, more than 50% of cases with laparoscopy-proven endometriosis have normal findings on preoperative pelvic examination [55].

• *Surgery as the only possibility for histologically confirmed diagnosis:* diagnostic laparoscopy and excisional biopsy, which is the gold standard for a histologically confirmed diagnosis [56], are invasive procedures with distinct morbidity and even mortality [54]. Diagnostic laparoscopy carries an estimated risk of death of 0.1/1000 and the risk of injury to bowel, bladder, or blood vessel of 2.4%, of which two-thirds will require a laparotomy [57,58]. Consequently, medical healthcare providers hesitate to decide in favor of surgery when they are confronted with menstrual pain.

One-third of all diagnostic laparoscopies reveal endometriosis, one-third reveal no visible pathology, and the remaining third demonstrate other gynecological conditions [59–61]. Thus, two-thirds of these patients do not have endometriosis and it is questionable whether such outcome is adequate to justify laparoscopy [54]. Even when endometriosis is found, there is no guarantee that it is the cause of pain. In addition, a negative result from diagnostic laparoscopy may be detrimental to women's emotional well-being [62].

• *Lack of histological confirmation of diagnosis:* recent guidelines in the UK [63] and in the USA [64–66] suggest performing laparoscopy for pelvic pain as a second-line investigation in the event of failed therapeutic intervention. The response to gonadotropin releasing hormone (GnRH) agonists is considered to be sufficient for (preliminary) diagnosis. As there is no histological confirmation of endometriosis, some women may not experience this approach as a reliable diagnosis and therefore feel insecure.

Doctor and patient contribution to diagnostic delay

With respect to who is responsible for the delay, study results are controversial. One study shows that the major part of the diagnostic delay takes place after the woman has consulted a physician [39], but opposite results, i.e. patients and physicians contributing equally to the delay, have been reported too [42,56]. Even if women belatedly seek medical care, it has to be discussed critically how far doctors add to this delay by lacking adequate support in interpreting and investigating clinical symptoms of endometriosis.

Psychosomatic/psychosocial effects of diagnostic delay and potential advantages of early diagnosis

The increasing knowledge about psychosomatic aspects of endometriosis highlights the importance of an early diagnosis for women who suffer at physical, emotional, and social levels when they remain undiagnosed [40,47,67]. The absence of a specific diagnosis leaves women fearful about the cause of their pain [39,54,68]. Suspicion about life-threatening diseases such as cancer or rare/unknown disease without any established medical cure may increase anxiety [47,48]. Reality is often less frightening than introspection about the nature and extent of disease [67].

A concrete diagnosis enables women to communicate their difficulties to others, particularly their employers, and may therefore improve access to social support [39,47,54]. Diagnosis also legitimizes absences from social and role/work obligations. Moreover, an early diagnosis allows initiation of specific treatment and therefore increases a sense of control over the condition, helps to reduce pain as well as absenteeism at school or work and makes sexual intercourse more enjoyable for those with pelvic pain [39,40,47]. In addition, gynecologists can give advice about family planning, including a selection of contraceptive methods [39]. If it comes to management of fertility problems, adequate therapy could be initiated earlier [53].

Women suffering from (undiagnosed) endometriosis-associated pain will continue their attempts to receive adequate treatment which will result in a higher number of physicians seen before a definite diagnosis, with all the resulting costs for the patients as well as for the general healthcare system [56].

However, not all women may benefit from early diagnosis. For the proportion of patients with severe invasive disease, early diagnosis and institution of appropriate treatments will probably minimize the severity and consequences of the disease.

Doctor–patient relationship

The doctor–patient relationship is increasingly recognized as a critical component of effective healthcare [8,69,70]. In addition to its impact on comfort and satisfaction, a functioning doctor–patient rapport can augment motivation for adequate medical and psychological healthcare [8]. Physician attention may operate in various ways. On the one hand, listening more intently to patients provides more information. On the other hand, patients may interpret this attention either as an indication of respect or of being interested in their welfare, and thus be more motivated to seek high-quality care [8].

Qualitative research using interviews shows that encounters with healthcare professionals in the context of endometriosis are often experienced as inadequate [48]. A major point of criticism is that symptoms of endometriosis are trivialized, not taken seriously or dismissed [4,48,71–73]. As endometriosis causes major physical and psychological problems, the relationship between doctor and patient is under considerable strain. The currently limited and often not satisfying surgical and/or hormonal options may cause feelings of helplessness in physicians, which may interfere with adequate medical care [45]. An extensive workload, lack of experience, limited medical knowledge, the impression that information could have a negative effect on the patient's well-being and the avoidance of their own stress can be reasons to prevent physicians providing adequate medical counseling.

Despite the difficulties in the doctor–patient relationship, gynecologists are considered a main source of support for women with endometriosis. Endometriosis patients seem to desire a close relationship and expect psychological support from their doctor. Surprisingly, support from third parties, i.e. psychologists, self-help groups, patient seminars, and counselors, seems to be less important [74].

Psychosomatic and psychosocial consequences of diagnosed endometriosis

The following text provides information on psychosomatic/psychosocial effects experienced in women with chronically relapsing endometriosis, which, due to symptoms of the disease such as pain, infertility, etc., results in reduced quality of life. Pain is not a mandatory symptom of endometriosis; many women

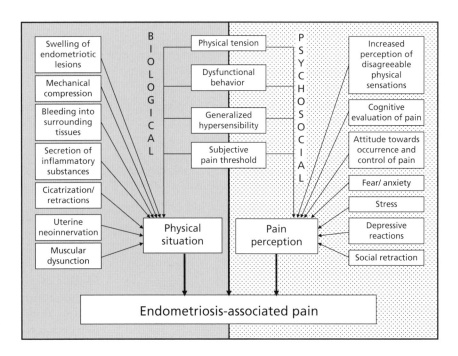

Figure 53.1 Biopsychosocial model of endometriosis-related pain.

experience either infrequent pain or a lesser intensity of pain and other endometriosis-associated symptoms vary in each individual case [75,76]. Therefore the described effect cannot be extrapolated to any woman with endometriosis. However, this chapter aims to give a complete overview of potential psychosomatic and psychosocial consequences of endometriosis, so that physicians can adapt this spectrum for any individual patient.

Factors influencing the development of psychosomatic and psychosocial consequences of endometriosis
Pain
Chronic pelvic pain is a frequent symptom of women with pelvic endometriosis and often increases with the course of disease. Endometriosis-associated pain includes dyspareunia, pelvic pain independent of the menstrual cycle, dysmenorrhea, pain after sexual intercourse, pain on defecation and pain-associated limitations of everyday activities. At the same time, up to 30% of women with confirmed endometriosis do not present any pain [77]. Duration and intensity of the pain are the distinctive factors determining effects on physical as well as psychosocial well-being. Secondary effects such as nausea, fainting or sleeping disorders may further increase the impact of pain on women's lives.

The underlying pathophysiological mechanisms of endometriosis-associated pain have not been fully illuminated. The perception and regulation of pain are determined by a complex system of somatic and psychosomatic factors (Fig. 53.1). From a somatic point of view, swelling of endometriotic lesions, bleeding into surrounding tissues, uterine dyssynergia, secretion of inflammatory mediators such as prostaglandins, cytokines, leukines or tumor necrosis factor (TNF), uterine neo-innervation as part of a chronic pain state, neo-innervation of peritoneum around implants, genetic predisposition to visceral pain and/or somatosensory

disorders, reactive spasm/dysfunction of pelvic floor and hip muscular system as well as mechanical pressure and a reduction of tissue elasticity (retractions) are discussed [67,77–81]. Moreover, there is a modulation of pain by the shifting hormonal milieu of the menstrual cycle [82]. In contrast to earlier assumptions, newer results suggest that there is a correlation between pain and increased stage of disease. At the same time, the discrepancy between clinical findings of endometriosis and pain perception raises the question of which factors do further determine pain perception.

Affective state, attention, current (mental) health status including emotional and cognitive factors, interpretations, beliefs about the pain (e.g. about its cause, duration, curability, and controllability), and history of sexual abuse are important elements of pain perception, which modify pain experience and ability to cope with pain [18,83,84]. The attentive observation of physical symptoms is often combined with cognitively false assessments. A pessimistic attitude regarding pain control is associated with a reduced pain threshold and may consequently increase symptoms [36,85]. Several results from human as well as animal research emphasize the hypothesis that a generalized hypersensibility is involved in endometriosis-related pain [85–87]. Further, segmentary inhibitory systems seem to be activated at the lower back (T10–L1) [86,87]. In rats, connections between reproductive organs, bladder, and colon seem to influence the pathophysiology in one organ through the (patho)physiology in others [88]. Similar effects of peripheral sensitization are likely to occur in women [89]. However, the impact of pain anticipation on such correlations has to be investigated carefully. Furthermore, the permanently increased stress level in chronic pain patients may influence pain reactions.

Women with chronic pain states seem to have a failing awareness of their own body, which is probably part of a defense mechanism [90–92]. Consequently, treatment modalities aimed at improving body awareness and positive body perceptions may be useful. Specific respiration patterns in the context of an inadequate body tension have been described in the context of chronic pelvic pain [90]. As diaphragmal breathing is involved in the normal lymphatic drainage from the muscles and intestines of the pelvic region [90] and as abnormal amounts of tissue edema in the hypogastric, inguinal, and pelvic regions have been demonstrated in women with chronic pelvic pain [93], it seems likely that such patterns may attribute to endometriosis-associated pain. Furthermore, there is a relationship between the experience of pain and the ability to relax [94]. Previous pain experiences may add to chronification of pain perception [36], i.e. physiological stress reactions such as vascular adaptations and muscular tension are involved in the chronification of pain [36,95]. Persistent pain is associated with despair, resignation, hopelessness, helplessness and depressive mood, which may form a vicious cycle [36,95]. The complex interactions between psychological strain and pain show that this symptom of endometriosis is strongly determined by psychosomatic factors.

Fatigue

Fatigue is subjectively perceived as one of the main burdens associated with endometriosis [96]. On the one hand, this seems to be a primary symptom of endometriosis while on the other, chronic pain adds to fatigue and lack of prospects. Fatigue may be aggravated by sleeplessness resulting from pain [97,98]. A further contributing factor is a general increased stress level due to endometriosis-related symptoms.

Infertility and adverse pregnancy outcome

Endometriosis represents a major cause of infertility [99–101]. As motherhood is perceived as a central factor in female biographies, infertility may seriously interfere with adequate self-esteem. Often such concerns represent an important strain upon relationships [45]. In many cultures, the woman is held responsible for her inability to conceive [7,102]. Also, despite significant advances in reproductive medicine, the management of infertility remains stressful [7,103].

Adverse pregnancy outcomes, such as pregnancy loss, preterm delivery, preeclampsia, and intrauterine growth restriction, have been demonstrated to occur more frequently in women with endometriosis [104] and may therefore increase endometriosis-associated strain.

Focusing on the disease

Women suffering from chronic endometriosis naturally deal with disease symptoms and options to improve well-being quite intensively. Consequently, their daily life is focused on endometriosis and potential positive aspects of human life receive less attention. Such a concentration on disease may interfere with everyday life, professional activity, partnership, social life, etc.

Treatment side-effects

Side-effects of surgical interventions and/or medical treatments further add to the strain associated with endometriosis.

Recurrence risk

As the recurrence risk of endometriosis is high, regardless of the type of treatment received, fear about relapses, especially when they have already occurred, represents an additional burden.

Personal coping resources

Personal coping resources, for example interpretation and perception of symptoms, will affect the impact of endometriosis. Besides the natural coping skills resulting from the personality as well as former life experiences, coping skills can be improved by psychosomatic training programs.

Doctor–patient relationship

In addition, an adequate doctor–patient relationship will positively influence endometriosis-associated symptoms (see above).

Specific consequences (Box 53.1)
Health-related quality of life

As in any chronic disease, endometriosis-related disorders essentially determine long-term quality of life [12,23,28,44,77,105,106]. Consequences are a result of disease severity, effects of the disease on everyday life, frequency and intensity of recurrence,

---

Box 53.1 Psychosocial consequences of chronic endometriosis

Factors associated with endometriosis such as:

- pain
- fatigue
- infertility and adverse pregnancy outcome
- focusing on endometriosis
- treatment side-effects
- personal coping resources
- inadequate doctor–patient relationships

Endometriosis-associated morphological, endocrinological and immunological changes may lead to:

- reduced health-related quality of life
- impaired educational achievement and professional activity
- perturbed body perception/female identity
- difficulties in partnership, realizing the wish for children and further social contacts
- limited performance of leisure activities
- disturbances of role performance/physical functioning
- diminished self-esteem
- sexual disorders
- reduced control over life
- limited perspectives for the future
- psychosomatic and psychiatric symptoms: depression, aggressiveness, fear/anxiety

---

impairment of short- and long-term personal aims and the medical as well as psychosocial support the patient receives from healthcare providers, her family, and friends.

Educational achievement and professional activity

Endometriosis-associated pain and the need for frequent surgery may impair education and professional activity [4,71,95,107]. Disease symptoms interfere with day-to-day life at work and may result in sick leave, lay-offs, and change of jobs [108]. Severe pain usually entails being unable to perform the job adequately, while taking strong analgesia limits the type of work and working effectiveness [71,107]. Data from a North American study show that during a period of 12 months, half of the women with endometriosis were not able to practice their profession during an average of 17.8 days [6]. Often the illness is disbelieved or trivialized by employers and colleagues, which compounds job-related problems, especially in workplaces that give no sickness benefit beyond the statutory minimum [71]. Many women feel embarrassed about having an attack of endometriosis at work [45]. They describe feeling guilty for having time off work as well as being anxious about not meeting the expectations of colleagues and superiors [45,95,109]. Although experiences in the workplace are quite diverse [71], these issues are felt more strongly if women work in a male-dominated environment or if they have a male boss [45]. However, reliable data on the quantitative dimension of these correlations are lacking.

A loss of social and economic status may occur because of changes in physical performance [110]. The reduced ability to work during education and in professional life will lead to financial burden for the employer, the public health system and the woman herself [95]. The endometriosis-associated costs to society are considerable but currently poorly identified, as are the costs to the individual.

Role performance/physical functioning

Role performance is defined as a person's ability to continue with daily commitments in life, e.g. household activities such as cooking, shopping, going to work, looking after children, etc. Severe chronic pain causes problems with mobility, i.e. walking, standing, sitting, exercising or even driving a car. In one study all women with endometriosis and only dysmenorrheal symptoms reported impaired ability to participate in gardening, housework, sports, and leisure activities [107]. Eating may be impaired because pain leads to loss of appetite and nausea [45]. Often women describe negative effects on sleeping, which are responsible for low energy levels during the day [45]. As would be expected, complaints related to physical limitations increase in parallel with the intensity of pain [28].

Self-esteem

Consequences of pain may lead to an important reduction of self-esteem [95]. In severe forms of endometriosis, a woman experiences the loss of a healthy active body and proceeds to a state of dependency and limitations [110]. Disease symptoms such as pain and infertility can induce feelings of worthlessness, powerlessness, reduced resilience, and ineffectiveness, as well as guilt towards partner, family, and colleagues [95]. In cases of infertility, the judgment that women with no children are not real women and that they have failed in life's purpose may have a negative impact on self-esteem [48]. Often women with endometriosis feel that they are being perceived as hypochondriacs [48]. Disbelief of health professionals who could legitimize their symptoms may lead to further reduced self-esteem [48]. Aggressive feelings towards others and oneself as well as loneliness may represent further factors [109].

Body perception/female identity

Often endometriosis is associated with a negative female body perception [109]. Pain and treatment side-effects may turn skin white, pale, bloated, greasy or spotty and lead to weight gain [45]. Hysterectomy, i.e. the removal of an organ which represents femininity, as well as infertility, may impair female identity [48,95,111]. In addition, diagnostic delay with a long-term trivialization or false attribution of disease symptoms may affect the woman's confidence in her own body [4].

Partnership/social relationships/leisure activities

The continuous presence of pain and fatigue may cause changes in a woman's affective, family, and social life [77,95,110]. In cases of severe pain, partners and/or family members have to take over duties and responsibilities for housework, leisure activities, family income, childcare, etc. [109]. While some women mention their friends and family as a source of emotional and practical support, others report that social contacts diminish as illness forces them to cancel appointments and social events [45,71,95]. Tiredness and lack of energy prevent normal participation in social events. Many of the women describe feeling worried about the pain starting in public [45].

While the social environment often provides support at diagnosis and during the first surgical interventions, partners, family, and friends often fail to offer ongoing aid in the long term. Women with endometriosis may prefer to hide some physical and psychosocial consequences, as they experience that some people are unable to understand how endometriosis influences their everyday lives. In addition, attempts to help of those not experienced in dealing with endometriosis and/or chronic pain are frequently perceived as counterproductive; for example, many women detest being pitied. Therefore talking to other people about their condition is often perceived as difficult. Consequently, endometriosis may result in social isolation [45].

Due to disease symptoms and eventual infertility, women may perceive themselves as an inadequate partner [95], which can disturb established and future affectionate relationships. While partners are described as the greatest source of support for most women [71], not all partners are able to stand the constant burden of endometriosis, which results in an increased rate of separations and marriage breakdown [48,71]. In contrast, in one study investigating women 15 years after diagnosis, only 7.7% reported endometriosis-related causes for break-ups [105]. Yet, it is difficult to differentiate between the unspecific effects of endometriosis and other causes leading to marriage breakdown.

Control over life

Many women with endometriosis feel that pain controls their lives, which causes feelings of powerlessness and frustration [45]. They report struggling to lead normal lives, for example attempting to arrange holidays or social events at times when their pain is expected to be less severe [45,48]. The unpredictability of the pain adds to the frustration. Participation in medical decisions may help to increase a feeling of control. In some instances, complementary therapies with more or less proven effects allow control to be regained. Such a decision to pursue complementary and/or alternative medicine is often taken when conventional medicine does not provide sufficient support in dealing with the disease [4].

Perspective on the future

At present, no treatment modality has been proven to prevent recurrence [112]. Consequently, the future is often viewed with a mixture of optimism and pessimism. The majority of women with chronic endometriosis worry that symptoms will return and question their ability to cope with the disease in the long term [71]. A major factor is that the clinical course can never be predicted, which hampers the development of long-term plans.

Psychological consequences

The absence of a correlation between the extent of endometriosis and the presence and intensity of pain suggests a possible link between the personality of the affected woman and her manifestation of pain [113]. A few studies of psychological characteristics in women diagnosed with endometriosis have been carried out, with contradictory results. One study found elevated levels of neuroticism, psychiatric morbidity, psychoticism, and introversion in women with endometriosis compared to healthy women or women with benign gynecological symptoms [29]. In addition, women with endometriosis seem to be characterized by a higher level of emotional suppression [16]. Although no prospective studies have been conducted, is seems likely that such correlations rather represent a consequence than a cause of the disease [28].

Fear/anxiety

Anxiety is typically observed in patients with chronic pain. Pain intensity correlates positively with the degree of anxiety symptoms [28]. With a background of endometriosis symptoms and the prognosis of the disease, an increased level of anxiety is easy to understand. In one study, 87.5% of endometriosis patients presented anxiety, with 63.5% showing an intense degree [28]. Accordingly, such women may show increased health concerns [11,45]. As endometriosis patients present an augmented anxiety when compared with other chronic pelvic pain patients [29,114], it can currently not be excluded that there are primary differences regarding anxiety between these groups. One factor might be that pain is often reported to be more severe in endometriosis [13]. However, results are controversial [115].

Depression

Depression is one of the psychological factors most studied and is found in about 80% of women with chronic pain [110]. Nevertheless, depression is still underdiagnosed and poorly treated, especially when it is present in conjunction with other clinical conditions. Depression results from the interaction between the predisposed factors of each patient, her cognitive structures, the stress factor, the disease, and its symptoms. Therefore, it is not surprising that endometriosis is associated with an increase of depressive symptoms [4,11,26,115]. Prevalence studies in endometriosis are scarce. Of endometriosis patients evaluated in one study, 86.5% presented depressive symptoms, with 22.1% suffering from a mild, 31.7% from a moderate, and 32.7% from a severe form [28].

Pain seems to play an important role in the onset of depression. In a study from 2006, depression was diagnosed in 86% of endometriosis patients with chronic pelvic pain, compared to 38% of those without [110]. Nevertheless, the quantitative effect of pain on the prevalence of depression in endometriosis is still unclear [83,110]. It is possible that the intensity of the pain is related to the degree of depression [116] but there are also opposite results [83]. Research results did not demonstrate any clear correlation between the disease stage of endometriosis and depression [115,117]. There is evidence that depression is a consequence of chronic pain but there is no consensus with regard to which condition comes first [116,118,119].

Work issues and family judgment of being a hypochondriac are mentioned as main factors contributing to depression [4]. Furthermore, women may become depressed knowing that they suffer from a chronic disease with an uncertain prognosis concerning fertility and quality of life [39]. Also, a loss of female organs may add to the risk for depression. Further potential factors are side-effects of hormonal treatment, especially GnRH analogs and progesterone [120–122], but results are controversial [121,123]. Advancing age is related to an increase in severity of emotional suffering caused by the disease, which may manifest as depressive symptoms [28].

Depressive reactions impair a patient's adherence to treatment, repeatedly leading to unsatisfactory results in the control of the disease. Furthermore, depression can interfere with a woman's perceived sense of control, handling of adverse situations, and resourcefulness [96].

Aggressiveness

In qualitative studies, women also report feelings of aggressiveness resulting from the secondary effects of endometriosis [4,45]. Such feelings are a normal part of the mourning process and are not surprising given the background of limitations that endometriosis imposes on these women's lives. Also, aggressiveness may be a symptom of depression which is more often seen in men than in women, but which can occur in women too.

Co-morbidity with psychosomatic disorders

Some studies show an association of endometriosis with diseases where psychosomatic factors are involved in the genesis of the disease, such as irritable bowel syndrome, interstitial cystitis, chronic fatigue syndrome or fibromyalgia [42,85]. Women with endometriosis suffer significantly more often from migraine than those without endometriosis [124]. On the one hand, similarities in prostaglandin and nitric oxide production/pathways may contribute to co-morbidity [124]. On the other hand, psychosomatic factors are known to influence the onset and intensity of clinical symptoms in both diseases.

Specific psychosomatic features in adolescents

The burden of endometriosis in the adolescent population is considerably underappreciated and the health-related quality of life impact of endometriosis in this younger population has not been widely studied [89,112]. In an Endometriosis Association survey, the majority of 4334 respondents reported first symptoms as adolescents, and their diagnostic experience seemed much more difficult than for those women who first experienced symptoms as adults [56]. Each step of the diagnostic experience, i.e. seeking medical help and receiving diagnosis, took longer for the adolescent-onset group. They were also more likely to report not being taken seriously by their physicians overall or to be told that nothing was wrong, which, despite the fact that this study group is not representative, reflects that many physicians fail to consider endometriosis as a diagnosis in adolescents [125,126].

Endometriosis may keep an adolescent out of school and prevent her from participating in extracurricular sporting and social activities [127]. It often causes skepticism and criticism among friends, teachers, family, and doctors, and if left undiagnosed or misdiagnosed, results in questioning of one's own validity and worth [127]. As adolescence is an important time for developing not only the future personality but also the basis for later professional activity, symptoms of endometriosis with resulting secondary effects may seriously interfere with normal adolescent development.

Psychosomatic therapeutic options

Psychosomatic management in endometriosis aims to restore normal function by giving the patient insight into her condition, reducing her emotional distress, developing strategies to deal with chronic pain as well as other disease-associated symptoms and by generating long-term concepts for a fulfilling life with endometriosis [128]. See Box 53.2. Today, patients frequently ask for a holistic approach in gynecological care. Fortunately, an increasing number of departments of gynecology seem to aim for such an approach, but the integration of psychosomatic counseling is currently hampered by a lack of adequately trained gynecologists [129]. Consequently, despite a high motivation of doctors and other healthcare providers, actual offers remain far below the effective needs [129].

Communication

Over half of the doctor's time is spent talking with patients [130]. Time spent taking a detailed history, including discussions of

---

Box 53.2 Psychosocial support options

Basics
- Adequate doctor–patient relationship
- Patient-centered communication aiming at shared decisions

Diagnostic approach
- Listening and taking women's descriptions of clinical symptoms seriously
- Accurate early (preliminary) diagnosis of physical and psychosocial disease symptoms/effects

Therapeutic approach
- Meticulous information about the patient and important persons on clinical and psychosocial aspects of the disease
- Instructions and/or mediation of:
  – medical/surgical treatment options
  – pain management against a background of a biopsychosocial model of pain
  – coping strategies including relaxation techniques and where applicable support in dealing with losses (mourning process)
- Sexual counseling/sexual therapy
- Aiming for a holistic concept to integrate endometriosis into private/professional life
- Proposal of contact with self-help groups

---

social, psychological and sexual issues, is likely to be worthwhile, as a doctor and patient may then consider the pain and its management in a wider psychosocial context and be therefore more effective. Practitioners should use patient-centered communication [7]. The ideal doctor providing support for women with endometriosis is described as being sympathetic to their plight, listening and taking complaints seriously without giving the impression that women have to legitimize their disease [4,130]. Because physicians are more powerful than their patients and have more authority, they must be vigilant about not abusing their power. Positive communication may also increase patient perceptions of physician competence [8,70,131].

Diagnostic approach

In adolescents younger than 18 years, a direct evaluation by laparoscopy is recommended, as the long-term effects of GnRH agonist medication on bone formation and density remain unknown [64,65]. In women older than 18 years, a differentiated diagnostic approach should be discussed with the patient. As there are advantages and disadvantages of a laparoscopic diagnosis, a potential solution would be a "working diagnosis," involving patients in the decision about diagnostic and therapeutic interventions [47]. This would allow women to choose between a histologically confirmed diagnosis with the risks of laparoscopy, on the one hand, and a less reliable diagnosis without the risks of surgery on the other. It would provide a provisional language with which women could articulate their experiences and legitimate absence from normal social and work roles when necessary. If pain symptoms can be relieved effectively by medical treatment without harmful side-effects, then whether endometriosis was ever present or even the cause of the pain will remain irrelevant for many women [132]. At the same time, women who need a concrete diagnosis could decide in favor of laparoscopy.

Medical information

In gynecology, the importance of adequate medical information to improve coping is well known for genetic counseling and cancer. Although the desire for medical information can change during the course of the disease, it is often generally underestimated by physicians [106]. Information on causes and course of a disease is crucial for the feeling of being able to control health and well-being. Uncertainty and insufficient information may increase fear. Patients with little knowledge on their (suspected) disease suffer more often from depression compared to well-informed patients. Furthermore, education is essential to improve patients' treatment adherence [112]. Only with detailed medical information can patients and doctors become partners in dealing with the disease.

As there is no universally valid way of optimal counseling, patients' needs have to be explored carefully. The patient's wish to be informed is often not identical with the patient's expression to be informed and can therefore not always be recognized by the medical team. An analysis by Raspe [133] showed that 20% of the patients investigated do not want any detailed information, 35% would like to know more but do not ask for detailed information, and the remaining 45% want to know more and succeed in asking for more information. Fear of making oneself appear ridiculous and the impression that the doctor is short of time may lead to patients abandoning any supplementary questions. Therefore doctors should actively and repeatedly offer to inform their patient.

Adequate medical information is important throughout the diagnostic process and after diagnosis has been confirmed. Thoughtful pre- and postoperative patient education is essential to place laparoscopic findings in the appropriate clinical context. Use of information brochures and DVDs can help patients to prepare for consultations [74]. For some women, photography or video images of endometrial lesions may be important to induce a feeling of legitimization of their pain experience [50]. Currently women with endometriosis do often feel insufficiently informed, especially about potential coping strategies and possibilities to improve pain management [95].

In addition to the patient, their social contacts, especially the partner, should be informed about the potential physical and psychological consequences of the disease as well as how to deal with the woman's symptoms.

Medical decisions

By providing relevant information on diagnostic as well as therapeutic possibilities, physicians enable their patients to develop their own way of dealing with the disease. While it is the responsibility of physicians to make sure that medical information is reliable, only the patient can adapt this information to her individual needs. Such an approach allows doctors and patients to consolidate their resources in finding solutions to reducing the impact of endometriosis. A shared decision treatment approach may reduce patient confusion, non-adherence, and treatment avoidance.

Psychosomatic aspects of pain management

Surgical treatment of endometriosis helps to reduce pain, but about 33% of those treated do not improve [4,5,134]. With this background, the relevance of endometriotic implants as causes for pain should be investigated critically, i.e. other reasons for pelvic pain should be taken into account [89]. On the other hand, psychosomatic therapeutic options for pain management have to be considered. The few studies investigating the efficacy of combined approaches suggest a positive synergy of physical and psychological treatment [135]. Repeated solely somatically oriented treatment attempts confirm the patient's convictions that pain has exclusively to be attributed to physical aspects [36]. Such an attitude promotes chronification and renders the use of efficient psychosomatic therapeutic options more difficult [36]. Therefore it is crucial for the long-term well-being of women with endometriosis to differentiate between physical and psychological factors and to deal adequately with both. At the same time, it is important not to interpret disease symptoms as psychosomatic when they should be attributed to somatic disease [49].

An important method in psychological pain management is to change dysfunctional behaviors, for example inappropriate relieving postures, avoidance of physical activities and/or social avoidance [36]. Pain-associated negative thoughts may be modified by cognitive therapy [36]. Common techniques include positive self-verbalization, cognitive restructuring and changing the focus of attention on the background of pain symptoms, accompanying symptoms and individual psychosocial burden [36].

Relaxation techniques can interrupt the cycle of pain and increasing body tension and therefore reduce pain intensity. In addition to progressive muscular relaxation and autogenous training, different concepts for body therapy have recently been implemented [36,91,92,136]. Body therapies increase body awareness. Also Mensendieck somatocognitive therapy, a therapy aimed at improving body awareness, balanced posture and controlled movement, awareness of tension and relaxation as well as functional respiration, succeeded in ameliorating the pain experience in women with chronic pelvic pain when compared to gynecological treatment alone [90,137,138]. Lateral inhibition brought about by alternative stimuli, for example touching, manual release of muscles that changes the focus of pain to other body sensations, and coping may be used to reduce endometriosis-associated pain [90]. Psychosomatic techniques, including depth psychotherapy, systemic psychotherapy, hypnotherapy, psychodynamic-interpersonal therapy, just to give some examples as well as acupuncture, biofeedback, and counselling or prescribing antidepressants, as indicated, may help to diminish symptoms of endometriosis [7,93,139].Therapies may be designed as single, partner or group activities [135].

One important factor probably contributing to reduction of pain is the emotional support resulting from frequent contact with the therapist. Although psychosomatic techniques proved to have a significant effect in a variety of diseases leading to chronic pain [92,139], currently only clinical experiences of specialized therapists are available to confirm their effect in endometriosis. Even if quantitative effects remain to be confirmed by well-designed intervention studies, such options should be integrated into patient counseling when developing a plan for dealing with endometriosis.

Women with endometriosis have to face and mourn endometriosis-associated losses, including the lack of children, the changes of a former dream of life, untroubled leisure activities, partnership, social contacts and/or career, in order to adapt everyday activities to their personal actual physical and psychological possibilities [95].

Self-help organizations

Often partners, family, and friends lack understanding of what living with endometriosis feels like. Exchange with other endometriosis patients may represent an opportunity to improve skills in dealing with the disease. Women living with endometriosis have an intense experience of how to integrate the disease into everyday life and may enrich the possibilities of therapeutic options. In this context, support provided by self-help organizations may open new opportunities [95]. Studies show that women value the knowledge of such organizations about endometriosis, being listened to and believed, and having support from others who understand their symptoms [140].

Future research into psychosomatic/ psychosocial aspects of endometriosis

As the correlation between stage of disease and actual well-being is only weak, it remains to be clarified which factors do indeed determine well-being. Further studies should focus on behavioral interactions between pain beliefs, coping styles, and levels of functioning. To date, no evaluation of possible burn-out or post-traumatic stress syndrome has been made. Future research projects should include financial burden and interviews with family members. Several European projects from university hospitals in Leuven, Belgium, and Zürich, Switzerland, in co-operation with national and international self-help organizations, are currently under way to address some of these questions. However, once the potential psychosomatic consequences of endometriosis are confirmed by well-designed studies, research projects will have to investigate the benefit of reinforcing individual resources and active pain-coping skills [83].

Conclusion

Despite recent advances in medical science, endometriosis continues to negatively affect the lives of affected women. However, the disease does not always cause pain, treatment is effective in many cases, and infertility might be overcome in up to two-thirds of patients. The main clinical symptoms, i.e. pain, fatigue, and infertility, are strongly influenced by psychosocial factors and have an important effect on the health-related private as well as professional quality of life. Unlike many other chronic conditions, the experience of endometriosis is likely to be dismissed or normalized in dealings with healthcare professionals.

With this background, adequate treatment of endometriosis can only be realized when psychosomatic aspects of the disease are integrated into medical care. A greater awareness of the multidimensional impact of endometriosis from gynecologists and other healthcare professionals would be beneficial for the women concerned. Doctors and patient organizations both play a role in ensuring that any fears concerning chronic conditions are alleviated by providing factual information and setting expectations for treatment outcome. Future efforts should be directed toward improving the level of awareness of endometriosis and optimizing treatment effectiveness and side-effect profiles.

References

1. Ozkan S, Murk W, Arici A. Endometriosis and infertility: epidemiology and evidence-based treatments. Ann N Y Acad Sci 2008;1127:92–100.
2. Eskenazi B, Warner ML. Epidemiology of endometriosis. Obstet Gynecol Clin North Am 1997;24(2):235–258.
3. Hurd WW. Criteria that indicate endometriosis is the cause of chronic pelvic pain. Obstet Gynecol 1998;92(6):1029–1032.
4. Cox H, Henderson L, Wood R, Cagliarini G. Learning to take charge: women's experiences of living with endometriosis. Complement Ther Nurs Midwifery 2003;9(2):62–68.
5. Waller KG, Shaw RW. Gonadotropin-releasing hormone analogues for the treatment of endometriosis: long-term follow-up. Fertil Steril 1993;59(3):511–515.
6. Kjerulff KH, Erickson BA, Langenberg PW. Chronic gynecological conditions reported by US women: findings from the National Health Interview Survey, 1984 to 1992. Am J Public Health 1996;86(2):195–199.
7. Lal M. Psychosomatic approaches to obstetrics, gynaecology and andrology – a review. J Obstet Gynaecol 2009;29(1):1–12.
8. Moore PJ, Sickel AE, Malat J, Williams D, Jackson J, Adler NE. Psychosocial factors in medical and psychological treatment avoidance: the role of the doctor–patient relationship. J Health Psychol 2004;9(3):421–433.
9. Collins ML. Personality correlates of endometriosis. Doctoral thesis. Michigan: Western Michigan University. 1979.
10. Roth H. Psychosomatische Aspekte der Endometriose. Kiel: Universität Kiel, 1996.

11. Strauss B, Didzus A, Speidel H. A study concerning the psychosomatics of endometriosis. Psychother Psychosom Med Psychol 1992;42:242–252.

12. Lutje W, Brandenburg U. [Psychosomatic aspects of endometriosis]. Zentralbl Gynakol 2003;125(7–8):281–285.

13. Peveler R, Edwards J, Daddow J, Thomas E. Psychosocial factors and chronic pelvic pain: a comparison of women with endometriosis and with unexplained pain. J Psychosom Res 1996;40(3):305–315.

14. Paras ML, Murad MH, Chen LP et al. Sexual abuse and lifetime diagnosis of somatic disorders: a systematic review and meta-analysis. JAMA 2009;302(5):550–561.

15. Tietjen GE, Brandes JL, Peterlin BL et al. Childhood maltreatment and migraine (Part III). Association with comorbid pain conditions. Headache 2010;50(1):42–51.

16. Thomas E, Moss-Morris R, Faquhar C. Coping with emotions and abuse history in women with chronic pelvic pain. J Psychosom Res 2006;60(1):109–112.

17. Belaisch J, Allart JP. [Endometriosis and surviving adolescence]. Gynecol Obstet Fertil 2006;34(3):242–247.

18. Harrop-Griffiths J, Katon W, Walker E, Holm L, Russo J, Hickok L. The association between chronic pelvic pain, psychiatric diagnoses, and childhood sexual abuse. Obstet Gynecol 1988;71(4):589–594.

19. Rubin JJ. Psychosomatic pain: new insights and management strategies. South Med J 2005;98(11):1099–1110; quiz 1111–1112, 1138.

20. Harrison V, Rowan K, Mathias J. Stress reactivity and family relationships in the development and treatment of endometriosis. Fertil Steril 2005;83(4):857–864.

21. Glaser R, Kiecolt-Glaser JK. Stress-induced immune dysfunction: implications for health. Nat Rev Immunol 2005;5(3):243–251.

22. Seli E, Arici A. Endometriosis: interaction of immune and endocrine systems. Semin Reprod Med 2003;21(2):135–144.

23. Petrelluzzi KF, Garcia MC, Petta CA, Grassi-Kassisse DM, Spadari-Bratfisch RC. Salivary cortisol concentrations, stress and quality of life in women with endometriosis and chronic pelvic pain. Stress 2008;11(5):390–397.

24. Jerjes WK, Peters TJ, Taylor NF, Wood PJ, Wessely S, Cleare AJ. Diurnal excretion of urinary cortisol, cortisone, and cortisol metabolites in chronic fatigue syndrome. J Psychosom Res 2006;60(2):145–153.

25. Fries E, Hesse J, Hellhammer J, Hellhammer DH. A new view on hypocortisolism. Psychoneuroendocrinology 2005;30(10):1010–1016.

26. Lewis DO, Comite F, Mallouh C et al. Bipolar mood disorder and endometriosis: preliminary findings. Am J Psychiatry 1987; 144(12):1588–1591.

27. Walker E, Katon W, Jones LM, Russo J. Relationship between endometriosis and affective disorder. Am J Psychiatry 1989;146(3):380–381.

28. Sepulcri RP, do Amaral VF. Depressive symptoms, anxiety, and quality of life in women with pelvic endometriosis. Eur J Obstet Gynecol Reprod Biol 2009;142(1):53–56.

29. Low WY, Edelmann RJ, Sutton C. A psychological profile of endometriosis patients in comparison to patients with pelvic pain of other origins. J Psychosom Res 1993;37(2):111–116.

30. Simon G. Psychiatric disorder and endometriosis. Am J Psychiatry 1988;145(8):1040–1041.

31. Houston DE, Noller KL, Melton LJ 3rd, Selwyn BJ. The epidemiology of pelvic endometriosis. Clin Obstet Gynecol 1988;31(4):787–800.

32. Low WY, Edelmann RY. Psychosocial aspects of endometriosis: a review. J Psychosom Obset Gynaecol 1991;12:3–12.

33. Vigano P, Parazzini F, Somigliana E, Vercellini P. Endometriosis: epidemiology and aetiological factors. Best Pract Res Clin Obstet Gynaecol 2004;18(2):177–200.

34. Missmer SA, Cramer DW. The epidemiology of endometriosis. Obstet Gynecol Clin North Am 2003;30(1):1–19, vii.

35. Houston DE. Evidence for the risk of pelvic endometriosis by age, race and socioeconomic status. Epidemiol Rev 1984;6:167–191.

36. Greimel ER, Thiel I. [Psychological treatment aspects of chronic pelvic pain in the woman]. Wien Med Wochenschr 1999;149(13):383–387.

37. Taylor RN, Lebovic DI, Mueller MD. Angiogenic factors in endometriosis. Ann N Y Acad Sci 2002;955:89–100; discussion 118, 396–406.

38. Hadfield R, Mardon H, Barlow D, Kennedy S. Delay in the diagnosis of endometriosis: a survey of women from the USA and the UK. Hum Reprod 1996;11(4):878–880.

39. Husby GK, Haugen RS, Moen MH. Diagnostic delay in women with pain and endometriosis. Acta Obstet Gynecol Scand 2003;82(7): 649–653.

40. Arruda MS, Petta CA, Abrao MS, Benetti-Pinto CL. Time elapsed from onset of symptoms to diagnosis of endometriosis in a cohort study of Brazilian women. Hum Reprod 2003;18(4):756–759.

41. Dmowski WP, Lesniewicz R, Rana N, Pepping P, Noursalehi M. Changing trends in the diagnosis of endometriosis: a comparative study of women with pelvic endometriosis presenting with chronic pelvic pain or infertility. Fertil Steril 1997;67(2):238–243.

42. Sinaii N, Cleary SD, Ballweg ML, Nieman LK, Stratton P. High rates of autoimmune and endocrine disorders, fibromyalgia, chronic fatigue syndrome and atopic diseases among women with endometriosis: a survey analysis. Hum Reprod 2002;17(10):2715–2724.

43. Whelan E. Putting pain to paper: endometriosis and the documentation of suffering. Health Interdiscip J Soc Stud Health Illness Med 2003;7:463–482.

44. Garry R, Clayton R, Hawe J. The effect of endometriosis and its radical laparoscopic excision on quality of life indicators. Br J Obstet Gynaecol 2000;107(1):44–54.

45. Jones G, Jenkinson C, Kennedy S. The impact of endometriosis upon quality of life: a qualitative analysis. J Psychosom Obstet Gynaecol 2004;25(2):123–133.

46. Ballard KD, Seaman HE, de Vries CS, Wright JT. Can symptomatology help in the diagnosis of endometriosis? Findings from a national case-control study Part 1. Br J Obstet Gynaecol 2008; 115(11):1382–1391.

47. Ballard K, Lowton K, Wright J. What's the delay? A qualitative study of women's experiences of reaching a diagnosis of endometriosis. Fertil Steril 2006;86(5):1296–1301.

48. Cox H, Henderson L, Andersen N, Cagliarini G, Ski C. Focus group study of endometriosis: struggle, loss and the medical merry-go-round. Int J Nurs Pract 2003;9(1):2–9.

49. Ballweg ML. Blaming the victim. The psychologizing of endometriosis. Obstet Gynecol Clin North Am 1997;24(2):441–453.

50. Denny E. "You are one of the unlucky ones": delay in the diagnosis of endometriosis. Div Health Soc Care 2004;1:39–44.

51. Hillier SG, Scambler G. Women as patients and providers. In: Scambler G, editor. Sociology in Applied to Medicine. Edinburgh: WB Saunders, 1997, pp.121–134.

52. Kessler LG, Burns BJ, Shapiro S et al. Psychiatric diagnoses of medical service users: evidence from the Epidemiologic Catchment Area Program. Am J Public Health 1987;77(1):18–24.

53. Matsuzaki S, Canis M, Pouly JL, Rabischong B, Botchorishvili R, Mage G. Relationship between delay of surgical diagnosis and severity of disease in patients with symptomatic deep infiltrating endometriosis. Fertil Steril 2006;86(5):1314–1316; discussion 1317.

54. Garry R. Diagnosis of endometriosis and pelvic pain. Fertil Steril 2006;86(5):1307–1309; discussion 1317.

55. Eskenazi B, Warner M, Bonsignore L, Olive D, Samuels S, Vercellini P. Validation study of nonsurgical diagnosis of endometriosis. Fertil Steril 2001;76(5):929–935.

56. Greene R, Stratton P, Cleary SD, Ballweg ML, Sinaii N. Diagnostic experience among 4,334 women reporting surgically diagnosed endometriosis. Fertil Steril 2009;91(1):32–39.

57. Jansen S, Jorgensen J, Caplehorn J, Hunt D. Preoperative ultrasound to predict conversion in laparoscopic cholecystectomy. Surg Laparosc Endosc 1997;7(2):121–123.

58. Chapron C, Querleu D, Bruhat MA et al. Surgical complications of diagnostic and operative gynaecological laparoscopy: a series of 29,966 cases. Hum Reprod 1998;13(4):867–872.

59. Kresch AJ, Seifer DB, Sachs LB, Barrese I. Laparoscopy in 100 women with chronic pelvic pain. Obstet Gynecol 1984;64(5):672–674.

60. Kang SB, Chung HH, Lee HP, Lee JY, Chang YS. Impact of diagnostic laparoscopy on the management of chronic pelvic pain. Surg Endosc 2007;21(6):916–919.

61. Cox L, Ayers S, Nala K, Penny J. Chronic pelvic pain and quality of life after laparoscopy. Eur J Obstet Gynecol Reprod Biol 2007;132(2):214–219.

62. Moore J, Ziebland S, Kennedy S. "People sometimes react funny if they're not told enough": women's views about the risks of diagnostic laparoscopy. Health Expect 2002;5(4):302–309.

63. Royal College of Obstetricians and Gynaecologists. The initial management of chronic pelvic pain. RCOG Guidelines 2005;41.

64. American College of Gynecologists. Endometriosis in adolescents. Commitee Opinion No. 310. Obstet Gynecol 2005; 105:921–927.

65. Medical management of endometriosis. Am J Obstet Gynecol 1999;11:706–718.

66. Gambone JC, Mittman BS, Munro MG, Scialli AR, Winkel CA. Consensus statement for the management of chronic pelvic pain and endometriosis: proceedings of an expert-panel consensus process. Fertil Steril 2002;78(5):961–972.

67. Steege JF. Too soon, too late, too often, too seldom? Fertil Steril 2006;86(5):1310–1311; discussion 1317.

68. Zondervan KT, Yudkin PL, Vessey MP et al. The community prevalence of chronic pelvic pain in women and associated illness behaviour. Br J Gen Pract 2001;51(468):541–547.

69. McManus IC, Gordon D, Winder BC. Duties of a doctor: UK doctors and good medical practice. Qual Health Care 2000;9(1):14–22.

70. Moore PJ, Adler NE, Robertson PA. Medical malpractice: the effect of doctor–patient relations on medical patient perceptions and malpractice intentions. West J Med 2000;173(4):244–250.

71. Denny E. Women's experience of endometriosis. J Adv Nurs 2004;46(6):641–648.

72. Carlton D. Awareness of endometriosis. Practice Nurse 1996;12:514–515.

73. Denny E, Mann CH. Endometriosis and the primary care consultation. Eur J Obstet Gynecol Reprod Biol 2008;139(1):111–115.

74. Bitzer J, Greiner Mai E, Skott F. Endometriosis – quality of life and doctor patient relationship. J Fertil Reprod 1999;9:27–32.

75. Kennedy S, Bergqvist A, Chapron C et al. ESHRE guideline for the diagnosis and treatment of endometriosis. Hum Reprod 2005;20(10): 2698–2704.

76. Moen MH, Stokstad T. A long-term follow-up study of women with asymptomatic endometriosis diagnosed incidentally at sterilization. Fertil Steril 2002;78(4):773–776.

77. Adamson GD. A 36-year-old woman with endometriosis, pelvic pain, and infertility. JAMA 1999;282(24):2347–2354.

78. Atwal G, du Plessis D, Armstrong G, Slade R, Quinn M. Uterine innervation after hysterectomy for chronic pelvic pain with, and without, endometriosis. Am J Obstet Gynecol 2005;193(5): 1650–1655.

79. Berkley KJ, Dmitrieva N, Curtis KS, Papka RE. Innervation of ectopic endometrium in a rat model of endometriosis. Proc Natl Acad Sci USA 2004;101(30):11094–11098.

80. Diatchenko L, Slade GD, Nackley AG et al. Genetic basis for individual variations in pain perception and the development of a chronic pain condition. Hum Mol Genet 2005;14(1):135–143.

81. Tu FF, As-Sanie S, Steege JF. Musculoskeletal causes of chronic pelvic pain: a systematic review of existing therapies: part II. Obstet Gynecol Surv 2005;60(7):474–483.

82. Riley JL 3rd, Robinson ME, Wise EA, Price DD. A meta-analytic review of pain perception across the menstrual cycle. Pain 1999;81(3):225–235.

83. Eriksen HL, Gunnersen KF, Sorensen JA, Munk T, Nielsen T, Knudsen UB. Psychological aspects of endometriosis: differences between patients with or without pain on four psychological variables. Eur J Obstet Gynecol Reprod Biol 2008;139(1):100–105.

84. Hartmann KE, Ma C, Lamvu GM, Langenberg PW, Steege JF, Kjerulff KH. Quality of life and sexual function after hysterectomy in women with preoperative pain and depression. Obstet Gynecol 2004;104(4): 701–709.

85. Audebert A. [Women with endometriosis: are they different from others?]. Gynecol Obstet Fertil 2005;33(4):239–246.

86. Bajaj P, Madsen H, Arendt-Nielsen L. Endometriosis is associated with central sensitization: a psychophysical controlled study. J Pain 2003;4(7):372–380.

87. Giamberardino MA, Berkley KJ, Affaitati G et al. Influence of endometriosis on pain behaviors and muscle hyperalgesia induced by a ureteral calculosis in female rats. Pain 2002;95(3):247–257.

88. Berkley KJ. A life of pelvic pain. Physiol Behav 2005;86(3):272–280.

89. Stratton P. The tangled web of reasons for the delay in diagnosis of endometriosis in women with chronic pelvic pain: will the suffering end? Fertil Steril 2006;86(5):1302–1304; discussion 1317.

90. Haugstad GK, Haugstad TS, Kirste UM, Leganger S, Klemmetsen I, Malt UF. Mensendieck somatocognitive therapy as treatment approach to chronic pelvic pain: results of a randomized controlled intervention study. Am J Obstet Gynecol 2006;194(5):1303–1310.

91. Grahn B, Ekdahl C, Borgquist L. Motivation as a predictor of changes in quality of life and working ability in multidisciplinary rehabilitation. A two-year follow-up of a prospective controlled study in patients with prolonged musculoskeletal disorders. Disabil Rehabil 2000;22(15):639–654.

92. Mattson M, Wikman M, Dahlgren L, Mattssson B. Physiotherapy as empowerment – treating women with chronic pelvic pain. Adv Physio 2000;2(3):125–143.

93. Stones RW, Cheong YC, Howard FM. Interventions for treating chronic pelvic pain in women. Cochrane Database Syst Rev 2005;4:CD000387.

94. Kvale A, Ljunggren AE, Johnsen TB. Examination of movement in patients with long-lasting musculoskeletal pain: reliability and validity. Physiother Res Int 2003;8(1):36–52.

95. Weinstein K. The emotional aspects of endometriosis: what the patient expects from her doctor. Clin Obstet Gynecol 1988;31(4):866–873.

96. Lemaire GS. More than just menstrual cramps: symptoms and uncertainty among women with endometriosis. J Obstet Gynecol Neonatal Nurs 2004;33(1):71–79.

97. Hawkridge C. Living with Endometriosis: A Practical Guide to the Causes and Treatments. London: Vermillion, 1996.

98. Huntington A, Gilmour JA. A life shaped by pain: women and endometriosis. J Clin Nurs 2005;14(9):1124–1132.

99. Smith S, Pfeifer SM, Collins JA. Diagnosis and management of female infertility. JAMA 2003;290(13):1767–1770.

100. D'Hooghe TM, Debrock S, Hill JA, Meuleman C. Endometriosis and subfertility: is the relationship resolved? Semin Reprod Med 2003;21(2):243–254.

101. Meuleman C, Vandenabeele B, Fieuws S, Spiessens C, Timmerman D, D'Hooghe T. High prevalence of endometriosis in infertile women with normal ovulation and normospermic partners. Fertil Steril 2009;92(1):68–74.

102. Noorbala AA, Ramezanzadeh F, Abedinia N, Yazdi SAB, Jafarabadi M. Study of psychiatric disorders among fertile and infertile women and some predisposing factors. J Fam Plan Reprod Health Care 2007;1(1):6–11.

103. Chen TH, Chang SP, Tsai CF, Juang KD. Prevalence of depressive and anxiety disorders in an assisted reproductive technique clinic. Hum Reprod 2004;19(10):2313–2318.

104. Stephansson O, Kieler H, Granath F, Falconer H. Endometriosis, assisted reproduction technology, and risk of adverse pregnancy outcome. Hum Reprod 2009;24(9):2341–2347.

105. Fagervold B, Jenssen M, Hummelshoj L, Moen MH. Life after a diagnosis with endometriosis – a 15 years follow-up study. Acta Obstet Gynecol Scand 2009;88(8):914–919.

106. Leeners B, Imthurn B. [Psychosomatic aspects of endometriosis – current state of scientific knowledge and clinical experience]. Gynakol Geburtshilfliche Rundsch 2007;47(3):132–139.

107. Oehmke F, Weyand J, Hackethal A, Konrad L, Omwandho C, Tinneberg HR. Impact of endometriosis on quality of life: a pilot study. Gynecol Endocrinol 2009;25(11):722–725.

108. Bianconi L, Hummelshoj L, Coccia ME et al. Recognizing endometriosis as a social disease: the European Union-encouraged Italian Senate approach. Fertil Steril 2007;88(5):1285–1287.

109. Bodden-Heidrich R, Hilberink M, Frommer J et al. Qualitative research on psychosomatic aspects of endometriosis. Zsch Psychosom Med 1999;45:372–389.

110. Lorencatto C, Petta CA, Navarro MJ, Bahamondes L, Matos A. Depression in women with endometriosis with and without chronic pelvic pain. Acta Obstet Gynecol Scand 2006;85(1):88–92.

111. Flory N, Bissonnette F, Binik YM. Psychosocial effects of hysterectomy: literature review. J Psychosom Res 2005;59(3):117–129.

112. Gao X, Yeh YC, Outley J, Simon J, Botteman M, Spalding J. Health-related quality of life burden of women with endometriosis: a literature review. Curr Med Res Opin 2006;22(9):1787–1797.

113. Gomibuchi H, Taketani Y, Doi M et al. Is personality involved in the expression of dysmenorrhea in patients with endometriosis? Am J Obstet Gynecol 1993;169(3):723–725.

114. Renaer M, Vertommen H, Nijs P, Wagemans L, van Hemelrijck T. Psychological aspects of chronic pelvic pain in women. Am J Obstet Gynecol 1979;134(1):75–80.

115. Waller KG, Shaw RW. Endometriosis, pelvic pain, and psychological functioning. Fertil Steril 1995;63(4):796–800.

116. Doan BD, Wadden NP. Relationships between depressive symptoms and descriptions of chronic pain. Pain 1989;36(1):75–84.

117. Sinaii N, Plumb K, Cotton L et al. Differences in characteristics among 1,000 women with endometriosis based on extent of disease. Fertil Steril 2008;89(3):538–545.

118. Ward NG. Pain and depression. In: Bonica JJ, editor. The Management of Pain, 2nd edn. Philadelphia: Lea and Febuger, 1990, pp. 310–319.

119. Fishbain DA, Cutler R, Rosomoff HL, Rosomoff RS. Chronic pain-associated depression: antecedent or consequence of chronic pain? A review. Clin J Pain 1997;13(2):116–137.

120. Warnock JK, Bundren JC, Morris DW. Depressive symptoms associated with gonadotropin-releasing hormone agonists. Depress Anxiety 1998;7(4):171–177.

121. Warnock JK, Bundren JC, Morris DW. Sertraline in the treatment of depression associated with gonadotropin-releasing hormone agonist therapy. Biol Psychiatry 1998;43(6):464–465.

122. Warnock JK, Bundren JC, Morris DW. Depressive mood symptoms associated with ovarian suppression. Fertil Steril 2000;74(5):984–986.

123. Steingold KA, Cedars M, Lu JK, Randle D, Judd HL, Meldrum DR. Treatment of endometriosis with a long-acting gonadotropin-releasing hormone agonist. Obstet Gynecol 1987;69(3 Pt 1):403–411.

124. Ferrero S, Pretta S, Bertoldi S et al. Increased frequency of migraine among women with endometriosis. Hum Reprod 2004;19(12): 2927–2932.

125. Kontoravdis A, Hassan E, Hassiakos D, Botsis D, Kontoravdis N, Creatsas G. Laparoscopic evaluation and management of chronic pelvic pain during adolescence. Clin Exp Obstet Gynecol 1999;26(2):76–77.

126. Vercellini P, Fedele L, Arcaini L, Bianchi S, Rognoni MT, Candiani GB. Laparoscopy in the diagnosis of chronic pelvic pain in adolescent women. J Reprod Med 1989;34(10):827–830.

127. Ballweg ML, Campbell PF. Psychosocial aspects of teen endo. J Pediatr Adolesc Gynecol 2003;16(3 Suppl):S13–15.

128. Montenegro ML, Vasconcelos EC, Candido Dos Reis FJ, Nogueira AA, Poli-Neto OB. Physical therapy in the management of women with chronic pelvic pain. Int J Clin Pract 2008;62(2):263–269.

129. Leeners B, Imthurn B, Hugi A, Neises M, Delex-Zaiontz N. Gyneco-psychosomatic counseling in Germany and Switzerland – aims and state of the art. J Psychosom Res 2006;61(1):91–94.

130. Alldrich CK. The Medical Interview: Gateway to the Doctor–Patient Relationship, 2nd edn. New York: Parthenon Publishing Group, 1999.

131. Schuth W, Richter K, Schertel K, Kieback D. "Erwartet hab'ich eigentlich …" Erfahrungen gynäko-onkologischer Patientinnen mit dem behandelnden Arzt im Vergleich zu ihren Erwartungen. In: Neises M, editor. Psychosomatische Gynäkologie und Geburtshilfe. Geissen: Psychosozial Verlag, 2000.

132. Kennedy S. Should a diagnosis of endometriosis be sought in all symptomatic women? Fertil Steril 2006;86(5):1312–1313; discussion 1317.

133. Raspe H-H. Aufklärung und Information im Krankenhaus. Göttingen: Vandenhoeck + Ruprecht, 1983.

134. Sutton CJ, Ewen SP, Whitelaw N, Haines P. Prospective, randomized, double-blind, controlled trial of laser laparoscopy in the treatment of pelvic pain associated with minimal, mild, and moderate endometriosis. Fertil Steril 1994;62(4):696–700.

135. Albert H. Psychosomatic group treatment helps women with chronic pelvic pain. J Psychosom Obstet Gynaecol 1999;20(4):216–225.

136. Richmond J. NIH Technology Assessment Panel: integration of behavioural and relaxation approaches into the treatment of chronic pain and insomnia. JAMA 1996;276:313–318.

137. Mensendieck B. Look Better, Feel Better. New York: Harper, 1954.

138. Haugstad GK, Haugstad TS, Kirste U et al. Reliability and validity of a standardized Mensendieck physiotherapy test (SMT). Physiother Theory Pract 2006;22(4):189–205.

139. Henningsen P, Zipfel S, Herzog W. Management of functional somatic syndromes. Lancet 2007;369(9565):946–955.

140. Whitney ML. Importance of lay organizations for coping with endometriosis. J Reprod Med 1998;43(3 Suppl):331–334.

54 Endometriosis in the Adolescent Patient

Claire Templeman

Department of Obstetrics and Gynecology and Surgery, University of Southern California and Children's Hospital Los Angeles, Los Angeles, CA, USA

Introduction

The prevalence of endometriosis in adults varies depending upon the population studied. To date, there have not been any population-based prevalence studies investigating endometriosis in adolescents. However, Parker et al, in the Menstrual Disorders of Teenagers (MDOT) study [1], conducted their research with the aim of establishing parameters for menstrual disturbance in Australian teenagers. These authors reported on menstrual symptoms in 1051 adolescents. They found that although 75% of their population reported typical menstrual symptoms, described as mild dysmenorrhea with a low interference in life activities, there was a subgroup of girls, consisting of 10% of their population, who had severe dysmenorrhea, reported a low effectiveness of over-the-counter medications and a high rate of interference with life activities secondary to pain. It is this group that the authors strongly suggest should be evaluated by gynecologists for endometriosis.

Studies evaluating girls with these atypical symptoms via laparoscopy report high rates of endometriosis. Goldstein et al [2] reported a 47% incidence of disease in adolescent females undergoing laparoscopy for chronic pelvic pain, with 58% of these girls having minimal disease. Laufer et al [3] reported finding endometriosis at the time of surgery in 67% of adolescents who had pain refractory to simple medical treatments like non-steroidal anti-inflammatory agents (NSAIDs) or oral contraceptive pills (OCP). They also observed that all adolescents had stage I or II disease as described by the American Fertility Society's (AFS) classification [4]. Similiarly, Reese et al [5] found that 73% of the adolescents with chronic pain refractory to simple analgesia and oral contraceptives had endometriosis at the time of laparoscopy, most commonly AFS stage I red colored lesions.

Gao et al [6] have produced some data that highlight the economic importance of endometriosis among adolescents.

These authors assessed the direct and indirect costs of endometriosis and concluded that as endometriosis-related hospital length of stay steadily declined from 1993 to 2002, per-patient cost increased 61%. In addition, adolescents (aged 10–17 years) had endometriosis-related hospitalizations and females 23 years or younger constituted >20% of endometriosis-related outpatient visits [6]. The direct economic impact of endometriosis on adolescents is poorly understood currently, but given that the symptoms and treatment modalities are very similar, the direct costs may be even greater in this age group than adults, since younger patients are likely to be treated for a relatively longer time period [6]. This is an area that requires further research.

Pathophysiology of endometriosis in adolescence

The pathogenesis of endometriosis remains an enigma, and as a result no single theory can explain the development of endometriosis in all patients. Retrograde menstruation with transplantation and implantation of endometrial tissue and cells into the peritoneal cavity were suggested as a possible etiology for endometriosis by Sampson [7]. Retrograde menstruation has been reported in women at the time of laparoscopy during menstruation; however, this observation is often made from a single menstrual cycle since women are unlikely to undergo serial laparoscopies. However, D'Hooghe et al [8] in their primate studies showed that recurrent retrograde menstruation during two subsequent cycles was observed in all baboons with spontaneous endometriosis but only in 25% of baboons with either a normal pelvis or experimentally induced endometriosis. Retrograde menstruation as an etiology for endometriosis appears to be particularly important in adolescents with obstructive müllerian anomalies [9]. In baboons with experimentally induced obstructed

Endometriosis: Science and Practice, First Edition. Edited by Linda C. Giudice, Johannes L.H. Evers and David L. Healy.
© 2012 Blackwell Publishing Ltd. Published 2012 by Blackwell Publishing Ltd.

menstruation, endometriosis has been shown to develop within 3 months [10] and there is a positive correlation between the weight of endometrial tissue used for intrapelvis seeding and the extent of the resulting peritoneal endometriosis [11].

There are specific defects in the endometrium of women with endometriosis that include a decrease in endometrial cell apoptosis [12] and decreased sensitivity to progesterone, resulting in increased matrix metalloproteinase activity [13]. The effect of these defects is an increase in the number of cells with invasive capacity that are refluxed through the fallopian tubes and into the peritoneal cavity. In addition, neo-angiogenesis as the result of cytokine and vascular endothelial growth factor secretion may also play an important role in the establishment of endometriosis [14]. Another focus of research is in the area of environmental toxins and oxidative stress. In particular, dioxin has been implicated in the pathophysiology of endometriosis [15]. However, studies of eutopic endometrium of adolescents with endometriosis or of endocrine-disrupting chemicals in this age group are lacking.

Investigation into the genetics of endometriosis is being undertaken in several centers [16]. This focus includes linkage analysis for sibling pairs where first-degree relatives of patients with surgically confirmed endometriosis are evaluated. These data have demonstrated a 6.9% relative risk of the disease in comparison with controls [17]. In addition, microarray [18] and epigenetic evaluation of DNA [19] are techniques aimed at determining important genes in pivotal molecular pathways that may be associated with the development of endometriosis.

The finding of predominantly smooth muscle endometriotic lesions in the rectovaginal septum [20] of some women has led to the theory of embryonic müllerian rests [21] as an etiology for endometriosis. This theory is also supported by the finding of endometriosis in the pelvis of premenarchal girls [22]. Still other patients will develop endometriosis in surgical site wounds such as cesarean section wounds or episiotomy sites. Since hematogenous and lymphatic spread to a single site is unlikely, this has lead to the unintentional surgical transplantation theory of endometriosis.

That endometriosis diagnosed in adolescence may progress is a concern for many patients and their families. In primate studies, D'Hooghe et al [8] evaluated the hypothesis that spontaneous endometriosis may be a progressive disease. Using serial laparoscopy where stage, number, size, and type of endometriosis lesions were noted on a pelvic map, these authors have shown that over 24 months the number of new subtle surface lesions increased by 69%. In association with this, they also found that 10% of the lesions were undergoing remodeling and 21% were unchanged. How these results from baboons kept in captivity, without intervening pregnancy and subjected to serial laparoscopy, are applicable to humans has not yet been established. However, they have led to the suggestion that endometriosis may be a progressive disease in some patients.

Sutton et al [23] have produced some evidence about the natural history of endometriosis. In their randomized, placebo-controlled trial evaluating the laparoscopic treatment of endometriosis, these authors demonstrated that equal numbers of placebo patients had disease that progressed, regressed and remained static at second-

look laparoscopy. Konnickx also found that the only significant correlate with pain symptoms was the depth of endometriosis invasion [24]. This would suggest that the more superficial red and atypical lesions present in adolescents should not be painful. However, it has become clear that there are alternative mechanisms for the production of pain in endometriosis and that red lesions in particular are very active in the synthesis of prostaglandins [25], which are likely to be important in pain symptomatology. In addition, several other mechanisms may be important in the production of pain in patients with endometriosis and these include cytokine production, bleeding within the implant itself, as well as stimulation of neural tissue both within the lesion [26,27] and within the endometrium of patients with endometriosis [28].

Endometriosis lesions themselves appear to have a developmental pathway. Several authors [29] have found that the typical lesions of endometriosis, black and white scarred areas along with endometriomas, appear to increase with age. This is consistent with other authors who have found that red flame-like and atypical clear vesicular lesions are more prominent in younger patients [30,31]. This knowledge is important since atypical disease may be missed if the surgeon is only looking for the black lesions associated with typical endometriosis. This may partially explain the phenomenon of "negative laparoscopy" in young patients and underlies the importance of biopsy for any suspicious lesions in these patients.

Endometriosis epidemiology

Age at menarche and menstrual cycle patterns in women have been investigated as potential risk factors for endometriosis. However, the studies are inconsistent with Missmer et al [32] finding early age at menarche and shorter menstrual cycle lengths as risk factors for the development of endometriosis while other authors found no relationship [33].

Relative weight in childhood as a risk factor for the development of endometriosis has been recently investigated by Nagel et al [34] in a case–control study. These authors asked participants to recall their relative weights between the ages of 10 and 16 years. This was categorized as "underweight," "average weight" and "overweight". The authors found that women who reported being overweight at age 10 years were more likely to be diagnosed with endometriosis later in life. They propose that overweight girls reach menarche earlier than their thin peers, such that being "overweight" during childhood could be assumed to increase exposure to menstrual flow and subsequently increase the risk of endometriosis. However, in a prospective cohort study that examined the relationship between childhood body size (assessed by showing participants a nine-level figure drawing of body sizes) and endometriosis risk, the authors found a significant reduction in the incidence of endometriosis with increasing body size at all the age endpoints studied (age 5, 10 and 20 years) [35]. This relationship persisted when adjusted for Body Mass Index (BMI), birthweight, parity, age at menarche, and oral contraceptive use. The authors suggest that obesity in adolescent women in association with insulin resistance results in disruption of ovulation and ultimately oligoamenorrhea.

Presentation and diagnosis

Dysmenorrhea in adolescents may be primary or secondary to endometriosis. The true prevalence of primary dysmenorrhea is difficult to assess since many girls do not seek medical attention, with one study revealing that 98% of adolescents used non-pharmacological means to address their symptoms [36].

Dysmenorrhea is reported to have a significant impact on school absenteeism and quality of life in Caucasian adolescents, with recent reports confirming a very similar pattern among African American and Hispanic girls [36].

In an Australian study [1], menstruation in adolescence was found to be associated with pain defined as dysmenorrhea in 93% of those girls surveyed. These authors also confirmed significant associations between increasing severity of menstrual pain and interference with life activities, with 25% of study participants reporting pain severe enough to be absent from school on a recurrent basis.

Endometriosis should be considered in girls who do not respond to simple NSAIDs and OCPs, since two-thirds of girls who are investigated with laparoscopy in this clinical setting have been found to have endometriosis [3].

Recent data from the Endometriosis Association suggest that patients who have symptoms suggestive of endometriosis as an adolescent wait longer to be surgically diagnosed than women who are first symptomatic as adults [36]. Indeed, these authors report that each step of the diagnostic experience takes longer for the adolescent: adolescents wait longer to seek medical advice and take longer to receive a diagnosis once they do present. In addition, girls who saw a physician other than a gynecologist have a longer time to definitive diagnosis [37]. Some of this delay may be explained by the diversity of symptoms that patients with endometriosis experience, in addition to the fact that laparoscopy is required for a definitive diagnosis.

A detailed history and physical examination is critical in the assessment of adolescents presenting with pain symptomatology. If appropriate, pelvic examination for signs of uterosacral nodularity and levator tenderness may point to the diagnosis of endometriosis. However, in virginal patients this exam is likely to be omitted. External genital inspection with labial traction and rectal exam should be considered if there is suspicion of an obstructive anomaly.

Rare cases of vulvar endometriosis have also been reported, and thus biopsy of suspicious lesions should be considered [38]. Rackow *et al* [39] have also suggested that in adolescents with urinary frequency associated with chronic pelvic pain, the diagnosis of interstitial cystitis should be considered and cystoscopy performed once urinary tract infection is excluded.

Abdominal wall assessment for signs of muscle injury and trigger points is helpful as this indicates that physical therapy is very likely to be useful in the management of pain symptoms [40].

Imaging with pelvic ultrasound is useful to exclude the possibility of an endometrioma or to confirm the presence of a uterine anomaly. Tumor markers such as CA-125 are unlikely to be helpful in adolescents since they have early-stage disease and rarely have endometriomas [3,5].

Management strategies

The history and physical examination should help the treating physician to develop a strategy about the likely cause of the pain symptomatology. Often, what began as pain secondary to endometriosis has progressed to involve a component of musculoskeletal pain with associated depression and anxiety [41]. Therefore it is important to recognize that for treatment to be effective, the managing physician must seek and address all these issues, if present.

The treatment algorithms used to manage adolescents are largely based upon research performed in adults. Typically, medical management is used initially, although surgical intervention may be required if a müllerian anomaly is suspected or the endometriosis is of advanced stage. If the adolescent has persistent pain despite intervention with medical therapy, she should be offered laparoscopy for definitive diagnosis.. Empiric gonadotropin releasing hormone agonist therapy has been utilized in adults with chronic pelvic pain and a suspected diagnosis of endometriosis. This approach (detailed below) may be considered in adolescents, but with special consideration to patient age.

In the absence of a clinically useful marker of endometriosis, the challenge is distinguishing which patients may have pain and progressive disease from those whose disease will remain the same or even regress. Clinically, however, the physician is often confronted with an adolescent in chronic pain and therefore intervention to relieve symptoms becomes a priority.

Medical therapy

Non-steroidal anti-inflammatory drugs are often the first-line medication used to treat dysmenorrhea, and many adolescents have used these at the time of presentation. The American College of Obstetricians and Gynecologists (ACOG) has issued a statement supporting the empiric use of NSAIDs for dysmenorrhea [42].

These drugs act through inhibition of the cyclo-oxygenase (COX) enzyme pathway which is responsible for the production of prostaglandins and leukotrienes. Some drugs in this family may also act through promotion of prostaglandin (PG) E_2, a vasodilator. In placebo-controlled trials, NSAIDs have been found to significantly decrease menstrual loss and improve primary dysmenorrhea [43]. In endometriotic lesions there is a positive feedback loop between prostaglandins and estrogen production through aromatase production. In addition, in mouse models of endometriosis, COX-2 inhibitors have been found to decrease both the size and the microvessel density within endometriotic lesions [44].

Other medical treatments for endometriosis are aimed at suppressing pituitary gonadotropin secretion and/or steroid hormone production by the ovary. This results in atrophy of the endometrial implants, at least while the patient is taking the medication. Oral contraceptives (OCs) are used empirically to treat both primary dysmenorrhea and dysmenorrhea secondary to endometriosis [45] and despite the paucity of randomized trials demonstrating effectiveness, the ACOG also supports the use of OCs in this setting [42].

Perhaps the major reason why OCs are so commonly used as first-line therapy in this age group is their relatively low incidence of side-effects and the ease with which they can be stopped should the patient wish to change medications. In addition, a trial of OCs either after or concurrent with NSAIDs is helpful in assessing the likelihood that the adolescent has endometriosis [3]. Tokushige et al [46] have shown that the administration of oral progestogens and continuous oral contraceptive pills reduces nerve fiber density and growth factor receptors in the eutopic endometrium of women with endometriosis. However, the suppressive effect of these drugs was lower on the nerve fibers in peritoneal endometriosis lesions [47]. Further research is required in this area to determine whether these findings correlate with objectively measured symptoms.

Progestins have been shown to be effective in reducing pain symptoms in patients with endometriosis [48]. Possible mechanisms for this include downregulation of estrogen receptors and a reduction in matrix metalloproteinases in endometriosis tissue [49], with the added benefit of amenorrhea particularly with the depot injections and medicated intrauterine device delivery systems [50]. Depot medroxyprogesterone acetate (DMPA) is a monthly injection that has been used in adolescents with endometriosis as a method of treating pain symptoms with the added benefit of being a very effective contraceptive. A subcutaneous, monthly formulation has been introduced, with comparable efficacy to the intramuscular injection but less impact on bone mineralization [51].

Although the medicated intrauterine device (IUD) is not FDA-approved for the treatment of endometriosis, a Cochrane review suggested that this system does reduce painful periods in women who have had surgery for endometriosis. However, this review was based upon one small study and the authors also comment on the need for further well-designed randomized controlled trials in this setting [52]. Of note, the ACOG in a technical bulletin supports the use of IUDs in an adolescent population [53]. This Committee Opinion addresses the use of IUDs for contraception both in the emergency setting and for long-term preventive use; however, it does not specifically discuss the use of the levonorgestrel-containing IUD (LNG-IUD) for the treatment of pelvic pain and possible endometriosis. If this is considered for use in an adolescent, the ACOG recommends that all adolescents are screened for chlamydia and gonorrhea prior to insertion.

Paterson et al [54] surveyed gynecologists in New Zealand about their use of the LNG-IUD in adolescents. Of interest, the two most common reasons for using this treatment were the management of menorrhagia in adolescents with intellectual disability, and endometriosis. Another interesting approach to the use of progestins in adolescents has been reported by Al-Jefout

et al [55]. These authors report on an adolescent patient refractory to all other medications who was successfully treated with a LNG-IUD and an etonogestrel subdermal implant. The rationale for this approach was to target the endometrium locally with the LNG-IUD and to suppress the more distant ectopic implants with a constant dose of systemic progestogen.

Newer drugs, available in experimental protocols in adults, include aromatase inhibitors [56]. However, there are no data on the use of this medication in adolescents, and aromatase inhibitors are not FDA-approved for treatment of endometriosis-related pain.

Gonadotropin releasing hormone agonists (GnRHa) have been shown to be effective in reducing pain associated with endometriosis [57]. They are effective by suppressing the hypothalamic-pituitary axis which results in a hypoestrogenic environment and side-effects such as hot flushes and mood changes. Empiric use of GnRHa has been advocated for adults with chronic pain but should *not* be used in adolescents under 18 years of age due to detrimental effects on bone density [42]. They may be considered in adolescents as young as 16 years with known endometriosis who are refractory to other medical therapies, with some special considerations. These include the use of add-back therapy, typically norethisterone acetate 5 mg daily, vitamin D and calcium along with appropriate monitoring of bone mineral density via age-matched Z-scores at least every 2 years [42,58]. These measures are aimed at maximizing the effect of GnRHa and minimizing the side-effects.

The effect of norethindrone acetate (NTA) "add-back" therapy given in conjunction with GnRHa on bone mineral density (BMD) in adolescents has been evaluated by Divasta et al [59]. In this retrospective study, adolescents with endometriosis diagnosed surgically (mean age 17.7 years, range 13–21) were treated with GnRHa and 5 mg NTA, with BMD measured after a minimum of 4 months of GnRHa administration. These authors found that BMD at the hip was preserved but it was decreased at the lumbar spine in one-third of adolescents. These results require further evaluation in a prospective trial with BMD measured before treatment and longitudinal follow-up data.

Laparoscopic surgery remains the gold standard for the diagnosis of endometriosis. This is typically performed in adolescents who have pain symptoms refractory to medical treatment or if there is concern about a müllerian anomaly. In looking for endometriosis in adolescents at the time of surgery, it is important to be aware that the disease is most commonly located in the cul-de-sac and is atypical in appearance [60]. Two randomized controlled trials in adults have established a relationship between surgical intervention and reduction of pain in patients with endometriosis. Sutton et al [23] demonstrated a significant reduction in pain, lasting up to 6 months, in patients who underwent resection of their disease when compared to those who had diagnostic laparoscopy alone. Interestingly, these results were poorer for stage I than III disease. Abbott et al [61] confirmed these results and included quality of life measures, which were also improved at 6 months follow-up. Whether such intervention changes the natural history of the disease or improves future reproductive potential in adolescents is unknown. In terms of long-term follow-up, Abbott et al [62] have shown that the improvement in pain may last up to 5 years but the risk of further intervention is higher in younger patients and those in whom disease resection is suboptimal. Nerve ablation techniques including presacral neurectomy and uterine nerve ablation techniques have not been studied in the adolescent population.

Pre- and postoperative hormonal suppression in general has not been shown to be of benefit in terms of decreasing the number of patients with symptom recurrence over time [63]. However, there is a paucity of randomized trials in this area and further research is needed. Recently, there has been a report of a significant reduction in endometrioma recurrence at 36 months in adult women who take the oral contraceptive pill after surgery compared to those who do not [64].

There is a paucity of data on the outcome of therapy for endometriosis in adolescents. A recent retrospective study examined the outcome of surgery and postoperative medical therapy in this population [65]. Over a 12-year period, 90 eligible patients were evaluated in this study with laparoscopy and postoperative medical treatment: either OCs or GnRHa in addition to add-back therapy with NTA. Stage at initial surgery and subsequent surgeries (if performed) were recorded. The authors conclude that there was no change in endometriosis stage in 70% of patients between the first and second surgery (median 29 months) and an improvement in 19% of patients. Hence they suggest that combined medical and surgical treatment retards disease progression in this population. However, there are several significant limitations to this study, including the lack of a control group, lack of routine biopsy to confirm diagnosis at the time of surgery, and the retrospective nature of the study. Further research involving a prospective randomized, placebo-controlled trial is needed to answer this question definitively.

Complementary management

In treating adolescents with endometriosis, it is important to realize that chronic pain is often multifactorial. Behavioral modification techniques such as relaxation and biofeedback as well as cognitive therapy aimed at improving coping skills can be helpful. In addition, physical therapy may be helpful in patients for whom musculoskeletal conditions of the abdominal wall and pelvic floor are contributing to their symptoms [66].

Among patients in whom dysmenorrhea is a primary component of their pain symptomatology, Chinese herbal medicine (CHM) may offer an alternative to pain medications or hormonal manipulation. Although not specifically studied in adolescents, among adult women, a Cochrane review found this treatment promising and in need of further rigorous study [67]. In addition, CHM has also been investigated as treatment in women diagnosed with endometriosis [68]. Based upon two randomized controlled trials with a total of 158 women in which CHM was administered to patients post surgery for a diagnosis of endometriosis, Flower et al found that CHM was as effective as gestinone and more effective than danazol in relieving dysmenorrhea, with

a lower incidence of side-effects [68]. Once again, the authors conclude that more research is required to determine the place of this treatment in the management of endometriosis.

Wayne et al [69] have reported on a small RCT using Japanese acupuncture. A total of 18 patients were enrolled and 14 completed the study treatments over 8 weeks. Pain was reduced in the treatment group but there was no statistically significant difference between the groups after 4 weeks. Larger trials in this area are needed.

Conclusion

The natural history of endometriosis in an individual patient remains largely unknown and therefore it is difficult to determine whether early intervention in adolescents enhances future fertility or improves long-term disease outcome. The most immediate issue is a young woman in pain and a physician who needs to make a diagnosis and manage the symptoms. Laparoscopy remains the gold standard for establishing the diagnosis and long-term control of symptoms in adolescents requires medical management often in combination with complementary therapies. Current research focused on the pathophysiology of endometriosis is likely to add to our understanding of the natural history of the disease, allowing future studies to better assess therapeutic outcomes in adolescents. The place of alternative therapies such as CHM and acupuncture remains to be determined but they appear to be promising adjuncts to the management of pain in this population.

References

1. Parker MA, Sneddon AE, Arbon P. The menstrual disorder of teenagers (MDOT) study: determining typical menstrual patterns and menstrual disturbance in a large population-based study of Australian teenagers. Br J Obstet Gynaecol;117(2):185–192.
2. Goldstein DP, de Cholnoky C, Emans SJ. Adolescent endometriosis. J Adolesc Health Care 1980;1(1):37–41.
3. Laufer MR, Goitein L, Bush M, Cramer DW, Emans SJ. Prevalence of endometriosis in adolescent girls with chronic pelvic pain not responding to conventional therapy. J Pediatr Adolesc Gynecol 1997;10(4):199–202.
4. American Society for Reproductive Medicine. Revised classification of endometriosis. Fertil Steril 1996;67:817–821.
5. Reese KA, Reddy S, Rock JA. Endometriosis in an adolescent population: the Emory experience. J Pediatr Adolesc Gynecol 1996;9(3):125–128.
6. Gao X, Outley J, Botteman M, Spalding J, Simon JA, Pashos CL. Economic burden of endometriosis. Fertil Steril 2006;86(6):1561–1572.
7. Sampson J. The development of the implanation theory for the origin of peritoneal endometriosis. Am J Obstet Gynecol 1940;40:549–557.
8. D'Hooghe TM, Bambra CS, Raeymaekers BM, Koninckx PR. Development of spontaneous endometriosis in baboons. Obstet Gynecol 1996;88(3):462–466.

9. Sanfilippo JS, Wakim NG, Schikler KN, Yussman MA. Endometriosis in association with uterine anomaly. Am J Obstet Gynecol 1986;1 54(1):39–43.

10. D'Hooghe TM, Bambra CS, Suleman MA, Dunselman GA, Evers HL, Koninckx PR. Development of a model of retrograde menstruation in baboons (Papio anubis). Fertil Steril 1994;62(3):635–638.

11. D'Hooghe TM, Bambra CS, Raeymaekers BM, de Jonge I, Lauweryns JM, Koninckx PR. Intrapelvic injection of menstrual endometrium causes endometriosis in baboons (Papio cynocephalus and Papio anubis). Am J Obstet Gynecol 1995;173(1):125–134.

12. Harada T, Kaponis A, Iwabe T et al. Apoptosis in human endometrium and endometriosis. Hum Reprod Update 2004; 10(1):29–38.

13. Osteen KG, Yeaman GR, Bruner-Tran KL. Matrix metalloproteinases and endometriosis. Semin Reprod Med 2003;21(2):155–164.

14. Di Carlo C, Bonifacio M, Tommaselli GA, Bifulco G, Guerra G, Nappi C. Metalloproteinases, vascular endothelial growth factor, and angiopoietin 1 and 2 in eutopic and ectopic endometrium. Fertil Steril 2009;91(6):2315–2323.

15. Bruner-Tran KL, Yeaman GR, Crispens MA, Igarashi TM, Osteen KG. Dioxin may promote inflammation-related development of endometriosis. Fertil Steril 2008;89(5 Suppl):1287–1298.

16. Montgomery GW, Nyholt DR, Zhao ZZ et al. The search for genes contributing to endometriosis risk. Hum Reprod Update 2008;14(5):447–457.

17. Simpson JL, Elias S, Malinak LR, Buttram VC Jr. Heritable aspects of endometriosis. I. Genetic studies. Am J Obstet Gynecol 1980; 137(3):327–331.

18. Mettler L, Salmassi A, Schollmeyer T, Schmutzler AG, Pungel F, Jonat W. Comparison of c-DNA microarray analysis of gene expression between eutopic endometrium and ectopic endometrium (endometriosis). J Assist Reprod Genet 2007;24(6):249–258.

19. Guo SW. Epigenetics of endometriosis. Mol Hum Reprod 2009;15(10):587–607.

20. Nisolle M, Donnez J. Peritoneal endometriosis, ovarian endometriosis, and adenomyotic nodules of the rectovaginal septum are three different entities. Fertil Steril 1997;68(4):585–596.

21. Batt RE, Smith RA. Embryologic theory of histogenesis of endometriosis in peritoneal pockets. Obstet Gynecol Clin North Am 1989;16(1):15–28.

22. Marsh EE, Laufer MR. Endometriosis in premenarcheal girls who do not have an associated obstructive anomaly. Fertil Steril 2005;83(3):758–760.

23. Sutton CJ, Ewen SP, Whitelaw N, Haines P. Prospective, randomized, double-blind, controlled trial of laser laparoscopy in the treatment of pelvic pain associated with minimal, mild, and moderate endometriosis. Fertil Steril 1994;62(4):696–700.

24. Koninckx PR, Meuleman C, Demeyere S, Lesaffre E, Cornillie FJ. Suggestive evidence that pelvic endometriosis is a progressive disease, whereas deeply infiltrating endometriosis is associated with pelvic pain. Fertil Steril 1991;55(4):759–765.

25. Wu MH, Shoji Y, Chuang PC, Tsai SJ. Endometriosis: disease pathophysiology and the role of prostaglandins. Expert Rev Mol Med 2007;9(2):1–20.

26. Tokushige N, Markham R, Russell P, Fraser IS. Nerve fibres in peritoneal endometriosis. Hum Reprod 2006;21(11):3001–3007.

27. Tokushige N, Russell P, Black K et al. Nerve fibers in ovarian endometriomas. Fertil Steril 2010;94(5):1944–1947.

28. Tokushige N, Markham R, Russell P, Fraser IS. Different types of small nerve fibers in eutopic endometrium and myometrium in women with endometriosis. Fertil Steril 2007;88(4):795–803.

29. Redwine DB. The distribution of endometriosis in the pelvis by age groups and fertility. Fertil Steril 1987;47(1):173–175.

30. Davis GD, Thillet E, Lindemann J. Clinical characteristics of adolescent endometriosis. J Adolesc Health. 1993;14(5):362–368.

31. Redwine DB. Age-related evolution in color appearance of endometriosis. Fertil Steril 1987;48(6):1062–1063.

32. Missmer SA, Cramer DW. The epidemiology of endometriosis. Obstet Gynecol Clin North Am 2003;30(1):1–19, vii.

33. Templeman C, Marshall SF, Ursin G et al. Adenomyosis and endometriosis in the California Teachers Study. Fertil Steril 2008; 90(2):415–424.

34. Nagle CM, Bell TA, Purdie DM et al. Relative weight at ages 10 and 16 years and risk of endometriosis: a case-control analysis. Hum Reprod 2009;24(6):1501–1506.

35. Vitonis AF, Baer HJ, Hankinson SE, Laufer MR, Missmer SA. A prospective study of body size during childhood and early adulthood and the incidence of endometriosis. Hum Reprod 2010; 25(5):1325–1334.

36. Harel Z. Dysmenorrhea in adolescents and young adults: etiology and management. J Pediatr Adolesc Gynecol 2006;19(6):363–371.

37. Greene R, Stratton P, Cleary SD, Ballweg ML, Sinaii N. Diagnostic experience among 4,334 women reporting surgically diagnosed endometriosis. Fertil Steril 2009;91(1):32–39.

38. Eyvazzadeh AD, Smith YR, Lieberman R, Quint EH. A rare case of vulvar endometriosis in an adolescent girl. Fertil Steril 2009;91(3):929.

39. Rackow BW, Novi JM, Arya LA, Pfeifer SM. Interstitial cystitis is an etiology of chronic pelvic pain in young women. J Pediatr Adolesc Gynecol 2009;22(3):181–185.

40. Schroeder B, Sanfilippo JS, Hertweck SP. Musculoskeletal pelvic pain in a pediatric and adolescent gynecology practice. J Pediatr Adolesc Gynecol 2000;13(2):90.

41. Sinaii N, Cleary SD, Younes N, Ballweg ML, Stratton P. Treatment utilization for endometriosis symptoms: a cross-sectional survey study of lifetime experience. Fertil Steril 2007;87(6):1277–1286.

42. American College of Obstetricians and Gynecologists. Endometriosis in adolescents. Committee Opinion No. 310.Obstet Gynecol 2005;105(4):921–927.

43. Roy SN, Bhattacharya S. Benefits and risks of pharmacological agents used for the treatment of menorrhagia. Drug Saf 2004; 27(2):75–90.

44. Ozawa Y, Murakami T, Tamura M, Terada Y, Yaegashi N, Okamura K. A selective cyclooxygenase-2 inhibitor suppresses the growth of endometriosis xenografts via antiangiogenic activity in severe combined immunodeficiency mice. Fertil Steril 2006;86(4 Suppl):1146–1451.

45. Davis L, Kennedy SS, Moore J, Prentice A. Modern combined oral contraceptives for pain associated with endometriosis. Cochrane Database Syst Rev 2007;3:CD001019.

46. Tokushige N, Markham R, Russell P, Fraser IS. Effects of hormonal treatment on nerve fibers in endometrium and myometrium in women with endometriosis. Fertil Steril 2008;90(5):1589–1598.

47. Tokushige N, Markham R, Russell P, Fraser IS. Effect of progestogens and combined oral contraceptives on nerve fibers in peritoneal endometriosis. Fertil Steril 2009;92(4):1234–1239.

48. Prentice A, Deary AJ, Bland E. Progestagens and anti-progestagens for pain associated with endometriosis. Cochrane Database Syst Rev 2000;2:CD002122.

49. Rodgers AK, Falcone T. Treatment strategies for endometriosis. Expert Opin Pharmacother 2008;9(2):243–255.

50. Vercellini P, Frontino G, de Giorgi O, Aimi G, Zaina B, Crosignani PG. Comparison of a levonorgestrel-releasing intrauterine device versus expectant management after conservative surgery for symptomatic endometriosis: a pilot study. Fertil Steril 2003;80(2):305–309.

51. Schlaff WD, Carson SA, Luciano A, Ross D, Bergqvist A. Subcutaneous injection of depot medroxyprogesterone acetate compared with leuprolide acetate in the treatment of endometriosis-associated pain. Fertil Steril 2006;85(2):314–325.

52. Abou-Setta AM, Al-Inany HG, Farquhar CM. Levonorgestrel-releasing intrauterine device (LNG-IUD) for symptomatic endometriosis following surgery. Cochrane Database Syst Rev 2006; 4:CD005072.

53. American College of Obstetricians and Gynecologists. Intrauterine device and adolescents. Committee Opinion No. 392. Obstet Gynecol 2007;110(6):1493–1495.

54. Paterson H, Miller D, Devenish C. A survey of New Zealand RANZCOG Fellows on their use of the levonorgestrel intrauterine device in adolescents. Aust N Z J Obstet Gynaecol 2009; 49(2):220–225.

55. Al-Jefout M, Palmer J, Fraser IS. Simultaneous use of a levonorgestrel intrauterine system and an etonogestrel subdermal implant for debilitating adolescent endometriosis. Aust N Z J Obstet Gynaecol 2007; 47(3):247–249.

56. American College of Obstetricians and Gynecologists. Aromatase inhibitors in gynecologic practice. Obstet Gynecol 2008; 112(2 Pt 1):405–407.

57. Dlugi AM, Miller JD, Knittle J. Lupron depot (leuprolide acetate for depot suspension) in the treatment of endometriosis: a randomized, placebo-controlled, double-blind study. Lupron Study Group. Fertil Steril 1990;54(3):419–427.

58. Laufer MR. Current approaches to optimizing the treatment of endometriosis in adolescents. Gynecol Obstet Invest 2008; 66(Suppl 1):19–27.

59. Divasta AD, Laufer MR, Gordon CM. Bone density in adolescents treated with a GnRH agonist and add-back therapy for endometriosis. J Pediatr Adolesc Gynecol 2007;20(5):293–297.

60. Laufer MR. Identification of clear vesicular lesions of atypical endometriosis: a new technique. Fertil Steril 1997;68(4):739–740.

61. Abbott J, Hawe J, Hunter D, Holmes M, Finn P, Garry R. Laparoscopic excision of endometriosis: a randomized, placebo-controlled trial. Fertil Steril 2004;82(4):878–884.

62. Abbott JA, Hawe J, Clayton RD, Garry R. The effects and effectiveness of laparoscopic excision of endometriosis: a prospective study with 2–2 year follow-up. Hum Reprod 2003;18(9):1922–1927.

63. Yap C, Furness S, Farquhar C. Pre and post operative medical therapy for endometriosis surgery. Cochrane Database Syst Rev 2004; 3:CD003678.

64. Vercellini P, Somigliana E, Daguati R, Vigano P, Meroni F, Crosignani PG. Postoperative oral contraceptive exposure and risk of endometrioma recurrence. Am J Obstet Gynecol 2008;198(5):504.

65. Doyle JO, Missmer SA, Laufer MR. The effect of combined surgical-medical intervention on the progression of endometriosis in an adolescent and young adult population. J Pediatr Adolesc Gynecol 2009;22(4):257–263.

66. Greco CD. Management of adolescent chronic pelvic pain from endometriosis: a pain center perspective. J Pediatr Adolesc Gynecol 2003;16(3 Suppl):S17–19.

67. Zhu X, Proctor M, Bensoussan A, Wu E, Smith CA. Chinese herbal medicine for primary dysmenorrhoea. Cochrane Database Syst Rev 2008;2:CD005288.

68. Flower A, Liu JP, Chen S, Lewith G, Little P. Chinese herbal medicine for endometriosis. Cochrane Database Syst Rev 2009;3:CD006568.

69. Wayne PM, Kerr CE, Schnyer RN et al. Japanese-style acupuncture for endometriosis-related pelvic pain in adolescents and young women: results of a randomized sham-controlled trial. J Pediatr Adolesc Gynecol 2008;21(5):247–257.

55 Fertility Preservation in Patients with Endometrioma

Jennifer Hirshfeld-Cytron[1,2], Candace Tingen[2,3] and Teresa K. Woodruff[2,3]

[1] Department of Obstetrics and Gynecology, Division of Reproductive Endocrinology and Infertility, Feinberg School of Medicine, Northwestern University, Chicago, IL USA

[2] Center for Reproductive Science, Northwestern University, Evanston, IL, USA

[3] Department of Obstetrics and Gynecology, Division of Fertility Preservation, Feinberg School of Medicine, Northwestern University, Chicago, IL, USA

Introduction

Endometriosis is an estrogen-dependent, progesterone-resistant inflammatory disorder that affects 5–10% of women of reproductive age [1,2]. It is defined by endometrial tissue that lies outside the uterine cavity, most often on the pelvic peritoneum and ovaries. Clinically, it presents as a constellation of symptoms including chronic pelvic pain, dyspareunia, and infertility [1]. The origin of endometriosis remains unknown; one theory suggests that retrograde menstruation through the fallopian tubes leads to the implantation of eutopic endometrium on peritoneal surfaces [1,3]. However, a large number of women with retrograde menstruation do not develop endometriosis [1]. Identifying the factors that predispose a patient to developing the disease is an active area of research [4].

Endometriosis has three distinct clinical presentations: peritoneal endometriosis, ovarian endometrioma, and rectovaginal endometriotic nodules. It is unclear whether these forms represent the same disease process or arise as a result of different pathophysiological mechanisms [5,6]. One possibility is that endometriomas result from an invagination of the ovary with coelomic metaplasia and clonality, which supports the classification of endometriomas as a distinct disease entity. Endometriosis contributes to infertility in multiple ways, including tubal blockage, impaired tubal function, decreased receptivity of the endometrium, and decreased oocyte and embryo quality. Endometriomas are believed to affect infertility by decreasing ovarian reserve, caused either by the mass itself or its surgical removal, or perhaps, by inflaming the ovary.

Endometriomas

The management of endometriomas greater than 3 cm is predominantly surgical, and is performed to improve patient pain and other symptoms. An increase in conception has been shown following laparoscopic removal of endometriomas greater than 3 cm, with 60% of pregnancies occurring spontaneously [7]. In patients with impaired fertility, removal of larger cysts can improve the outcome of assisted reproductive technologies (ART). Yet, there is disagreement on the optimal treatment of infertility in patients with endometriomas; an individualized approach is most often recommended [8–10]. Furthermore, it does not appear that surgical management improves gonadotropin doses used for ovarian stimulation [11] and following cystectomy, patients may actually present with diminished ovarian reserve [12], defined as the number of good-quality, gonadotropin-responsive follicles present in the ovary.

A relationship between decreased ovarian reserve and decreased pregnancy rate following cystectomy has not been demonstrated by retrospective analysis [12]. A reduction in ovarian reserve after cystectomy may be due to the inadvertent removal of healthy ovarian tissue and thermal damage from excessive cautery [13,14]. It is further debated whether ablative or excisional procedures are more likely to contribute to a loss of ovarian reserve [15,16]. Some recommend a three-step procedure while others have shown in retrospective analysis that excision with minimal use of thermal energy is superior for minimizing the effect on fertility [15–17]. More specifically, the three-step procedure, first described by Donnez, involves diagnostic laparoscopy with cyst drainage followed by 3 months of gonadotropin releasing hormone (GnRH) agonist therapy. A second laparoscopy is then performed with CO_2 laser ablation of the cyst wall. There is a need for

Endometriosis: Science and Practice, First Edition. Edited by Linda C. Giudice, Johannes L.H. Evers and David L. Healy.
© 2012 Blackwell Publishing Ltd. Published 2012 by Blackwell Publishing Ltd.

prospective, randomized trials to address the use of surgical management versus expectant management for endometriomas prior to undergoing *in vitro* fertilization (IVF).

Follicle counts in ovarian masses have shown that mass histology, and not solely patient age, dictates the number of follicles within a specimen (Tingen and Woodruff, unpublished results). Although similar data have not been collected extensively from patients with endometriosis, some work has suggested that the ovaries of patients with endometriomas, versus those with teratoma or cystadenoma histology, have significantly less normal ovarian cortex surrounding the cyst [18,19]. Furthermore, one study demonstrated that the remaining ovarian cortex surrounding endometriomas is associated with microscopic stromal implants; in contrast, the residual cortex around teratomas or benign cystadenomas was not morphologically altered [18]. Compared with other benign cysts, endometriomas may have a broader impact on follicular density within the remainder of the affected ovary, and histology type may determine the number of available "recruitable" follicles that determine ovarian reserve. Thus, the endometriomas *per se* may affect ovarian reserve, independent of the potential negative effects of surgery.

Current and emerging treatments for fertility preservation

Fertility preservation includes a wide range of options [20–21]. With diminished ovarian reserve due either to endometrioma histology or secondary to cystectomy, patients with endometriomas may benefit from some of these fertility preservation procedures. Recent advances in fertility preservation techniques may give these patients the option for future child bearing.

Fertility preservation for patients with cancer is beginning to be implemented on a larger scale, with both traditional and investigational options being offered to patients prior to undergoing fertility-threatening chemotherapy or radiation therapy. Though fertility preservation work has been focused on the cancer patient cohort [21], patients with certain non-malignant diseases may also be good candidates for fertility preservation. Several diseases and their treatments also affect the reproductive axis, including gastrointestinal diseases, rheumatological disorders, non-malignant hematological conditions, and neurological and renal disorders. The detrimental effects of these diseases and their therapies on reproductive function are only now being appreciated.

Other disease processes – including cancer and endometrioma– or their treatments can affect fertility by directly impairing ovarian function. Strategies to protect ovarian function in these patient groups have focused on decreasing ovulation and decreasing ovarian blood flow [22] prior to gonadotoxic therapy. The use of oral contraceptives and progestins has shown minimal effect on preserving fertility [22]. In cohort studies of patients with hematological malignancy, systemic lupus erythematosus (SLE), and glomerulonephritis, GnRH agonists in the setting of alkylating agent-based chemotherapies have shown some benefit [22–26]. In a cohort study of women with severe SLE, the rate of premature ovarian failure (POF) with GnRH agonist therapy was 5% (1 of 20) versus 30% (6 of 20) in matched controls [23]. The interpretation of these studies has been controversial, however, and therapy with GnRH agonists is still considered experimental [27]. GnRH agonist therapy also carries a risk of impaired bone health. A major criticism of the cohort analysis is the shorter follow-up times in control patients (range of 2–15-year follow-up), which was felt to be insufficient to document POF and could influence the perceived benefits of therapy. A prospective study of GnRH agonists in SLE patients is needed to validate the prior cohort studies.

The benefit of using GnRH agonists, as part of the Donnez three-step procedure for endometrioma resection discussed above, may be based on a suppression of follicle recruitment and subsequent protection from ablative injury, thereby maintaining the primordial follicle pool [17]. Research into the optimal use of GnRH agonists for fertility preservation continues, but a definitive randomized trial is urgently needed to ensure this medical treatment can be appropriately used or abandoned.

In vitro fertilization followed by embryo cryopreservation is the most widely available and well-established fertility preservation strategy for all young women with a fertility-threatening treatment. Reported survival rates per thawed embryo from young women after cancer treatment range from 35% to 90%, and implantation rates range between 8% and 30% [20,28]. The technology has been steadily improving over the past several years [20]. Potential obstacles to embryo cryopreservation are the requirement for a male partner or sperm donor, the time needed for ovarian hormonal stimulation prior to oocyte retrieval, and whether the patient is a candidate for hormone treatment. It is debated whether patients with estrogen-sensitive cancers, such as breast or endometrial cancer, should undergo ovarian stimulation where peak estrogen levels can reach up to 10 times that seen in the natural cycle [20,28]. Some believe there is no direct evidence to suggest that peak estrogen levels for a short time have a negative effect on these patients [28]. Furthermore, pregnancy, during which peak estrogen levels are even higher and for a more extended period of time, does not seem to have increased disease progression or recurrence in breast cancer patients [29,30].

Some advocate the use of ovarian stimulation with aromatase inhibitors, which have significantly lower estrogen levels but similar oocyte retrieval rates [31,32]. Long-term study is needed to address the impact of aromatase inhibitors and gonadotropin stimulation on embryo development, disease progression, recurrence, and survival. SLE can also flare in response to estrogen. Of note, available data have not suggested that high estrogen levels seen during ovarian stimulation affect endometriosis recurrence or growth of endometriomas [33–34]. In patients with endometriomas, a poor response to ovarian stimulation and decreased number of oocytes retrieved are seen [35–37]. In particular, following surgery, patients have demonstrated a markedly decreased response to gonadotropin stimulation [38]. These characteristics have not translated into worse IVF outcomes in retrospective analysis [35–37]. Prospective studies are needed to more directly address this question. Oocyte retrieval in a patient with endometrioma is also problematic, as it increases the risk of developing other morbidities, including infection [39,40]. The concern about infection at the time of oocyte retrieval is based on the blood content of the cysts, which serves as an ideal culture medium for bacteria, although one study has reported low rates of pelvic infection [8].

Oocyte cryopreservation is an option for patients without current partners or who do not wish to use donor sperm to create embryos. However, ovarian stimulation is required and so this option may not be as successful in patients with endometriosis. Current oocyte freezing techniques have limited the success of this procedure, with a mean oocyte survival rate of 47%, fertilization rate of 52%, and pregnancy rate per thawed oocyte of 1.52% based on 21 studies [20]. Utilization of an alternative freezing technique, vitrification, has resulted in reported rates of 81% survival and 45% clinical pregnancies per cycle [41]. Yet, oocyte cryopreservation is still considered experimental by the American Association of Reproductive Medicine and must be performed under ethics committee protocols at many centers [42].

Ovarian tissue cryopreservation and transplantation of the thawed tissue at a later date is a fertility preservation option for patients without a partner or who cannot undergo hormonal stimulation. This option may be optimal for patients with endometriomas, as ovarian tissue retrieval can be performed during cystectomy. Since a mass effect on the affected ovary can negatively impact the ability to remove viable tissue strips, obtaining tissue from the contralateral ovary may be the most prudent approach in patients with endometriomas. Transplantation of thawed ovarian tissue can be performed orthotopically, by placing the tissue in the ovarian fossa, or heterotopically, by placing the tissue subcutaneously. The heterotopic approach requires subsequent IVF embryo transfer, but theoretically it is minimally invasive, reversible, repeatable, and allows for easier access [43]. This approach has produced human fertilized oocytes that develop into four-cell embryos, but successful pregnancy has only been achieved in animals thus far [44,45]. The approach has yet to result in a livebirth and thus has been less actively pursued.

Successful livebirths from orthotopic transplantation have been described for cancer patients following treatment-induced ovarian failure, and in at least nine sets of twins, in which one twin donated ovarian tissue to a sister, who had been diagnosed with POF [46–50]. The technique remains investigational, with concerns regarding long-term viability of the grafts as well as the potential risk of transmission of cancer cells, particularly in patients with systemic blood-borne cancers [41]. For instance, a patient had an ovary removed at the time of chronic myeloid leukemia diagnosis, and the ovary had no evidence of cancer by histology, but RT-PCR demonstrated a small amount of tumor cells present in the ovary [51]. This risk may be particularly relevant in patients with endometriomas, where there may be a risk of reseeding diseased cells within the transplanted tissue.

Finally, the *in vitro* growth of immature ovarian follicles, obtained by enzymatic isolation either from cryopreserved tissue or from tissue collected at time of surgery, is being investigated as a fertility preservation option. As described above, ovarian tissue retrieval from the contralateral ovary in patients with endometriomas can be performed during cystectomy; however, unlike tissue transplantation, *in vitro* follicle culture avoids the risk of reintroducing malignant cells. Novel, three-dimensional culture systems are being developed that allow granulosa cell expansion and growth of immature follicles to the antral stage, at which point the oocyte is extracted for *in vitro* maturation and IVF [52–56]. *In vitro* maturation of immature oocytes retrieved from aspirated follicles at the time of tissue collection is also being investigated. Successful livebirths have been achieved with *in vitro* cultured murine follicles [57].

Fertility preservation strategies for patients with fertility-threatening diseases or who must undergo gonadotoxic treatments range from well-established, widely available techniques to investigational techniques being conducted at specialized centers. Awareness among internists, family physicians, pediatricians, and surgeons about the reproductive consequences of certain medical conditions and their treatments, appropriate and timely referral of patients to fertility-sparing or restorative programs and comprehensive patient education are three major actions needed to ensure that medical intervention does as much good as possible while avoiding or correcting any harm to future fertility. Efforts to raise the awareness of clinicians about the available options and the pathways of referral are starting to make an impact on patient care, not only for those diagnosed with cancer but also for patients with non-malignant but equally fertility-threatening diseases, including endometriomas, inflammatory bowel disease, thalassemia, sickle cell anemia, Fanconi anemia, hemochromatosis, SLE, juvenile SLE, chronic renal disease, and multiple sclerosis.

Fertility preservation for patients with endometriomas (see Box 55.1)

The benefit of extending fertility preservation options to patients with endometriomas remains unclear and further studies need to be done to identify the best strategies for this cohort. Fertility preservation may be appropriate in young patients diagnosed with an endometrioma, who may not yet be planning to start a family but who are scheduled to undergo surgical treatment. At the minimum, a discussion with patients about the effects of the endometrioma and/or surgical treatment on ovarian reserve and future fertility is warranted. Ovarian tissue retrieval at the time of cystectomy may be an option, but the benefits and success rate of this strategy in this patient population are not known. Studies are needed to evaluate the ovarian reserve of patients with recurrent endometriomas, or who have undergone surgical management of endometriomas over time. These studies may form the rationale for actively investigating the use of fertility preservation techniques or development of new approaches to patients diagnosed with endometriosis and/or endometriomas.

Box 55.1 Evidence to support use of fertility preservation for endometrioma patients

- Clinical evidence suggests a poor response to ovarian stimulation following surgical removal

- Histology of ovaries removed with endometrioma suggests a negative effect to the surrounding cortex not involved in the lesion, which is not seen with other histology. The number of follicles is decreased throughout the entire ovary involved with endometrioma

- Anecdotal evidence and case reports suggest that endometrioma may make ART techniques difficult and/or more likely to have infectious co-morbidity

---

Acknowledgments

This work is supported by the following funding sources: NIHUL1:8UL1DE019587 and RL1 (RO1): 5RL1HD058295

References

1. Bulun SE. Endometriosis. N Engl J Med 2009;360(3):268–279.

2. Giudice LC. Clinical Practice. Endometriosis. N Engl J Med 2010:362(25):2389–2398.

3. Sampson J. Peritoneal endometriosis due to menstrual dissemination of endometrial tissue into the peritoneal cavity. Am J Obstet Gynecol 1927;14:422–469.

4. Witz CA. Pathogenesis of endometriosis. Gynecol Obstet Invest 2002;53(Suppl 1):52–62.

5. Brosens I. Endometriosis rediscovered? Hum Reprod 2004; 19(7):1679–1680; author reply 80–81.

6. Garry R. Is insulin resistance an essential component of PCOS? The endometriosis syndromes: a clinical classification in the presence of aetiological confusion and therapeutic anarchy. Hum Reprod 2004;19(4):760–768.

7. Fuchs F, Raynal P, Salama S et al. [Reproductive outcome after laparoscopic treatment of endometriosis in an infertile population]. J Gynecol Obstet Biol Reprod (Paris) 2007;36(4):354–359.

8. Benaglia L, Somigliana E, Iemmello R, Colpi E, Nicolosi AE, Ragni G. Endometrioma and oocyte retrieval-induced pelvic abscess: a clinical concern or an exceptional complication? Fertil Steril 2008;89(5): 1263–1266.

9. Garcia-Velasco JA, Arici A. Surgery for the removal of endometriomas before in vitro fertilization does not increase implantation and pregnancy rates. Fertil Steril 2004;81(5):1206.

10. Gibbons WE. Management of endometriosis in fertility patients. Fertil Steril 2004;81(5):1204–1205.

11. Demirol A, Guven S, Baykal C, Gurgan T. Effect of endometrioma cystectomy on IVF outcome: a prospective randomized study. Reprod Biomed Online 2006;12(5):639–643.

12. Esinler I, Bozdag G, Aybar F, Bayar U, Yarali H. Outcome of in vitro fertilization/intracytoplasmic sperm injection after laparoscopic cystectomy for endometriomas. Fertil Steril 2006;85(6):1730–1735.

13. Hachisuga T, Kawarabayashi T. Histopathological analysis of laparoscopically treated ovarian endometriotic cysts with special reference to loss of follicles. Hum Reprod 2002;17(2):432–435.

14. Somigliana E, Ragni G, Benedetti F, Borroni R, Vegetti W, Crosignani PG. Does laparoscopic excision of endometriotic ovarian cysts significantly affect ovarian reserve? Insights from IVF cycles. Hum Reprod 2003;18(11):2450–2453.

15. Tsolakidis D, Pados G, Vavilis D et al. The impact on ovarian reserve after laparoscopic ovarian cystectomy versus three-stage management in patients with endometriomas: a prospective randomized study. Fertil Steril 2010;94(1):71–77.

16. Hart RJ, Hickey M, Maouris P, Buckett W. Excisional surgery versus ablative surgery for ovarian endometriomata. Cochrane Database Syst Rev 2008;2:CD004992.

17. Donnez J, Nisolle M, Gillet N, Smets M, Bassil S, Casanas-Roux F. Large ovarian endometriomas. Hum Reprod 1996;11(3):641–646.

18. Maneschi F, Marasa L, Incandela S, Mazzarese M, Zupi E. Ovarian cortex surrounding benign neoplasms: a histologic study. Am J Obstet Gynecol 1993;169(2 Pt 1):388–393.

19. Schubert B, Canis M, Darcha C et al. Human ovarian tissue from cortex surrounding benign cysts: a model to study ovarian tissue cryopreservation. Hum Reprod 2005;20(7):1786–1792.

20. Sonmezer M, Oktay K. Fertility preservation in female patients. Hum Reprod Update 2004;10(3):251–266.

21. Jeruss JS, Woodruff TK. Preservation of fertility in patients with cancer. N Engl J Med 2009;360(9):902–911.

22. Dooley MA, Nair R. Therapy Insight: preserving fertility in cyclophosphamide-treated patients with rheumatic disease. Nat Clin Pract Rheumatol 2008;4(5):250–257.

23. Somers EC, Marder W, Christman GM, Ognenovski V, McCune WJ. Use of a gonadotropin-releasing hormone analog for protection against premature ovarian failure during cyclophosphamide therapy in women with severe lupus. Arthritis Rheum 2005;52(9):2761–2767.

24. Blumenfeld Z, Shapiro D, Shteinberg M, Avivi I, Nahir M. Preservation of fertility and ovarian function and minimizing gonadotoxicity in young women with systemic lupus erythematosus treated by chemotherapy. Lupus 2000;9(6):401–405.

25. Sinha R, Dionne JM. Should gonadotropin releasing hormone analogue be administered to prevent premature ovarian failure in young women with systemic lupus erythematosus on cyclophosphamide therapy? Arch Dis Child 2008;93(5):444–445.

26. Cigni A, Faedda R, Atzeni MM et al. Hormonal strategies for fertility preservation in patients receiving cyclophosphamide to treat glomerulonephritis: a nonrandomized trial and review of the literature. Am J Kidney Dis 2008;52(5):887–896.

27. Oktay K, Sonmezer M, Oktem O, Fox K, Emons G, Bang H. Absence of conclusive evidence for the safety and efficacy of gonadotropin-releasing hormone analogue treatment in protecting against chemotherapy-induced gonadal injury. Oncologist 2007;12(9):1055–1066.

28. Klock SC, Zhang JX, Kazer RR. Fertility preservation for female cancer patients: early clinical experience. Fertil Steril 2010;94(1):149–155.

29. Blakely LJ, Buzdar AU, Lozada JA et al. Effects of pregnancy after treatment for breast carcinoma on survival and risk of recurrence. Cancer 2004;100(3):465–469.

30. Kroman N, Jensen MB, Melbye M, Wohlfahrt J, Mouridsen HT. Should women be advised against pregnancy after breast-cancer treatment? Lancet 1997;350(9074):319–322.

31. Azim AA, Costantini-Ferrando M, Oktay K. Safety of fertility preservation by ovarian stimulation with letrozole and gonadotropins in patients with breast cancer: a prospective controlled study. J Clin Oncol 2008;26(16):2630–2635.

32. Azim A, Oktay K. Letrozole for ovulation induction and fertility preservation by embryo cryopreservation in young women with endometrial carcinoma. Fertil Steril 2007;88(3):657–664.

33. Benaglia L, Somigliana E, Vighi V, Nicolosi AE, Iemmello R, Ragni G. Is the dimension of ovarian endometriomas significantly modified by IVF-ICSI cycles? Reprod Biomed Online 2009;18(3):401–406.

34. Benaglia L, Somigliana E, Vercellini P et al. The impact of IVF procedures on endometriosis recurrence. Eur J Obstet Gynecol Reprod Biol 2010;148(1):49–52.

35. Tsoumpou I, Kyrgiou M, Gelbaya TA, Nardo LG. The effect of surgical treatment for endometrioma on in vitro fertilization outcomes: a systematic review and meta analysis. Fertil Steril 2009: 92(1):75–87.

36. Gupta S, Agarwal A, Agarwal R, Loret de Mola JR. Impact of ovarian endometrioma on assisted reproduction outcomes. Reprod Biomed Online 2006;13(3):349–360.

37. Suzuki T, Izumi S, Matsubayashi H, Awaji H, Yoshikata K, Makino T. Impact of ovarian endometrioma on oocytes and pregnancy outcome in in vitro fertilization. Fertil Steril 2005;83(4):908–913.

38. Benaglia L, Somigliana E, Vighi V, Ragni G, Vercellini P, Fedele L. Rate of severe ovarian damage following surgery for endometriomas. Hum Reprod 2010;25(3):678–682.

39. Chen MJ, Yang JH, Yang YS, Ho HN. Increased occurrence of tubo-ovarian abscesses in women with stage III and IV endometriosis. Fertil Steril 2004;82(2):498–499.

40. Moini A, Riazi K, Amid V et al. Endometriosis may contribute to oocyte retrieval-induced pelvic inflammatory disease: report of eight cases. J Assist Reprod Genet 2005;22(7–8):307–309.

41. Tulandi T, Huang JY, Tan SL. Preservation of female fertility: an essential progress. Obstet Gynecol 2008;112(5):1160–1172.

42. Ethics Committee of the American Society for Reproductive Medicine. Fertility preservation and reproduction in cancer patients. Fertil Steril 2005;83(6):1622–1628.

43. Roberts JE, Oktay K. Fertility preservation: a comprehensive approach to the young woman with cancer. J Natl Cancer Inst Monogr 2005; 34:57–59.

44. Lee DM, Yeoman RR, Battaglia DE et al. Live birth after ovarian tissue transplant. Nature 2004;428(6979):137–138.

45. Oktay K, Buyuk E, Veeck L et al. Embryo development after heterotopic transplantation of cryopreserved ovarian tissue. Lancet 2004;363(9412):837–840.

46. Meirow D, Levron J, Eldar-Geva T et al. Pregnancy after transplantation of cryopreserved ovarian tissue in a patient with ovarian failure after chemotherapy. N Engl J Med 2005;353(3):318–321.

47. Demeestere I, Simon P, Emiliani S, Delbaere A, Englert Y. Fertility preservation: successful transplantation of cryopreserved ovarian tissue in a young patient previously treated for Hodgkin's disease. Oncologist 2007;12(12):1437–1442.

48. Silber SJ, Grudzinskas G, Gosden RG. Successful pregnancy after microsurgical transplantation of an intact ovary. N Engl J Med 2008;359(24):2617–2618.

49. Donnez J, Dolmans MM, Demylle D et al. Livebirth after orthotopic transplantation of cryopreserved ovarian tissue. Lancet 2004; 364(9443):1405–1410.

50. Silber S, Kagawa N, Kuwayama M, Gosden R. Duration of fertility after fresh and frozen ovary transplantation. Fertil Steril 2010; 94(6):2191–2196.

51. Courbiere B, Prebet T, Mozziconacci MJ, Metzler-Guillemain C, Saias-Magnan J, Gamerre M. Tumor cell contamination in ovarian tissue cryopreserved before gonadotoxic treatment: should we systematically exclude ovarian autograft in a cancer survivor? Bone Marrow Transplant 2010;45(7):1247–1248.

52. West-Farrell ER, Xu M, Gomberg MA, Chow YH, Woodruff TK, Shea LD. The mouse follicle microenvironment regulates antrum formation and steroid production: alterations in gene expression profiles. Biol Reprod 2009;80(3):432–439.

53. West ER, Shea LD, Woodruff TK. Engineering the follicle microenvironment. Semin Reprod Med 2007;25(4):287–299.

54. Xu M, Banc A, Woodruff TK, Shea LD. Secondary follicle growth and oocyte maturation by culture in alginate hydrogel following cryopreservation of the ovary or individual follicles. Biotechnol Bioeng. 2009;103(2):378–386.

55. Xu M, West E, Shea LD, Woodruff TK. Identification of a stage-specific permissive in vitro culture environment for follicle growth and oocyte development. Biol Reprod 2006;75(6):916–923.

56. Xu M, Woodruff TK, Shea LD. Bioengineering and the ovarian follicle. Cancer Treat Res 2007;138:75–82.

57. Xu M, Kreeger PK, Shea LD, Woodruff TK. Tissue-engineered follicles produce live, fertile offspring. Tissue Eng 2006;12(10):2739–2746.

56 Eye to the Future: Research, Diagnostics, and Therapeutics

Peter A. W. Rogers and Gareth C. Weston

Centre for Women's Health Research, Department of Obstetrics and Gynaecology, Monash University, Melbourne, Australia

Future directions in endometriosis research

Future gazing can be a risky occupation, especially when dealing with a complex disease like endometriosis, where significant breakthroughs are often unpredictable and unplanned. Having said this, it is also true that the chance of a research-driven breakthrough occurring rises in direct proportion to the size of the research effort being made. This latter issue is a matter of concern in the field of endometriosis, where the broadly held view is that research is significantly underfunded relative to the cost of endometriosis to society. This chapter will examine the immediate challenges facing endometriosis research, and look forward to some of the potential advances that may be on the horizon in diagnosis and therapy for this costly disease.

Endometriosis-related research faces significant hurdles that are inherent to any complex, chronic disease, with numerous factors contributing to the difficulties that researchers face. These problems include, but are not limited to the following.
- Endometriosis is poorly defined as a disease with multiple types, grades, and symptoms. This makes disease classification a key issue when selecting groups of patients for clinical or basic studies.
- Diagnosis typically occurs many years after symptoms first occur, making study of factors involved in the initiation of the disease process very difficult.
- From our current knowledge, it appears that several different genes have contributory effects, with the assumption that there are also multiple interacting environmental triggers. It is unlikely that any single key event will be identified that causes endometriosis; rather, an interaction of multiple events that may not be identical from woman to woman.
- Experimental models for studying endometriosis are limited and inadequate. This in turn creates difficulties for the design of good experiments or preclinical testing of potential new therapeutics.

- Endometriosis research has been a low priority for funding, presumably in part because the disease is non-fatal, can more often than not be treated surgically, and until quite recently public awareness has been limited. While public awareness is now increasing due to the efforts of well-organized patient advocate groups, funding for endometriosis research is still low in many countries.
- Understanding of the pathophysiology of endometriosis and improving treatment options require input across many disciplines, including surgery, reproductive medicine, endocrinology, pathology, oncology, epidemiology, genetics, immunology, toxicology, and pain. A multidisciplinary approach is likely to provide the best prospect of improving outcomes but large teams require large budgets and bringing the necessary clinical and research expertise together in one place presents significant logistical challenges.

Despite the impediments to endometriosis research discussed above, significant progress is being made on several fronts, both in improving understanding of the basic disease mechanisms and in new approaches to diagnosis and treatment. Priority areas for endometriosis research were recently identified at an international workshop endorsed by the World Endometriosis Society and the World Endometriosis Research Foundation [1]. At this meeting a group of international experts made 25 recommendations for research that were collectively identified as priorities. The need for a multidisciplinary approach to research on endometriosis was one of the key initial recommendations from the workshop [1].

One problematic aspect of endometriosis research is the difference between nearly all animal models, where endometriosis is induced, and humans where it occurs spontaneously. The current inability to study spontaneous induction of endometriosis seriously limits our ability to identify the pathophysiological mechanisms involved or the reasons for increased susceptibility in some women. One avenue for investigating this problem is genetic studies aimed at identifying genes or single nucleotide polymorphisms (SNPs) that are linked to or associated with increased risk of endometriosis. This topic has

Endometriosis: Science and Practice, First Edition. Edited by Linda C. Giudice, Johannes L.H. Evers and David L. Healy.
© 2012 Blackwell Publishing Ltd. Published 2012 by Blackwell Publishing Ltd.

been covered in detail elsewhere in this book but it is relevant to note that as the technology for rapid mass sequencing of DNA and RNA improves, so too does the prospect that a number of genes or SNPs that increase susceptibility to endometriosis will be identified. This is both exciting and challenging. It is exciting because for the first time we will know the identity of genes that play a role in the establishment and growth of spontaneous endometriotic lesions in humans, and it is challenging because there is a high probability that we will have a lot of fundamental biological work to do before we understand the functional role of many of the genes or SNPs identified.

An intriguing aspect of endometriosis is that despite the fact that current studies suggest it is a polygenic disease (i.e. there are likely to be multiple genes that can influence disease initiation and/or progression), and despite several different forms of disease (ovarian, deep infiltrating, diffuse, peritoneal), there is a commonality in pathways that results in ectopic growth and invasion of tissues of endometrial appearance. This may not be particularly surprising given the phenomenal regenerative capabilities of endometrium, but it does suggest that the difference between a disease-free state and growth of ectopic lesions is finely balanced, and that any one of a number of relatively minor biological events could tip the balance towards disease. Events known to increase or suspected of increasing the risk of endometriosis include presence of increased menstrual debris in the peritoneal cavity, excessive exogenous estrogenic stimulation, aberrant estrogen metabolism or signaling in the endometrium, reduced immune surveillance in the peritoneal cavity, or increased endometrial oncogene expression. The discovery that increased induction of the oncogene k-ras in ovarian surface epithelium in a mouse model results in a condition similar to peritoneal endometriosis [2] supports the thesis that relatively minor changes in the invasive potential of reproductive tract cells can lead to inappropriate ectopic growth. If this is indeed the case, then presumably there are also numerous cellular processes that can be targeted to tip the balance back towards a less invasive endometrial phenotype. Whether this is the case and, if it is, whether such processes can be harnessed for therapeutic purposes are key questions for future research.

The majority of endometriosis research has traditionally been performed by groups with a background in reproductive medicine. This is understandable given that endometriosis patients are normally seen by this clinical discipline, and subjects and tissues for research are therefore readily available. However, the primary symptom of endometriosis is pain, and it is increasingly being recognized that more research is required to better understand and treat endometriosis-associated pain. As previously stated, multidisciplinary collaboration is the ideal approach for bringing reproductive and pain research experts together, and remains a priority for future research.

The ultimate goals of endometriosis research are better diagnostics, especially for early stage and mild disease, and of course, effective medical therapies that cure the disease. New candidate targets for diagnostics and therapeutics are most likely to be identified from fundamental research into the pathophysiology of endometriosis. Future directions in diagnosis and therapy of endometriosis are discussed further in the following sections.

Future directions in diagnosis of endometriosis

The most pressing issue in the diagnosis of endometriosis is to find a non-invasive diagnostic test. The current gold standard diagnostic test is visualization of the pelvis directly via a surgical procedure – laparoscopy. As the symptoms of endometriosis are neither sensitive nor specific for the condition, the diagnosis of endometriosis at present requires excessive use of laparoscopy. This is not only financially costly, but laparoscopy has a 1 in 10,000 mortality risk, as well as a risk of damage to bowel, bladder, or major blood vessels of approximately 2.4 in 10,000, a complication often requiring a laparotomy for surgical repair [3]. Many of the types of non-invasive or minimally invasive diagnostic tests showing future promise have been covered in more detail in previous chapters. What follows is a summary of current research and future directions in research into new diagnostic tests.

The most well-known serum marker for endometriosis is the glycoprotein CA-125. However, its widespread expression in most tissues derived from coelomic epithelium, including many tissues from the female pelvis [4], impair its usefulness as a diagnostic test. It has been proposed that a better screening test may be formed by combining a number of serum markers, in a similar way to the triple or quadruple serum test [5] for Down syndrome screening. In one of the more recent attempts, D'Hooghe's group in Belgium combined the inflammatory markers interleukin (IL)-6, IL-8, tumor necrosis factor (TNF)-α, and hsCRP with CA-125 and CA-19-9 [6]. While the sensitivity was acceptable, the specificity of the combined plasma test was 61–63%, limiting its clinical applicability as a non-invasive test if a reduction in unnecessary laparoscopies is the chief aim. Preliminary work from Italy has evaluated the use of diamide-induced oxidative stress in erythrocytes from peripheral blood in addition to CA-125 and HE4 (human epididymal secretory protein E4), and initial results appear promising [7], although the technique may be technically challenging.

No doubt, further potential biomarkers will continue to emerge from the many genomic and proteomic analyses under way, and new combinations of serum biomarkers will be evaluated. However, it is essential, for any diagnostic tests to be accepted, that the test undergoes evaluation at multiple centers, in prospective trials, and that such trials adhere to the principles outlined in the Standards for the Reporting of Diagnostic Accuracy Trials statement [8].

The role of imaging tests for the diagnosis of endometriosis is reviewed extensively elsewhere. It is well known that ultrasound is a poor diagnostic test for peritoneal endometriosis, but a reasonable one for ovarian endometriomas. There continue to be reports of the use of ultrasound (either vaginal or rectal) or magnetic resonance imaging (MRI) for the detection of deep infiltrating rectovaginal endometriosis [9]. The trouble with ultrasound is that considerable expertise not available in most centers is required, subjective elements (i.e. eliciting of pain) are involved, and it is technically difficult (i.e. vaginal saline instillation). The problem with MRI is its high cost and low availability, combined with the need for considerable expertise in the interpretation of MRI scans of the female reproductive tract.

The eutopic endometrium from women with endometriosis has molecular and cellular differences to that of women without endometriosis [10]. There are an increasing number of both genomic [11,12] and proteomic [13,14] studies of differences in mRNA and protein expression from eutopic endometrium of women with and without endometriosis that demonstrate this. These differences may explain why 90% of women have retrograde flow of endometrial tissue through the fallopian tubes during menstruation, but only 8–10% of women develop the disease. Characteristics of the retrogradely shed endometrium make it more likely to implant, or more resistant to clearance by the immune system.

Efforts have been made to try to exploit differences in eutopic endometrium, from women with and without endometriosis, to form a diagnostic test. Presumably, a pipelle sample of endometrium performed in the office setting could be used as a minimally invasive test for endometriosis in the peritoneal cavity. One of the most promising diagnostic tests of this kind is the finding, by Ian Fraser's group in Sydney, of small unmyelinated nerve fibers in the eutopic endometrium of women with endometriosis, but not in the endometrium of women without endometriosis [15]. Not only does the presence of these nerve fibers present a possible screening test for endometriosis, but they may be involved in the pain symptoms of endometriosis. There has now been a prospective double-blind trial assessing the utility of the test [16]. It was shown to have 98% sensitivity, 83% specificity, 91% positive and 96% negative predictive values in 99 consecutive women presenting for a laparoscopy for pelvic pain in a tertiary hospital. However, calls have been made for the test to be studied in larger prospective trials outside a tertiary hospital setting [17]. Nonetheless, this test shows considerable promise.

Differences in protein expression have also been studied via proteomics to search for diagnostic protein markers for endometriosis in peripheral blood serum [18] and in peritoneal fluid [19]. The advantage of screening via a blood test is obvious, although peritoneal fluid would be more difficult to obtain without a laparoscopy. The work so far has been very preliminary.

Some very recent work has reported differences in the urine of women with endometriosis compared to controls. Using mass spectroscopy of gel-separated proteins, pilot studies have identified cytokeratin 19 as a urinary marker for the presence of endometriosis [20]. If confirmed, this novel finding could rapidly lead to a home use diagnostic kit for endometriosis. The biological reason for elevated cytokeratin 19 in the urine of women with endometriosis is less clear at the present time.

Future directions in treatment of endometriosis

Most of the treatment types available for endometriosis have been discussed in much more detail in prior chapters. Here we will explore in brief some of the future directions in the treatment of endometriosis.

The treatment of endometriosis depends on whether the patient is presenting for relief of pain symptoms or for infertility. Where there is a desire for pregnancy, the types of treatments that can be delivered are limited, either because the treatments themselves have a contraceptive effect (e.g. progestins, Mirena-IUD) or because their possible teratogenic effects are unknown (e.g. angiogenesis inhibitors).

At present, laparoscopic surgical resection/removal of endometriosis lesions continues to be the mainstay of treatment. Medical treatments have side-effects, and their benefits are usually reversible on cessation of therapy. However, medical therapies may have a role in preventing or delaying recurrence of endometriotic lesions. There are currently very few RCTs examining either surgical or medical treatment for treatment of pain or infertility associated with endometriosis, making most treatment regimes heavily influenced by the individual bias/preference of the gynecologist.

Treatment of infertility associated with endometriosis still needs to be individualized. Whether a woman is encouraged to try naturally for a pregnancy following laparoscopic excision of lesions depends not only on the semen analysis and tubal patency, but also on her age. The older the woman, the more likely she will be referred for infertility treatment earlier. With earlier diagnosis, and with the advent of oocyte freezing, young single women with endometriosis now have the option of oocyte cryopreservation as an "insurance" against progression of the disease later [21,22]. Many women are now taking these steps to preserve their fertility in the face of known endometriosis disease. Where women are trying to achieve a pregnancy using *in vitro* fertilization, they face a reduced pregnancy rate per cycle of treatment compared with women without endometriosis. This has been attributed to reduction in both egg quality [23] and implantation potential of the eutopic endometrium [24]. Becoming increasingly acceptable to patients with multiple cycle failure in these situations is the use of donor eggs to overcome reduced egg quality, and gestational surrogates to improve embryo implantation.

There are several issues associated with the treatment of pain with endometriosis. Laparoscopic surgical treatment can be technically challenging. Surgeons treating endometriosis need to have appropriate levels of laparoscopic surgical training, and training programs need to provide adequate exposure for junior trainees to provision them with such skills. For rectovaginal endometriosis, a colorectal surgeon with experience in operating on endometriosis in conjunction with a gynecologist may be required. Patients should have a frank discussion with their gynecologist regarding fertility preservation, given the potential threat to ovarian reserve by extensive pelvic surgery. They may wish to have oocyte or embryo cryopreservation prior to undergoing surgery. The role of robotic surgery in the treatment of endometriosis continues to be explored [25]. There continues to be a lack of RCT data regarding the use of adjuvant medical therapy either before or after surgery to reduce recurrence rates [26].

There are an increasing number of potential medical treatments for endometriosis. The use of a Mirena IUD [27] has become increasingly popular to treat endometriosis, as well as the more established hormonal therapies for endometriosis. Other medical treatments undergoing various phases of investigation include progesterone and estrogen receptor modulators (SPRMs and SERMs), statins, aromatase inhibitors, antiangiogenic agents, and immune modulators such as anti-TNF-α. None of these medical treatments has yet supplanted surgical excision of endometriotic lesions as the gold standard for treatment. The Holy Grail of endometriosis treatment is to find a medical therapy with few or no side-effects that is effective and safe for use in pregnancy. This appears to be a far-off prospect at present.

In conclusion, current basic research on endometriosis holds significant hope for new diagnostics and therapeutics in the foreseeable future. The length of time before advances become available for clinical treatment will depend to a significant extent on the funding that is made available for research on endometriosis, as well as the ability of researchers to maximize resources through collaboration and multidisciplinary approaches. Current endometriosis awareness campaigns and lobbying remain essential components of the path forward.

References

1. Rogers PA, D'Hooghe TM, Fazleabas A et al. Priorities for endometriosis research: recommendations from an international consensus workshop. Reprod Sci 2009;16:335–346.

2. Dinulescu DM, Ince TA, Quade BJ, Shafer SA, Crowley D, Jacks T. Role of K-ras and Pten in the development of mouse models of endometriosis and endometrioid ovarian cancer. Nat Med 2005;11:63–70.

3. Xu M, Vincent K, Kennedy S. Diagnosis of endometriosis. In: Rombauts L, Tsaltas J, Maher P, Healy D, editors. Endometriosis. Melbourne: Blackwell Publishing, 2008, pp.133–148.

4. Weston GC, Rogers PAW. Diagnosis of endometriosis: pitfalls of current methods. In: Garcia-Velasco JA, Rizk B, editor. Endometriosis: Current Management and Future Trends. New Delhi: Jaypee Medical Publishers, 2010, pp.93–99.

5. Ndumbe FM, Natvi O, Chilaka VN, Konje JC. Prenatal diagnosis in the first trimester of pregnancy. Obstet Gynecol Surv 2008;63:317–328.

6. Mihalyi A, Gevaert O, Kyama CM et al. Non-invasive diagnosis of endometriosis based on a combined analysis of six plasma biomarkers. Hum Reprod 2010;25:654–664.

7. Bordin L, Fiore C, Dona G et al. Evaluation of erythrocyte band 3 phosphotyrosine level, glutathione content, CA-125, and human epididymal secretory protein E4 as combined parameters in endometriosis. Fertil Steril 2010;94(5):1616–1621.

8. Bossuyt PM, Reitsma JB, Bruns DE et al. The STARD statement for reporting studies of diagnostic accuracy: explanation and elaboration. Ann Intern Med 2003;138:W1–12.

9. Grasso RF, di Giacomo V, Sedati P et al. Diagnosis of deep infiltrating endometriosis: accuracy of magnetic resonance imaging and transvaginal 3D ultrasonography. Abdom Imaging 2010;35(6):716–725.

10. Matsuzaki S, Canis M, Pouly JL et al. Endometrial dysfunction in endometriosis – biochemical aspects. In: Rombauts L, Tsaltas J, Maher P, Healy D, editors. Endometriosis. Melbourne: Blackwell Publishing, 2008, pp.89–100.

11. Kao LC, Germeyer A, Tulac S et al. Expression profiling of endometrium from women with endometriosis reveals candidate genes for disease-based implantation failure and infertility. Endocrinology 2003;144:2870–2871.

12. Matsuzaki S, Canis M, Vaurs-Barriere C, Boespflug-Tanguy O, Dastugue B, Mage G. DNA microarray analysis of gene expression in eutopic endometrium from patients with deep endometriosis using laser capture microdissection. Fertil Steril 2005;84(Suppl 2):1180–1190.

13. Zhang H, Niu Y, Feng J, Guo H, Ye X, Cui H. Use of proteomic analysis of endometriosis to identify different protein expression in patients with endometriosis versus normal controls. Fertil Steril 2006;86:274–282.

14. Stephens AN, Hannan NJ, Rainczuk A et al. Post-translational modifications and protein-specific isoforms in endometriosis revealed by 2D DIGE. J Proteome Res 2010;9(5):2438–2449.

15. Tokushige N, Markham R, Russell P, Fraser IS. High density of small nerve fibres in the functional layer of the endometrium in women with endometriosis. Hum Reprod 2006;21:782–787.

16. Al-Jefout M, Dezarnaulds G, Cooper M et al. Diagnosis of endometriosis by detection of nerve fibres in endometrial biopsy: a double blind study. Hum Reprod 2009;24:3019–3024.

17. Evers JLH, van Steirteghem AC. All that glistens is not gold. Hum Reprod 2009;24:2972–2973.

18. Zhang H, Niu Y, Feng J, Guo H, Ye X, Cui H. Use of proteomic analysis of endometriosis to identify different protein expression in patients with endometriosis versus normal controls. Fertil Steril 2006;86:274–282.

19. Hou Z, Sun L, Gao L, Liao L, Mao Y, Liu J. Cytokine array analysis of peritoneal fluid between women with endometriosis of different stages and those without endometriosis. Biomarkers 2009;14:604–618.

20. Tokushige N, Markham R, Fraser IS et al. The discovery of a highly upregulated protein in the urine of women with endometriosis. Society for Gynecologic Investigation Annual Scientific Meeting, Orlando, Florida, March 2010. Abstract 702.

21. Oktay K, Cil AP, Bang H. Efficiency of oocyte cryopreservation: a meta-analysis. Fertil Steril 2006;86:70–80.

22. Lamar CA, DeCherney AH. Fertility preservation: state of the science and future research directions. Fertil Steril 2009;91:316–319.

23. Falconer H, Sundqvist J, Gemzell-Danielsson K, von Schoultz B, D'Hooghe TM, Fried G. IVF outcome in women with endometriosis in relation to tumour necrosis factor and anti-Mullerian hormone. Reprod Biomed Online 2009;18:582–588.

24. Kao LC, Germever A, Tulac S et al. Expression profiling of endometrium from women with endometriosis reveals candidate genes fro disease-based implantation failure and infertility. Endocrinology 2003;144:2870–2881.

25. Oehler MK. Robot-assisted surgery in gynaecology. Aust NZ J Obstet Gynaecol 2009;49:124–129.

26. Yap C, Furness S, Farquhar C. Pre and post operative medical therapy for endometriosis surgery. Cochrane Database Syst Rev 2004;3:CD003678.

27. Shimoni N. Intrauterine contraceptives: a review of uses, side effects, and candidates. Semin Reprod Med 2010;28:118–125.

Index

Endometriosis: Science and Practice, First Edition. Edited by Linda C. Giudice, Johannes L.H. Evers and David L. Healy.
© 2012 Blackwell Publishing Ltd. Published 2012 by Blackwell Publishing Ltd.